# Register Now for Online Access to Your Book!

SPRINGER PUBLISHING CONNECT™

AF768748

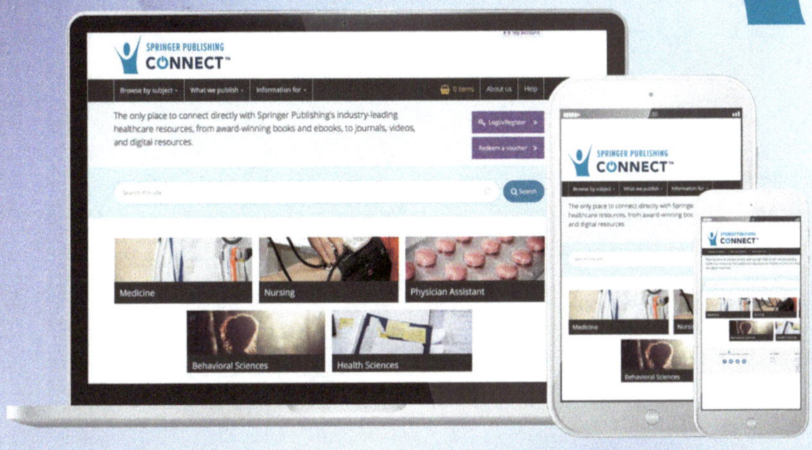


Your print purchase of *Comprehensive Neonatal Nursing Care*, Seventh Edition, **includes online access to the contents of your book**—increasing accessibility, portability, and searchability!

**Access today at:**
**http://connect.springerpub.com/content/book/978-0-8261-4972-5**
or scan the QR code at the right with your smartphone. Log in or register, then click "Redeem a voucher" and use the code below.

**994FN2AN**

*Scan here for quick access.*

**Having trouble redeeming a voucher code?**
**Go to https://connect.springerpub.com/redeeming-voucher-code**

**If you are experiencing problems accessing the digital component of this product, please contact our customer service department at cs@springerpub.com**

The online access with your print purchase is available at the publisher's discretion and may be removed at any time without notice.

**Publisher's Note:** New and used products purchased from third-party sellers are not guaranteed for quality, authenticity, or access to any included digital components.

# Comprehensive Neonatal Nursing Care

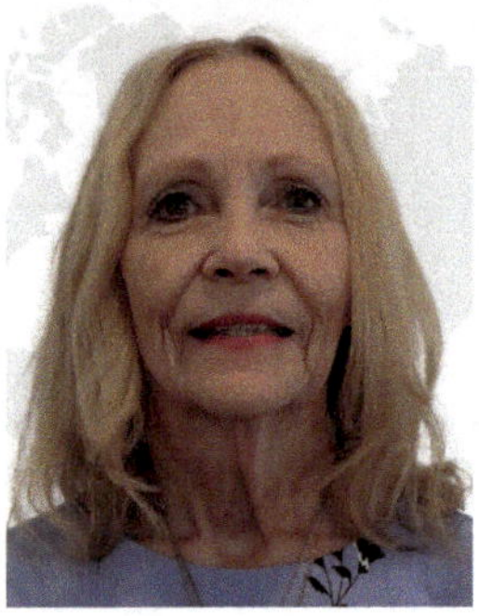

**Carole Kenner, PhD, RN, FAAN, FNAP, ANEF, IDFCOINN**, is the Carol Kuser Loser Dean/Professor of the School of Nursing and Health Sciences at The College of New Jersey. Dr. Kenner received a Bachelor of Science in Nursing from the University of Cincinnati and her master's and doctorate degrees in nursing from Indiana University. She specialized in neonatal/perinatal nursing for her master's degree and obtained a minor in higher education for her doctorate. She has authored more than 200 journal articles and 40 textbooks.

Her career is dedicated to nursing education and to the health of neonates and their families, as well as educational and professional development of healthcare practices in neonatology. Her dedication includes providing a healthcare standard for educating neonatal nurses nationally and internationally. Her passion led her to begin the journal *Newborn and Infant Nursing Reviews*, in which she served as editor and then associate editor. She worked with the National Coalition on Health Professional Education in Genetics (NCHPEG) and the American Nurses Association to develop genetic competencies. She helped develop the End-of-Life Nursing Education Consortium (ELNEC) Neonatal/Pediatric modules. She served as the co-chair of the Oklahoma Attorney General's Task Force on End of Life/Palliative Care. She also helped develop program recommendations for perinatal/neonatal palliative care as part of a family-centered/developmental care project sponsored by the National Perinatal Association. She serves on the Consensus Committee of Neonatal Intensive Care Design Standards, which sets recommendations for Neonatal Intensive Care Unit designs; the March of Dimes Nursing Advisory Committee; and the Consensus Committee of the Standards, Competencies, and Best Practices for Infant and Family-Centered Developmental Care in the Intensive Care Unit. Dr. Kenner is also Co-Vice Chair of Healthcare Professional Associations of the Partnership for Maternal, Newborn, Child, and Adolescent Health (PMCH); on the Leadership Team of the International Neonatal Consortium; and is a Board Member for the following organizations: Vermont Oxford Network, Preemie World, and Books for Healing and a member of the Every Woman Every Newborn Everywhere Management Team. She is a fellow of the American Academy of Nursing (FAAN), a fellow in the National Academies of Practice, a fellow in the Academy of Nursing Education, past president of the National Association of Neonatal Nurses (NANN), and founding president and Chief Executive Officer of the Council of International Neonatal Nurses (COINN), the first international organization representing neonatal nursing and setting standards globally. She is the 2011 recipient of the Audrey Hepburn Award for Contributions to the Health and Welfare of Children Internationally.

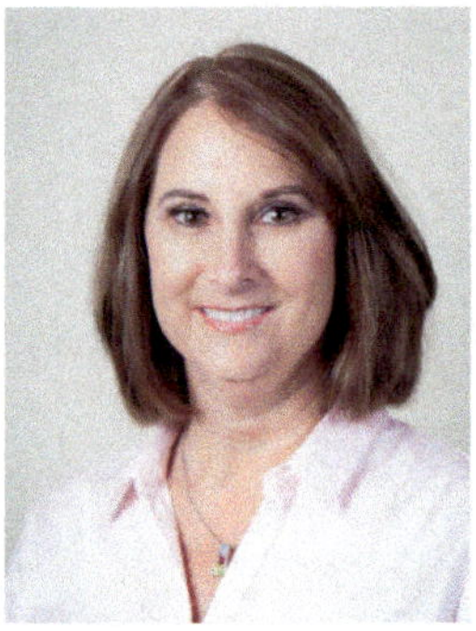

**Leslie B. Altimier, DNP, RN, MSN, NE-BC**, is the Regional Director of Neonatal Services at SSM Health: Cardinal Glennon Children's & St. Mary's Hospitals in St. Louis, Missouri. She received her Bachelor of Science in Nursing from Kent State University, her Master's of Science in Nursing from the University of North Carolina, Greensboro, and her Doctor of Nursing Practice from Northeastern University in Boston. Dr. Altimier completed a postdoctoral fellowship in compassionate healthcare through Northeastern University in collaboration with the Schwartz Center for Compassionate Healthcare and the Jonas Center for Nursing and Veterans Healthcare.

Dr. Altimier is a renowned clinician who lectures nationally and internationally and has published over 200 articles, chapters, and books on the care of neonates and families, NICU design, and organizational leadership. She was the editor-in-chief of *Newborn and Infant Nursing Reviews (NAINR)* journal and, is currently the editor-in-chief of the *Journal of Neonatal Nursing (JNN)*, the official journal of the Neonatal Nurses Association (NNA), and is on the advisory board for neonatal intensive care journal. She is a member of the National Association of Neonatal Nurses (NANN), the Council of International Neonatal Nurses, Inc. (COINN), the International Academy of Nurse Editors (INANE), and the American Organization for Nursing Leadership (AONL).

Dr. Altimier has contributed to nursing through practice, education, leadership, research, and publications. She is passionate about neuroprotective developmental care, family-integrated care, and compassionate care and has earned the Neonatal Developmental Care Specialist Designation from NANN. Her goal is to create a culture of change in healthcare worldwide.

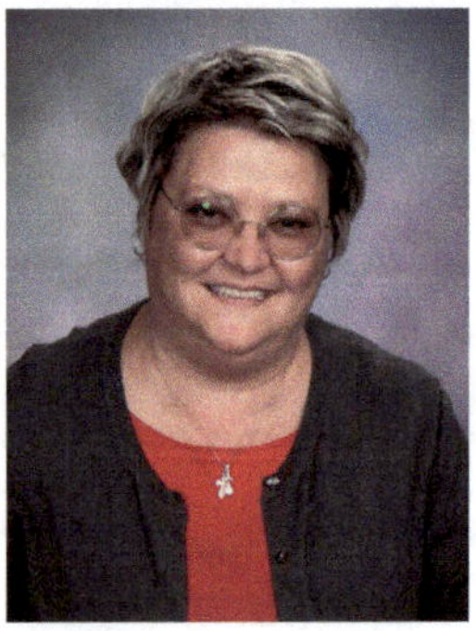

**Marina V. Boykova, PhD, RN, FNAP**, is an associate professor of nursing in the School of Nursing and Health Sciences, Holy Family University, Philadelphia, Pennsylvania. Dr. Boykova received her Diploma in Nursing Practice from the School of Nursing #3, Saint Petersburg, Russia; a Certificate in Theory and Practice of Nurse Education, Medical College #1, Saint Petersburg, Russia; a Certificate in Theory and Practice of Nurse Education, Chester, United Kingdom; a Bachelor of Science with Honors in Professional Practice (Nursing), University of Liverpool, Chester, United Kingdom; a Diploma of Higher Education in Nursing, Novgorod University of Y. Mudrogo, Novgorod, Russia; a Master's of Science in Health Promotion (Distinction), University of Liverpool, Chester, United Kingdom; and a Doctor of Philosophy in Nursing, University of Oklahoma, Oklahoma City, Oklahoma. She is a member of Sigma Theta Tau International, the Council of International Neonatal Nurses (COINN), the National Association of Neonatal Nurses (NANN), the National Academies of Practice (NAP), the Eastern Nursing Research Society, and the American Nurses Association (ANA). She serves as a nonexecutive director for the Council of International Neonatal Nurses, Inc. (COINN). She is a member of the COINN Research Committee and the World Health Organization (WHO) STAGE Midwifery Working Group on Transitioning to Midwifery Models of Care. She is a fellow in the National Academies of Practice (NAP). Dr. Boykova's clinical background is neonatal intensive care nursing. Her research interests center on transition from hospital to home and to primary care for parents of preterm infants. She has published over 40 journal articles, over 20 book chapters, and co-edited three textbooks. She coauthored a policy brief on Reducing Preterm Births for the American Academy of Nursing.

# Comprehensive Neonatal Nursing Care

Seventh Edition


*Carole Kenner, PhD, RN, FAAN, FNAP, ANEF, IDFCOINN*

*Leslie B. Altimier, DNP, RN, MSN, NE-BC*

*Marina V. Boykova, PhD, RN, FNAP*

Editors


SPRINGER PUBLISHING

First Springer Publishing edition 978-0-8261-0975-0 (2013); subsequent edition 2019



Springer Publishing Company, LLC
902 Carnegie Center/Suite 140, Princeton, NJ 08540
www.springerpub.com
connect.springerpub.com

*Acquisitions Editor*: John Zaphyr
*Senior Development Editor*: Julia Curcio
*Production Editor*: Toni Brokaw
*Compositor*: S4Carlisle Publishing Services

*ISBN*: 978-0-8261-4743-1
*e-book ISBN*: 978-0-8261-4972-5
*DOI*: 10.1891/9780826149725

26 27 28 29 / 5 4 3 2 1



Library of Congress Cataloging-in-Publication Data

Names: Kenner, Carole author | Altimier, Leslie B. author | Boykova, Marina V. author
Title: Comprehensive neonatal nursing care / [edited by] Carole Kenner, PhD, RN, FAAN, FNAP, ANEF, IDFCOINN, Leslie B. Altimier, DNP, RN, MSN, NE-BC, Marina V. Boykova, PhD, RN, FNAP.
Description: Seventh edition. | Princeton, New Jersey : Springer Publishing Company, [2026] | Includes bibliographical references and index. |
Identifiers: LCCN 2025032334 (print) | LCCN 2025032335 (ebook) | ISBN 9780826147431 paperback | ISBN 9780826149725 ebook
Subjects: LCSH: Neonatal nursing | Neonatology
Classification: LCC RJ253 .C66 2026 (print) | LCC RJ253 (ebook)
LC record available at https://lccn.loc.gov/2025032334
LC ebook record available at https://lccn.loc.gov/2025032335



Printed in the United States of America by Gasch Printing.

*I wish to first express my appreciation for the love and support of my parents who always loved to see a new text.*
*—Carole*

*Thank my children, Jen, Julie, and Kevin, for their love, support, and encouragement for me as a mom and professional.*
*—Leslie*

*For my mom, whose love and support were endless.*
*—Marina*

*Together we would like to express our appreciation for the assistance of John Zaphyr and Julia Curcio, from Springer Publishing Company, who guided this project. Thank you for believing in this project. We want to thank the professionals across the globe who take care of the babies and their families.*
*—Carole Kenner, Leslie Altimier, and Marina Boykova*

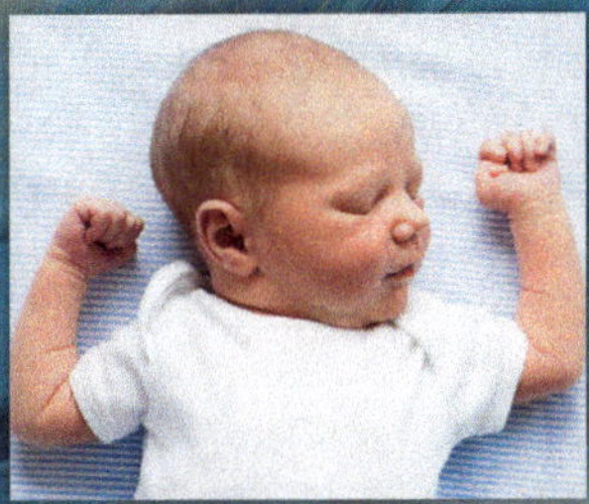

Source: Famveldman/Adobe Stock.

# Contents

## UNIT IV: SPECIAL CONSIDERATIONS



## UNIT V: ENVIRONMENTAL HEALTH AND FAMILY-CENTERED CARE IN THE NEONATAL INTENSIVE CARE UNIT AND BEYOND



**The sections VI and VII for this title may be accessed by visiting www.springerpub.com/courseconnect.**

**See inside front cover and tear-out card for CourseConnect details.**

## UNIT VI: SPECIAL TOPICS IN NEONATAL CARE

## UNIT VII: NEONATAL DIAGNOSTIC AND CARE PROTOCOLS

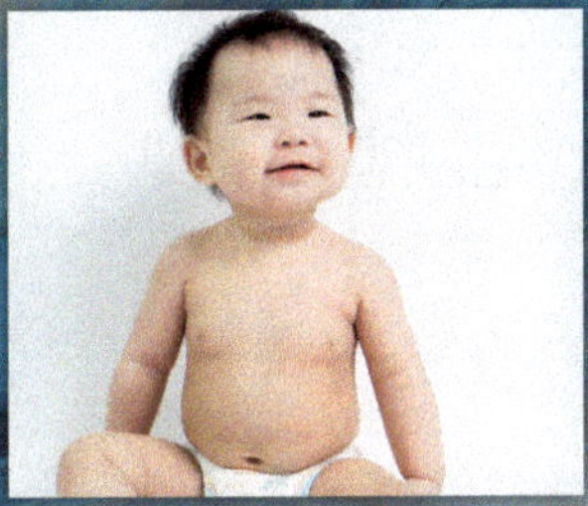

Source: Kenishirotie/Adobe Stock.

# Contributors

**Leslie B. Altimier, DNP, RNC, MSN, NE-BC**
Regional Director of Neonatal Services
SSM Health, Cardinal Glennon Children's Hospital & St. Mary's Hospital
Fetal Care Institute
St. Louis, Missouri

**Gail A. Bagwell, DNP, APRN, CNS, FAAN, FNAP**
Immediate Past President at National Association of Neonatal Nurses (NANN)
Clinical Nurse Specialist for Perinatal Outreach
Nationwide Children's Hospital Division of Neonatology
Columbus, Ohio

**Morgan Baldwin, MSN, RN, CPNP**
SSM Health Cardinal Glennon Pediatrics Specialty Services
Grand Boulevard, St. Louis, Missouri

**Marina V. Boykova, PhD, RN**
Assistant Professor
School of Nursing and Allied Health
Holy Family University
School of Nursing and Allied Health
Philadelphia, Pennsylvania

**Caitlin Bradley, PhD, RN, NNP-BC**
Lead APRN, NICU
Boston Children's Hospital
Boston, Massachusetts

**Jennifer M. Burford, RN, MSN, FNP-C**
Pediatric Palliative Care
Cardinal Glennon Children's Hospital
St. Louis, Missouri

**Marsha Campbell-Yeo, PhD, NNP-BC, RN**
Professor and Clinician Scientist
School of Nursing
Department of Pediatrics, Psychology and Neuroscience
Dalhousie University
IWK Health
Halifax, Nova Scotia, Canada

**Ashlea D. Cardin, OTD, OTR/L, BCP, CNT**
Aota Board Certification in Pediatrics
Missouri State University
Springfield, Missouri

**Waldemar A. Carlo, MD**
Co-Director of Neonatology
University of Alabama at Birmingham
Birmingham, Alabama

**Terri A. Cavaliere, DNP, NNP-BC, FAANP**
Clinical Associate Professor
Stony Brook University
School of Nursing
Stony Brook, New York

**Robin D. Clark, MD**
Professor of Pediatrics
Chief, Division of Pediatric Genetics
Loma Linda University School of Medicine
Loma Linda, California

**Mary Coughlin, MS, NNP-NCC-E**
Trauma Informed Professional™
Caritas Coach®
Founder and President
Caring Essentials Collaborative, LLC
Boston, Massachusetts

**Lorelei Crowder, RN, BSN**
President
HI Healthcare
Honolulu, Hawaii

**Deborah A. Discenza, MA**
Founder and President
PreemieWorld, LLC
Springfield, Virginia

**Dolores R. Dzubaty, PhD, MSN, RNC-OB**
Faculty Emeritus
The College of New Jersey
Ewing Township, New Jersey

**Taryn M. Edwards, MSN, APRN, NNP-BC**
Nemours Children's Health Delaware
Children's Hospital of Philadelphia
Wilmington, Delaware

**Wakako Eklund, DNP, APRN, NNP-BC, FAANP, FAAN**
Pediatrix Medical Group of Tennessee
Nashville, Tennesse

**Mats Eriksson, PhD, RN**
Department of Pediatrics
Faculty of Medicine and Health
Örebro University Hospital
Örebro, Sweden
Faculty of Medicine and Health
School of Health Sciences
Örebro University
Örebro, Sweden

**Genevra Galura, PharmD, BCPPS**
Clinical Pharmacy Specialist
Neonatal Intensive Care Unit
Rush University Medical Center
Chicago, Illinois

**Samuel Gentle, MD**
Assistant Professor
Neonatology
Department of Pediatrics
Yale University School of Medicine
New Haven, Connecticut

**Megan E. Glemza, DNP, NNP-BC**
University of Florida
Gainesville, Florida

**Donna A. Goff, MD, MS**
Medical Director
Fetal and Pediatric Cardiology
Pediatrix Medical Group Houston, Texas

**Georgia Haas, MS, RD, LD**
NICU Dietitian
SSM Health Cardinal Glennon Children's Hospital
St. Louis, Missouri

**Kathryn Hanson, MS, MD, FAAP**
Assistant Professor
Division of Neonatal-Perinatal Medicine
Department of Pediatrics
St. Louis University School of Medicine
SLUCare at SSM Health
St. Louis, Missouri

**Pamela A. Harris-Haman, DNP, CRNP, NNP-BC**
Neonatal Nurse Practitioner
University of Pennsylvania Medical Center-Susquehanna
Vising Professor
Chamberlain University
Middletown, Pennsylvania

**Jacqueline Hoffman, APRN, NNP-BC**
Associate Professor
Oregon Health & Science University
Portland, Oregon
Assistant Professor
Rush University
Chicago, Illinois

**Gloria Johnson, NP**
Pediatrix Medical Group
Houston, Texas

**Jocquelin V. Jones, DNP, APRN, NNP-BC**
Assistant Professor and NNP Track Lead
Creighton University College of Nursing
Omaha, Nebraska

**Leilani Kahoano**
Founder/President/Kumu Hula
Caring For Hawai'i Neonates aka Mālama o Nā Keiki
Honolulu, Hawaii

**Susan Kau, BSN, RNC-NIC**
Neonatal Intensive Care Unit Staff Nurse
Kapi'olani Medical Center for Women and Children/Caring for Hawaii Neonates
Honolulu, Hawaii

**William Keenan, MD**
Saint Louis University School of Medicine
St. Louis, Missouri

**Carole Kenner, PhD, RN, FAAN, FNAP, ANEF, IDFCOINN**
Carol Kuser Loser Dean/Professor
The College of New Jersey
School of Nursing and Health Sciences
Ewing Township, New Jersey

**Miki Konishi, PhD, RN, PHN**
Professor
School of Nursing
Dokkyo Medical University
Tochigi, Japan

**Mike Kurz, DNP, APRN, NNP-BC**
Community Medical Center
Neonatology
Missoula, Montana

**David Lebanon, DNP, NNP-BC, NPT-BC, VA-BC, NNIC**
University of Texas Southwestern Medical Center
Dallas, Texas

**Carolyn Houska Lund, MS, RN, FAAN**
Associate Clinical Professor
Adjunct Faculty
University of California School of Nursing
San Francisco, California

**Christina Mahoney, BSN, RN**
Staff Nurse
Neonatal Intensive Care Unit
Boston Children's Hospital
Boston, Massachusetts

**Maureen F. McCourt, MS, RN, NNP-BC, PNP**
Instructor
NNP Program
Northeastern University
Boston, Massachusetts
Neonatal Nurse Practitioner Supervisor
Women and Infants Hospital
Providence, Rhode Island

**Denise McFadden, DNP, MSN, RNC-MNN**
Associate Professor
School of Nursing
Holy Family University
Philadelphia, Pennsylvania

**Jacqueline M. McGrath, PhD, RN, FAAN**
Professor Emeritus
School of Nursing
University of Texas at San Antonio
San Antonio, Texas

**Tamara M. Meeker, MSN, CRPN, NNP-BC**
Surgical Nurse Practitioner
Newborn Intensive Care Unit
Children's Hospital of Philadelphia
Philadelphia, Pennsylvania

**Samual Mooneyham, MSN, RN**
Clinical Nurse Manager
Brookline Pediatrics
Brookline, Massachusetts

**Monica Muir, DO**
Physician/Assistant Professor of Pediatrics
SSM Health Cardinal Glennon Children's Hospital
St. Louis, Missouri

**Masahiko Murase, PhD, MD**
Associate Professor
Children's Medical Center
Showa University Yokohama Northern Hospital
Yokohama Kanagawa, Japan

**Vivek Narendran, MD, MBA, MRCP**
Medical Director
Neonatal Intensive Care Unit
University of Cincinnati Medical Center
Medical Director
Cincinnati Perinatal Outreach Project
Department of Pediatrics
University of Cincinnati
Cincinnati Children's Hospital Medical Center
Cincinnati, Ohio

**Susan K. Newbold, PhD, RN, NI-BC, FAAN, FHIMSS, FAMIA**
Director
Nursing Informatics Boot Camp
Franklin, Tennessee

**Khiet D. Ngo, DO, MS**
Assistant Professor of Basic Sciences & Clinical Medicine
Department of Medical Education & Pediatrics
Loma Linda University School of Medicine
Loma Linda University Children's Hospital
Loma Linda, California

**Justine Parsons, RN, BN, MN, Grad Dip Education**
Clinical Nurse Consultant
John Hunter Children's Hospital
Newcastle, NSW, Australia

**Raylene M. Phillips, MD, FAAP, FABM, IBCLC**
Associate Professor of Pediatrics/Neonatology
Loma Linda University School of Medicine
Loma Linda, California

**Geralyn Sue Prullage, DNP, APN, NNP-BC**
Director of Education
Council of International Neonatal Nurses
Chicago, Illinois

**Eric A. Raynal, MD, MEd**
Assistant Professor, Department of Pediatrics
University of Cincinnati
Attending Physician
Division of Neonatology and Pulmonary Biology
Cincinnati Children's Hospital Medical Center
Cincinnati, Ohio

**Lori Baas Rubarth, PhD, APRN, NNP-BC**
Professor Emeritus & NNP Track Faculty
Creighton University College of Nursing
Omaha, Nebraska

**Manoj Shah, MD**
Associate Professor
Pediatric Gastroenterology & Nutrition
Loma Linda University School of Medicine
Loma Linda, California

**Elizabeth L. Sharpe, DNP, APRN, NNP-BC, VA-BC, FAANP, FAAN**
Associate Clinical Professor
The Ohio State University
Columbus, Ohio

**Jordan A. Sullivan, BSN, RNC-NIC**
NRP/BLS Coordinator for Neonatal Services
Neonatal Intensive Care Unit
Nationwide Children's Hospital
Columbus, Ohio

**Colin Travers, MD**
Associate Professor
Diversion of Neonatology
Heersink School of Medicine
University of Alabama-Birmingham
Birmingham, Alabama

**Dorothy Vittner, PhD, RN, FAAN**
Assistant Professor
Director Post Masters DNP Program
Fairfield University
Egan School of Nursing & Health Studies
Fairfield, Connecticut

**Robert D. White, MD**
Director
Regional Newborn Program
Beacon Children's Hospital
South Bend, Indiana

**Valerie Willis, PhD**
Adjunct Clinical Assistant Professor
Department of Medical and Molecular Genetics
Indiana University School of Medicine
Indianapolis, Indiana

**Rita Wyrebek, MD, MS**
Neonatologist
Assistant Professor of Pediatrics
SSM Health Cardinal Glennon Children's Hospital
University School of Medicine
Saint Louis, Missouri

## PARENT VOICES CONTRIBUTORS

**Amy Blanchard**
Graham's Foundation
Perrysburg, Ohio

**Jennifer Canvasser, MSW**
NEC Society
Davis, California

**Katie Reginato Cascamo, MA**
Courageous Steps
Stillwater, Maine

**Jennifer Degl**
Mahopac Falls, New York

**Deborah A. Discenza**
PreemieWorld, LLC
Springfield, Virginia

**Jennifer M. Driscoll**
Lily's Hope Foundation
Allentown, Pennsylvania

**Crystal Duffy**
Twin to Twin
Houston, Texas

**Ali Dunn**
MeTwo Books
Indianapolis, Indiana

**Jimena Guild**
Graham's Foundation
Perrysburg, Ohio

**Laural Kapferer, MS**
Team Grayson
Boston, Massachusetts

**Jenny R. McCormick**
PreemieWorld, LLC
Springfield, Virginia

**Heather McKinnis**
Graham's Foundation
Perrysburg, Ohio

**Farrin Moreno**
The University of Texas at San Antonio
San Antonio, Texas

**Tracy Pella**
Connected Forever
Tecumseh, Nebraska

**Keira Sorrells**
Preemie Parent Alliance
Madison, Mississippi

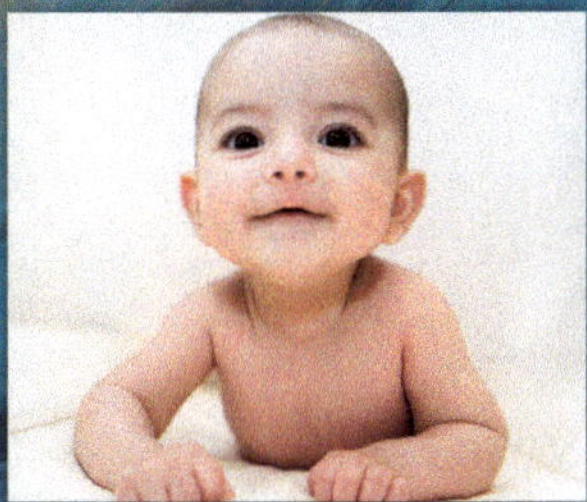

*Source:* Franco Deriu/Adobe Stock.

# Past Contributors to the Sixth Edition

**Diane M. Anderson, PhD, RD**
Associate Professor
Department of Pediatrics, Section of Neonatology
Baylor College of Medicine
Houston, Texas

**Shreyas Arya, MD, MBBS**
Clinical Fellow
Division of Neonatology and Pulmonary Biology
Cincinnati Children's Hospital Medical Center
Cincinnati, Ohio

**Susan Tucker Blackburn, PhD, RN, FAAN**
Professor Emeritus
Department of Family and Child Nursing, School of Nursing
University of Washington
Seattle, Washington

**Mary Beth Bodin, DNP, CRNP, NNP-BC**
Neonatal Consultant
Tuscaloosa, Alabama

**Robin Dawn Clark, MD**
Professor of Pediatrics in Medical Genetics
Loma Linda University Health
Loma Linda, California

**Amy D'Agata, PhD, MS, RN**
Assistant Professor, College of Nursing
University of Rhode Island
Kingston, Rhode Island
Adjunct Assistant Professor, Department of Pediatrics
Brown University
Providence, Rhode Island

**Georgia R. Ditzenberger, PhD, NNP-BC, APNP**
Assistant Professor, CHS
Neonatology Division, Department of Pediatrics, University of Wisconsin, School of Medicine and Public Health
Madison, Wisconsin

**Jenna L. Dobry, BSc (Hon)**
Clinical Research Coordinator
Section of Neonatology, Department of Pediatrics
Cummings School of Medicine
University of Calgary
Calgary, Alberta, Canada

**Kelly Benham French**
Parent and Professor of Practice in Journalism
The Media School
Indiana University
Bloomington, Indiana

**Kathleen Haubrich, PhD, RN**
Associate Professor, Department of Nursing
Miami University
Hamilton, Ohio

**Stephanie Hoe, BSN, RN**
Neonatal Staff Nurse
Kapiolani Medical Center for Women & Children
Caring for Hawai'i Neonates
Honolulu, Hawaii

**Joanne McManus Kuller, RN, MS**
Neonatal Clinical Nurse Specialist
University of California at San Francisco Benioff Children's Hospital Oakland
Oakland, California

**Abhay Lodha, DM, MD, MBBS, MSC**
Associate Professor
Department of Pediatrics
Cumming School of Medicine, University of Calgary
Calgary, Alberta, Canada

**Kathryn R. McLean, MSN, RN, NNP-BC**
Neonatal Nurse Practitioner
Women and Infants Hospital
Providence, Rhode Island

**Mary E. Coughlin McNeil, MS, NNP, RNC-E**
President and Founder
Caring Essentials Collaborative, LLC
Boston, Massachusetts

**Merry-K. Moos, BSN, FNP, FAAN**
Research Professor (retired)
Department of Obstetrics and Gynecology
University of North Carolina at Chapel Hill
School of Medicine
Consultant, Center for Maternal and Infant Health
Lead Nurse Planner, National March of Dimes
President, MK Moos, Inc.
Chapel Hill, North Carolina

**Dorothy M. Mullaney, DNP, MHSc, ANPRN, NNP-BC, RN**
Director, Associate Providers
Dartmouth Hitchcock Medical Center
Assistant Professor of Pediatrics
Geisel School of Medicine at Dartmouth
Hanover, New Hampshire

**Debra M. Parker, MSN, APRN-NP**
Lead Neonatal Nurse Practitioner
Methodist Women's Hospital
Omaha, Nebraska

**Leslie A. Parker, PhD, NNP-BC, FAAN**
Associate Professor
University of Florida
Gainesville, Florida

**Lyn S. Prater, PhD, RN**
Senior Lecturer and Undergraduate Clinical Coordinator
Baylor University, School of Nursing
Dallas, Texas

**Shahirose S. Premji, PhD, MScN, BSc, BScN, RN, FAAN**
Director and Professor
School of Nursing, Faculty of Health
York University
Toronto, Ontario, Canada

**Jana L. Pressler, PhD, RN**
Assistant Dean and Professor
University of Nebraska Medical Center College of Nursing
Lincoln Division
Lincoln, Nebraska

**Cheryl Riley, DNP, RN, NNP-BC**
Clinical Associate Professor and NNP Program Coordinator
Baylor University, School of Nursing
Dallas, Texas

**Donna J. Ryan, DNP, RN, CNE**
Assistant Professor, Nurse Educator
Elmira College
Elmira, New York

**Beth Shields, PharmD**
Associate Director of Operations
Pediatric Clinical Specialist
Rush University Medical Center
Chicago, Illinois

**Kaye Spence, AM, RN, MN**
Adjunct Associate Professor
Clinical Nurse Consultant—Neonatology
Grace Centre for Newborn Care
The Children's Hospital at Westmead
Westmead, Australia

**Becky Spencer, PhD, RN, IBCLC**
Assistant Professor
Texas Woman's University
College of Nursing
Denton, Texas

**Carol Turnage Spruill, MSN, APRN-CNS, CPHQ, NTMNC**
Clinical Nurse Specialist
Department of Women, Infants and Children
University of Texas Medical Branch
Galveston, Texas

**Deborah K. Steward, PhD, RN**
Faculty Emeritus
Ohio State University
College of Nursing
Columbus, OH

**Valerie Boebel Toly, PhD, RN, CPNP**
Assistant Professor
Frances Payne Bolton School of Nursing
Case Western Reserve University
Cleveland, Ohio

**Marlene Walden, PhD, RN, NNP-BC, CCNS, FAAN**
Nurse Scientist Manager
Arkansas Children's Hospital
Adjunct Associate Professor
University of Arkansas for Medical Sciences
Little Rock, Arkansas

**Karen Walker, PhD, RN**
Clinical Associate Professor, University of Sydney
Research Manager, Grace Centre for Newborn Care
Senior Research Fellow, IMPACT for Cerebral Palsy
President, Australia College of Neonatal Nurses
Vice President, Council of International Neonatal Nurses, Inc. (COINN)
Westmead, Australia

**Tami Wallace, DNP, APRN, NNP-BC**
Neonatal Nurse Practitioner and Educator Nationwide Children's Hospital
Columbus, Ohio

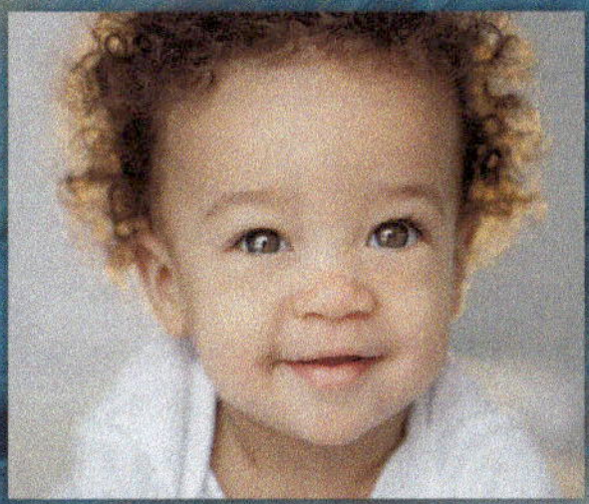

*Source:* Miramiska/Adobe Stock.

# Preface

One of the most complex issues in healthcare is the care of sick or premature infants and those with multiple, severe congenital anomalies. Despite advanced technology and knowledge, preterm delivery continues to be a significant problem in the United States. Maternal risk factors have changed over the past decade. For example, more women with congenital heart anomalies and chronic illnesses, such as diabetes or sickle cell anemia, are giving birth to infants with consequent health problems. The rise of in vitro fertilization has resulted in increased multiple births and prematurity. Many infants in neonatal intensive care units (NICUs) have been exposed to substances or are born to mothers with other risk factors such as delayed childbearing or childhood cancers.

The care of these at-risk infants requires the use of more and more complex technology. Surfactant administration, nitric oxide administration, high-frequency jet ventilators, neurally adjusted ventilatory assist (NAVA) (Stein & Firestone, 2014), and new hybrid ventilators providing high-frequency and conventional modes of ventilation are being used in Europe and are likely to be brought to the United States for Food and Drug Administration (FDA) approval. New technologies now can provide continuous, noninvasive monitoring of endotracheal tube position and obstruction (Hütten et al., 2015). Servo-controlled oxygen administration, which leads to greater compliance with targeted oxygen saturation ranges, is being developed (Claure & Bancalari, 2015). Near-infrared spectroscopy (NIRS), amplitude-integrated EEGs (aEEGs), dialysis, organ transplantation, and other extraordinary measures are becoming commonplace. Better integration of technologies (both electronic medical records [EMRs] and medical devices) will be the basis for decision support and predictive analytics. However, in the midst of these high-tech interventions, neuroprotective developmentally supportive care interventions such as olfactory and gustatory support, using visible rather than audible alarms, music therapy, cycling lights, using more physiologically and developmentally appropriate positioning, and skin-to-skin contact (SSC) are being recognized as evidence-based neuroprotective interventions, due to increasing evidence regarding the importance of maintaining a developmentally supportive NICU environment for improved long-term infant/child and family outcomes. Some consequences of prematurity are caused by early parent–infant separation and a lack of parents' participation in the care of their infant during traditional neonatal intensive care. The family is an essential partner in decision making and care for their infant, and family-centered care is being expanded to family-integrated care, a paradigm shift from nurse caring to nurse coaching for parents providing the care.

Providers of neonatal care need up-to-date accurate and comprehensive information as a basis for providing care to newborns. A thorough understanding of normal physiology as well as the pathophysiology of disease processes is necessary for well-designed care practices. Knowledge about associated risk factors, genetics, critical periods of development, principles of nutrition and pharmacology, and current neonatal research findings are all essential in providing optimal care for neonates. A newer concept called *de-implementation* refers to the science of abandoning and unlearning practices built on the scaffolding of habit. Practices that are novel but yet not fully tested, unproven practices (those that lack supporting evidence), and practices of habit (practices that continue despite contradictory evidence) should go through the process of de-implementation. Care practices need to be based on the best evidence-based practices available, rather than on tradition and habits.

A multidisciplinary approach has been replaced by an integrated interprofessional approach to care. All these elements form the foundation for assessment, planning, implementation, and evaluation of the effectiveness of neonatal care. The nurse plays a vital role in the provision of integrated healthcare to newborns. During the past decade, the nurse's role has included added responsibilities, which are recognized at both the staff and advanced practice levels. For the purposes of this book, we define the roles of the neonatal staff nurse, clinical nurse specialist (CNS), and neonatal nurse practitioner (NNP).

## NEONATAL STAFF NURSE

The neonatal staff nurse role requires accurate and thorough assessment skills, excellent ability to communicate with other health professionals and patients' families, and a broad understanding of physiology and pathophysiology on which to base management decisions. It requires highly developed technical skills as well as critical decision-making skills. With healthcare delivery changes, the role also requires supervision of ancillary personnel and an informed delegation of certain patient-oriented tasks. These changes require the staff nurse to possess even better assessment skills and sound knowledge of physiology and pathophysiology than in the past because some decision making will be done in concert with other, less highly trained personnel. Additionally, the neonatal nurse is an essential contributor to the decision-making process surrounding the care of the critically ill neonate, including involvement in the ethical challenges that may occur regarding the level of care provided. In a recent position statement (#3067) by the National Association of Neonatal Nurses (NANN) (Conway-Orgel, 2016), it was recommended that nursing be a part of the multidisciplinary team that facilitates decision making affecting the health and well-being of the infant throughout the hospital stay.

In 2014, as the professional voice of neonatal nurses, NANN published a position statement (#3061) recommending that subspecialty NICUs (Level II, III, and IV NICUs) be staffed with a sufficient number and an appropriate mix of qualified registered nurses to attend to the emergent and complex care requirements of critically ill and convalescent infants (NANN, 2021).

## CLINICAL NURSE SPECIALIST

CNSs are advanced practice registered nurses (APRNs) who have graduate preparation (master's or doctorate) in nursing. Like other APRNs, they are trained in physiology, pharmacology, and physical assessment in addition to their particular areas of specialty. CNSs are expert clinicians with advanced education and training in a specialized area of nursing practice who work in a wide variety of healthcare settings. Regardless of specialty or setting, CNSs provide leadership in clinical expertise, nursing practice, and systems innovation. CNSs provide for the diagnosis, treatment, and ongoing management of patients. CNSs diagnose, develop plans of care for, treat, and provide ongoing management of complex patients. In many states, the CNSs can prescribe medications and offer durable medical equipment and therapies. They also provide expertise and support to nurses caring for patients at the bedside, help drive practice changes throughout the organization, and ensure the use of best practices and evidence-based care to achieve the best possible patient outcomes. Research and demonstration projects have shown that the CNS role is uniquely suited to lead implementation of evidence-based quality improvement actions that also reduce cost throughout the healthcare system (National Association of Clinical Nurse Specialists, 2016).

## NEONATAL NURSE PRACTITIONER

The NNP is a registered nurse with clinical expertise in neonatal nursing who has received formal education at either the master's or doctoral level, with supervised clinical experience in the management of sick newborns and their families. The NNP manages a caseload of neonatal patients with consultation, collaboration, and general supervision from a physician; however, many state legislatures are following the Institute of Medicine's (IOM's) recommendation for autonomous NNP practice by repealing restrictive practice laws, thereby increasing healthcare access for millions of patients (American Association of Nurse Practitioners, 2018; Barton Associates, 2019). As a result, NNPs have increasing authority and responsibility. Using extensive knowledge of pathophysiology, pharmacology, and physiology, the NNP exercises independent or intradependent (in collaboration with other health professionals) judgment in the assessment, diagnosis, and initiation of certain delegated medical processes and procedures. As an advanced practice neonatal nurse, the NNP is additionally involved in education, consultation, and research at various levels.

NANN and the National Association of Neonatal Nurse Practitioners (NANNP), a division of NANN, published position paper #3059, a synthesis of previous efforts, which discusses the role, preparation, and scope of practice of the neonatal APRN (NANN, 2024). NANN and NANNP define the educational and preparation standards for those pursuing the NNP role. NANN published a position statement in 1990, reaffirmed the definition of the NNP in 2000, and in 2009 issued another position statement that defined the NNP competencies (NANN, 2009). NANN (2023) reaffirmed these core competencies for NNPs in its *Education Standards and Curriculum Guidelines for Neonatal Nurse Practitioner Programs* in 2014, which were further elaborated upon by NANNP in the development and revision of its *Competencies and Orientation Toolkit for Neonatal Nurse Practitioners* (NANNP, 2014). In 2017, NANN and NANNP published a document describing the minimum standards necessary for preparation of NNPs, titled *Education Standards and Curriculum Guidelines for Neonatal Nurse Practitioner Programs* (NANN, 2023).

In the current practice environment, outcome measures specific to the NNP must now be incorporated into professional requirements. To guide the process of continuous practice evaluation, individual practice standards have been provided by The Joint Commission in the form of ongoing professional practice evaluation or as focused professional practice evaluation (The Joint Commission, 2015). To accomplish this goal, NNPs must participate, direct, and develop performance metrics to evaluate their individual (direct) and collaborative (aggregate) contributions to improving patient and family care and outcomes while demonstrating decreased healthcare expenditures (Snapp et al., 2017). Developing these outcome evaluation tools and processes will assist in the benchmarking and validation of care provided by NNPs.

The American Association of Colleges of Nurses (AACN) has proposed a change in the educational preparation for APRNs. The proposal recommends that the nurse practitioner be prepared at a "doctor of nursing practice" (DNP) level. This will likely affect the NNP role, as well as other APRNs, over the next few years.

## PURPOSE AND CONTENT

The book's seventh edition provides a comprehensive assessment and examination of the care of neonates from a physiologic and pathophysiologic approach appropriate for any health professional concerned with neonatal care.

This text provides a complete physiologic and embryologic foundation for each neonatal body system. Additionally, it includes medical, surgical, and psychosocial care because the integrative management approach is absolutely imperative to the well-being of the newborn and family. Appropriate diagnostic tests and their interpretation are included in each organ-system chapter. There is extensive use of research findings in the chapters to provide evidence to support practice strategies and demonstrate the rationale for clinical decision making. Complete references for more in-depth reading are found at the end of each chapter so that the reader may pursue more specific information on a topical area. Use of tables and illustrations further supports material that is presented in the narrative portions. New to this edition are special emergency alerts, quality and/or safety issues, and parent voices, which are infused into applicable chapters. New chapters include Neonatal Abstinence Syndrome, and Touch a Life, Affect a Lifetime: Trauma-Informed Care in the NICU.

In the United States, the economic effect of preterm births is well over $25 billion per year (Behrman & Butler, 2007). Greater cost savings can be derived from technology that reduces labor costs, because NICU RN and respiratory therapy labor expenses account for over 60% of total neonatal care (Rhine, 2016). Now more than ever, neonatal care providers must examine patient, family, and staff outcomes to meet the demands for providing cost-effective and high-quality care. Research is critical to support both the art and science of neonatal care. Whenever possible, the contributors remind the reader of areas in need of further study. This book is not a quick reference: It provides comprehensive, in-depth discussions along with detailed physiologic principles and collaborative management strategies. It provides a sound basis for safe and effective neonatal care; however, the format should make the information easier to find.

We begin the seventh edition with the effect of environmental influences and critical periods on the developing fetus. This transitions into the aspects of perinatal care, the high-risk pregnancy, the effects of labor on the fetus, and postpartal risk factors. The text then focuses on more specific neonatal topics, starting with resuscitation and stabilization of the newborn, assessment of the newborn and infant, followed by the normal term infant. Each organ system is discussed in depth, including the respiratory system and its complications and new technologies, followed by assessment of, and management strategies for, the cardiovascular, gastrointestinal, metabolic, endocrine, immunologic, integumentary, hematopoietic, musculoskeletal, neurologic, auditory, ophthalmic, and genitourinary systems. The thread of integrative management is interwoven throughout the text. Foundational topics such as fluids, electrolytes, and acid–base balance; nutrition management; pharmacology; pain management; as well as emerging technologies and healthcare simulation are included, in addition to fetal therapy, surgical considerations, and emerging infections. Vulnerable populations cared for frequently in NICU settings are included, such as infants undergoing transplants, extremely low birth weight (ELBW) infants, late preterm infants, and infants withdrawing from opioids/neonatal abstinence syndrome. Chapters addressing environmental health and family-centered care in the NICU and beyond include neurobehavioral development, management of the NICU environment, trauma-informed care, family partnerships, palliative and end-of-life care, postdischarge care of the newborn, and, the NICU through a mother's eyes. The final group of chapters covers neonatal care in the new millennium with topics including trends in neonatal care delivery, informatics, human genetics and genomics, trends in neonatal research and evidence-based practice, legal issues, global perspectives in neonatal care, and competency-based education and continuous competency. The seventh edition recognizes that neonatal nursing and care are global issues. The last section includes neonatal diagnostic and evidence-based care protocols pulled out separately, so that they are easy to find and use.

To provide depth to these topical areas, physicians, nurses, infant developmental specialists, and other health professionals concerned with neonatal care from across the country and around the world have contributed in all editions. The attempt was made not only to tap the experts in the neonatal field but also to have them represent as wide a geographic area as possible. We hope that the broad geographic distribution of contributors and reviewers will help minimize the effect of regional differences in clinical practice.

We hope that you will find the text's information very useful and helpful to you in providing high-quality care to newborns and their families.

*Carole Kenner*
*Leslie B. Altimier*
*Marina V. Boykova*

## RECOMMENDED READINGS


American Nurses Association. (2015). *Code of ethics for nurses with interpretive statements*. Author.

Institute of Medicine. (2011). *The future of nursing: Leading change, advancing health* (pp. 163–220). National Academies Press.

National Governors Association. (2012). *Nurse practitioners have potential to improve access to primary care*. https://classic.nga.org/cms/home/news-room/news-releases/page_2012/col2-content/nurse-practitioners-have-potenti.html

Prasad, V., & Ioannidis, J. P. (2014). Evidence-based de-implementation for contradicted, unproven, and aspiring healthcare practices. *Implementation Science, 9*, 1. https://doi.org/10.1186/1748-5908-9-1

## REFERENCES


American Association of Nurse Practitioners. (2018). *State practice environment*. https://www.aanp.org/legislation-regulation/state-legislation/state-practice-environment

Barton Associates. (2019). *Nurse practitioner scope of practice laws*. https://www.bartonassociates.com/nurse-practitioners/nurse-practitioner-scope-of-practice-laws

Behrman, R. E., & Butler, A. S. (Eds.). (2007). *Preterm birth: Causes, consequences, and prevention*. National Academies Press.

Claure, N., & Bancalari, E. (2015). Oxygen saturation targeting by automatic control of inspired oxygen in premature infants. *NeoReviews, 16*, e406–e412. https://doi.org/10.1542/neo.16-7-e406

Conway-Orgel, M. (2016). *Position statement #3067: NICU nurse involvement in ethical decisions (treatment of critically ill newborns)*. National Association of Neonatal Nurses. https://nann.org/wp-content/uploads/2025/04/NICU-Nurse-Involvement-in-Ethical-Decisions-fb3.pdf

Hütten, M. C., Goos, T. G., Ophelders, D., Nikiforou, M., Kuypers, E., Willems, M., Niemarkt, H. J., Dankelman, J., Andriessen, P., Mohns, T., Reiss, I. K., & Kramer, B. W. (2015). Fully automated predictive intelligent control of oxygenation (PRICO) in resuscitation and ventilation of preterm lambs. *Pediatric Research, 78*, 657–663. https://doi.org/10.1038/pr.2015.158

The Joint Commission. (2015). *Standards BoosterPak™ for focused professional practice evaluation/ongoing professional practice evaluation (FPPE/OPPE)*. Author.

National Association of Clinical Nurse Specialists. (2016). *Key findings from the 2016 Clinical Nurse Specialists Consensus*. https://nacns.org/wp-content/uploads/2016/11/2016-CNS-Census-Findings.pdf

National Association of Neonatal Nurse Practitioners. (2014). *Competencies & orientation toolkit for neonatal nurse practitioners* (2nd ed.). National Association of Neonatal Nurses.

National Association of Neonatal Nurses. (2009). Position statement #3042: Requirements for advanced neonatal nursing practice in neonatal intensive care units. *Advances in Neonatal Care, 9*(4), 190–194. https://doi.org/10.1097/ANC.0b013e3181b0129a

National Association of Neonatal Nurses. (2021). *Position statement #3074: RN staffing in the neonatal intensive care unit*. Author. https://nann.org/wp-content/uploads/2025/04/updated_RN_nicu_staffing-ad7.pdf

National Association of Neonatal Nurses. (2023). *Education standards and curriculum guidelines for neonatal nurse practitioner programs*. Author. https://nann.org/all-new-curriculum-guidelines-and-education-competencies-for-neonatal-nurse-practitioner-programs

National Association of Neonatal Nurses. (2024). *Advanced practice registered nurses practicing within the neonatal population: Role, preparation, and scope of practice*. Author. https://nann.org/wp-content/uploads/2025/04/APRN_Scope_FINAL_May2024-d7c.pdf

Rhine, W. D. (2016). Technology—Considerations for the NICU of the future. *Newborn and Infant Nursing Reviews, 16*(4), 208–212. https://doi.org/10.1053/j.nainr.2016.09.005

Snapp, B., Wilson, J., Puchalski, M., Wallace, T., & Task Force Leader (2017). Quality metrics: executive summary of position statement 3068: From the national association of neonatal nurses. *Advances in neonatal care : official journal of the National Association of Neonatal Nurses, 17*(1), 9. https://doi.org/10.1097/ANC.0000000000000356

Stein, H., & Firestone, K. (2014). Application of neurally adjusted ventilatory assist in neonates. *Seminars in Fetal and Neonatal Medicine, 19*, 60–69. https://doi.org/10.1016/j.siny.2013.09.005

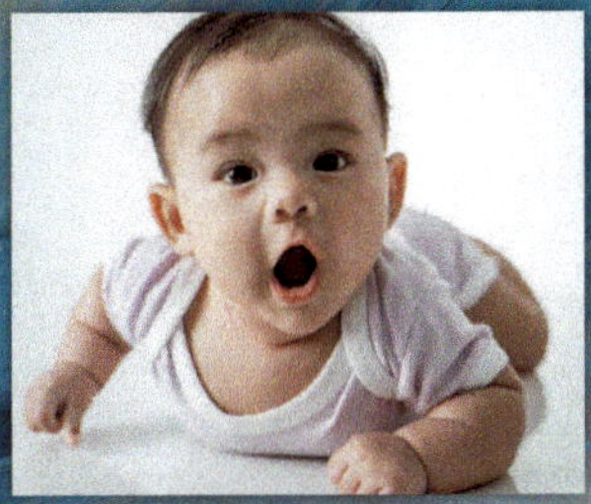

Source: Odua Images/Adobe Stock.

# Acknowledgments

The idea for this book was born in the basement office of the lead editor (Dr. Carole Kenner) in Cincinnati, Ohio. In 1992, we recognized there was not a comprehensive book about nursing care for neonates. The first edition of the book was created in 1993. Over the course of the next three decades, we have refined the content to reflect new trends in neonatal care. I am grateful to Drs. Leslie Altimier and Marina Boykova for taking this journey with me.

*Carole Kenner*

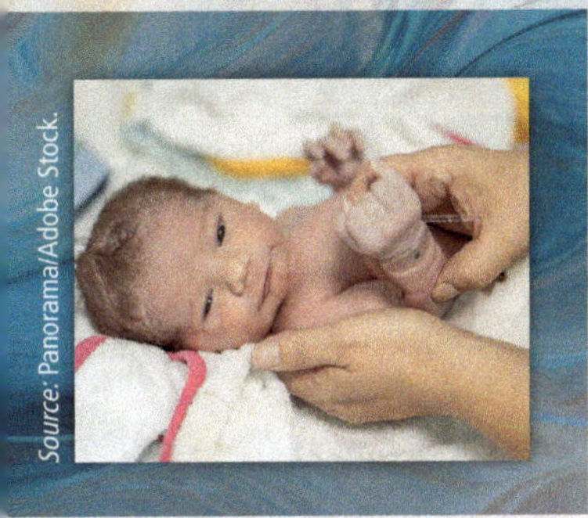


Unit I: Prenatal Considerations and Care

CHAPTER 1

# Fetal Development: Environmental Influences and Critical Periods

Carole Kenner

## INTRODUCTION

In this chapter, the major events of prenatal development are described, and critical development periods for the major organ systems are identified. A brief review of the events beginning with fertilization is included. Human genetics is discussed in Chapter 34, "Human Genetics and Genomics: Impact on Neonatal Care".

## EARLY FETAL DEVELOPMENT

Human development begins with the fertilization of an ovum (female gamete) by a spermatocyte (male gamete). The fusion of the ovum and sperm initiates a sequence of events that causes the single-celled zygote to develop into a new human being. During the 38 to 42 weeks of gestation, dramatic growth and development occur that are unequaled during any other period of life.

### Fertilization

Large numbers of spermatozoa are necessary to increase the chances for conception because the spermatozoa must traverse the cervical canal, uterus, and uterine (fallopian) tubes to reach the ovum; approximately 200 to 600 million sperm are deposited in the posterior fornix of the vagina during ejaculation. The usual site of fertilization is in the ampulla, the widest portion of the uterine tubes, located near the ovaries. Sperm are propelled by the movement of the tails, aided by muscular contractions of the uterus and fallopian tubes. The spermatozoa undergo two physiologic changes to penetrate the corona radiata and zona pellucida, the barriers around the secondary oocyte. The first change is capacitation, an enzymatic reaction that removes the glycoprotein coating from the spermatozoa and plasma proteins from the seminal fluid. Capacitation generally occurs in the uterus or uterine tubes and takes about 7 hours. The second change, the acrosome reaction, occurs when a capacitated sperm passes through the corona radiata, causing structural changes that result in the fusion of the plasma membranes of the sperm and the oocyte. Progesterone released from the follicle at ovulation stimulates the acrosome reaction. Three enzymes are released from the acrosome to facilitate entry of the sperm into the ovum. Hyaluronidase allows the sperm to penetrate the corona radiata, whereas trypsin-like enzymes and zona lysin digest a pathway across the zona pellucida (Persaud & Torchia, 2025; Sadler, 2023).

Only about 300 to 500 spermatozoa reach the ovum. When a spermatozoon encounters the ovum, the zona pellucida and the plasma membrane fuse, preventing entry by other sperm. After penetration by a single sperm, the oocyte completes the second meiotic cell division, resulting in the haploid number of chromosomes (22, X) and the second polar body. The chromosomes are arranged to form the female pronucleus (Persaud & Torchia, 2025; Sadler, 2023).

As the spermatozoon moves close to the female pronucleus, the tail detaches, and the nucleus enlarges to form the male pronucleus. The male and female pronuclei fuse, forming a diploid cell called the *zygote*. The zygote contains 23 autosomes and 1 sex chromosome from each parent (46, XX or 46, XY). The genetic sex of the new individual is determined at fertilization by the contribution of the male parent. The male parent (XY) may contribute either an X or a Y chromosome. If the spermatozoon contains an X chromosome, the offspring is female (46, XX). If the spermatozoon receives one Y chromosome, the offspring is male (46, XY). Individual variation is the result of random or independent assortment of the autosomal chromosomes (Persaud & Torchia, 2025; Sadler, 2023).

### Cleavage

Mitotic cell division occurs after fertilization as the zygote passes down the uterine tube, resulting in the formation of two blastomeres (Figure 1.1). The cells continue to divide, increasing in number, although decreasing in size. The term *cleavage* is used to describe the mitotic cell division of the zygote (Figure 1.2). When the number of cells reaches approximately 16 (usually on the third day), the zygote is called a

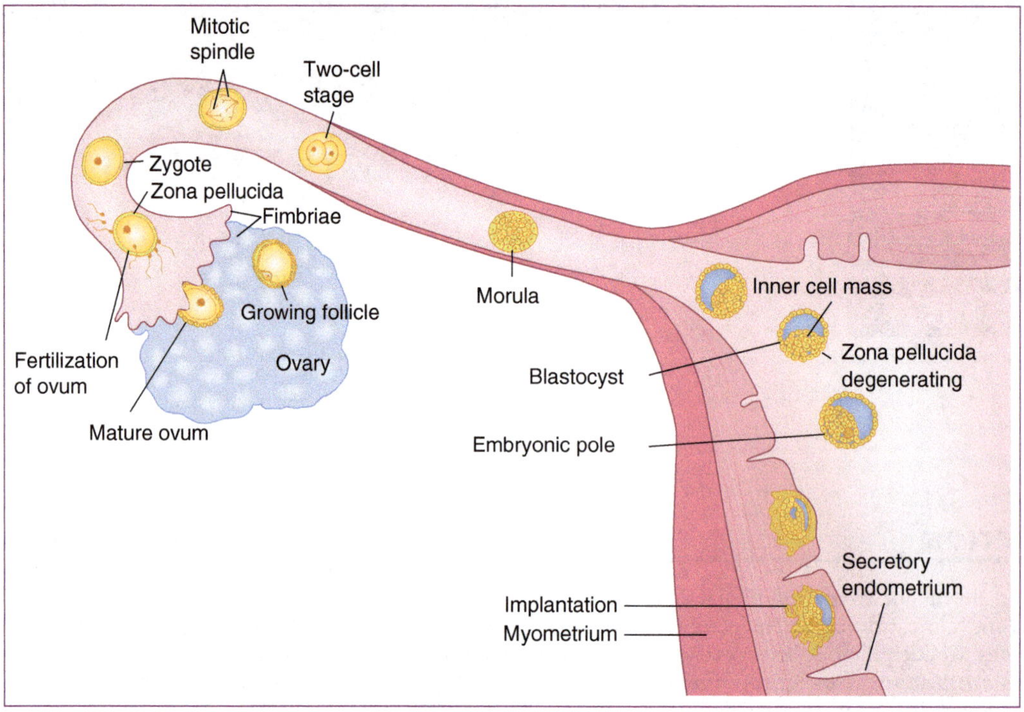


**FIGURE 1.1 Fantastic voyage.** From fertilization to implantation. The journey through the fallopian tubes takes approximately 4 days. During this time, mitotic cell division occurs. Implantation occurs on about day 9 through 12.

*morula*, because of its resemblance to a mulberry. The zygote reaches the morula stage about the time it enters the uterus. The morula consists of groups of centrally located cells called the inner cell mass and an outer cell layer. At this stage, the individual cells are called *blastomeres*. The outer cell layer forms the trophoblast, from which the placenta develops. The inner cell mass, called the *embryoblast*, gives rise to the embryo (Persaud & Torchia, 2025; Sadler, 2023).

After the morula penetrates the uterine cavity, fluid enters through the zona pellucida into the intercellular spaces of the inner cell mass. The fluid-filled spaces fuse, forming a large cavity known as the *blastocyst cavity* about the fourth day after fertilization. The morula is now called the *blastocyst*. This outer cell layer, known as the *trophoblast*, forms the wall of the blastocyst, which later becomes the placenta, and the embryoblast projects from the wall of the blastocyst into the blastocyst cavity. The uterine secretions nourish the blastocyst until implantation occurs (Persaud & Torchia, 2025; Sadler, 2023).

## Implantation

Degeneration of the zona pellucida occurs on about the fifth day after fertilization, allowing the blastocyst to attach to the endothelium of the endometrium on about the sixth day. The trophoblasts then secrete proteolytic enzymes that destroy the endometrial endothelium and invade the endometrium. Two layers of trophoblasts develop; the inner layer is made up of cytotrophoblasts, and the outer layer is composed of syncytiotrophoblasts. The syncytiotrophoblast has finger-like projections that produce enzymes capable of further eroding the endometrial tissues. By the end of the seventh day, the blastocyst is superficially implanted (Figure 1.3).

## Formation of the Bilaminar Disk

Implantation is completed during the second week. The syncytiotrophoblast continues to invade the endometrium and becomes embedded. Spaces in the syncytiotrophoblast, called *lacunae*, fill with blood from ruptured maternal capillaries and secretions from eroded endometrial glands. This fluid nourishes the embryoblast by diffusion. The lacunae give rise to the uteroplacental circulation. The lacunae fuse to form a network that then becomes the intervillous spaces of the placenta. The endometrial capillaries near the implanted embryoblast become dilated and eroded by the syncytiotrophoblast. Maternal blood enters the lacunar network and provides circulation and nutrients to the embryo. Maternal embryonic blood circulation provides the developing embryo with nutrition and oxygenation and removes waste products before the development of the placenta. Finger-like projections, primary chorionic villi, of the chorion develop into the chorionic villi of the placenta at about the same time (Moore et al., 2015; Sadler, 2015).

The inner cell mass differentiates into two layers: the hypoblast (endoderm), a layer of small cuboidal cells, and the epiblast (ectoderm), a layer of high columnar cells. The two layers form a flattened, circular bilaminar embryonic disk. The amniotic cavity is derived from spaces within the epiblast. As the amniotic cavity enlarges, a thin layer of epithelial cells covers the amniotic cavity. During the development of the amniotic cavity, other trophoblastic cells form a thin extracoelomic membrane, which encloses the primitive yolk sac.

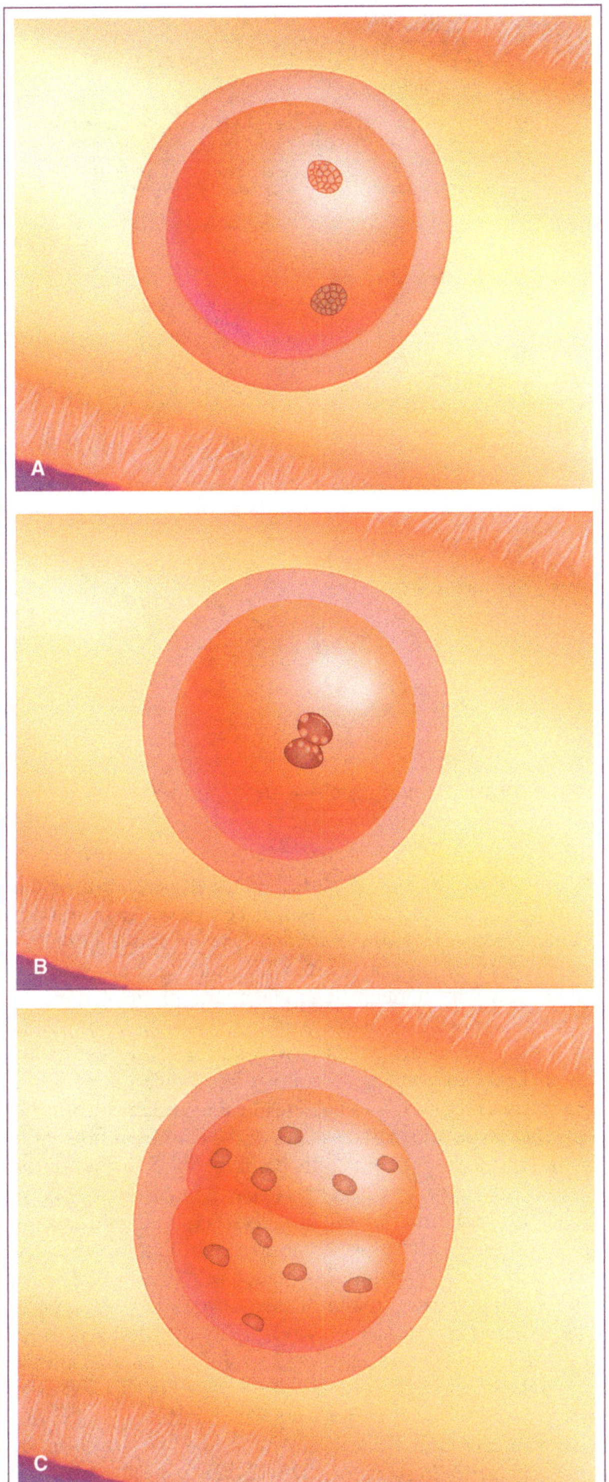


**FIGURE 1.2 Stages of cell division: cleavage.** (A) Zygote. (B) Zygote undergoing first cleavage. (C) Two-cell blastomere state.

The yolk sac produces fetal red blood cells (RBCs). Other trophoblastic cells form a layer of mesenchymal tissue, called the *extraembryonic mesoderm*, around the amnion and primitive

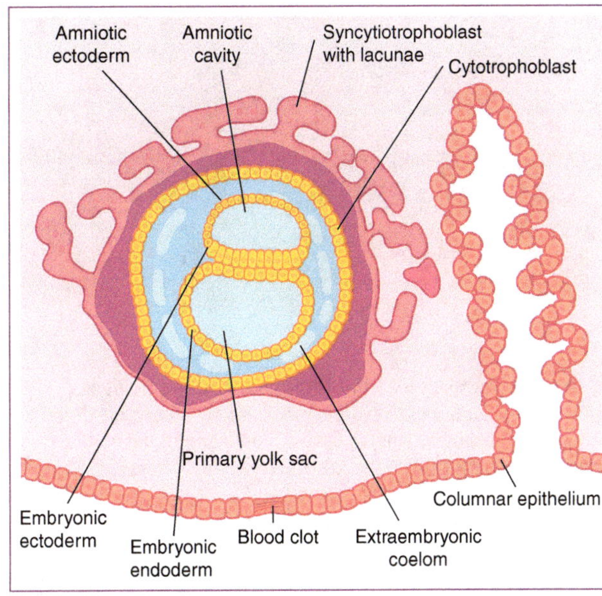


**FIGURE 1.3 Cross section of a blastocyst at 11 days.** Two germ layers are present. The trophoblast has differentiated into the syncytiotrophoblast and the cytotrophoblast.

yolk sac. Isolated coelomic spaces in the extraembryonic mesoderm fuse to form a single, large, fluid-filled cavity surrounding the amnion and yolk sac, except for the area where the amnion is attached to the chorion by the connecting stalk. The primitive yolk sac decreases in size, creating a smaller secondary yolk sac (Persaud & Torchia, 2025; Sadler, 2023).

Two layers of extraembryonic mesoderm result from the formation of the extraembryonic cavity. The extraembryonic somatic mesoderm lines the trophoblast and covers the amnion, and the extraembryonic splanchnic mesoderm covers the yolk sac. The chorion is made up of the extraembryonic somatic mesoderm, the cytotrophoblast, and the syncytiotrophoblast. The chorion forms the chorionic sac, in which the embryo, the amniotic sac, and the yolk sac are located. By the end of the second week, there is a slightly thickened area near the cephalic region of the hypoblastic disk, known as the *prochordal plate*, which marks the location of the mouth (Persaud & Torchia, 2025; Sadler, 2023).

## Formation of the Trilaminar Embryonic Disk: The Third Week of Development

The third week of development is marked by rapid growth, the formation of the primitive streak, and the differentiation of the three germ layers, from which all fetal tissue and organs are derived (Persaud & Torchia, 2025; Sadler, 2023; Figure 1.4).

**Gastrulation.** Gastrulation is the process through which the bilaminar disk develops into a trilaminar embryonic disk. Gastrulation is the most important event of early fetal formation; it affects the remainder of embryologic development. During the third week, epiblast cells separate from their original location and migrate inward, forming the mesoblast, which spreads cranially and laterally to form a layer between

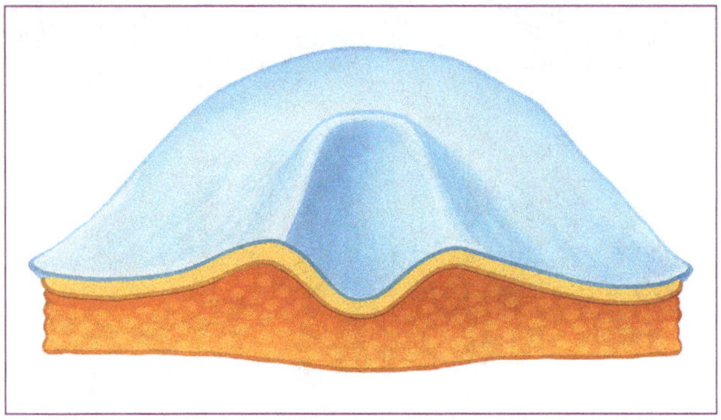

**FIGURE 1.4 Formation of the trilaminar embryonic disk: gastrulation.** During gastrulation, the bilaminar embryonic disk changes to a trilaminar embryonic disk, consisting of the epiblast (ectoderm), hypoblast (endoderm), and mesoblast (mesoderm).

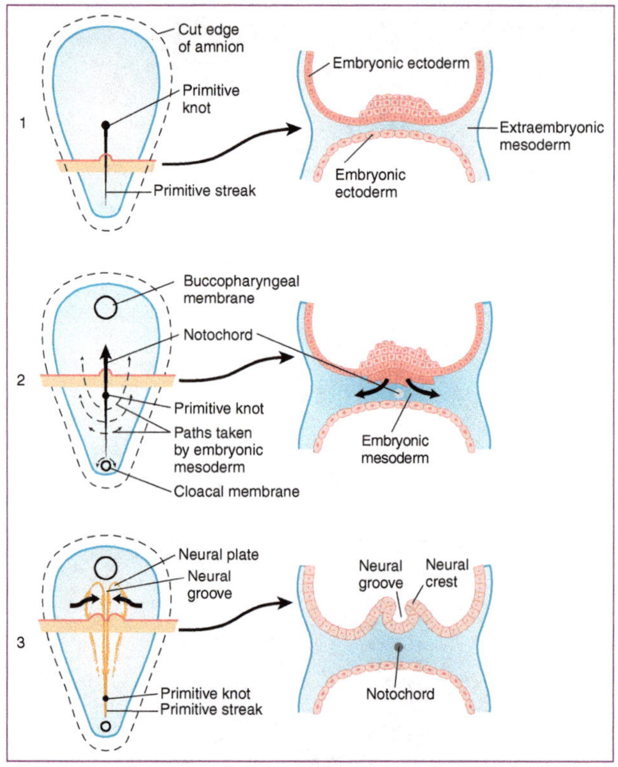


**FIGURE 1.5 Formation of primitive streak, primitive knot, notochord, and neural groove.**

the ectoderm and the endoderm called the *intraembryonic mesoderm*. Other mesoblastic cells invade the endoderm, displacing the endodermal cells laterally, forming a new layer, the embryonic ectoderm. Thus, the hypoblastic ectoderm produces the embryonic ectoderm, embryonic mesoderm, and most of the embryonic endoderm. These three germ layers are the source of the tissue and organs of the embryo (Persaud & Torchia, 2025; Sadler, 2023).

**Primitive Streak.** Over days 14 and 15, a groove and thickening of the ectoderm (epiblast), called the *primitive streak*, appears caudally in the center of the dorsum of the embryonic disk. The primitive streak results from the migration of ectodermal cells toward the midline in the posterior portion of the embryonic disk. The primitive groove develops in the primitive streak. When the primitive streak begins to produce mesoblastic cells that become intraembryonic mesoderm, the epiblast is referred to as the *embryonic ectoderm* and the hypoblast is referred to as the *embryonic mesoderm* (Persaud & Torchia, 2025; Sadler, 2023).

**Notochordal Process.** Cells from the primitive knot migrate cranially and form the midline cellular notochordal process. This process grows cranially between the ectoderm and endoderm until it reaches the prochordal plate, which is attached to the overlying ectoderm, thus forming the oropharyngeal membrane. The cloacal membrane, caudal to the primitive streak, develops into the anus (Persaud & Torchia, 2025; Sadler, 2023).

The primitive streak produces mesenchyme (mesoblasts) until the end of the fourth week. The primitive streak does not grow as rapidly as the other cells, making it relatively insignificant in size when compared with the other structures that continue to grow. Persistence of the primitive streak or remnants is the cause of sacrococcygeal teratomas (Persaud & Torchia, 2025; Sadler, 2023).

The notochord, a cellular rod that develops from the notochordal process, is the structure around which the vertebral column is formed. It forms the nucleus pulposus of the intervertebral bodies of the spinal column (Figure 1.5; Persaud & Torchia, 2025; Sadler, 2023).

**Neurulation.** Neurulation is the process through which the neural plate, neural folds, and neural tube are formed. The developing notochord stimulates the embryonic ectoderm to thicken, forming the neural plate. The neuroectoderm of the neural plate gives rise to the central nervous system (CNS). The neural plate develops cranial to the primitive knot. As the neural plate elongates, it gets wider and extends cranially to the oropharyngeal membrane. The neural plate invaginates along the central axis to form a neural groove with neural folds on each side. The neural folds move together and fuse, forming the neural tube, which shows the first indication of brain development (Figure 1.6). The neural tube detaches from the surface ectoderm, and the free edges of the ectoderm fuse, covering the posterior portion of the embryo. With formation of the neural tube, nearby ectodermal cells lying along the crest of each neural fold migrate inward, invading the mesoblast on each side of the neural tube. These irregular, flattened masses are called the *neural crest*. This structure's cells give rise to the spinal ganglia, the ganglia of the autonomic nervous system (ANS), and cranial nerves V, VII, IX, and X. Neural crest cells also form the meningeal covering of the brain and spinal cord and the sheaves that protect nerves. The neural crest cells contribute to the formation of pigment-producing cells, the adrenal medulla, and skeletal and muscular development in the head (Persaud & Torchia, 2025; Sadler, 2023).

**Development of Somites.** Another important event of the third week is the development of somites, which give rise to most of the skeleton and associated musculature and much of the dermis of the skin. During formation of the neural tube, the intraembryonic mesoderm on each side thickens, forming longitudinal columns of paraxial mesoderm. At about 20 days, the paraxial mesoderm begins to divide into paired cuboidal

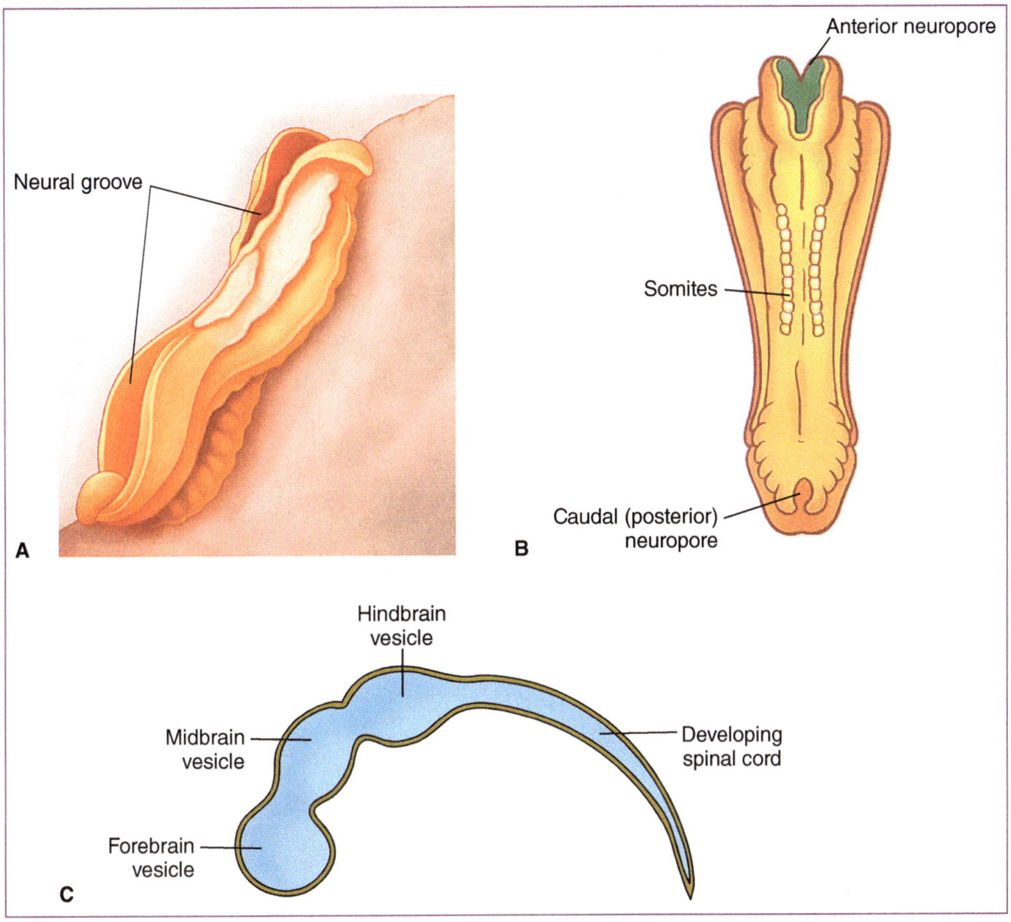


**FIGURE 1.6 Formation of the neural tube.** (A) Neural groove. (B) Closure of the neural tube almost completed. (C) Dilation of the neural tube forms the forebrain, midbrain, and hindbrain.

bodies known as *somites*. In all, 42 to 44 somites develop, in a craniocaudal sequence, although only 38 develop during the "somite" period. These somite pairs can be counted and give an estimate of fetal age before a crown-to-rump (C-R) measurement is possible (Persaud & Torchia, 2025; Sadler, 2023).

**Intraembryonic Cavity.** Another significant process is the formation of the intraembryonic cavity. This structure first appears as several small spaces within the lateral mesoderm and the cardiogenic mesoderm. These spaces combine to form the intraembryonic cavity; it is horseshoe shaped and lined with flattened epithelial cells that eventually line the peritoneal cavity. The intraembryonic cavity divides the lateral mesoderm into the parietal (somatic) and visceral (splanchnic) layers. It gives rise to the pericardial cavity, the pleural cavity, and the peritoneal cavity (Persaud & Torchia, 2025; Sadler, 2023).

## PLACENTAL DEVELOPMENT AND FUNCTION

The rudimentary maternal fetal circulation is intact by the fourth week of gestation. Growth of the trophoblast results in numerous primary and secondary chorionic villi, covering the surface of the chorionic sac until about the eighth week of gestation. At about the eighth week, the villi overlying the conceptus (decidua capsularis) degenerate, leaving a smooth area (smooth chorion). The villi underlying the conceptus (decidua basalis) remain and increase in size, producing the chorion frondosum, or fetal side of the placenta. The maternal side of the placenta is made up of the chorion and the chorionic villi. On implantation of the conceptus, maternal capillaries of the decidua basalis rupture, causing maternal blood to circulate through the developing fetal placenta (chorion frondosum). As growth and differentiation progress, extensions from the cytotrophoblast invade the syncytial layer and form a cytotrophoblastic shell, surrounding the conceptus and chorionic villi. This shell is continuous but has communications between maternal blood vessels in the decidua basalis and the intervillous spaces of the chorion frondosum. The latter is attached to the maternal side of the placenta (decidua basalis) by the cytotrophoblastic shell and anchoring villi. The placenta is mature and completely functional by 16 weeks of development (Figure 1.7). If the corpus luteum begins to regress prior to the 16th week and fails to produce enough progesterone (the hormone responsible for readying the uterine cavity for the pregnancy), the pregnancy is aborted because the placenta is not capable of supporting the pregnancy on its own until about this time (Persaud & Torchia, 2025; Sadler, 2023).

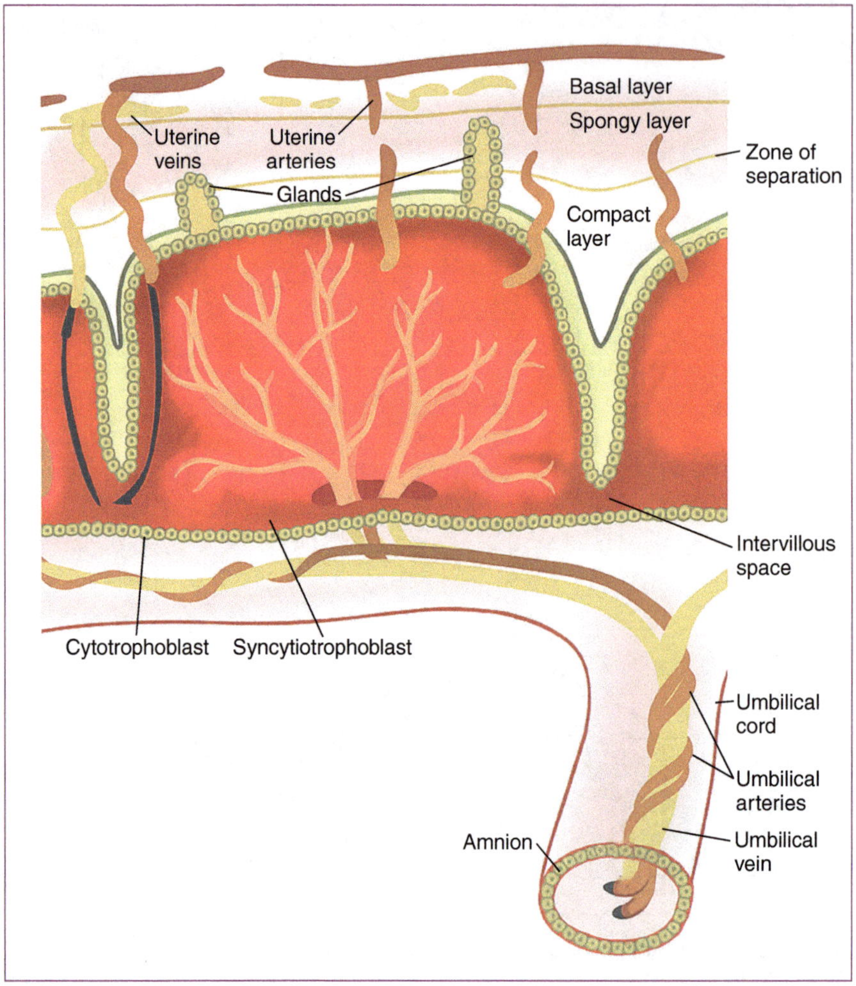


**FIGURE 1.7 Formation of the placenta.** The fetal and maternal sides of the placenta. Separation of the placenta from the uterus occurs at the site indicated by the gray line labeled zone of separation.

## Placental Fetal Circulation

A simple ebb-and-flow circulation is present in the embryo, yolk sac, connecting stalk, and chorion by 21 days of gestation. By 28 days, unidirectional circulation is established. Deoxygenated fetal blood leaves the fetus via the umbilical arteries and enters the capillaries in the chorionic villi, where gaseous and nutrient exchanges take place. Oxygenated blood returns to the fetus through the umbilical veins. At first, there are two arteries and two veins, but one vein gradually degenerates, leaving two arteries and one vein. If only one artery is present, a congenital anomaly, especially a renal one, should be suspected (Persaud & Torchia, 2025; Sadler, 2023).

## Placental Function

Normal growth and development of the embryo depend on adequate placental function. The placenta is responsible for oxygenation, nutrition, elimination of wastes, production of hormones essential for maintenance of the pregnancy, and transportation of substances. In addition, the placenta synthesizes glycogen, cholesterol, and fatty acids, which provide nutrients and energy for early fetal development. Transportation across the placental membrane occurs primarily through simple and facilitated diffusion, active transport, and pinocytosis. Oxygen, carbon dioxide, and carbon monoxide cross the placenta through simple diffusion. The fetus depends on a continuous supply of oxygenated blood flowing from the placenta (Persaud & Torchia, 2025; Sadler, 2023).

Water and electrolytes cross the placenta freely in both directions. Glucose is converted to glycogen in the placenta as a carbohydrate source for the fetus. Amino acids move readily across the placental membranes for protein synthesis in the fetus. Free fatty acids are transferred across the placenta by pinocytosis. There is limited or no transfer of maternal cholesterol, triglycerides, and phospholipids. Water- and fat-soluble vitamins cross the placenta and are essential for normal development (Persaud & Torchia, 2025; Sadler, 2023).

The placenta produces and transports hormones that maintain the pregnancy and promote growth and development of the fetus. Human chorionic gonadotropin (hCG), a protein hormone produced by the syncytiotrophoblast, is excreted in maternal serum and urine. The presence of hCG is used as a test for pregnancy. Human placental lactogen, also a protein hormone produced by the placenta, acts as a fetal growth–promoting hormone by giving the fetus priority for receiving maternal glucose (Persaud & Torchia, 2025; Sadler, 2023).

The placenta also produces steroid hormones. Progesterone, produced by the placenta throughout gestation, is responsible for maintaining the pregnancy. Estrogen production by the placenta depends on stimulation by the fetal adrenal cortex and liver. Placental transport of maternal antibodies provides the fetus with passive immunity to certain viruses. Immunoglobulin G (IgG) antibodies are actively transported across the placental barrier, providing humoral immunity for the fetus. IgA and Immunoglobulin M (IgM) antibodies do not cross the placental barrier, placing the neonate at risk for neonatal sepsis. However, failure of IgM antibodies to cross the placental membrane explains the lower incidence of a severe hemolytic process in ABO blood type incompatibilities when compared with Rh incompatibilities. The latter result when an Rh-negative mother has an Rh-positive fetus. If the mother is sensitized to the Rh-positive fetal blood cells, the mother produces IgG antibodies. IgG is transferred from the maternal to fetal circulation, and hemolysis of fetal RBCs occurs (Persaud & Torchia, 2025; Sadler, 2023).

The placenta is selective in the transfer of substances across the placenta; however, this selectivity does not screen out all potentially harmful substances. Viral, bacterial, and protozoal organisms can be transferred to the fetus through the placenta. Toxic substances such as drugs and alcohol can also be transferred to the fetus. The effects of these substances depend on the stage of gestation and type and duration of exposure, as well as the interaction of these and other factors, such as nutrition.

## EMBRYONIC PERIOD: WEEKS 4 THROUGH 8

The embryonic period lasts from the beginning of gestational week four through the end of week eight. Organogenesis, which is the formation of all major organs, occurs during this period. The shape of the embryo changes as the organs develop, taking a more human shape by the end of the eighth week. The major events of the embryonic period are the folding of the embryo and organogenesis.

### Folding of the Embryo

In the trilaminar embryonic disk, the growth rate of the central region exceeds that of the periphery so that the slower growing areas fold under the faster growing areas, forming body folds. The head fold appears first because of craniocaudal elongation of the notochord and growth of the brain, which projects into the amniotic cavity. The folding downward of the cranial end of the embryo forces the septum transversum (primitive heart), the pericardial cavity, and the oropharyngeal membrane to turn under onto the ventral surface. After the embryo has folded, the mass of mesoderm cranial to the pericardial cavity, the septum transversum, lies caudal to the heart. The septum transversum later develops into a portion of the diaphragm. Part of the yolk sac is incorporated as the foregut, lying between the heart and the brain. The foregut ends blindly at the oropharyngeal membrane, which separates the foregut from the primitive mouth cavity (stomodeum) (Persaud & Torchia, 2025; Sadler, 2023).

The tail fold occurs after the head fold because of craniocaudal growth progression. Growth of the embryo causes the caudal area to project over the cloacal membrane. During the tail folding, part of the yolk sac is incorporated into the embryo as the hindgut. After completion of the head and tail folding, the connecting stalk is attached to the ventral surface of the embryo, forming the umbilical cord. Folding also occurs laterally, producing right and left lateral folds. The lateral body wall on each side folds toward the median plane, causing the embryo to assume a cylindrical shape. During the lateral body folding, a portion of the yolk sac is incorporated as the midgut. The attachment of the midgut to the yolk sac is minimal after this fold develops. After folding, the amnion is attached to the embryo in a narrow area in which the umbilical cord attaches to the ventral surface (Persaud & Torchia, 2025; Sadler, 2023).

### Organogenesis: Germ Cell Derivatives

The three germ cell layers (ectoderm, mesoderm, and endoderm) give rise to all tissues and organs of the embryo. The germ cells follow specific patterns during the process of organogenesis. The main germ cell derivatives are listed in Box 1.1. The development of each major organ system is discussed separately. The embryonic period is the most critical period of development because of the formation of internal and external structures. The critical periods of development for the organs are also discussed in the section on specific organ development.

**BOX 1.1**

**GERM CELL DERIVATIVES**

**Ectoderm**

CNS (brain, spinal cord)

PNS

Sensory epithelia of eye, ear, and nose

Epidermis and its appendages (hair and nails)

Mammary glands

Subcutaneous glands

Teeth enamel

Neural crest cells

Spinal, cranial, and autonomic ganglia cells

Nerve sheaths of PNS

Pigment cells

Muscle, connective tissue, and bone of branchial arch origin

Adrenal medulla

Meninges

*(continued)*

**BOX 1.1**

**GERM CELL DERIVATIVES (*continued*)**

**Mesoderm**

Cartilage

Bone

Connective tissue

Striated and smooth muscle

Heart, blood, and lymph vessels and cells

Gonads

Genital ducts

Pericardial, pleural, and peritoneal lining

Spleen

Cortex of adrenal gland

**Endoderm**

Epithelial lining of respiratory and gastrointestinal tracts

Parenchyma of tonsils, thyroid, parathyroid, liver, thymus, and pancreas

Epithelial lining of bladder and urethra

Epithelial lining of tympanic cavity, tympanic antrum, and auditory tube

CNS, central nervous system;
PNS, peripheral nervous system.

## DEVELOPMENT OF SPECIFIC ORGANS AND STRUCTURES

### Nervous System

The origin of the nervous system is the neural plate, which arises as a thickening of the ectodermal tissue about the middle of the third week of gestation. The neural plate further differentiates into the neural tube and the neural crest. The neural tube gives rise to the CNS. The neural crest cells give rise to the peripheral nervous system (PNS) (Figure 1.8; Persaud & Torchia, 2025; Sadler, 2023).

The cranial end of the neural tube forms the three divisions of the brain: the forebrain, the midbrain, and the hindbrain. The cerebral hemispheres and diencephalon arise from the forebrain; the pons, cerebellum, and medulla oblongata arise from the hindbrain. The midbrain makes up the adult midbrain (Persaud & Torchia, 2025; Sadler, 2023).

The cavity of the neural tube develops into the ventricles of the brain and the central canal of the spinal column. The neuroepithelial cells lining the neural tube give rise to nerves and glial cells of the CNS. The PNS consists of the cranial, spinal, and visceral nerves and the ganglia. The somatic and visceral sensory cells of the peripheral nervous system arise from neural crest cells. Cells that form the myelin sheaths of the axons, called *Schwann cells*, also arise from the neural crest cells (Persaud & Torchia, 2025; Sadler, 2023).

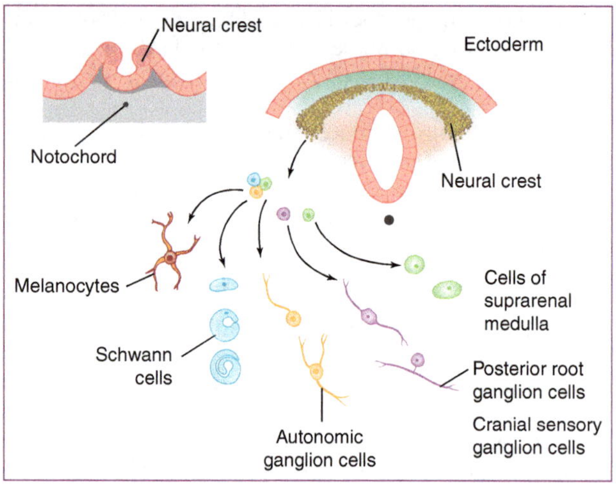


**FIGURE 1.8 Differentiation of the nervous system.** The cells of the neural crest differentiate into the cells of the ganglia, Schwann cells, and the cells of the suprarenal medulla and melanocytes.

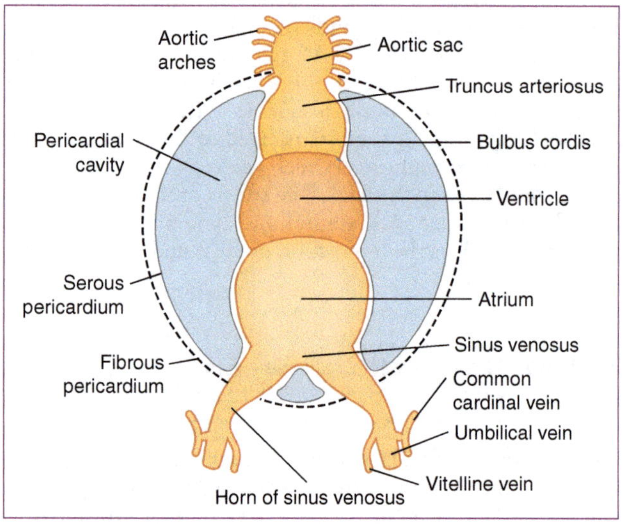


**FIGURE 1.9 Formation of the single heart tube.** The appearance of the single heart tube inside the pericardial cavity. Note that the atrium and sinus venosus are outside the pericardial cavity.

### Cardiovascular System

The fetal cardiac system appears at about 18 to 19 days of gestation, and circulation is present by about 21 days. The cardiovascular system is the first organ system to function in utero. The heart starts to beat at the beginning of the fourth week. The heart and blood develop from the middle layer (mesoderm) of the trilaminar embryonic disk. Tissue from the lateral mesoderm migrates up the sides of the embryonic disk, forming a horseshoe-shaped structure that arches and meets above the oropharyngeal membrane. With further development, paired heart tubes form, which then fuse into a single heart tube (Figure 1.9). The vessels that make up the vascular system throughout the body develop from mesodermal cells that connect to each other, with the developing heart tube and the placenta. Thus, by the end of the third week of gestation, there is a functional cardiovascular system (Moore et al., 2015; Sadler, 2015).

As the heart tube grows, the folding of the embryonic disk results in the movement of the heart tube into the chest cavity. The heart tube differentiates into three layers: the endocardial layer, which becomes the endothelium; the cardiac jelly, which is a loose tissue layer; and the myoepicardial mantle, which becomes the myocardium and pericardium. The single heart tube is attached at its cephalic end by the aortic arches and at the caudal end by the septum transversum. The attachments limit the length of the heart tube. Continued growth results in dilated areas and bulges, which become specific components of the heart. The atrium, ventricle, and bulbus cordis can be identified first, followed by the sinus venosus and truncus arteriosus. To accommodate continued growth, two separate bends in the heart occur—first to the right to form a U shape, the next resulting in an S-shaped heart. Bending of the heart is responsible for the typical location of cardiac structures (Figure 1.10; Persaud & Torchia, 2025; Sadler, 2023).

Initially, the heart is a single chamber; partitioning of the heart into four chambers occurs from the fourth to sixth weeks of gestation. The changes that cause the partitioning of the heart occur simultaneously. The atrium is separated from the ventricle by endocardial cushions, which are thickened areas of endothelium that develop on the dorsal and ventral walls of the open area between the atrium and ventricle. The endocardial cushions fuse with each other to divide the atrioventricular canals into right and left atrioventricular canals. Partitioning of the atrium occurs through invagination of tissue toward the endocardial cushions, forming the septum primum. As the septum primum grows toward the endocardial cushions, it becomes very thin and perforates, becoming the foramen ovale. The septum primum does not fuse completely with the endocardial cushions; it has a lower portion that lies beside the endocardial cushions. Overlapping of the septum primum and the septum secundum forms a wall if the pressure in both atria is equal. In utero, the pressure on the right side is increased, allowing blood to flow across the foramen ovale from the right side of the heart to the left side (Figure 1.11; Persaud & Torchia, 2025; Sadler, 2023).

The ventricle is also partitioned by a membranous and muscular septum. The muscular portion of the septum develops from the fold of the floor of the ventricle. With blood flowing through the atrioventricular canal, ventricular dilation occurs on either side of the fold or ridge, causing it

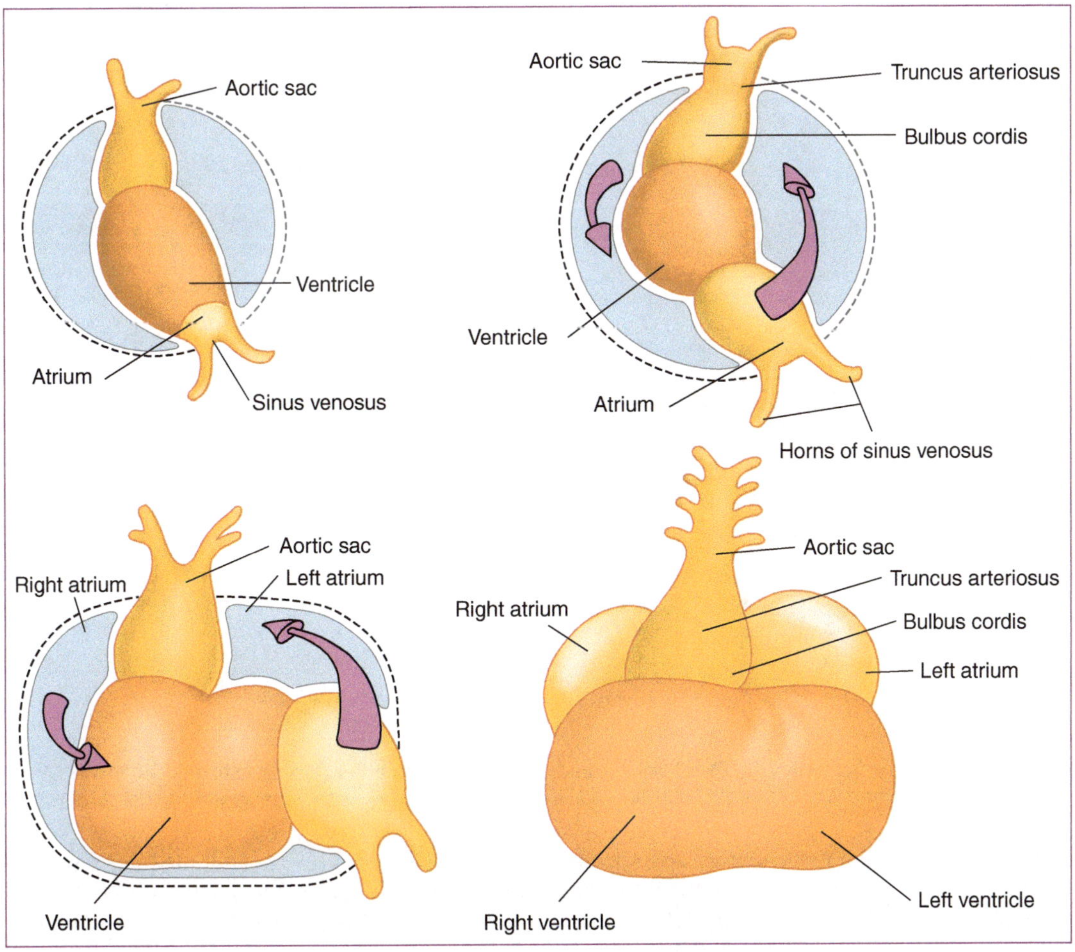


**FIGURE 1.10 Bending of the heart tube inside the pericardial cavity.** The bending of the heart tube brings the atrium into the pericardial cavity. The sinus venosus is taken into the right atrium and the coronary sinus.

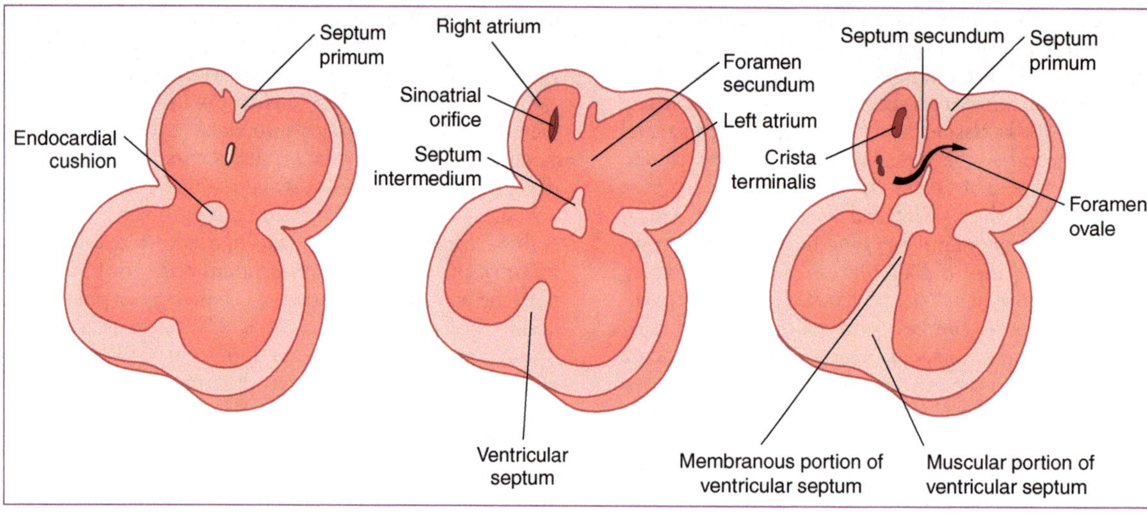


**FIGURE 1.11 Partitioning of the atrium.** The partitioning of the atrium into the right and left atria through septation.

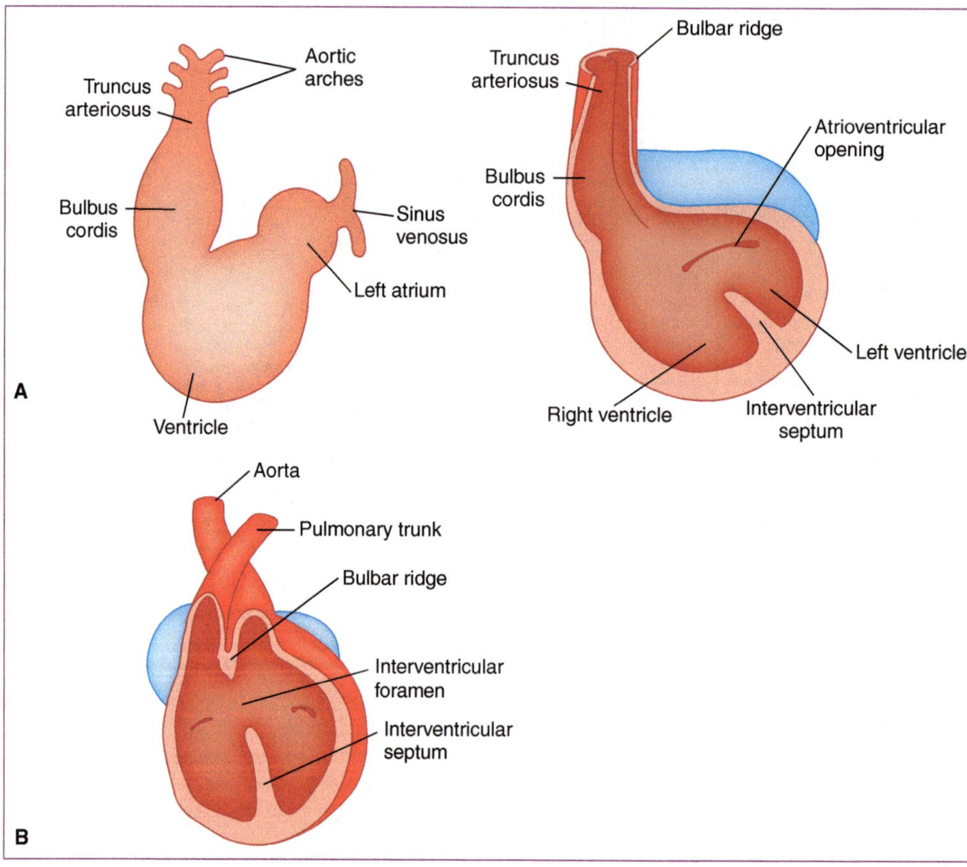


**FIGURE 1.12 Partitioning of the ventricles.** (A) Five chambers are present in the heart at 5 weeks' gestation. (B) At 6 weeks, the bulbus cordis has been taken into the ventricles and the interventricular septum has partitioned the ventricles into right and left sides.

to become a septum. The membranous septum arises from ridges inside the bulbus cordis. These ridges, continuous into the bulbus cordis, form the wall that divides the bulbus cordis into the pulmonary artery and the aorta. The bulbar ridges fuse with the endocardial cushions to form the membranous septum. The membranous and muscular septa fuse to close the intraventricular foramen, resulting in two parallel circuits of blood flow. The pulmonary artery is continuous with the right ventricle, and the aorta is continuous with the left ventricle (Figure 1.12; Persaud & Torchia, 2025; Sadler, 2023).

The blood flowing through the bulbus cordis and truncus arteriosus in a spiral causes the formation of ridges. The ridges fuse to form two separate vessels that twist around each other once. Thus, the pulmonary artery exits the right side of the heart and is in the left upper chest; the aorta exits the left side of the heart and is located close to the sternum (Persaud & Torchia, 2025; Sadler, 2023).

The pulmonary veins grow from the lungs to a cardinal vein plexus. Concurrently, a vessel develops from the smooth wall of the left atrium. As the atrium grows, the pulmonary vein is incorporated into the atrial wall. The atrium and its branches give rise to four pulmonary veins that enter the left atrium. These pulmonary vessels, connected to the plexus of the cardinal vein, provide a continuous circulation from lung to heart. The pulmonary and aortic valves (semilunar valves) develop from dilations within the pulmonary artery and aorta. The ebb-and-flow circulation through these structures causes them to hollow out to form the cusps of the valves. The tricuspid and mitral valves develop from tissue around the atrioventricular canals that thicken and then thin out on the ventricular sides, forming the valves (Figure 1.13; Persaud & Torchia, 2025; Sadler, 2023).

## Respiratory System

The development of the respiratory system is linked to the development of the face and the digestive system. The respiratory system is composed of the nasal cavities, nasopharynx, oropharynx, larynx, trachea, bronchi, and lungs (Figure 1.14). Development of the lungs occurs in four overlapping stages, which extend from the fifth week of gestation until about 8 years of life (Table 1.1). At term birth, the normal respiratory system functions immediately. For adequate functioning of the respiratory system, there must be enough alveoli, adequate capillary blood flow, and an adequate amount of surfactant produced by the secretory epithelial cells or the type II pneumatocytes. It is the surfactant that prevents alveolar collapse and aids in respiratory gas exchange. Production of surfactant begins around 20 weeks but does not reach adequate levels until late in gestation. In addition, work to identify the role of epidermal growth factor (EGF) in the development of the fetal respiratory system has determined that EGF indirectly promotes branching morphogenesis of the lung epithelium through a direct effect on the mesenchyme (Persaud & Torchia, 2025; Sadler, 2023).

## Muscular System

The muscular system develops from mesodermal cells called *myoblasts*. Striated skeletal muscles are derived from myotomal mesoderm (myotomes) of the somites. Most striated skeletal muscle fibers develop in utero. Almost all striated skeletal muscles are formed by 1 year of age. Growth is achieved by an increase in the diameter of the muscle fibers, rather than the growth of new muscle tissue. Smooth muscle fibers arise from the splanchnic mesenchyme surrounding the endoderm

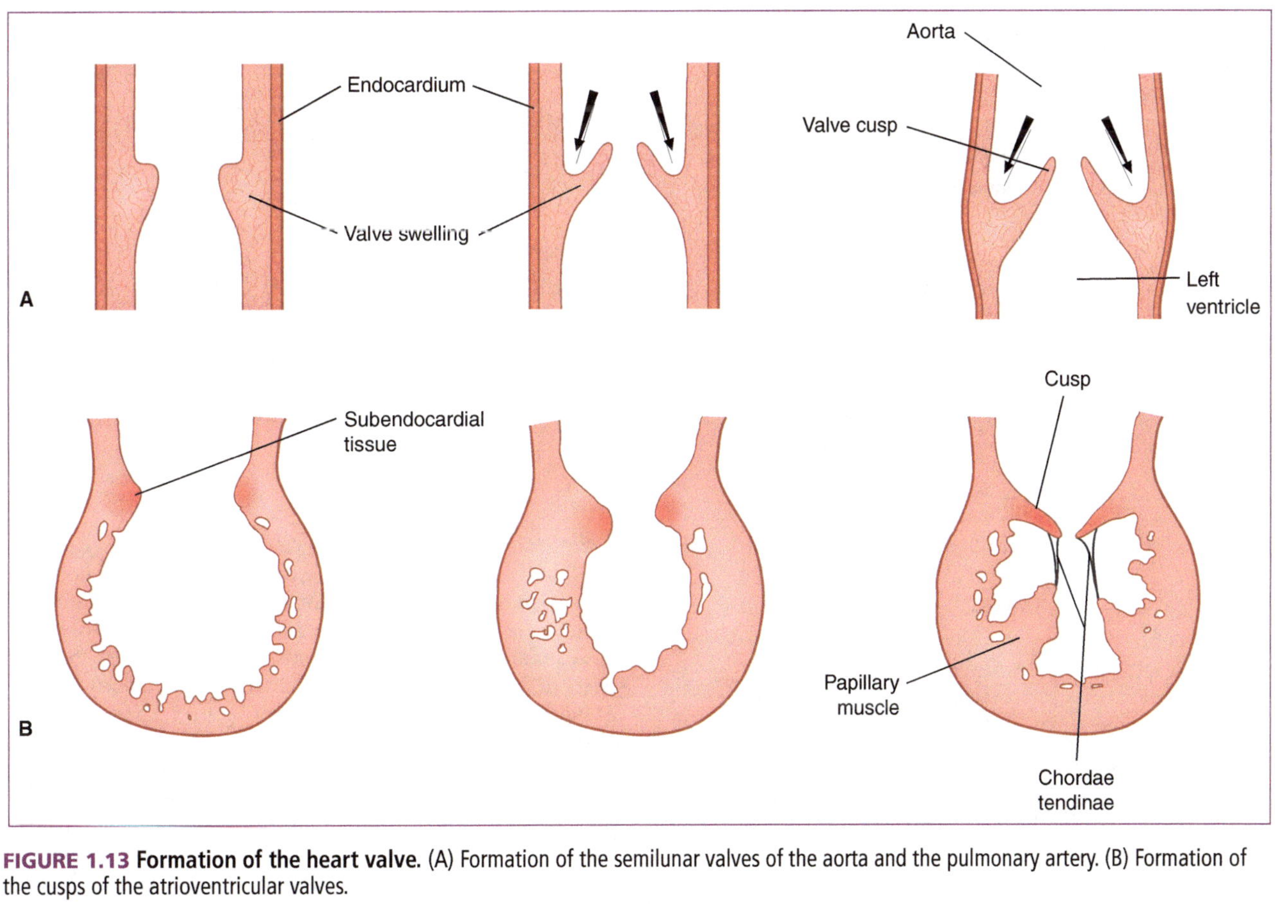


**FIGURE 1.13 Formation of the heart valve.** (A) Formation of the semilunar valves of the aorta and the pulmonary artery. (B) Formation of the cusps of the atrioventricular valves.

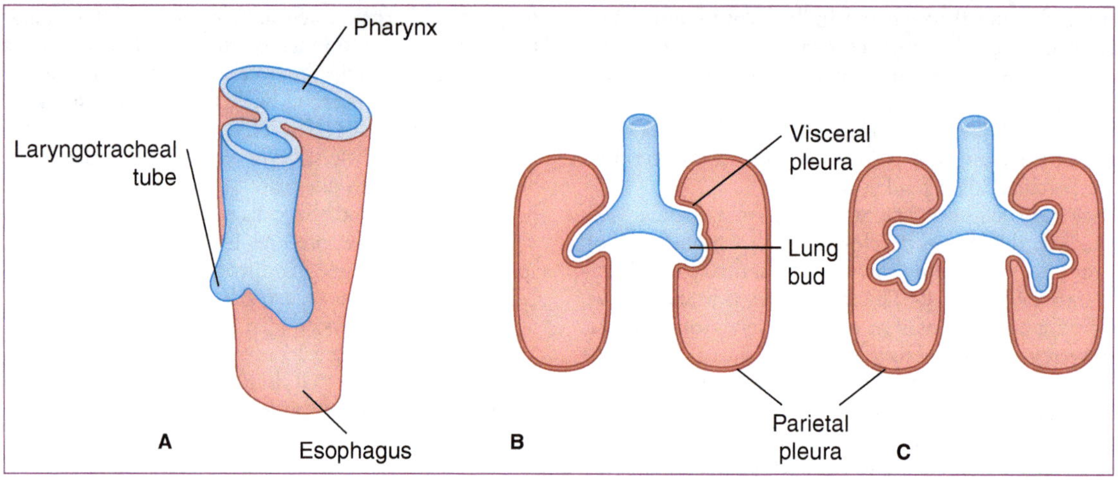


**FIGURE 1.14 Development of the pulmonary system.** (A) The laryngotracheal groove and tube have formed; the margins of the laryngotracheal groove fuse, forming the laryngotracheal tube. (B) Invagination of the lung buds into the intraembryonic cavity. (C) Division of the lung buds into the right and left mainstem bronchi.

**TABLE 1.1**

**STAGES OF LUNG DEVELOPMENT**

| Stage | Critical Events |
|---|---|
| Stage 1: Pseudoglandular period: weeks 5–7 | Development of the conducting airway |
| Stage 2: Canalicular period: weeks 13–25 | Enlargement of the bronchial lumina and terminal bronchioles<br>Vascularization of lung tissue<br>Development of respiratory bronchioles and alveolar ducts<br>Development of a limited number of primitive alveoli |
| Stage 3: Terminal sac period: week 24 to birth | Development of primitive pulmonary alveoli from alveolar ducts<br>Increased vascularity<br>Type II pneumatocytes begin to produce surfactant by about 24 weeks |
| Stage 4: Alveolar period: late fetal period until about 8 years of age | Pulmonary alveoli formed by thinning of terminal air sac lining<br>One-eighth to one-sixth of adult number of alveoli present at term birth<br>Alveoli increase in number until age 8 years |

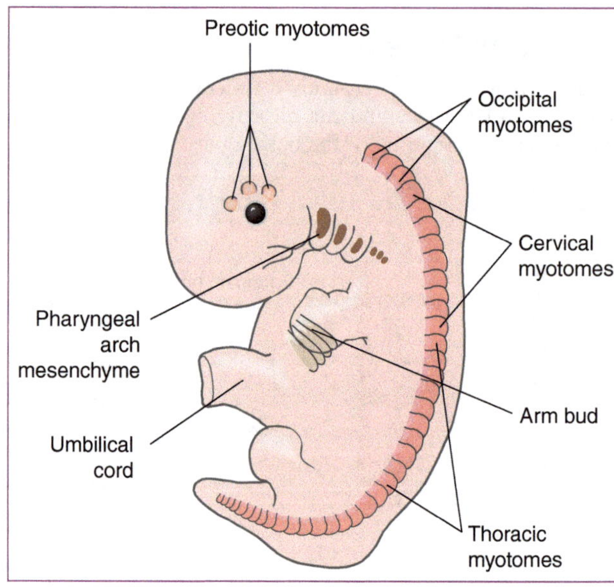


**FIGURE 1.15 Origin of the muscles of the head and neck.**

of the primitive gut. Smooth muscles lining vessel walls of blood and lymphatic systems arise from somatic mesoderm. As smooth muscle cells differentiate, contractile filaments develop in the cytoplasm, and the external surface is covered by an external lamina. As the smooth muscle fibers develop into sheets or bundles, the muscle cells synthesize and release collagenous, elastic, or reticular fibers (Figure 1.15; Persaud & Torchia, 2025; Sadler, 2023).

Cardiac muscle develops from splanchnic mesenchyme from the outside of the endocardial heart tube. Cells from the myoepicardial mantle differentiate into the myocardium. Cardiac muscle fibers develop from differentiation and growth of single cells rather than fusion of cells. Cardiac muscle growth occurs through the formation of new filaments. The Purkinje fibers develop late in the embryonic period. These fibers are larger and have fewer myofibrils than other cardiac muscle cells. The Purkinje fibers function in the electrical conduction system of the heart (Persaud & Torchia, 2025; Sadler, 2023).

## Skeletal System

The skeletal system develops from mesenchymal cells. In the long bones, condensed mesenchyme forms hyaline cartilage models of bones. By the end of the embryonic period, ossification centers appear, and these bones ossify by endochondral ossification. Other bones, such as the skull bones, are ossified by membranous ossification in which the mesenchyme cells become osteoblasts (Figure 1.16).

The vertebral column and the ribs arise from the sclerotome compartments of the somites. The spinal column is formed by the fusion of a condensation of the cranial half of one pair of sclerotomes with the caudal half of the next pair of sclerotomes. The skull can be divided into the neurocranium and the viscerocranium. The neurocranium forms the protective covering around the brain. The viscerocranium forms the skeleton of the face. The neurocranium is made up of the flat bones that surround the brain and the cartilaginous structure, or chondrocranium, that forms the bones of the base of the skull. The neurocranium (chondrocranium) is made up of several separate cartilages, which fuse and ossify by endochondral ossification to form the base of the skull (Persaud & Torchia, 2025; Sadler, 2023).

## Gastrointestinal System

The gastrointestinal system is primarily derived from the lining of the roof of the yolk sac. The primitive gut, consisting of the foregut, midgut, and hindgut, is formed during the fourth gestational week (Figure 1.17). The structures that arise from the foregut include the pharynx, esophagus, stomach, liver, pancreas, gallbladder, and part of the duodenum. The esophagus and trachea have a common origin, the laryngotracheal diverticulum. A septum, formed by the growing tracheoesophageal folds, divides the cranial part of the foregut into the laryngotracheal tube and the esophagus. Smooth muscle develops from the splanchnic mesenchyme that surrounds the esophagus. The epithelial lining of the esophagus, derived from the endoderm, proliferates, partially obliterating the esophageal lumen. The esophagus undergoes recanalization by the end of the embryonic period (Persaud & Torchia, 2025; Sadler, 2023).

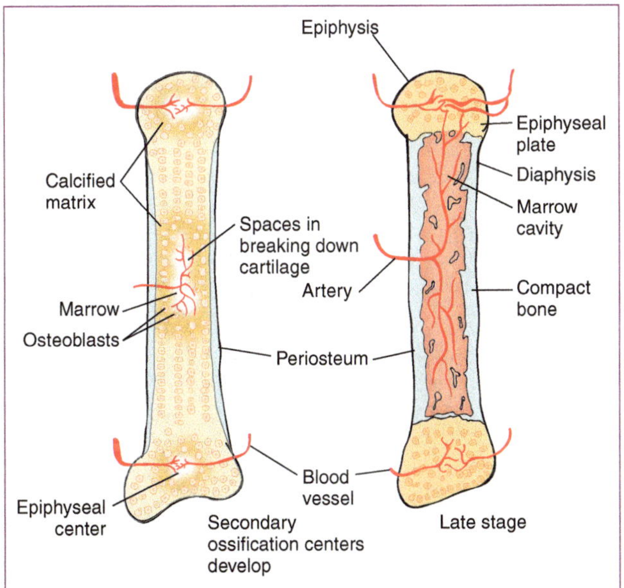


**FIGURE 1.16 Endochondral ossification of bones.**

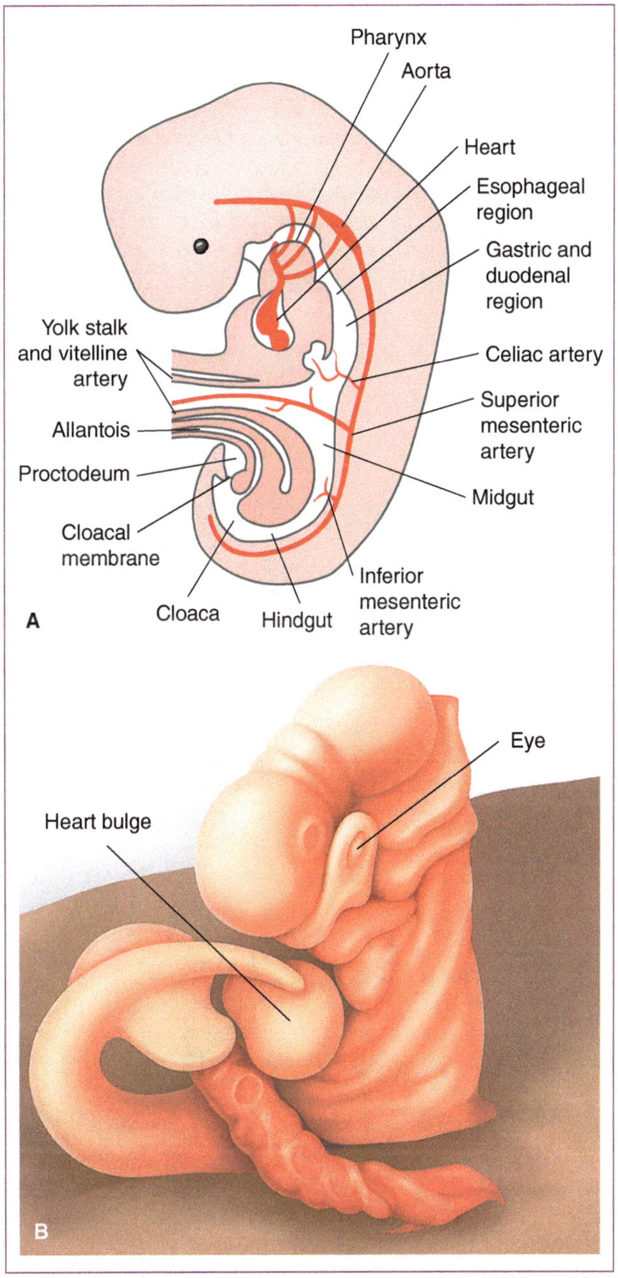


**FIGURE 1.17 (A, B). The primitive gut.** The early gastrointestinal system presents in an embryo at about 4 weeks' gestation.

The stomach originates as a dilation of the caudal portion of the foregut. The characteristic greater curvature of the stomach develops because the dorsal border grows faster than the ventral border. As the stomach develops further, it rotates in a clockwise direction around the longitudinal axis. The duodenum is derived from the caudal and cranial portions of the foregut and the cranial portion of the midgut. The junction of the foregut and midgut portions of the duodenum is normally distal to the common bile duct (Persaud & Torchia, 2025; Sadler, 2023).

The liver, gallbladder, and biliary ducts originate as a bud from the caudal end of the foregut. The liver is formed by growth of the hepatic diverticulum, which grows between the layers of the ventral mesentery, forming two parts. The liver forms from the largest cranial portion. Hepatic cells originate from the hepatic diverticulum. Hematopoietic tissue and Kupffer cells are derived from the splanchnic mesenchyme of the septum transversum. The liver develops rapidly and fills the abdominal cavity. The liver begins its hematopoietic function by gestational week six (Persaud & Torchia, 2025; Sadler, 2023).

The smaller portion of the hepatic diverticulum forms the gallbladder. The common bile duct is formed from the stalk connecting the hepatic and cystic ducts to the duodenum. By the 12th week, bile formation begins by the hepatic cells. The pancreas is derived from the pancreatic buds that arise from the caudal part of the foregut. Insulin secretion begins at week 10 (Persaud & Torchia, 2025; Sadler, 2023).

The structures that are derived from the midgut include the remainder of the duodenum, the cecum, the appendix, the ascending colon, and most of the transverse colon. The intestines undergo extensive growth during the first weeks of development. The liver and kidneys occupy the abdominal cavity, restricting the space available for intestinal growth. The growth of the intestines is accommodated through a migration out of the abdominal cavity via the umbilical cord. A series of rotations occurs before the intestines return to the abdomen. The first rotation is counterclockwise, around the axis of the superior mesenteric artery. At about the 10th week, the intestines return to the abdomen, undergoing further rotation. When the colon returns to the abdomen, the cecal end rotates to the right side, entering the lower right quadrant of the abdomen. The cecum and appendix arise from the cecal diverticulum, a pouch that appears in gestational week five on the caudal limb of the midgut loop (Figure 1.18; Persaud & Torchia, 2025; Sadler, 2023).

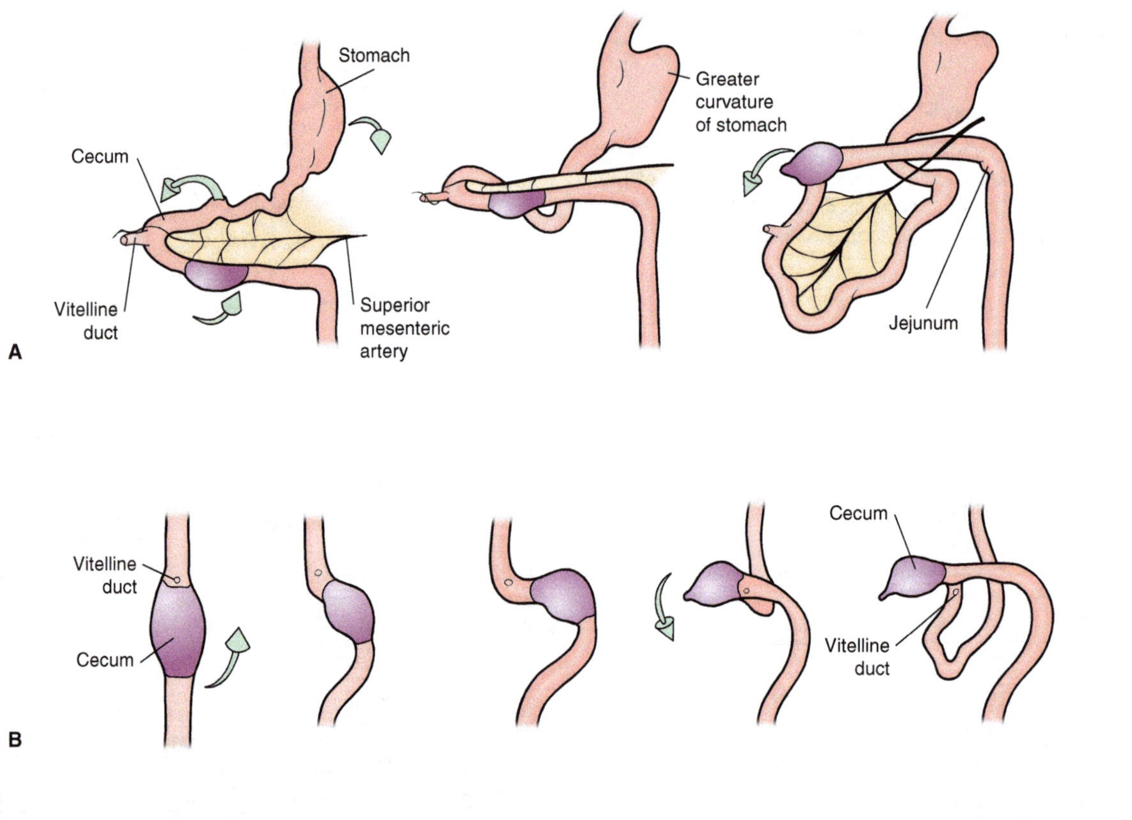


**FIGURE 1.18 Migration and rotation of the midgut.** (A) Counterclockwise 90° rotation of midgut loop and "herniation" into extraembryonic cavity. (B) Counterclockwise 180° rotation of midgut loop on return to the abdominal cavity.

The hindgut is that portion of the intestines from the midgut to the cloacal membrane. The latter structure consists of the endoderm of the cloaca and the ectoderm of the anal pit. The cloaca is divided by the urorectal septum. As the septum grows toward the cloacal membrane, folds from the lateral walls of the cloaca grow together, dividing the cloaca into the rectum and upper anal canal dorsally and the urogenital sinus ventrally. By the end of the sixth week, the urorectal septum fuses with the cloacal membrane, forming a dorsal anal membrane and a larger ventral urogenital membrane. At about the end of the seventh gestational week, these two membranes rupture, forming the anal canal (Persaud & Torchia, 2025; Sadler, 2023).

### Urogenital System

The development of the urinary and genital systems is closely related. The urogenital system develops from the intermediate mesenchyme, which extends along the dorsal body wall of the embryo. During embryonic folding in the horizontal plane, the intermediate mesoderm is moved forward and is no longer connected to the somites. This mesoderm forms the urogenital ridge on each side of the primitive aorta. Both the urinary and genital systems arise from this urogenital ridge. The area from which the urinary system is derived is called the *nephrogenic cord*. The genital ridge is the area from which the reproductive system is derived (Persaud & Torchia, 2025; Sadler, 2023).

There are three stages of development of the kidney: the pronephros, the mesonephros, and the metanephros. The pronephros, a nonfunctional organ, appears in the first month of gestation and then degenerates, contributing only a duct system for the next developmental stage. The mesonephros uses the duct of the pronephros and develops caudally to the pronephros (Figure 1.19). The mesonephros begins to produce urine during development of the metanephros. The mesonephros degenerates by the end of the embryonic period. Remnants of the mesonephros persist as genital ducts in males or vestigial structures in females. The metanephros appears in the fifth week of gestation and becomes the permanent kidney. The metanephros begins to produce urine by about week 11. The number of glomeruli increases until week 32, when the fetal kidney becomes subdivided into lobes. The urinary bladder and the urethra arise from the urogenital sinus and the splanchnic mesenchyme. The caudal portion of the mesonephric ducts is incorporated into the bladder, giving rise to the ureters (Persaud & Torchia, 2025; Sadler, 2023).

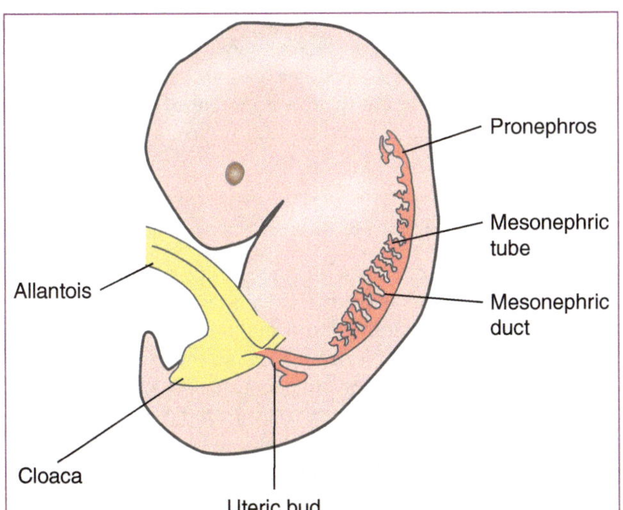


**FIGURE 1.19 Development of the kidney.** The locations of the pronephros and mesonephros.

Although the genetic sex of the embryo is determined at conception, the early development of the genital system is indistinguishable until the seventh week of gestation. In the seventh week, the gonads begin to differentiate. The ovaries and the testes are derived from the coelomic epithelium, the mesenchyme, and the primordial germ cells. Development of female sexual organs occurs in the absence of hormonal stimulation precipitated by the H-Y antigen gene carried on the Y chromosome. If the Y chromosome is present, testes develop; otherwise, ovaries develop (Persaud & Torchia, 2025; Sadler, 2023).

## FETAL PERIOD: WEEK NINE THROUGH BIRTH

The fetal period begins at the start of week nine following conception and continues through the duration of pregnancy. It is characterized by further growth and development of the fetus and the organs formed during the embryonic period.

### Weeks 9 to 12

At the beginning of this period, the head is large, and the body begins growing faster than the head. The face is broad and characterized by a wide nose and widely spaced eyes. The mouth is formed, and palate formation is complete. Tooth buds appear for the baby teeth. Fingernails are present, and the fetus can curl its fingers to make a fist. The intestines enter the abdomen from the umbilical cord. By the end of the 12th week, blood formation shifts from the liver to the spleen. The fetus can produce urine and excretes it into the amniotic fluid. By the end of the 12th week, the sex of the fetus can be identified by appearance of the external genitalia. By week 12, the fetus weighs 45 g (1.6 oz) and has a C-R length of 8 cm (3.2 in.; Persaud & Torchia, 2025; Sadler, 2023).

### Weeks 13 to 16

During this time of rapid growth, the fetal head becomes smaller in proportion to the body. The appearance of hair patterning is forming on the head, and *lanugo*, a fine downy hair, is found on the body. Fingerprints are now developed. The fetus can now open its mouth, make a sucking motion, and swallow amniotic fluid. Ossification of the fetal skeleton is active during this time. Reflex response and muscular activity begin. The lower limbs lengthen during this time, and limb movement is more coordinated. In females, the ovaries differentiate and contain primordial follicles. At 16 weeks, the fetal weight is about 200 g (7 oz) and the C-R length is 13.5 cm (5.4 in.; Persaud & Torchia, 2025; Sadler, 2023).

### Weeks 17 to 20

This marks a period of slower growth. The skin is covered in a fatty, cheese-like substance called *vernix caseosa* that protects it from exposure to amniotic fluid. The limbs are in proportion to the rest of the body and muscles are well developed. Myelination of the spinal cord begins at 20 weeks. Lanugo now covers the body, and brown fat begins to form at the base of the neck, behind the sternum, and around the kidneys. Fetal movement is usually felt by the mother around 18 weeks. The uterus is formed in the female fetus by 18 weeks, and at 20 weeks the testes begin to descend in the male fetus. At 20 weeks, the fetus has a crown-to-heel (C-H) length of 25 cm (10 in.) and a weight of 435 g (15 oz; Persaud & Torchia, 2025; Sadler, 2023).

### Weeks 21 to 25

During this period, there is substantial weight gain, but the fetus is thin and has little subcutaneous fat. The skin is wrinkled and translucent red because the capillaries are close to the surface of the skin. The fetus has a grasp, and startle reflex and rapid eye movements begin. Eyebrows and eyelashes are fully formed. Teeth that will become second molars are forming. At 24 weeks, the lungs begin to produce surfactant. IgG levels reach maternal levels. At 24 weeks, the fetus has a C-H length of 28 cm (11.2 in.) and a weight of 780 g (1 lb 11½ oz; Persaud & Torchia, 2025; Sadler, 2023).

### Weeks 26 to 29

The fetal lungs, pulmonary capillaries, and CNS are more mature, and the fetus is likely to survive if born after 24 to 25 weeks. Blood formation (erythrocyte production) shifts from the spleen to the bone marrow. The CNS is now mature enough to direct breathing movements and control body temperature. There is now enough subcutaneous fat to help maintain body temperature. The eyelids that have been closed since 9 weeks' gestation start to open. In males, the testes descend into the inguinal canal and upper scrotum. At 28 weeks, the fetus has a C-H length of 35 cm (14 in.) and a weight of 1,200 to 1,250 g (2 lb 12 oz; Persaud & Torchia, 2025; Sadler, 2023).

### Weeks 30 to 34

This period marks a rapid increase in body fat and muscle. Bones are fully developed but are soft and pliable. The lungs are not yet mature but developed enough to provide gas exchange if the fetus were to be born during this period. Surfactant production is not quite at mature levels. The fetus exhibits rhythmic breathing movements because of a more mature CNS. The pupillary light reflex is present at 30 weeks. The fetal skin is smooth and pigmented, and the fingernails reach the fingertips. At 32 weeks, the fetus has a C-H length of 38 to 43 cm (15.2 to 17.2 in.) and weighs 2,000 g (4 lb 7 oz; Persaud & Torchia, 2025; Sadler, 2023).

### Weeks 35 to 36

Growth of all body systems continues until birth but at a slower rate. The circumference of the head and abdomen is approximately equal by 36 weeks. The fetus starts to look "plump" and the skin is less wrinkled. Lanugo is disappearing. In males, the testes are in the scrotum. In both males and females, breasts are enlarged. At 36 weeks, the fetus has a C-H length of 42 to 48 cm (16.8 to 17.2 in.) and a weight of 2,500 to 2,750 g (5 lb 8 oz to 6 lb 1 oz; Persaud & Torchia, 2025; Sadler, 2023).

### Weeks 37 to 40

The fetus is considered *full term* between 38 and 40 weeks. During the last few weeks of gestation, the fat increases in the fetus at a rate of 14 g/day; however, white fat makes up 16% of its total weight. Amniotic fluid decreases to 500 ml or less as the fetal mass fills the uterus. The measurement of the fetal foot is slightly larger than the femur and this is used as an alternate measurement to confirm fetal age. The chest is more prominent but slightly smaller than the diameter of the head. The earlobes are firm, and the skin has a smooth, polished appearance. Vernix caseosa is present in the deep folds and creases of the skin. The lungs are well developed and can exchange gases. The lecithin-sphingomyelin (L/S) ratio is approaching 2:1, indicating lung maturity. At term, the fetus weighs 3,200 g or more and is 48 to 52 cm (19 to 21 in.) long (Persaud & Torchia, 2025; Sadler, 2023).

## DEVELOPMENTAL RISKS

The fetus is at less risk for structural defects caused by teratogenic factors than is the embryo; however, there is still a risk for functional impairment of existing structures. This risk is addressed in the section on environmental factors. Changes in specific organs or organ systems during the fetal period are discussed in the section on the development of specific organs (Persaud & Torchia, 2025; Sadler, 2023). Box 1.2 summarizes prenatal development.

### Congenital Defects

Congenital defects or anomalies are structural or anatomic abnormalities present at birth. Congenital defects vary in severity and location, ranging from minor insignificant defects to major organ system defects and are attributed to genetic or chromosomal abnormalities or to maternal or environmental factors. Most congenital defects result from an interaction between genetic and environmental factors, or multifactorial inheritance. Congenital defects caused by single-gene disorders and chromosomal abnormalities are discussed in Chapter 34, "Human Genetics and Genomics: Impact on Neonatal Care". The influence of the environment on embryonic development is discussed in this section.

**BOX 1.2**

**THREE PERIODS OF FETAL DEVELOPMENT**

**Embryonic Period**

Extends from the fertilization of the ovum

**Period 1: Preembryonic Period**

Extends from the fertilization of the ovum to the formation of the embryonic disk with three germ layers—weeks 1–3.

**Period 2: Embryonic Period**

Period of rapid growth and differentiation; formation of major organ systems occurs—weeks 4–8.

**Period 3: Fetal Period**

Further growth and development of organ systems—extends from weeks 9–40 (term).

*Source:* Data from Moore, K. L., & Persaud, T. V. N. (2008). *The developing human: Clinically oriented embryology* (8th ed.). Saunders.

Moore and Persaud (2008) listed six mechanisms that can cause congenital defects: (a) too little growth, (b) too little resorption, (c) too much resorption, (d) resorption in the wrong location, (e) normal growth in an abnormal position, and (f) overgrowth of a tissue or structure. Embryonic organs are most sensitive to noxious agents during a period of rapid cell growth and differentiation. Damage to the primitive streak at about 15 days of gestation could cause severe congenital malformations of the embryo because of its role in the production of intraembryonic mesoderm, from which all connective tissue is formed. Biochemical differentiation occurs before morphologic differentiation, so organs or structures are sensitive to the action of teratogens before they can be identified.

## Critical Periods of Human Development

Environmental influences during the first 2 weeks after conception may prevent successful implantation of the blastocyst and cause spontaneous abortion of the embryo. The most sensitive period for the embryo, known as the *critical period*, is the period of organogenesis, during the first 8 weeks of development. Each organ has a critical period during which its development is most likely to be adversely affected by the presence of teratogenic agents; however, some organs such as the brain are sensitive throughout fetal development (Persaud & Torchia, 2025).

The terms *congenital anomaly*, *congenital malformation*, and *birth defect* are used synonymously to describe structural abnormalities (cleft lip/palate, heart defects, clubfoot, neural tube) but they can also refer to functional problems (developmental or behavioral disorders including seizures; trisomy; fragile X; and sensory, metabolic, or degenerative disorders) (U.S. Department of Health and Human Services, n.d.). Usually, a malformation is a defect of a morphogenic or developmental field and may result in complex or multiple malformations. A disruption is an interruption of a normal developmental process. This may be caused by a teratogen such as a drug or virus; however, it is not inherited. A deformation is an alteration in form or shape that results from mechanical forces in otherwise healthy tissue. Dysplasia is abnormal development of tissue and may affect several organs.

Birth defects occur in about 3% of all live births in the United States (March of Dimes, 2025). They account for about 20.7% of all U.S. deaths under 1 year of age (U.S. EPA, 2022).

## Environmental Factors

The effects of stress, climate change (including excessive heat exposure, pollution, and excessive noise during pregnancy) all are known to affect fetal growth and development. Epigenetic changes in the placenta can result from environmental exposures. They can affect brain development (Kidd et al., 2023). Rani and Dhok (2023) present an excellent overview of environmental contaminants including pesticides, heavy metals, dioxin derivatives, and polychlorinated diphenyl compounds and substances including alcohol, narcotics, and tobacco. They point out that the effect depends on the stage of fetal development at the time of the exposure.

## Infectious Agents

Several viral agents including rubella, cytomegalovirus (CMV), herpes simplex virus (HSV), and HIV have been positively identified as teratogenic to the developing fetus. Rubella (German measles) is a viral infection spread through the air or by close contact. The virus can cross the placenta, and during the first trimester can cause cataracts, permanent hearing loss, cardiac malformations (especially patent ductus arteriosus and pulmonary stenosis), and congenital rubella syndrome in the fetus. If exposed in the second or third trimester, the fetus can develop learning disabilities or speech and hearing problems. Prevention is the goal; however, women should be tested to determine if the rubella antibody is present; if not, they should be vaccinated as long as they are not pregnant and will avoid pregnancy for at least 6 months.

CMV is a virus belonging to the herpes family. It is transmitted by direct contact of body fluids including urine, saliva, blood, semen, and breast milk. Approximately 30% to 50% of women have never been infected with CMV, and infected women have no symptoms (Sadler, 2015). One in 200 infants is CMV infected, but only one in five will become ill (Centers for Disease Control and Prevention [CDC], n.d.-a). If exposed in early gestation, the embryo will likely spontaneously abort. A small number of infants who are infected will have microcephaly, meningoencephalitis, hearing and vision loss, mental retardation, and/or seizures (CDC, n.d.-a).

HSV is one of the most common sexually transmitted infections (STIs) among adult women and is transmitted across broken skin and mucous membranes by direct exposure to the virus. There is a 30% to 50% risk of transmission to the fetus when there is a primary outbreak late in pregnancy. Fetal infection is transmitted during birth 85% of the time. An infected fetus has a 50% mortality rate. Infants who survive may have significant neurologic defects, blindness, and seizures (Moore et al., 2015; Sadler, 2015).

HIV is the virus that causes AIDS. HIV is transmitted through body fluids—blood, semen, genital fluids, and human milk—and can cross the placenta in pregnancy. Almost all pediatric cases of HIV are acquired in utero or through breastfeeding. Women who are treated in pregnancy with an antiretroviral medication reduce the risk of transmission to 2% (Peterson, 2019). Anomalies associated with HIV are microcephaly, growth factor, and craniofacial features.

Toxoplasmosis is caused by a protozoan, *Toxoplasma gondii (T. gondii)*, and when exposed in utero can cause hydrocephalus, cerebral calcification, microphthalmia, and ocular defects in the fetus. *T. gondii* can be contracted from raw or undercooked meat, by handling feces of infected cats, or from the soil. The risk and severity depend on the timing of the exposure in pregnancy (Moore et al., 2015; Sadler, 2015).

Untreated primary maternal infections of *Treponema pallidum*, the spirochete that causes syphilis, can result in serious congenital anomalies or stillborn infants. Congenital syphilis is classified as early or late. Early congenital syphilis is defined as in the first 3 months of life and may cause vesiculobullous lesions, rash, lymphadenopathy, hepatosplenomegaly, and a mucopurulent nasal discharge known as "snuffles". Late congenital syphilis occurs around or after age 2 and includes symptoms such as gummatous ulcers on the nose, septum, and palate; bossing of frontal and parietal bones; optic atrophy leading to blindness; interstitial keratitis; and sensorineural deafness. Treatment must be done as early as possible to prevent complications and transmission of the infection to the fetus (Moore et al., 2015).

Zika virus is a growing public health problem. When a fetus is exposed to Zika, resultant malformations may occur. The most common effects are microcephaly, macular scarring and retinal changes, contractures, clubfoot, arthrogryposis, and hypertonia (CDC, n.d.-c).

Other viral agents have been implicated as causes of congenital malformations. Such malformations have been reported following maternal infection with mumps, varicella, echovirus, coxsackie virus, and influenza virus. The incidence of congenital malformations following these infections is unknown, but is suspected to be low (Sadler, 2015). More information can be found in Chapter 11, "Immune System".

## Drugs/Medications

Drug safety is a primary concern during pregnancy, especially in women with pregestational disease. Safety of a medication cannot be tested on pregnant women for obvious ethical reasons because it could expose a fetus to possible teratogens.

Few drugs are known to be teratogenic; however, no drug can be considered completely safe. The U.S. Food and Drug Administration (FDA) as of June 2015 established three labels for prescription drugs used in pregnancy or preconception. They are 8.1 Pregnancy (including during labor); 8.2 Lactation; and 8.3 Females and Males of Reproductive Potential (FDA, 2014). Over-the-counter medications are not included in this labeling nomenclature (FDA, 2014). The FDA established a pregnancy exposure registry to maintain up-to-date information on the medication along with a risk summary (FDA, 2014).

Drugs that are known teratogens that can cause birth defects include antibiotics streptomycin and tetracycline; antineoplastic agents; anticoagulants, anticonvulsants; hormones such as adrenocorticoids and diethylstilbestrol (DES); antithyroid drugs; psychotropics; antianxiety agents such as diazepam; and retinoic acid (a metabolite of vitamin A).

Hormonal agents are also implicated in the incidence of congenital defects. Androgenic agents (progestins) may cause masculinization of female fetuses. DES, a synthetic estrogen used to prevent abortion in the 1940s and 1950s, has been found to cause an increased incidence of vaginal and cervical cancer in female children exposed to the drug in utero. There are also associated abnormalities of the reproductive system, often causing reproductive dysfunction (Moore et al., 2015; Sadler, 2015).

Amphetamines are associated with oral clefts and heart defects. Salicylates (aspirin), a commonly used medication during pregnancy, may be harmful to the fetus if taken in large amounts or may lead to bleeding problems. Isotretinoin, a drug used to treat acne, causes craniofacial abnormalities, cleft palate, thymic aplasia defects, and neural tube defects (Sadler, 2015).

Opioids, often prescribed for pain relief, if used in pregnancy can result in a premature birth, intrauterine growth restriction (IUGR), and the infant may experience withdrawal, referred to as *neonatal abstinence syndrome* (NAS; March of Dimes, 2025). NAS secondary to in-utero opioid exposure increased fivefold in the United States from 2000 to 2012, and has continued to rise with recent rates reported as high as 20 per 1,000 live births (Milliren et al., 2018). For more information on NAS, please see Chapter 24, "Neonatal Abstinence Syndrome".

## Illicit Drugs

Social or recreational drugs are highly suspected of contributing to congenital defects and the risk of spontaneous abortion. Drugs such as lysergic acid diethylamide (LSD) have been associated with limb abnormalities and CNS abnormalities. Other drugs that may be teratogenic include phencyclidine and marijuana. "Crack" cocaine has been associated with preterm birth (PTB), low birth weight (LBW), premature rupture of membranes (PROM), placental abruption, and sudden infant death syndrome (SIDS; Gouin et al., 2011). The tendency of drug users to use multiple drugs, combined with poor nutritional habits and lack of prenatal care, makes it difficult to establish the effects of the drugs individually.

**Marijuana.** Cannabis (marijuana, hashish, or sensimilla, all products of the *Cannabis sativa* or *Cannabis indica* plant) is the most commonly used psychoactive substance in the United States with an estimated 1 in 5 adults aged 18 to 25 years reporting use in the past month in 2015 (Center for Behavioral Health). Recent estimates of the prevalence of cannabis use among pregnant women in the United States range between 3% and 16%—The National Survey on Drug Use and Health suggests that it has increased as much as 62% between 2002 and 2014 (Brown et al., 2017).

As yet, no teratogenic effects of marijuana have been reported; yet, research on the teratogenicity of marijuana is difficult because it remains illegal in many states. Co-use of other substances is common among prenatal and postpartum marijuana users.

Evidence is inconclusive as to its effect on premature birth or LBW; however, there is evidence to suggest a potential effect on fetal brain development (National Institute on Drug Abuse, 2018). Ko et al. (2018) found that prenatal marijuana use was not independently associated with lower average birthweight or gestational age; however, postpartum marijuana use was associated with depressive symptoms and shorter breastfeeding duration. Growing evidence suggests prenatal cannabis exposure has a detrimental impact on offspring neurocognitive function starting in the toddler years (Wu et al., 2011). More research is needed, especially as marijuana becomes legal in many states.

**Alcohol.** The term *fetal alcohol syndrome* (FAS) is used to describe the cluster of defects characteristic of maternal ingestion of alcohol. A major factor in the development of FAS is timing, amount, and frequency of alcohol consumption during pregnancy. Infants with FAS may exhibit craniofacial abnormalities, microcephaly, limb deformities, smooth philtrum, thin upper lip, small palpebral fissures, and short nose. They may have visual impairment. They may exhibit cognitive impairment; impaired fine motor skills; developmental disabilities; attention deficit disorder; and seizure disorder as well as alcohol-related birth defects (ARBD) such as heart and kidney defects, malformations of the bone, and hearing (CDC, n.d.-b). Fetal alcohol spectrum disorder (FASD) is a modern term that describes the range of permanent effects of alcohol use in pregnancy. This cluster of conditions is preventable if pregnant women do not consume alcohol (CDC, n.d.-b). There is no known safe level of alcohol consumption during pregnancy, and even low levels of prenatal alcohol exposure have been found to cause adverse fetal effects, and not just in the brain (Sarman, 2018)

**Tobacco.** The dangers of smoking cigarettes in pregnancy have been well documented. Use of tobacco during pregnancy can lead to PTB, LBW, PROM, placenta previa, placental abruption, or stillbirth. The fetus can suffer from growth restriction because of the vasoconstrictive properties of nicotine, which decreases oxygenated blood to the fetus. Damage to fetal lung and brain tissue is also possible (CDC, n.d.-f). Katoka et al. (2018) demonstrated that newborn weight decreased as the category of number of cigarettes per day increased, with a significant reduction at the 6 to 10 cigarettes. Based on the study results and the principle of harm reduction, if a pregnant woman is unable to quit smoking, she should be encouraged to reduce consumption to less than six cigarettes per day.

**E-Cigarettes.** Electronic nicotine delivery systems (ENDS), a comparatively new phenomenon, are gaining in popularity, especially among adolescent nonsmokers, and are frequently perceived as being safer than regular cigarettes (Dutra & Glantz, 2014; Grana et al., 2014). Because ENDS emissions have been found to have lower levels and overall numbers of toxins compared with tobacco cigarettes, they are commonly marketed as safer alternatives without regard to the intrinsic adverse effects of nicotine (Grana et al., 2014). If pregnant women perceive ENDS as safer than tobacco cigarettes, there is potential for unrealized harm because current tobacco-smoking pregnant women may use ENDS to decrease the amount of tobacco cigarettes smoked during pregnancy (England et al., 2016; Wigginton et al., 2017). This perceived harm reduction strategy could result in continued nicotine exposure and associated complications, as well as currently undetermined additional maternal–fetal risks (Bhandari et al., 2018). The variety of flavorings offered may also put the fetus at risk for damage to the lungs and brain (CDC, n.d.-d). Another potential ENDS-associated issue important to expecting mothers is the possibility of unintentional ingestion of ENDS liquids by young children at home (American Association of Poison Control Centers, n.d.). In addition to the perception of lower health risks, the relative lesser cost of e-cigarettes compared with tobacco cigarettes could encourage their use. As such, for women who already smoke and are facing financial hardship during pregnancy, e-cigarettes may seem like a rational solution.

**Ionizing Radiation.** There is no established "safe" level for radiation. Large amounts of exposure during pregnancy can be detrimental to the fetus; however, this is a rare occurrence. The severity of radiation-induced defects depends on the duration and timing of exposure. Radiation exposure during the first trimester of pregnancy most likely will result in loss of the embryo. High levels of radiation can cause microcephaly, microphthalmia, growth restriction, skeletal and visceral abnormalities, retinal changes, cataracts, and cleft palate. There is no evidence that the small amount of radiation required for modern radiographic studies is harmful; however, caution is used to minimize the exposure to the fetus because of the potential for cumulative effects of radiation exposure throughout the lifespan (Groen et al., 2012). Low-dose ionizing radiation (LDIR) is known to promote oxidative stress; however, these levels may not be large enough to result in genomic mutations. There is emerging evidence that oxidative stress causes epigenetic modifications, which can result in permanent cellular transformations without altering the underlying DNA nucleotide sequence. Intrauterine fetal development is highly susceptible to oxidative stress-induced epigenetic programming when exposed to LDIR during pregnancy (Tharmalingam et al., 2017).

**Heavy Metals.** Heavy metals such as lead (Pb), cadmium (Cd), cobalt, manganese (Mn), and mercury (Hg) during pregnancy put the developing fetal brain at risk (CDC, n.d.-e). More specifically, high maternal second-trimester blood levels of Pb and Mn during pregnancy are associated with neural tube defects (NTDs) in the newborn (Özel et al., 2018). Ingestion of predatory fish (e.g. shark, swordfish, king mackerel, tilefish) while pregnant may damage the developing fetal brain and CNS (Mayo Clinic, 2016).

**Bisphenol-A.** Bisphenol-A (BPA) is an organic compound used to make polycarbonate plastic, epoxy resins, and dental sealants. BPA can be found in plastic baby bottles, plastic lining in canned foods, and polycarbonate plastic containers. The chemical structure of BPA is similar to estrogen and may have the same effect on the body. High levels of BPA found in blood have been associated with recurrent miscarriages, preeclampsia, IUGR, and PTB. Fetal exposure to BPA may result in the development of diabetes or heart disease when the child is older (Endocrine Society, 2015).

## Maternal Disease

Pregestational maternal disease can be teratogenic to a fetus. Women with poorly controlled pregestational diabetes have a three to four times higher risk of having a fetus with a birth defect than women in the general population. Anomalies typically occur between weeks five and eight and can include brain anomalies, skeletal defects, developmental abnormalities, and congenital heart defects.

Thyroid deficiency during the last two trimesters of pregnancy and first months after birth can result in intellectual disability or other neurologic deficits in the neonate. Hypothyroidism or hyperthyroidism during pregnancy can have an adverse effect on fetal growth and result in neonatal hypothyroidism or hyperthyroidism.

Women with phenylalanine hydroxylase deficiency (phenylketonuria [PKU]) and hyperphenylalaninemia are at risk of having a fetus with congenital anomalies if the phenylalanine levels are elevated in pregnancy. High maternal levels of phenylalanine during pregnancy can result in microcephaly, delayed speech, mental retardation, neurologic damage, congenital heart defects, facial anomalies, microcephaly, and delayed development (Mayo Clinic, 2018).

## Other

Another teratogenic factor is hyperthermia caused by maternal use of hot tubs or saunas or by maternal febrile illness during pregnancy. Hyperthermia can increase the incidence of embryonic resorption and malformations. The type and severity of congenital defect depend on the amount of temperature elevation, duration of the exposure, and stage of embryonic development. If the mother is exposed during the critical period (the first 8 weeks) when the CNS is particularly vulnerable to hyperthermia, congenital defects of the CNS may occur (Tobah, n.d.).

Good nutrition has long been considered essential for proper growth and development of the fetus. Dietary habits have a profound effect on pregnancy outcomes. However, with the exception of folic acid, in which there is evidence that deficiencies are causally related to defects of the neural tube, there is little known about the role of micronutrients on fetal development. Supplementation of vitamins and minerals must occur within the appropriate critical period of development to be effective. Finally, advanced paternal age has recently been associated with an increased risk of complex disorders such as autism, schizophrenia, autism spectrum disorder, and achondroplasia (Kaltsas et al., 2023).

## SUMMARY

This chapter has provided an overview of embryologic and fetal development, outlined the critical periods of development, and described the more common congenital defects. Knowledge of embryologic and fetal development is essential as a foundation for understanding the role of environment, genetics, physical, or other factors that may have an effect upon anatomy, physiology, or pathophysiology of the organism. The future health of the individual in large part depends on numerous events that take place during gestation. As knowledge of genetics, development, and human pathophysiology improves, better healthcare technologies may emerge that can significantly reduce morbidity and mortality and improve quality of life.

## CASE STUDY

**Identification of the Problem.** A 19-year-old female at approximately 19 weeks of gestation presents to the high-risk clinic by referral from her primary obstetrician. She had a morphology scan at her doctor's office at 18 weeks with intracranial calcifications noted as well as a probable hyperechogenic bowel. She and her husband had moved to North Carolina from a small town in Mississippi. They had married immediately after graduation from high school and he had joined the Army. They had neither family in the area nor any other social support systems.

**Assessment: History and Physical Examination.** The patient's primary obstetrician had forwarded prenatal records that described a 24 to 48 hour viral illness between 16 and 17 weeks with a fever of 102°F (38.9°C) and flu-like symptoms including myalgia and malaise. Detailed ultrasounds demonstrated numerous intracranial calcifications, microcephaly, pleural effusions, and decreased amniotic fluid. The perinatologist discussed with the couple the probability that she had been exposed to and developed CMV, which was passed on to the fetus. The couple refused amniocentesis following a prolonged discussion with family members in Mississippi because they had decided to continue with the pregnancy regardless of the outcome. The infant was born at 37 weeks and was diagnosed with blindness, deafness, and is likely to have severe mental disabilities.

**Diagnostic Tests and Working Diagnosis.** When a woman is infected with CMV for the first time during pregnancy (primary infection), the risk that her baby will get infected is as high as 50%. Primary maternal CMV infections occur in 0.15% to 2.0% of all pregnancies. Infants born with CMV are at risk for long-term disabilities such as mental retardation, learning disabilities, epilepsy, cerebral palsy, hearing impairment or deafness, and visual impairment or blindness. Congenital CMV infection is transmitted to the fetus by maternal viremia and placental infection. Maternal IgG transports the virus across the placental syncytiotrophoblast. In a primary infection in which the placenta becomes infected with CMV, the ability to provide nutrients and oxygen to the fetus is impaired. The placenta becomes enlarged, and tissue damage occurs due to viral placentitis and revascularization. Many symptoms in the newborn are due to the infection of the placenta rather than the direct effect of the virus on the fetus. A primary CMV infection in the first trimester is associated with the worst outcomes. A maternal infection that occurs prior to conception is unlikely to pass to the fetus.

Although the majority (85% to 90%) of congenital infections are asymptomatic, 5% to 20% of infants born to mothers with primary CMV infection are overtly symptomatic. Only 10% to 15% of these babies will show symptoms of infection at birth. Symptoms may include petechia, jaundice, hepatosplenomegaly, microcephaly, IUGR, chorioretinitis, thrombocytopenia, and anemia. Babies born with CMV are also at risk for long-term effects such as sensorineural hearing loss, vision problems, and psychomotor development delay. CMV-infected children have a mortality rate of about 5%, and severe neurologic morbidity occurs in 50% to 60% of survivors. Asymptomatic infants are also at risk of developing long-term neurodevelopmental morbidity, but the risk is much lower than in symptomatic neonates.

Diagnosis is made by viral culture of amniotic fluid and by ultrasound examination. Amniocentesis is essential for prenatal diagnosis and CMV isolation from amniotic fluid is the gold standard for prenatal diagnosis. A high viral load in the amniotic fluid may indicate a poor outcome; however, it may also be related to gestational age at the time of sampling. Once a fetal infection has been diagnosed, the fetus should be closely monitored by ultrasound. Abnormal ultrasound findings include abnormalities in amniotic fluid such as polyhydramnios or oligohydramnios, IUGR, hydrocephaly or microcephaly, intracranial calcifications, cerebral ventriculomegaly or atrophy, hyperechogenic bowel, pseudomeconium ileus, hepatosplenomegaly, ascites or hydrops, and/or necrotic, cystic, or calcified lesions in the brain or liver. Some babies that have been infected with CMV during pregnancy will show signs of problems on ultrasound; however, the absence of sonographic findings does not guarantee a normal outcome. Some fetuses with CMV will not show any signs of infection on ultrasound. Once a fetus is diagnosed with a CMV infection, ultrasounds should be done every 2 to 4 weeks to watch for signs that may predict the outcome. Routine serologic testing is not recommended and should be used only when a pregnant woman develops a flu-like illness or if a CMV infection is suspected following an ultrasound.

**Development of Management Plan and Implementation.** Currently, there is no effective therapy for CMV infection, and women can be offered the option of pregnancy termination once a fetal infection is detected by ultrasound or amniocentesis and once a fetus is determined or suspected to be affected. Research on the use of CMV-specific hyperimmune globulin in pregnant women with a primary infection has been reported to improve outcomes; however, further studies are needed. There is also some evidence that ganciclovir treatment of babies with symptoms of congenital CMV may be beneficial for prevention or amelioration of hearing loss.

There are currently no vaccines for CMV and no clinical trials of new vaccines. Prevention of congenital CMV infection by practicing good personal hygiene is crucial. Pregnant women should avoid intimate contact with saliva and urine from young children and use good handwashing after changing diapers and wiping secretions. At least one-third of women in the United States have direct contact with children less than 3 years old. Children and staff who care for children in day care centers are especially likely to be infected; therefore, pregnant women who have children in day care settings are especially vulnerable. One should assume that all children under age 3 have CMV in their urine and saliva. Other recommendations include not sharing cups, plates, or toothbrushes; not kissing children on or near the mouth; and not sharing towels or washcloths with a young child.

## ONLINE RESOURCES

CourseConnect

Resources for this chapter are online and available at www.springerpub.com/courseconnect.

## REFERENCES

References for this chapter are online and available at www.springerpub.com/courseconnect.

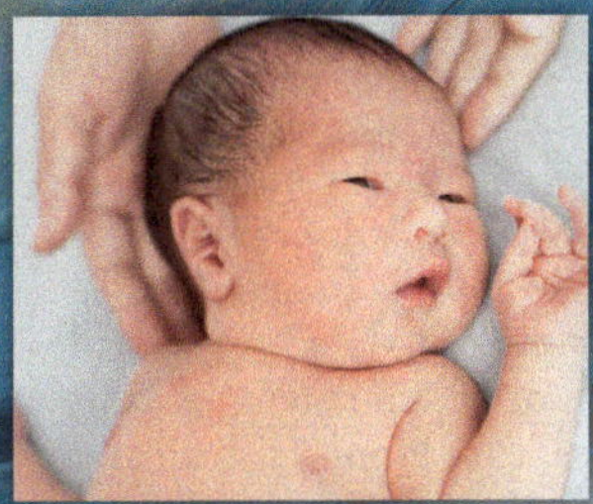

Source: Jirasaki/Adobe Stock.

CHAPTER 2

# Prenatal, Intrapartal, and Postpartal Risk Factors

Dolores R. Dzubaty

## INTRODUCTION

Women who discover they are pregnant expect to experience an uneventful pregnancy and deliver a healthy term newborn. However, women and their partners are exposed to a myriad of physical, environmental, psychological, genetic, and behavioral factors that influence pregnancy and the outcome. Women with access to excellent prenatal care may be unknowingly exposed to factors that are detrimental to a fetus. The result may be a pregnancy that is completed preterm and an infant affected by the complications of prematurity, low birth weight (LBW), or possibly congenital disorders. Preterm birth (PTB) and the resultant health complications not only cause neonatal morbidity and mortality but can affect the newborn throughout the life span.

Perinatal providers assess and identify patient risk factors that may result in poor pregnancy outcomes. Ideally, education can be provided prenatally so that patients enter the pregnancy in a state of good health, minimize their exposure to known teratogens, and are knowledgeable about lifestyle changes that may need to occur. Identifying risk factors and developing education for all women is a global, national, and local concern. Many organizations have contributed to the knowledge utilized by healthcare practitioners caring for women before, during, and after pregnancy. This chapter presents information on the risk factors contributing to complications in pregnancy and possible changes that can increase healthy outcomes. The perspective will be global and national in recognizing the multicultural patient population.

## GLOBAL

In October 2015, the United Nations General Assembly adopted the document "Transforming Our World: 2030 Agenda for Sustainable Development" (United Nations [UN], 2015). Within this document, the General Assembly advanced a commitment to:

> *build on the Millennium Development Goals and complete what they did not achieve. They seek to realize the human rights of all and to achieve gender equality and the empowerment of all women and girls. They are integrated and indivisible and balance the three dimensions of sustainable development: the economic, social, and environmental* (p. 5).

The Resolution stating the 17 new Sustainable Development Goals (SDG) set forth went into effect on January 1, 2016 (UN, 2015). The assembly recognized in this document that different nations would have dissimilar challenges in meeting the goals set forth. Implementation of action to reach the SDG and targets would occur on national levels. The commitment to maternal, newborn, and child health remains embedded in these new goals.

## NATIONAL

At the national level, member nations have committed to the 2030 Agenda (UN, 2015) and adopted policies and procedures, as well as support efforts to improve and sustain the conditions of their populations. In low-resource countries, there are challenges of infrastructure deficiencies. Fewer healthcare facilities, farther distances to travel to obtain care, and lack of transportation means to obtain care all adversely affect pregnancy outcomes. Cultural practices that are not recognized to support healthy outcomes may still be prevalent in some regions of countries with modern services. The result is healthcare disparity based on geographic location, adherence to cultural beliefs, and socioeconomic status.

Disparity in healthcare can also be found in more developed countries based on geographic location, socioeconomic status, and personal belief system. Healthcare provider groups such as the Association of Women's Health, Obstetric, and Neonatal Nursing (AWHONN, 2023) and the Royal College of Nurse-Midwives (2024) have developed standards of care and educational offerings for nurses and midwives. The purpose is to ensure care delivery at all levels to support healthy pregnancy outcomes, reduce prematurity, and provide consistent care. The International Confederation of Midwives (2024) seeks to educate, empower, and provide care to women globally. Despite all the efforts put forth by these groups, healthcare disparity and poor perinatal outcomes persist. A review of the National Vital Statistics System (NVSS) and the National Center for Health Statistics by Joseph et al. (2023) reveals maternal death rates in the United States are increasing across all races and ethnic groups. This investigation also exhibited inconsistencies in reporting factors.

## PERINATAL OUTCOMES INDICATORS

As healthcare delivery differs between countries, common indicators must be chosen to compare the improvement or worsening of prenatal outcomes. PTB rate, LBW, and neonatal and infant mortality are three indicators that can be compared.

### Preterm Birth

From 2021 to 2022, the neonatal mortality rate in the United States increased by 3% after a 20-year downward trend. Among the five leading causes of neonatal mortality, PTB and LBW accounted for 14% of infant deaths (Ely & Driscoll, 2024). This increase was not consistent across all races and ethnicities.

PTBs range from 5% to 16.2% worldwide, with most births occurring between 32 and 37 weeks of pregnancy gestation (World Health Organization [WHO], 2023). Approximately 13.4 million babies are *Born Too Soon*, as their document is titled, and more than a million infants die due to complications of prematurity (WHO, 2023). The outcomes for premature infants born in low-income countries are not as favorable as those born in high-income countries. Many preterm infant survivors are left with hearing, vision, or intellectual problems that last a lifetime (WHO, 2023).

The definition of PTB distinguishes the level of prematurity by weeks of gestational age. Survival rates of infants born at less than 28 weeks are very low. Determining gestational age to classify a neonate in any subcategory in developed countries uses a combination of early ultrasound and the mother's menstrual history. When ultrasound is unavailable, or only ultrasound but not menstrual history, the determination of gestational age may not be as accurate and result in statistical differences when studying outcomes of PTB. In clinical practice, assigning an infant to the wrong subcategory of prematurity may result in following a different standard of care. In 2020, the WHO put forth recommendations for perinatal care in any setting, including educating care providers. The objective is to provide care that would possibly reduce PTB and educate the caregiver to be able to provide care to an infant born preterm. Through the education provided, caregivers learn physical assessment techniques that can be used in low-income, low-resource settings.

There is no single cause of preterm labor. Preterm labor may result from intraamniotic inflammation (Gomez-Lopez et al., 2022) or placental factors (Jaiman et al., 2022). A meta-analysis by Mitrogiannis et al. (2023) identified factors considered highly likely and most probable, such as amphetamine use by the mother, maternal personality disorder, history of prior termination of pregnancy, and current placenta previa. The occurrence of preterm labor is not always predictable, and the interplay of multiple factors may occasionally result in preterm labor. As a result, prenatal care may include fetal fibronectin testing when appropriate, observation for shortened cervical length by ultrasound, prior pregnancy history, presence of infection or inflammatory conditions, and known environmental exposures, all of which may help identify women who are at risk for premature labor. Historically, some women even with several risk factors may not deliver prematurely.

Screening tools, ultrasounds, and other testing can only be effective if available and accessible. Lack of insurance, transportation, literacy, and immigration status have been identified as some of the reasons Latino women do not obtain prenatal care in the Midwest United States (Camargo et al., 2023). Utilizing available prenatal care is a global problem, as evidenced in Ethiopia, where factors of equipment shortages, access, and issues within the healthcare system have been identified as hindrances for pregnant women (Tamiso et al., 2023). Problems within any healthcare system may include a lack of appropriate healthcare facilities, trained caregivers, or equipment.

Preterm infants require specialized care to survive. There is significant variation in the methods and effectiveness of care delivered to preterm infants between high- and low-income countries as well as within geographic areas of the same country. The cost of providing neonatal intensive care for vulnerable preterm infants adds a financial burden for the family (Lambiase et al., 2024), the workplace through parental leaves (Patel et al., 2024), and the healthcare system beyond birth (Hua et al., 2023). The overall costs of care increase for neonates of extreme prematurity due to more diagnostic or medical procedures, medications, longer hospital stays, and long-term care. Preterm infants are also at higher risk for hospital readmission, adding more to the financial burden (Moreno et al., 2024). The reality is that not all countries have the infrastructure or finances to treat all preterm infants aggressively. However, some initial interventions can be performed in any setting, which can increase the chances of survival for many premature infants, even in low-resource nations.

### Birth Weight

Regardless of gestational age, birth weight is also an important determinant of neonatal survival. LBW is defined as an initial birth weight of less than 2,500 g and is further categorized as either very low birth weight (VLBW) or extremely low birth weight (ELBW). VLBW is defined as an initial birth weight of less than 1,500 g, and ELBW is defined as a birth weight of less than 1,000 g. Ideally, birth weight should be measured within the first hour of birth before significant postnatal losses occur. In some cases, when the infant is distressed, the birth weight may be estimated until an accurate weight can be determined. LBW infants are at higher risk for neonatal and postnatal morbidity and mortality. While survival for VLBW infants has improved with advances in neonatal care, there is a risk for increased morbidity (Vanhaesebrouck et al., 2023). Children born in any category of LBW may have residual effects of prematurity and require treatment for neurologic, cognitive, and physical problems in the future (Dhivar et al., 2024). Appropriate support in the future for this population can be costly and problematic, especially in countries challenged with meeting the costs of adequate prenatal care.

The macrosomic or large for gestational age (LGA) fetus also has risks. Pregnancy risk factors for being LGA include maternal obesity, maternal age older than 35, maternal diabetes, prolonged pregnancy longer than 41 weeks, abnormally tall or short maternal stature, and male fetus. LGA is defined as greater than the 90th percentile for weight adjusted for gender and gestational weeks at delivery. Potential complications for the mother include prolonged labor with increased risk for cephalopelvic disproportion (CPD) and the need for cesarean section. During vaginal delivery, the LGA infant is at significant risk for birth trauma. In the period immediately following delivery, the macrosomic infant is at risk for hypoglycemia, polycythemia, and hyperbilirubinemia (Sousa et al., 2024).

Determination of gestational age can be estimated prior to delivery or upon examination of the newborn. Additional physical measurements are obtained to determine if the infant's weight and size are appropriate for the gestational age obtained. Gestational age can be based on maternal history, ultrasound when available, or physical assessment. After birth, the neonate's weight, frontal occipital head circumference, and length at birth are plotted on a graph to evaluate the appropriateness of growth based on gestational age. The infant is categorized as appropriate for gestational age (AGA) if birth weight falls between the 10th and 90th percentile for his or her gestational age; small for gestational age (SGA) if birth weight falls into the lower 10th percentile for weight based upon gestational age; or LGA if birth weight is greater than 90th percentile for weight based upon gestational age, or more than 4,000 g at any gestational age (Wu et al., 2022). Identification of infants who are SGA or LGA helps ensure they receive proper monitoring of blood glucose and early feedings if indicated.

In developed countries where bariatric surgery is available, micro and macronutrient deficiency has been associated with SGA due to lower food intake (Burlina et al., 2023). The SGA neonate does not have the risk for poor perinatal outcomes as the LBW neonate. However, some fetuses may, in fact, have increased perinatal risk due to fetal growth restriction (FGR) or intrauterine growth restriction (IUGR). FGR and IUGR can be caused by maternal, fetal, or placental problems (Tsikouras et al., 2024). Maternal causes include conditions such as preeclampsia, smoking, or taking certain drugs can result in progressive uteroplacental insufficiency and limit the normal delivery of oxygen and nutrients to the fetus. Inadequate maternal nutrition, low prepregnancy weight, low weight gain in pregnancy, or inadequate prenatal care are other maternal causes of FGR. Fetal conditions that can contribute to FGR include fetal genetic factors, congenital infection, intrauterine crowding from multiple pregnancies, Rh isoimmunization, or twin-to-twin transfusion. Abnormal placental pathophysiology resulting in poor perfusion through the placenta includes abnormal cord insertion, placental infarcts, or implantation issues such as placenta previa or abruptio placenta, which are also causes of FGR (Tsikouras et al., 2024). Severe uteroplacental insufficiency restricts blood flow to the fetus and affects fetal growth and oxygenation. To spare the function of vital organs, the fetus enters a brain-sparing mode, accounting for fetal growth changes. Although oxygen and nutrients are prioritized by the brain, heart, and adrenals, the chronic hypoxia and hypoglycemia experienced by the FGR fetus cause asymmetrical growth and development as well as organ, motor, and cognitive disabilities after birth (Wu et al., 2023).

Fetuses with FGR must be identified and closely monitored with non-stress testing, biophysical profiles, amniotic fluid volume estimates, contraction stress tests, and Doppler studies of maternal and umbilical vessels when available. Infants may be subject to preterm delivery and FGR due to altered placental implantation and function (Tsikouras et al., 2024). **Emergency Alert:** **Preterm delivery is indicated if signs of fetal stress or distress are present.** After birth, infants with FGR often have problems with low blood glucose or thermoregulation due to a lack of subcutaneous fat. An FGR infant born preterm is at increased risk for necrotizing enterocolitis, thrombocytopenia, retinopathy of prematurity (ROP), neonatal jaundice, and renal failure because blood is shunted away from the gastrointestinal and renal system to the brain, heart, and other vital organs as a protective mechanism during fetal development (Raffa et al., 2024). Prematurity and LBW, when occurring together, have also been identified as having an effect on neurodevelopment, resulting in developmental disabilities and cognitive impairments (Vanhaesebrouck et al., 2023). **Emergency Alert:** **Infants with low birth weight have also been found to be more at risk of developing a metabolic syndrome with insulin resistance, hypertension, hypercholesterolemia, and heart disease (Jańczewska et al., 2023; Talarico et al., 2023; Zamir et al., 2024).**

## Neonatal & Infant Mortality Rates

Neonatal deaths during the first 28 days of life accounted for 46% of deaths of children under age 5 in 2022 (United Nations Children's Fund [UNICEF], 2024). International disparities exist, with some countries below or meeting the SDG for 2030, whereas others are still well above the goal. PTB complications are responsible for most neonatal deaths worldwide (UNICEF, 2024). The world infant mortality rate (IMR) ranges from < 5 to > 35 deaths per 1,000 live births (UNICEF, 2024). Infants from low- or middle-income countries represent a higher percentage of neonatal deaths than infants from industrialized nations. PTB complications, intrapartum events, and neonatal infections represent the causes of 47% of neonatal deaths (UNICEF, 2019). PTBs and the resulting complications contribute to higher neonatal mortality. Preterm birth rates have declined in the United States between 2010 and 2020; however, the United States remains in the top eight countries, accounting for 50% of preterm births in 2020 (Ohuma et al., 2023). Differences in the interpretation of what constitutes fetal viability can account for some differences in how neonatal deaths are reported. Neonatal mortality in the United States was reported to be 3.59% (Ely & Driscoll, 2024). In contrast, postneonatal mortality, which occurs between 28 days and 1 year, is reported at 1.94% as of June 2024 (Driscoll & Ely, 2024). Most of the recorded infant deaths are attributed to prematurity followed by underlying perinatal causes responsible for birth defects, sepsis, cord or placental complications, maternal complications, and respiratory distress.

IMRs differ in the United States by race, ethnicity, and geographic region. The highest IMR was reported in infants born to non-Hispanic Black (NHB) mothers (10.90 deaths per 1,000 live births) compared with infants born to non-Hispanic White (NHW) mothers (4.52 per 1,000 live births) (Ely & Driscoll, 2024). Based on 2022 birth data in the United States, NHB mothers had a higher rate of delivering infants of LBW (< 2,500 g) compared with infants of NHW mothers (Osterman et al., 2024). Ethnic disparities are also evidently related to neonatal mortality during the first 28 days of life. Comparison rates for NHB and NHW infants for the three leading causes of neonatal death demonstrate that disparities in infant outcomes persist across populations. Infants of NHB mothers had a higher rate of neonatal deaths related to congenital malformations, prematurity or LBW, and being affected by maternal complications of pregnancy compared with infants of NHW mothers (Osterman, 2025).

## Epidemiologic Paradox

Pregnancy outcomes, such as risk for preterm labor, cannot always be predicted by the presence of maternal risk or sociodemographic factors. Screening tools that may be useful in predicting preterm labor are not available for all populations (Cresswell et al., 2023). For example, Mexican women who immigrate to the United States have demographic and socioeconomic factors such as high rates of teen pregnancy, less education, and higher rates of no prenatal care or late prenatal care in the third trimester that put them at high risk for poor perinatal outcomes. However, Asian Indian women who immigrate to the United States have demographic and socioeconomic risk factors like White women that put them at low risk. Asian Indian women have higher education levels with more college graduates, less teen pregnancy, and are more likely to initiate prenatal care in the first trimester. However, an "epidemiologic paradox" transpires, and outcomes do not occur as predicted. NHB women have the highest incidence of LBW, SGA, and fetal and neonatal deaths in the United States (Ely & Driscoll, 2024). Foreign-born Mexican women with demographic and socioeconomic risk factors comparable to Black women have better than expected perinatal outcomes, including less LBW and fewer neonatal deaths (Ely & Driscoll, 2024). In comparison, Asian women in the United States initiate prenatal care later, have lower incidences of preterm delivery, and have higher incidences of LBW and VLBW than White women (Ely & Driscoll, 2024). This "epidemiologic paradox" suggests that other factors might give foreign-born women either a perinatal advantage or disadvantage when assessing for preterm delivery risk (Barreto et al., 2024; Yang, et al., 2024a).

# MATERNAL RISK FACTORS

Evaluation of maternal risk factors may help anticipate many of the neonates who will be at increased risk for problems at birth. There is no way to accurately predict every neonate who will be at risk because a cause-and-effect relationship between high-risk maternal characteristics or behaviors and poor outcomes is not always clearly defined. For example, there have been cases of identical twins where one twin was born healthy, and the other one required admission to the neonatal intensive care unit (NICU). Although both babies had similar genetic makeup, gestational age, and exposure to the same in-utero environment, only one had problems.

One of the most essential ways to decrease problems of prematurity, LBW, and perinatal death is to promote optimal pregnancy health. The ideal state is for all women considering pregnancy to seek preconception counseling. During the preconception visit, the woman can learn about risk factors that could potentially cause birth defects or problems with pregnancy. Risk factors may be either modifiable or nonmodifiable. Examples of modifiable risk factors that can be changed include diet, smoking, alcohol use, and substance use or abuse. Nonmodifiable risk factors are intrinsic factors that cannot be changed, such as maternal age, ethnicity, genetic inheritance, or preexisting health problems. Risk factors usually do not occur in isolation. The presence of multiple risk factors has an additive effect. For example, a pregnant woman who lacks financial resources might also have a poor obstetric history, inadequate nutritional intake, increased stress, and poor coping behaviors. Some maternal risk factors can be modified through patient education, counseling, lifestyle changes, and support. The purpose of preconception care is to help the woman who is contemplating pregnancy get into optimal physical condition for childbearing before conception. Unfortunately, preconception counseling is not the norm. Therefore, all women of childbearing age must be encouraged to live healthy lifestyles and to seek early prenatal care in the first trimester of pregnancy. Even the first trimester of pregnancy is not too late to implement interventions or modify lifestyle risk factors to maximize positive pregnancy outcomes.

Maternal risk factors include demographic, behavioral, and psychosocial factors, as well as maternal medical and pregnancy-related conditions. Demographic risk factors include ethnicity, age, socioeconomic status, occupation, and environmental or work-related exposures. Psychosocial risk factors include social, behavioral, stress-related, or maternal psychological conditions. Medical risk factors for prematurity that are unalterable can vary by population and can consist of previous obstetric events or pregnancy-related conditions such as multiple gestation, pregnancy-induced hypertension (PIH), or gestational diabetes. Modifiable risk factors include low prepregnancy weight, low or high body mass index (BMI), and behavioral risk factors the mother has before or during pregnancy. Examples of behavioral risk factors that can be harmful to the fetus include inadequate dietary intake, smoking, or substance use (drugs or alcohol). A complete maternal history at the first prenatal visit will help identify important demographic and medical risk factors that might influence the pregnancy outcomes for both the mother and neonate. The presence of risk factors should serve as a warning.

## Maternal Age

Maternal age is a risk factor for poor perinatal outcomes at either end of the childbearing age spectrum. The maternal childbearing age range has widened over the past decade partially due to advances in assisted reproductive technology (ART) that have made it possible for women to achieve pregnancy, even into the fifth or sixth decade of life, if desired. Worldwide, the maternal age at the time of the first child's birth ranges from a mean of 18.1 years in less developed populations to a mean of 32.2 years in more industrialized nations (Central Intelligence Agency, n.d.).

There is evidence that pregnancy during adolescence increases the risk of adverse outcomes. Demonstrated complications of adolescent pregnancy include increased risk of anemia, preterm delivery, postpartum hemorrhage, and preeclampsia (İşgüder et al., 2024). Adolescent pregnancy has also resulted in a higher risk of fetal malformations; hemolysis, elevated liver enzymes, low platelets (HELLP) syndrome; and FGR neonates. Mothers younger than age 20 are especially high risk because they are biologically immature and have not had the chance to complete their own physical growth and reproductive development, and typically have poor healthcare decision-making skills (Ursache et al., 2023). Reproductive immaturity can increase risks of fetal loss, PTB, or infant death.

In 2023, the U.S. teen birth rates for ages 15 to 19 years declined to 13.1 births per 1,000 births, representing a decline of 6% since 2021 (Martin et al., 2024). Even so, the United States has one of the highest teen birth rates worldwide compared with other developed nations. The numbers of teen and adolescent births globally are challenging to estimate, but rates are higher in countries where child marriage is allowed. Child marriage rates are declining in many countries due to the efforts of numerous stakeholders guided by the newly introduced Sustainable Goals affecting women and children (WHO, 2015). The United Nations report (2024) states that maternal mortality has decreased only slightly, with a slight decrease in the adolescent birth rate. However, insignificant improvements in other areas affect pregnancy, such as available clean water and adequate food supplies. Lack of attainment of the SDGs is thought to be due to the economic downturn many countries experienced during and after the COVID-19 pandemic, resulting in less government financial commitment. Teen mothers and their infants have increased perinatal risks, including a higher risk of dying during childbirth compared with 20-year-old women. Maternal age is a risk factor for the survival of infants born to teen mothers (UNICEF, 2019). There are also lifelong disadvantages for younger teen mothers with fewer formal education years. Education is known to be a factor related to the promotion of positive pregnancy behaviors. Pregnant adolescents who are less educated most likely will not use contraception, may not recognize danger signs in pregnancy that something is wrong, or may not even seek prenatal care. On a global level, there are many programs directed at preventing teen pregnancy, which focus on physical and sexual education in general and pregnancy prevention (Myat et al., 2024). Pregnant adolescents face medical challenges due to physical immaturity, high risk of sexually transmitted infections (STIs), and poor nutrition. Adolescents are also emotionally immature and may not cope well with the pregnancy itself and the sequelae of being socially unaccepted, financially unstable, and unable to identify support resources (Pietras et al., 2024). Preexisting maternal disadvantages, such as medical conditions, drug use, and poor relationships, are more likely to account for adverse outcomes of teen parenting for mothers and infants (Ursache, 2023; WHO, 2022). A need has been identified for improved education and healthcare during the preconception, perinatal, and postdelivery periods for the benefit of teens and their infants (Padhani et al., 2024).

*Advanced maternal age* refers to women older than 35 at the estimated delivery date. Women may have problems conceiving secondary to infertility or may choose to delay childbearing. The resulting trend has been an increase in the number of pregnant women of advanced maternal age. Advances in reproductive science have made it possible for women who are postmenopausal in their 50s or 60s to conceive. The birth rate for women ages 40 to 44 was 12.6 births per 1,000 women, and the birth rate for women ages 45 to 49 increased in 2023 to 1.1 births per 1,000 women (Hamilton et al., 2024). Advanced maternal age poses increased risks for decreased fertility, chromosomal abnormalities in the infant, spontaneous abortion, and preterm delivery (Frederiksen et al., 2024; Pathare et al., 2023). Late fetal and early perinatal death rates are higher for pregnant women 40 and older than for any other age group. Women older than 35 are at increased risk for perinatal morbidity and mortality; however, the increased risk appears to be related to previous obstetric and medical comorbidities more than age alone (Johal et al., 2024). Although fertility tends to decline with advanced maternal age, women between the ages of 35 and 39 have an increased risk of conceiving twins without the assistance of fertility treatments. Current guidelines suggest practitioners screen for maternal genetic disorders and medical disorders and avoid multifetal implantation while attempting single-gestation pregnancies (American Society for Reproductive Medicine, 2024).

Older pregnant women with prior medical diseases, such as chronic hypertension, are at an increased risk for adverse outcomes of pregnancy (Masembe et al., 2024). The rates of prenatal medical complications, including diabetes, cardiac disease, and hypertension in pregnant women, increase as maternal age advances. Pregnancy at an advanced maternal age can also contribute to increased risks of gestational hypertension, gestational diabetes, and placenta previa (Zhou et al., 2023).

Advanced maternal age creates genetic risks. The prevailing theory is that all females are born with all of the oocytes they will ever have, which contain the genetic material they will pass on to their progeny. According to maternal aging theory, as a woman ages, her oocytes and the genetic material contained within her also age. Aging genetic material is more likely to have errors during cell division and migration during meiosis that can result in aneuploidy (an abnormal number of chromosomes), lower implantation rates, decreased fertility, or increased risk of spontaneous abortion (Frederiksen, 2024). Although chromosomal disorders can occur at any maternal age, there is an increased risk after age 35. **Quality and Safety:** **Advances in screening tests now allow practitioners the advantage of offering testing appropriate to a patient's low- or high-risk status (Cornel et al., 2024).**

## PATERNAL FACTORS

Paternal age does not appear to be an independent factor in adverse pregnancy outcomes such as disparities in placental growth or maternal outcomes (Kaltsas et al., 2024). However, the use of assisted reproductive technology (ART) increased as paternal age increased. The use of ART has also been associated with cord insertion abnormalities (Fukuda et al., 2023a), ovarian hyperstimulation, and placental complications (Heshmatnia et al., 2023). Sociodemographic differences in paternal age demonstrated increased risk of preterm birth, LBW, gestational diabetes, and gestation hypertension (Ha et al., 2024). **Quality and Safety: A careful assessment of the family history of both parents will help alert the healthcare provider to potential risks.**

## LIFE COURSE DETERMINANTS OF BIRTH OUTCOMES AND WEATHERING

The life course theory (LCT) is an approach used to explain health, disease, and health disparities across populations and over time. LCT focuses on social, economic, and environmental factors as key determinants that help shape health or disease in communities and populations. Intergenerational preprogramming (i.e., maternal preconception health) and prenatal preprogramming (i.e., the in-utero environment) are recognized as an influence on fetal and child health. While health can be affected at any time, there are critical and sensitive periods when events can have a maximal effect on lifetime health, such as during fetal development, early childhood, or adolescence. The goal would be to promote interventions during these sensitive times to maximize health (WHO, 2021).

Applying the LCT perspective to preterm delivery would imply that reproductive and birth outcomes are the product of circumstances and events that occur not only during pregnancy but throughout the life of the mother, beginning either before or at the time when she was conceived. The LCT perspective acknowledges that early-life experiences can shape health across an entire lifetime and could potentially influence the health of future generations (Wagner et al., 2024). According to the LCT perspective, assessing the woman's experiences during the immediate preconception and prenatal period is insufficient to determine risks for poor outcomes. Assessment of major events during her entire life course and the effects of material deprivation, social disadvantage, discrimination, and marginalization must be explored (Wagner et al., 2024). The health consequences of poverty and race-based discrimination and the health effects of chronic stress must also be considered. For example, exposure to poor nutrition as a child or even as a developing fetus could affect a woman's pregnancy outcomes. The life course perspective aligns with the developmental origins of the health and disease approach, which posits the vital role of the fetus in the utero environment in the development of the structure and functions of the body's organs. For example, a lack of folic acid during development can lead to neural tube defects (Liu et al., 2024); exposure to tobacco can lead to LBW or short gestation (Meaton et al., 2023); and exposure to maternal antidepressants may cause PTB and increased risk of neonatal morbidity (Wecker et al., 2024). Components of a perinatal life course risk assessment and prevention tool are under development and activation, promising to decrease healthcare disparities (LaFave et al., 2024).

## PSYCHOLOGICAL STRESS IN PREGNANCY

Maternal mental health and psychological stress are increasingly being studied as possible sources of adverse perinatal outcomes. Stress is an interaction between the person and environment in which there is a perceived discrepancy between the demands of the environment and the individual's resources (i.e., psychological, social, or biologic) for dealing with it. During pregnancy, women may experience many types of stressors. Chronic life stressors include stress about finances, work situations, difficult relationships, health concerns of self or other family members, or other factors. Acute stressors during pregnancy include situational crises or natural disasters. There is a growing body of evidence related to the effects of acute and chronic maternal stress during pregnancy.

Chronic stress results in physiologic dysfunction over time that impairs the immune response and produces metabolic and cardiovascular changes that create illness. Chronic stressors can harm pregnancy and result in LBW (Matsas et al., 2023). Increased stress during pregnancy can result in normal stress reactions, causing increased physiologic response, which harms the pregnancy. A woman may be entering her pregnancy unknowingly in a poor physiologic state and at risk for hypertension and diabetes due to these changes. Pregnancy, labor, and delivery may trigger a response in women who experience posttraumatic stress disorder (PTSD) resulting from prior adverse pregnancy outcomes or sexual assault. Healthcare providers should evaluate all patients who exhibit signs of depression in pregnancy to rule out PTSD so the patient receives the proper psychological support (Horsch et al., 2024). The diagnosis of PTSD and its effect on pregnancy outcomes can be found in all countries, ethnic groups, and socioeconomic levels.

Pregnancy-related anxiety is a form of anxiety specific to pregnant women. It includes (a) fear of pain; (b) concerns about the health of the baby, labor, and delivery; (c) pregnancy-specific support and giving birth; and (d) negative interactions with care providers (Hildingsson & Johansson, 2024). The exact mechanism by which maternal stress causes preterm labor is not fully understood, but it is thought to occur by one of two mechanisms. A corticotropin-releasing hormone released as a by-product of maternal stress could stimulate neuroendocrine pathways within the maternal-fetal–placental unit that trigger labor, or maternal stress could cause increased maternal and fetal susceptibility to inflammation and infection, triggering labor through an immune-inflammatory pathway (Bergeron et al., 2024). These interactions between neuroendocrine, immune, and behavioral processes may be tempered by maternal resilience resources. Some accepted methods of stress reduction used in the general population have been attempted with pregnant populations. A study was conducted that introduced clients to the use of tele-yoga with results demonstrating a decrease in participants' stress levels (Ganjekar et al., 2024).

Not all women are affected in the same way by stress, which could account for difficulty predicting outcomes. Critical periods may occur during pregnancy where there is altered vulnerability to the effects of prenatal stress. The cumulative effects of lifetime exposure to acute stress and experiences of chronic day-to-day stress increase the risk of stress-related disease during pregnancy. They may help explain some ethnic disparities in birth outcomes. Just as it is difficult to predict the consequences related to stress, it is imperative to assess the methods pregnant women may use to cope with stress prenatally. Social support in the healthcare setting utilized by at-risk patients may prevent adverse outcomes in the pregnancies of the patient population (Houston et al., 2024; Rex et al., 2024).

Smoking, alcohol use, and drug abuse have been cited by many as methods used to deal with stress. Care providers can advise alternative stress-reduction measures to improve pregnancy outcomes. Care providers need to make an individual assessment of the suitability of stress reduction activities for patients. Physical activity, such as walking, can reduce the incidence of gestational hypertension and diabetes (Taliento et al., 2024). In identifying a safe area for the patient to walk prenatally, the provider has also informed the patient of a possible safe area to bring the infant. Yoga is another intervention that some women may already practice and is useful in the treatment of anxiety and depression in the general population (Datta et al., 2023). Many of the moves and poses can be adapted for pregnancy. In addition to alternatives, providers can offer smoking cessation programs and support to mothers because quitting at any time during pregnancy will improve neonatal outcomes (Ganjekar et al., 2024; Lučovnik et al., 2024). The success of any intervention will depend on the appropriateness for the individual client.

## OBSTETRIC FACTORS

Obstetric history is a good indicator of the presence of maternal risk factors. Women with previous obstetric complications are more at risk for problems with the current pregnancy. Previous obstetric history of infertility, stillbirth, preterm infant, infant with growth restriction or congenital anomalies/genetic problems, complications during pregnancy or birth, or other poor outcomes are clues that indicate that the pregnancy must be closely monitored. Prepregnancy health status is another factor associated with the risk of preterm delivery. Wu et al. (2024) identified women at risk for preterm labor and delivery to include those under 25 years of age and over 35 years, lower socioeconomic status, prior chronic disease, and a history of gynecologic disorders. Important obstetric factors that can compound pregnancy risk are the timing and adequacy of prenatal care and the multiparity of the mother (Başkiran et al., 2023; Saaka & Sulley, 2023).

## PRENATAL CARE

Prenatal care that begins in the first trimester of pregnancy and continues until birth helps promote good birth outcomes. In the United States, 7% of women started prenatal care during the last trimester or received no prenatal care, with higher rates of late or no prenatal care seen in NHB and Hispanic women compared with NHW women (Osterman et al., 2024). The WHO has set a worldwide goal for at least eight focused antenatal care visits during pregnancy (WHO, 2016). Inadequate prenatal care increases the risk for LBW, PTB, and undiagnosed complications in pregnancy, such as gestational diabetes (Camargo et al., 2023; Fente et al., 2023). Neonatal deaths are seen in infants of women who may not have received prenatal care with causes including sepsis, respiratory distress, intrauterine hypoxia, and asphyxia occurring during the birth process (Kochanek et al., 2024).

The decision to seek prenatal care is influenced by the woman's attitudes toward pregnancy, cultural preference, or lifestyle factors. Access to prenatal care may be limited due to financial constraints or geographic availability of a trained practitioner. Eight prenatal visits prior to delivery are considered a protective factor against LBW and prematurity. Current recommendations by the WHO (2016) encourage group antenatal care contact and private contact to encourage pregnant women to engage in antenatal care, improve satisfaction, and decrease adverse pregnancy outcomes.

Providing care to the mother at delivery by a skilled birth attendant could also improve outcomes through early recognition of problems during labor and intervention. Worldwide, there are many countries where most women deliver at home with or without the assistance of a trained practitioner. Countries with high rates of births attended by untrained practitioners also have high rates of infant mortality (Khalida et al., 2023; Zegeye et al., 2023). The United Nations SDG 3 (2015) seeks to provide universal access for all women to reproductive care, including access to prenatal care and family planning information.

## PARITY

Parity or number of previous deliveries has been considered another risk factor for preterm delivery, LBW infant, and abnormal placental implantation. Parity is difficult to disassociate from age, because women with higher parity are usually older. In an age-matched case-control study, Zhou et al. (2023) found adverse pregnancy outcomes appeared to be related to maternal age rather than grand multiparity. In general, primiparous women older than 35 years of age and multiparous teens younger than 18 years of age have an increased risk for PTB at any gestational length (Osterman et al., 2024). Primiparous teenagers tend to have the highest risk of having an extremely PTB (EPTB). The incidence of EPTB is higher in older primiparous Black and Hispanic women compared with teenagers. On the other hand, in White women, EPTB risk is highest at either end of the age spectrum for both teens and older primiparas. However, for all races, the risks for any PTB increase in women who are older than 40 years of age (Osterman et al., 2024).

## INTERPREGNANCY LEVEL

Interpregnancy level is defined as the amount of time between the delivery of a baby and the subsequent conception of another child. A short interpregnancy level of less than

6 months increases the risk for maternal complications, including third-trimester bleeding, premature rupture of membranes (PROM), puerperal endometritis, anemia, and maternal death. Women with more prolonged interpregnancy levels have the highest risk for preeclampsia, eclampsia, and gestational diabetes, which may be related to older maternal age (Ni et al., 2023). The risk for prematurity is increased when the interpregnancy level is less than 18 months and should be considered when providing postpartum care (Hassen et al., 2024).

## ASSISTED REPRODUCTIVE TECHNOLOGY

ART is any procedure or medical treatment used to assist a woman to achieve pregnancy. ART is an option for many couples who have a history of infertility. Methods used include medications to stimulate ovulation and release of eggs or procedures where eggs and sperm are removed and mixed outside the body to achieve fertilization. In some cases, the eggs, sperm, or embryos might be frozen for later use or manipulated with instrumentation during the earliest stages of cell formation.

According to the CDC, about 2.3% of U.S. pregnancies are conceived using ART (CDC, n.d.-a). ART increases the risk for multiple pregnancies, prematurity, and LBW. Multiple embryos may be implanted to maximize the chance for success. More recent statistics in the United States demonstrate a higher rate of singletons and very few triplets (CDC, n.d.-b). The risk of prematurity increases with multiple gestation pregnancy. The American Society for Reproductive Medicine (ASRM) advises that providers limit the number of embryos transferred and educate clients regarding the risks inherent in higher-order multiple gestation (ASRM, 2021). However, the risk for prematurity and LBW exists for even singleton pregnancies conceived with ART, possibly due to other comorbidities (Jiang et al., 2023). Women who use ART due to infertility remain at risk for developing gestational hypertension, gestational diabetes, and delivering preterm (Ban et al., 2024; Moramezi et al., 2023). Clients conceiving using in vitro fertilization (IVF) had the additional increased risk of fetal malpresentation, placenta previa, placental abruption, and delivery by cesarean section.

## POSTTERM PREGNANCY

Postterm pregnancy is a pregnancy that continues past 42 weeks (294 days) or 14 days past the estimated due date (American College of Obstetricians and Gynecologists, 2023). The cause of postterm pregnancy is not known, but it occurs more often with male fetuses and may have a genetic basis. Some cases of postterm pregnancy can be attributed to inaccurate dates used to calculate the estimated date of confinement. Ultrasound dating of pregnancy is accurate if done during the first trimester; however, ultrasound dating of pregnancy has a margin of error.

Postterm infants are more likely to have macrosomia, with increased risks for prolonged labor or CPD with increased risk for cesarean section, or shoulder dystocia with increased risks of possible musculoskeletal injury (i.e., fractured clavicle or brachial plexus injury). These infants are more at risk for cord compression due to oligohydramnios and meconium-stained amniotic fluid (Shiferaw et al., 2024). Postterm pregnancy has also been related to increased incidence of chorioamnionitis and more frequent NICU admissions (Budal et al., 2024). There is a risk of cesarean section and associated complications with postterm pregnancy to both the mother and neonate (Place et al., 2024). Close surveillance of postterm pregnancies is needed due to increased risks of complications as gestational age advances. Postterm fetuses should be evaluated by non-stress testing or biophysical profiles. Cervical ripening and induction of labor at 41 weeks is an alternative approach for the management of postterm pregnancies when combined with appropriate fetal assessments (Place et al., 2024).

## UNFAVORABLE HEALTH BEHAVIORS

Personal habits such as smoking, illicit drug use, or alcohol use can compromise overall maternal health during pregnancy and can negatively influence fetal well-being. Prepregnancy maternal health status and poor health behaviors can play a role in PTL risk. Babies born to mothers who smoke, drink alcohol, or use drugs are at higher risk of LBW and PTB (Arabzadeh et al., 2024; Silveira et al., 2024). Inadequate nutrition, over-the-counter or prescribed drug consumption, and environmental factors may represent other HCBs and increase risks during pregnancy.

### Smoking

Smoking is a significant predictor of LBW, possibly due to impaired oxygen delivery (hypoxia) and nutrient delivery from the mother to the fetus (Meaton et al., 2023). The combination of PTB and LBW leaves the neonate at higher risk for NICU admission. The risk of adverse effects on fetal outcomes decreases with smoking cessation. Earlier smoking cessation during pregnancy reduces the risk of the adverse effects of LBW (Tatsuta et al., 2023). The recent popularity of nicotine delivery systems such as e-cigarettes results in delivering the same neurotoxic effects as tobacco smoking. Unfortunately, some pregnant women have the perception that using e-cigarettes is less harmful than regular cigarettes and can be used to help in smoking cessation. Quite the contrary, e-cigarette use has been demonstrated to increase the risk of both PTB and LBW (Ammar et al., 2023). Women who smoke are more likely to use alcohol or illicit drugs during pregnancy than those who do not smoke. The effect of smoking on pregnancy outcomes is also dose dependent, with increased risk for PTB and LBW when smoking and exposure to smoking occur throughout the pregnancy consistently (Selvaratnam et al., 2023). The smoking rate in the United States during pregnancy has been estimated to be 9.5% in 2022, with ethnic variations. More NHW women (5.4%) smoked during pregnancy as compared with NHB women (3.1%) and Hispanic women (1.0%) (Osterman et al., 2024).

## Substance Use or Abuse

Substance use and abuse is a concern for childbearing women of all ages. Marijuana smoking has been associated with an increased risk of fetal death and LBW adjusted for the effect of confounding factors (Habersham et al., 2024). Women using multiple substances, such as marijuana, smoking, and alcohol, are more likely to make choices that put themselves and the fetus at increased risk for LBW, PTB, and STIs (Silveira et al., 2024). Additional studies have identified marijuana, when used alone or combined with cigarette smoking, to be significant in increased risk of PTB and LBW (Crosland et al., 2024). The effect of marijuana on pregnancy outcomes will become more apparent as more states legalize medicinal and recreational use.

Maternal alcohol ingestion during pregnancy can result in fetal alcohol spectrum disorders (FASD). The incidence of FASD may be related to environmental exposure and genetic susceptibility. Alcohol is believed to have a direct teratogenic effect that limits fetal growth and brain growth. The fetal effects of drinking are most pronounced if the fetus is exposed during the first trimester of pregnancy. The minimum amount of alcohol that is harmful to the fetal brain is not known. Higher amounts of alcohol are absorbed by women with lower body fat and poor diets, which in turn increases the amount absorbed by the fetus (Grzywacz et al., 2023). It is known that binge drinking (ingestion of more than five drinks on one occasion) leads to higher levels of blood alcohol. Binge drinking is a particular concern during early pregnancy because it raises risks to the fetus at the same level as exposure throughout the pregnancy by the chronic drinker (Grzywacz et al., 2023). In addition to being SGA, the neonate exposed to alcohol prenatally may have a greater risk for respiratory distress syndrome, hyperbilirubinemia, and NICU admission (Popova et al., 2024). Neonates who have been exposed to alcohol at any time prenatally can develop symptoms of FASD. Healthcare providers need to accurately assess women prenatally for alcohol use to be more prepared for possible adverse outcomes. Research has identified the combined use of alcohol, smoking, and illicit drug use in multiple populations of pregnant women (Ragsdale et al., 2024).

Illicit drug use in pregnant women is inclusive of misuse or abuse of prescription drugs and use of illegal substances. Illegal drug use crosses all socioeconomic sectors, with the prevailing drug of choice initially being what is available and affordable. The use of crack cocaine has been more prevalent among more marginalized populations. Neonates of mothers who use crack cocaine are at higher risk for placental abnormalities affecting neonatal outcomes (Hirschel et al., 2024). Pregnant women using illicit drugs also tend to enter prenatal care later in their pregnancy. Research that focuses on smoking, alcohol, and illicit drug use often relies on self-reporting by subjects, which may not be consistent across all demographic groups and may lead to some inaccuracy in findings (Murnan et al., 2024). However, the result of polypharmacy habits of the mother can result in PTB, LBW, and possible neonatal abstinence syndrome or neonatal opioid withdrawal syndrome in the neonate (Crosland et al., 2024; Dumbhare & Taksande, 2023; Phyu et al., 2024; Silveira et al., 2024). Opioid use, both prescribed and illicit, has increased in the United States and resulted in multiple methods of treatment for mothers and infants. Neonatal outcomes related to exposure to opioids may differ based on the drug of choice, resulting in congenital heart defects, neural tube defects, or cleft palate (Wouldes & Lester, 2023). There are challenges to treating the mother for addiction during pregnancy without having detrimental effects on the neonate (Kanervo et al., 2024). Treatment options for the neonate presenting with neonatal abstinence syndrome also vary based on the severity of symptoms and provider preference (Phyu et al., 2024).

## Nutrition

Adequate nutrition prior to conception and during pregnancy is important for maternal and fetal health. The pregnant woman needs to consume enough calories and nutrients to meet her and the developing fetus's physiologic needs. Nutritional risks include inadequate or excessive weight gain; medical conditions that complicate pregnancy, such as hyperemesis gravidarum; dental conditions that compromise the ability to take in food; or insufficient resources to access food. Lack of adequate nutrients before or during early pregnancy can lead to birth defects. The importance for all women of childbearing age (between 15 and 45) to consume at least 400 mcg of folic acid daily to help prevent neural tube defects has been well established. Adequate folic acid intake, either through diet or supplements, has been demonstrated to decrease the risk of neural tube defects and perinatal mortality (Liu et al., 2024) and reduce the risk of developing Kawasaki disease (Fukuda et al., 2023b). However, due to food fortification with synthetic folic acid in developed countries, care must be taken to stay within the folic acid intake recommendations through diet and supplements. Conditions resulting from excess folic acid intake include increased risk of gestational diabetes in mothers and increased insulin resistance in children (Fardous & Heydari, 2023). The WHO continues to recommend supplemental iron and folic acid daily, beginning prenatally if possible (WHO, 2024a), to prevent maternal anemia and neural tube defects.

Anemia is a serious problem affecting about half of pregnant women worldwide. It is more prevalent in nonindustrialized nations due to poor nutrition, iron-deficient diets, the presence of parasitic diseases, and the incidence of HIV and AIDS. Women who are anemic are less likely to withstand blood loss during delivery and have increased risks of perinatal death, LBW, stillbirths, and prematurity. Promoting adequate nutrition before pregnancy is key to improving pregnancy outcomes. WHO (2024a) recommendations in nonindustrialized nations encourage the intervention of 30 to 60 mg of elemental iron and 0.4 mg of folic acid weekly to prevent anemia if daily dosing is not acceptable. Unfortunately, not all women take the recommended supplements, possibly due to lack of education.

Inadequate nutrition may be another risk factor for prematurity, LBW, or pregnancy loss, especially in teen pregnancy or for women at risk for not eating due to food scarcity or conditions such as anorexia nervosa or depression. Many women do not eat an adequate diet, even when not pregnant. During pregnancy, they may not consume adequate trace elements or antioxidant micronutrients (i.e., selenium, copper, zinc, manganese, and vitamins C and E). Although micronutrients are essential in the promotion of adequate placental development, prevention of FGR, and prevention of fetal mortality and morbidity, excess intake has also been associated with adverse pregnancy outcomes (Prabhu et al., 2024). However, without specific guidelines recommending dosing of micronutrients, providers may not provide clear advice (Buhling et al., 2023) or limit recommendations for supplementation with only folic acid, iron, vitamin D, and iodine, depending on the country (Saros et al., 2024). Women who do not consume enough nutrients to maintain their growth, as measured by gains in BMI or height, are more at risk of having LBW infants compared to adequate-weight mothers. Both high and low maternal BMI, and associated high and low weight gain during pregnancy, have been associated with poor pregnancy outcomes for both mother and neonate (Yin et al., 2023). Obesity rates have been steadily increasing in industrialized nations with the result of increased risk of preeclampsia (Das et al., 2024), macrosomia and preterm birth (Yin et al., 2023), and infertility (Wang et al., 2024). In response to the risks of poor pregnancy outcomes while obese, many women of childbearing age have chosen bariatric surgery for weight reduction before conception. While this procedure has decreased the risk of complications associated with obesity, there is an increased possibility of complications related to poor nutritional intake due to the malabsorption of micronutrients needed to support healthy pregnancy and normal fetal growth (Huluţă et al., 2024).

Conditions in many countries contribute to chronic undernutrition throughout the lifespan, resulting in poor pregnancy outcomes. Girls are more at risk for nutritional deprivation in some countries due to girl gender bias. Chronic undernutrition can delay menarche in young girls. In some cultures, predominantly rural, underdeveloped populations, early adolescent marriage and pregnancy are permissible. A secondary analysis of data obtained by the Nepal Demographic and Health Surveys demonstrated that adolescents of disadvantaged or differing ethnic groups were more at risk for anemia (Rai et al., 2023). A review of adolescent pregnancies in Turkey revealed findings of maternal anemia and FGR to be more prevalent among adolescents than pregnant adults (İşgüder et al., 2024). Food insecurity can not only increase the risk for an LBW infant but can also increase the risk of birth defects. Interventions that can help improve the nutritional status of pregnant women in food-insecure locations are also aimed at increasing infant birth weight, which can markedly decrease infant mortality. Interventions, including providing fresh food, cooking and storage instructions, and case management, have decreased maternal depression, LBW, and PTB (Ferris et al., 2024).

Even in high- to moderate-income nations, some pregnant women living on low incomes do not get adequate nutrition. In the United States, nutritional support during pregnancy, along with nutritional education and participation in programs such as the Supplemental Nutrition Assistance Program (SNAP) for women, infants, and children, have been demonstrated to increase the mean birth weight and reduce the odds for LBW for infants of low-income women on Medicaid. Food banks are increasing in middle- and higher-income countries as food insecurity increases in rural and urban areas and families face the challenges of meeting multiple monetary and social needs (Mossenson et al., 2024). Unfortunately, the use of the SNAP program and food banks as a nutrition resource has not improved the nutritional intake of pregnant women as expected due to the availability of primarily processed foods with low nutritional value. Highly processed foods are associated with increased intake of sugars, fats, and sodium, increasing risks of gestational diabetes and gestational hypertension (Granich-Armenta et al., 2024). Fresh fruits and vegetables, considered more nutritious, are limited in food deserts of urban areas, contributing to the continued risk of PTB and maternal gestational hypertension (Haley et al., 2024).

Maternal foodborne illness or ingestion of toxic substances during pregnancy can be harmful to the fetus. *Listeria monocytogenes,* though rare, is a special concern in pregnancy because 1 in 25,000 pregnant women are infected with this, and 1 in 4 will spontaneously abort or lose their infant soon after birth (CDC, 2024). Women who ingest food contaminated with *Listeria* do not usually feel ill; however, the fetus can be significantly affected. Eating food contaminated by microorganisms such as *Listeria* or substances such as heavy metals can cause abortion, stillbirth, preterm delivery, neonatal infections, fetal brain or kidney problems, or even maternal death. While *Listeria* and other food contaminants are found in many foods, teaching pregnant women simple basic precautions such as handwashing when preparing food, avoiding cross-contamination of meat dishes or other prepared foods, and avoiding nonpasteurized milk may help prevent infection (CDC, 2024a).

Pica is a dietary practice seen in almost every culture. Substances such as starch, ice, clay, or dirt are ingested as a craving to increase iron or calcium intake possibly. The harmfulness of pica in pregnancy is dependent on the substance and amount ingested by the pregnant woman. Women who practice pica tend to have lower hemoglobin (Hb) and hematocrit (Hct) levels and micronutrient deficiencies (Ashraf et al., 2024). One concern if the mother eats dirt or paint chips is that they could be contaminated with lead or heavy metals, which could be harmful and cause anemia or lead poisoning. Contamination of soil and water increases the risk of elevated lead and other heavy metal levels in women, which can then result in increases in spontaneous abortion, fetal deaths, or PTB (Hoover et al., 2023; Zhang et al., 2023).

The influence of cultural dietary practices and basic food preparation knowledge as potential risk factors must be addressed and assessed. Healthcare practitioners must become familiar with the food and complementary medicine cultural practices of local ethnic groups, because they may affect pregnancy outcomes. Exposure to possible food contaminants can have adverse consequences on pregnancy. Education needs to be provided so women know the potential sources of food contamination and possible recalls of food products during pregnancy and when preparing infant formula or food.

## Over-the-Counter and Complementary Drugs

Drugs taken during pregnancy can have harmful effects on the fetus, whether they are controlled substances or over-the-counter medications. Despite warnings that pregnant women should not take any medications without consulting with their healthcare provider, many pregnant women take over the counter or nonprescribed medications during pregnancy, including complementary therapies they might not consider to be harmful. According to the CDC (2024b), 9 in 10 women take some medication during pregnancy. Of those women, 70% report taking prescription medications. Findings of a study by Thunbo et al. (2024) on the prevalence of prescription medication use by primiparous pregnant women reported that 63.3% of women used at least one medication between 1998 and 2018. Using more than one medication during pregnancy was reported by 35.2% of the same cohort. Prescribed antidepressants and asthma medications are among the most prescribed used during pregnancy. Many women regularly take over-the-counter drugs such as cold remedies, aspirin, nonsteroidal anti-inflammatory drugs (NSAIDs), or herbal teas. Some women might take medications that could be harmful to the fetus before they know that they are pregnant. Even vitamins and dietary supplements taken in excessive dosages can be harmful to the fetus. Pregnant women with preexisting medical problems such as asthma, arthritis, heart problems, diabetes, or epilepsy who must continue to take their prescribed medications during pregnancy should check with their healthcare provider to determine if the prescribed medication will need to be changed to one that is less harmful to the fetus. Communication between patient and provider is essential because some women stop taking their prescribed medications when they discover they are pregnant.

Healthcare providers must be cognizant of Food and Drug Administration (FDA) pregnancy categories and drugs that must be used cautiously or contraindicated in pregnancy. Thalidomide was withdrawn from the market in the 1960s after it was linked to fetal limb-shortening birth defects when it was used during pregnancy. Currently, thalidomide is used to treat certain types of beta thalassemia (Yang et al., 2024b) and relapses of multiple myeloma (Nadeem et al., 2024). Both conditions can occur in women of childbearing age. There are stringent educational requirements, warnings about the risks of pregnancy, and mandatory contraception for both men and women who use thalidomide. It is possible that pregnancy could occur despite these measures.

## Environmental Influences

Every individual is conceived with a unique genetic makeup called a *genotype*. The *phenotype*, or the person's ultimate physiologic and psychological makeup, is determined during the postconception period until after birth. The expression of the genetic inheritance (i.e., the actual physiologic and psychological makeup of the person) results from complex gene–gene interactions and environmental influences upon genes that occur at the molecular level. Exposure by the mother to environmental toxicants either before or during pregnancy can precipitate gene-environment interactions that can alter these molecular interactions, especially if the exposure to harmful substances occurs at critical periods of fetal development. Two critical periods when gene–gene-environment interactions can be most harmful are during organogenesis (when fetal organs are being formed) and during the fetal period, when there is rapid growth of all systems. Spina bifida is an example of a gene-environment interaction. A fertilized egg might inherit the genes to have an intact neural tube at conception. Neural tube defects occur when there is a lack of adequate folic acid at a critical stage of development while in utero. Exposure to teratogens, substances that are known to cause birth defects, during these times can result in birth defects or other adverse outcomes. Two pregnant women could be exposed to the same toxicants at the same point during pregnancy and could have infants with different outcomes. For example, two infants could inherit the genetic trait of sickle cell disease (SCD). Yet, when born, they could have different expressions of the disease based upon other complex molecular interactions within genes, which the environment could influence. It is recognized that factors outside the cell DNA influence functional and developmental outcomes throughout the person's life (Lossi et al., 2024). The study of epigenetics is an evolving science that looks at factors such as genetic inheritance, imprinting, or nutritional factors that are hypothesized to mediate genetic interactions at the molecular level and that may one day provide more insight into these complex processes.

Environmental hazards are found in air, water, and food. Environmental changes have increased health risks related to increases in air pollution, water contamination, and the effect of extreme weather events (Conway et al., 2024). Maternal exposure to air pollutants during pregnancy has been associated with decreased fetal birth weight (Bartha et al., 2023). Exposure to increased particulate matter in outdoor or indoor air, has been associated with increases in PTB, LBW, and incidence of gestational diabetes (GDM) (You et al., 2024). Poor or socially disadvantaged women, especially women of color, are more often exposed to environmental hazards because they tend to live in older sections of towns or work in areas with high exposure. Older homes may increase the risk of lead paint exposure. Impoverished parts of cities and villages are often located close to working or abandoned factories where pregnant women are exposed to incinerator emissions or other air, soil, and water pollution sources. Maternal exposure to air pollution during pregnancy has also been associated with adverse effects on in-utero lung development, resulting in reduced lung function in young children (Usemann et al., 2024). Fine particulate air pollution, such as that produced by passive exposure to cigarette smoke, organic pollutants, and motor vehicles, can have detrimental effects on pregnancy outcome and early childhood health concerns related to lung development and fetal size (Bartha et al., 2023; Usemann et al., 2024; You et al., 2024). Sun et al. (2024) have also identified an increased risk for preeclampsia among mothers in urban settings due to intensified perinatal exposure to air pollution resulting from increased motor vehicle traffic.

Suburban and rural populations are more likely to be exposed to agricultural pesticides or chemicals because they are more likely to garden and do yard work. Another population at risk for pesticide and chemical exposure is those who work on farms or as migrant workers. Both maternal and paternal exposure to environmental toxins can be contributors to fetal risk and result in alterations in neurodevelopment and IQ (Wang et al., 2023). The disadvantaged might be more likely to be exposed to multiple pollutants, which, as an aggregate, would affect an SGA neonate even if born at term (Eick et al., 2024). Birth outcomes can also be affected by natural or manmade disasters such as hurricanes, severe ice storms, earthquakes, chemical spills, or terrorism. The occurrence of a disaster alters the availability of safe food and water or adequate prenatal care, which may increase risks for PTB. Increased maternal stress could cause mothers to use substances such as alcohol or tobacco for stress management. There have been some studies linking certain disasters with outcomes such as increased rates of spontaneous abortion, congenital anomalies, decreased fetal growth, and changes in maternal mental health status. However, disasters do not seem to cause PTB.

### Emerging Risk Factors

Sleep problems during pregnancy have been linked to an increased risk for GDM during pregnancy (Eleftheriou et al., 2023). This risk may be related to increased BMI and insulin resistance in women with some sleep disturbances. An increase in fasting blood sugars between 34 and 36 weeks' gestation was also found in a study by Akbari et al. (2024). Obstructive sleep apnea (OSA) during pregnancy has been associated with numerous maternal complications, such as gestational hypertension, gestational diabetes, and preeclampsia (Maniaci et al., 2024). There is also an increased prevalence of OSA during pregnancy, possibly due to the physiologic changes that support weight gain, resulting in the narrowing of the airways. Fetal complications such as FGR and preterm labor have not been identified as complications of sleep disturbances consistently through numerous studies.

## MATERNAL MEDICAL AND OBSTETRIC CONDITIONS

Diabetes, hypertension, and bleeding disorders are some of the most common maternal complications of pregnancy. These complications can lead to preterm delivery and perinatal death or can influence fetal morbidity. The WHO (2024b) has identified severe bleeding after childbirth, infections after childbirth, and hypertension as three of the major causes of maternal mortality worldwide. Recommendations for antenatal care include assessment for anemia, asymptomatic bacteriuria, and intimate partner violence (WHO, 2016).

### Diabetes

Women with known pregestational diabetes should seek preconception care. The conceptual visit should include a complete physical examination with an evaluation of blood glucose levels, cardiovascular and renal health, gastrointestinal system, an eye examination to check for diabetic retinopathy, and an assessment of neuropathy. A team approach with a diabetes nurse educator and dietitian can teach the woman how to implement the dietary and lifestyle changes needed for a healthy pregnancy. Oral hypoglycemic medication may be continued in pregnancy by monitoring maternal glucose levels. Metformin can be used safely in the preconception period and during pregnancy for women with type 2 (Paschou et al., 2024). Metformin may be used in combination with insulin during pregnancy if necessary or when the woman cannot obtain insulin (Wu et al., 2023). Ideally, the woman with diabetes should maintain euglycemia for several months before pregnancy, because hyperglycemia in early pregnancy has been associated with an increased risk for pregnancy loss, especially in women developing diabetic ketoacidosis (DKA) (Coetzee et al., 2023). Regulation of blood glucose is sometimes tricky during pregnancy because pregnancy creates a state of insulin resistance, and insulin needs change with each trimester. Glycosylated hemoglobin (HbA1c) levels should be maintained as close to the normal range as possible during pregnancy, especially during fetal organogenesis.

The worldwide prevalence of GDM is difficult to establish because there are no international guidelines. Individual countries and organizations have established their own criteria and testing schedules, sometimes based on the availability of testing resources and maternal access to care. Comparative studies have been undertaken utilizing the International Association of Diabetes and Pregnancy Study Group (IADPSG) and WHO (2013) criteria and the Diabetes in Pregnancy Study Group of India (DIPSI) criteria to better assess and intervene with diverse populations (Bakshi et al., 2023). In the United States, there are ethnic variations in the prevalence of GDM, with Asian Indian, non-Hispanic Native American, non-Hispanic Native Hawaiian or Pacific Islander, and Hispanic women having higher rates than NHB and NHW women (CDC, 2022). Identification and treatment of women with gestational diabetes is the key to promoting positive neonatal outcomes. The most essential principle of diabetes management for all pregnant women is to maintain tight glycemic control. Prolonged and frequent exposure to hyperglycemia increases the risks for birth defects (i.e., cardiovascular, musculoskeletal, and central nervous system [CNS] anomalies), hypoglycemia, respiratory complications, shoulder dystocia, and NICU admission (Karkia et al., 2023). Maternal complications can include an increased risk of gestational hypertension, preeclampsia, and rectal sphincter injury (Karkia et al., 2023).

Currently, pregnant women in the United States are screened for gestational diabetes following current Association of Obstetricians and Gynecologists (ACOG) recommendations. Screening begins with reviewing patient history, clinical risk factors, and administering a 50 g 1-hour oral glucose tolerance test (OGTT) at 24 and 28 weeks' gestation (ObG Project, n.d.). Physicians may decide to screen earlier for those with a history of previous GDM, previous neonate weighing more than 4,000 g, or having a first-degree relative with diabetes mellitus or a woman they suspect will not return for regular care. The American Diabetes Association (ADA) recommends a 75 g OGTT at 24 to 28 weeks with blood glucose measurement when fasting and 1 and 2 hours after blood glucose administration. The diagnosis of gestational diabetes is based on the results of two abnormal values with the blood glucose screening for the ACOG and ADA criteria (El Sayed et al., 2023; ObG Project, n.d.). Current WHO (2013) recommendations follow the IADPSG guidelines.

Diabetes during pregnancy is frequently accompanied by maternal vascular changes that can compromise uteroplacental circulation; therefore, fetal non-stress testing is recommended in the last trimester. If early delivery is indicated, amniocentesis can be done to determine fetal lung maturity; however, results of the lecithin sphingomyelin (L/S) ratio are often inaccurate for infants of mothers with diabetes. Infants of diabetic mothers generally have macrosomia. These large babies have increased risks for birth injuries due to shoulder dystocia, including fractured clavicles or nerve palsies. Large infants are more likely to be delivered by cesarean section. Infants of diabetic mothers should be closely monitored for hypoglycemia in the immediate postbirth period and until feeding is well established.

## Hypertension in Pregnancy

Approximately 13% of pregnancies in the United States between 2017 and 2019 were complicated by hypertensive disorders (Ford et al., 2022). The four identified categories of hypertension in pregnancy are: chronic hypertension, gestational hypertension, preeclampsia and eclampsia, and gestational hypertension superimposed on chronic hypertension (Ford et al., 2022). Chronic hypertension exists when there is a history of hypertension before the pregnancy, or it can also be diagnosed during pregnancy for the first time. Some women with preexisting hypertension develop superimposed preeclampsia during their pregnancy (Sweeney et al., 2024). Women with chronic hypertension who develop superimposed preeclampsia are at increased risk for fetal complications (Sweeney et al., 2024). Gestational hypertension is diagnosed during pregnancy and usually disappears within 12 weeks after delivery. Preeclampsia is a pregnancy-specific disease that generally occurs after 20 weeks of pregnancy. It is characterized by hypertension, thrombocytopenia, and signs of renal impairment (Khosla et al., 2024). As the condition progressively worsens, maternal laboratory work indicates elevations in liver enzymes and low platelets. HELLP syndrome occurs in about 20% of pregnancies complicated by preeclampsia. Hemolysis, elevated liver enzymes, and low platelets characterize this syndrome. Approximately half of women with HELLP syndrome are preterm.

Hypertension in pregnancy causes vasoconstriction with subsequent poor maternal circulatory and placental perfusion. Decreased uteroplacental circulation compromises the fetus; therefore, it is more likely to be growth restricted, SGA, or at increased risk for stillbirth (Anh et al., 2024). Women with gestational hypertension are also at increased risk for abruptio placenta. Delivery is the definitive treatment and is generally recommended even before 34 weeks' gestation in the event of severe preeclampsia (Walia et al., 2023). Early delivery will be based on the stability of the mother and the outcomes of fetal testing. A serious risk for the mother with preeclampsia is the possibility of eclamptic seizures due to cerebral edema and central nervous system excitability or progression to HELLP syndrome. Seizures increase the risk of a placental abruption. Therefore, if the mother's condition worsens, early delivery will be elected; however, the ability of the fetus to survive must be considered. Corticosteroid administration is advised and may be beneficial if the fetus is between 24 and 34 weeks of gestational age and if the mother has never had them (Dong et al., 2024). Women with severe gestational hypertension (defined as blood pressure > 160/110 mm Hg) without proteinuria can quickly develop severe complications of preeclampsia, such as thrombocytopenia and pulmonary edema, affecting neonatal outcomes (Odunvbun et al., 2023). The earlier hypertensive disease occurs in pregnancy, the more likely complications will develop, reinforcing the need for early and consistent prenatal care (Anh et al., 2024; Barda et al., 2023).

If preeclampsia worsens, the pregnant woman is admitted to the hospital for stabilization and delivery. If the woman has a seizure, oxygen should be provided during and immediately following the seizure, and the fetus should be monitored for signs of distress. Magnesium sulfate is the drug of choice to prevent central nervous system excitability from cerebral edema. Infants rarely have harmful effects from in-utero exposure to magnesium sulfate prior to delivery but should be monitored for signs of respiratory depression or hypotonia after birth.

Ethnic differences in the progression of hypertensive disorders in pregnancy have been noted. NHB women were hospitalized earlier in the pregnancy for treatment of gestational hypertension. Their babies had lower gestational age and birth weight. NHB women also had a higher incidence of maternal and neonatal deaths than other ethnic groups despite starting prenatal care in the first trimester (Ford et al., 2022).

## Prelabor Rupture of Membranes

PROM is a cause of preterm delivery and can occur at any time during a pregnancy. Following the rupture of membranes, the fetus is at increased risk for problems related to oligohydramnios, cord compression, chorioamnionitis, and abruptio placenta. Women with PROM may report that they are leaking fluid from the vagina or may have experienced a gush of fluid. Sterile speculum examination, nitrazine testing, and microscopic examination of fluid for ferning are methods to evaluate if membranes have ruptured. The decision of whether to deliver or to use expectant management must weigh the advantage of postponing delivery until gestational age increases against the risk for maternal or fetal sepsis. Current guidelines recommend expectant management when premature prelabor rupture of membranes (PPROM) occurs at less than 34 weeks' gestation if no maternal or fetal contraindications are present. When PPROM occurs between 24 and 34 weeks' gestation, a single course of corticosteroids is recommended. PPROM prior to 32 weeks, which exhibits signs of possible delivery, should be treated with magnesium sulfate for the neuroprotective effect on the neonate. A course of antibiotics may also be considered to prevent infection. Signs of intrauterine infection include fever greater than 100.4°F (38.0°C), uterine tenderness, and maternal or fetal tachycardia. The white blood cell count test results should be used judiciously as an indicator of infection, especially if steroids have been given within the previous 5 to 7 days. Management of PPROM at 34 to 37 weeks' 6 days' gestation would not include tocolysis. Management would remain the same if there is no indication of infection (Garg & Jaiswal, 2023).

Fetal outcomes after PPROM are related to gestational age at the time of membrane rupture and whether the infant is delivered without complications of infection or asphyxia from cord compression or prolapse. Neonates born at 22 weeks' gestation after PPROM have lower survival rates. As gestational age increases from 23 to 32 weeks' gestation, outcomes after PPROM improve. Survival of preterm infants who are delivered after spontaneous PPROM is dependent on factors such as weeks of gestation at delivery, if they experience other complications, and if delivery is spontaneous or induced (Kim et al., 2023). Sometimes, in the absence of other indications, a wait-and-see approach might be taken where delivery is not expedited. If PROM occurs at earlier gestational ages, the risk for chorioamnionitis increases. At delivery, infants of women with chorioamnionitis tend to be of younger gestational age and weigh less than infants of women who do not have chorioamnionitis.

## Maternal Infections

Infections are a major risk factor for maternal and fetal health during pregnancy. Women may be infected before pregnancy or acquire the infection during pregnancy. Maternal infections can be transmitted to the infant while in utero across the placenta, as an ascending infection of vaginal origin, during the birth process, or even during the postpartum period. Fetal infections can cause congenital anomalies, LBW, respiratory illness after birth, or even death. Infectious agents include protozoal, helminthic, STIs, viruses, and bacterial organisms.

Infectious diseases, such as STIs, HIV/AIDS, tuberculosis (TB), and malaria are preventable causes of perinatal morbidity and mortality. Adverse pregnancy outcomes can include spontaneous abortion, PTB, and PROM. Coinfections with these diseases during pregnancy can increase maternal risk of morbidity and mortality. For example, syphilis with overlapping infections of HIV and hepatitis B can result in liver damage to the mother and vertical transmission to the fetus (Gedefie et al., 2024). In northeast Ethiopia, methods of transmission of overlapping infections include receiving piercings and tattoos as well as unsafe sex practices (Gedefie et al., 2024). HIV infection and weakening of the immune system increases susceptibility to active tuberculosis infection among those with latent TB infection (Navasardyan et al., 2024). The combination of antiretroviral medications to treat HIV and anti-TB medications to treat TB can result in multidrug interactions. HIV and anti-TB treatment continue during pregnancy. Maternal antibodies to both maternal infections pass through the placenta to the fetus. During follow-up antibody testing, Hjelmar et al. (2024) found that infants demonstrated decreasing HIV-IgG antibodies over time, but TB-specific IgG antibodies increased. The cause of increased TB IgG antibodies could not be identified explicitly due to infants receiving the Bacille Calmette-Guerin (BCG) vaccine at birth or postnatal exposure to environmental cases of TB.

Malaria is another infection found in pregnant women in Africa, South America, and Asian-Pacific countries. Currently, numerous vaccines are developing to combat this infection (Stanisic & Good, 2023). Several strategies have been used to lessen or eradicate malaria infections in the general population and pregnant women. Prevention measures include education and insecticide-treated mosquito netting (Onyinyechi et al., 2024). Intermittent dosing with sulfadoxine-pyrimethamine (IPTp-SP) has been used for prevention. Still, the medication is contraindicated in women who are HIV positive, and use is becoming limited due to parasitic resistance (Eisenberg & Krieger, 2023). An alternative medication is being considered, but it is more costly than the current IPTp-SP.

Vaccine-preventable infections kill more women and babies in low-income nations because basic immunization practices, such as tetanus or rubella vaccination, may be unavailable to them. Tetanus, a disease that can be easily prevented, still accounts for neonatal deaths in developing nations. Tetanus develops in newborns due to unclean cord-handling practices, including instrumentation and the use of traditional cord salves that can cause infection. Once infected, the infant loses the ability to suck within a few days of exposure and progresses through stiffness, seizures, and death (WHO, 2018). Rubella in pregnancy can result in miscarriages, stillbirths, or severe defects in the surviving fetus. Symptoms of rubella may include hearing impairment, congenital cataracts, microcephaly, and congenital heart defects.

During 2015 and 2016, the Zika virus (ZIKV), a mosquito-borne illness that can enter the placenta and pass to the fetus, was identified. The movement of the virus transplacentally resulted in congenital malformations (Elliott & Mattapallil, 2024). Microcephaly and ocular damage were identified as neonatal outcomes. Follow-up studies of infants born affected by maternal ZIKV have identified infants born with microcephaly to have a higher incidence of damage to structures of the brain, resulting in epilepsy, motor impairments, and hearing abnormalities, among other deficits (Martelli et al., 2024). Unfortunately, many mothers who are infected are asymptomatic or mistake the flu-like symptoms for minor ailments. The virus can also be transmitted through intercourse (Bhandari et al., 2023). Prevention measures advised include topical insect repellent sprays and controlling mosquito populations. There are vaccines in development, and research is being conducted to alter the genetic code and structure of the flaviviruses (Martelli et al., 2024). Prevention of sexually transmitted ZIKV may be more challenging because the carrier would have to be identified and willing to use barrier methods of birth control.

The United Nations SDG 3 focuses on combating HIV/AIDS, malaria, TB, and other infectious diseases and on the prevention and treatment before and during pregnancy of communicable and noncommunicable diseases known to increase the risk of PTB (UN, 2015). Every pregnant woman must be screened for risk factors for infection. Early identification and treatment of women with infections will improve maternal and neonatal outcomes.

## Abruptio Placenta

Abruptio placenta, or premature separation of the placenta prior to delivery, is a leading cause of stillbirth and neonatal mortality. Placental separation is thought to be due to changes in placental vasculature, thrombosis, and reduced placental perfusion. A genetic basis for abruptio placenta has been speculated to cause these changes. Placental separation occurs in several ways. In marginal separation, the edges of the placenta separate, and bright red bleeding is present. Occult or hidden abruptio placenta occurs when the edges of the placenta are intact, but the central part of the placenta detaches from the uterus, allowing blood loss to accumulate behind the placenta without any outward signs of bleeding. Complete abruptio placenta occurs when the placenta completely detaches, a situation that is incompatible with fetal survival. There is a four to six times higher risk of premature delivery when there is a diagnosis of abruptio placenta. Premature delivery increases the risk of infant mortality. **Quality & Safety: Infants of mothers with abruptio placenta who survive must be closely monitored for signs of blood loss and shock.**

Risk factors for abruptio placenta include smoking, multiple pregnancy, and maternal age greater than 50. Increased risk in older women could be related to increased rates of chronic hypertensive disorders or aging of the uterine blood vessels. The risk of abruptio placenta increases with multiple pregnancies as the number of fetuses increases from singleton to triplet pregnancies. The risk of perinatal complications such as preterm delivery, intraventricular hemorrhage, and death increases in the presence of abruptio placenta (Farghaly et al., 2024; Zhang et al., 2024).

## POSTPARTUM RISK FACTORS

After birth, the leading causes of infant death are congenital anomalies, complications of prematurity and LBW, sudden infant death syndrome (SIDS), now called sudden unexpected infant death (SUID), and perinatal complications (Kochanek et al., 2024). Congenital anomalies account for most neonatal deaths in the first month of life. Infants who are LBW are more likely to die from complications of prematurity (i.e., respiratory distress, infections, or anemia), maternal complications in pregnancy, or placenta/cord conditions. In addition to these leading causes of death, other risk factors such as maternal smoking or drug usage could affect the health of the neonate or cause injury. Providing information and anticipatory guidance to the parents to increase awareness of these factors might be enough to protect the infant and promote positive outcomes.

### Drugs Excreted in Maternal Milk

Maternal medications taken while lactating are a concern because medications may alter the milk supply or cross to the infant through the milk supply. While many medications have been demonstrated to be safe, others have not been reported in the literature. Psychotropic drugs pose a particular concern because there has been an increase in their use. These drugs and their metabolites have long half-lives and are detectable in infant tissues and the developing brain. The long-term consequences of this exposure have not been thoroughly studied. As new drugs are placed on the market, their safety for the infant must be evaluated. Some untoward effects on the infant from the use of prescribed maternal drugs include possible immune suppression, neutropenia, skin rash, central nervous system changes including irritability, restlessness, sleepiness, lethargy, or convulsions, and gastrointestinal effects such as feeding problems, vomiting, diarrhea, slow weight gain, blood in stool, jaundice, or dark urine. A comprehensive list of drugs, foods, and environmental agents that are excreted in human milk and that could be potentially harmful to neonates is available from the American Academy of Pediatrics (AAP).

The AAP recommendations include using the LactMed Bookshelf provided by the National Library of Medicine (LactMed@NIH) (NIH, n.d.-a) as a resource for current toxicology and information on medications. The Bookshelf resource can be accessed for free and downloadable to any device. Professionals, as well as the public, can use the resource. Medication information is updated frequently. When drugs are prescribed for lactating women, the following factors should be considered. When a medication is necessary, the neonate's neonatologist or pediatrician and the mother's physician should consult together to select the most appropriate drug for the mother, with minimal effects upon lactation and minimal transfer to the neonate. Consider measuring the neonate's blood concentration with the drug to see if there are potential risks from the drug for the neonate. Advise the nursing mother to take the medication immediately after breastfeeding the neonate or pumping to minimize infant drug exposure.

### Sudden Unexpected Infant Death Syndrome

Sudden unexpected infant death syndrome (SUIDS) or sudden unexpected infant death (SUID) is a leading cause of death in infants in the postneonatal period in the United States as well as in other developed countries. SUIDS is broken down into SIDS, unexplained deaths, and accidental strangulation/suffocation in bed. Programs such as the AAP Back to Sleep campaign urged parents to place their infants on their backs instead of prone to sleep, which dramatically lowered infant deaths from SIDS. In the United States, the SIDS death rate declined between 1990 and 2022. However, a slight increase has been noted between 2018 and 2022 (CDC, n.d.-c). Despite these advances, disparities in SIDS rates exist. Infants born to Black, American Indian, or Alaskan Native mothers have the highest rates of death from SIDS at twice the rate of infants of White mothers. Infants of Hispanic and Asian or Pacific Islander mothers have the lowest rates (CDC, 2024c). Maternal risk factors include young single mothers with a history of prenatal smoking or substance abuse. One of the causes of the recent increase in infant deaths has been attributed to maternal drug use (Kitsantas et al., 2024). Prenatal education regarding preterm birth and the resulting sequelae of health issues and practicing safe sleep habits have been recognized as factors that would slow the increase in infant mortality (Ramos et al., 2023).

Over 70 causes of SIDS have been proposed. SIDS has been blamed on environmental factors such as soft bedding, overheating, entanglement in blankets, immunizations, tobacco smoke exposure, or bed sharing with parents or siblings, especially if a bed partner consumes alcohol (Pease et al., 2023). Genetic factors have also been blamed for the findings. Possible structural defects in the brain that control cardiac and respiratory function might explain the diminished arousal response in infants with SIDS that precedes death. Genetic mutations resulting in cardiomyopathies and cardiac arrhythmias changes have been identified in ~11% to 13% of SIDS victims (Puckelwartz et al., 2024). Genome sequencing has also identified ~5% of reviewed SIDS cases to have an epilepsy gene variant (Puckelwartz et al., 2024). In reality, the cause of SIDS is probably multifactorial. The triple risk theory proposes that multiple complex factors (including genetics, prenatal risk factors, and environmental risk factors) make some babies more vulnerable to environmental triggering events and unable to respond to these events through usual homeostatic mechanisms (Renz-Polster et al., 2024). Preterm or LBW infants are at increased risk for SIDS (Habich et al., 2024). Term infants with a history of apnea are also at risk. The peak age at death from SIDS is between 1 and 4 months, with most deaths occurring before 6 months of age (NIH, n.d.). No definitive link between SIDS and immunizations has been established.

Sleeping in the prone position has been highly associated with SIDS and is one reason the Back to Sleep campaign was successful in reducing SIDS death rates. The rate of SIDS increases for preterm infants who are placed in a prone position. Many parents of premature infants place their infant to sleep on his or her stomach or side once at home. Neonatal care practices place preterm infants in prone or side-lying positions at times. When parents see their baby in a prone or side-lying position while in the hospital, education should be provided explaining the reason. Infants may become habituated to the prone position for sleeping, especially if they have had a prolonged hospitalization. Nurses need to educate parents and encourage them to share information with their childcare providers about placing the baby on the back to sleep (Ramos et al., 2023). Neonatal nurses must continue to educate each parent about the risk factors for SIDS and remind parents that the safest place for a baby is in its crib in the parent's room for the first 6 months.

## Child Abuse

Child abuse in infants is sometimes challenging to identify. Parents of an injured infant arrive for emergency treatment and seem severely distraught about their child's injuries. They often offer reasonable explanations for the injury that must be ruled out with medical tests. The victims, the babies, cannot speak for themselves to describe what happened. New parents are subject to many stressors that could trigger child abuse, such as lack of sleep, financial strain, and dealing with inconsolable infants (Loiseau et al., 2023). Healthcare providers have a legal and ethical duty to report cases of suspected child abuse to child protective services but may be very conflicted about the interactions with those agencies (Johnsen et al., 2024). Two forms of child abuse are discussed further: abusive head trauma (AHT), a subset of shaken baby syndrome (SBS); and medical child abuse (MCA), previously Munchausen syndrome by proxy (MSBP).

## Abusive Head Trauma/Shaken Baby Syndrome

AHT describes a serious form of head trauma caused by several mechanisms, including abusive shaking of an infant causing a whiplash-type injury, blunt trauma, or a combination of both (Hartman & Greene, 2024). It is a public health issue and the leading cause of death due to child abuse. When the infant is shaken, the head flops back and forth, causing rapid acceleration, deceleration, and/or rotational forces of the brain within the skull, causing stretching, shearing, and tearing of blood vessels of the brain. Several types of injuries occur with AHT/SBS. Intracranial injuries cause direct brain injury and damage to the axons. Shearing forces exerted on the veins that bridge from the dura to the brain cause intracranial bleeding. During shaking, there is a lack of oxygen in the brain, further compounded by chemical processes within the damaged cells. These injuries lead to swelling of the brain and increased intracranial pressure (ICP) that further compromises brain oxygenation. Even one year after injury, children with AHT may have retinal hemorrhages, seizures, and signs of other injuries. External signs of injury to the face or head may be present, and injuries or bruising of the long bones, thorax, or abdomen may occur because of firmly grasping the infant during the shaking episode (Hartman & Greene, 2024).

AHT/SBS most often results when a parent becomes frustrated with an infant who is crying and inconsolable. Parents who are stressed with the parenting role, parents of premature infants, those who are sleep deprived, or parents who do not have support or help to care for their baby's needs may have low tolerance for infant crying. Obtaining a careful obstetric history may lead to the discovery of a difficult or premature delivery. Poverty and stress are risk factors for abuse. In frustration, they may pick up the baby and shake it to quiet it. Newborns are more susceptible to the forces of shaking and may sustain injury even if not shaken as roughly as an older child. Once parents shake their infant and get a response, they might shake the infant again over time, causing the infant to be injured repeatedly. Because the intracranial bleeding can be slow initially, the infant might not manifest symptoms until 48 to 72 hours after the injury. Children who appear to have mild injury may not be brought to the hospital by their parents immediately and be misdiagnosed by healthcare providers (Hartman & Greene, 2024).

When parents seek medical attention for the infant, the history of events that preceded the infant's symptoms is often vague. Signs of AHT/SBS vary based on the extent of the injury and are sometimes subtle, such as feeding difficulties, vomiting, lethargy, hypothermia, failure to thrive, and increased somnolence. These vague symptoms may make diagnosis difficult. More life-threatening signs include seizures, bulging fontanelle, apnea, coma, bradycardia, or complete cardiovascular collapse. Outcomes are poor for children who present with coma. Survivors of coma may have severe neuromotor impairment, visual impairment, and developmental delay. They may require shunting for hydrocephalus. Long-term occupational therapy, physical therapy, and speech therapy will be needed to help the children achieve their maximum potential. Seizures, apnea, and cardiac arrest can occur suddenly in an infant brought to the hospital with vague symptoms. These infants are at higher risk of mortality even without having seizures (Chou et al., 2024). A small percentage of children will have no outward ill effects from the shaking. The remaining children have long-term sequelae, including ongoing neurologic injuries and visual impairment.

New parents need to be taught not to shake their infant at any time. Prior to discharge, time should be spent exploring parents' concerns about taking a newborn home, their sources of support, and their coping strategies under stress. Nurses should assess the parents' knowledge about normal infant crying patterns and teach them how to handle stress or frustration due to prolonged periods of infant crying (Bater et al., 2024). Referral for stress management techniques, anger management, and provision of a parenting hotline number might help prevent this devastating injury. Parent education of normal infant development may be effective in reducing the occurrence of AHT/SBS in high-risk neonatal populations.

### Medical Child Abuse

MCA, formerly known as MSBP, is a rare form of child abuse where a parent, usually a mother, fabricates illness in a dependent child to draw attention to themselves as the parent of a sick child. Four criteria are required for a diagnosis: (a) a parent or guardian fabricates illness in the child, (b) the child is presented for medical care, (c) the perpetrator denies knowledge of the cause of the child's illness, and (d) the signs and symptoms subside if the child is separated from the perpetrator (Goulbourne & Huber, 2024). The diagnosis of MCA includes two diagnoses: one for the child and one for the parent. The parent's response might range from fabricating the illness of a child, exaggerating symptoms of the sick child, to inducing the symptoms in the child, such as by attempts to suffocate or poison the child. Some of the most common types of fabrications include gastrointestinal (diarrhea), neurologic (seizures), infections (fevers), dermatologic (strange rashes), and cardiopulmonary (acute life-threatening events). Some children will die because of the parent's abuse or ministrations. Unwittingly, physicians or healthcare workers can be drawn into the situation attempting to help the child based upon the parent's description of what is occurring. Healthcare professionals might prescribe unnecessary diagnostic tests or treatments for the child (Goulbourne & Huber, 2024). Healthcare professionals need increased awareness of MCA and should question cases where children are seen constantly for parent-reported conditions not witnessed by anyone else or if siblings of the child have had similar hospitalizations or have died from SIDS or under suspicious circumstances. Cases where infants who are not gaining weight begin to gain during hospitalization are also suspect. If the parent is approached and refuses to get psychological help, or if the child has been subjected to a major illness because of the parent, then the child may need to be placed in a protective environment. MCA has long-term psychological implications for the child, including PTSD, behavioral problems, and depression (Goulbourne & Huber, 2024).

## PERINATAL CARE IN DEVELOPING NATIONS

Pregnant women in developing nations have many of the same risk factors for prematurity and LBW as women in the United States. Poor prepregnancy physical condition, inadequate spacing between pregnancies, inadequate nutrition, decreased weight gain during pregnancy, maternal anemia, and lack of access for perinatal care are global issues. Availability of safe clean water is becoming a global problem. Poverty and lack of education about pregnancy health are sometimes compounded by lack of skilled care providers, lack of transportation to healthcare centers, issues of war, civil unrest, and low status of women (Tamiso et al., 2023; WHO, 2023).

Decreasing worldwide maternal and neonatal mortality rates is a priority of the United Nations SDGs. Maternal mortality rates have declined 34% between 2000 and 2020 in response to global efforts toward achieving the Millennial Development Goals (currently Sustainable Development Goals). Partnership programs have developed in many countries to improve access to birth control and prenatal care. Management of chronic diseases such as HIV and malaria, efforts to ensure a skilled attendant at delivery, and evidence-based practices are beginning to make a positive difference (UNICEF, 2024). However, the number of maternal deaths is still too high; approximately 287,000 mothers died worldwide due to complications of pregnancy and childbirth in 2020. Almost 99% of these deaths occurred in developing countries, with the highest rates in Africa and South Asia (UNICEF, 2024).

Globally, the neonatal mortality rate declined more slowly and fell from 37 per 1,000 births in 1990 to 17 per 1,000 births in 2022 (UNICEF, 2024a). Neonatal mortality fell by 53% between 1990 and 2022 but still accounts for more than 47% of deaths in children younger than age 5 worldwide, representing an increase. The worldwide average is 17 neonatal deaths per 1,000 live births, ranging from < 5 neonatal deaths per 1,000 live births for high-income countries to > 35 neonatal deaths per 1,000 live births in low-income countries. Stillbirth rates globally average 13.9 stillbirths per 1,000 live births in 2021, with a range from 1.6 per 1,000 live births in high-income countries to 31.2 per 1,000 in low-income countries in 2021 (UNICEF, 2024a). Improved prenatal care, having a skilled attendant at delivery, enhanced use of hygienic practices for clamping and care of the umbilical cord, and concerted efforts to provide basic resuscitation equipment and training in neonatal resuscitation have had good results in some countries; however, much work still needs to be done (WHO, 2023).

Many neonates worldwide have died from preventable conditions. Some congenital anomalies could have been prevented with maternal folic acid supplementation. Many newborns die from birth asphyxia, which might have been prevented with timely neonatal resuscitation at delivery. Some deaths from prematurity might have been prevented with adequate prenatal care or a system of basic neonatal care for premature infants. Some deaths from infections could have been prevented with the use of hygienic practices at birth, patient teaching about cord care, immunizations, maternal screening for infectious disease risks, or treatment for HIV during pregnancy. Keys to making changes include creating funding partnerships, improving infrastructure and professional education, and implementing culturally appropriate evidence-based care.

The WHO and United Nations Children's Fund (UNICEF) provided a report in 2022 regarding the efforts to improve birth outcomes and decrease neonatal loss in developing nations and globally. These efforts were conceived and attempted as part of the SGD 2030 Agenda in 2015 by the

WHO, UNICEF, the United States Agency for International Development (USAID), and organizations of UN member nations. Perinatal programs can be tailored to meet the specific needs of each country and are meant to improve perinatal care, lower mortality of mothers and infants, and improve perinatal outcomes. As stated in the report, many challenges have held back the accomplishment of meeting the stated goals because of climate change, wars, and a global pandemic. In this report, António Guterres, Secretary General of the United Nations (2022 Progress Report on the EWEC Global Strategy), said:

> *Sadly, this report shows that regarding the health and rights of women and children, that promise is not being kept. Far from a progress report, this document describes a reversal. Women's and children's health and rights are threatened to a degree not seen in more than a generation. (Forward, p.vi)*

Recommendations are made within the report to work globally toward Every Woman Every Child SGD goals.

Antenatal care is implemented on a local level not only to screen for possible problems but also to educate women about how to promote a healthy pregnancy. Optimal timing and spacing of pregnancy are important parts of prenatal care to encourage mothers who are in the best physical condition prior to conception. Prevention and control of infection are also important during the prenatal period. Proper medical treatment of women who are infected with STIs or HIV/AIDS during pregnancy will increase the infant's chances of healthy survival.

Antenatal screening alone cannot predict or prevent most problems during pregnancy or delivery; therefore, all pregnant women should be considered high risk and must have access to skilled birth attendants and timely emergency obstetric care. Nations with the highest rates of neonatal and maternal mortality are those that have the lowest number of births attended by a skilled birth attendant. In some countries, access to medical care is difficult due to living in remote village locations, lacking basic transportation, or with poor infrastructure, making transporting women or infants with problems to specialized centers difficult. Sometimes, developing nations' policies interfere with providing safe obstetric care. The current WHO (2020) recommendations for antenatal care stress the differences in expected care with diverse populations.

Basic training and equipment for infant resuscitation at birth will help prevent some of the poor birth outcomes related to birth asphyxia. Many facilities in developing nations are working with antiquated equipment as they attempt to provide care for neonates. Textbooks are often outdated or are not written in the healthcare provider's native language. The AAP Neonatal Resuscitation Program (NRP) is an effective method to provide immediate resuscitative care to neonates. This program has been translated into at least 24 languages and taught in over 130 countries through formally organized courses through the AAP or by independent efforts of NRP instructors (AAP, 2025). The Helping Babies Survive program is a suite of evidence-based infant resuscitation programs designed for settings where human or technological resources are limited. It is not intended to replace NRP but serves as an adjunct for training birth attendants to assess and stimulate breathing during the initial Golden Minute of life. Neonatal mortality is lower when the mother has received professional care during the antenatal period and during childbirth.

Postpartum care includes parent teaching about infant care and family planning services to help prevent short intervals between pregnancies, which can increase the risk of poor perinatal outcomes (Hassen et al., 2024; Sevoyan et al., 2024). Strategies for successful breastfeeding, proper cord care, recognition of signs of illness, and promotion of psychosocial well-being are all skills parents need to have to promote optimal newborn health. Women of childbearing age need to learn the importance of being in optimal physical condition before and during pregnancy. Family planning services will help women become empowered to make choices about when to have children and will help prevent unnecessary abortions.

## SUMMARY

This chapter has presented some prenatal, intrapartum, and postpartum risk factors that influence neonatal health, especially prematurity and LBW. The perinatal nurse must be aware of potential risk factors when screening pregnant women and providing counseling and support. The presence of risk factors can raise suspicion that a baby might have problems after delivery; however, many more babies will be born healthy even in the presence of multiple risk factors. Anticipation of neonates at risk helps ensure that adequate personnel and equipment are available at birth to manage problems should they occur. Patient education about modifiable risk factors and support for altering detrimental healthcare behaviors can help prevent some adverse neonatal outcomes.

Some inroads have been made to improve maternal and child health internationally. Many nations still have many barriers, including creating the infrastructure needed to support the WHO United Nations goals outlined in the SDG (UN, 2015). Recommendations and training of adequate healthcare professionals to provide care will take multiple nations' commitment and monetary resources. Some countries are beginning to see success in reducing maternal and infant mortality. A sustained worldwide effort is needed to continue to improve these outcomes.

## CASE STUDY

**Identification of the Problem.** A 29-year-old woman arrives at the clinic reporting she had a positive home pregnancy test. The last menstrual period (LMP) was 4 months ago, March 10. The provider assesses potential antepartum risk factors during the first prenatal visit.

**Assessment: History and Physical Examination.**

- Menstrual History. Menarche at age 12. Regular periods every 30 days with a duration of 4 to 5 days, LMP 3/10.
- *Obstetric History.* G4T3P0A0L3, all vaginal deliveries. First pregnancy term, 12 years ago. The female infant weighed 3,570 g at birth and is in good health today. Second a vaginal delivery 6 years later, term male born

at 40w 4d gestation weighing 3,830 g. He is now 5 years old and in good health. Third vaginal delivery, term male infant at 40w 2d gestation and weighed 3,800 g. The child is now 3 years old and reported to be in good health. The current expected date of confinement (EDC) is December 17.

- *Past Gynecologic History.* Uses no contraception currently. Has a past history of multiple sexual partners, currently in a monogamous relationship. STI and HIV status is negative. The blood type is O+.
- *Past Medical History.* History of acute idiopathic pancreatitis at 15. Avoids any symptoms or "flare-ups" during her previous pregnancies by watching her diet. She reports mild hypertension in the last trimester of the previous pregnancy that was managed by decreasing her work hours.
- *Drug/Substance Abuse History.* Denies taking any prescription, over-the-counter, homeopathic, or street drugs. Has not taken prenatal vitamins. She smokes 10 to 12 cigarettes a day. Alcohol: consumes two to three beers a week. She denies alcohol use since she found out she was pregnant.
- *Family/Social History.* Lives with a husband, the baby's father. Denies familial history of genetic problems. Employed part-time as waitstaff in a casual dining restaurant. Reports husband yells at her a lot and gets angry easily. Reports they are getting along great now.

## Assessment: Physical Examination.

- *Neurologic.* Alert & oriented (A&O) × 4; pupils equal, round, and reactive to light and accommodation (PERRLA); deep tendon reflexes (DTRs) 2+ bilaterally without clonus
- *Head and Neck.* Neck supple, thyroid examination unremarkable; denies headache, blurred vision, flashing lights in eyes, or scotoma
- *Cardiovascular.* Heart rate regular without murmur; denies palpitations, chest pain
- *Respiratory.* Lungs clear to auscultation; denies history of asthma, TB, or bronchitis; reports chronic smoker's cough; denies thick sputum
- *Abdomen/Gastrointestinal.* Gravid abdomen, distended, fundal height 20 cm, uterine fundus at umbilicus; bowel sounds present, active; denies problems with constipation or diarrhea; reports appetite is fair, occasional nausea and vomiting
- *Genitourinary.* Denies vaginal spotting or cramping; reports urinary frequency during the day; denies burning with urination
- *Extremities.* No edema noted in pretibial area. DTRs 2+
- *Other.* Reports backache when standing for prolonged periods at work; reports breast tenderness; no colostrum noted

## Diagnostic Tests

- *Blood type:* O+
- Hb: 10.9; Hct: 34%
- *HIV test:* Negative
- *Vaginal Cultures:* Negative
- *50 g 1-hour GTT Results:* 150 mg/dl
- *100 g 3-hour GTT Results:*
  - Fasting: 130 mg/dl
  - 1 hour: 190 mg/dl
  - 2 hours: 155 mg/dl
  - 3 hours: 138 mg/dl

## Working Diagnosis

- Increased risk for prematurity due to a history of smoking
- Increased risk for gestational diabetes due to previous pregnancy and medical history
- Increased risk for PIH due to previous history
- Increased risk for injury due to anemia
- Increased risk for injury related to potential physical abuse from significant other
- Increased risk to fetus for FAS due to report of maternal drinking
- Increased risk for SGA infant due to maternal smoking
- Increased risk for LGA infant due to previous history

## Development of Management Plan

1. Counsel regarding alcohol use in pregnancy, consider outpatient treatment.
2. Provide contact information for emergency women's shelter.
3. Teach danger signs during pregnancy and symptoms of PTL and when to notify the practitioner.
4. Encourage smoking cessation and provide resources.
5. HIV testing, screening/treatment for STIs
6. Obtain glucose challenge test (GCT) at 24 and 28 weeks, follow blood glucose closely.
7. Dietary counseling for iron, diabetic diet, limiting fats
8. Promote breastfeeding.
9. Serial ultrasounds to monitor infant growth

**Implementation.** The patient and nurse discussed needed lifestyle modifications during pregnancy and developed a plan to support the patient's counsel and refer them to a support group for smoking cessation. The patient agreed to attend a smoking cessation group for pregnant women. The patient decided to refrain from alcohol usage during pregnancy. HIV testing completed. Completed GCT at 28 weeks and patient was referred for nutritional counseling for GDM and sources of iron in the diet. Daily iron supplementation was provided. Fetal growth was monitored with serial ultrasounds. The patient was instructed on how to monitor daily fetal kick counts at 34 weeks.

**Evaluation of Effectiveness.** The patient attended a smoking cessation group and reported that she cut down her smoking while pregnant to two to three cigarettes a day. She also noted she refrained from the use of alcohol during the remainder of the pregnancy and avoided second-hand smoke outside at the workplace. GTT was positive for GDM, but she could maintain control of blood glucose with diet and exercise. She also developed mild hypertension and 3+ proteinuria during the last weeks of pregnancy, which was managed with bed rest in the last 2 weeks of pregnancy.

**Outcome.** The patient had labor induced at 38 weeks' gestation and delivered a 3,860 g girl. Her Apgar scores at 1 and 5 minutes were 8 and 9. Infant had no hypoglycemia after birth. No signs of FAS noted on admission physical examination. The mother decided to use an intrauterine device (IUD) for birth control following this delivery. Mother was discharged breastfeeding the infant and scheduled for follow-up postpartum visit and IUD insertion in 6 weeks.

## PARENT VOICES

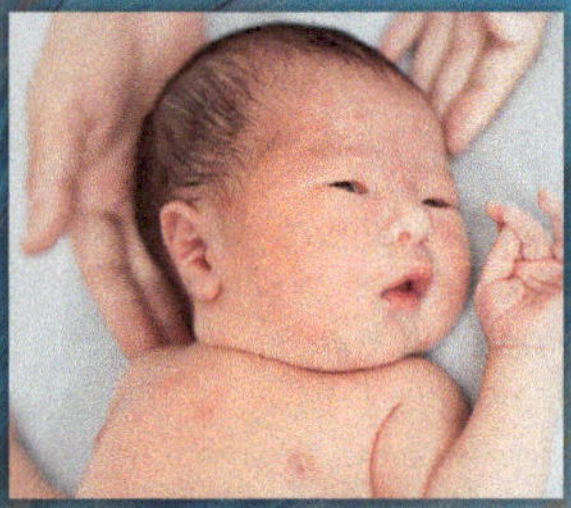

Source: Jirasaki/Adobe Stock.

### Ali Dunn

**After 3.5 years of infertility and multiple rounds of IVF, finding out I was pregnant was a surprise. Finding out I was expecting twins was shocking, even though I was well aware that the incidence of multiples increases with fertility treatments. Having a high-risk pregnancy due to twins can create additional stress and anxiety. Additional monitoring, appointments with specialists, and careful assessment of the risks involved can take a very natural experience and make it quite medical. Personally, my twin pregnancy started and ended with extreme medical interventions. While it was necessary and lifesaving, it also left me feeling disappointed that my pregnancy experience and birth plans were left unrealized.**

### Keira Sorrells

**Because we did fertility treatments and I was being monitored closely, we knew at our 6-week ultrasound that we were expecting multiples. We were told very quickly that triplets had (at the time) an 85% chance of a successful outcome, meaning little or no NICU time. Our goal was 32 to 34 weeks with the understanding being that they may need a little bit of oxygen, a little help learning how to suck, and a little time to grow. There was very little information shared on the possibility of our babies being born far earlier than 32 weeks. When I was admitted with preeclampsia at 25 weeks, I was totally unprepared, terrified, and sure none of my daughters would survive delivery. I had never seen the inside of the NICU, nor had I ever laid eyes on a baby that weighed just 1 lb 4 oz and still had her eyes fused shut. The shock of seeing my three girls as three fetuses outside the womb is something I will not soon forget.**

## ONLINE RESOURCES

**CourseConnect**

Resources for this chapter are online and available at www.springerpub.com/courseconnect.

## REFERENCES

References for this chapter are online and available at www.springerpub.com/courseconnect.

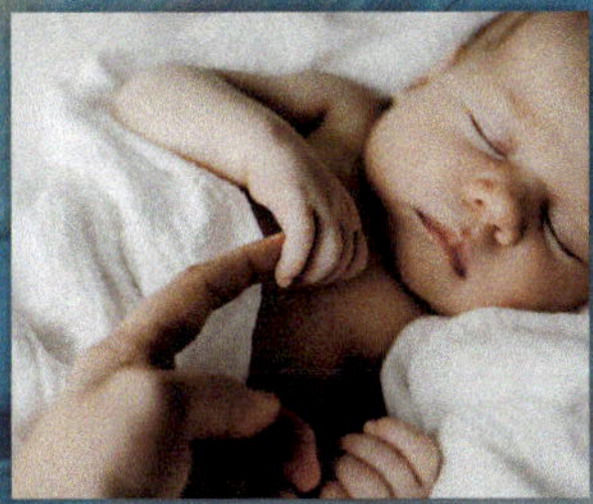
Source: Bostan Natalia/Adobe Stock.



CHAPTER 3

# Resuscitation and Stabilization of the Newborn and Infant

Gail A. Bagwell and Jordan A. Sullivan

## INTRODUCTION

The vulnerable and sick infant requires the healthcare professional to quickly assess and take action when signs of cardiac or respiratory depression are present. This chapter begins with a discussion of risk factors that predispose the newborn to cardiorespiratory depression followed by a description of the actions to be taken to avoid this depression or to alleviate the symptoms and reverse a downward spiral. The chapter then concludes with a short discussion on the stabilization of the ill neonate.

## CAUSES OF CARDIORESPIRATORY DEPRESSION IN THE NEWBORN

The combined effects of numerous maternal, fetal, and intrauterine factors determine the condition of an infant at birth (some of these factors are listed in Table 3.1). Although some of these factors emerge only during labor and delivery (e.g., cord prolapse), most arise during gestation (e.g., placenta previa) or even before conception (e.g., maternal diabetes). Regardless of the site or time of origin, the influence of each of these problems can manifest as cardiorespiratory depression in the newborn.

To provide effective care, the nurse must be able not only to recognize potential risk factors but also to understand the ways in which they disrupt cardiorespiratory function. Ideally, the healthcare professional determines that cardiorespiratory depression may occur and is thoroughly prepared to intervene. Although many risk factors come into play, the underlying pathogenic processes can be divided into six major categories. The mnemonic TAMMSS can be used as a simple but effective means of remembering these etiologic groups:

*T* Trauma
*A* Asphyxia (intrauterine)
*M* Medication
*M* Malformation
*S* Sepsis
*S* Shock (hypovolemia)

### Trauma

Traumatic injury to the central or peripheral nervous system of the newborn is an uncommon occurrence that can result in immediate or delayed respiratory depression. Because the skull is incompletely mineralized and has open sutures, it can undergo considerable distortion without fracture. The underlying membranes and vessels are, however, much less resilient and are easily stretched or torn (subgaleal hemorrhage) if overly compressed, particularly if the pressure is abruptly applied. Similarly, forced traction or torsion of the neck during delivery may damage the spinal cord or the phrenic nerve, with consequent paralysis of the diaphragm or brachial plexus nerve group. An unusually long and difficult delivery, multiple gestation, abnormal presentation (especially breech), cephalopelvic disproportion (secondary to macrosomia or a small or contracted pelvis), shoulder dystocia, or rapid extraction by forceps or vacuum extraction (as may be required for fetal distress) are frequently involved. Despite their generally low birth weight, premature infants also may be at risk because of the unusual compliance of their skulls.

### Asphyxia (Intrauterine)

The most common cause of cardiorespiratory depression at birth is fetal hypoxia and asphyxia. Any condition that reduces oxygen delivery to the fetus may be the cause. Such conditions include maternal hypoxia (from hypoventilation and hyperventilation, respiratory or heart disease, anemia, postural hypotension), maternal vascular disease that results in placental insufficiency (from preexisting or pregnancy-induced diabetes, primary or pregnancy-induced hypertension), and accidents involving the umbilical cord (compression, entanglement, or prolapse). Pos-term pregnancies also are at risk, perhaps because of placental aging and progressive placental insufficiency. An asphyxia episode occasionally may trigger the passage and aspiration of meconium in utero for term and postterm infants.

**TABLE 3.1**

**CONDITIONS ASSOCIATED WITH ASPHYXIATION OF NEWBORNS**

| Source of Problem | Conditions |
|---|---|
| Maternal | Amnionitis; anemia; gestational or insulin-dependent diabetes; gestational hypertension; preeclampsia or eclampsia; chronic maternal hypertension; maternal cardiac, pulmonary, renal, thyroid, neurologic, or genetic disease; maternal deformities; hypotension; infection; polyhydramnios; oligohydramnios; drug therapy such as magnesium sulfate; adrenergic agonists; maternal substance abuse; no prenatal care; mother older than 35 years of age; previous fetal or neonatal death. |
| Uterine | Preterm labor, prolonged labor, PROM, multiple gestation, breech or other abnormal fetal presentation, precipitous delivery, uterine tachysystole with fetal heart rate changes. |
| Placental | Placenta previa, abruption placentae, any second- or third-trimester bleeding, other significant intrapartum bleeding, placental insufficiency, postterm gestation. |
| Umbilical | Cord prolapse, entanglement, compression, or rupture. |
| Fetal | Category 2 or 3 fetal heart rate patterns, cephalopelvic disproportion, size date discrepancy, macrosomia, prematurity, intrauterine growth retardation, congenital abnormalities, fetal anemia or isoimmunization, erythroblastosis fetalis, intrauterine infection, decreased fetal activity, narcotics administered to the mother within 4 hours of delivery, meconium-stained fluid. |
| Iatrogenic | Mechanical (difficult forceps or vacuum delivery), emergency cesarean section, drugs–general anesthesia. |

## Medication

Pharmacologic agents given to the mother during labor and delivery may affect the fetus both directly and indirectly. Indirectly, these agents may cause maternal hypoventilation and hypotension or adversely affect placental perfusion. Hypnotic, analgesic, or anesthetic drugs may depress maternal respirations, resulting in reduced oxygen intake and delivery to the tissues and organs, including the uterus and placenta. Anesthetic agents, because of their effect on the sympathetic nervous system, may also cause peripheral vasodilation, diminished cardiac output, and hypotension with decreased placental perfusion. Narcotic analgesics, which rapidly cross the placenta, may directly depress the neonatal respiratory drive. Oxytocin (Pitocin), may cause uterine hyperstimulation and shorten placental perfusion time. Each of these conditions places the fetus at greater risk of fetal hypoxia and asphyxia. Prescription and nonprescription medications, herbs, and essential oils that the mother may take prior to delivery may also affect the fetus. Many street drugs, especially opiate derivatives, are known to cause infants to deliver prematurely, be small for gestational age (SGA), have congenital anomalies, and have respiratory depression on delivery.

## Malformation

Infants may have one of many congenital anomalies, but the ones that cause the most problems during the first few minutes of life are those associated with facial or upper airway deformities and conditions that lead to pulmonary hypoplasia. Many of these conditions can be diagnosed through antenatal ultrasonographic examinations and other screening techniques, but suspicion also should be raised if oligohydramnios or polyhydramnios is reported.

Oligohydramnios is seen with prolonged rupture or leakage of membranes and neonates with renal agenesis or dysplasia or urethral obstruction. If fluid is lost or diminished, the developing fetal structures may be compressed, leading to characteristic Potter facies (including micrognathia) or pulmonary hypoplasia. Polyhydramnios is seen in infants with impaired swallowing ability (as in anencephaly, neuromuscular disorders), in those with real or functional obstruction high in the gastrointestinal tract (as with esophageal atresia), and in those with profuse leakage of cerebrospinal fluid (as in neural tube defects), which contributes to the volume of amniotic fluid. Polyhydramnios is also noted with diaphragmatic hernia and hydrops fetalis.

## Sepsis

The fetus may acquire bacterial or viral agents from infected amniotic fluid, from maternal blood crossing the placenta, or from direct contact on passage through the birth canal. An infant is especially susceptible to infection if born prematurely (because these infants are relatively immunocompromised) or if born to a mother who had a premature rupture of membranes (PROM) or a history of infection or chorioamnionitis. If infection is acquired in utero, the lungs tend to be heavily involved, and the alveoli may be filled with exudate. The infant may be apneic at birth, may be slow to establish a spontaneous and regular breathing pattern, or may show frank signs of respiratory distress.

### Shock (Hypovolemia)

Most of the blood lost during delivery is from the maternal side of the placenta; therefore, it is of no consequence to the newborn. Blood loss from the fetal side of the placenta as a result of abruptio placenta or placenta previa can, however, lead to acute hypovolemia and cardiovascular collapse. Normally the umbilical cord is unusually strong, but ruptures are possible if cord tension increases suddenly, as in a precipitous delivery, or if the vessels are superficially implanted in the placenta (velamentous insertions). In rare cases, acute hypovolemia may occur without frank hemorrhage. With severe cord compression, for example, blood flow to the fetus is impeded. The umbilical arteries, however, are much more resistant to compression and continue to pump blood back to the placenta. In this case, the effects of hypovolemia and asphyxia may be superimposed. Infants with chronic blood loss (as in fetal–maternal hemorrhage or twin-to-twin transfusions) are generally asymptomatic immediately after delivery.

## PREPARATION FOR DELIVERY

While the majority of deliveries will result in a healthy neonate where delayed cord clamping can occur and then the infant can go immediately to the mother's chest for skin-to-skin care, healthcare professionals must always be prepared for a problem to arise. The general consensus is that approximately 10% of all births will require some assistance to begin breathing at birth, 5% will require positive pressure ventilation (PPV), 2% will require intubation, and only 1 to 3 babies per 1,000 births will require compressions and emergency medications (Weiner & Zaichkin, 2021).

**Quality and Safety: The success of resuscitative efforts depends on multiple factors: (a) anticipation of the need, (b) the presence of trained personnel, (c) ready availability of necessary equipment and supplies, and (d) strong communication and teamwork.** The most competent personnel and the finest equipment are useless if they are not present in the delivery room. Frantic calls for assistance or a scavenger hunt for equipment should never occur; they needlessly delay intervention and can compromise the patient's outcome.

The antepartum and intrapartum history of each pregnant woman must be carefully reviewed to identify those at risk of delivering a depressed infant. Especially worrisome is a fetus that clinically demonstrates the effects of asphyxia (i.e., an indeterminate/abnormal fetal heart rate pattern, particularly bradycardia and persistently minimal or loss of fetal heart rate variability; acidosis, as determined by fetal scalp blood sampling; or meconium-stained amniotic fluid).

### Personnel

Although most risk factors can be identified at some time during the pregnancy, many may not become apparent until birth. Delivery through meconium-stained amniotic fluid and unexpected diaphragmatic hernia are just two cases in point. At least one person competent in neonatal resuscitation should be present at every delivery. Each institution that delivers babies needs to have a plan in place on how to mobilize a full neonatal resuscitation team in an emergency such as the delivery of a depressed newborn (Aziz et al., 2020; Weiner & Zaichkin, 2021).

When a team is required, the role each member is to play in the resuscitative effort should be predetermined, including the head of the team. The head of the team, who has a complete set of resuscitation skills, will be the one to position the baby, open the airway and intubate the trachea if necessary, and evaluate and direct the resuscitation efforts. A second person will assist with positioning, suctioning, and drying, as well as giving oxygen and PPV. A third person is responsible for monitoring the heart rate (HR) and for initiating chest compressions, if needed. If intravenous (IV) medications are required, two additional individuals are needed, one to catheterize the umbilical vein and administer the drugs and the other to pass equipment and prepare the medications. The person who passes the equipment and prepares the medications may also be responsible for documenting the resuscitation process, but a sixth person is preferable to do this because minute-to-minute notations must be made. The individual delivering the baby is not considered part of this resuscitative team, because his or her main concern is the mother.

**Quality and Safety: All team members should be trained in neonatal resuscitation via an evidence-based program such as the American Academy of Pediatrics (AAP) Neonatal Resuscitation Program (NRP) for high-resource areas or inpatient facilities or Helping Babies Breathe (HBB) for low-resource areas or rural community settings.** Both the programs emphasize the importance of strong communication skills of team members for the team to be effective and provide the highest level of care possible.

### Equipment and Supplies

A newly born infant is predisposed to heat loss (particularly evaporative and radiant losses), and, if unprotected, can quickly become cold stressed. The consequences of such stress include hypoxemia, metabolic acidosis, and rapid depletion of glycogen stores with hypoglycemia. All are conditions that may exacerbate asphyxia and thus complicate resuscitation. Clearly, measures to prevent hypothermia must be part of any resuscitative effort. The delivery room should be kept warm, and the radiant bed should be preheated, if possible. Prewarming of linens, towels, and caps or other head coverings is also helpful.

A new systemic review of randomized and nonrandomized clinical trials was done looking at hypothermia in late preterm (> 34 weeks) and term infants. The review found that a delivery room temperature of 73.4°F (23°C) versus the traditional 68°F (20°C) resulted in newborns being able to maintain a normal temperature. For those infants at low risk for resuscitation, skin-to-skin care needs to be done and for those needing resuscitation in this age group the use of a polyethylene bag/wrap will help to maintain an normal temperature (Berg et al., 2023; Wyckoff et al., 2022).

For a premature baby of less than 32 weeks' gestation, the use of a polyethylene bag or wrap up to the baby's neck, without drying, in addition to a warm cap will reduce convective and evaporative heat loss. The use of the polyethylene bag or wrap will also help maintain the infant's body temperature in the delivery room as well as decrease hypernatremia at 24 to 48 hours of life due to transepidermal water loss. In addition, it has been found that a delivery room of at least 78.8°F (26°C) assists with maintaining a premature infant's (< 32 weeks' gestation) body temperature in combination with the use of a polyethylene bag or wrap. Because of this finding, all delivery room temperatures should be at least 78.8°F (26°C) when delivering a baby less than 32 weeks' gestation. Other interventions for preventing heat loss in infants less than 32 weeks' gestation are the use of a prewarmed hat and a thermal mattress (Aziz et al., 2020; Berg et al., 2023; Perlman et al., 2015; Weiner & Zaichkin, 2021; Wyckoff et al., 2022).

Possible exposure to blood and body fluids is of particular concern in the delivery room. Gloves, gowns, masks, and protective eyewear should be worn in the delivery room because procedures are likely to generate droplets or splashes of blood or other body fluids.

The additional equipment and supplies needed to carry out a full resuscitation (Box 3.1) should be checked as part of the daily routine. Small supplies should be organized according to frequency of use and may be displayed on a wall board, kept in the radiant warmer (if there is sufficient drawer space), or stored in a cart or specially designed tackle box. Breakaway security clips may be used to safeguard materials when they are not in use, but foolproof or locking closures that require a key or a code are not appropriate in delivery rooms, birthing rooms, or nurseries. A bedside table or flat surface (other than the bed) should be within reach to provide space for catheter trays and medication preparation.

As the delivery nears, the team should be assembled with the identified team leader. A preresuscitation briefing should occur, and all equipment and supplies should be double checked to ensure they are in working order. Having an organized routine of checking the equipment will ensure that all equipment is present and in working order. Hospital infection control policies dictate how far in advance packaged supplies can be opened, connected to tubing, and otherwise prepared. A backup or duplicate set of materials should be maintained in case of equipment failure, contamination, or multiple births. All items used should be restocked as soon as possible after the resuscitation.

## Good Communication and Teamwork

Communication and teamwork are behavior skills that are essential to a successful neonatal resuscitation. The best clinicians working together in resuscitation will not work effectively together if they do not possess the skills to communicate and coordinate with each other. Learning to communicate and assign tasks is as essential to a neonatal resuscitation as the ability to perform bag/mask ventilation or cardiac compressions. Key behavioral skills that

### BOX 3.1

### NEONATAL RESUSCITATION SUPPLIES AND EQUIPMENT

**Suction Equipment**

Bulb syringe

Mechanical suction and tubing

Suction catheters, 5F or 6F, 8F, 10F, 12F or 14F

8F feeding tube and 20-mL syringe

Meconium aspirator

**Bag-and-mask Equipment**

Device for delivering positive-pressure ventilation, capable of delivering 90% to 100% oxygen

Face masks, newborn and premature sizes (cushioned-rim masks preferred)

Oxygen source

Compressed air source

Oxygen blender to mix oxygen and compressed air with flowmeter (flow rate up to 10 L/min) and tubing

Pulse oximeter and oximeter probe

**Intubation Equipment**

Laryngoscope with straight blades, No. 0 (preterm) and No. 1 (term)

Extra bulbs and batteries for laryngoscope

Endotracheal tubes, 2.5-, 3.0-, 3.5-, 4.0-mm internal diameter (ID)

Stylet (optional)

Scissors

Tape or securing device for endotracheal tube

Alcohol sponges

$CO_2$ detector or capnograph

Laryngeal mask airway

**Medications**

Epinephrine 1:10,000 (0.1 mg/mL)—3-mL or 10-mL ampules

Isotonic crystalloid (normal saline or Ringer's lactate) for volume expansion—100 or 250 mL

Dextrose 10%, 250 mL

Normal saline for flushes

**Umbilical Vessel Catheterization Supplies**

Sterile gloves

Scalpel or scissors

Antiseptic prep solution

*(continued)*

**BOX 3.1**

### NEONATAL RESUSCITATION SUPPLIES AND EQUIPMENT (*continued*)

Umbilical tape

Umbilical catheters, 3.5F, 5F

Three-way stopcock

Syringes, 1, 3, 5, 10, 20, 50 mL

Needles, 25, 21, 18 gauge, or puncture device for needleless system

**Miscellaneous**

Gloves and appropriate personal protection

Radiant warmer or other heat source

Firm, padded resuscitation surface

Clock with second hand (timer optional)

Warmed linens

Stethoscope (with neonatal head)

Tape, 1/2 or 3/4 inch

Cardiac monitor and electrodes or pulse oximeter and probe (optional for delivery room)

Oropharyngeal airways (0, 00, and 000 sizes or 30-, 40-, and 50-mm lengths)

**For Very Preterm Babies**

Size 00 laryngoscope blade (optional)

Reclosable, food-grade plastic bag (1-gallon size) or plastic wrap

Chemically activated warming pad (optional)

Transport incubator to maintain baby's temperature during move to the nursery

*Source:* Adapted from Weiner, G. M., & Zaichkin J. G. (Eds.). (2021). *Textbook of neonatal resuscitation* (8th ed.). American Academy of Pediatrics, and American Heart Association.

are needed during a resuscitation are knowing your environment, using all available information, anticipating and planning, clearly identifying the team leader, communicating effectively, delegating the workload optimally, allocating time wisely, using resources wisely, calling for additional help when needed, and maintaining professional behavior (Weiner & Zaichkin, 2021).

For the majority of healthcare professionals, these behavioral skills do not come naturally in an emergency situation, so practicing these skills along with technical skills, such as bag/mask ventilation, on a regular basis is important. While the AAP only requires a healthcare provider to take the NRP course every 2 years, studies have shown that skills, knowledge, and self-confidence declined within 3 to 13 months after completing the training (Arlington et al., 2017; Bang et al., 2016; Soar, et al., 2010) Studies have shown that when training occurred at least every 6 months or more frequently in a simulation lab or at the bedside, there was improvement in skills, knowledge, and self-confidence (Matterson et al., 2018; Mosley & Shaw, 2013; Reisman et al., 2016; Surcouf et al., 2013). Simulation-based training on a regular basis should be done at all facilities to help healthcare providers maintain their cognitive, technical, and behavioral skills.

## GENERAL CONSIDERATIONS

The two goals of resuscitation are (1) to remove or ameliorate the underlying cause of asphyxia and (2) to reverse or correct the associated chain of events (hypoxia, hypercarbia, acidosis, bradycardia, and hypotension). To achieve these ends, resuscitation management should be centered on attempts to expand, ventilate, and oxygenate the lungs, with cardiac assistance provided as necessary. Intervention must, however, be specific to each infant in extent and form and must be determined by appropriate assessment.

The Apgar score provides a shorthand description of the neonate's condition at specific intervals after birth and may be useful as a rough prognostic indicator of long-term outcome; however, it does have limitations. Although it is a quantitative tool, the scoring often is subjectively or retrospectively applied. It often is poorly correlated with other indicators of well-being, such as cord pH. Its usefulness is suspect with extremely preterm infants, who may have poor respiratory drive and who may be relatively hyporeflexive and hypotonic because of immaturity rather than distress. Finally, waiting until the first Apgar score is assigned at 1 minute of age causes unnecessary delay in care. For these reasons, the Apgar score should not be used to determine the need for, or course of, resuscitation, but it may have a role in the determination of the continuation of resuscitation.

Delayed cord clamping for greater than 30 seconds in vigorous term and preterm newborns that have an intact placental circulation has been shown to be advantageous to the newborn. Preterm newborns who had delayed cord clamping for 30 to 60 seconds had higher blood pressure, higher blood volume, decreased need for blood transfusion, and decreased incidence of intraventricular hemorrhages (IVHs) and necrotizing enterocolitis (ACOG, 2020; Aziz et al., 2020; Liyanage, et al., 2020; Weiner & Zaichkin, 2021). For the term neonate, the advantage is less incidence of iron-deficiency anemia, although it may increase the amount and severity of jaundice (ACOG, 2020; Liyanage, et al., 2020). The determination of whether delayed cord clamping should occur in the delivery room should be discussed between the obstetrical and neonatal providers prior to the delivery of the infant. The condition of the neonate at birth will determine if delayed cord clamping can occur. Umbilical cord milking has been studied but at this time there is not sufficient evidence to support this practice in term and preterm infants (Liyanage, et al., 2020; Weiner & Zaichkin, 2021; see Figure 3.1).

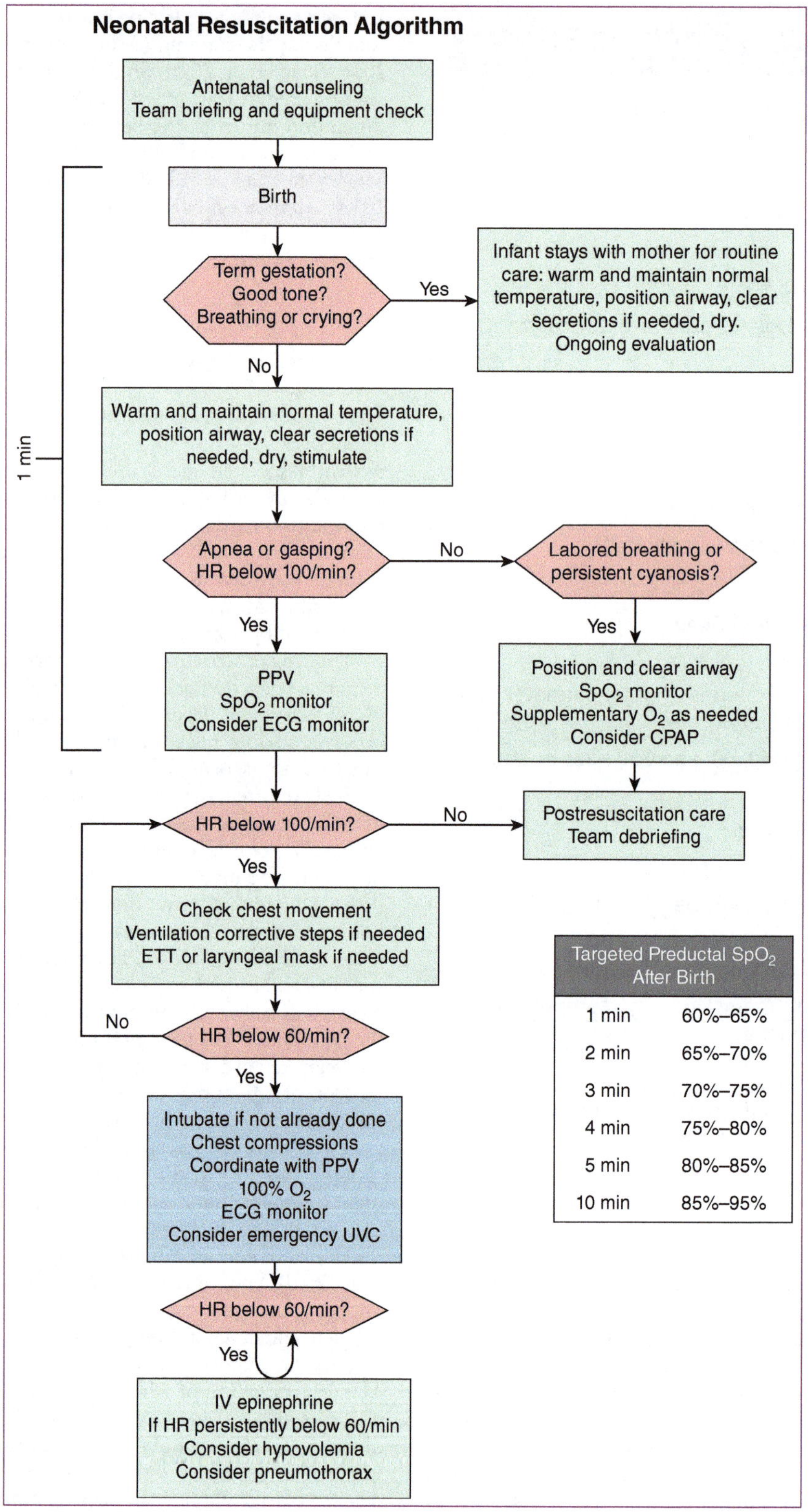


**FIGURE 3.1 American heart association neonatal resuscitation algorithm (2020).**

CPAP, continuous positive airway pressure; ETT, endotracheal tube; HR, heart rate; IV, intravenous; PPV, positive pressure ventilation; UVC, umbilical venous catheter.

*Source:* With permission from American Heart Association. (n.d.). *Guidelines for cardiopulmonary resuscitation and emergency cardiovascular care. Part 13: Neonatal resuscitation.* https://eccguidelines.heart.org/index.php/circulation/cpr-ecc-guidelines-2/part-13-neonatal-resuscitation/?strue=1&id=2.

As soon as the need for resuscitation is determined, the initiation of resuscitation is based on two signs: HR and respirations. HR is the most sensitive indicator of resuscitation efforts. In the review of literature it was found that the use of a three-lead electrocardiography (ECG) was more accurate than auscultation, palpation of the umbilical cord, or the use of a pulse oximeter in determining the neonate's HR (Aziz et al., 2020; Berg et al., 2023; Weiner & Zaichkin, 2021). Studies have demonstrated that healthcare providers could not palpate the umbilical cord accurately or that they underestimated the HR when auscultating the heart with a stethoscope. The three-lead ECG was quicker and more reliable than the pulse oximeter (Dawson et al., 2013; Iglesias et al., 2018; Katheria et al., 2012; Mizumoto et al., 2012; van Vonderen et al., 2015). Pulseless electrical activity (PEA) in newborns at one time was thought to not occur; but, more recently, PEA has been described in newborns (Patel et al., 2019: Sillers et al., 2019). For this reason, the NRP recommends that when a baby continues to deteriorate or not improve, auscultation and/or umbilical palpation should be used to assess if the heart is pumping blood (Berg et al., 2023; Weiner & Zaichkin, 2021).

As the resuscitation progresses, oxygenation is added to the signs that are assessed to determine the effectiveness of the resuscitation. Visual assessment of cyanosis is not a reliable method for judging a neonate's color or oxygen saturation in the delivery room and should not be used. In addition, with studies demonstrating that hyperoxia is as detrimental as hypoxia at the cellular and functional levels, the most accurate way of determining a neonate's oxygen saturation is to use a pulse oximeter in the delivery room (Weiner & Zaichkin, 2021). When placing a pulse oximeter, place it on the neonate's right hand or wrist, because preductal values are higher than postductal values. Always place the probe on the neonate prior to connecting the probe to the machine to produce quicker and more reliable values.

As soon as the infant has been positioned under a radiant warmer, thoroughly dried, airway cleared if necessary, and stimulated, the assessment of these three signs is to occur at 30-second intervals until compressions begin, at which time assessment will occur in 60-second intervals and interventions are carried out as needed. The basics of neonatal resuscitation are as easy as ABCD: *airway, breathing, circulation, and drugs*. These are the critical elements of any resuscitative effort.

## Airway Control

**Positioning.** Airway control is a fundamental prerequisite for effective oxygenation and ventilation. To achieve this, the infant should be placed in a flat supine position unless there is spinal deformity; then, the neonate would be placed in a side-lying position. The practice of placing the infant in a slight head-down tilt (Trendelenburg position) has been abandoned. This maneuver historically was used under the presumption that fluids from the lower extremities would be redistributed to the intrathoracic compartment. Studies with healthy adults in the Trendelenburg position have demonstrated improvement, albeit transient (lasting < 10 minutes), in the stroke volume of the heart, but these studies have also indicated that a tilt as slight as 10°C may cause blood to pool in the dependent cerebrovascular bed. Infants have only a limited ability to increase the stroke volume of their heart but are at greater risk than older children and adults for IVHs secondary to rupture of the vulnerable microvessels of the germinal matrix; consequently, the potential benefit, if any, of the head-down tilt position is not believed to be worth the risk.

Once the infant is in the supine position, the neck is placed in a neutral or slightly extended *sniffing* position that aligns the posterior pharynx, larynx, and trachea (Aziz et al., 2020; Weiner & Zaichkin, 2021). Compared with the adult tongue, an infant's tongue is relatively large in proportion to the mouth, and this slight extension moves the tongue and epiglottis away from the posterior pharyngeal wall and opens the airway. Care must, however, be taken to avoid full extension, which reduces the circumference of the airway and increases airway resistance. The reasonably safe extension posture appears to be no more than 15°C to 30°C from neutral. An oral airway should be placed if the tongue is unusually large (as in the Beckwith–Wiedemann syndrome) or if the chin is unusually small, causing posterior displacement of the tongue (as in the Pierre Robin sequence or the Potter association). Because newborns also have a relatively large head in comparison with the chest and tend naturally to fall into a flexed position, a shoulder roll made of a blanket or small towel may be used to raise the chest and align the cervical vertebrae. This roll may be particularly helpful if the occiput is exaggerated in size by molding, edema, or prematurity. If these procedures fail to provide an unobstructed airway, the placement of a laryngeal mask airway (LMA) or intubation is indicated (Weiner & Zaichkin, 2021).

**Suctioning.** Routine suctioning of neonates on the perineum was a standard of care for all deliveries whether the amniotic fluid was clear or meconium stained. There was no evidence to support this practice, so routine intrapartum oropharyngeal and nasopharyngeal suctioning for babies born with either clear or meconium-stained amniotic fluid was discontinued in 2011 as a recommendation for neonates at birth. After delivery, the infant is placed on the warming bed, quickly dried and positioned, and the airway is cleared by wiping the nose and mouth with a towel or by suctioning with a bulb syringe, or suction catheter if necessary. Increasing amounts of evidence show that suctioning, either bulb or mechanical, of the nasopharynx can create bradycardia during resuscitation; therefore, in 2010 the recommendations for suctioning (including bulb suction) immediately following birth changed. Suctioning is now reserved for only those neonates who have an obvious obstruction to spontaneous breathing or for those babies requiring PPV (Weiner & Zaichkin, 2021; Wyckoff et al., 2022). When the need for suctioning occurs, the mouth should always be suctioned before the nose, *M* before *N*, because suctioning may cause inadvertent stimulation and gasping. Mechanical suction is often mentioned as an alternative to the bulb syringe, but it generally should not be used immediately after delivery. If infants are suctioned vigorously within the first 5 minutes of life, apnea or arrhythmias may follow. These symptoms probably are due to vagal stimulation, with reflex bradycardia.

If a bulb syringe can be used instead of a suction catheter, this situation can usually be avoided. If mechanical suction is required, it should be applied for no longer than 5 seconds at a time with an 8 or 10 French suction catheter and with the equipment set to produce no more than 100 mm Hg (136 cm $H_2O$) negative pressure (Weiner & Zaichkin, 2021). To assist with the removal of a large amount of secretions from the mouth, turn the baby's head to the side, which will allow for the secretions to pool in the baby's cheek, where they can be more easily removed.

If meconium is present in the amniotic fluid and the baby is vigorous (strong respiratory effort, good muscle tone, and HR > 100 beats/min), the baby should be treated as a non-meconium baby and remain with the mother doing skin-to-skin care, although gentle bulb suctioning of the baby's mouth and nose may be needed. If meconium is present and the baby is non-vigorous (depressed respirations, decreased muscle tone, and/or a HR below 100 beats/min), proceed with the initial steps of resuscitation. Routine direct suctioning of the trachea before beginning the steps of resuscitation to decrease the chance of the baby aspirating the meconium is no longer recommended, because there is insufficient evidence to continue the practice (Aziz et al., 2020; Weiner & Zaichkin, 2021).

**Tactile Stimulation.** In a mildly depressed infant, drying and suctioning will usually be enough stimulation to induce effective respirations. If the respiratory rate and depth are nevertheless diminished, rubbing the back, trunk, or extremities as well as slapping or flicking the soles of the feet briefly will stimulate the infant to breathe. If the infant's reflexes are intact, 10 to 15 seconds of stimulation should be sufficient to elicit a response. Longer and more vigorous methods of stimulation should be avoided. Never spend more than 30 seconds to further stimulate an infant, because it is a waste of valuable time. Remember that the first 60 seconds after birth are referred to as the *Golden Minute*, so if clearing the airway and stimulating the neonate to breathe does not result in improvement after 60 seconds, PPV should be started (Weiner & Zaichkin, 2021).

## VENTILATION AND OXYGENATION

The most important and effective action in a neonatal resuscitation is ventilation of the compromised neonate. In fact, most infants who require resuscitation can be revived with ventilation and oxygen as needed, alone. Even when more aggressive therapies are required, they ultimately are undertaken to support oxygen delivery to the tissues, either by optimizing the airway (i.e., LMA or intubation) or by supporting the heart, which *pushes* oxygen to the periphery (i.e., chest compressions, medications).

### Free Flow Administration of Oxygen

Blow-by of 100% oxygen given at delivery was a common intervention in the past, but as stated earlier, increasing numbers of research studies show that increasing the compromised neonate's oxygen saturation more quickly than a normal healthy term neonate can be toxic and detrimental to not only a preterm infant, but to term infants as well. Studies have shown that giving a neonate 100% oxygen with PPV demonstrated no advantage in improvement when compared to neonates given PPV with room air (RA), and actually delayed the time to the first breath and/or cry in term infants. Because of the increasing evidence from randomized controlled trials and meta-analyses of the studies demonstrating the detriments of hyperoxia, such as increased incidence of chronic lung disease and changes in the cerebral blood flow, especially in preterm babies, the use of RA at the beginning of resuscitation has been recommended since 2010. If there is no improvement, however, in HR or oxygenation by pulse oximetry despite adequate ventilation, increasing the amount of oxygen the neonate is receiving should be considered (Aziz et al., 2020; Weiner & Zaichkin, 2021). An infant who is breathing spontaneously but fails to maintain its oxygen saturation ($SpO_2$) within the range for the age of the infant, in RA (Table 3.2), needs supplemental oxygen. The oxygen can be provided directly from the end of the oxygen tube held in a cupped hand, by a funnel or face mask attached to the tubing, by a flow-inflating ventilation bag, by a T-piece resuscitator, or by the tail of a self-inflating bag. The blender attached to a flowmeter should be set to deliver to 10 L/min, and the tubing, funnel, or mask should be held close to the infant's face to maximize the inhaled concentration of oxygen, but not so close that pressure would build up (Weiner & Zaichkin, 2021).

The NRP guidelines changed in 2010 to reflect the use of RA initially on both free-flow ventilation and PPV for term infants and the use of RA to 30% oxygen for preterm infants. During resuscitation, start with RA (21%) at sea level for term infants, and then, using the preductal pulse oximeter as your guide, increase your oxygen concentration as

**TABLE 3.2**

**TARGETED PREDUCTAL $SPO_2$ AFTER BIRTH**

| Age in Minutes | $SpO_2$ Range (%) |
|---|---|
| 1 | 60–65 |
| 2 | 65–70 |
| 3 | 70–75 |
| 4 | 75–80 |
| 5 | 80–85 |
| 10 | 85–95 |

*Source:* Modified from Weiner, G. M., & Zaichkin, J. (Eds.). (2021). *Textbook of neonatal resuscitation* (8th ed.). American Academy of Pediatrics and American Heart Association.

necessary to maintain the appropriate oxygen saturation for the infant's age in minutes after birth. When determining the amount of oxygen to use in preterm infants, several studies were analyzed that looked at preterm infants younger than 35 weeks' gestation who were resuscitated using either RA or oxygen concentrations of 65% or greater. The studies showed no difference in long-term outcomes of bronchopulmonary dysplasia, retinopathy of prematurity, or IVHs, but because of concerns of the effects of hyperoxia the recommendation is to start with a low range of oxygen, between RA and 30%, when resuscitating preterm infants younger than 35 weeks' gestation (Aziz et al., 2020; Weiner & Zaichkin, 2021).

## VENTILATION

If after the initial steps of resuscitation, the infant is not spontaneously breathing, gasping, or has a HR less than 100 beats/min, then PPV should be immediately instituted. Begin PPV with a pressure of 20 to 25 cm $H_2O$ to inflate the lungs on all neonates, although term neonates may require higher pressures for the first few breaths to inflate the lungs. After the initial breaths, reassess the need for the higher pressures on a term neonate, realizing that you may need to adjust the pressure as needed to achieve a rising HR, chest expansion, and audible breath sounds. Occasionally, it may become necessary to increase the positive pressure if no improvement occurs. Positive end expiratory pressure (PEEP) has been shown to achieve lung inflation quicker, remove the fetal lung fluid more rapidly, and prevent collapse of the alveoli between breaths. When using PEEP, set the PEEP to 5 cm because this has been found to be beneficial for both term and preterm infants requiring PPV. A ventilation rate of 40 to 60 breaths/min should be used when ventilating the newborn (Aziz et al., 2020; Weiner & Zaichkin, 2021).

### Continuous Positive Airway Pressure

The use of continuous positive airway pressure (CPAP) in the delivery room is an option for all neonates who are spontaneously breathing and have a HR greater than 100 beats/min. When CPAP is provided, it decreases the work of breathing for the neonate by keeping the alveoli stinted open on exhalation and helps to establish the functional residual capacity. This is especially helpful for preterm babies who are surfactant deficient, making it difficult for the alveoli to stay open upon exhalation. Studies have been conducted to assess the outcomes for preterm neonates who had CPAP in the delivery room versus being intubated and given PPV. Several studies have demonstrated that spontaneously breathing infants younger than 30 weeks' gestation given CPAP had reduced rates of intubation, decreased length of time on mechanical ventilation, and possibly decreased incidence of death and development of bronchopulmonary dysplasia (BPD) with no increase in the development of air leaks or IVHs. Taking the results of these and other studies into consideration, the recommendation now is that spontaneously breathing preterm neonates with respiratory distress may be supported initially with CPAP rather than intubation and PPV. The one caveat to using CPAP is that the risk of developing a pneumothorax is increased, so providers must be prepared to deal with the air leak if it should occur (Aziz et al., 2020; Weiner & Zaichkin, 2021).

### Positive Pressure Devices

Three types of ventilation devices are available for neonatal use: the self-inflating bag, the flow-inflating bag, and the T-piece resuscitator. Whichever device is used, it should have the capability of delivering an oxygen concentration between 21% and 100%.

*Self-inflating bags* do not require gas flow but do require a reservoir to deliver high concentrations of oxygen. Traditionally, these bags have been fitted with a pressure-release *popoff* valve preset at 30 to 40 cm $H_2O$ to prevent overinflation of the lungs and the risk of pneumothorax. Most self-inflating bags must be squeezed to move gas through the circuit and are not capable of passive, free-flow oxygen delivery.

*Flow-inflating bags*, on the other hand, are closed systems and therefore must be connected to a compressed gas source. Although self-inflating bags have the advantages of being both easy to operate and gas-flow independent, flow-inflating bags provide more reliable oxygen concentrations (particularly at low flow rates), better control of inspiratory times, and a greater range of peak inspiratory pressures, as well as free-flow oxygen.

A *T-piece resuscitator* is a mechanical device that provides flow-controlled and pressure-limited breaths. Like the flow-inflating bag, it requires a compressed gas source to operate. The peak inspiratory pressure and end expiratory pressure are set manually with adjustable controls and the breaths are delivered manually when the operator alternately occludes and opens the aperture on the tubing attached to the mask, LMA, or endotracheal tube (ET).

All three of the devices can be used to provide ventilation by mask, LMA, or ET tube. Both types of ventilation bags can be equipped with a manometer to monitor airway pressure as well. Though a manometer is important, visualization of the chest is equally, if not more, important. The degree of chest rise should simulate that seen when a normal newborn takes an easy breath. Excessive chest rise reflects overzealous delivery of tidal volume; if there is no movement, delivery is inadequate. A self-inflating or flow-inflating bag that has a regulatory valve with a minimum volume of 200 ml and a maximum volume of 750 ml should be used in resuscitating neonates. Term newborns require only 10 to 25 ml with each ventilation (4–6 ml/kg). A bag larger than this makes delivering the correct size breath difficult (Weiner & Zaichkin, 2021).

### Methods of Ventilation

For mask ventilation, a face mask is used to provide an oxygen-enriched *microenvironment*. An anatomically shaped mask with a cushioned rim is preferred for this purpose. Because masks are available in a variety of sizes, care must be taken to select one that covers the tip of the chin, the mouth, and the nose but not the eyes. Mask ventilation is a simple, noninvasive method of oxygen delivery that can be initiated without delay but the use of a mask has disadvantages. First, it may be difficult to obtain and maintain a good seal between the mask and the infant's face, particularly around the infant's nose. Any leakage of air results in underventilation, which is aggravated if low lung compliance or high airway resistance is a factor. The seal should be *airtight* without excessive pressure applied. Second, the mask itself has a considerable amount of dead space. Consequently, a sufficient tidal volume must be delivered to prevent accumulation and rebreathing of carbon dioxide. Masks used for neonatal resuscitation ideally should have a dead space of less than 5 ml. Finally, prolonged bag and mask ventilation may produce gastric distention from swallowed gas, which in turn impedes diaphragmatic excursions and places the infant at risk of regurgitation and aspiration. This problem can be easily avoided, however, by inserting an 8 French orogastric tube if mask ventilation continues beyond several minutes. The gastric contents should be suctioned, and the tube left in place as a vent as long as mask ventilation or CPAP is provided (Weiner & Zaichkin, 2021).

Mask ventilation suffices for most infants, but if it proves ineffective (as evidenced by poor chest rise or continuing bradycardia) or if prolonged ventilation is expected, an LMA or ET tube should be inserted. Premature infants (certainly those weighing < 1,000 g) who have diminished lung compliance, immature respiratory musculature, and decreased respiratory drive may also benefit from early intubation (Weiner & Zaichkin, 2021).

Infants suspected of having a diaphragmatic hernia, hydrops fetalis, or certain airway or gastrointestinal abnormalities also benefit from immediate intubation. Uncuffed ET tubes with a uniform internal diameter should be used. The proper tube size and depth of insertion are determined by the infant's size, weight, gestational age, and nasal–tragus length (NTL; Table 3.3). Most neonatal ET tubes have a set of black lines (vocal cord guide) near the tip of the tube that serve as a guide for insertion. When the vocal cords are situated between the two lines, the tube should be properly positioned with its tip in the midtrachea. In the past, the distance from the midtrachea (tube tip) to the infant's upper lip was used to determine proper tube placement, but it was not always accurate. A more accurate method for determining the proper depth of an ET tube is to measure the NTL in a neonate and add 0.39 in. (1 cm). This method has been shown to be more accurate in both term and preterm infants. Gestational age has also been shown to be accurate in determining insertion tube depth (Weiner & Zaichkin, 2021).

When the tube is properly situated, the centimeter marking on the side of the tube at the level of the upper lip should be at or near NTL. Tubes with metallic markers or fiber-optic illumination at the tip may make it possible to determine the depth of the tube transdermally (i.e., by observing a circle of light on the skin or by hearing an audible signal from a transcutaneous locator instrument), but these modifications do not allow differentiation between ET intubation and esophageal intubation, and therefore offer no advantage in an emergency situation. Similarly, capnometers used during resuscitation to measure end-tidal carbon dioxide, and thus confirm tube placement in the trachea, may be inaccurate when pulmonary blood flow is poor or absent (Weiner & Zaichkin, 2021).

Correct placement is best demonstrated by the tried-and-true methods: improved clinical signs (HR, improving oxygenation, and activity), symmetric chest rise, bilateral and equal breath sounds (as auscultated in the axillae), and fogging of the tube on exhalation. Air should not be heard entering the stomach, and the abdomen should not be distended. If any doubts exist, tube placement can be checked by repeated laryngoscopy; the tube should be clearly seen passing through the glottic opening (Weiner & Zaichkin, 2021).

**TABLE 3.3**

**ENDOTRACHEAL TUBE SIZE AND PLACEMENT**

| Infant's Weight (g) | Infant's Gestational Age (weeks) | Tube Size (mm) | Insertion Depth (cm) |
|---|---|---|---|
| 500–600 | 23–24 | 2.5 | 5.5 |
| 700–800 | 25–26 | 2.5 | 6.0 |
| 900–1,000 | 27–29 | 2.5 | 6.5 |
| 1,100–1,400 | 30–32 | 3.0 | 7.0 |
| 1,500–1,800 | 33–34 | 3.0 | 7.5 |
| 1,900–2,400 | 35–37 | 3.5 | 8.0 |
| 2,500–3,100 | 38–40 | 3.5 | 8.5 |
| 3,200–4,200 | 41–43 | 3.5 or 4.0 | 9.0 |

*Source:* Adapted from Weiner, G. M., & Zaichkin, J. (Eds.). (2021). *Textbook of neonatal resuscitation* (8th ed.). American Academy of Pediatrics and American Heart Association.

ET intubation is the definitive technique for airway management and ventilation. Agility and accuracy in placement, however, require continual practice. Also, many hospital personnel are restricted by policy or statute from learning or using this skill. The LMA, which was approved by the U.S. Food and Drug Administration (FDA) in 1991, has been enthusiastically accepted in some settings as an alternative that offers most of the advantages of intubation but does not require laryngoscopy for placement.

The LMA (Figure 3.2) is a relatively long tube with a bag connector and an inflation port at one end and an inflatable soft cuff at the other. The tube is blindly passed into the hypopharynx so that the tip of the cuff lodges in the esophageal opening. Inflated, the cuff creates a seal around the larynx. The tube then is connected to a bag that delivers oxygen by ventilation through the central aperture of the laryngeal mask.

Since the LMA was approved for use by the FDA, research has been done to assess effectiveness in neonates.

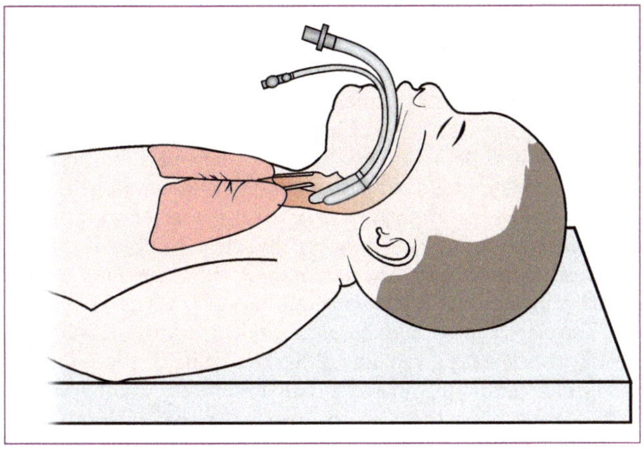

**FIGURE 3.2 LMA inserted in neonate.**

*Source:* Adapted from Weiner, G. M., & Zaichkin, J. (Eds.). (2021). *Textbook of neonatal resuscitation* (8th ed., p. 87). American Academy of Pediatrics and American Heart Association.

For ventilation purposes, the LMA is as effective, but never more effective, as intubation. Placement of the LMA has been studied in neonates who are 34 weeks and older or who weigh more than 2,000 g, and case reports have shown LMAs to be an effective alternative when mask ventilation and intubation were unsuccessful. These studies also showed that effective ventilation was achieved quickly using an LMA (Wyckoff et al., 2022). An advantage of LMA is that it can be placed by a registered nurse (RN), respiratory therapist (RT), or an advance practice provider or physician, making providing an airway to neonates in distress easier in facilities where a physician might not be in-house 24 hours a day. Training healthcare professionals to place an LMA can be done using a manikin. Studies have shown it to be an effective training tool (Gandini & Brimacombe, 2004; Micaglio et al., 2006).

Situations where an LMA may be useful include those where a neonate has a congenital anomaly of the mouth, lip, or palate; anomalies of the head, neck, tongue, or pharynx; a small mandible; or when ventilation with a mask is ineffective and intubation is not feasible. A disadvantage of an LMA is that even with successful placement, nearly a quarter of infants with an LMA subsequently develop airway obstruction, probably because of displacement during patient movement. The cuff provides only a low-pressure seal around the larynx, which limits the airway pressures that can be achieved during ventilation. The risks of gastric insufflation and regurgitation of gastric contents are reduced but not eliminated. Because of its size, the LMA is currently restricted to infants greater than 34 weeks' gestation or 2 kg, although there have been anecdotal reports of successful use in very small infants (1–1.5 kg). The LMA also does not provide access to the lower airway, and therefore, is not suitable for meconium removal or drug administration, nor does it preserve the airway during laryngospasm. Its usefulness in neonates who require chest compressions or with the use of emergency medication administration still needs to be assessed (Weiner & Zaichkin, 2021; Wyckoff et al., 2022).

**Chest Compressions.** Chest compressions are rarely required for resuscitation in the delivery room. They are performed in only 1 to 3 of every 1,000 deliveries but probably are avoidable even in most of these cases. According to some authorities, approximately one-third of the infants who received chest compressions showed biochemical evidence of asphyxia (acidemia), but the remaining two-thirds were found to have a malpositioned ET tube or inadequate ventilatory support (i.e., insufficient rate or pressure). Clearly, the airway should be reassessed, and respiratory support should be optimized before chest compressions are initiated. Assuming that these components are satisfactory, chest compressions are begun if the HR drops below 60 beats/min after 30 seconds of *effective* ventilation (Weiner & Zaichkin, 2021).

Chest compressions provide temporary support for circulation and oxygen delivery. Pressing on the sternum has two effects: It compresses the heart against the vertebral column, and it increases intrathoracic pressure. Both effects cause blood to be pushed out of the heart into the arterial circulation. When the sternal pressure is released, the ventricles return to their original shape, intrathoracic pressure falls toward zero, and venous blood is pulled into the heart by a suction effect (Weiner & Zaichkin, 2021).

There are two techniques to perform chest compressions, but the thumb method is preferred by the AAP. For the thumb method, both hands encircle the chest; the fingers support the back, and the thumbs (pointing cephalad either side by side or one on top of the other, depending on the infant's size) are used to press the sternum downward. The two-finger method should only be used if the compressor's hands are too small to encircle the neonate's chest. In this method, one hand supports the back from below while two fingers of the free hand are held perpendicular to the chest and the fingertips are used to apply downward pressure on the sternum. The two-thumb method is preferred because comparative studies have shown that higher systolic blood pressure, higher diastolic blood pressure, higher mean arterial pressure, and higher coronary perfusion pressure are generated with less external compression force when the thumb method is used. This method also has had fewer reports of trauma to the liver and other abdominal organs. Moreover, the thumb method is perhaps easier and certainly less tiring to perform. If access to the umbilicus is needed to facilitate placement of an umbilical venous catheter (UVC) for administration of emergency drugs, the compressor should move to the head of the bed next to the person providing ventilation and continue compressing with the two-thumb method, though the thumbs will now be pointing caudally (Weiner & Zaichkin, 2021).

For both methods, the pressure is applied to the lower-third of the sternum (just below the nipple line but above the xiphoid process), where the right ventricle lies closest to the sternum. Just enough force is used to depress the sternum one-third of the anterior/posterior chest wall diameter (Weiner & Zaichkin, 2021). To obtain the most optimal myocardial and cerebral blood flows, the downward stroke and release phases of the compression should be equal in time. This equalization is best accomplished with a smooth stroke and release rhythm.

No matter which method of compression is utilized, compressing the heart for a full 60 seconds with coordinated ventilation is essential prior to reassessing the HR. Studies have demonstrated that it takes at least a minute for the diastolic pressure to increase enough to begin perfusing the coronary arteries. For this reason, the recommendations are for a full 60 seconds of coordinated compressions and ventilation before reassessing the HR (Aziz et al., 2020; Weiner & Zaichkin, 2021).

PPV with 100% oxygen must be given while chest compressions are performed. The most recent guidelines recommend interposing chest compressions with ventilations at a 3 to 1 ratio. Every fourth compression is dropped to allow delivery of a single effective breath. During the course of a full minute, 90 compressions and 30 ventilations are given (Weiner & Zaichkin, 2021). In order to provide an adequate number of compressions without simultaneous compression/ventilation, the ventilation rate is dropped to 30 from the 40 to 60 that was done with ventilation alone.

Faster rates were recommended in the past, but they only increase the chance of administering simultaneous compressions and ventilations. Most studies indicate that simultaneous delivery increases the intrathoracic pressure to a level at which ventilation is impeded and coronary perfusion is reduced. Whether there is any effect on cerebral blood flow is equivocal, but there have been other reports of lower survival rates when simultaneous compression and ventilation were used.

Experimental techniques, such as external circulatory assist devices (e.g., mechanical *thumpers*, pneumatic vests, and abdominal binders), counterpoint abdominal compressions (e.g., cough cardiopulmonary resuscitation), and active decompression (e.g., plumber's plunger), have shown promise in animal studies. Only a few large-scale clinical trials have been conducted, however, and most of those used adults. Consequently, these methods cannot be advocated for neonatal resuscitation at this time.

## Medications

Medications are rarely used in neonatal resuscitation, and if they are needed, only two are used: epinephrine and normal saline. Sodium bicarbonate and other medications are no longer used in the immediate resuscitative period but may be considered in postresuscitation care.

**Epinephrine.** Epinephrine is a direct-acting catecholamine with both alpha-adrenergic and beta-adrenergic effects. These effects lead to peripheral vasoconstriction, acceleration of the HR, and an increase in the forcefulness of cardiac contractions. The net effect is a sharp rise in blood pressure (pressor effect) and an increase in cardiac output. The marked pressor effect combined with the increased aortic diastolic pressure increases the cerebral and myocardial perfusion pressures, maintaining blood flow to these critical organs during resuscitation. Epinephrine is, therefore, considered the drug of choice with asystole or persistent bradycardia (HR < 60 beats/min) despite effective ventilation with 100% oxygen and chest compressions for 60 seconds. For newborns, the recommended dosage is 0.01 to 0.03 mg/kg or 0.1 to 0.3 ml/kg of 0.1 mg/ml (1 mg/10 ml concentration) intravenously (Aziz et al., 2020; Weiner & Zaichkin, 2021). The drug is rapidly inactivated by an enzymatically driven process known as *sulfoconjugation*, in which the active compound is conjugated with sulfate. The half-life of infused epinephrine is approximately 3 minutes. Consequently, the dose may be repeated every 3 to 5 minutes as clinically indicated.

Epinephrine ideally should be administered via the IV/UVC/IO route. Because IV/UVC placement may be difficult and time-consuming during resuscitation and not all neonates are candidates for an intraosseous (IO) placement, an initial dose of epinephrine can be given by the ET tube. Unfortunately, absorption into the circulation from the pulmonary capillary bed may be highly variable because of the low blood-flow state associated with resuscitation. In addition, much of the ET-instilled drug remains along the walls of the ET tube and in the conducting airways, with a relatively small amount finding its way into the deep absorptive surfaces of the alveoli. If epinephrine is given by the ET tube, a higher dose of 0.05 to 0.1 mg/kg or 0.5 to 1.0 ml/kg of 0.1 mg/ml (1 mg/10 ml concentration) should be given (Aziz et al., 2020; Weiner & Zaichkin, 2021). If ET epinephrine is given prior to the establishment of vascular access and the neonate continues with a HR < 60 beats/min, giving an IV dose of epinephrine immediately after establishment of a vascular access should be done (Aziz et al., 2020; Weiner & Zaichkin, 2021).

A number of steps can be taken to aid delivery when the ET route is necessary. First, to optimize blood flow to the lungs, every effort must be made to ensure that chest compressions are performed effectively. Second, epinephrine may be dispersed more quickly to deeper pulmonary tissues by following the instillation with a few forceful ventilations. Administering epinephrine via the ET tube will deliver higher doses, which will lead to increased volume of fluid of up to 1 ml, so dilution is no longer needed (Weiner & Zaichkin, 2021).

Although higher doses of epinephrine administered by the ET route may have a role in exceptional situations, routine IV/UVC administration of high-dose epinephrine is not recommended in newborns. Studies with adults and older children have shown a dose–response relationship, with higher doses bringing about greater improvements in coronary and cerebral blood flow; in neonates, however, the efficacy and safety of high-dose IV/UVC epinephrine have not been adequately evaluated. Most of these studies have been conducted with patients with a history of coronary artery disease who demonstrate ventricular fibrillation. Neonates, however, more commonly have bradycardia caused by hypoxia. These pathophysiologic differences prevent the extrapolation of findings. Furthermore, administration of high doses has generally been followed by a prolonged period of hypertension. Because the newborn, particularly the prematurely born, has a vascular germinal matrix, the risk may be greater for intraventricular hemorrhage. In fact, this area of the brain is most susceptible to hemorrhage when hypertension is preceded by hypotension, which is the case with resuscitation. For this reason, only the standard dose of epinephrine (0.01–0.03 mg/kg) should be given by the IV/UVC route.

**Volume Expanders.** Volume expanders are indicated with evidence or suspicion of acute blood loss with signs of hypovolemia. These signs include pallor despite oxygen therapy, hypotension with weak pulses despite a normal HR, delayed capillary refill, and failure to respond to resuscitation (Aziz et al., 2020; Weiner & Zaichkin, 2021). Low hematocrit and hemoglobin concentrations are diagnostic of blood loss, but the levels may be misleadingly normal immediately after acute loss. In general, it takes about 3 hours for a sufficient amount of fluid to shift from the interstitial to the intravascular space to produce the degree of compensatory hemodilution reflected by a fall in laboratory values.

The basic requirement for any replacement solution is that the electrolyte and protein composition be roughly equivalent to that which was lost. Otherwise, an osmotic pressure gradient is created, and fluids are driven out of the capillaries into the interstitial tissue. The expansion of circulatory volume is only transient, and the infant is put at risk for secondary problems, particularly pulmonary edema. Clearly, whole blood is the fluid of choice for volume replacement, and it offers the added benefit of oxygen-carrying capacity. Fresh O-negative blood cross-matched against the mother should be used. When blood is not readily available, isotonic fluids, such as 0.9% normal saline, may also be used (Weiner & Zaichkin, 2021). Glucose-containing fluids (e.g., $D_5W$ or $D_{10}W$) should not be given by bolus because of the risk of profound hyperglycemia. Hyperglycemia with untreated asphyxia may aggravate metabolic acidosis.

For emergency treatment of hypovolemia, 10 ml/kg of volume expander is given slowly over 5 to 10 minutes by the IV/UVC/IO route (Weiner & Zaichkin, 2021). Rapid infusion must be avoided because abrupt changes in vascular pressure in the vulnerable germinal matrix capillaries place the infant (especially a preterm infant) at greater risk of IVH. The response is usually dramatic, with a prompt improvement in blood pressure, pulses, and color. If the signs of hypovolemia continue, however, a second volume replacement may be given. Persistent failure beyond this point probably indicates some degree of *pump failure*, and further improvement is not likely until cardiac function is improved.

**Naloxone.** In the past, naloxone was used for the infant of the mother who received a narcotic analgesic for pain control during labor, because these lipid-soluble drugs rapidly cross the placenta within 2 minutes of administration and can cause neonatal respiratory depression. Peak fetal narcotic levels occur 30 minutes to 2 hours after administration to the mother. The degree and duration of depression shown by the newborn depend on the dose, the route, and how soon before delivery the drug was given. Affected neonates show decreased respiratory effort and muscle tone but typically have a good HR and perfusion. Due to insufficient evidence regarding the safety and efficacy of this drug in the neonate and animal studies that report complications, the use of this drug is, however, no longer recommended (Weiner & Zaichkin, 2021).

**Other Drugs.** Sodium bicarbonate, dopamine, atropine, and calcium were at one time used routinely in the acute phases of neonatal resuscitation but are no longer used because they are rarely very useful. These drugs, along with glucose boluses, are more commonly used now in the postresuscitation period in the neonatal special care or intensive care unit.

**Special Circumstances.** For some infants, changes in or variations of the usual resuscitative measures are needed. Most of these infants are extremely premature, have congenital anomalies, structural defects, or conditions that compromise the cardiovascular system, such as neural tube defects, abdominal wall defects, diaphragmatic hernias, hydrops fetalis, esophageal atresia, pneumothorax, choanal atresia, and laryngeal anomalies. Resuscitative measures with these disorders are discussed in greater detail elsewhere in this textbook.

**Withholding or Discontinuing Resuscitation.** The law and its underlying ethical principles require that treatment be provided and continued as long as it is judged to be effective in ameliorating or correcting an underlying pathophysiologic process. Unfortunately, the data is insufficient to allow a general recommendation for how long resuscitation should be performed before continuation can be deemed futile and efforts are terminated. There is evidence that survival is unlikely at any birth weight if the Apgar score remains 0 after 20 minutes of resuscitation that has effective ventilation, coordinated with chest compressions and administration of medication, but recently some controversy has arisen with the standard of stopping resuscitation on a neonate at 20 minutes because reports have emerged regarding intact survival in infants who have received therapeutic hypothermia after birth (Aziz et al., 2020). Taking into consideration this evidence, NRP still recommends that it may be reasonable to stop resuscitation at 20 minutes if the Apgar score is 0 and the resuscitative efforts have been effective, but each resuscitation should be individualized to the situation at hand and the wishes of the family (Aziz et al., 2020; Weiner & Zaichkin, 2021).

In the past, NRP made recommendations on when noninitiation of resuscitation would be appropriate, but the current NRP recommendation is to follow the AMA Code of Medical Ethics on determining whether noninitiation should occur. The AMA states that five factors need to be weighed to make that determination. **Emergency Alert:** **Per the AMA Code of Medical Ethics, the five factors for determining whether noninitiation should occur are (1) the chance that the therapy will succeed, (2) the risks involved with treatment and nontreatment, (3) the degree to which the therapy, if successful, will extend life, (4) the pain and discomfort associated with the therapy, and (5) the anticipated quality of life for the newborn with and without the treatment.** This information would need to be discussed with the parents prior to the delivery of the neonate, if time allows. If time does not allow or sufficient information is not available, then initiation of resuscitation should occur, and discontinuation can occur as more information becomes available (Weiner & Zaichkin, 2021).

Although many hospitals have guidelines for withholding full resuscitation for extremely low-birth-weight (ELVW) infants and those with lethal anomalies, early and well-documented discussion with parents is recommended when such events are anticipated prenatally. If the event was not anticipated, great attention should be given to postmortem evaluation. Blood for chromosome examination and other pertinent laboratory work, radiographs, and an autopsy are important both for family counseling and for evaluation of the resuscitation process.

**Postresuscitation Management.** A successfully resuscitated neonate requires special consideration and care postresuscitation. The goal of care of stabilization is to reverse the causes of cell death and tissue injury (hypoxia, ischemia, and acidosis) and avoid or treat any exacerbating conditions (hypothermia, hypoglycemia, respiratory failure, infection). The level of neonatal care for which the facility is designated and the baby's condition will help determine whether the baby should be kept at the same facility as the mother or transported from the facility to a tertiary or quaternary referral center. When transporting a baby from one facility to another, a dedicated neonatal transport team should be used to improve the outcomes for the neonate because adult transport teams do not have the knowledge or skill set to care for the critically ill neonate.

Because newly born infants that required resuscitation are at risk for further deterioration, the main goal for the newly resuscitated neonate is to prevent future complications if at all possible. A concept that originated in the emergency medicine domain and is being adopted in the neonatal domain due to improved outcomes is the *Golden Hour* concept. In trauma medicine, it was found that if a patient was treated in the first 60 minutes following the accident, then irreversible internal damage was prevented, and survival improved. In recent years, this concept has been applied to the newly resuscitated neonate, especially the extremely premature neonate, and refers to the first hour of a neonate's life. Principles of the Golden Hour include the standardization of treatment protocol during and after resuscitation of the neonate, improving teamwork, maintaining thermoregulation, the administration of glucose-containing fluids to prevent hypoglycemia, and providing appropriate developmental support for the neonate. By standardizing how care is implemented, both short- and long-term outcomes related to thermoregulation, hypoglycemia, respiratory complications, sepsis, and IVHs in the neonate may be decreased (Castrodale & Rinehart, 2014; Lambeth et al., 2016). Infants who are 36 weeks of gestation or greater who had advance resuscitation are at risk for developing hypoxic-ischemic encephalopathy (HIE) and should be closely monitored. For those who exhibit signs of HIE, determining if they meet criteria for therapeutic cooling should be done in a timely manner to help improve outcomes (Aziz et al., 2020; Weiner & Zaichkin, 2021).

There are several postresuscitation programs available to train healthcare providers in the care of the recently resuscitated neonate. The Perinatal Continuing Education Program and the S.T.A.B.L.E. Program are two such programs that are available to assist healthcare professionals with learning the skills necessary to stabilize the successfully resuscitated neonate. Both programs cover fluid administration, maintenance of the glucose levels, temperature regulation, airway management, blood pressure stabilization, laboratory work needed, antibiotic administration, parental support, and skills acquisition in the form of simulation. All of these topics are discussed in detail in other sections of this textbook.

**Documentation.** No resuscitative event can go unrecorded. Unfortunately, the circumstances surrounding resuscitation are fraught with medicolegal hazards. Assessment of the infant is generally limited to the most basic measurements (respiratory rate, HR, and oxygenation). Immediate response may be affected by many factors unrelated to professional competence. Furthermore, the ultimate outcome may not become apparent for years. Even the best, most appropriate care can look *bad* in retrospect if documentation is incomplete or inaccurate. Yet no area of the hospital is perhaps less conducive to quality documentation than the delivery room, where a variety of professionals (nurses, physicians, and respiratory therapists) from different clinical areas (obstetrics, neonatology, anesthesiology), each with a unique perspective on the situation, are brought together in an emergency. Notes are jotted on bed linen, scrub clothes, paper towels, or anything at hand. More often than not, these brief notes are so hastily written that they are little more than a list of the medications given. When transcribed, the events may be documented in two totally separate charts, one for the mother and another for the infant. Great care must be taken with record keeping so that events and actions can be accurately reconstructed many years into the future.

Descriptive charting is most appropriate in this situation. The record should include the pertinent perinatal factors, the physical findings, the activities performed, and the infant's response, but definitive diagnoses should not be offered. It is particularly important that information concerning the pregnancy, labor, and delivery be based on fact and not hearsay. Terms such as *fetal distress* and *asphyxia* tend to take on a life of their own once they have been committed to paper, even if they are not supported by clinical evidence. It is best to record factual data, such as vital signs and blood gas determinations, without adding an interpretation. Ventilation, chest compressions, and administration of medications are essential items for documentation, but the basics should not be dismissed. It is just as important to note that attempts were made to keep the infant dry and warm.

Accurate timing of notes can be critical, because actions are judged by the minute-to-minute changes noted in the chart. A preprinted recording form or an electronic form not only helps in this regard but can also provide a structure for evaluation and decision making.

## Care of the Family During Resuscitation and Stabilization

An ill neonate is a crisis for families because no one expects their baby to be born prematurely or ill. When risk factors are known that could result in a neonate needing to be resuscitated (i.e., extremely premature baby), the physician should discuss with the parents prior to the delivery, if time allows, the options available as well as survival rates of the diagnosed condition of the infant. Parents have a role in deciding the goals of the care to be delivered to their baby, but they cannot make an informed decision unless they have been presented complete and reliable information. Unfortunately, many times this type of information may not be available until after the initial resuscitation or many hours later.

During resuscitation and stabilization, healthcare professionals should keep the parents informed of what is occurring to their newborn. Parents' wishes should be honored, if appropriate. Parents may wish to be present during resuscitation efforts. In a systematic review of research studies published in 2021 supported this presence of parents from both a health professional's and parent's point of view (Dainty et al., 2021). Some professionals are concerned about legal ramifications of the family's presence during cardiopulmonary resuscitation but the positives for both the family and healthcare team outweigh the negatives (Jones et al., 2011; Oczkowski et al., 2015).

## Resuscitation and Stabilization in Low-Resource Settings

The content of this chapter has focused on resuscitation and stabilization in high-resource settings. With the globalization of healthcare and the increase in healthcare providers from developed countries traveling to countries with limited resources to teach neonatal resuscitation and care to improve neonatal survival, it has, however, become evident that our care practices do not translate to the low-resource settings where medical equipment, supplies, personnel, and even electricity are limited. Because of this, AAP joined with the United States Agency for International Development, Laerdal Global Health, Johnson & Johnson, Save the Children, and other global organizations to develop an educational program to teach healthcare providers in a limited resource setting to resuscitate and care for term and preterm newborns. The program is called Helping Babies Survive and consists of three educational suites: Helping Babies Breathe (HBB), Essential Care for Every Baby (ECEB), and Essential Care for Small Babies (ECSB). HBB was launched in 2010 and was the first of the three educational programs. The HBB goal is to give every baby born in the world a chance to take its first breath and focuses on resuscitation. Since it has been in use, HBB has been translated into over 25 languages and has helped improve neonatal care in over 80 countries. The other two educational suites, ECEB and ECSB, were launched in 2014 and 2015, respectively, to help improve care after the birth of the baby (AAP, 2023).

The HBB is an evidence-based hands-on training tool that uses the same evidence incorporated into NRP. NRP and HBB are not interchangeable courses, though, and the main difference between the two is that HBB was designed for resource-limited (equipment and personnel) settings and uses different educational methodology, mentorship, and quality improvement components. Since HBB was launched in 2010, a 47% reduction in neonatal mortality and a 24% reduction in fresh stillbirths has been documented in areas that have implemented the program (AAP, 2023). Because of the success of HBB, ECEB and ECSB were developed to help with the postdelivery care of the neonate. The same methodology of education is used with both ECEB and ECSB as in HBB.

## SUMMARY

Although most depressed infants respond to drying, warming, positioning, suctioning, and tactile stimulation, every obstetric and neonatal unit should be adequately equipped and well prepared to handle neonatal emergencies. To provide neonatal care effectively, nurses must understand the cardiorespiratory transition and must be able to identify factors that may interfere with successful transition, comprehend the principles of resuscitation, and intervene on the basis of assessment of respirations, HR, and color.

## CASE STUDY

**Identification of the Problem.** A 40-year-old is admitted to labor & delivery (L&D) for preterm labor and imminent emergency cesarean section requiring resuscitation of the preterm infant.

**Assessment: History and Physical Examination.** A 40-year-old Caucasian female is admitted to the labor and delivery unit via the emergency squad. The mother states she is approximately 28 weeks' gestation, she reports contractions, and she noticed a gush of blood-tinged fluid at home an hour ago when voiding. She has had regular prenatal examinations and is negative on all serologies. She denies taking any prescription, nonprescription, or over-the-counter medications except for a multivitamin with iron. A urine toxicology screen on the mother was negative; a glucose tolerance test was negative.

On examination, membranes are noted to be ruptured with bloody amniotic fluid, the cervix is dilated to 8 cm and 100% effaced. Fetal heart tones are audible but faint and a category III fetal HR pattern is demonstrated on the fetal monitor. The mother is taken for an emergency cesarean birth.

**Differential Diagnosis**

a. Preterm infant
b. Respiratory distress
c. Hypothermia due to prematurity
d. Potential for hypovolemia due to bleeding

**Development of Management Plan.** *Preparation for Delivery*: Increase the delivery room temperature to 78°F (25.5°C) and 82°F (27.8°C), preheat radiant warmer in manual mode, place chemical thermal mattress between mattress and blanket with plastic side down (do not activate until the baby is born), place a polyethylene bag/wrap on top of blanket. Assemble personal protective equipment (PPF) and ensure a neonatal stethoscope is present. A bulb syringe should be present as well as a suction catheter with tubing connected to wall suction set at 100 mm Hg. For intubation, a properly functioning laryngoscope with an appropriate size blade (0 or 00), a 2.5 ET tube with stylet, a pulse oximeter, and cardiac monitor should be at the bedside. An umbilical cord insertion tray with a 3.5 umbilical catheter should be present as well as epinephrine at 0.1 mg/ml (1 mg/10 ml) and normal saline. In addition, appropriately sized syringes for ET and IV epinephrine and normal saline fluid bolus should be available. A minimum of 2 NRP-trained personnel will be needed for resuscitation with one of them able to intubate and place an umbilical line. Additional personnel may be required to assist with resuscitation.

At delivery, the baby is pale blue and limp with minimal respiratory effort, so immediate cord clamping is done and the neonate is taken to the warming bed for resuscitation. The baby appears to be an AGA 28-week infant and approximately 850 g.

**Implementation.** Warm and dry: Place on preheated radiant warmer and into the polyethylene bag, place temperature probe on the infant (titrate as necessary); place hat on baby's head, stimulate baby, place head in sniffing position and open mouth, suction infant's mouth and then nose with bulb suction. Place cardiac leads and pulse oximeter on right hand.

Infant remains apneic with HR 40 and pulse oximeter is not reading.

Start bag/mask ventilation with oxygen at 30% $F_IO_2$ at a rate of 40 to 60 breaths/min (one breath every 2 to 3 seconds).

No chest rise observed. Perform "MR SOPA" steps:

- Mask.
- Reposition airway.
- Attempt to ventilate, no chest rise.
- Suction.
- Open airway.
- Attempt to ventilate, no chest rise.
- Increase pressure (PIP).
- Place alternate airway.

The baby is intubated orally with a 2.5 ET tube on the first attempt. There are no spontaneous respirations, and the HR improved slightly to 55 beats/min and oxygen saturation 50 after 30 seconds of PPV.

Begin cardiac compressions at a ratio of 3 compressions to 1 breath. Increase $F_IO_2$ to 100% with compressions. Begin to prepare for line insertion. After 60 seconds of chest compressions and breaths, the HR remains at 55 beats/min. An initial dose of epinephrine 0.1 mg/kg (1 ml/kg) of the 0.1 mg/ml to 1 mg/10 ml concentration is given via the ET tube while line placement occurs.

The umbilical cord is tied, cleaned, cut, and a 3.5 UVC is advanced 2 to 4 cm with blood return and is secured. The HR remains at 55 beats/min and epinephrine 0.2 mg/kg (0.2 ml/kg) of the 0.1 mg/ml = 1 mg/10 ml concentration is given via the UVC and followed with a 3 ml normal saline (NS) flush. After 60 seconds, HR has increased to 70 beats/min and the oxygen saturation is now 66. Pulses are weak and baby is still very pale. A 10 ml/kg dose of normal saline is administered over 5 and 10 minutes with the neonate HR increasing to 115 and oxygen saturation rising to 98% on 100% oxygen at 10 minutes of age. Begin to wean $F_IO_2$ in 5% increments to keep $O_2$ saturations no > 95%.

**Working Diagnosis (unknown diagnosis).** Premature infant 28 weeks' gestation, postresuscitation. **Evaluation of Effectiveness**

Neonate HR and pulse oximetry readings in normal limits with respirations being supported.

**Outcome.** Infant transferred to NICU for further care and treatment.

**Diagnostic Tests.** No diagnostic tests in the delivery room but once in the NICU, chest/abdominal x-ray, complete blood count (CBC) with differential and platelets, blood cultures, IV fluids started and placed on a ventilator and cardiac monitor in the NICU.

## ONLINE RESOURCES

CourseConnect

Resources for this chapter are online and available at www.springerpub.com/courseconnect.

## REFERENCES

References for this chapter are online and available at www.springerpub.com/courseconnect.

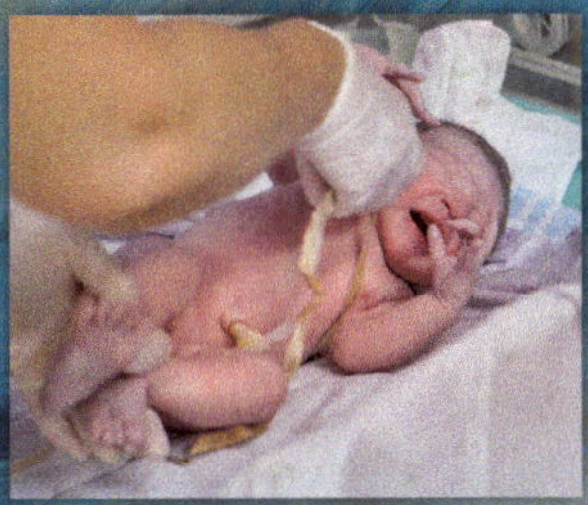

Source: Андрей Журавлев/Adobe Stock.

CHAPTER 4

# Assessment of the Newborn and Infant

Terri A. Cavaliere

## INTRODUCTION

Assessment is a continuous evaluation process throughout the neonatal period. Physical examinations are performed for many reasons and at various times. They can be brief checks or more structured, comprehensive analyses to determine wellness or evaluate specific problems. The results serve as platforms for clinical judgments about diagnoses and treatments. This chapter addresses various aspects of comprehensive physical assessments of the neonate.

## FIRST NEONATAL ASSESSMENT AND THE APGAR SCORE

The initial assessment occurs immediately after delivery with the allocation of Apgar scores. Virginia Apgar developed this tool to indicate the clinical status of infants immediately after delivery (Apgar, 1953). The score consists of five elements, assigned at 1 and 5 minutes, with each component receiving 0, 1, or 2 points, which are then tallied to provide a total score (Table 4.1). It should be performed at 1 and 5 minutes; however, if the total score is below 7 at 5 minutes, the assessment is repeated every 5 minutes for up to 20 minutes.

The Apgar score is a rapid means of evaluating a neonate's clinical condition and/or the response to resuscitation. Although the Apgar score was initially designed to assess the need for intervention to establish breathing at 1 minute, the score should not be used to determine the initial need for intervention, what interventions are required, or when to intervene, because resuscitation must begin before the 1-minute Apgar score is assigned (Simon et al., 2024).

Apgar scores should not be used to predict morbidity or mortality but to convey information about the newborn's response to resuscitation (Goldsmith, 2025). If assigned during resuscitation, it is not equivalent to one given to a spontaneously breathing infant. No accepted standard exists for assigning an Apgar score during resuscitation after birth; many of the elements contributing to the score are affected by resuscitation (Simon et al., 2024).

**TABLE 4.1**

**APGAR SCORING SYSTEM**

| Component | Assigned Score | | |
|---|---|---|---|
| | 0 | 1 | 2 |
| Heart rate (beats/min) | Absent | < 100 (slow) | 100 |
| Respiratory effort | None | Weak cry; hypoventilation | Good, strong cry |
| Muscle tone | Limp | Some flexion | Active motion |
| Reflex irritability | No response | Grimace | Cough or sneeze |
| Color | Blue or pale | Extremities blue | Completely pink |

*Source:* Adapted from Goldsmith, J. P. (2025). Overview and initial management of delivery room resuscitation. In R. J. Martin, A. A. Fanaroff, & M. C. Walsh (Eds.), *Fanaroff & Martin's neonatal-perinatal medicine: Diseases of the fetus and infant* (12th ed., Vol. 1, pp. 530–544). Elsevier.

## OTHER CONSIDERATIONS FOR THE INITIAL NEONATAL ASSESSMENT

Before the infant leaves the delivery area, a brief physical examination should be performed. Components include inspection for birth injuries, major congenital anomalies, and evaluation of pulmonary and cardiovascular adjustment to extrauterine life. Appraisal of early transition to extrauterine life includes observation of color, adequacy of perfusion and oxygenation; assessment of respiratory effort; auscultation of breath sounds and heart sounds; and inspection of the amount, color, and consistency of secretions. Tone, activity, and appropriateness of state should also be noted. A cursory inspection of all external areas is necessary before the infant leaves the delivery area, including a general evaluation of the external genitalia and, in males, palpation for testes in the scrotum. The entire examination should be performed under a radiant heat source to prevent significant heat loss from the infant.

## Evaluation of Transition

Adaptation to both intrapartum and neonatal events is reflected in the transition from a fetal to an extrauterine environment. These events result in sympathetic activity that affects the infant's color, respiration, heart rate, behavioral state, gastrointestinal (GI) function, and temperature (Gardner, 2020). Physiologic and biochemical changes characteristic of transition affect the physical findings of early examinations. The examination performed during transition is described separately because findings that are normal during transition may be abnormal if they appear at other times.

As the neonate's circulation adjusts to the extrauterine pathway, there may be a period in which pulmonary vascular resistance remains greater than systemic vascular resistance, resulting in a right-to-left shunt across the ductus arteriosus. Higher preductal oxygen saturation causes the neonate's face and upper body to appear pink while the lower body and legs appear pale or blue, creating a visible demarcation across the chest. Transitional differential cyanosis subsides as circulation changes from the fetal to the neonatal pathway. Acrocyanosis is common during this period. To evaluate babies with deeper skin pigmentation, the nurse should observe the color of the mucous membranes. When the neonate is stimulated, the skin may appear blushed or bright red; this color change is called *erythema neonatorum*, or generalized hyperemia, which develops a few hours after birth. It generally resolves within several minutes to an hour and rarely appears with the same intensity (Gomella, 2020). Erythema neonatorum is not synonymous with erythema toxicum neonatorum.

The neonatal heart rate may range from 160 to 180 beats per minute (beats/min) in the first 15 minutes; it slowly falls to a baseline rate of 100 to 120 beats/min by 30 minutes. The heart rate is labile, and brief periods of asymptomatic, irregular heart rates are not pathologic. Murmurs are common, because the ductus arteriosus may still be patent. Respirations are also irregular during the first 15 minutes, ranging from 60 to 100 breaths per minute (breaths/min). Grunting, flaring, retractions, and brief periods of apnea may also be seen. Crackles may be present on auscultation (Gardner, 2020).

Despite the changes in the heart and respiratory rates during the initial 15 to 30 minutes of life, healthy-term infants are awake and alert. They may rest quietly, cry periodically, startle spontaneously, and breastfeed during this period. Full-term babies often show flexed posture with good muscle tone; preterm newborns, in comparison, have less flexion and tone. Temperature has decreased, and gastrointestinal (GI) activity includes the establishment of bowel sounds and the production of saliva. This first period of reactivity may be prolonged in infants who have experienced difficult labor and delivery, in sick term infants, and well premature infants (Gardner, 2020).

After the first period of reactivity, the infant is relatively unresponsive or sleeping, and the heart rate drops to a baseline of 100 to 120 beats/min. This interval, approximately 60 to 100 minutes in length, is followed by a second period of reactivity, which lasts anywhere from 10 minutes to several hours. During this time the infant may show rapid color changes, intermittent tachypnea and tachycardia, and changes in tone. A healthy infant may have periods during which the respiratory rate is considerably higher than 60 breaths/min; however, the infant does not appear distressed and can slow this rate enough to nipple feed successfully. Meconium often is passed during this period (Gardner, 2020). Figure 4.1 summarizes some of the physical changes seen during the transition period.

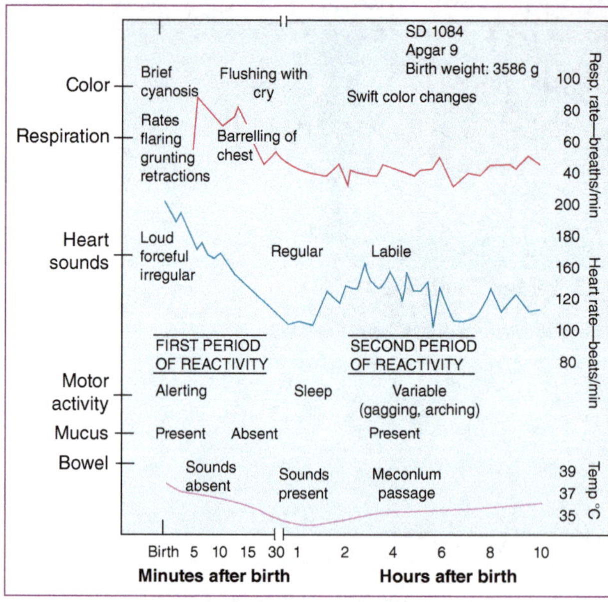


**FIGURE 4.1 Normal transition period.**

*Source:* Based on Desmond, M. M., Rudolph, A. J., & Phitaksphraiwan, P. (1966). The transitional care nursery. A mechanism for preventive medicine in the newborn. *Pediatric Clinics of North America, 13*(3), 651–668. https://doi.org/10.1016/S0031-3955(16)31875-2.

## Newborn Examination

The comprehensive newborn examination should be performed within the first 12 to 18 hours of life after transition has been completed successfully. The examination should be initiated when the infant is quiet and should progress from assessments that are least likely to disturb the infant to those that are most irritating. An examination sequence based on the infant's state is outlined in Table 4.2.

**TABLE 4.2**

## EXAMINATION SEQUENCE BASED ON INFANT'S STATE

| Assessment Technique | Required State | Arousing Maneuver | Equipment |
|---|---|---|---|
| Observe general appearance | | | |
| Observe color | | | |
| Observe resting posture | Quiet | | |
| Observe spontaneous activity | Active | | |
| Count respirations | Quiet | | Clock |
| Count heartbeats | Quiet | | Clock |
| Inspect facies at rest | Quiet | | |
| Auscultate heart sounds | Quiet | | Stethoscope |
| Auscultate breath sounds | Quiet | | Stethoscope |
| Measure blood pressure | Quiet | | Blood pressure cuff |
| Inspect head and neck region | | | |
| Stimulate response to sound | Quiet | | Calibrated noise maker |
| Inspect trunk anteriorly | | | |
| Palpate abdomen, cardiac impulse | Quiet | | |
| Feel pulses | | | |
| Examine genitalia | | | Lubricant for rectal examination |
| Inspect trunk posteriorly | | | |
| Inspect arms and hands | | | |
| Inspect legs and feet | | | |
| Assess passive tone | | | |
| Assess active tone | Active | X | |

(*continued*)

**TABLE 4.2**

**EXAMINATION SEQUENCE BASED ON INFANT'S STATE (*continued*)**

| Assessment Technique | Required State | Arousing Maneuver | Equipment |
|---|---|---|---|
| Elicit primitive reflexes | Active | X | |
| Assess muscle strength | Active | X | |
| Assess GA | | | |
| Test range in major joints | | X | |
| Manipulate hips | | X | |
| Measure temperature | | | Thermometer |
| Examine ears | | | Otoscope |
| Determine pupil response | | | Bright light |
| Examine fundi | Quiet | X | |
| Elicit tendon reflexes | | X | Percussion hammer |
| Stimulate response to pain | | X | |
| Weigh infant | Quiet | X | Scales, growth chart |
| Measure length, head, chest, and abdominal circumferences | | X | Tape measure, growth chart |
| Transilluminate head | | X | High-intensity light |
| Percuss abdomen and lungs | Quiet | | |

*Source:* Data from Fletcher, M. A. (1998). *Physical diagnosis in neonatology*. Lippincott-Raven.

## Discharge Examination

The discharge examination is to assess the neonate's ability to be cared for outside the controlled environment of the hospital. The needs of a healthy, full-term infant being discharged home with the mother are different from those of a growing, preterm infant who has been hospitalized for weeks or months and who has significant sequelae. Evaluating the caretaker's capability to care for and observe changes in the infant is an important aspect of the discharge assessment and follow-up plan. Anticipatory guidance regarding feedings, sleeping position and environment, skin care, safety practices, and recognition of signs and symptoms of illness should be provided.

## Outpatient Examination

The first outpatient examination focuses on the infant's adaptation to the home environment, including evaluation of any issues noticed at discharge. Some factors to be considered are temperature stability, ability and success at feeding and elimination, sleep patterns, normal color, condition of the umbilical stump, reassessment of hip stability, and state and behavior. Any inaccessible areas during earlier examinations should be included (eyes, ear canals, and eardrums) (Fletcher, 1998).

The birth history, including birth and discharge weights, gestational age (GA), and any problems, should be reviewed. As part of the complete physical examination, height, weight, and head circumference should be plotted and developmental progress observed. The results of newborn metabolic screening (if available) and the infant's immunization status should be reviewed. Anticipatory guidance issues include nutrition, elimination, sleep patterns, development and behavior, social and family relationships, and injury prevention.

### Environment

This should take place in a quiet, warm environment. The room should be well lit, yet the light should not be so strong that the infant is deterred from opening the eyes. Prevention of heat loss is critical to the comfort and the maintenance of thermal neutrality and glucose homeostasis. Most healthy-term infants can tolerate being undressed in a reasonably warm room for the 5 to 10 minutes required to perform the physical assessment. If the environment is cool or drafty, an external heat source should be provided.

A placid infant provides the best opportunity for gathering meaningful data. Extraneous environmental noise hampers auscultation and assessment of bodily sounds and may be overwhelming, causing changes in state and cardiovascular status (Honeyfield, 2025). Handling the infant gently and speaking in a soothing voice allows the examiner to complete most of the assessment without distressing the infant. Disturbing components of the examination, such as deep palpation of the abdomen and assessment of the hips, should be performed last.

Having one or both parents present during the routine neonatal assessment offers the opportunity to judge their competence in caregiving and to educate them about their infant's unique physical traits, behavior, and coping skills. The examiner may also use this time to build rapport and trust with the parents, to listen to their concerns, and to offer pertinent information. Some issues may require privacy for discussion; therefore, confidentiality should be considered when conversing with parents in the presence of others.

## COMPREHENSIVE HISTORY

The neonatal history is very similar to that of an older child or adult, including information about the past medical history, the current condition, and the family. For a newly delivered infant, the initial neonatal assessment probably will be conducted before speaking to the parents. Basic information about pregnancy and delivery should be available in the maternal records; a complete history lays the foundation for the comprehensive newborn examination and should be elicited directly from the parents.

The components of a complete history are summarized in Table 4.3. After the data collected from the complete history and physical assessment are organized and all expected and

**TABLE 4.3**

**COMPONENTS OF A COMPREHENSIVE NEONATAL HISTORY**

| Component | Data Required |
|---|---|
| Identifying data | Infant's name; parents' names; parents' telephone numbers (home and work); infant's date of birth, gender, and race; and source of referral (obstetric or pediatric provider) if any. |
| Chief complaint | Statement of initial known status (age, gender, birth and current weights, and GA by dates and examination) and any problems. |
| Interim history/history of newborn | Chronologic record of newborn's history delivery to present should answer questions related to where (location), what (quality, factors that aggravate or relieve symptoms), when (onset, duration, frequency), and how much (intensity, severity). |
| Antepartum history | Historical data about the pregnancy, including maternal age, gravidity, parity, last menstrual period, and estimated delivery date. Date and GA at which prenatal care began, provider of care, and number of visits should be recorded here. Maternal health during pregnancy, infections, medications taken, use of illicit drugs or alcohol, abnormal bleeding, and results of prenatal screening tests should also be included. |
| Obstetric history | Significant history regarding previous pregnancies; neonatal problems or subsequent major medical problems of previous children and current age and health status of living children should be noted. |

*(continued)*

**TABLE 4.3**

**COMPONENTS OF A COMPREHENSIVE NEONATAL HISTORY (*continued*)**

| Component | Data Required |
|---|---|
| Intrapartum history | Duration of labor, whether spontaneous or induced, duration of rupture of membranes, type of delivery, complications; infant's birth weight, presentation at delivery, and Apgar scores; resuscitative measures if required and response to those measures. |
| Past medical history | Significant maternal history of chronic health problems or diseases treated in the past or during the pregnancy, including surgical procedures and hospitalizations before or during the pregnancy. |
| Family medical history | Significant family medical history of chronic disorders, disabilities, known hereditary diseases, or consanguinity. Incorporation of a family history tool may reveal genetic conditions. |
| Social history | Parents' marital status, paternal involvement, occupations, and educational level; sources of financial support, housing accommodations, and insurance status must be noted, as well as any support agencies involved. Family units should be defined and religious and cultural affiliations noted, along with the number of individuals living in the home. Plans for childcare should be elicited, as well as any current family stressors (e.g., moving, death in the family). |

unexpected findings have been reviewed, areas of concern are identified and prioritized for further evaluation and attention. This forms the framework for a clinical diagnosis and plan of care.

It is vital that, in communicating with parents from diverse cultures, nurses appreciate and respect differences in communication patterns and in childbearing and health practices. Knowledge of cultural variations in family and health practices assists nurses in developing sensitivity to differences; however, the family must be observed carefully for cues to family practices and relationships with children and one another.

## Physical Assessment Techniques

The techniques used for physical assessment are inspection, palpation, percussion, and auscultation. Learning these skills requires patience and practice, and the inability of the newborn to provide verbal cues presents an additional challenge. With experience, the practitioner learns to process a multitude of observations while assessing individual systems and then to use these data to form a clinical impression and plan of care. (Honeyfield, 2025)

**Inspection.** Inspection is the simple yet intricate use of the auditory and visual senses to evaluate state, color, respiratory effort, posture, and activity, as well as the shape and symmetry of various body regions. It is a crucial skill in the physical assessment of neonates, but it is also a difficult one to master. The sense of smell may be used to note unusual odors. Impressions acquired from methodical observation establish priorities for the remainder of the systematic assessment. In the physical examination, thoughtful observation, rather than simple looking, is the most efficient means of detecting changes. Inspection should be used throughout the physical assessment and should continue if the infant remains in the nurse's care.

**Auscultation.** Auscultation involves listening for bodily sounds (Honeyfield, 2025). The bell of the stethoscope is used for low-pitched sounds (e.g., cardiovascular sounds) and the diaphragm for higher pitched sounds (e.g., lung and bowel sounds). The stethoscope should be placed lightly but firmly against the wall of the body part being assessed. A calm infant and quiet environment facilitate auscultation. Practice in recognizing normal body sounds is required before abnormal sounds can be identified accurately

**Palpation.** Here, touch is used to determine hydration, texture, tension, pulsation, vibration, amplitude, and tenderness, as well as the depth, size, shape, and location of deep structures. Palpation must be gentle and is performed with the flats of the finger pads rather than the fingertips (Honeyfield, 2025). To gather the most accurate information, the infant should be calm at the onset of the abdominal examination. Relaxing the abdominal musculature by flexing the infant's knees and with one hand facilitates palpation of the liver and spleen. Gentle pressure is necessary during palpation of sensitive organs (e.g., liver, spleen, and skin) at risk for injury and bleeding. Warm hands, use of a pacifier, and progression from superficial to deep palpation help maintain the infant's comfort throughout most of the examination. Tender areas should always be palpated last.

**Percussion.** Percussion, direct or indirect, is the use of tapping to produce sound waves that may be assessed according to intensity, pitch, duration, and quality (Table 4.4). Direct percussion targets the body part with the tip of the middle

TABLE 4.4

PERCUSSION SOUNDS

| Type of Sound | Intensity | Pitch | Duration | Quality | Common Locations |
|---|---|---|---|---|---|
| Tympany | Loud | High | Moderate | Drum like | Gastric air-filled intestine (tapping puffed out cheeks) |
| Resonance | Moderate to loud | Low | Long | Hollow | Lungs |
| Hyperresonance | Very loud | Very low | Long | Booming | Lungs with trapped air; lungs of a young child |
| Dullness | Soft to moderate | High | Moderate | Thud like | Liver, fluid-filled space (e.g., stomach) |
| Flatness | Soft | High | Short | Flat | Muscle |

*Source:* Data from Engel, J. (2006). *Pocket guide to pediatric assessment* (5th ed.). Mosby.

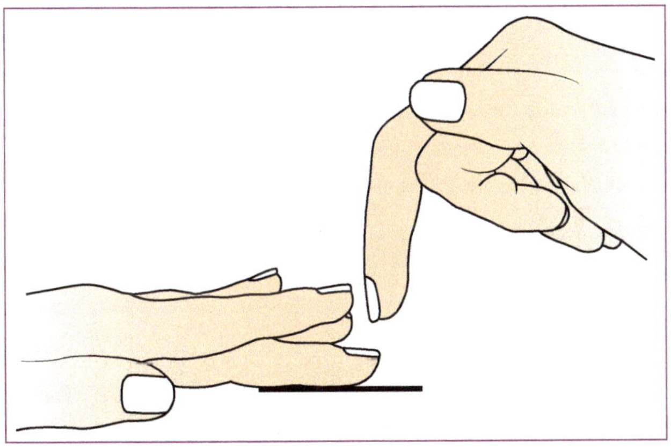

**FIGURE 4.2 Percussion technique. Note the position of the fingers.**

*Source:* From Engel, J. (2006). *Pocket guide to pediatric assessment* (5th ed.). Mosby.

right finger, while with indirect percussion, the examiner places the middle finger of the nondominant hand against the skin of the body part to be assessed and strikes the distal joint of the nondominant hand. Vibrations are transmitted from the bones of the finger joint touching the infant's body to the underlying tissue. See Figure 4.2.

## Assessment of Size and Growth

Well-being in the fetal and neonatal periods is reflected by a normal growth pattern. Fetal and neonatal growth rates are predictable and can be measured by various methods. To determine if growth is adequate, an appropriate standard must be used with which the child's measurements can be compared. The growth curves used must match the patient as closely as possible in gender, race, GA, genetic potential, and environmental factors, such as altitude. A discussion of the techniques used to estimate and assess fetal growth is beyond the scope of this chapter and can be found elsewhere in this text

## Assessment of Gestational Age

A determination of GA is part of the assessment of every newborn; although formal assessments of GA may be unnecessary for routine newborn examinations (Griswold & Srinivas, 2025). According to these authors, the most useful tools for GA estimates of normal, healthy, term neonates are "early antenatal ultrasound evaluation combined with information about the mother's last menstrual period" (p. 470).

Classification of newborns by GA enables healthcare providers to identify possible disorders and initiate intervention or screening. Table 4.5 presents terms used in GA assessment and in determining the adequacy of in utero growth.

Neonates with the lowest risk of problems associated with morbidity and mortality are term infants who developmentally are appropriate for GA. Risks associated with categories of GA and intrauterine growth restriction (IUGR) are shown in Table 4.6.

GA is determined by the evaluation of physical, neurologic, and neuromuscular characteristics. The New Ballard score (NBS) is a widely used assessment tool (Figure 4.3; Table 4.7). It includes six neurologic and six physical criteria and permits assessment of extremely premature infants. Despite its advantages over the other scoring systems, the NBS is accurate only to within 2 weeks and tends toward overestimating the GA of extremely premature neonates (Griswold & Srinivas, 2025). Performing the examination as soon as possible in the first 12 hours of life enhances its accuracy.

**TABLE 4.5**

**TERMS AND ABBREVIATIONS USED IN ASSESSMENT OF GA AND ADEQUACY OF INTRAUTERINE GROWTH**

| Term and Abbreviation | Description |
|---|---|
| Low birth weight (LBW) | Infant weighing < 2,500 g |
| Very low birth weight (VLBW) | Infant weighing < 1,500 g |
| Extremely low birth weight (ELBW) | Infant weighing < 1,000 g |
| AGA | Parameter (weight) within the 10th–90th percentile for GA |
| LGA | Parameter above the 90th percentile for GA |
| SGA | Parameter below the 10th percentile for GA |
| IUGR | Slowing of intrauterine growth documented by ultrasound; a neonate may be IUGR without being SGA |
| Symmetric IUGR | Measurements for weight, length, and head circumference all within the same growth curve even if neonate is AGA, LGA, or SGA |
| Asymmetric IUGR | Measurements for weight, length, and head circumference in different growth curves |
| Early term gestation | Neonate delivered between 37 0/7 and 38 6/7 weeks |
| Term gestation | Neonate born between 37 and 42 weeks' gestation |
| Preterm gestation | Neonate delivered before completion of week 37 of gestation |
| Late preterm | Neonate delivered between 34 0/7 and 36 6/7 weeks |
| Postterm gestation | Neonate delivered after completion of week 42 of gestation |

AGA, appropriate for gestational age; IUGR, intrauterine growth restriction; LGA, large for gestational age; SGA, small for gestational age.

**TABLE 4.6**

**RISKS ASSOCIATED WITH GESTATIONAL AGE AND INTRAUTERINE GROWTH RESTRICTION**

| Category | Risks |
|---|---|
| SGA, LGA, IUGR | Perinatal and long-term problems |
| Preterm SGA | Problems associated with immaturity of body systems and placental insufficiency |
| Preterm | Problems associated with immaturity of body systems |
| Postterm | Problems associated with placental insufficiency |
| Term LGA | Risks are greatest in perinatal period, but long-term problems can develop |

IUGR, intrauterine growth retardation/restriction; LGA, large for gestational age; SGA, small for gestational age.

**Neuromuscular Maturity**

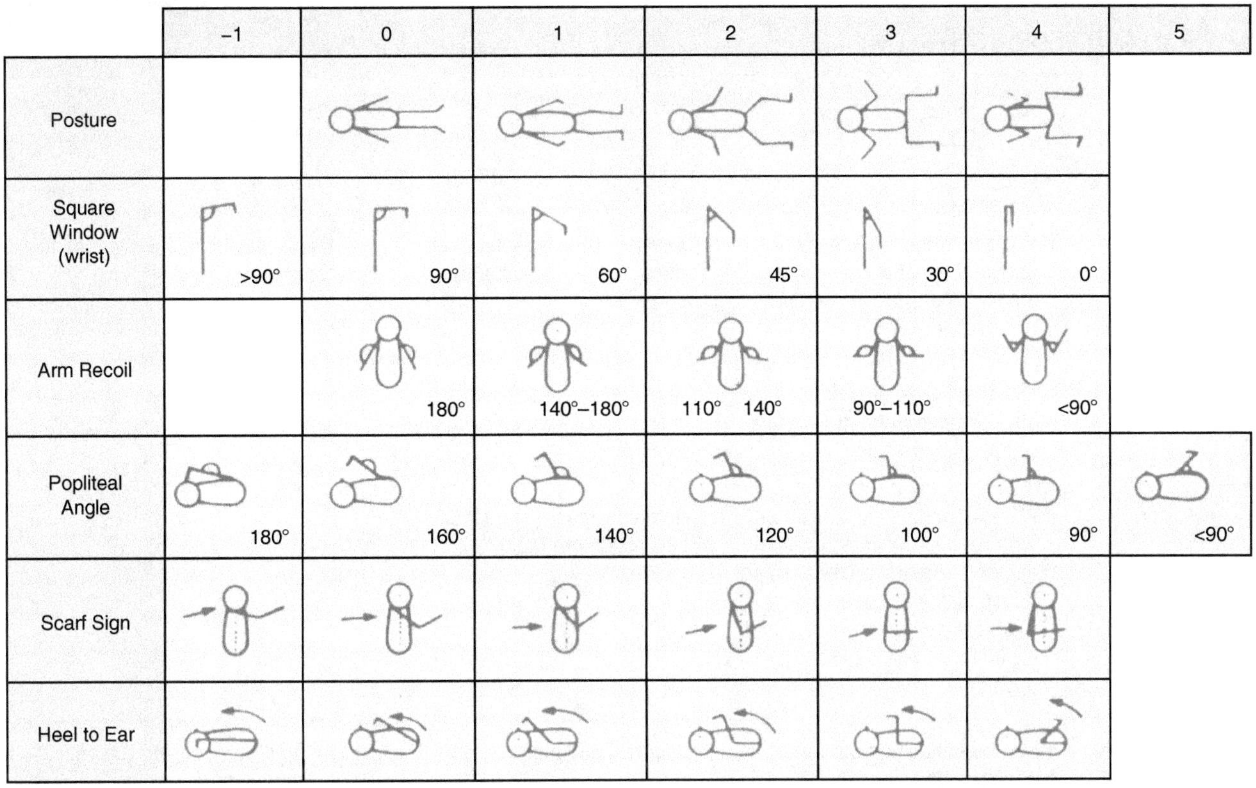


**Physical Maturity**

| | | | | | | | |
|---|---|---|---|---|---|---|---|
| Skin | sticky friable transparent | gelatinous red, translucent | smooth pink, visible veins | superficial peeling and/ or rash few veins | cracking pale areas rare veins | parchment deep cracking no vessels | leathery cracked wrinkled |
| Lanugo | none | sparse | abundant | thinning | bald areas | mostly bald | |
| Plantar Surface | heel-toe 40–50 mm: –1 <40 mm: –2 | >50 mm no crease | faint red marks | anterior transverse crease only | creases ant. 2/3 | creases over entire sole | |
| Breast | imperceptible | barely perceptible | flat areola no bud | stippled areola 1–2 mm bud | raised areola 3–4 mm bud | full areola 5–10 mm bud | |
| Eye/Ear | lids fused loosely: –1 tightly: –2 | lids open pinna flat stays folded | sl. curved pinna; soft; slow recoil | well-curved pinna; soft but ready recoil | formed and firm instant recoil | thick cartilage ear stiff | |
| Genitals (male) | scrotum flat smooth | scrotum empty faint rugae | testes in upper canal rare rugae | testes descending few rugae | testes down good rugae | testes pendulous deep rugae | |
| Genitals (female) | clitoris prominent labia flat | prominent clitoris small labia minora | prominent clitoris enlarging minora | majora and minora equally prominent | majora large minora small | majora cover clitoris and minora | |

**Maturity Rating**

| score | weeks |
|---|---|
| –10 | 20 |
| –5 | 22 |
| 0 | 24 |
| 5 | 26 |
| 10 | 28 |
| 15 | 30 |
| 20 | 32 |
| 25 | 34 |
| 30 | 36 |
| 35 | 38 |
| 40 | 40 |
| 45 | 42 |
| 50 | 44 |

**FIGURE 4.3 Components of New Ballard score.**

*Source:* From Ballard, J. L., Khoury, J. C., Wedig, K., Wang, L., Eilers-Walsman, B. L., & Lipp, R. (1991). New Ballard score, expanded to include extremely premature infants. *Journal of Pediatrics, 119*, 417–423. https://doi.org/10.1016/S0022-3476(05)82056-6.

## TABLE 4.7

### NEW BALLARD SCORING SYSTEM

| Component | Assessment Technique | Effect of Maturity | Comments |
|---|---|---|---|
| ***Neuromuscular Maturity*** | | | |
| Posture | Observe infant while baby is unrestrained and supine; note amount of flexion and extension of extremities. | Extensor tone is replaced by flexor tone in a cephalocaudal progression. | Knees may be hyperextended in a frank breech delivery. |
| Square window | Flex wrist; measure minimum angle formed by ventral surface of forearm and palm. | Angle decreases; at term, there is no space between palm and forearm. | Response depends on muscle tone and intrauterine position. |
| Arm recoil | Place infant in supine position with head in midline; flex elbow and hold forearm against arm for 5 seconds; fully extend elbow, then release; note time required for infant to resume flexed position. | Angle decreases and recoil becomes more rapid. | |
| Popliteal angle | Flex hips, placing thighs on abdomen; keeping hips on surface of bed, extending the knee as far as possible until resistance is met; estimate popliteal angle. | Popliteal angle decreases. | Amount of extension can be beyond point where resistance is first met; this assessment also is affected by intrauterine position and hip dislocation. |
| Scarf sign | With head in midline, pull hand across chest to encircle neck; note position of elbow relative to midline. | Increased resistance to crossing the midline. | Reflects muscle tone; response is altered by obesity, hydrops, or fractured clavicle. |
| Heel to ear | Keep infant supine with pelvis on mattress; press feet as far as possible toward head, allowing knees to be positioned beside abdomen; estimate angle created by arc from back of heel to mattress. | Angle decreases; hip flexion decreases toward term. | Reflects muscle tone. |
| ***Physical Maturity*** | | | |
| Skin | Observe translucency of skin over abdominal wall. | Skin becomes thicker and ultimately dry and peeling; pigmentation increases. | Skin becomes drier hours after birth; phototherapy or sunlight enhances pigmentation. |

(*continued*)

**TABLE 4.7**

## NEW BALLARD SCORING SYSTEM (*continued*)

| Component | Assessment Technique | Effect of Maturity | Comments |
|---|---|---|---|
| Lanugo | Assess for presence and length of hair over back. | Lanugo emerges at 19–20 weeks and is most prominent at 27–28 weeks; then gradually disappears, first from the lower back and then from at least half of the back. | The degree of pigmentation and quantity of hair are related to race, nutritional status. |
| Plantar surface | Measure length of foot; determine presence or absence of true deep creases (not merely wrinkles). | Early in gestation, foot length correlates with fetal growth; creases develop from toes to heel, and absence of creases correlates with immaturity. | Plantar creases also reflect intrauterine fetal activity; accelerated creasing is seen with oligohydramnios; diminished creasing suggests lack of activity in a mature fetus. |
| Breast | Estimate diameter of breast bud; assess color and stippling of areola. | Definition and stippling of areola and pigmentation are evident near term; bud size increases because of maternal hormones and fat accumulation. | With intrauterine growth restriction, breast tissue may be diminished, but development of areola proceeds regardless of malnutrition. |
| Ear cartilage | Fold top of auricle; observe speed of recoil. | Cartilage becomes stiff, and the auricle thickens. | Compression in utero and absence or dysfunction of auricular muscles diminishes firmness. |
| Eyelid opening | Without attempting to separate eyelids, evaluate the degree of fusion. | Opening begins at 22 weeks; lids are completely unfused by 28 weeks. | Fused eyelids should not be considered a sign of nonviability; lids may be fused at term with anophthalmia. |
| ***External Genitalia*** | | | |
| Male | Palpate scrotum to assess degree of descent of testes; observe rugae and suspension (cryptorchidism). | At 27–28 weeks, testes begin to descend into scrotum; rugae formation of scrotum begins at about 28 weeks; by term, rugae are well defined, and scrotum is pendulous. | Rugae are decreased with scrotal edema; testes may be absent. |
| Female | Assess size of labia minora and labia majora. | Labia minora increase in size before labia majora; at term, labia majora cover labia minora completely. | Size of labia majora depends on amount of body fat; with malnutrition, size may be diminished; edema may increase size of labia majora. |

*Source:* Adapted from Trotter, C. W. (2025). Gestational age assessment. In C. L. Witt & C. M. Wallman. (Eds.), *Tappero & Honeyfield's Physical assessment of the newborn* (7th ed., pp. 39–58). Springer Publishing Company.

## Clinical Assessment of Nutritional Status

GA assessment does not identify all infants with intrauterine malnutrition. Although the terms *small for gestational age* (SGA) and *intrauterine growth retardation/restriction* (IUGR) are related, they are not synonymous. IUGR represents a reduction in the expected fetal growth pattern, whereas SGA refers to an infant whose birth weight is less than population norms. Not all IUGR infants are SGA, and not all SGA infants are IUGR (Devaskar et al., 2025).

Many, but not all infants, who are either SGA or IUGR are malnourished in utero. However, malnutrition can occur in neonates of any birth weight. Because malnutrition alters body composition and can prevent adequate brain growth, it is important to identify infants who have been affected in utero. These infants may be at risk for problems associated with aberrant growth (Devaskar et al., 2025).

## Measurement Techniques

For most infants, the parameters of weight, length, and occipitofrontal circumference (OFC) are adequate for the basic physical assessment. These measurements are compared against standard growth curves. If the infant has any abnormalities in the size of a body component or if the infant shows disproportionate growth, further examination is warranted.

**Weight and Length.** Weight can be falsely increased by several factors, including clothing and infant motion. The weight of the average full-term infant who is appropriate for gestational age (AGA) is 3.5 kg, with a range of 2,700 to 4,000 g (Tappero, 2025). Birth weights are affected by genetics and geographic location. For instance, African American, Hawaiian, and Asian neonates weigh less than White infants (Tappero, 2025) and populations that live in high altitudes have babies that are normally smaller than cohorts born at sea level. It is helpful to use growth graphs that are specific for populations and locations if they are available.

The crown-to-heel length can be obtained using a measurement board or a standard tape measure. With the infant supine and legs extended, a line is drawn on the bed at the baby's head and another at the heels, then the distance between these two points is measured (Figure 4.4). The average full-term newborn is 50 cm long with a range of 48 to 53 cm (Tappero, 2025). Other measurement techniques are described in the appropriate sections.

## Physical Examination of the Neonate

The following sections describe the newborn examination beyond the transition period.

**Vital Signs.** Once transition is complete, the respiratory rate ranges between 40 and 60 breaths/min and may be irregular. Respirations are easy and unlabored; breath sounds should be clear on auscultation. The heart rate varies from 100 to 160 beats/min, depending on the infant's state and GA (Vargo, 2025). Premature neonates have a higher baseline heart rate. The resting heart rate is the most representative of any baby.

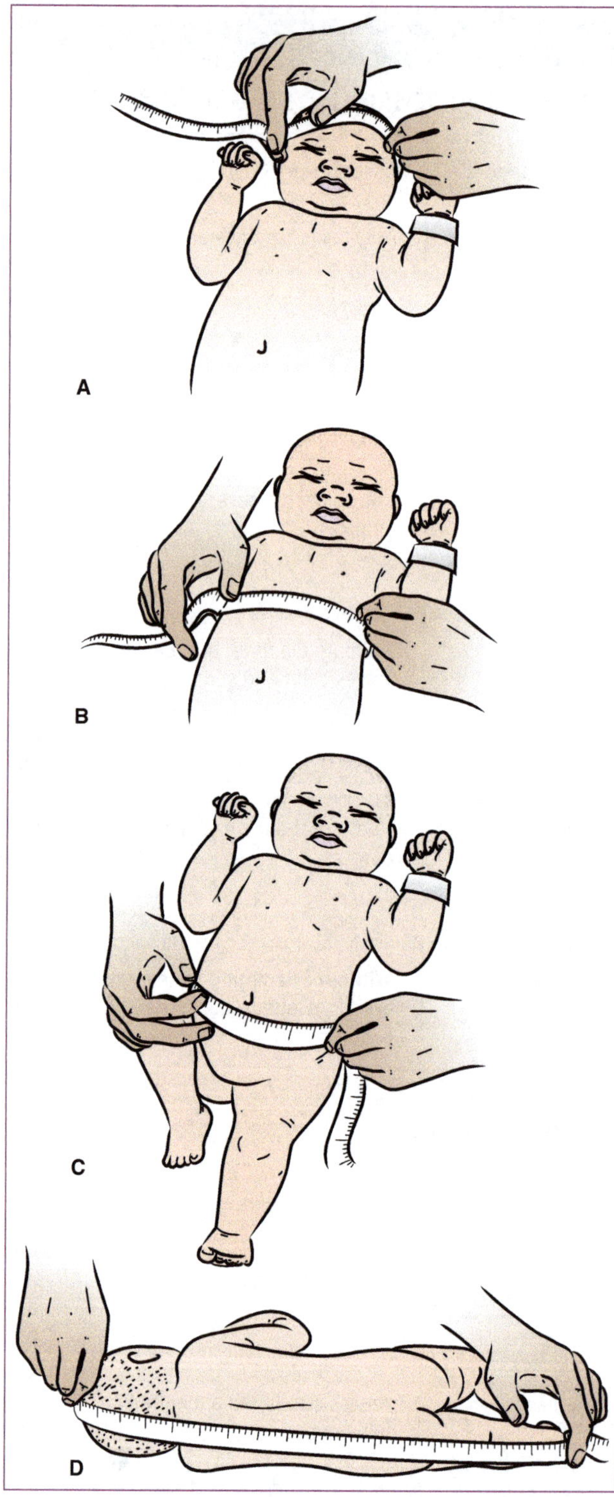


**FIGURE 4.4** Newborn measurements.

Bamba, V., & Kelly, A. (2025) Assessment of growth. In Robert M. Kliegman, Joseph W. St Geme, Nathan J. Blum, et al. (Eds.), *Nelson textbook of pediatrics*, (21st ed., pp. 172–178) Elsevier.

Normal blood pressure ranges depend on GA, chronologic age, methods used, and other variables. It should be assessed starting at routine well-child visits, at 3 years of age, and more frequently or earlier for children identified as high risk for hypertension (Hegyi et al., 1994). Temperature is determined by axillary measurement; acceptable values range from 95.9°F (35.5°C) to 99.5°F (37.5°C) (Gardner & Hernandez, 2016).

The heart is assessed for rate, rhythm, character of heart sounds, and presence of murmurs. In the first few days of life, the point of maximal impulse (PMI) is located at the fourth intercostal space at or to the left of the midclavicular line. Auscultation should be performed at the second and fourth intercostal spaces, cardiac apex, and axilla (Vargo, 2025). Murmurs are commonly heard before the ductus arteriosus is completely closed. Persistent murmurs may not be normal and require evaluation. Brief asymptomatic irregularities in rate and rhythm are not uncommon, especially in the preterm baby. The most common benign dysrhythmias are sinus bradycardia or tachycardia, and premature atrial or ventricular contractions (Vargo, 2025). Exact identification of the abnormality cannot be made solely by auscultation. An electrocardiogram (ECG) or heart monitor is needed to properly identify the abnormality.

A precordial impulse may be visible along the left sternal border during the first 6 hours (Vargo, 2025). Due to the thin skin and absence of subcutaneous fat in premature neonates, the precordial impulse may be visible for a longer period. Pulses are palpated for rate, strength, and synchrony. Radial or brachial pulses are compared for timing and intensity, and the same is done for bilateral femoral pulses. Finally, the pre- and postductal pulses are examined.

Perfusion is assessed by checking the capillary refill, depressing the skin over the abdomen or on an extremity until the area blanches. The capillary refill time is the number of seconds that elapse until the color returns to the area. This should be less than 3 seconds.

**General Appearance.** General appearance reflects nutritional status, maturity, and overall well-being. Term neonates normally are well formed and have stores of subcutaneous fat, assuming the fetal position at rest. Premature babies display less flexion than those born at term. Movement should be spontaneous and tremulous. Neonates range in mood from quiet to alert; they are consolable when crying. A normal cry is strong and sustained.

**Skin.** The skin is assessed for maturity, consistency, and color. Discolored areas, variations, or abnormalities are noted for size and location. The skin of a full-term newborn contains subcutaneous fat that provides insulation against heat loss. It is smooth, pink, and wrinkle free. Premature infants lack subcutaneous fat; their skin is thinner than that of term babies and has visible blood vessels over the chest and abdomen. Extremely immature babies often have a gelatinous appearance with transparent skin. They commonly have a red, ruddy color caused by underdevelopment of the stratum corneum. Subcutaneous fat also is lacking in neonates who are IUGR. This group of babies may have loose skin folds, particularly around the knees.

Vernix is the greasy yellow or white substance found on fetal skin, particularly in the axillary, nuchal, and inguinal folds. Composed of sebaceous gland secretions, lanugo, and desquamated epithelial cells, it protects against fluid loss and bacterial invasion (Witt, 2025). Vernix is most abundant during the third trimester and decreases in amount as the fetus approaches 40 weeks.

Lanugo is fine, downy hair that first appears on the fetus at 19 to 20 weeks' gestation and becomes most prominent at 27 to 28 weeks. It begins to disappear from the lower back and usually is not present at term.

**Head.** The head is inspected for shape, symmetry, bruises, and lesions. Neonates delivered by cesarean section generally have a rounded head. Infants born vaginally in vertex position can have overriding sutures; this results in an irregularly shaped head that persists only for a few days in full-term neonates but may be evident for several weeks in premature babies (Griswold & Srinivas, 2025). The head circumference is measured in the occipitofrontal plane and is the largest diameter around the head. The average OFC in a full-term neonate is 35 cm, ranging from 31 to 38 cm (Johnson, 2025). See Figure 4.5.

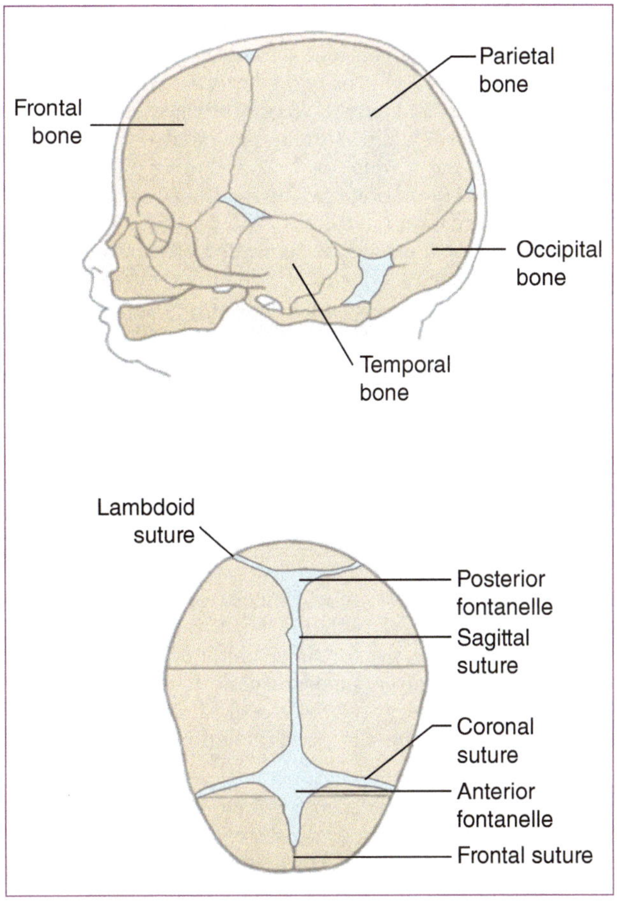


**FIGURE 4.5 Major bones of the head in the newborn with sutures and fontanelles.**

*Source:* Modified from Fletcher, M. A. (1998). *Physical diagnosis in neonatology*. Lippincott-Raven.

Palpate to assess the firmness of bone, the size, configuration of fontanelles and sutures, and to detect swelling, masses, or bony defects. The degree of overlap of sutures may vary, depending on the extent of molding. Normally, the sutures should move freely when gentle pressure is applied to the bones on opposite sides of the suture lines (Johnson, 2025). Directly after birth, it may be difficult to determine if the sutures are fused or merely overlap. Reevaluation when molding and overlap have resolved may yield more reliable information about the presence of craniosynostosis (Johnson, 2025).

The anterior fontanelle is 2 to 3 cm wide, 3 to 4 cm long, and diamond shaped (see Figure 4.5). It should be flat and soft; tense, bulging fontanelles may be reflective of intracranial pressure, while a sunken fontanelle can signify dehydration (Johnson, 2025). The posterior fontanelle is 1 to 2 cm wide and triangular. It may be difficult to palpate the fontanelles directly after birth because of cranial molding. Tension in the fontanelle should be assessed with the infant in recumbent and upright positions. Serial measurements of the width of the anterior fontanelle are more helpful than a single measurement (Fletcher, 1998).

Hair is evaluated for several characteristics. Term newborns have fine hair with identifiable individual strands; premature neonates have hair that is more widely dispersed and described as "fuzzy." One or two whorls are considered normal, while abnormally placed whorls, absence of a whorl or sporadic patches of white hair may be a familial trait and is a benign finding, but a white forelock and other pigmentation defects in the eyes or skin may be associated with deafness or mental retardation (Fletcher, 1998). The anterior hairline varies, with normal growth of pigmented hair onto the forehead of hirsute babies. The posterior hairline ends at the neck crease. Usually, one off-center hair whorl is present in the parietal region (Johnson, 2025).

**Face and Neck.** Inspect the face for shape, symmetry, and bruising or dysmorphic features. The overall facial configuration should be evaluated; the features should be proportional and symmetric. Unusual facial features may be familial or pathognomonic of a malformation syndrome. Gag, sucking, and rooting reflexes should be evaluated.

The newborn has a relatively short neck that should be palpated or observed for symmetry, appearance of the skin, range of motion, masses, and fistulous openings. The neck should be symmetrical with the head, demonstrating full range of motion (Keeton & Duderstadt, 2025). In utero positioning can cause an asymmetric neck. Redundant skin or webbing may be evident (Gontasz et al., 2024). The clavicles can be palpated at this time, and should be intact, without crepitus or swelling.

**Ears.** The ears are evaluated and compared for shape, configuration, position, amount of cartilage, and signs of trauma. The position of the ears at term should be similar bilaterally; approximately 30% of the pinna should lie above a line from the inner and outer canthi of the eye toward the occiput. The rotation of the ears should also be assessed; the long axis of the pinna should lie approximately 15° posterior to the true vertical axis of the head (Fletcher, 1998; Figure 4.6).

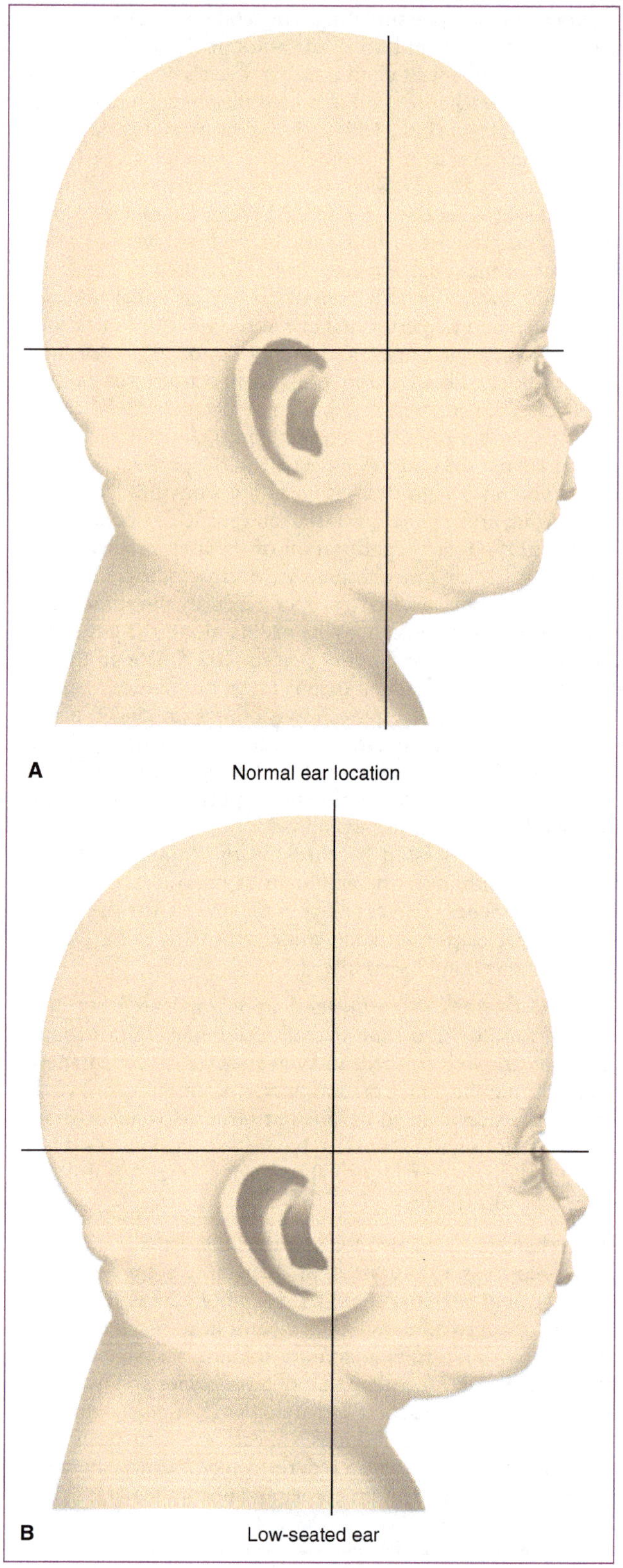


**FIGURE 4.6** Normal (left) and low-seated (right) ear positions.

Abnormalities of the external ear may be associated with syndromes, but often they represent minor structural variations and may be within the normal range (Johnson, 2025).

The presence and patency of the auditory canal can be documented by inspection. Otoscopic examination is not usually part of the examination in the newborn period because the ear canals are filled with vernix, amniotic debris, and blood. This condition clears in approximately 60% of term infants by 1 week of age but may persist for weeks. Less debris is seen in preterm babies, whose canals may clear more quickly.

Because infants frequently remain hospitalized beyond the neonatal period and because evaluation of the middle ear is part of a health maintenance examination, it is appropriate to include otoscopic examination in this section. In a neonate, the ear lobe is pulled toward the chin, and the speculum is directed toward the face. The ear canals of preterm babies are prone to collapse because they are more pliable. Positive pressure applied through the pneumatic otoscope prevents the cartilaginous ear canal from obscuring the view (Fletcher, 1998). The neonatal tympanic membrane is thicker, grayer, and more vascular than that of an adult or older child (Figure 4.7). Universal hearing screening programs are mandated by law in all 50 states (Centers for Disease Control and Prevention, n.d.).

**Eyes.** The eyes should show a spontaneous range of motion and conjugate movements. The lids should be symmetric in both horizontal and vertical placement, and the lashes should be directed outward in an orderly fashion. The eyes should be clear and should have an evenly colored iris, which may be dark gray, blue, or brown, depending on race. Pigmentation should be similar between the two eyes. Permanent eye color is not established for several months, but darker races may show permanent pigmentation in the first week of life. The surface of the conjunctiva should be smooth. During the first few days of life, the cornea may appear slightly hazy because of corneal edema, but thereafter the cornea should be clear and shiny. The sclerae normally are white, but a bluish coloration may be noted in premature and other small infants because their sclerae are thinner (Fletcher, 1998; Orge & Salem, 2025).

An ophthalmoscope is used to assess the pupillary and red reflexes. The light should be directed on the pupils from approximately 6 inches. The pupils should be round and equal in diameter and should constrict equally in response to light (pupils equal and reactive to light [PERL]; Johnson, 2025). The beam of light illuminating the retina causes the red reflex. The retina (fundus) appears as a yellowish white/gray or red background, depending on the amount of melanin in the pigment epithelium. The pigment varies with the complexion of the baby; in dark-skinned infants, the reflex will be pale or cloudy (Griswold & Srinivas, 2025; Honeyfield, 2025).

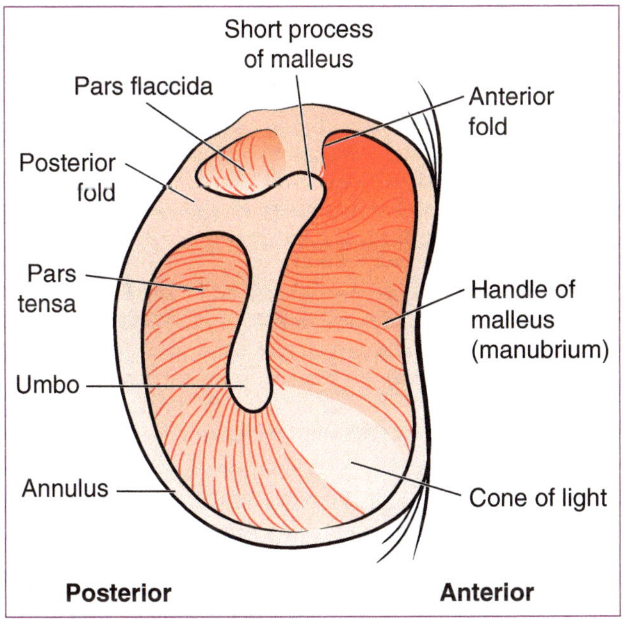


**FIGURE 4.7 Normal landmarks of the right tympanic membrane as seen through an otoscope.**

*Source:* Modified from Lewis, S. M., Bucher, L., Heitkemper, M. M., Harding, M. M, Kwong, J., & Roberts, D. (2017). *Medical-surgical nursing: Assessment and management of clinical problems* (10th ed.). Elsevier.

**Nose.** The nose should be evaluated for shape and symmetry, patency of nares, skin lesions, or signs of trauma. The nasal mucosa should be pink and slightly moist; secretions should be thin, clear, and usually scanty (Fletcher, 1998). The nose should be midline. Immediately after birth, the nose may be misshapen because of compression in utero, but this should correct spontaneously in a few days (Fletcher, 1998). Obstructions and deformities may denote anatomic malformations or congenital syndromes. The patency of the nares can be demonstrated by alternate occlusion of each naris using gentle pressure (Fletcher, 1998). Nasal flaring may be indicative of respiratory distress, but in an otherwise healthy newborn it does not indicate respiratory distress when it appears as the only symptom (Gardner, 2020).

**Mouth.** Inspect the mouth for size, shape, color, and abnormal structures and masses. It should be evaluated both at rest and while the infant is crying. The speed of response and intensity of neonatal reflexes, such as rooting, gagging, and sucking, are also assessed. The mouth is a midline structure symmetric in shape and movement. The mouth, chin, and tongue should be proportionate with fully formed lips (Fanning, 2025; Johnson, 2025).

The mucous membranes should be pink and moist, and oral secretions should be thin and clear. Excessive secretions or drooling suggests inability to swallow or esophageal or pharyngeal obstruction. Both the hard and soft palates should be inspected and palpated to rule out clefts. A high-arched palate may be seen in malformation syndromes, but it generally is insignificant if it appears as an isolated characteristic (Griswold & Srinivas, 2025).

The tongue should be smooth on all surfaces; the lingual frenulum may be short but not so short as to restrict tongue movement. Limitation of movement would be obvious on crying, when the tip of the tongue would form an inverted *V* (Fletcher, 1998; Johnson, 2025).

**Thorax.** The chest is evaluated for size, symmetry, musculature, bony structure, number and location of nipples, and ease of respiration. It should be symmetric in shape and movements. Because the anteroposterior diameter is approximately equal to the transverse diameter, the chest appears round. The chest circumference of a term infant should be about 2 cm smaller than the head circumference (Fraser, 2025). At all GAs, the chest measurement normally is smaller than the OFC (Keeton & Duderstadt, 2025).

Occasional mild subcostal retractions may be seen in healthy newborns because of decreased compliance of the ribs. During sleep, a paradoxical breathing pattern is typical of newborns. On inspiration, the chest wall is drawn in and the abdomen protrudes; the reverse occurs on expiration (Fletcher, 1998). However, in neonates with respiratory distress, this may be indicative of inadequate lung compliance and deficiency of lung volume (Fraser, 2025).

The amount of breast tissue depends on the GA and birth weight, whereas areolar development reflects only GA. Two nipples should be present in equal alignment. The internipple distance varies by GA and chest circumference, but the distance from the outer edge of one areola to the outer edge of the other should be less than 25% of the circumference of the chest (Fraser, 2025). Widely spaced nipples are associated with a variety of congenital syndromes (Fraser, 2025).

Newborn breast tissue may hypertrophy because of the influence of maternal hormones. A milky substance (witch's milk) may appear toward the end of the first week of life, and this discharge may persist for a few weeks to several months (Fraser, 2025).

**Abdomen.** The abdomen is inspected for contour and size, symmetry, skin character, umbilical cord location, and anatomy. Palpation yields information about muscle mass and tone of the abdominal wall, location and size of viscera, tenderness, and masses (Bohara, 2025). Bowel sounds are detected on auscultation; they are relatively quiet in newborns until feedings are established. Compared with term babies, preterm neonates have less active bowel sounds. Evaluating changes in bowel sounds from the infant's baseline is more clinically useful than an isolated assessment (Fletcher, 1998).

The normal abdomen in an infant is round and soft, protruding slightly. The umbilical cord should be bluish-white, shiny, and moist with two arteries and one vein. To facilitate palpation, the knees and legs should be flexed toward the hips, allowing the abdominal muscles to relax. The edge of the liver can be palpated 1 to 2 cm below the right costal margin at the midclavicular line; this edge should be smooth, firm, and well defined (Bohara, 2025). The tip of the spleen can be felt below the left costal margin in newborn infants. The size of the spleen depends on variables such as circulating blood volume, day of life, method of delivery, and type of therapy, which must be considered when interpreting the significance of mild enlargement (Fletcher, 1998).

The kidneys are in the flanks. The lower pole of both kidneys should be palpable because of the reduced tone of neonatal abdominal muscles (Vogt, 2025). The kidneys should be smooth and firm. Enlarged kidneys are somewhat easy to detect, but normal-size neonatal kidneys may be more difficult to find. The presence of renal tissue is confirmed when voiding has occurred (Cavaliere, 2025).

**Anogenital Area.** The anogenital area should be examined with the infant supine. GA affects the appearance of the external genitalia. Maturational changes are described in Figure 4.3 and Table 4.7. The genitalia should be readily identifiable as male or female.

- *Males:* The normal length of the penis at term is 3.5 cm (± 0.7 cm; Fletcher, 1998). Gentle traction is applied on the foreskin to visualize the urethral meatus; the opening should be at the central tip of the glans. Physiologic phimosis, a nonretractable foreskin, normally is seen in newborns. The opening in the prepuce should be large enough to allow urination. The urine stream should be forceful and straight. The inguinal area and scrotum should be palpated for masses, swelling, and the presence of testes. The testes should be firm, smooth, and comparatively equal in size. Testicular descent begins at approximately 27 weeks' gestation. At term both testes should be in the scrotum, which should be fully rugated. The scrotum should be more deeply pigmented than the surrounding skin (Cavaliere, 2025).
- *Females:* The labial, inguinal, and suprapubic areas are inspected and palpated to detect masses, swelling, or bulges. The clitoris should be located superior to the vaginal opening. Hymenal tags and mucous/bloody vaginal discharges are benign, transient findings (Cavaliere, 2025).

Edema of the genitalia is common in both sexes in breech deliveries. It may also be because of transplacentally acquired maternal hormones. The perineum should be smooth and should have no dimpling, fistulae, or discharges (Cavaliere, 2025, Gardner, 2020).

The anus is evaluated for patency and tone. Patency can be documented by gentle insertion of a soft rubber catheter. The passage of meconium does not confirm a patent anus, because meconium may be passed through a fistulous tract (Dingeldein, 2025). Gentle stroking of the anal area should produce constriction of the sphincter, known as the anal wink (Bohara, 2025).

**Back.** The infant should be placed in the prone position while the back is examined for curvature, patency, and presence of structural abnormalities. Vertebrae are palpated for enlargement and pain. Symmetry should be seen on both sides of the back and between the two scapulae. The spine should be straight and flexible and should have no visible defects, such as pits, hair tufts, or dimples (Tappero, 2025).

**Extremities and Hips.** The extremities are observed for symmetry, degree of flexion, and presence of defects and fractures. Full range of motion should be present, and the extremities should move symmetrically. Although symmetry of gluteal skin folds suggests normal hips, the Ortolani and Barlow maneuvers should be performed to confirm the stability of the hips (Figure 4.8). The Ortolani maneuver reduces a dislocated femoral head into the acetabulum, and the Barlow maneuver reflects the ability of femoral head to be dislocated (Tappero, 2025).

The limbs should be equal in length and be proportional to the body; they also should be straight and without edema or crepitus. Palpation or movement of the limbs should not produce a painful response. The digits should be equally spaced and have no webbing or fusion. The nails should extend to the end of the nail beds.

**Reflexes.** The most common neonatal reflexes are presented in Table 4.8.

### Variations and Abnormal Findings on Physical Examination

Minor variations and abnormal findings of the physical examination are presented in Table 4.9.

## HEALTH MAINTENANCE IN THE FIRST YEAR OF LIFE

The goal of health maintenance, or primary care, is to provide consistent preventive healthcare for the infant and education for the parents. In addition to the basic surveillance provided for all infants, high-risk infants have other needs that must be addressed. Primary care for these infants often requires a multidisciplinary approach, and the healthcare provider is responsible for coordinating medical, developmental, and social services. Because high-risk infants face the possibility of developmental delays, neurologic sequelae, and nutritional deficits, follow-up must include formal developmental, neurologic, and nutritional assessments in addition to routine screening tests. The healthcare provider may need to schedule longer and more frequent visits to evaluate the infant adequately and to assess the family's adjustment to caring for the child. They need to provide parental guidance.

There are published guidelines for health supervision (Bellflower, 2017; Dunn, 2016; Hagan et al., 2017). These guidelines indicate the elements that can be included in office visits for patients from birth to 18 years of age. They are intended to be used for those infants and children whose health needs are within the normal range. In the current healthcare arena, information is updated rapidly, and readers are encouraged to use the most recently updated guidelines.

### Immunizations

For information on immunizations, please see Chapter 28, "Postdischarge Care of the Infant, Newborn, and Families". The necessity of continuing or modifying the feeding plan according to the adequacy of growth, the need for dietary supplements (vitamins, minerals, human milk fortifier), medications (ranitidine, metoclopramide), and biochemical monitoring (e.g., for rickets or osteopenia) should also be addressed.

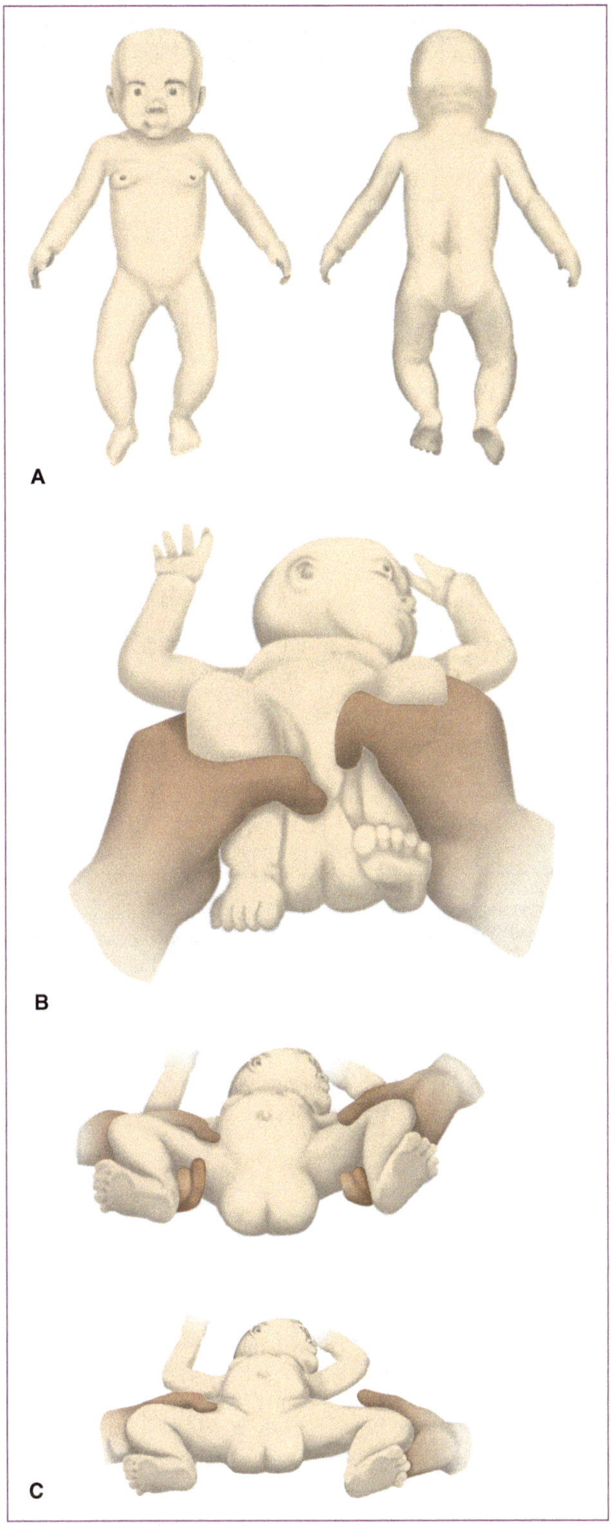


**FIGURE 4.8 Signs of congenital dislocation of hip.** (A) Asymmetry of gluteal and thigh folds, (B) Barlow maneuver, and (C) Ortolani maneuver.

*Source:* Based on Lewis, S. M., Bucher L., Heitkemper, M. M., Harding, M. M., Kwong, J., & Roberts, D. (2017). *Medical-surgical nursing: Assessment and management of clinical problems* (10th ed.). Elsevier.

TABLE 4.8

ASSESSMENT OF NEONATAL REFLEXES

| Reflex | Technique | Response | Comments |
|---|---|---|---|
| Asymmetric tonic neck | With infant supine and in light sleep or quiet awake state, turn head to right until jaw is over shoulder; hold for 15 seconds, then release. | Occipital flexion and mental extension; right arm and leg are extended; left arm and leg are flexed. Premature neonates may lie at rest in this position for extended periods. | Reflex appears at 35 weeks' gestation and disappears by 6–7 months of age. |
| Babinski | Using thumbnail, scratch sole of foot at lateral side from toes to heel. | Dorsal flexion of great toe with extension of other toes. | Care must be taken not to elicit plantar grasp by stimulating sole of foot. Reflex appears at 34–36 weeks' gestation, is well established at 38 weeks, and disappears at 12 months of age. |
| Doll's eyes | Rotate head from side to side, observing eye movement. | As head is moved to right or left, eyes move in opposite direction. | Lack of eye movement with head rotation or movement of eyes in same direction as head may indicate brainstem or oculomotor nerve dysfunction. Reflex is well established and may even be exaggerated at 24–25 weeks' gestation. |
| Galant (truncal incurvation) | Place infant prone, either lying on flat surface or in suspension; lightly stroke along either side of spinal column from shoulder to buttocks. | Normal response is strong incurvation of whole vertebral column toward stimulated side. | Reflex is first seen at 28 weeks' gestation. |
| Glabellar | Hold head firmly and tap forehead just above nose. | Normal response is tighter closure of both eyes and wrinkling of brow. | Asymmetry, absent or exceptionally strong response (closure longer than 1 second), or generalized startle is abnormal. |
| Moro | Hold infant suspended over mattress, supporting head with one hand and body with other hand; rapidly lower both hands 10–20 cm without flexing neck, but do not allow baby to drop back to mattress. | Symmetric abduction of arms and extension at elbows with hands open completely, followed by adduction of arms and flexion at elbows with curling of fingers; infant cries or grimaces at conclusion. | Response attenuates and ultimately disappears with repetition as habituation occurs. No response is seen at < 26 weeks' gestation; extension only at 30 weeks; variable adduction at 34 weeks; complete response at 38 weeks. Reflex disappears at 6 months of age. |
| Palmar grasp | Stimulate palmar surface of hand with a finger. | Neonate grasps finger: grasp tightens with attempt to remove finger. | Reflex appears at 28 weeks' gestation, is well established after 32 weeks, and disappears at 2 months of age. |

(continued)

**TABLE 4.8**

**ASSESSMENT OF NEONATAL REFLEXES (*continued*)**

| Reflex | Technique | Response | Comments |
|---|---|---|---|
| Pupillary | Elicit in darkened environment by presenting bright, sharply focused light from periphery. | Pupils constrict equally. | Reflex is sluggish but present between 28 and 32 weeks' gestation in healthy neonates; it is fully present after 34 weeks. |
| Rooting | Stroke cheek and corner of mouth. | Mouth opens and head turns toward stimulus. | Reflex appears at 28 weeks' gestation, followed by long latency period beginning at 30 weeks; it is well established at 32–34 weeks and disappears by 3–4 months of age. |
| Stepping | Hold neonate upright and allow feet to touch flat surface. | Alternating stepping movements. | Reflex appears at 35–36 weeks' gestation, is well established at 37 weeks, and disappears at 3–4 months of age. |
| Sucking | Touch or stroke lips. | Mouth opens, and neonate begins to suck. | Reflex appears at 28 weeks' gestation, is well established by 32–34 weeks, and disappears at 12 months of age. |

*Sources:* Data from Fanning, B. A. (2025). Neurologic assessment. In C. L. Witt & C. M. Wallman (Eds.), *Tappero & Honeyfield's physical assessment of the newborn* (7th ed., pp. 181–206). Springer Publishing Company; E. P. Tappero & M. E. Honeyfield (Eds.), *Physical assessment of the newborn* (7th ed., pp. 167–192). Springer Publishing Company.

**TABLE 4.9**

**ABNORMALITIES AND VARIATIONS FOUND ON PHYSICAL EXAMINATION OF NEWBORNS AND INFANTS**

| Finding | Definition/Description | Comments |
|---|---|---|
| ***Skin*** | | |
| Color | Acrocyanosis (blue discoloration of the hands, feet, and perioral area), commonly seen in the first 6–24 hours of life. | Occurs when blood flow to an area is sluggish and all available oxygen has been extracted; exacerbated by cooling and diminished by warming; normal variation but abnormal if persists beyond the first 24 hours of life. |
| | Cutis marmorata (mottling of the skin in response to cold or other stressful stimuli); caused by dilation of capillaries, usually greatest on the extremities but may be seen on the trunk. | May be suggestive of other conditions (e.g., cardiovascular hypertension, hypothyroidism) if mottling is extensive, shows no improvement with warming, or persists beyond first few months (Fletcher, 1998; Vargo, 2025). |

(*continued*)

## TABLE 4.9

### ABNORMALITIES AND VARIATIONS FOUND ON PHYSICAL EXAMINATION OF NEWBORNS AND INFANTS (*continued*)

| Finding | Definition/Description | Comments |
|---|---|---|
| | Cyanosis (blue discoloration of the skin, tongue, and mucous membranes). | Caused by an excess of desaturated hemoglobin (Hb) in the blood (cardiopulmonary disease) or a structural defect in the Hb molecule (methemoglobin); always an abnormal finding. |
| | Jaundice (yellow coloring of the skin, mucous membranes, and sclerae). | Caused by deposition of bilirubin; may be physiologic. |
| | Pallor (absence of color or paleness of the skin). | Caused by a decrease in cardiac output, subcutaneous edema, anemia, or asphyxia (Griswold & Srinivas, 2025). |
| | Plethora (ruddy skin coloration in the newborn). | Caused by high circulating red blood cell volume (abnormal finding). |
| Lesions | Café au lait spots (light tan or brown macules with well-defined borders, representing areas of increased epidermal melanosis); except for deeper pigmentation, appearance is not different from that of surrounding skin. | More common in normal infants of color. Six or more macules, regardless of spots' size or infant's race, may be pathologically significant, especially if located in the axilla. |
| | Cutis aplasia (localized or widespread foci of absence of some or all layers of skin); defect may be covered by a thin, translucent membrane or scar tissue, or area may be raw and ulcerated. | Occurs predominantly on the scalp and less frequently on the limbs and trunk (Narendran, 2025). |
| | Ecchymosis (purple or blue-black macule larger than 2 mm in diameter); represents extravasation of blood into subcutaneous tissue. | Results from trauma to underlying blood vessels or fragility of the vessel walls. |
| | Erythema toxicum (white or yellow papules on red macular base), commonly found on face, trunk, or proximal extremities but not on hands or feet. | Common, benign finding; vesicles are rare, sterile, and composed primarily of eosinophils (Witt, 2025). When vesicles are pronounced or coalescent, they may mimic postural infectious rash. |
| | Harlequin fetus (most severe form of congenital ichthyosis; skin is completely covered with thick, horny scales resembling armor that are divided by deep red fissures). | Most such infants die of dehydration, infection, or respiratory insufficiency within a few hours or days (Narendran, 2025). |
| | Harlequin sign (vascular phenomenon represented by distinct midline demarcation in side-lying infants; dependent half is deep red, upper half is pale). | Benign finding that lasts a few seconds to 30 minutes, occasionally reverses when position is changed. The physiologic basis is unknown and without pathologic significance. Occurs most frequently in LBW neonates (Narendran, 2025; Witt, 2025). |

(*continued*)

**TABLE 4.9**

## ABNORMALITIES AND VARIATIONS FOUND ON PHYSICAL EXAMINATION OF NEWBORNS AND INFANTS (*continued*)

| Finding | Definition/Description | Comments |
|---|---|---|
| | Strawberry hemangioma (red, raised, circumscribed, soft, compressible, lobulated tumor; may occur anywhere on the body). | Benign tumor of the vascular endothelium that has a proliferative and an involutional phase, most involute spontaneously. Treatment is unnecessary unless vital functions are affected (Narendran, 2025; Witt, 2025). |
| | Cavernous hemangioma (similar to strawberry hemangioma; involves dermis and subcutaneous tissue and is soft and compressible on palpation; overlying skin is bluish red in color). | Cavernous lesions may cause thrombocytopenia (Kasabach–Merritt syndrome) or hypertrophy of bone and soft structures of extremities (Klippel-Trenaunay-Weber syndrome; Narendran, 2025; Witt, 2025). |
| | Mongolian spot (blue-black macule, lacking a sharp border, most frequently seen on sacrum, buttocks, flanks, or shoulders). | Benign lesion, common in dark-skinned neonates, resulting from delayed disappearance of dermal melanocytes; lesion gradually disappears during the first years of life (Witt, 2025). |
| | Milia (1 mm, pearly white or yellow papules without erythema; in the mouth these are called *Epstein's pearls*). | Epidermal inclusion cysts caused by blockage of sebaceous glands; a benign finding that resolves during the first weeks of life (Witt, 2025). |
| | Miliaria—three types:<br>1. Crystallina (1–2 mm, thin-walled vesicles with non-erythematous and nonpigmented base [without inflammation]).<br>2. Rubra—small, erythematous, grouped papules [prickly heat]).<br>3. Pustulosis or profunda (non-erythematous pustules). | Lesions caused by blockage of sweat glands. They are exacerbated by a warm, humid environment and most frequently develop in intertriginous areas and over the face and scalp. They resolve when the environmental factors are eliminated (Narendran, 2025; Witt, 2025). |
| | Neonatal pustular melanosis (small, superficial vesiculopustules with little or no surrounding erythema; crusted or scaly collarettes appear after vesicles rupture; lesions eventually resolve into hyperpigmented areas). | Transient and benign; frequently confused with infectious lesions. Smears of pustular material reveal predominant neutrophils and no bacteria. (Witt, 2025). |
| | Salmon patch nevus; dull, pink, irregularly shaped macules that blanch on pressure; commonly found on nape of neck [stork bite], glabella, forehead, eyelids, and upper lip). | Benign finding: lesions are composed of distended, dilated capillaries, and most lesions (except those on the neck) disappear by 1 year of age (Witt, 2025). |
| | Port wine stain (nevus, macular lesion; present at birth but may be pale and hard to discern; initially pink in color with sharply delineated borders; progresses to dark red/purple; some develop small, angiomatous nodules). | Developmental vascular malformation that occurs mostly on the face; does not increase in size but grows with the infant; may occur alone or with structural anomalies (e.g., Sturge–Weber syndrome; Narendran, 2025; Witt, 2025). |

(*continued*)

**TABLE 4.9**

**ABNORMALITIES AND VARIATIONS FOUND ON PHYSICAL EXAMINATION OF NEWBORNS AND INFANTS (*continued*)**

| Finding | Definition/Description | Comments |
|---|---|---|
| | Petechiae (tiny red or purple, nonblanching macules that range from pinpoint to pin head size). | Caused by minute hemorrhages in the dermal or submucosal layers; may be benign and self-limiting or pathognomonic of serious underlying conditions. They are benign when found on presenting part and when localized areas appear at the same time; progressive, widespread areas require evaluation (Fletcher, 1998; Witt, 2025). |
| Redundant skin | More skin than is necessary or normally present in a particular area. | Seen in the neck after resolution of cystic hygroma or in the abdomen in a neonate with prune belly syndrome. |
| Sclerema neonatorum | Diffuse, stone-hard, nonpitting cutaneous induration; overlying skin appears pale and waxy; face has a masklike appearance; joints are stiff. | Occurs in debilitated neonates; diffuse systemic process with grave prognosis (Narendran, 2025). |
| Subcutaneous fat necrosis | Firm, nonpitting, poorly circumscribed, reddish violet lesions appearing in the first weeks of life on the face, arms, trunk, thighs, and buttocks. Affected areas may be slightly elevated above adjacent skin (Prazad et al., 2025). | Most often seen in areas where a fat pad is present. May occur secondary to cold or trauma and sometimes accompanied by hypercalcemia (Narendran, 2025). |
| ***Head and Neck*** | | |
| Acrocephaly | Congenital malformation of the skull caused by premature closure of the coronal and sagittal sutures; accelerated upward growth of the head gives it a long, narrow appearance with a conic shape at the top (also called *oxycephaly*). | May be associated with premature closure of sutures; found with certain syndromes (e.g., Crouzon, Apert) (Zhou & Tomei, 2025). |
| Anencephaly | Failed closure of the anterior neural tube without skull formation; the brain is severely malformed, lacking definable structure, although a rudimentary brainstem usually is present. | Most affected neonates (75%) are stillborn; without intervention; the remainder die in the neonatal period (Zhou & Tomei, 2025). |
| Brachycephaly | Congenital malformation of the skull caused by premature closure of the coronal suture; excessive lateral growth of the head gives it a short, broad appearance. | Condition found with certain syndromes (e.g., trisomy 21, Apert) (Zhou & Tomei, 2025). |
| Bruit | Abnormal murmur-like sound heard on auscultation of an organ or gland that is caused by dilated, tortuous, or constricted vessels. The specific character of the bruit, its location, its association with other clinical findings, and the time of occurrence in a cycle of other sounds is of diagnostic importance. | Bruits heard over the fontanelle or lateral skull associated with signs of congestive heart failure may denote intracranial arteriovenous malformation (Fanning, 2025; Johnson, 2025). |

(*continued*)

## TABLE 4.9

### ABNORMALITIES AND VARIATIONS FOUND ON PHYSICAL EXAMINATION OF NEWBORNS AND INFANTS (*continued*)

| Finding | Definition/Description | Comments |
|---|---|---|
| Caput succedaneum | Vaguely demarcated pitting edema of the scalp that may extend across suture lines and can shift in response to gravity. | Benign finding that appears at birth (from pressure of the maternal cervix on the fetal skull) and resolves in a few days (Prazad et al., 2025). |
| Cephalohematoma | Extradural fluid collection caused by bleeding between the skull and periosteum; generally occurs over one or both parietal bones and does not cross the suture lines; has distinct margins and may be fluctuant or tense. | 1. May form during labor and enlarges for the first 12–24 hours; most resolve spontaneously over several weeks to months (Johnson, 2025; Stark et al., 2022a).<br>2. Linear skull fracture is found in 5% of unilateral and 18% of bilateral lesions (Stark et al., 2022a; Stark et al., 2022b; Johnson, 2025).<br>3. May result in hyperbilirubinemia (Stark et al., 2022a). |
| Craniosynostosis | Premature closure of one or more cranial sutures, causing abnormal skull shape and possibly a palpable ridge along the suture line. | Head growth is restricted in the area perpendicular to the stenotic suture and is excessive in unrestricted areas. Most cases are isolated events, but the condition can occur in some syndromes (Zhou & Tomei, 2025). |
| Craniotabes | Congenital thinness of bone at the top and back of the head. Bones may collapse with gentle pressure and recoil (ping-pong). | 1. May be a normal variant if present to a mild degree near suture lines. May be caused by the pressure of the skull against the maternal pelvic brim; spontaneous resolution usually occurs in a few weeks (Fletcher, 1998).<br>2. May be associated with congenital syphilis and other congenital conditions (osteogenesis imperfecta); due to bone resorption or delay in ossification (Gontasz et al., 2024). |
| Dolichocephaly or scaphocephaly | Congenital malformation of the skull in which premature closure of the sagittal suture results in restricted lateral growth. | Long, narrow head (Zhou & Tomei, 2025). |
| | Skull shape, often seen in premature babies as a result of prolonged positioning with head turned to the side. | |
| Encephalocele | Protrusion of brain tissue through a congenital defect in the cranium; most often occurs in the occipital midline but may also be seen in the frontal, temporal, or parietal areas. | Other cranial defects, congenital anomalies (hydrocephalus, microcephaly, craniosynostosis), and autosomal recessive syndromes (Walker–Warburg) are frequently seen (Gressens & Huppi, 2025). |
| Hair whorls | Two or more hair whorls, or abnormally placed whorls (other than parietal area). | May indicate brain anomaly; it has been postulated that the pattern of hair development correlates with underlying brain development (Johnson, 2025). |

(*continued*)

**TABLE 4.9**

**ABNORMALITIES AND VARIATIONS FOUND ON PHYSICAL EXAMINATION OF NEWBORNS AND INFANTS (*continued*)**

| Finding | Definition/Description | Comments |
|---|---|---|
| Macrocephaly | Excessive head size compared to weight, length, and GA. OFC is over 90th percentile. | 1. Familial; facial features usually are normal.<br>2. May reflect pathologic condition (e.g., hydrocephaly, hydranencephaly) or chromosomal or neuroendocrine disorder (Dean & Doherty, 2024). |
| Microcephaly | Abnormally small head size relative to weight, length, and GA. OFC is under 10th percentile. | Associated with either microcephaly (marked reduction in size of brain or cerebral hemispheres) or acquired brain atrophy. |
| Molding | Process by which the head shape is altered as the fetus passes through the birth canal. The biparietal diameter becomes compressed, the head is elongated, and skull bones may overlap at the suture lines. | Benign finding: condition usually resolves during the first few postnatal days. |
| Neck masses | May be detected on palpation or inspection. | Most common neck mass: caused by development of sequestered lymph channels, which dilate into cysts (Griswold & Srinivas, 2025; Johnson, 2025). |
| | Cystic hygroma (soft, fluctuant mass that is easily transilluminated; usually laterally placed or over clavicles). | |
| | Goiter (anterior mass caused by hypothyroidism). | Rare in neonates (Johnson, 2025). |
| | Thyroglossal duct cyst/branchial cleft cyst; a mass may be found high in the neck. | Rare in neonates (Johnson, 2025). |
| Plagiocephaly | Asymmetry of the skull due to flattening of the occiput. Can be deformational (positional) or due to premature or irregular closure of the coronal or lambdoidal sutures. | 1. Posterior plagiocephaly almost always due to mechanical forces (positional; "back to sleep").<br>2. Anterior plagiocephaly is most commonly due to premature fusion of the sutures (Zhou & Tomei, 2025). |
| Subgaleal | Bleeding into the potential space between the epicranial aponeurosis and the periosteum of the skull; manifests as a firm to fluctuant scalp mass with poorly demarcated borders that may extend onto the face, forehead, or neck and may be accompanied by signs of hypovolemia. | May be a life-threatening condition; can be caused by hemorrhage coagulopathy, asphyxia, or vacuum extraction (Prazad et al., 2025). |
| Webbed neck | Redundant skin at posterolateral region of neck. | Found with Turner, Noonan, and Down syndromes (Meier & Mestas, 2025). |

(*continued*)

**TABLE 4.9**

**ABNORMALITIES AND VARIATIONS FOUND ON PHYSICAL EXAMINATION OF NEWBORNS AND INFANTS (*continued*)**

| Finding | Definition/Description | Comments |
|---|---|---|
| ***Face*** | | |
| Asymmetry | Unequal appearance or movement of mouth and lips; unequal closure of eyes; uneven appearance of nasolabial folds. | Often caused by in utero positioning but may be due to facial nerve paresis; in mild cases may be evident only with crying (affected side fails to move or moves less when infant cries). |
| ***Ears*** | | |
| Auricular appendage | Accessory tragi, most commonly in pretragal areas, may occur within or behind the ear. These structures contain cartilage and are not truly skin tags. | Primarily of cosmetic significance unless accompanied by other diffuse malformations. Seen in certain congenital syndromes (e.g., Goldenhar, Treacher Collins); hearing assessment is indicated when other anomalies are present (Johnson, 2025; Mitchell, 2025). |
| Auricular sinus | Narrow, fistulous tract most often located directly anterior to helix. | May be familial or may be associated with microtia, auricular appendage, facial cleft syndromes, and syndromic anomalies of the outer ear (Mitchell, 2025). |
| Low-set ears | Superior attachment of pinna lies below imaginary line drawn between both inner canthi and extended posteriorly. | May be associated with chromosomal or renal anomalies (Lewis, 2014a, 2014b). |
| Microtia | Severely misshapen, dysplastic external ear. | Frequently associated with other malformations that result in conductive hearing loss (i.e., atresia of auditory meatus, abnormalities of middle ear; Gontasz et al., 2024; Mitchell, 2025). |
| ***Eyes*** | | |
| Blepharophimosis | Narrow palpebral fissures in the horizontal measurement; also known as *short palpebral fissures.* | Usually caused by lateral displacement of the inner canthi; seen in certain dysmorphic or chromosomal syndromes (Fletcher, 1998; Orge & Salem, 2025). |
| Brushfield spots | Pinpoint white or pale-yellow spots on the iris. | Seen in 75% of neonates with Down syndrome but may also be a normal variant; not always visible at birth (Johnson, 2025; Orge & Salem, 2025). |
| Coloboma | Cleft-shaped defect in ocular tissue (eyelid, iris, ciliary body, retina, or optic nerve). | Result of incomplete embryologic closure of ocular structures; may be an isolated finding or part of a malformation syndrome (CHARGE, trisomy 13, 18, 22) (Bennett & Meier, 2019; Orge & Salem, 2025). |

(*continued*)

## TABLE 4.9

### ABNORMALITIES AND VARIATIONS FOUND ON PHYSICAL EXAMINATION OF NEWBORNS AND INFANTS (*continued*)

| Finding | Definition/Description | Comments |
|---|---|---|
| Ectropion | Eversion of the margin of the eyelid, which leaves the conjunctiva exposed. | Seen in facial nerve paralysis, in certain syndromes, and in harlequin fetus and collodion baby (Fletcher, 1998; Orge & Salem, 2025). |
| Entropion | Inversion of the eyelid; eyelashes may be in contact with the cornea and conjunctiva. | Congenital condition that usually resolves spontaneously without damage (Fletcher, 1998; Griswold & Srinivas, 2025; Orge & Salem, 2025). |
| Epicanthal folds | Vertical fold of skin at the inner canthus on either side of the nose. | A feature of normal fetal development and may be present in normal infants. Characteristic of trisomy 21 but may occur in malformation syndromes, especially those with a flat nasal bridge; may also be a physical manifestation of in utero compression (Potter facies; Mitchell, 2025). |
| Exophthalmos | Abnormal displacement of the eye characterized by protrusion of the eyeball. | May be caused by increased volume of the orbit (tumor), swelling secondary to edema or hemorrhage, endocrine disorder (e.g., Graves' disease, hyperthyroidism); known as *proptosis* when accompanied by shallow orbits (Crouzon disease; Fletcher, 1998; Orge & Salem, 2025). |
| Hypertelorism | Increased distance between the orbits, observed clinically as a large interpupillary distance (see Telecanthus) (Parikh & Mitchell, 2015). | Frequently seen in craniofacial syndromes (Orge & Salem, 2025). |
| Hypotelorism | Decreased distance between the orbits, observed clinically as smaller-than-normal interpupillary distance (Parikh & Mitchell, 2015). | Frequently seen in trisomies 13 and 21 and in other syndromes (Orge & Salem, 2025). |
| Leukocoria | White pupil, denoting an abnormality of the lens, vitreous, or fundus; an indication for further evaluation (Orge & Grigorian, 2015). | May be seen on direct visualization, or as absence of a red reflex; most seen in cataracts; also found in retinoblastoma, retinal detachment, and vitreous hemorrhage. |
| Microphthalmia | Small eye; diameter measures less than two-thirds of the normal 16 mm at birth (Orge & Grigorian, 2015). | Can be hereditary or caused by chromosomal anomalies and environmental influences during development. Associated with multisystem conditions or syndromes (e.g., CHARGE, trisomy 13, fetal rubella effects). |
| Nystagmus | Involuntary, rhythmic movements of the eye; may be horizontal, vertical, rotary, or mixed. Optokinetic nystagmus reflexive response to a moving target. | Occasional, intermittent nystagmus in an otherwise healthy newborn may be normal in the neonatal period; however, it must be evaluated if frequent or persistent (or both). Pathologic forms may be due to ocular, neurologic, or vestibular defects (Orge & Salem, 2025). |

(*continued*)

**TABLE 4.9**

**ABNORMALITIES AND VARIATIONS FOUND ON PHYSICAL EXAMINATION OF NEWBORNS AND INFANTS (*continued*)**

| Finding | Definition/Description | Comments |
|---|---|---|
| Ptosis (blepharoptosis) | Abnormal drooping of one or both upper eyelids; lid does not rise to normal level. | Caused by congenital or acquired weakness in the levator muscle or paralysis of the third cranial nerve; may be difficult to detect in neonates unless unilateral with asymmetry between the eyelids (Orge & Salem, 2025). |
| Strabismus | Misalignment of the visual axes:<br>Esotropia—crossed eyes<br>Exotropia—wall eye. | Refer for ophthalmologic evaluation if present by third month of age. Results from inheritance, paralysis of the lateral rectus muscle, or refractive errors; may be due to diseases that reduce visual acuity in one eye (Orge & Salem, 2025). |
| Subconjunctival hemorrhage | Bright red area on sclerae. | Caused by rupture of a capillary in the mucous membrane that lines the conjunctiva; commonly seen after vaginal delivery, does not reflect ocular trauma unless massive and associated with other findings; usually resolves in 7–10 days (Prazad et al., 2025). |
| Synophrys | Meeting of the eyebrows in the midline. | Seen in multisystem conditions or syndromes (e.g., Cornelia de Lange, congenital hypertrichosis) (Mitchell, 2025). |
| Telecanthus | Lateral displacement of the inner canthi; eyes appear too widely set because of a disproportionate increase between the inner canthi; interorbital distance is appropriate (Mitchell, 2025). | Evident in fetal alcohol syndrome (FAS) and other syndromes; not synonymous with hypertelorism, although its presence can lead to a false impression of hypertelorism (Sharma, 2014). |
| *Nose* | | |
| Choanal atresia | Obstruction of posterior nasal passages. | Patency is assessed in quiet states. If condition is bilateral, neonate is cyanotic at rest and pink when crying; if unilateral, baby is unable to breathe if mouth is held closed and unaffected naris is occluded with examiner's finger. Atresia/stenosis may be confirmed by passing a catheter. |
| Nasal deformation | May result from pressure in utero. | Benign condition that resolves in a few days. |
| | May be due to dislocation of the septal cartilage. | Attempts to restore normal anatomy are unsuccessful; nares remain asymmetric when tip of nose is compressed (Johnson, 2025; Prazad et al., 2025). |

(*continued*)

## TABLE 4.9

### ABNORMALITIES AND VARIATIONS FOUND ON PHYSICAL EXAMINATION OF NEWBORNS AND INFANTS (*continued*)

| Finding | Definition/Description | Comments |
|---|---|---|
| *Mouth* | | |
| Cleft lip/palate | Failure of midline fusion during first trimester. | May occur alone or with other malformations. |
| Epstein's pearls | Small, white, pearl-like inclusion cysts that appear on the palate and gums. | Benign finding that disappears spontaneously by a few weeks of age (Johnson, 2025). |
| Micrognathia | Underdevelopment of the jaw, especially the mandible. | Dysmorphic feature seen in certain malformation syndromes (e.g., Pierre Robin sequence) (Meier & Mestas, 2025; Johnson, 2025). |
| ***Thorax/Chest*** | | |
| Asymmetry | May be unequal in shape or excursion. | 1. Asymmetric shape caused by positioning in utero or presence of air trapping or space-occupying lesions.<br>2. Unequal excursion caused by diaphragmatic hernia, phrenic nerve damage, or air leakage or trapping (Fraser, 2025). |
| Auscultation | Adventitious breath sounds | Fraser (2025). |
| | Crackles | Discrete, noncontinuous bubbling sounds during inspiration; classified as fine, medium, or coarse. Previously called *rales*. |
| | Rhonchi | Continuous, nonmusical, low-pitched sounds occurring on inspiration and expiration; caused by secretions or aspiration in large airways. |
| | Stridor | Rough, harsh sounds caused by narrowing of upper airways; present during both phases of respiratory cycle but worse during inspiration; common with laryngomalacia, subglottic stenosis, and vascular ring. |
| | Wheezes | Musical, high-pitched sound generated by air passing at high velocity through a narrowed airway; heard most often on expiration but can be noted during both phases of respiratory cycle if airway diameter is restricted and fixed. |
| | Grunting | Sound produced by forceful expiration against a closed glottis; compensatory mechanism to prevent or reverse alveolar collapse. |

(*continued*)

**TABLE 4.9**

**ABNORMALITIES AND VARIATIONS FOUND ON PHYSICAL EXAMINATION OF NEWBORNS AND INFANTS (*continued*)**

| Finding | Definition/Description | Comments |
|---|---|---|
| | Murmur | Grades I through VI assigned depending on intensity and presence of thrill. |
| Barrel chest | Increased anteroposterior diameter of the chest. | Result of air trapping in the pleural space (pneumothorax) or distal airways (aspiration or pneumonia), space-occupying lesions, or overdistention from mechanical ventilation (Fletcher, 1998; Fraser, 2025). |
| Heave | Diffuse, gradually rising impulse seen in the anterior chest overlying the ventricular area. A *parasternal heave* is a precordial impulse that may be felt (palpated) in patients with cardiac or respiratory disease. Precordial impulses are visible or palpable pulsations of the chest wall that originate on the heart or the great vessels. | Can be associated with hypertrophied ventricles or volume overload (Felner, 1990). |
| Pectus carinatum | Deformation of chest wall caused by protuberant sternum; also called *pigeon chest*. | May be associated with Marfan, Noonan, and other syndromes (Fraser, 2025). |
| Pectus excavatum | Deformation of chest wall caused by depressed sternum; also called *funnel chest*. | May be associated with Marfan, Noonan, and other syndromes (Fraser, 2025); may develop after birth in neonates with laryngomalacia. |
| Retractions | Drawing in of the soft tissues of the chest between and around the firmer tissue of the cartilaginous and bony ribs; seen in intercostal, subcostal, substernal, and suprasternal areas. | Mild subcostal retractions may be seen in healthy newborns; intercostal, substernal, and suprasternal retractions reflect increased breathing and suggest respiratory distress. |
| Supernumerary nipples (polythelia) | Extra nipples: may appear as slightly pigmented linear dimples or may be more defined, with palpable breast nodules. | Normal variant: nipples appear along the mammary line. Prospective studies have refuted the association with renal anomalies; no indication for further evaluation based solely on the presence of supernumerary nipples. |
| ***Abdomen*** | | |
| Abdominal wall defects | Exstrophy of the bladder (protrusion and eversion of the bladder through an embryologic defect, resulting in absence of muscle and connective tissue on the anterior abdominal wall). | Often associated with other defects of the genitourinary (GU) and musculoskeletal systems and the GI tract (Cavaliere, 2025; Rowe & Merguerian, 2024). |
| | Gastroschisis (protrusion of viscera through an abdominal wall defect arising outside the umbilical ring; the cord therefore is not inserted on the defect, and the herniated organs are not covered by peritoneum). | Defect usually is to the right of the umbilicus (Bohara, 2025; Dingeldein, 2025). |

(*continued*)

**TABLE 4.9**

**ABNORMALITIES AND VARIATIONS FOUND ON PHYSICAL EXAMINATION OF NEWBORNS AND INFANTS (*continued*)**

| Finding | Definition/Description | Comments |
|---|---|---|
| | Omphalocele (herniation of viscera through an abdominal wall defect within the umbilical ring; defect usually is covered by a translucent, avascular sac at the base of the umbilicus). | Umbilical cord always inserts into the sac; occasionally, the sac may rupture. Defect usually is larger than 4 cm and may be associated with other congenital defects and chromosomal anomalies (Bohara, 2025; Dingeldein, 2025). |
| | Umbilical hernia (failure of the umbilical ring to contract, allowing protrusion of bowel or omentum through the abdominal wall). | Characterized by a fascial defect smaller than 4 cm and intact umbilical skin (Dingeldein, 2025; Fletcher, 1998). |
| Bruit | See section under Head and Neck. | Persistence after a position change may indicate abnormalities of the umbilical vein or hepatic vascular system, hepatic hemangioma, or renal artery stenosis (Bohara, 2025). |
| Diastasis rectus | Midline bulge from xiphoid to umbilicus, seen when abdominal muscles are flexed. | Caused by separation of the two rectus muscles along the median line of the abdominal wall; a common benign finding in newborns that has no clinical significance; resolves without intervention (Bohara, 2025). |
| Distention | Increase in abdominal girth caused by an increase in the volume of intraperitoneal, thoracic, or pelvic contents. | May be pathologic or benign. Pathologic causes include GI obstruction, ascites, abdominal mass, organomegaly, and depression of the diaphragm (tension pneumothorax). Benign causes include postprandial state, crying, swallowing of air with feedings, air leakage with mechanical ventilation, and administration of continuous positive airway pressure (CPAP). |
| Patent urachus | Postnatal persistence of communication between the urinary bladder and the umbilicus; may result in passage of urine from the umbilicus, which otherwise appears normal. Other signs are a large, edematous cord that fails to separate after the normal interval and retraction of the umbilical cord during urination. | Lower urinary tract obstruction should be considered (Cavaliere, 2025). |
| Prune belly syndrome | Congenital deficiency of abdominal musculature, characterized by a large, flaccid, wrinkled abdomen, cryptorchidism, and GU malformations. | Almost always seen in males (Vogt, 2025). |
| Scaphoid abdomen | Abdomen with a sunken anterior wall. | May be present with a diaphragmatic hernia or malnutrition. |

(*continued*)

**TABLE 4.9**

## ABNORMALITIES AND VARIATIONS FOUND ON PHYSICAL EXAMINATION OF NEWBORNS AND INFANTS (*continued*)

| Finding | Definition/Description | Comments |
|---|---|---|
| Single umbilical artery | | Seen in fewer than 1% of neonates; ~40% of affected newborns have other major congenital malformations. When this condition occurs without other abnormalities, it usually is a benign finding (Griswold & Srinivas, 2025). |
| ***Genitalia/Perineum*** | | |
| Ambiguous | Presence of a phallic structure not discretely male or female, abnormally placed urethral meatus, and inability to palpate one or both gonads in a male. | May be associated with serious endocrine disorders; rapid evaluation and diagnosis are critical (Cavaliere, 2025; Thompson & Wherrett, 2025). |
| Anal atresia | Absence of an external anal opening; imperforate anus. | Infant may fail to pass meconium; however, meconium may be passed through a rectovaginal or rectovestibular fistula in a female or rectoperineal or rectourethral fistula in a male (Bohara, 2025). |
| Chordee | Ventral or dorsal curvature of the penis; most evident on erection. | May occur alone but often accompanies hypospadias (Cavaliere, 2025; Palmer & Palmer, 2016). |
| Clitoromegaly | The appearance of an enlarged clitoris, with no regard to cause (Al Remeithi & Wherrett, 2015); it may be swollen, enlarged, widened, or merely prominent, as in premature females. | May be a normal finding in a premature female or may represent masculinization from exposure to excess androgens during fetal life. |
| Cryptorchidism | Testis or testes in extrascrotal location (undescended testis or testes); characterized by empty, hypoplastic scrotal sac. | In most cases descent occurs spontaneously by 6–9 months of age; descent after 9 months is rare. Bilateral cryptorchidism occurs in up to 30% of patients; consider disorder of sexual differentiation until proven otherwise (Cavaliere, 2025; Palmer & Palmer, 2016; Thompson & Wherrett, 2025). |
| Epispadias | Abnormal location of urethral meatus on the dorsal surface of the penis; abnormal urine stream may be seen. | Varies in severity from mild (glanular) to complete version seen in exstrophy of the bladder; all forms are associated with dorsal chordee; may require evaluation by a urologist before circumcision (Palmer & Palmer, 2016; Vogt, 2025). |

(*continued*)

## TABLE 4.9

### ABNORMALITIES AND VARIATIONS FOUND ON PHYSICAL EXAMINATION OF NEWBORNS AND INFANTS (*continued*)

| Finding | Definition/Description | Comments |
|---|---|---|
| Hydrocele | Nontender scrotal swelling caused by fluid collection; arises from passage of peritoneal fluid through patent processus vaginalis. | May be seen with inguinal hernia but can be distinguished from hernia because hydrocele appears translucent on transillumination; entire circumference of testis may be palpated; and it cannot be reduced (Cavaliere, 2025; Elder, 2016; Palmer & Palmer, 2016). |
| Hydrocolpos/ hydrometrocolpos | Manifests as suprapubic mass or protruding perineal mass because of accumulation of secretions in vagina or vagina and uterus. | Caused by excessive intrauterine stimulation by maternal estrogens, with obstruction of the genital tract by an intact hymen, hymenal bands, vaginal membrane, or vaginal atresia (Cavaliere, 2025; Karfer, 2016). |
| Hymenal tag | Redundant tissue manifesting as an annular tag protruding from the vagina. | Benign finding: most disappear during the first year of life. |
| Hypospadias | Abnormal location of urethral meatus on the ventral surface of the penis; caused by incomplete development of the anterior urethra; abnormal urine stream may be seen. | Urethral opening may be found on the glans, scrotum, or perineum. Infants with penoscrotal or perineal type or with glanular form and other genital anomalies or dysmorphic features should be evaluated to rule out disorders of sexual differentiation (Thompson & Wherrett, 2025). Evaluation by a urologist may be required before circumcision. |
| Inguinal hernia | Scrotal mass caused by the presence of loops of intestines in the scrotal sac; arises from persistence of processus vaginalis, often associated with hydrocele. | On examination, the entire circumference of the testis is not palpable, and the scrotum cannot be transilluminated. Unless incarcerated, hernias are reducible (Cavaliere, 2025). |
| Micropenis/ microphallus | Abnormally short or thin penis. | Penis more than two standard deviations below the mean of length and width for age according to standard charts; frequently requires evaluation by an endocrinologist and a geneticist (Thompson & Wherrett, 2025). |
| Phimosis | Intractable foreskin. | Must be differentiated from physiologic phimosis, a nonretractable foreskin that is a normal finding in neonates (Cavaliere, 2025). |
| Priapism | Constantly erect penis. | Abnormal finding in neonate (Broderick, 2016; Cavaliere, 2025). |
| Retractile testis | Normally descended testis that recedes into the inguinal canal because of activity of the cremaster muscle. | May not be seen in the newborn period because of lack of cremaster reflex in this age group; however, some newborns do demonstrate this response (Cavaliere, 2025; Elder, 2016). |

(*continued*)

## TABLE 4.9

### ABNORMALITIES AND VARIATIONS FOUND ON PHYSICAL EXAMINATION OF NEWBORNS AND INFANTS (*continued*)

| Finding | Definition/Description | Comments |
|---|---|---|
| Testicular torsion | Twisting of the testis or testes on the spermatic cord; manifests as a swollen, red or bluish-red scrotum; may be painful, but this is not a universal symptom in the neonate. | Urgent evaluation and management are required, because the blood supply to the testis is compromised, which results in irreversible ischemic damage to the testis; condition may occur in utero (Griswold & Srinivas, 2025; Prazad et al., 2025). |
| ***Musculoskeletal System*** | | |
| Arachnodactyly | Unusually long, spiderlike digits. | Characteristic of, but not universally present in, Marfan syndrome and homocystinuria (Mitchell, 2025). |
| Arthrogryposis | Persistent flexure or contracture of one or more joints. | May be associated with oligohydramnios or an underlying neuromuscular disorder (Mitchell, 2025). |
| Brachydactyly | Shortening of one or more digits because of abnormal development of phalanges, metacarpals, or metatarsals. | Benign trait if an isolated finding; may be a component of skeletal dysplasias (achondroplasia) and syndromes (trisomy 21) (Mitchell, 2025). |
| Calcaneus foot | Abduction of the forefoot with the heel in valgus position (turned outward). | Associated with external tibial torsion; often caused by in utero positioning. |
| Camptodactyly | Congenital flexion deformity of the finger; bent finger. | Usually involves the little finger; can be a minor variant, familial trait, or part of a syndrome (Mitchell, 2025). |
| Clinodactyly | Lateral angulation deformity of a finger with either radial or ulnar deviation. | Usually involves the little finger; may be a benign finding if occurring alone but can be associated with congenital syndromes (Mitchell, 2025). |
| Crepitus | Crackling sensation produced by the presence of air in tissues (subcutaneous emphysema) or the movement of bone fragments (clavicular fracture). | |
| Genu recurvatum | Abnormal hyperextensibility of the knee, allowing the knee to bend backward. | May be due to trauma, prolonged intrauterine pressure, or general joint laxity. May be a feature of other disorders (Ehlers-Danlos, Marfan syndromes) (Hardesty, 2025; Gontasz et al., 2024). |
| Kyphosis | Round shoulder deformity; forward bending of the spine. Caused by congenital failure of formation of all or part of the vertebral body, with preservation of the posterior elements and failure of the anterior segmentation of the spine. | Severe deformities may be apparent at birth; less severe abnormalities may not appear until several years later; a progressive deformity can result in paraplegia (Mitchell, 2025; Son-Hing & Hardesty, 2025). |

(*continued*)

## TABLE 4.9

### ABNORMALITIES AND VARIATIONS FOUND ON PHYSICAL EXAMINATION OF NEWBORNS AND INFANTS (*continued*)

| Finding | Definition/Description | Comments |
|---|---|---|
| Lordosis | Exaggeration of the normal curvature in the cervical and lumbar spine. | Caused by a bony abnormality of the spine (Meier & Mestas, 2025). |
| Lymphedema | Puffiness of the dorsum of the hands or feet. | Characteristic of Noonan or Turner syndrome (Mitchell, 2025). |
| Meningocele | Saclike protrusion of the spinal meninges through a congenital defect in the spinal column. | Herniated cyst is filled with cerebrospinal fluid but does not contain neural tissue; affected infants usually do not show neurologic deficits (Nguyen & Tomei, 2025). |
| Metatarsus valgus | Congenital deformity of the foot in which the forepart rotates outward away from the midline and the heel remains straight. | Fixed deformity of the foot, which cannot be brought into neutral position; compare with metatarsus adductus, a functional deformity in which the foot can be brought into neutral position (Son-Hing & Hardesty, 2025). |
| Metatarsus varus | Congenital bony abnormality of the foot in which the forepart rotates inward toward the midline and the heel remains straight. | Fixed deformity: the foot cannot be brought into neutral position. Compare with metatarsus adductus, a functional deformity in which the foot can be brought into neutral position (Son-Hing & Hardesty, 2025). |
| Myelomeningocele | Defect identical to meningocele but with associated abnormalities in the structure and position of the spinal cord. | Affected infants usually show neurologic deficits below the level of the abnormality (Nguyen & Tomei, 2025). |
| Polydactyly | Presence of more than the normal number of digits; there may be a complete extra digit (preaxial) that is normal in appearance, or a skin tag (postaxial). | May be an isolated finding, inherited as an autosomal dominant trait, or may occur in a variety of syndromes (trisomy 13, Meckel–Gruber syndrome) (Mitchell, 2025; Son-Hing & Hardesty, 2025). |
| Rachischisis | Congenital fissure of the spinal cord in which the incompletely folded cord is splayed apart and exposed along the back. | Caused by incomplete neurulation; often accompanied by anencephaly (Fletcher, 1998; Gressens & Huppi, 2025). |
| Rocker bottom feet | Deformity of the foot in which the arch is disrupted, giving a rounded appearance (rocker bottom) to the sole. | Usually seen in conjunction with congenital syndromes (trisomies 13 and 18) (Mitchell, 2025; Son-Hing & Hardesty, 2025). |
| Scoliosis | Failure of formation or segmentation of the vertebrae; manifests as lateral (side-to-side) curvature of the spine. | May be congenital or acquired; may occur as part of another condition or may be idiopathic (Son-Hing & Hardesty, 2025). |

(*continued*)

## TABLE 4.9

### ABNORMALITIES AND VARIATIONS FOUND ON PHYSICAL EXAMINATION OF NEWBORNS AND INFANTS (*continued*)

| Finding | Definition/Description | Comments |
|---|---|---|
| Simian crease | Single transverse line in the palm. | May be benign, but when accompanied by other dysmorphic features (e.g., incurving fifth finger, epicanthal folds, low-set thumb), it may be a sign of trisomy 21 (Mitchell, 2025). |
| Spinal dimple, dermal sinus | Pit or depression that occurs along the midline of the back, often at the base of the spinal cord in the lumbosacral area; may be accompanied by tufts of hair. | May be a benign finding, especially if the base of the defect can be visualized; however, defect can extend into the spinal cord, representing a neural tube defect and tethered spinal cord (Fanning, 2025; Liu & Glotzbecker, 2025). |
| Syndactyly | Fusion of two or more digits; may involve only soft tissue (simple) or may include bone or cartilage (complex). | May occur as an isolated defect or as part of a syndrome (e.g., Cornelia de Lange, Smith-Lemli-Opitz) (Son-Hing & Hardesty, 2025). |
| Talipes equinovarus | Clubfoot; congenital deformity of the foot and lower leg marked by adduction of the forefoot (turned inward and pointed medially), varus position of the heel (turned inward), and downward pointing of the toes. | May be congenital (isolated deformity), teratologic (associated with underlying neuromuscular disorder), or positional (normal foot held in equinovarus position in utero) (Son-Hing & Hardesty, 2025). |
| Tibial torsion | Abnormal rotation of the feet while the knees are pointing forward; maybe internal (toes in) or external (toes out). | Often caused by in utero positioning; resolves spontaneously (Son-Hing & Hardesty, 2025). |
| Torticollis | Shortening of the sternocleidomastoid muscle, resulting in head tilt toward the affected muscle and chin rotation toward the unaffected muscle; a palpable mass may appear during the first few weeks of life. | May be due to birth trauma, intrauterine malposition, muscle fibrosis, venous abnormalities in the muscle, or congenital cervical vertebral abnormalities (Liu & Glotzbecker, 2025). |
| ***Neurologic Examination*** | | |
| Brachial plexus injuries | Peripheral damage to the network of spinal nerves supplying the arm, forearm, and hand. | Multifactorial etiology; interaction between characteristics of the brachial plexus, maternal and fetal risk factors, and birth trauma (Liu & Glotzbecker, 2025). |
| | Erb–Duchenne palsy (upper arm paralysis): Arm is adducted and internally rotated, with elbow extension, flexion of the wrist, and pronation of the forearm. The arm falls to the side of the body when passively abducted, and the Moro reflex is absent on the affected side but the grasp is intact. | Arises from injury to the fifth and sixth cervical roots; most common brachial plexus injury (Liu & Glotzbecker, 2025; Prazad et al., 2025). |

(*continued*)

**TABLE 4.9**

**ABNORMALITIES AND VARIATIONS FOUND ON PHYSICAL EXAMINATION OF NEWBORNS AND INFANTS (*continued*)**

| Finding | Definition/Description | Comments |
|---|---|---|
| | Klumpke palsy (lower arm paralysis): Hand is paralyzed, and voluntary movement of the wrist and grasp reflex *are* absent. | Rare; results from injury to the eighth cervical and first thoracic roots; usually Horner syndrome (ptosis, miosis, and enophthalmos) is present on the affected side; delayed pigmentation of the iris may be seen (Liu & Glotzbecker, 2025; Prazad et al., 2025). |
| | Paralysis of the entire arm: Arm is completely motionless, flaccid, and powerless and hangs limply; all reflexes are absent, and sensory deficit may extend to the shoulder. | Liu & Glotzbecker (2025). |
| Facial nerve palsy | Facial weakness or paralysis arising from compression of the seventh cranial nerve, caused by intrauterine position or forceps delivery; characterized by asymmetry of facial movement (most evident on crying), ptosis, and unequal nasolabial folds. | Prazad et al. (2025). |
| Phrenic nerve injury | Cause of respiratory distress secondary to paralysis of the diaphragm; arises from upper brachial plexus injury. | Rarely occurs as an isolated phenomenon; accompanies signs and symptoms of Erb–Duchenne palsy (Prazad et al., 2025). |

GA, gestational age; OFC, occipitofrontal circumference.

## SUMMARY

The comprehensive history and physical assessment create the framework for identifying problems and planning interventions. Assessment allows the nurse to gather information and evaluate and integrate that information as the infant's care proceeds. Although careful attention to the obvious is important, subtle findings detected by an experienced practitioner may also play a crucial role in the continuing care of the infant and family.

## ONLINE RESOURCES

**CourseConnect**

Resources for this chapter are online and available at www.springerpub.com/courseconnect.

## REFERENCES

References for this chapter are online and available at www.springerpub.com/courseconnect.

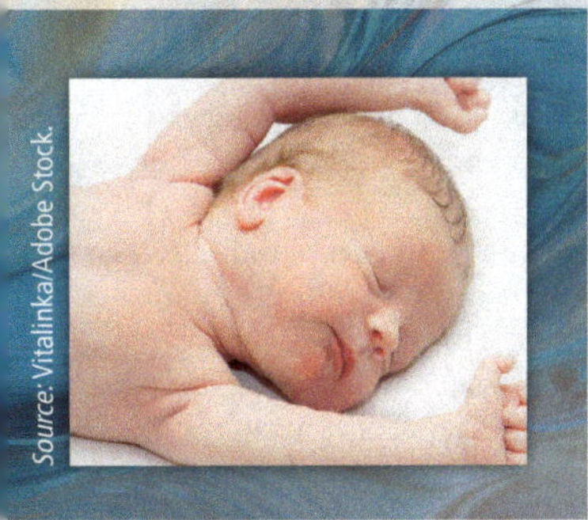


CHAPTER 5

# Term Newborn

Miki Konishi and Masahiko Murase

## INTRODUCTION

The nurse caring for the newborn plays a unique role in providing care and assisting in integrating the baby into the family. Understanding of the newborn is optimized when a maternal/family history is known. This information, including previous health issues and prenatal, intrapartum, and postpartum histories, is critical for assessing adaptation to extrauterine life. It gives insight into the newborn's environment and helps determine the nurse's care plan. The skills of assessment, analysis, planning, implementation, and evaluation of both mother and newborn are critical. They must occur synchronously for the nurse to assist the newborn's transition from birth to discharge.

## ADMISSION

Providing the optimal environment for the newborn begins at birth. As a major concept of neonatal resuscitation, the primary goal of neonatal care at birth is to facilitate the establishment and maintenance of cardiovascular and temperature stability and promote mother–infant bonding, and breastfeeding is recognized as a healthy baby transition (AHA, 2020). If the baby cries and has good muscle tone immediately after birth, infants should stay with the mother for routine care. "Mothers and newborns have an emotional and physiological need to be together at birth and during the following hours and days" (Crenshaw, 2019). Initial nursing interventions after birth, such as drying the infant, initial assessment, and Apgar scoring, should occur while the baby is skin-to-skin (kangaroo mother care). Nursing interventions, including birth weight, vitamin K, and ophthalmic antibiotic administration, should be delayed to allow at least 1 hour of uninterrupted skin-to-skin contact (SSC) and breastfeeding attempts. As the 10 steps to successful breastfeeding (WHO, 2024), nurses should support mothers in initiating breastfeeding as soon as possible after birth and assist with positioning and latching. This principle applies to all healthy babies, whether vaginal birth or cesarean section.

Babies having difficulty transitioning from intrauterine to extrauterine life may be placed in the radiant warmer and observed for further evaluation. The admission nurse receives a comprehensive report from the labor and delivery nurse, which includes the maternal history and the delivery summary.

### Vital Signs

A complete physical assessment of the newborn is done on admission (see Chapter 4, "Assessment of the Newborn and Infant"). The vital signs include temperature, respiratory rate, heart rate, and blood pressure (see Table 5.1). The American Pain Society (1995) in 1995 introduced the idea of pain as the fifth vital sign in the mid-1990s. Infants cannot raise their voices, so neonatal pain should be assessed by every vital sign using a pain scale. These are taken during the initial physical

**TABLE 5.1**

**NORMAL RANGE FOR VITAL SIGNS**

| Temperature | Respiratory Rate | Heart Rate | Blood Pressure Systolic | Blood Pressure Diastolic |
|---|---|---|---|---|
| 97.7°F–99.5°F (36.5°C–37.5°C) | 30–60 breaths/min | 100–160 beats/min | 60–80 mm Hg | 40–50 mm Hg |

assessment, repeated periodically according to the institution's protocol, and documented at every shift. Any abnormal value should be reported, and more frequent assessments of vital signs may be required.

The initial temperature gives the nurse a baseline from which to evaluate the thermoregulation ability of the newborn and is taken in the axilla. The acceptable range of values is from 97.7°F (36.5°C) to 99.5°F (37.5°C). The apical heart rate is counted for one full minute. When an infant moves and cries, the heart rate is between 140 and 160 beats per minute (beats/min), but when he/she sleeps, it may temporarily be below 100 beats/min. The acceptable range is from 100 to 160 beats/min. The respiratory rate is counted for one full minute, and the acceptable range of values is from 30 to 60 breaths per minute (breaths/min). However, it is common to have respiratory rates as high as 80 to 100 breaths/min within the first 12 minutes of life (Baixauli-Alacreu et al., 2020), most likely representing the normal transition to extrauterine life. Normal blood pressure depends on gestational age and day of life (See Chapter 4, "Assessment of the Newborn and Infant"); the acceptable range values are systolic 60 to 80 mm Hg and diastolic from 40 to 50 mm Hg. Oxygen saturation is adequate for evaluating oxygenation. Generally, the pulse oximeter probe should be placed on an infant's right hand, unaffected by the ductus arteriosus. It takes over 10 minutes for preductal oxygen saturation of healthy babies to be achieved above 95% (Gardner et al., 2021). Glucose screening should be performed only on at-risk infants, though no study has evaluated optimal timing and intervals; monitoring should begin within 60 minutes after birth for infants with suspected significant hyperinsulinemia and commence before the second feeding or 2 to 4 hours after birth, in other at-risk groups (Wight, 2021).

## Medications

The administration of vitamin K is given as a prophylaxis for hemorrhagic disease of the newborn by the intramuscular (IM) route using the vastus lateralis muscle. In some countries in Europe and Asia, vitamin K is administered orally. The CDC (2025b) and American Academy of Pediatrics (AAP) statement has not promoted oral medicine of vitamin K because IM injection is the most effective and is limited to parents who refuse IM injection. The Canadian Paediatric Society has recommended similar prophylactic treatment but also proposed that an acceptable alternative was a 2 mg dose of oral vitamin K administered within 6 hours of birth, then repeated at 2 to 4 weeks and 6 to 8 weeks of age. No reliable evidence compares the oral and IM route of administration of prophylactic vitamin K in newborns, and the efficacy of the oral regimen relies on compliance with the protocol of multiple doses (Jullien, 2021). Either way, vitamin K must be administered to newborns, especially breastfed babies, to prevent bleeding.

As a prophylaxis against neonatal ophthalmia due to organisms such as chlamydia, erythromycin ointment or drops are applied. This practice is mandated by state law and is required in most states in the United States. The Canadian Paediatric Society (2024) does not recommend the routine use of eye medicine in newborns immediately after birth because it may no longer be useful, but maternal screening for chlamydia is done. The U.S. Preventive Services Task Force (2019) recommends eye medicine, which is inexpensive, preventive, and less harmful because not all pregnant women have been screened.

Hepatitis B virus (HBV) is a serious viral disease that affects the liver. This virus is spread through contact with an infected person's blood or other body fluids. The vaccine can prevent HBV and the serious complications associated with it, including liver cancer and cirrhosis. Routine hepatitis vaccination in the United States began in 1991. Recommendations call for three doses of Hepatitis B vaccines for all babies. The first dose should be given shortly after birth, the second dose 1 through 2 months, and the third between 6 and 18 months of life. If the mother is HBV positive, both HBV vaccine and HBV immune globulin (HBIG) should be given in separate limbs within 12 hours of birth. The final is provided by 6 months of age, and $HB_sAg$ and anti-HBs are checked between 9 and 12 months. In the case of infants less than 2,000 g, an additional vaccination will be given at the beginning of 1 month after birth, so the total time of vaccinations is four doses (CDC, 2025a).

Japan started vaccination for children born to mothers who were HBV carriers in 1986 to prevent vertical transmission. Thus, even if all infants were not routinely vaccinated, the positive rate among children was considered low. However, epidemiologic surveys conducted from 2013 to 2015 showed that this did not necessarily mean the positive rate among children was not low, and some cases of horizontal transmission among them were also reported. Therefore, in 2016, HBV vaccinations for all children began on a schedule like that in the United States (Doi & Kanto, 2021).

## The First Bath

The WHO (2022) recommends delaying the first bath after 24 hours of birth because it reduces the mortality rate, prevents hypothermia, and increases exclusive breastfeeding. AWHONN and NANN (2018) also recommend that, ideally, the first bath should occur between 6 and 24 hours of age.

Before bathing, axillary temperature must be 98.2°F (36.8°C) or more on two consecutive measurements. The infant should be bathed every few days using appropriate safety measures for only 5 to 10 minutes. The bath water should be 100.4°F (38°C) to less than 104°F (40°C), and the room temperature should be between 79°F (26°C) and 81°F (28°C–). Shampoo once or twice a week by gently massaging the entire scalp, including the area over the fontanelles, using warm tap water with a neutral or weakly cleanser for bathing, not antimicrobial soaps or chlorhexidine products. After bathing, the newborn is dried with prewarmed towels or blankets and is put on the mother's chest. The bath equipment should be disinfected before and after each use.

The vernix on the skin provides a mechanical barrier with antimicrobial properties that protect the infant from infection and will be absorbed into the skin over 24 hours. Vernix is produced during the fetal period, and the fetus swallows it and amniotic fluid to protect the intestines. During parturition, it functions as a biofilm. The benefits of vernix are protection against infection, decreased skin permeability and transepidermal water loss (TEWL), moisturization of the skin surface, and pH development (AWHONN & NANN, 2018). Therefore, do not force it off; let it fall off naturally during regular care.

## Cord Care

Clean the umbilical cord and surrounding skin during the first bath to remove debris. Dry the cord with clean, absorbent gauze and leave it uncovered. Allow the cord to dry naturally. This means keeping the umbilical cord area clean and dry without topical agents. Keep the diaper folded to leave the cord uncovered to help prevent contamination with urine or stool. The routine use of antimicrobial agents such as isopropyl alcohol, povidone-iodine, topical antibacterial agents, and triple dye is not recommended (WHO, 2022; AWHONN & NANN, 2018). Redness, swelling, or drainage may be signs of infection and should be reported to the primary care provider.

The umbilical clip and the shrivel-up umbilicus must be placed so that they do not encounter the skin and not damage the skin. In Asian countries such as Japan and South Korea, there is a traditional culture of storing the umbilical cord with care, so it may be given to the parents.

# SECURITY

Safety and security measures are essential components of any environment providing newborn care. Institutions must have a safety and security system to ensure the infant's safety during its birth hospitalization. These systems also reassure parents that their baby is safe not only from internal threats but from external ones as well. Two identification bands are placed on each newborn. One should be worn on the arm and the other on the leg. The first one has the mother's identification (ID) number, which is given to the infant before cutting the umbilical cord. It is paired with the mother's ID band. This will ensure that the newborn is identified as the mother's. The other band includes date of birth, mother's name, and infant's sex. Products that do not come off easily and do not damage the babies' skin are chosen. Some products combine two baby bands and one for mothers.

Newborn abductions occur in hospitals around the world. Three hundred forty-five medical-related infant abductions of infants under 1 year of age in the United States were identified by the National Center for Missing & Exploited Children in the past 60 years, of which at least 140 have been taken from the hospital (NCMEC, 2025). To prevent babies from being taken away, visitors entering the maternal ward should have their names and health checked. They must then pass through a nurses' station to reach the nursery. Some hospitals are also implementing small sensors placed on babies' ankles. Tracking systems vary from institution to institution but are usually connected to the hospital's security systems. Whenever the alarm is set off or activated, a "Code Pink" is broadcast throughout the hospital, and security personnel are deployed to that area for follow-up.

NCMEC (2009) has published educational tools for parents. It is essential to share hospital safety policies with the parents. Most institutions now require an ID badge with the healthcare employee's picture and name while the employee is on duty. Mothers should be told not to leave the baby alone in the room, even if it is to use the bathroom. Kidnappers often pose as hospital staff, so mothers should check ID badges and know not to leave their children with suspicious people. All people in the hospital, including parents and medical staff, are prohibited from carrying the baby and moving around, and a crib is used. This not only prevents the baby from falling accidents but also from being abducted.

# BACK TO SLEEP

In 1994, the National Institute of Child Health and Human Development, along with the AAP, launched the Back to Sleep campaign to reduce the risk of sudden infant death syndrome (SIDS). The campaign was expanded and renamed Safe to Sleep® in 2012 to address not only SIDS, but also other sleep-related infant deaths. The WHO (2022, p. 124) says, "Putting the baby to sleep in the supine position during the first year is recommended to prevent SIDS and sudden unexpected death in infancy (SUDI)." In the 2022 update, the AAP recommends a safe sleep environment to reduce the risk of all sleep-related deaths.

A safe sleep environment includes placing the infant in a supine position on a firm, flat, non-inclined sleep surface (with an angle less than 10 degrees), room-sharing without bed-sharing for at least the first 6 months after birth, and avoiding soft bedding. Layers of clothing are preferable to blankets or coverings to keep infants warm. Not dressing babies too tightly or covering their faces and heads is important to prevent overheating. There is no evidence that a knit cap prevents hypothermia, so it is unnecessary to wear it indoors except for infants admitted to the NICU. The AAP (Moon, et al., 2022) further recommends avoiding exposure to smoke (nicotine), alcohol, and illicit drugs (including marijuana and opioids) and promoting breastfeeding, routine immunizations, and using a pacifier. Pacifiers help infants sleep; however, they must be used after breastfeeding is established.

In the newborn nursery, infants are placed on their backs in the cribs, and this practice is taught to parents as a part of the initial safety teaching protocol. The Safe to Sleep® campaign provides educational resources, including booklets, handouts, and infographics, to help people learn about safe infant sleep and share information with friends, family, and others.

# DAILY CARE

Medical records document routine daily care, including vital signs and physical assessments. Nurses must check the head circumference, condition of the fontanel, skin color (jaundice), and appearance of heart murmurs and report any abnormalities to the doctor.

Feeding is at least eight times a day, every 3 hours. If exclusive breastfeeding increases and the interval is shorter, the number of feedings increases. Lactation consultants should be available for all breastfeeding mothers. Weight is measured daily. Physiologic weight loss peaks 3 to 5 days after birth. If neonatal weight loss exceeds 7%, nurses must assess the infant's feeding status, considering the possibility of nutritional deficiencies.

It is usual for the baby to urinate within the first 24 hours of birth and have a urine output of 1 ml/kg/hr or more. Assess for signs of dehydration or cardiac failure when urine output is low. Reviewing intake and output is an essential parameter for measuring the nutritional status of the newborn.

Black-green sticky meconium is seen within 24 hours after birth. Gastrointestinal atresia is suspected if there is no excretion within 24 hours after birth. After going through granular stools, the stool becomes yellow. Defecation occurs two to five times a day, and the frequency of defecation is higher in breastfed infants than formula-fed infants. The white stool is a sign of biliary atresia. It is difficult for mothers to determine whether the stool is "white," so Japanese maternal and child health handbooks include a card that indicates the color of the stool. This leads to early diagnosis of biliary atresia (Gu et al., 2015).

## CIRCUMCISION

Circumcision is one of the most performed surgical procedures in the world. It is estimated that 13% of newborns around the world are circumcised (Prabhakaran et al., 2018). Established health benefits of circumcision include a reduced incidence of urinary tract infection (UTI), recurrent balanoposthitis, human immunodeficiency virus (HIV) and other sexually transmitted infections (STIs), and prevention of paraphimosis and penile carcinoma. On the other hand, there are complications associated with circumcision. Therefore, national guidelines recommend that circumcision should only be performed when the benefits outweigh the disadvantages, and routine circumcision for asymptomatic cases is not recommended (Prabhakaran et al., 2018). Newborns are generally asymptomatically circumcised. Therefore, medical professionals should share this information with families and allow parents to decide whether to perform preventive circumcision, considering their religious, cultural, and personal preferences.

The nurse caring for the newborn who is to be circumcised must ensure that the parent has signed the proper consent form, assembled the necessary equipment for the procedure, and then participated in the "time-out" surgical protocol before the care provider initiates the surgical procedure. Because circumcision is a painful procedure, pain management techniques must be implemented before, during, and after the procedure. Pain relief can be achieved using lidocaine/prilocaine cream applied to the foreskin 30 to 60 minutes before the procedure. Alternatively, nerve blocks can be performed about 5 minutes before the procedure using 1% lidocaine without epinephrine (Omole et al., 2020). Nerve blocks include the dorsal penile nerve block and ring block. Oral sucrose solution administered before circumcision can also be an effective analgesic. A recent randomized controlled trial showed that lidocaine/prilocaine cream, oral sucrose solution, and a ring block provided the best analgesic effect (Sharara-Chami et al., 2018). After the procedure, petroleum jelly and gauze are placed on the glans to prevent the diaper from sticking to the wound during healing. The newborn can be discharged from the hospital shortly afterward because there is no need to wait for the newborn to urinate. Parents are generally instructed to have a follow-up visit within 3 to 5 days and are advised to reapply the dressing at each diaper change until healing is complete or the Plastibell device naturally detaches, which typically occurs within 5 to 7 days (Omole et al., 2020). There are three types of circumcision devices in use in the United States today that are most common for basic circumcision methods: the Gomco or Yellen clamp, the Plastibell, and the Mogen clamp. Because these techniques are equally effective, the choice of the device should be guided by the physician's experience (Omole et al., 2020).

## NEONATAL THERMOREGULATION

Thermoregulation is the ability to balance heat production and heat loss to maintain normal body temperature. Normal adaptation to extrauterine life requires minimizing all the mechanisms for heat loss. The infant loses heat by evaporation, convection, conduction, and radiation. Evaporation is heat loss that occurs by water evaporation from the wet skin and mucous membrane. Evaporation of amniotic fluid from the infant's skin in the delivery room is the main source of heat loss in the initial newborn period. Convection is heat loss from cooling air movement. Conduction is heat loss to cooler objects that are in direct contact with the infant, such as a cold bed.

In contrast with conduction, radiation is heat loss to cooler objects without direct contact. On the other hand, neonates' main heat production method is nonshivering thermogenesis (NST). The heat production of neonates depends entirely on brown adipose tissue (BAT), deposited after 25 weeks' gestation and primarily found around the scapulae, kidneys, adrenals, neck, and axilla (Wood et al., 2022).

Care aims to arrange a thermoneutral environment (TNE) in which a neonate maintains a body temperature while minimizing energy expenditure and oxygen consumption. The presence of cold stress increases metabolic and physiologic demands on all infants (Gardner et al., 2021). Clinical symptoms of hypothermia are the following (Gardner et al., 2021; Wood et al., 2025):

- pale or mottled skin
- acrocyanosis
- central cyanosis
- irritability or lethargy
- weak cry
- respiratory distress
- apnea
- bradycardia
- feeding intolerance
- emesis
- hypoglycemia
- metabolic acidosis

### Management

In cases of mild hypothermia 96.8°F to 97.5°F (36.0°C–36.4°C), the infant can be rewarmed by SSC in a warm room. With moderate hypothermia 89.6°F to 96.6°F (32.0°C–35.9°C), the infant should be placed on a radiant warmer or a preheated incubator set at 95°F to 96.8°F (35.0°C–36.0°C). In cases of severe hypothermia (< 89.6°F [32°C]), the infant should be rewarmed on a radiant warmer over several hours. Feeding should be continued to provide calories and fluid to prevent hypoglycemia, which is common in infants experiencing hypothermia.

## Hyperthermia

Hyperthermia is defined as a body temperature greater than 99.5°F (37.5°C). The most common cause of hyperthermia is excess environmental heat. It is important to differentiate hyperthermia from fever, which is a raised body temperature in response to infection and inflammation. Although it is impossible to distinguish between fever and hyperthermia based on body temperature measurement alone, infection should always be considered first. It is necessary to assess the environmental factors, such as the mode and temperature that the radiant warmer is set on and the number of blankets in which the infant is swaddled. Steps should be taken to correct any environmental factors present. The clinical appearance of the infants often indicates the causative mechanism. Any signs and symptoms of infection should be reported to the healthcare provider.

# GLUCOSE HOMEOSTASIS

Glucose provides metabolic fuel for the developing fetus. In utero, the fetus receives a constant supply of glucose from the mother through facilitated diffusion across the placenta. Fetal blood glucose levels correlate with maternal blood glucose levels, fluctuating between 60% and 80% of maternal blood glucose levels. A large amount of glucose is accumulated and stored during the late stages of pregnancy. The umbilical cord is cut off at birth, cutting off the energy supply. Then, energy requirements increase due to cold stress, breathing movements, and muscle activity. Blood glucose levels drop rapidly within 1 to 2 hours after birth.

In contrast, newborns maintain blood glucose levels through insulin suppression, glucagon secretion, lipolysis, and the secretion of insulin antagonist hormones, catecholamines, and cortisol. Because the amount of glucose stored in newborns before birth is limited, there is a risk of hypoglycemia after birth. Newborn blood glucose levels rise within 18 hours after birth and remain stable until 48 hours after birth. It rises again after 72 hours, reaching adult levels after 96 hours (Harris et al., 2020).

Neonatal glucose requirements are 4 to 6 mg/kg/min, two to three times the adult requirement. This is due to a high brain-to-body weight ratio. During hypoglycemia, lactate and hydroxybutyrate act as alternative fuels. However, in recent years, it has been reported that these contribution rates are low (Harris et al., 2020). For this reason, management to prevent the onset of hypoglycemia is necessary.

The blood glucose level, the critical point for neurodevelopment, is not yet clear. Harris et al. (2020) found that 10% of newborns had blood glucose levels of 47 mg/dl or less within 48 hours of birth. Furthermore, when comparing groups randomly divided into those with hypoglycemia diagnostic thresholds of less than 36 mg/dl and those with less than 47 mg/dl, no significant difference was observed in neurodevelopment at 18 months of age (van Kempen et al., 2020).

## Screening

Screening for hypoglycemia should target infants with signs, symptoms, or high-risk factors, while routine screening is unnecessary for healthy-term newborns after a normal pregnancy and delivery. Signs of hypoglycemia include nervousness, cyanosis, seizures, apnea, tachypnea, weak or high-pitched cry, decreased tone, lethargy, poor feeding, and eye rolling. The critical period is 24 to 72 hours postbirth, and underlying conditions such as sepsis must be evaluated. Prolonged hypoglycemia under 10 mg/dl may lead to coma or seizures, necessitating vigilance for neurologic signs due to the risk of brain damage (Thornton et al., 2015).

Infants of diabetic mothers (IDMs) may develop asymptomatic hypoglycemia within 1 to 12 hours postbirth. Small-for-gestational-age (SGA) or large-for-gestational-age (LGA) infants can experience hypoglycemia as early as 3 hours after birth, with risks lasting up to 10 days. Screening for at-risk asymptomatic infants should start within hours of birth and continue through several feedings. SGA infants should be fed every 2 to 3 hours, with glucose checked before each feeding for the first 24 hours and extended if hypoglycemia occurs, because term or premature SGA infants are at risk.

Bedside blood glucose meters allow rapid detection and treatment but have limitations as point-of-care (POC) tools. Test strips correlate with plasma glucose but may deviate by 10 to 20 mg/dl, especially at low levels. No POC method is precise enough for standalone neonatal hypoglycemia (NH) screening, making laboratory confirmation essential when low glucose is suspected (Committee on Fetus and Newborn & Adamkin, 2011).

Definitions of hypoglycemia vary. The AAP recommends ≥ 40 mg/dl within 4 hours of birth and ≥ 45 mg/dl within 24 hours. The British Association of Perinatal Medicine defines it as < 36 mg/dl, the WHO as < 47 mg/dl, and the Pediatric Endocrine Society as < 50 mg/dl within 48 hours and < 60 mg/dl after 48 hours (Committee on Fetus and Newborn & Adamkin, 2011; Thornton et al., 2015). Higher thresholds and frequent measurements increase asymptomatic hypoglycemia diagnoses, potentially separating infants from mothers and hindering breastfeeding. Facilities must determine which criteria best balance accurate diagnosis and maternal–infant bonding.

## Management

The algorithm proposed by the AAP is shown in Figure 5.1 (Committee on Fetus and Newborn & Adamkin, 2011). IV glucose therapy is performed if the child has symptoms and the blood glucose level is < 40 mg/dl. If the child is asymptomatic, the criteria for hypoglycemia differ depending on whether the child is born to 4 hours of age or 4 to 24 hours of age. However, the target glucose screen is > 45 mg/dl before routine feeds.

## New Treatments

A group that used oral dextrose gel had a lower incidence of hypoglycemic events and mother–infant separation compared to the group that did not, and it was suggested that the breastfeeding rate after discharge was improved (Edwards et al., 2022). The group that used oral dextrose gel reduced the incidence of hypoglycemic events and the occurrence of mother–infant separation compared to the group that did not use it.

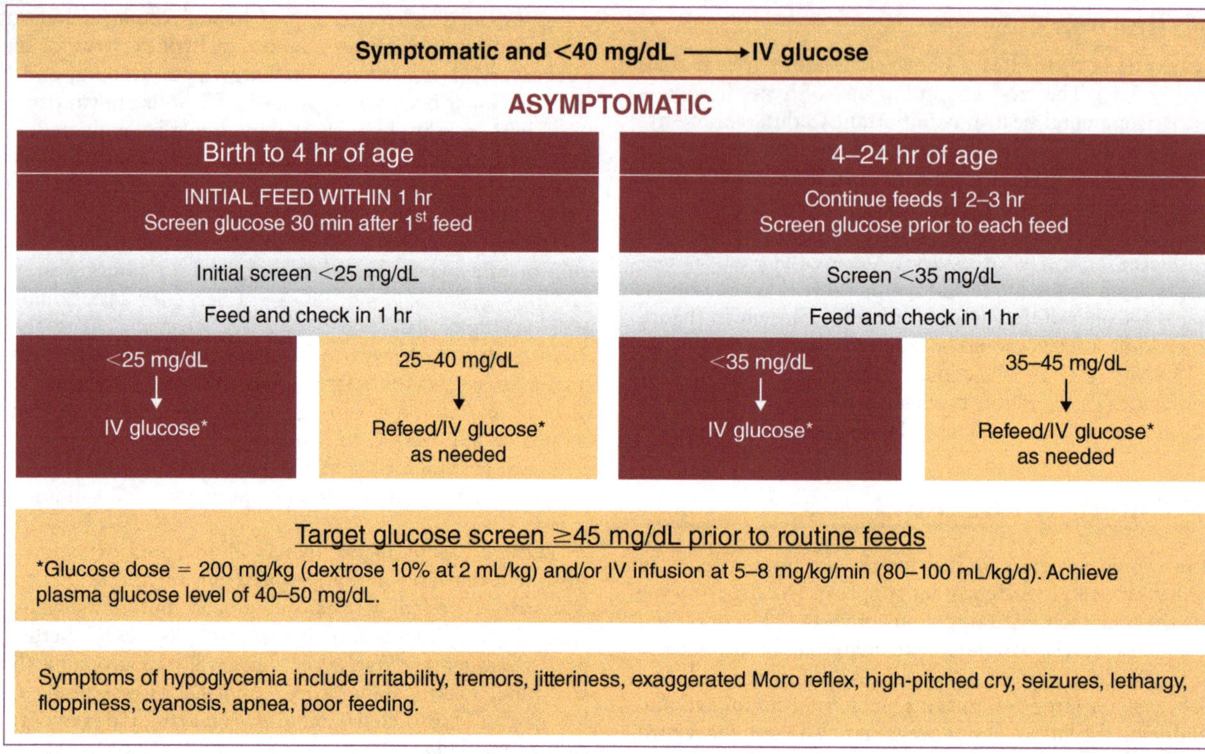


**FIGURE 5.1 Screening and management of postnatal glucose homeostasis in late preterm and term infants who are small for gestational age (SGA), large for gestational age (LGA), or are born to a diabetic mother (IDM).**

*Source:* From Adamkin, D. H. (2011). Postnatal glucose homeostasis in late-preterm and term infants. *Pediatrics, 127,* 575–579. https://doi.org/10.1542/peds.2010-3851.

It also suggests an improvement in breastfeeding rate after discharge (Edwards et al., 2022). In a randomized controlled trial (RCT) targeting asymptomatic hypoglycemia cases in SGA and IUGR, IDM, and LGA, and late preterm infants, the group that only breastfed and the group that used oral dextrose gel after breastfeeding were compared. As a result, the group that used oral dextrose gel after breastfeeding had a significantly lower frequency of IV therapeutic intervention than the group that used oral dextrose gel after breastfeeding (Gupta et al., 2022). No adverse events were reported in either study. From these results, oral dextrose gel used for term infants is probably an effective and safe first-line treatment. The effects on long-term neurodevelopment are unclear, and further research is needed.

## HYPERBILIRUBINEMIA

Neonatal jaundice is a condition in which the skin becomes yellowish due to increased bilirubin concentration in the body during the neonatal period. In general, visible jaundice occurs when the total bilirubin (TB) in the blood of a newborn exceeds 5.0 to 7.0 mg/dl. Jaundice begins on the face and spreads to the chest, abdomen, and lower limbs, but the yellowing of the bulbar conjunctiva is relatively easy to identify. Jaundice is caused by an elevation in unconjugated (indirect) and/or conjugated (direct) bilirubin levels. Bilirubin is an antioxidant at low levels and a potent neurotoxin at high levels. Elevations in bilirubin are either due to an increase in production (breakdown of heme-containing proteins) and/or a delay in the elimination or reabsorption of bilirubin.

Most bilirubin comes from the breakdown of red blood cells (RBCs), a smaller portion from ineffective erythropoiesis in the bone marrow, and the liver's breakdown of tissue heme and heme proteins. Heme is degraded by heme oxygenase, resulting in the release of iron and the formation of carbon monoxide and biliverdin. Biliverdin is then reduced to bilirubin by biliverdin reductase. The bilirubin that is formed is taken up by the liver, bound to protein Y or ligandin, and conjugated in the smooth endoplasmic reticulum with glucuronides to form bilirubin monoglucuronide in a reaction catalyzed by uridine diphosphate and monophosphate glucuronosyltransferase. The now water-soluble bilirubin glucuronide is excreted into the intestinal lumen to be eliminated in stool. The conjugated bilirubin can be deconjugated by the intestinal enzyme beta-glucuronidase and reabsorbed into circulation intestinally. This is the enterohepatic pathway (Ullah et al., 2016).

### Physiologic Jaundice

Physiologic jaundice in the healthy-term newborn follows a typical pattern and does not present within the first 24 hours of life. Two main factors contribute to the development of hyperbilirubinemia: high bilirubin production and low excretion. The bilirubin production capacity of newborns is about twice that of adults (Itoh et al., 2023). Relative polycythemia and shortened RBC lifespan are associated with increased production. Excretion capacity includes immature hepatic uptake and conjugation processes and increased enterohepatic circulation. The bilirubin conjugating capacity of the liver is only 1% at full term and 0.1% at 30 weeks of gestation. It then develops and becomes equivalent to adults at 3 months of age (Itoh et al., 2023). These causes make jaundice more likely to appear.

Factors that contribute to the development of hyperbilirubinemia include lower gestational age, a previous sibling with jaundice, isoimmune or other hemolytic anemia, scalp hematoma, Down syndrome (Trisomy 21), or diabetes. Kemper et al. (2022) showed that hyperbilirubinemia risk factors and children with these risk factors require closer monitoring than those without. Asian newborns typically have much higher peak serum bilirubin levels during physiologic jaundice than Caucasians, leading to increased neonatal hyperbilirubinemia. This difference necessitates race-specific hour-specific nomograms for transcutaneous bilirubin concentration. Using Caucasian-based nomograms for Asian infants could result in unnecessary blood sampling referrals, highlighting the importance of population-specific guidelines for jaundice management in newborns (Itoh et al., 2023).

Premature birth is also a factor that worsens neonatal jaundice. The risk of blood TB exceeding 17 mg/dl is 20.79 (2.3–187.7) at 35 to 36 weeks of gestation and 1.8 (1.0–115.4) at 37 weeks of gestation (odds ratio [95% confidential interval]) with 40 weeks of gestation as the reference. Neonates under 37 weeks of gestation are prone to hyperbilirubinemia (Maisels et al., 2009).

### Breastfeeding Jaundice

Breastfeeding jaundice typically occurs on days 2 to 5 after birth. Serum bilirubin concentrations are strongly associated with greater weight loss in breastfeeding infants with jaundice. This occurs due to insufficient feeding. Some infants who are thought to have breastfeeding jaundice may have pathologic jaundice. Therefore, mothers and infants need to be aware of the risk of developing hyperbilirubinemia. To prevent breastfeeding jaundice, it is necessary to initiate early breastfeeding, frequent breastfeeding (8–12 times or more in 24 hours), optimize early breastfeeding management, and provide education on early feeding cues and signs of suckling adequacy. To optimize early breastfeeding management, mothers ensure and evaluate comfortable positioning, effective latch, and adequate milk transfer from healthcare professionals trained in breastfeeding management, and healthcare providers support SSC for all mothers and infants. Early breastfeeding cues are moving about or restlessness, lip smacking, hand movements toward the mouth, and vocalizing (Flaherman et al., 2017). Signs of suckling adequacy include appropriate urine output and transitional stooling, normal weight loss by an hour of age and delivery method, absence of maternal discomfort, and audible swallowing as the mother's milk volumes increase (Kemper et al., 2022). If the infant is not receiving sufficient milk at the breast despite these interventions, supplement with small amounts of formula (Flaherman et al., 2017).

### Breastmilk Jaundice

The causes of breastmilk jaundice include the infant and the breastmilk components. The cause on the infant side is the inherently low activity of UGT1A1 and further activity reduction due to UGT1A1 gene polymorphism. UGT1A1*6 is a polymorphism present in East Asia, which is why neonatal jaundice is common in East Asia. Breastmilk includes inhibitors of hepatic UGT1A1 (prenatal and nonesterified fatty acid) (Itoh et al., 2023). Even in cases of breastmilk jaundice, high levels of indirect bilirubin can cause kernicterus. Therefore, phototherapy should be initiated once blood bilirubin levels reach a therapeutic threshold. In addition, in cases of breastmilk jaundice, blood bilirubin levels will decrease if breastfeeding is discontinued for 2 to 3 days. After that, blood bilirubin levels do not rise again even if breastfeeding is resumed but will gradually decrease. If blood bilirubin levels increase sharply or phototherapy cannot be used, discontinuing breastfeeding should be considered.

### Pathologic Jaundice

Pathologic jaundice in full-term infants is diagnosed when jaundice appears within 24 hours of birth or persists for 1 or more weeks after birth. A total serum bilirubin (TSB) of 5 mg/dl/day or higher, or an increase in TSB of 18 mg/dl or higher, is also considered pathologic. Treatment and management of pathologic jaundice vary depending on the condition. Therefore, when pathologic jaundice is found, a thorough examination is required. Hereditary diseases can also cause pathologic jaundice, so it is important to ask about the family history.

## ACUTE BILIRUBIN ENCEPHALOPATHY AND KERNICTERUS

Bilirubin is neurotoxic, and abnormal hyperbilirubinemia can cause acute bilirubin encephalopathy (ABE). Without timely medical intervention, ABE progresses to kernicterus, which leads to permanent symptoms. In the 20$^{th}$ century, kernicterus, or bilirubin encephalopathy stood out as a major cause of cerebral palsy (CP) among term infants in Japan (Morioka, 2018). Japan's contribution to the development of the transcutaneous bilirubin measurement technology as a noninvasive method of monitoring bilirubin level is significant globally (Yamanouchi, Yamauchi, & Igarashi, 1980).

While this chapter focuses on the normal term newborn, the premature infant's assessment and management must be considered in contrast. Due to the increase in hyperbilirubinemia-related neurodevelopmental outcomes among preterm infants in Japan, a specific guideline to manage the phototherapy or exchange transfusions were developed and updated for the Japanese neonatal population (Morioka, 2018). In Morioka's (2018) paper, table 4 provides the Japanese current guidelines for managing hyperbilirubinemia in the country's NICUs. This guideline provides lower thresholds for treatment accounting to the gestational age at birth, corrected gestational age, and hours since birth, directing the users to consider standard phototherapy, intense phototherapy, and exchange transfusion with or without albumin infusion. Due to the higher frequencies among Asian infants to present with hyperbilirubinemia, the specific protocol by Morioka is followed in Japan to prevent negative neurodevelopmental outcomes for infants who are born early and those born at term. This Japanese example is given to alert the reader to the need to consider their country's guidelines and the population that they serve. For a more in-depth discussion of hyperbilirubinemia and current guidelines recognized worldwide (Kemper et al., 2022), please see Chapter 13, "Hematologic System".

Early treatment is, therefore, crucial. In the United States, the incidence of kernicterus decreased from 0.7 to 0.2 per 100,000 between 2006 and 2016, with an overall rate of 0.5 per 100,000 (Bhatt et al., 2022). However, in low- and middle-income countries, the rate is approximately 73 per 100,000 and remains a significant problem (Greco et al., 2016). High neurotoxicity risk factors include gestational age under 38 weeks, albumin levels below 3.0 g/dl, isoimmune hemolytic disease, sepsis, and clinical instability in the previous 24 hours (Kemper et al., 2022). These cases require stricter management.

ABE symptoms vary by phase. In the early phase (1–3 days), symptoms include decreased alertness, poor feeding, mild hypotonia, and hyperreflexia. The middle phase (end of the first week) is marked by stupor, irritability, hypertonia of extensor muscles, opisthotonos, retrocollis, and high-pitched crying. The late phase (after the first week) presents with hypo- or hypertonia, pronounced opisthotonos-retrocollis, apnea, stupor or coma, fever, seizures, and high-pitched cries (Qian et al., 2022). Scoring systems such as bilirubin-induced neurologic dysfunction (BIND) and modified BIND (BIND-M) help diagnose and grade bilirubin encephalopathy. The BIND-M score assesses mental status, muscle tone, cry characteristics, and upward gaze paresis, categorizing ABE as subtle (1–3), moderate (4–6), or advanced (7–9) (Qian et al., 2022).

Kernicterus is classified into four subtypes: classic, auditory, motor, and subtle kernicterus. Classic kernicterus features auditory neuropathy and motor symptoms like dystonia, oculomotor paresis, and enamel dysplasia. Auditory kernicterus predominantly affects hearing, while motor kernicterus shows primarily motor symptoms. Subtle kernicterus, or bilirubin-induced neurological dysfunction (BIND), involves mild neurodevelopmental issues without classical kernicterus findings (Shapiro, 2010). Risk factors for hyperbilirubinemia neurotoxicity include gestational age under 38 weeks, low albumin, hemolytic disease, sepsis, and recent clinical instability (Kemper et al., 2022).

## Assessment

Transcutaneous bilirubin (TcB) measurement is a good screening tool for detecting hyperbilirubinemia in newborns. However, TcB does not directly measure bilirubin. There is a good correlation between TcB measures and TSB concentrations, with the TSB generally within 3 mg/dl of the TcB among newborns with TSB concentrations < 15 mg/dl. Therefore, phototherapy or exchange transfusion should not be initiated based on TcB results. Use TSB as the definitive test to guide phototherapy and escalation-of-care decisions, including exchange transfusion. TSB should be measured if the TcB exceeds or is within 3 mg/dl of the phototherapy treatment threshold or if the TcB is 15 mg/dl (Kemper et al., 2022). Screening tests for hyperbilirubinemia consist of assessing clinical risk factors and measuring bilirubin levels either by serum or TcB and plotting them on an age-in-hour-specific bilirubin nomogram. This range of TSB levels rather than one specific level provides the threshold for the onset of neurotoxicity.

Clinical practice guidelines for neonatal hyperbilirubinemia have been published in various regions. However there are a few differences among these regional guidelines regarding initiating TSB levels of phototherapy (Zhang et al., 2021). The AAP Subcommittee on Hyperbilirubinemia (2022), Canadian Paediatric Society (2007), National Association of Neonatal Nurses Board of Directors (2011), and Okwundu et al. (2023) recommend the following clinical practices:

- Successful breastfeeding should be promoted and supported to decrease the incidence of severe hyperbilirubinemia.
- Nursery protocols for the identification and evaluation of hyperbilirubinemia should be established.
- Hospitals should adopt facility-wide policies and procedures that maintain an adequate standard of care for all newborns to prevent ABE and kernicterus.
- TSB or TcB should be measured as soon as possible for infants who are jaundiced < 24 hours after birth.
- The TcB or TSB should be measured between 24 and 48 hours after birth or before discharge if that occurs earlier.
- Jaundice should be assessed regularly, at least every 8 to 12 hours, and nurses should have independent authority to obtain a TSB or TcB level.
- Education for healthcare providers must emphasize that visual inspection is unreliable as the sole method for assessing jaundice.
- The results should be plotted on the predictive nomogram if the TSB concentration does not require immediate intervention.
- Infants with a gestational age of less than 38 weeks are at higher risk for severe hyperbilirubinemia and require closer monitoring.
- Closer surveillance of infants with a gestational age of less than 38 weeks is necessary because of their higher risk for severe hyperbilirubinemia.
- All infants should be assessed for adequacy of breastfeeding and the risk of severe hyperbilirubinemia before discharge. Universal discharge screening should be combined with assessing clinical risk factors (of which gestational age and exclusive breastfeeding are the most important) and a targeted follow-up.
- Parents should receive written and verbal information about jaundice.
- If an appropriate follow-up cannot be arranged for an infant, it is recommended that an outpatient follow-up bilirubin measure be taken; discharge may be delayed.
- Phototherapy and exchange transfusion are to be used for treatment when indicated.
- All nurseries should have the equipment to provide intensive phototherapy.
- Breastfeeding should be encouraged for the infant receiving phototherapy or nutritional supplementation.
- Bilirubin levels must be evaluated according to the infant's age in hours, not days.
- There should be a systematic approach to the risk assessment of all infants before discharge and institution of follow-up care if the infant develops jaundice.

## Management

Phototherapy is used to decrease the TSB level and prevent the accumulation of bilirubin in the brain. The photoisomerization of bilirubin begins as soon as the light is turned on. The light causes the bilirubin molecules to undergo quick photochemical reactions that form nontoxic, excretable isomers. These isomers have different shapes when compared to the conjugated bilirubin. They can be excreted into the bile without conjugation or special transport carriers. This effective process has almost eliminated the need for exchange transfusions.

Factors that affect the dose of phototherapy include the light source's spectral qualities, the light's intensity, the distance between the light and the infant, and the amount of surface area exposed. Intensive phototherapy requires a narrow-spectrum LED blue light with an irradiance of at least 30 mW/cm$^2$ per nm at a wavelength of around 475 nm. Light outside the 460 to 490 nm range provides unnecessary heat and potentially harmful wavelengths. Phototherapy devices can be ordered as single, double, triple, or quadruple devices. Fiber-optic blankets may also be used. The pad containing fiber-optic fibers can be placed against the skin and remains cool to touch. Due to the spectral power of the pad alone, it is commonly used in combination with overhead lights (Kemper et al., 2022).

When administering phototherapy to newborns, proper positioning and exposure are crucial. The infant should be supine with maximum body exposure, eye shields, and minimal diaper coverage. The effectiveness of phototherapy depends on irradiance, exposed skin area, and treatment duration. To maximize results, healthcare providers should use light sources above and below the baby, expose as much skin as possible, and minimize interruptions, especially for infants with higher TSB levels. Opaque eye shields are required during phototherapy to protect the eyes from retinal damage. During the assessment of the infant, the phototherapy lights should be turned off and the eye shields removed to assess the eyes for drainage, edema, and redness. Complications of eye shields include eye irritation, corneal abrasion, blocked tear ducts, and conjunctivitis. Eye care should consist of cleaning the eyes with sterile water or saline. A separate cleaning pad should be used for each eye and cleaned from the inner canthus outward. Sterile gloves should be worn while providing eye care. Some phototherapy units produce heat, and the infant's temperature must be monitored to avoid overheating. Phototherapy can also cause diarrhea and water loss in stools. It is important to monitor for skin breakdown in the perianal area and use protective barriers if needed (Kemper et al., 2022).

During phototherapy, the infant is separated from the mother, which has the potential to interfere with lactation. As long as the hyperbilirubinemia is not severe, the phototherapy can be interrupted to allow for breastfeeding and skin-to-skin care. Eye shields should be removed if the phototherapy is not in use.

# FEEDING THE HEALTHY NEWBORN

Human milk provides optimal nutrition for infants. The AAP Policy Statement on Breastfeeding and the Use of Human Milk (Meek & Noble, 2022) recommends exclusive breastfeeding for 6 months and as long as mutually desired by mother and child for 2 years or beyond. This recommendation is consistent with the guidelines and policies of the WHO, American Academy of Family Physicians, and Canadian Paediatric Society.

Many health benefits for infants and children have been attributed to breastfeeding and are confirmed through systematic literature reviews and meta-analyses. Breastfeeding is associated with the following benefits for the term infant (Meek & Noble, 2022):

- protection against SIDS with breastfeeding for at least 2 months
- decreased infant mortality with exclusive breastfeeding
- protection against lower respiratory tract infection, with a longer duration of exclusive breastfeeding providing the strongest protection
- protection against severe or persistent diarrhea, with a longer duration of exclusive breastfeeding providing the strongest protection
- protection against otitis media
- protection against asthma, being the most protective against wheezing in the first 2 years
- protection against eczema in the first 2 years
- protection against Crohn disease and ulcerative colitis
- protection against childhood and adult obesity
- protection against types 1 and 2 diabetes
- protection against leukemia
- decreased caries (up to 12 months)

Breastfeeding is associated with the following benefits for the very low birth weight (VLBW) infant (Meek & Noble, 2022):

- reduced instances of necrotizing enterocolitis (NEC)
- reduced late-onset sepsis
- reduced chronic lung disease
- reduced retinopathy of prematurity (ROP)
- improved neurodevelopment

Breastfeeding also has economic and health effects. Previously, we could only focus on the cost effects of preventing acute illnesses that would occur if breastfeeding was not performed. However, the recent increase in the availability of longitudinal data and electronic health records and the ability to perform simulation modeling have made it possible to determine the long-term effects. The economic loss from not breastfeeding consistently exceeded \$100 billion annually for the United States and around \$300 billion annually in global studies (Jegier et al., 2024; Walters et al., 2019). This cost arises from the deaths of women and children and child cognitive losses.

A systematic review of 58 experimental and quasiexperimental studies that examined the effect of the Baby-Friendly Hospital Initiative (BFHI) 10 steps on breastfeeding intention, duration, and exclusivity was conducted in 2016 (Pérez-Escamilla et al., 2016). They found that hospitals that adhered to the BFHI 10 steps had mothers who breastfed longer, and there was a dose-response between the number of 10 steps implemented in hospitals and improved breastfeeding outcomes. WHO and UNICEF updated the *Ten Steps to Successful Breastfeeding* to include improved guidance for implementation within healthcare facilities (Table 5.2).

**TABLE 5.2**

**WHO/UNICEF BABY FRIENDLY HOSPITAL INITIATIVE**

| **Ten Steps to Successful Breastfeeding (Revised 2024)** | |
|---|---|
| **Critical management procedures** | 1a. Comply fully with the *International Code of Marketing of Breast-Milk Substitutes* and relevant World Health Assembly resolutions. |
| | 1b. Have a written infant feeding policy that is routinely communicated to staff and parents. |
| | 1c. Establish ongoing monitoring and data management systems. |
| | 2. Ensure that staff have sufficient knowledge, competence, and skills to support breastfeeding. |
| **Key clinical practices** | 3. Discuss the importance and management of breastfeeding with pregnant women and their families. |
| | 4. Facilitate immediate and uninterrupted skin-to-skin contact and support mothers to initiate breastfeeding as soon as possible after birth. |
| | 5. Support mothers to initiate and maintain breastfeeding and manage common difficulties. |
| | 6. Do not provide breastfed newborns any food or fluids other than breastmilk, unless medically indicated. |
| | 7. Enable mothers and their infants to remain together and to practice rooming-in 24 hours a day. |
| | 8. Support mothers to recognize and respond to their infants' cues for feeding. |
| | 9. Counsel mothers on the use and risks of feeding bottles, teats, and pacifiers. |
| | 10. Coordinate discharge so that parents and their infants have timely access to ongoing support and care. |

*Source:* From World Health Organization. (2018). *Ten steps to successful breastfeeding* (revised 2018). http://www.who.int/nutrition/bfhi/ten-steps/en.

## NURSING INTERVENTIONS THAT PROMOTE SUCCESSFUL BREASTFEEDING

### Skin-to-Skin Contact

Providing the optimal breastfeeding environment begins at birth. SSC improves breastfeeding rate. The healthy, stable newborn should be placed directly on the mother's bare chest immediately after birth. Initial nursing interventions after birth, including drying the infant, initial assessment, and Apgar scoring, should occur while the baby is skin to skin (kangaroo mother care) with the mother. Nursing interventions, including birth weight and vitamin K and ophthalmic antibiotic administration, should be delayed, allowing at least 1 hour of uninterrupted SSC and breastfeeding attempts. Nurses should remain with the mother and assist with breastfeeding positioning and latch. SSC should also be maintained during painful procedures, including heel sticks, venous punctures, and injections because SSC reduces the neonates' pain response (Johnston et al., 2017).

The 2016 Cochrane Review (Moore et al., 2016) regarding early SSC of mothers and healthy infants revealed empirical evidence that early and frequent SSC promotes stability of the cardiorespiratory system in the neonate and higher blood glucose levels. Neonates who received SSC had similar body temperatures when compared to infants who did not receive SSC. Women who experienced SSC after vaginal birth reported longer durations of breastfeeding and better success with exclusive breastfeeding compared to women who did not experience SSC. SSC in the operating room after a cesarean can safely occur and promote exclusive breastfeeding (Berg & Hung, 2011; Stone et al., 2014). Earlier onset of lactogenesis II (milk production), increased oxytocin release, and increased milk production as a result of frequent SSC are also suggested in the literature (Chen et al., 1998; Cong et al., 2015; Hemachandra et al., 2016). Inadequate positioning during SSC can increase the risk of SIDS and sudden unexpected infant death (SUID) in infants. Prone positioning and early SSC without proper supervision by trained staff are specifically recognized as risk factors. Safe sleep practices are recommended during the newborn's hospital stay, including parental education and frequent staff monitoring, particularly when the mother is drowsy or sedated (Feldman-Winter et al., 2016; Meek & Noble, 2022).

## CONTRAINDICATIONS TO BREASTFEEDING

Mothers should avoid breastfeeding in the following situations (Meek & Noble, 2022): if the infant has classic galactosemia; if the mother has an HIV infection, human T-cell lymphotropic virus type I or type II infection, untreated brucellosis, or suspected or confirmed Ebola virus disease; or if the mother is using illicit drugs, such as opioids, cocaine, or phencyclidine.

### Maternal–Infant Separation Only When Medically Necessary

Healthcare professionals should recommend 10 to 12 feedings at the breast per 24 hours during the first 3 to 5 days after birth. Milk production occurs through lactogenesis I and II. Lactogenesis I begins between the 10th and 22nd week of pregnancy and is hormonally mediated, leading to the development of glandular tissue and lactocytes. Lactogenesis II, the onset of milk production, starts after birth with the separation of the placenta, causing a drop in maternal progesterone levels. This process relies on frequent suckling, which stimulates prolactin release from the anterior pituitary for milk production and oxytocin release from the posterior pituitary for the milk ejection reflex (Wambach & Riordan, 2016). Mothers with diabetes, delivery-related stress, or retained placenta face risks of delayed lactogenesis and require close monitoring and timely intervention (Lawrence & Lawrence, 2022).

Extended separation between mother and infant in the hospital reduces breastfeeding opportunities. During the first few days, achieving a good latch may take multiple attempts, so uninterrupted mother–infant time is critical for recognizing hunger cues and practicing breastfeeding. Parents should be taught to identify early hunger cues, such as arm and leg movements, rooting, lip smacking, and fingers or fists-to-mouth actions, which may occur during light sleep with closed eyes. Late hunger cues include restlessness, crying, and screaming (Wambach & Riordan, 2016).

Mothers should be encouraged to continuously room-in with their infants to respond to hunger cues promptly and bond effectively. Infant assessments by healthcare providers should occur whenever possible in the mother's room. The breastfeeding mother–infant pair should only be separated for medical reasons.

### Pacifier Use

Pacifier use in healthy breastfed infants is somewhat controversial. Avoidance of pacifiers includes the implementation of baby-friendly hospital practices. A Cochrane review found that pacifier use in healthy term infants before and after lactation is established does not reduce the duration of breastfeeding up to 4 months of age. However, there was insufficient evidence on the potential harms of pacifiers on infants and mothers (Jaafar et al., 2016). Medical staff should educate parents on the possible risks of pacifier use and encourage them to decide on pacifier use for mothers who are well motivated to breastfeed (Jaafar et al., 2016; WHO, 2024).

The specific recommendations of the AAP regarding pacifier use and breastfeeding infants are to avoid pacifier use in the neonatal period until breastfeeding is well established. The AAP encourages pacifier use in infants undergoing painful procedures and during naps and sleep as potential protection against SIDS (Eidelman et al., 2012). One further recommendation is to discourage the use of pacifiers to rule out hunger or delay feeding; breastfeeding should occur before offering a pacifier. Parents must be educated on all the risks and benefits of pacifier use in breastfed infants to make an informed decision that best suits their needs and parenting philosophy.

## ADEQUACY OF BREASTFEEDING

The three leading indicators of adequate breastmilk transfer are audible swallowing by the infant, adequate urine and stool output, and weight gain. Healthcare professionals caring for breastfeeding mother–infant dyads must assess breastmilk transfer competency. At least one full breastfeeding session should be observed, ideally once per shift after birth and at least once before discharge. Mothers need guidance on infant positioning and achieving a deep latch. Typical positions include the football hold, cross-cradle hold, and side-lying position. Mothers should support the infant's head with one hand and their breast with the other, ensuring that fingers do not cover the areola. Hand-expressing drops of breastmilk onto the infant's lips can entice a wide-mouth gape. Once the gape is achieved, the infant should be brought quickly to the breast to feel the nipple on its palate, triggering the sucking reflex. The infant should take in most of the areola with lips flanged outward.

Healthcare providers should listen for audible swallowing during breastfeeding. Initially, the infant may take 5 to 10 sucks before a swallow, heard as a soft "k" sound. As milk production increases, swallowing becomes more frequent. Adequate breastfeeding involves sustained sucking and swallowing for 10 to 15 minutes on at least one breast. If the infant detaches, feeding can continue on the other breast, with mothers encouraged to alternate starting breasts. Sustained audible swallowing and signs of satiety, such as slower sucking, sleepiness, and self-detaching, are more critical indicators than feeding duration (Wambach & Riordan, 2016). Breastfeeding adequacy can be assessed using tools such as the LATCH assessment by Jensen et al. (1994), which scores five breastfeeding indicators from 0 to 10 (Table 5.3). A higher score indicates adequate latch, milk transfer, and maternal comfort.

TABLE 5.3

LATCH BREASTFEEDING ASSESSMENT TOOL

| | 0 | 1 | 2 |
|---|---|---|---|
| Latch | Too sleepy or reluctant<br>No latch achieved | Repeated attempts<br>Hold nipple in mouth<br>Stimulate suck | Grasps breast<br>Tongue down<br>Lips flanged<br>Rhythmic sucking |
| Audible swallowing | None | A few with stimulation | Spontaneous and intermittent < 24 hours old Spontaneous and frequent > 24 hours old |
| Type of nipple | Inverted | Flat | Everted (with stimulation) |
| Comfort of mother | Engorged<br>Cracked/bleeding/large blisters or bruises<br>Severe discomfort | Filling<br>Reddened/small blisters or bruises<br>Mild/moderate discomfort | Soft<br>Nontender |
| Hold or positioning | Full assist (staff holds infant at breast) | Minimal assist<br>Teach one side; mother does other<br>Staff holds and then mother takes over | No assist from staff<br>Mother able to position/hold infant |

*Source:* From Jensen, D., Wallace, S., & Kelsay, P. (1994). LATCH: A breastfeeding charting system and documentation tool. *Journal of Obstetric, Gynecologic, and Neonatal Nursing, 23*, 27–32. https://doi.org/10.1111/j.1552-6909.1994.tb01847.x.

The second indicator of adequate breastfeeding is urine and stool output. Breastfed infants should have one wet diaper on the first day of life, increasing by one diaper per day up to five to six wet diapers daily. Wet diapers should feel heavier, with light-colored urine and little odor. Reddish-colored urine in the first days is normal. Neonates should pass at least one green to black tarry stool on days one and two. By days three and four, stools transition to green and are looser as milk production increases. From days four to seven, stools become yellow, loose, and seedy, with one to four stools daily. By the second week, stools increase in volume and occur three to five times daily. It is normal for occasional stool-free days (Wambach & Riordan, 2016). If output is inadequate, breastfeeding should be evaluated for milk transfer and frequency, and neonates should be checked for jaundice or dehydration signs. Referrals to lactation consultants may be necessary for breastfeeding difficulties.

The third indicator of adequate breastfeeding is weight gain. Healthy neonates typically lose up to 5% of birth weight in the first 3 days due to evaporative loss. A 7% weight loss warrants breastfeeding, urine, and stool output evaluation. **Emergency Alert: Weight loss exceeding 7% with adequate breastfeeding and output may indicate fluid overload from maternal IV fluids during labor (Giudicelli et al., 2020).** A 10% weight loss requires intervention to support lactogenesis II and milk transfer. Mothers should pump both breasts for 10 to 15 minutes after feeding, at least eight times daily, using a hospital-grade pump, and feed expressed milk to the infant via cup, finger feeding, or the Supplemental Nursing System (SNS). If breastmilk is insufficient, expressed milk or pasteurized donor human milk (PDHM) is recommended over formula, provided in physiologic volumes, such as 5 to 10 ml on day 1 and 10 to 15 ml on day 2 (Meek & Noble, 2022).

## Breastfeeding Follow-Up After Discharge

Breastfed neonates should be seen by a healthcare provider within 3 to 5 days after discharge from the hospital to assess breastfeeding adequacy, the onset of mother's milk, jaundice or elevated bilirubin levels, and weight gain. Neonates with weight loss should regain birth weight by 14 days of age. Breastfeeding should be assessed at all subsequent infant healthcare provider visits to include the baby's health and growth and the mother's support systems and motivation to continue breastfeeding. Exclusive breastfeeding should be encouraged and promoted throughout the first 6 months of the infant's life, with continued breastfeeding and the addition of solid foods through the first year of life and beyond if mother and infant desire. Formula supplementation should be avoided unless medically indicated.

## Formula Feeding

If a mother chooses not to breastfeed or breastfeeding is contraindicated and banked milk is not available or feasible, then formula feeding may be an alternative. Commercially prepared cow's milk–based formulas are all relatively similar in their nutrients, vitamins, minerals, proteins, carbohydrates, and fat composition. Other formulas are soy-based, casein or whey-hydrolysate, and amino acid formulas. Soy formulas are generally recommended to mothers whose infants have a cow's milk intolerance, galactosemia, and hereditary lactase deficiency. Casein or whey-hydrolysate formulas are recommended for children who cannot tolerate cow's milk or soy-based formulas.

Formulas come in many forms and concentrations such as concentrate, ready-to-feed, or powder forms. Parents and caregivers need to be educated on preparing the formula correctly according to product package instructions. Formula or breastmilk should never be heated in a microwave because of uneven heating and the potential for burns. Term infants require about 100 to 120 kcal/kg daily. Newborns receiving formula should be fed 1 to 2 oz per feeding every 3 to 4 hours for the first week and advanced to 2 to 4 oz per feeding around 1 week of age. A general volume recommendation is 2.5 oz/lb per day. The prepared formula cannot sit at room temperature for more than 2 hours because bacteria can grow. The prepared formula can be refrigerated for 24 hours before consumption.

# DISCHARGE SCREENING

## Newborn Bloodspot Screening

Newborn bloodspot screening (NBS) includes tests for inborn errors in metabolism, inborn errors of immunity, congenital hypothyroidism, congenital adrenal hyperplasia, hemoglobinopathies, cystic fibrosis (CF), and spinal muscular atrophy. Early diagnosis of NBS allows for early treatment shortly after birth, enabling many affected infants to live normal, healthy lives. In high-income countries, NBS has been well established as an efficient disease prevention system but is not yet fully implemented in low- and middle-income countries. Thus, when NBS spreads in low- and middle-income countries, it reduces preventable deaths of infants and children.

**TABLE 5.4**

**NEWBORN SCREENING IN THE UNITED STATES**

| Organic Acid Disorders (OADs) | Amino Acid Disorders (AADs) | Fatty Acid Oxidating Disorders (FAODs) | Hemoglobinopathis (HGBs) | Other Clinically Significant Disorders | |
|---|---|---|---|---|---|
| Isovaleric acidemia | Phenylketonuria | Medium-chain acyl-CoA dehydrogenase deficiency | Hemoglobin S/S disease (sickle cell anemia) | Congenital hypothyroidism | Galactokinase |
| Glutaric acidemia-Type I | Maple syrup urine disease | Very long-chain acyl-CoA dehydrogenase deficiency | Hemoglobin S/ß-thalassemia | Biotinidase deficiency | Galactoepimerase |
| 3-Hydroxy 3-methyl glutaric aciduria | Homocystinuria | Long-chain L-3-OH acyl-CoA dehydrogenase deficiency | Hemoglobin S/C disease | Congenital adrenal hyperplasia | T-cell defect |
| Multiple carboxylase deficiency | Citrullinemia | Trifunctional protein deficiency | Variant hemoglobinopathies (including HbE) | Galactosemia (classical transferase deficiency) | T-cell defect |
| Methylmalonic acidemia (mutase deficiency) | Argininosuccinic acidemia | Carnitine update defect | Glucose-6-phosphate dehydrogenase Deficiency | Early hearing detection and intervention | Krabbe |

*(continued)*

**TABLE 5.4**

## NEWBORN SCREENING IN THE UNITED STATES (*continued*)

| Organic Acid Disorders (OADs) | Amino Acid Disorders (AADs) | Fatty Acid Oxidating Disorders (FAODs) | Hemoglobinopathis (HGBs) | Other Clinically Significant Disorders | |
|---|---|---|---|---|---|
| 3-Methylcrotonyl-CoA carboxylase deficiency | Tyrosinemia type I | Short-chain acyl-CoA dehydrogenase deficiency | Other hemoglobins | CF | Fabry |
| Methylmalonic acidemia (cobalamin A and B) | Benign hyperphenylalaninemia | Glutaric acidemia type II | | Severe combined immunodeficiency (SCID) | cCHD |
| Propionic acidemia | Tyrosinemia type II | Medium/short-chain L-3-OH acyl-CoA dehydrogenase deficiency | | Pompe | Gaucher Niemann–Pick disease |
| ß-Ketothiolase deficiency | Defects of biopterin cofactor biosynthesis | Medium-chain ketoacyl-CoA thiolase deficiency | | Mucopolysaccharidosis Type 1 | Formiminoglutamic aciduria/ hyperornithinemia-hyperammonemia-homocitrullinuria syndrome |
| Methylmalonic acidemia (cobalamin C and D) | Argininemia | Carnitine palmitoyl transferase II deficiency | | Adrenoleukodystrophy | HIV |
| Malonic acidemia | Tyrosinemia type III | Carnitine acylcarnitine translocase deficiency | | Spinal muscular atrophy | Congenital toxoplasmosis |
| Isobutyryl-CoA dehydrogenase deficiency | Defects of biotin cofactor regeneration | Carnitine palmitoyl transferase II deficiency (liver) | | Mucopolysaccharidosis Type 3 | Congenital cytomegalovirus |
| 2-Methyl 3-hydroxy butyric aciduria | Hypermethioninemia | Dienoyl-CoA reductase deficiency | | Guanidinoacetate methyltransferase deficiency | Pyroglutamic acidemia |
| 2-methylbutyryl-CoA dehydrogenase deficiency | Citrullinemia type II | | | | |
| 3-Methylglutaconic aciduria | | | | | |

*Source:* Data from Therrell, B. L., Padilla, C. D., Borrajo, G. J. C., Khneisser, I., Schielen, P. C. J. I., Knight-Madden, J., Malherbe, H. L., & Kase, M. (2024). Current status of newborn bloodspot screening worldwide 2024: A comprehensive review of recent activities (2020–2023). *International Journal of Neonatal Screening, 10*(2), 38. https://doi.org/10.3390/ijns10020038. 

NBS programs differ within and between countries. The diseases covered by NBS programs across U.S. states and territories are listed in Table 5.4. However, it is important to note that the specific diseases screened for vary significantly from one state to another (Therrell et al., 2024). For further details about the methods used for each screening condition, readers can visit the federal website at https://www.newsteps.org/data-center/state-profiles. This site provides specific information on procedures and analyses related to various screened disorders alongside other summary data. Readers can select a state on the site to view its screening profile. By selecting "Disorder" within the profile, they can access a list of screened conditions and additional details about methods and biomarkers. The timing of specimen collection also varies widely from country to country. Collecting the first specimen between 24 and 72 hours after birth is standard practice in many areas (Therrell et al., 2024).

Following is the newborn screen blood specimen collection and handling procedure:

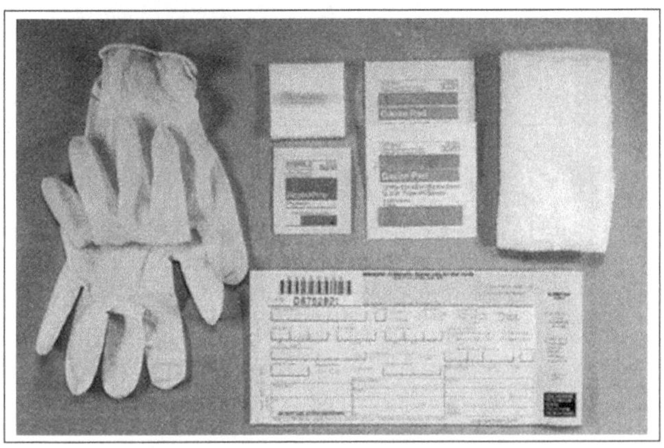

1. Required equipment includes a sterile lancet with tip less than 2.4 mm, sterile alcohol prep, sterile gauze pads, soft cloth, blood collection form, and gloves.

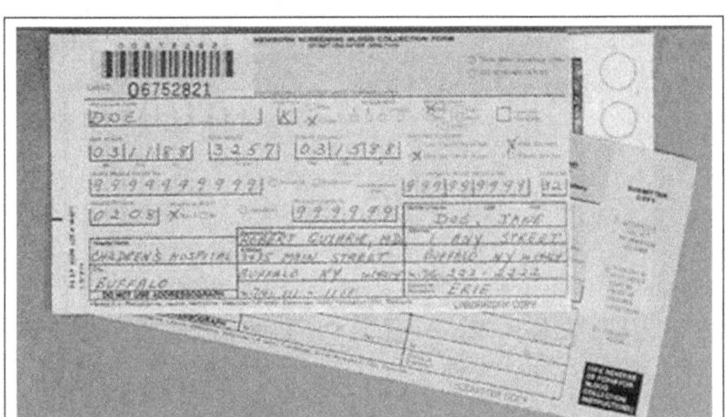

2. Complete all information. Do not contaminate filter paper circles by allowing the circles to come in contact with spillage or by touching them before or after blood collection.

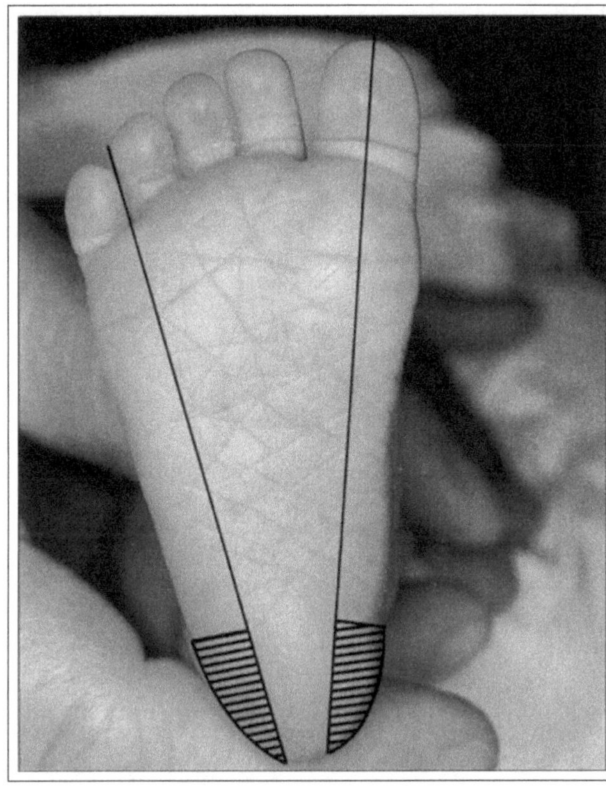

3. The hatched area indicates safe areas for the puncture site.

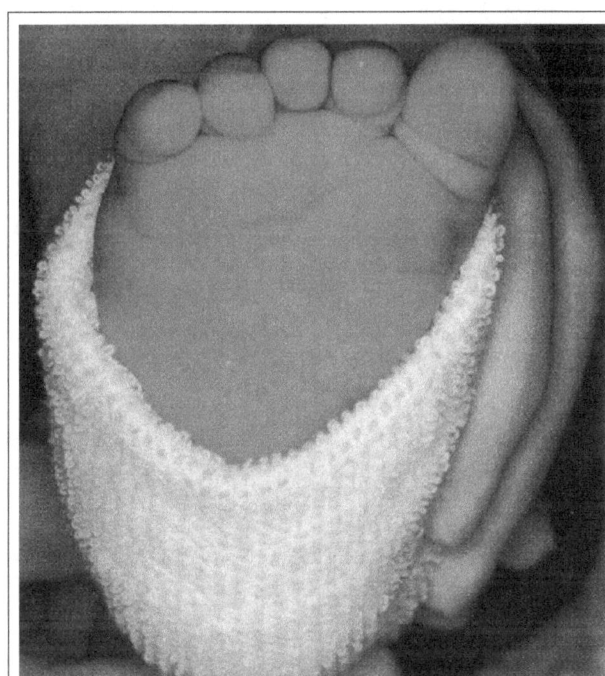

4. Warm the site with a soft cloth, moistened with warm water or a heel warmer for 3 to 5 minutes.

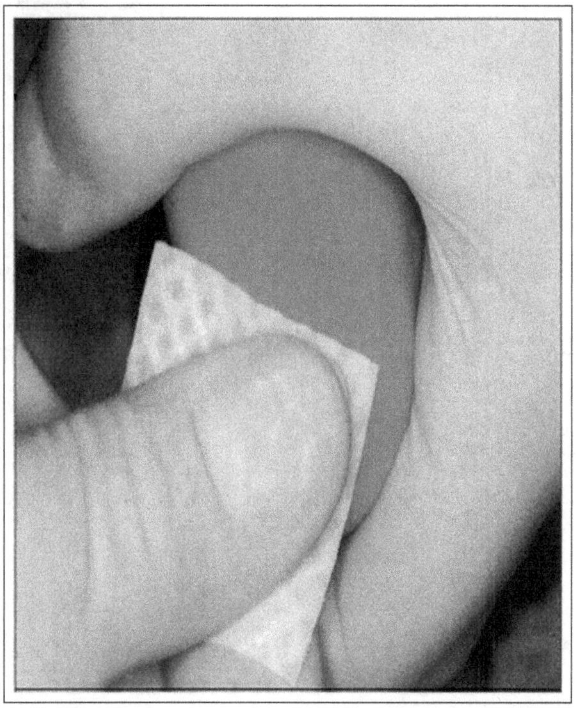

5. Cleanse the site with an alcohol prep pad. Wipe dry with a sterile gauze pad.

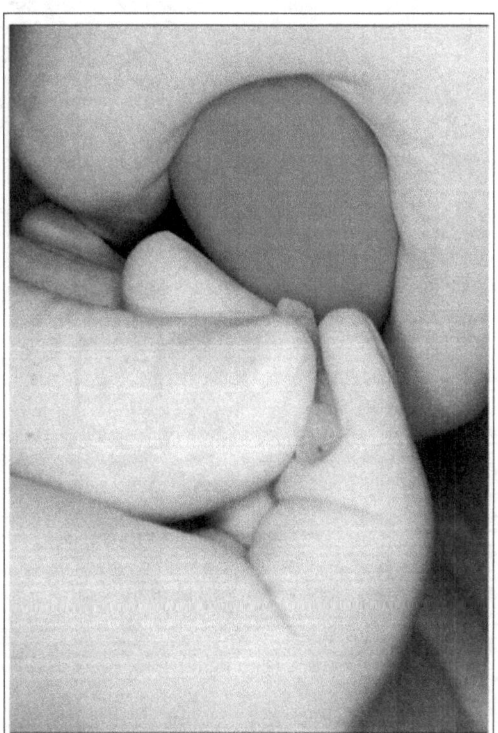

6. Puncture the infant's heel. Wipe away the first blood drop with a sterile gauze pad. Allow another large blood drop to form.

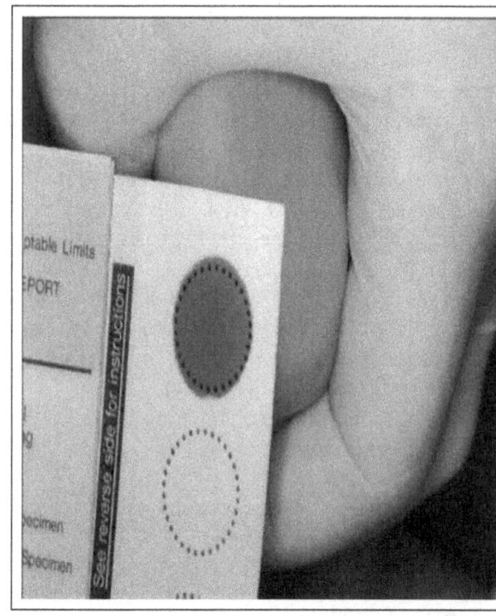


7. Lightly touch the filter paper to the large blood drop. Allow the blood to soak through and completely fill the circle with a single application to a large blood drop. (To enhance blood flow, gentle intermittent pressure may be applied to the area surrounding the puncture site.) Apply blood to one side of the filter paper only.

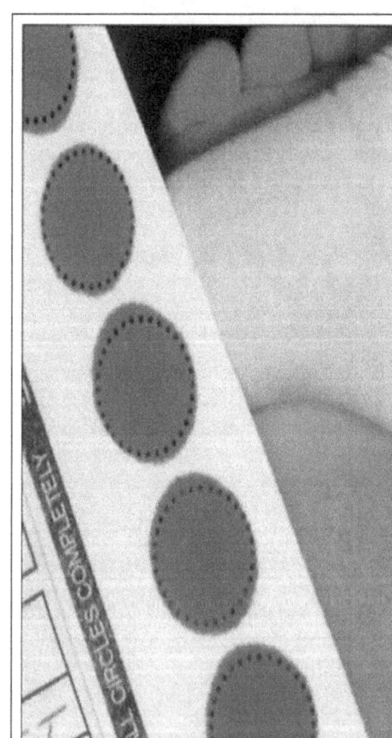

8. Fill the remaining circles in the same manner as in step 7 with successive blood drops. If blood flow is diminished, repeat steps 5 through 7. Care of the skin puncture site should be consistent with your institution's procedures.

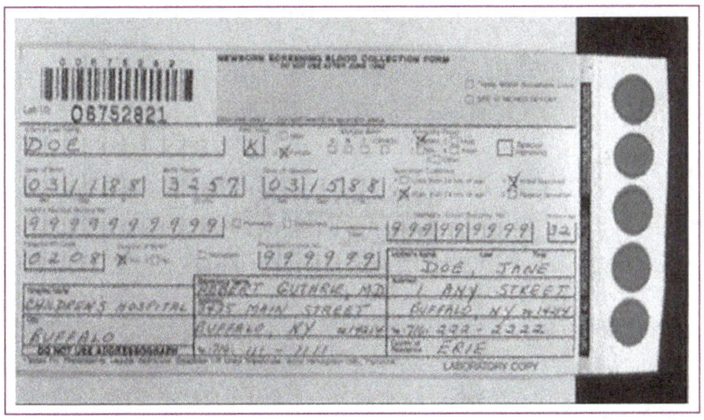


9. Dry the blood spots on a dry, clean, flat, and nonabsorbent surface for at least 4 hours.

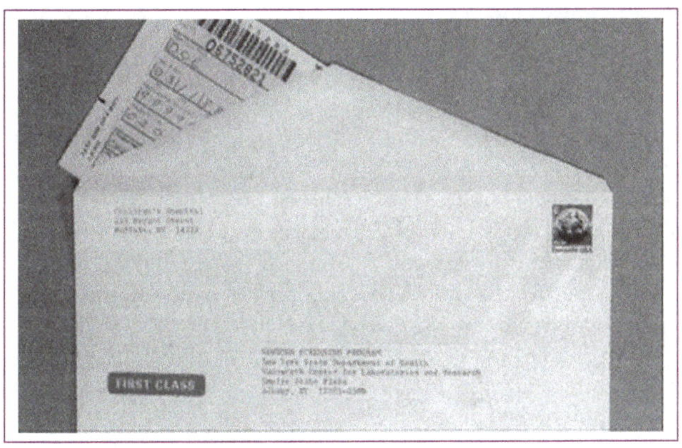


10. Mail the completed form to the testing laboratory within 24 hours of collection.

*Source:* Copyright © 2011, PerkinElmer, Inc. All rights reserved. PerkinElmer® is a registered trademark of PerkinElmer, Inc. All other trademarks are the property of their respective owners. Text and images reprinted with the permission of the New York State Department of Health.

## Newborn Hearing Screening

The Universal Newborn Hearing Screening (UNHS) commonly employs otoacoustic emissions (OAE) and automated auditory brainstem responses (AABR). OAE is a noninvasive, quick, and easy technique that uses a small probe to deliver sound into the ear canal and record responses from cochlear outer hair cells. It can be performed in less than 1 minute without specialized knowledge. OAE has limitations, such as high referral rates due to transient ear conditions, false positives from noise, and the inability to detect nerve dysfunction or auditory neuropathy caused by factors such as hyperbilirubinemia or ototoxic drugs.

AABR measures brain wave responses to sound stimuli using electrodes on the infant's head. It detects impairments in the cochlea, auditory nerve, and brainstem, distinguishing conductive from sensorineural hearing loss. AABR is particularly effective for identifying auditory neuropathy spectrum disorders, which OAE may miss. While AABR assesses a broader auditory range and has fewer false positives, it is more time consuming and costly (Wroblewska-Seniuk et al., 2017). Screening systems should be tailored to each facility's resources, including reexamination protocols.

Congenital cytomegalovirus infection (cCMV) contributes to approximately 10% of congenital hearing loss (Shearer et al., 2019). Diagnosis can be made via urine specimens from infants under 21 days old, and ganciclovir treatment has shown promise for improving hearing loss in affected children (Kimberlin et al., 2003). Targeted cCMV screening is now implemented for newborns who fail the UNHS in Japan and some states (Ito et al., 2024; Schleiss, 2024).

## Critical Congenital Heart Disease Screening

Pulse oximetry screening (POS) is a simple, rapid, accurate, and noninvasive method effective in detecting critical congenital heart disease (cCHD) in newborns (Girdhar & Ewer, 2024). Congenital heart disease (CHD) is the most common serious birth defect, affecting 4 to 10 per 1,000 newborns, with cCHD comprising 15% to 25% of cases (Girdher & Ewer, 2024). Duct-dependent defects can lead to acute cardiovascular collapse or death after ductus arteriosus closure. Early identification and cardiology consultation enable timely care and treatment. While antenatal ultrasound is widely used for CHD screening in high-income countries, its detection rates vary significantly. In settings without routine antenatal ultrasound, the risk of missed cCHD increases. POS is safe, noninvasive, easy, and cost effective. Early detection through POS could reduce CHD-related mortality, particularly in low-to-middle-income countries.

Because the algorithm has some variation within countries, screening should be performed according to the algorithm for each country. The algorithm in Figure 5.2 illustrates the steps to complete the screening recommended by the AAP. A screen is considered as passed if pulse oximetry is 95% or more in the right hand and foot and a difference of 3% or less between the 2. When pulse oximetry shows 90% to 94% in either the right hand or foot or a difference of 4% or more between the right hand and foot, the patient must repeat pulse oximetry measurements in 1 hour. A screen is considered as failed if pulse oximetry of 89% or less in either the right hand or foot in measurement 1, pulse oximetry shows 90% to 94% in either the right hand or foot or a difference of 4% or more between the right hand and foot in measurement 2 (Martin et al. 2020). The patient who fails the POS should undergo an echocardiogram at the hospital or birth center, or through a telemedicine platform for remote evaluation. If this option is unavailable, the patient should be transferred to another facility for appropriate treatment. The infant's healthcare provider must be notified immediately, and the infant may require follow-up care with a cardiologist.

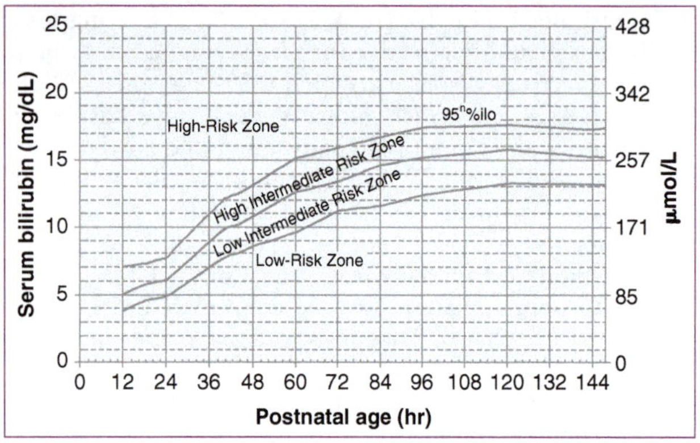


**FIGURE 5.2 Revised algorithm for cCHD screening with pulse oximetry.**

RH, right hand, cCHID, critical congenital heart disease.

*Source:* From Martin, G. R., Ewer, A. K., Gaviglio, A., Hom, L. A., Saarinen, A., Sontag, M., Burns, K. M., Kemper, A. R., & Oster, M. E. (2020). Updated strategies for pulse oximetry screening for critical congenital heart disease. *Pediatrics*, 146, e20191650. https://doi.org/10.1542/peds.2019-1650.

The overall sensitivity, specificity, and false positive rates of POS are 76.3%, 99.9%, and .1%, respectively (Plana et al., 2018). However, there is a difference in the detection rate for each particular CHD condition (Martin et al., 2020). Therefore, rather than relying solely on the POS, it is necessary to make a comprehensive judgment. Screening is done around 24 hours after birth. When POS is done in the first 24 hours, POS may detect serious noncardiac issues such as sepsis, pneumonia, and persistent pulmonary hypertension.

## DISCHARGE

Planning for discharge should begin at the time of admission. The nurse caring for the newborn and the primary care provider give discharge instructions to the parents. Nurses should increase opportunities for parents to care for their baby during hospitalization by supporting and interacting with them, teaching them appropriate ways to do so, and encouraging them. Even for healthy mothers and babies, the hospital stay should be long enough to allow the mother to recover sufficiently, be ready to care for herself and her newborn at home, and prevent the newborn from being readmitted. Benitz et al. (2015) stated that "Hospital Stay for Healthy Term Newborn Infants" includes the following criteria:

- The infant's physical examination, vital signs, excretion, and feedings are normal, and they do not have any excessive bleeding at the circumcision site, jaundice, or sepsis.
- Maternal and infant laboratory tests of infection and vaccination (hepatitis B and Tdap) and neonatal screenings were finished.
- The mother's knowledge, ability, and confidence to provide adequate care and safe sleep.
- Family, environmental, and social risk factors have been assessed.
- For newborns discharged before 48 hours after delivery, a healthcare practitioner made an appointment for the infant to be examined within 48 hours of discharge.

Research shows that strategic discharge teaching is effective. A unified intervention based on AAP guidelines, including checklists, demonstrations, staff education, and training videos, was developed to increase mothers' knowledge retention of neonatal teaching. Quality improvement (QI) methodologies were used to improve maternal knowledge retention. The process has been restructured and evaluated and has successfully continually improved mothers' knowledge (Hochreiter et al., 2022).

## SUMMARY

This chapter has outlined the basic information for assessing, managing, and discharging the normal newborn. There is a need for neonatal nurses to have a better understanding of the normal newborn as they care for the sick and/or preterm infant.

## CASE STUDY

**Identification of the Problem.** A term male infant presented at birth with 1- to 4-mm pustules covering his face, chest, trunk, and scrotum.

**Assessment: History and Physical Examination.** A term male infant, 39 + 4 weeks' gestation, weighing 3.6 kg, was born via a cesarean section for failure to progress. Apgar scores were 8 and 9 at 1 and 5 minutes, respectively. The mother was a 33-year-old G1 P0. The pregnancy was uncomplicated, the mother's blood type was A+, the syphilis screen was negative, the hepatitis screen was negative, the HIV screen was negative, and the rubella test was immune. The group B strep culture was negative. The mother received prenatal care. Medications during the pregnancy included prenatal vitamins. Complications during labor included failure to progress, which required a cesarean section.

**Physical Examination on Admission to the Newborn Nursery.**

- General: Appropriate for gestational age (AGA) term male infant in no distress with pustules covering his body. On admission to the newborn nursery, the infant was placed on a radiant warmer. Vital signs were stable: temperature 98.2°F (36.8°C), heart rate 158 beats/min, respirations 48 breaths/min, blood pressure 72/48 mm Hg, *m* = 52; blood sugar was 86.
- Head, ears, eyes, nose, and throat (HEENT): mild caput, anterior fontanelle soft and flat, sutures approximated and mobile, palate intact, ears appropriately placed; eyes normally spaced with red reflex bilaterally, pupils reactive, no hemorrhage noted; ears with ready recoil and symmetric
- RESPIRATORY: bilateral breath sounds clear and equal, with no grunting or retractions
- CARDIOVASCULAR (CV): regular rate and rhythm, good perfusion, brisk capillary refill, normal pulses × 4 extremities, and no murmur
- ABDOMEN: soft, flat, and nontender; active bowel sounds and no hepatomegaly
- GENITOURINARY (GU): normal male genitalia, testes descended bilaterally, rugae present, and anus patent

- NEUROLOGIC: awake and active, tone AGA; good suck and gag reflex
- SPINE: spine straight and intact, no dimples and neck supple, no masses
- EXTREMITIES: moving all extremities well with symmetric extremities; no hip clicks or clunks
- SKIN: warm and dry; moderate nonerythematous pustule approximately between 1 and 4 mm on the face, chest, trunk, scrotum, and thighs. The vesicle appears to contain milky, purulent exudate. The pustules rupture easily. Some appear superficial and are wiped off easily with vernix.

**Differential Diagnosis.**

- Acropustulosis
- Candidiasis
- Erythema toxicum
- Herpes simplex virus (HSV) infection
- Milia
- Miliaria
- Neonatal pustular melanosis
- *Staphylococcus aureus* infection

**Diagnostic Tests.** No further workup is indicated if the appearance is typical of transient neonatal pustular melanosis. If appearance is not typical, potassium hydroxide preparation, Gram stain, and Wright-Giemsa stain can be obtained to support other diagnoses in the differential. Bacterial and viral cultures can be done from the pustule. If pustules are clustered, a polymerase chain reaction (PCR) to identify possible herpes simplex should be considered.

**Working Diagnosis.** The working diagnosis is transient neonatal pustular melanosis, which is a benign, self-limiting rash of unknown etiology. In the United States, incidence has been reported to be 2.2% in White infants and as high as 4.4% in Black infants and infants with darker pigmentation.

The rash starts in utero, so eruptions are always present at birth, but the clinical appearance can vary. At first, the pustules appear uniform, round, 2- to 4-mm nonerythematous pustules that rupture easily. There is a thin white scale that is left around the perimeter of each denuded pustule. After a few hours, a central pigmented brown macule appears. This is smooth and has distinct borders that look like a freckle. The hallmark of this rash is the hyperpigmented spot that remains after the pustule has resolved. They may be profuse or sparse and typically are found under the chin and on the neck, upper chest, back, and buttocks. Occasionally, the palms, soles, and scalp are affected.

**Development of Management Plan.** No treatment is indicated. Parents will be anxious when they see pustules covering their baby and will need reassurance that neonatal pustular melanosis is a benign finding and that it fades and disappears over months.

### EVIDENCE-BASED PRACTICE

## Early Skin-to-Skin Contact in the Healthy Term Newborn

Kangaroo mother care (KMC) started at San Juan de Dios Hospital, Bogota, Colombia, because of the shortage of equipment and staff for premature infants and the frequency of cross-infection in the hospital. Whitelaw & Sleath (1985) and the WHO (2003) initially recommended it as an intervention for premature and low birth weight (LBW) infants. Recently, KMC has been widely implemented in healthy newborns and mothers immediately after birth.

SSC is one of the core elements of KMC, along with breastfeeding, follow-up, and early discharge (Chan et al., 2016). The AAP Policy Statement (Feldman-Winter et al., 2016), the Academy of Breastfeeding Medicine (Hernández-Aguilar et al., 2017; Kellams et al., 2018), and the AWHONN (2021) all have position statements and recommendations for policy regarding the implementation of SSC at birth. All healthy-term infants should be placed skin to skin immediately after delivery for at least 1 hour. Newborns should be placed naked or with diapers only and prone on the mother's chest. Mother and baby should be covered with a warm blanket.

There are many bio-psychosocial benefits of SSC for healthy-term newborns. Even in the case of cesarean section, SSC makes the mother feel a positive and natural birth experience and a sense of control (Deys et al., 2021). Intraoperative SSC is a safe and beneficial practice for mothers and newborns (Frederick et al., 2020).

While SSC has been safely implemented in hospitals worldwide, some rare adverse events have been documented. Andres et al. (2011) reviewed six cases of apparent life-threatening events (ALTEs) that occurred with infants in SSC within 2 hours after birth. In all six cases, the ALTE occurred with no apparent cause, and all six infants were born at term and were otherwise healthy. The common risk factors identified among the six cases were that the mothers were primiparous, in SSC with the infant in a prone position on the mother's chest, and the mother and infant were left alone in the delivery room.

Rodríguez-López et al. (2022) show the incidence of cardiorespiratory events during early SSC were more frequent in healthy-term newborns born during nighttime and to first-time mothers, mothers ≥ 35 years, and mothers with a gestational body mass index (BMI) > 25. To improve safe SSC practice, Feldman-Winter et al. (2016) suggest that continuous observation by staff and obtaining frequent vital signs of the newborn occur throughout SSC. The authors also suggest safe positioning of the newborn during SSC, including making sure the infant's face is visible with the mouth and nose not covered and the infant's head is in the sniffing position and turned to one side with a straight neck. The infant's shoulders and chest should face the mother, and the infant's legs should be flexed.

*(continued)*

## EVIDENCE-BASED PRACTICE (*continued*)

### References


Andres, V., Garcia, P., Rimet, Y., Nicaise, C., & Simeoni, U. (2011). Apparent life-threatening events in presumably healthy newborns during early skin-to-skin contact. *Pediatrics, 127*(4), e1073–e1076. https://doi.org/10.1542/peds.2009-3095

Association of Women's Health, Obstetric and Neonatal, Nurses. (2021). Immediate and sustained skin-to-skin contact for healthy late preterm and term newborns after birth: AWHONN practice brief number 14. *Journal of Obstetric, Gynecologic, & Neonatal Nursing, 50*(6): e13–e15. https://doi.org/10.1016/j.jogn.2021.07.007

Chan, G. J., Valsangkar, B., Kajeepeta, S., Boundy, E. O., & Wall, S. (2016). What is kangaroo mother care? Systematic review of the literature. *Journal of Global Health, 6*(1), 010701. https://doi.org/10.7189/jogh.06.010701

Deys, L., Wilson, P. V., & Meedya, D. S. (2021). What are women's experiences of immediate skin-to-skin contact at caesarean section birth? An integrative literature review. *Midwifery, 101*, 103063. https://doi.org/10.1016/j.midw.2021.103063

Feldman-Winter, L., & Goldsmith, J. P.; Committee on Fetus and Newborn; Task Force on Sudden Infant Death Syndrome. (2016). Safe sleep and skin-to-skin care in the neonatal period for healthy term newborns. *Pediatrics, 138*(3), e20161889. https://doi.org/10.1542/peds.2016-1889

Frederick, A., Fry, T., & Clowtis, L. (2020). Intraoperative mother and baby skin-to-skin contact during cesarean birth: Systematic review. *MCN: The American Journal of Maternal/Child Nursing, 45*(5), 296–305. https://doi.org/10.1097/NMC.0000000000000646

Hernández-Aguilar, M. T., Bartick, M., Schreck, P., Harrel, C., & Academy of Breastfeeding Medicine. (2018). ABM clinical protocol #7: Model maternity policy supportive of breastfeeding. *Breastfeed Medicine, 13*(9), 559–574. https://doi.org/10.1089/bfm.2018.29110.mha

Kellams, A., Harrel, C., Omage, S., Gregory, C., Rosen-Carole, R., & Academy of Breastfeeding Medicine. (2017). ABM Clinical Protocol #3: Supplementary feedings in the healthy term breastfed neonate, Revised 2017. *Breastfeed Medicine, 12*(3), 188–198. https://doi.org/10.1089/bfm.2017.29038.ajk

Rodríguez-López, J., Bértolo, J. D. C., Nadia Raquela García-Lara, N. R., Elorriaga, I. A., Echevarría, L. R., Vento, M., Parra-Llorca, A., Cabañas, F., Lozano, P., García-Algar, O., Martín-Ancel, A., Fernández, C. C., Carrasco, E. G., Arnal, I. O., Pellicer, A., Huarte, N. M., & Pallás-Alonso, C. R. (2022). Maternal and neonatal prognostic factors for cardiorespiratory events in healthy term neonates during early skin-to-skin contact. *Frontiers in Pediatrics, 10*, 907570. https://doi.org/10.3389/fped.2022.907570

Whitelaw, A., & Sleath, K. (1985). Myth of the marsupial mother: Home care of very low birth weight babies in Bogota, Colombia. *Lancet, 325*(8439), 1206–1208. https://doi.org/10.1016/s0140-6736(85)92877-6

World Health Organization. (2003). Kangaroo mother care: A practical guide. https://www.who.int/publications/i/item/9241590351


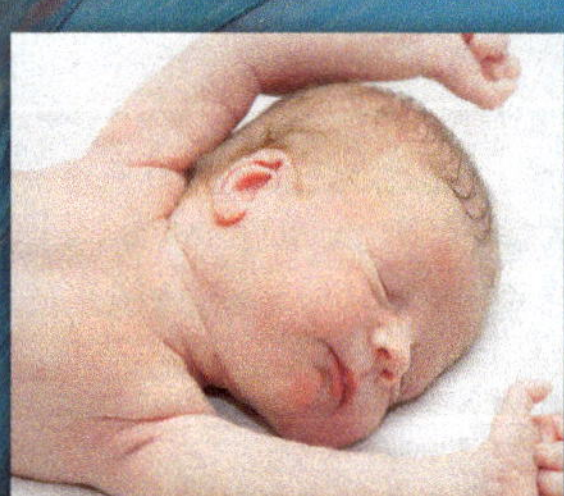

## PARENT VOICES

### Jennifer Canvasser, MSW

**My spouse and I struggled with infertility for 3 years before finding out we would be welcoming twins to the world. Despite our planning and best efforts, our twins, Micah and Zachary, were born at 27 weeks' gestation. Zachary spent 91 days in the NICU, while our son Micah was hospitalized for a total of 299 days due to developing NEC. Tragically, Micah died from complications of necrotizing enterocolitis (NEC) when the twins were 11 months old.**

**Three years after Micah and Zachary were born, we welcomed our rainbow baby, Elijah, to the world. Elijah was born weighing almost 9 lb at over 41 weeks' gestation. Thankfully, it was a healthy term pregnancy, yet I was constantly terrified and anxious of giving birth prematurely. It was most helpful when nurses would validate my feelings and recognize them as normal, given my past experience. Writing served as a helpful outlet for me during my pregnancy with Elijah, and I even wrote about it here: www.huffingtonpost.com/entry/5-ways-to-support-a-family-expecting-a-rainbow-baby_b_7222608.html**

**Number 3 in the blog really stands out for me as a bereaved mother: Get the birth order right. Death does not change birth order, simple as that.**

**Pregnancy after giving birth prematurely—or after a loss—is unique and these mothers deserve an empathetic, responsive care team tuned in to their needs and experiences.**

(*continued*)

## PARENT VOICES (*continued*)

### Heather McKinnis

**Our first baby came so early that deciding to give our micropreemie a sibling was a difficult decision. Each of our pregnancies after our preemie was emotionally and physically draining. Progesterone injections, countless ultrasounds, some bed rest, and early full-term scheduled C-sections became our normal. I had panic attacks, anxiety, and nightmares, although these decreased with each pregnancy. We never discovered the reason my first son came so early and each pregnancy was filled with the unknown. In the end, we were able to deliver three more beautiful babies close to full term. I was able to experience their deliveries, hear their cries, breastfeed, and hold them skin to skin. I finally felt like I was able to experience motherhood like everyone else around me. All those moments that my son's extremely premature delivery stole from us were given back three times over and I'll be forever grateful. After everything we went through with our 25-weeker, these experiences were incredibly healing.**

### Tracy Pella

**We gave birth to our twins at 23 + 4 weeks and one of our sons passed away the same day and our other son spent 134 days in the NICU. Post-NICU was filled with very much a "23-weeker life," including appointments, medications, and isolation. When our surviving twin was 4 years old, we were blessed to give birth to our daughter at 37 weeks during a planned C-section. Her birth may have been "normal" by standards of the baby world, but it was far from our normal. Remember, our normal was the 23-weeker life. Our first birth included saying goodbye to one of our sons and watching the other fight for his life for several months. That was our normal!**

**Being able to plan her arrival and the anticipation was exhausting. I often found myself waiting for the floor to drop from under me. It was almost like we wouldn't allow ourselves to believe we could have a normal delivery. Anxiety took over when I realized she wouldn't be monitored 24/7. I understood she was healthy, but it was more natural to think we wouldn't be able to take her home with us. Visitor after visitor commented that we must be elated she arrived full-term and healthy. Yes, we were happy, but we needed everyone to understand that this was new territory for us. We had put our defenses up and we had to get used to the idea that we got to leave the hospital doors with a baby. It was like experiencing birth and parenthood for the first time.**

## ONLINE RESOURCES

**CourseConnect**

Resources for this chapter are online and available at www.springerpub.com/courseconnect.

## REFERENCES

References for this chapter are online and available at www.springerpub.com/courseconnect.

UNIT III: Systems Assessment and Management of Disorders

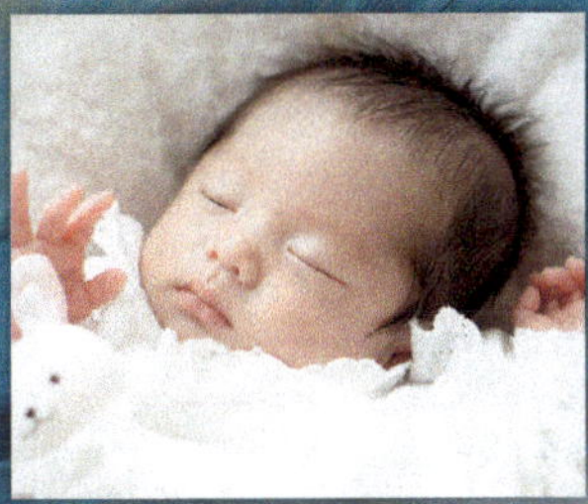

Source: Chihana/Adobe Stock.

CHAPTER 6

# Respiratory System

**Samuel Gentle, Colm Travers, and Waldemar A. Carlo**

## INTRODUCTION

The mechanisms that enable normal pulmonary function are complex. The clinician must fully comprehend the physiologic processes associated with neonatal respiratory diseases. Only through advanced knowledge can the clinician efficiently assess and evaluate the newborn's respiratory status. Systematic use of these assessment skills allows the clinician to positively affect patient outcomes as part of the collaborative team.

## EMBRYOLOGIC DEVELOPMENT OF THE LUNG

Typical pulmonary development of the embryo proceeds along a predetermined sequence throughout gestation (Greenough & Milner, 2005). Pulmonary development begins with the formation of an outpouching of the embryonic foregut during the fourth week of gestation. Sequential branching of the lung bud, which appears at about 4 weeks and is complete by the sixth week, marks the embryonic phase of lung development. Weeks 7 to 16, known as the *pseudoglandular phase*, are marked by the formation of conducting airways by branching of the aforementioned lung buds. This phase ends with the completion of the conducting airways. The canalicular phase follows through week 28, when gas exchange units, known as *acini*, develop. Surfactant-producing type II pneumocytes begin to form during the latter part of this phase. Mature, vascularized gas exchange sites form during the saccular phase, which spans the 29th through 35th weeks. During this phase, the interstitial space between alveoli thins, so respiratory epithelial cells tightly contact developing capillaries. The alveolar development phase, marked by expansion of the gas exchange surface area, begins at 36 weeks and extends into the postnatal period. Additional alveoli continue to develop well into childhood, perhaps as late as the seventh year of life (Table 6.1). The alveolar wall and interstitial spaces become very thin, and the single capillary network comes in close proximity to the alveolar membrane. No firm boundaries separate the phases of lung development, and gas exchange, albeit inefficient, is possible even before mature, vascularized gas exchange sites form. Lung development is a continuum that is marked by rapid structural changes. Interference at any time by premature birth or by disease introduces the possibility of inducing lung injury.

**TABLE 6.1**

**STAGES OF NORMAL LUNG GROWTH**

| Phase | Timing | Major Event |
|---|---|---|
| Embryonic | Weeks 4–6 | Formation of proximal airway |
| Pseudoglandular | Weeks 7–16 | Formation of conducting airways |
| Canalicular | Weeks 17–28 | Formation of acini |
| Saccular | Weeks 29–35 | Development of gas exchange sites |
| Alveolar | Weeks 36 through postnatal life | Expansion of surface area |

## NEWBORN PULMONARY PHYSIOLOGY AND THE ONSET OF BREATHING

The fetal lung is fluid filled, underperfused, and dormant with regard to gas exchange. The fetal lung receives only approximately 10% of the cardiac output (CO). Because the placenta is the gas exchange organ in fetal life, high blood flow is preferentially directed away from the lungs toward other developing body systems. The pulmonary vasculature maintains a high vascular resistance. Consequently, most of the right ventricular output is shunted from the pulmonary artery across the ductus arteriosus into the aorta, bypassing the pulmonary circulation. Before birth, the lungs are filled with fetal lung fluid, which is excreted into the lungs throughout the second and third trimester. Fetal lung fluid, together with fetal breathing movements, has an important function in maintaining mechanical strain on the developing lung that encourages normal lung growth.

Within moments after the umbilical cord is clamped, the newborn undergoes a transformation from a fetus floating in amniotic fluid to an air-breathing neonate. When normal breathing occurs after birth, the ensuing chain of events converts the fetal circulation to the neonatal pattern of circulation. Lung fluid is further absorbed and replaced with air, thus establishing lung volume and allowing for normal neonatal pulmonary function. The fetal lung fluid absorption process begins before birth when the rate of alveolar fluid secretion declines. Reabsorption accelerates during labor, with animal data suggesting that as much as two-thirds of the total clearance of lung fluid occurs during labor due to the cessation of active chloride secretion into the alveolar space. Perinatal fluid clearance is also related to epithelial sodium channels (ENaC) induced by increased serum cortisol after delivery (Janér et al., 2011). Oncotic pressure favors the movement of water from the air space back into the interstitium and into the vascular space. With the onset of breathing and lung expansion, water moves rapidly from the air spaces into the interstitium and is removed from the lung by lymphatic and pulmonary blood vessels. Because a large proportion of the clearance of lung fluid occurs during the labor process, primarily due to the release of hormones during labor, neonates born without labor after a scheduled cesarean delivery are at exceptionally high risk for delayed absorption of the fetal lung fluid and thus for transient tachypnea of the newborn (TTN). Late preterm infants whose mothers received betamethasone have lower rates of TTN, presumably due to the influence of corticosteroids on the upregulation of ENaC channels (Gyamfi-Bannerman et al., 2016). Birth prior to 38 weeks by elective scheduled cesarean delivery is significantly associated with an increased risk of respiratory disorders and an increased mortality risk (Tita et al., 2009).

Several cardiac changes must occur to complete the transition process from the intrauterine to the extrauterine environment. With the onset of breathing, highly negative intrathoracic pressures are generated with inspiratory efforts, filling the alveoli with air. Replacing alveolar fluid with air causes a precipitous decrease in hydrostatic pressure in the lung, leading to a decrease in pulmonary artery pressure. The resultant reduction in right atrial pressure and increase in pulmonary blood flow leads to an increase in alveolar oxygen tension ($PaO_2$), which causes constriction of the ductus arteriosus, which normally shunts right ventricular blood away from the lungs. Clamping of the umbilical cord removes the large, low-resistance, placental surface area from the circulation. This change in resistance causes an abrupt increase in systemic arterial pressure at the left atrium. As left atrial pressure rises, the flap valve opening between the atria, known as the *foramen ovale*, is closed. This closure prevents blood from bypassing the lungs by eliminating the shunt from the right to the left atrium. These simultaneous changes wherein the systemic vasculature resistance exceeds that of the pulmonary vasculature allow physiologic closure of both the foramen ovale and ductus arteriosus. The infant successfully transitions from the pattern of fetal circulation to neonatal circulation when blood coming from the right ventricle flows in its new path of least resistance (lower pressure) to the lungs instead of shunting across the foramen ovale to the left atrium or across the ductus arteriosus from the pulmonary artery to the aorta.

Understanding normal breathing and ventilation enables the clinician to assess the infant in respiratory distress and devise strategies for management. The respiratory system is composed of the following: (a) the pumping system (the chest wall muscles, diaphragm, and accessory muscles of respiration), which moves free gas into the lungs by creating a negative pressure gradient; (b) the bony rib cage, which provides structural support for the respiratory muscles and limits lung deflation; (c) the conducting airways, which connect gas-exchanging units with the outside but offer resistance to gas flow; (d) an elastic element, which offers some resistance to gas flow but provides pumping force for moving carbon dioxide–rich gas out of the system; (e) air-liquid interfaces, which generate surface tension that opposes lung expansion on inspiration but supports lung deflation on exhalation; and (f) the abdominal muscles, which aid exhalation by active contraction.

Limitations in the respiratory system predispose the newborn to respiratory difficulty. The circular, poorly ossified rib cage, with a flat instead of angular insertion of the diaphragm, is less efficient at generating negative intrathoracic pressure during inhalation. The highly compliant chest wall often moves in a contrary manner to the desired flow of air. Small muscles and a relative paucity of type I muscle fibers hinder the strength and endurance of respiratory muscles. The newborn has a relatively low functional residual capacity (lung volume at the end of exhalation) because the comparatively floppy chest wall offers little resistance to collapse, even when a normal amount of functional surfactant is present.

Surface tension is the force that arises from the interaction among the molecules of a liquid. Molecules in the interior of the liquid are attracted to each other, whereas molecules on the surface of the liquid are attracted to other molecules in the interior of the liquid, which results in the movement of the surface molecule toward the liquid. This explains why a droplet of water over a surface tends to adopt a given size and not continuously expand. If we think of the alveolus as a soap bubble, the molecules of the wall of the bubble are attracted to each other, which tends to collapse the bubble. The higher the surface tension, the faster the bubble collapses. The pressures across the wall of the bubble act against the surface tension and avoid the collapse of the bubble. The relationship between the surface tension and the distending pressures and the pressure across the wall of the bubble are described by Laplace's law, as shown in the following equation:

$$P = \frac{2ST}{r}$$

where $P$ is pressure, $ST$ is surface tension, and $r$ is radius of the alveolus. It is difficult to inflate a small or collapsed alveolus because it has a very small diameter. As its volume increases, the pressure needed to continue inflation becomes progressively less—that is, compliance of the alveolus and, thus, compliance of the lung, have improved. Coating the alveoli with an agent that decreases surface tension reduces the effort required to inflate the lungs from a low volume.

An alveolar cell known as the *type II pneumocyte* produces pulmonary surfactant. Surfactant is a mixture of proteins and phospholipids that naturally coats the mature alveoli, preventing alveolar collapse and loss of lung volume during exhalation—that is, as exhalation ensues and the lung deflates, the alveolar diameter becomes smaller. Surfactant coating of the alveolus reduces surface tension so that collapse is prevented and less pressure is required for reinflation with the next inspiration. Neonates with respiratory distress syndrome (RDS) have surfactant deficiency. In the absence of surfactant, surface tension is high, and the tendency is toward collapse of alveoli at end exhalation and resulting microatelectasis.

Compliance is the elasticity, or distensibility, of the lung. It is expressed as the change in volume caused by a change in pressure as follows:

$$CL = \frac{\Delta V}{\Delta P}$$

where CL is compliance of the lung; $V$ is change in volume, and $P$ is change in pressure. The higher the compliance, the larger the volume delivered to the alveoli per unit of applied inspiratory pressure. Surface tension and compliance are particularly important in the preterm infant with RDS. Surface tension is a force that opposes lung expansion. Surfactant deficiency increases surface tension in the alveoli, making it more difficult for the lungs to inflate. During exhalation, some alveoli collapse, resulting in decreased lung volume at the end of exhalation (low functional residual capacity). Clinically, the presence of retractions and other signs of respiratory distress, such as nasal flaring and grunting, manifest the effects of the respiratory muscles opposing increased surface tension. As the thoracic wall of the preterm infant lacks rigidity, the negative pleural pressure visibly deforms the chest in infants exhibiting RDS. When a preterm infant with RDS is intubated, a high peak inspiratory pressure (PIP) is required to expand the thorax (i.e., tidal volume is obtained only with a change in pressure). After surfactant is administered, the reduction in surface tension and increased compliance result in greater chest expansion with the same PIP due to the greater tidal volume obtained. Before surfactant is administered, it is difficult to inflate the lung because compliance is low.

*Resistance* is a term used to describe the characteristics of gas flow through the airways and pulmonary tissues. Resistance can be thought of as the capacity of the respiratory system to resist airflow. A substantial proportion of respiratory system resistance in infants is attributed to the nasal passages, as infants are primarily obligate nasal breathers. However, the principal component of lung resistance is determined by the small airways. Pressure is required to force gas through the airways (airway resistance) and to overcome the forces of the lung and chest wall, which work to deflate the respiratory system (tissue resistance). At a specific flow rate, resistance is described by the following equation:

$$R = \frac{p1 - p2}{F}$$

where $p1$ and $p2$ are pressures at opposite ends of the airway, and $F$ is the flow rate of gas (volume per unit of time). Resistance increases as airway diameter decreases. Because the airways of infants have a relatively small radius, the resistance to gas flow through those airways is high. Poiseuille's law recognizes that resistance to flow through a cylindrical object is inversely proportional to the fourth power of the radius.

In other words, if the radius of the airway is decreased by half, the resulting resistance to flow through the airway is increased 16-fold. Therefore, even minor obstructions of the airway can have a consequential effect on airflow.

The time constant is the time necessary for airway pressure to partially equilibrate throughout the respiratory system and equals the mathematical product of compliance and resistance. In other words, the time constant measures how quickly the lungs can inhale or exhale. It takes approximately five time constants to complete inhalation and exhalation. The time constant ($K_t$) is directly related to both compliance ($C$) and resistance ($R$). The following equation describes this relationship:

$$K_t = C \times R$$

An infant with RDS has decreased compliance, so the time constant of the respiratory system is relatively short. In such an infant, little time is required for the pressure must equilibrate between the proximal airway and the alveoli, resulting in the infant breathing rapidly with short inspiratory and expiratory times, which may be appropriate during mechanical ventilation. This allows the child with RDS to be ventilated at higher rates than would commonly be tolerated in most other populations. When compliance improves (increases), the time constant becomes longer. If sufficient time is not allowed for exhalation, the alveoli may become overdistended due to gas trapping, resulting in an air leak.

## Blood Gas Analysis and Acid–Base Balance

Oxygen diffuses across the alveolar-capillary membrane, moved by the difference in oxygen pressure between the alveoli and the blood. Most oxygen binds to hemoglobin in the blood, and a small proportion dissolves in the plasma. Thus, arterial oxygen content ($CaO_2$) is the sum of hemoglobin-bound oxygen and dissolved oxygen, as is shown by the following equation:

$$CaO_2 = (1.37 \times Hb \times SaO_2)\ (0.003 \times PaO_2)$$

where $CaO_2$ is arterial oxygen content (ml/100 ml of blood), 1.37 is the milliliters of oxygen bound to 1 g of hemoglobin at 100% saturation, Hb is hemoglobin concentration per 100 ml of blood (g/100 ml), $SaO_2$ is the percentage of hemoglobin bound to oxygen (%), 0.003 is the solubility factor of oxygen in plasma (ml/mm Hg), and $PaO_2$ is oxygen partial pressure in arterial blood (mm Hg).

In the equation for arterial oxygen content, the first term—(1.37 × Hb × $SaO_2$)—is the amount of oxygen bound to hemoglobin. The second term—(0.003 × $PaO_2$)—is the amount of oxygen dissolved in plasma. Most of the oxygen in the blood is carried by hemoglobin, with a minimal amount of oxygen dissolved in plasma. For example, if a premature infant has a $PaO_2$ of 60 mm Hg, a $SaO_2$ of 92%, and a hemoglobin concentration of 14 g/100 ml, then $CaO_2$ is the sum of oxygen bound to hemoglobin (1.37 × 14 × 0.92) = 17.6 ml and the oxygen dissolved in plasma (0.003 × 60) = 0.1 ml. In this typical example, only less than 1% of oxygen in the blood is dissolved in plasma; more than 99% is carried by hemoglobin. If the infant has a sudden decrease in the hemoglobin concentration to 10.5 g/dl but $PaO_2$ and $SaO_2$ remain the same, then $CaO_2$ (1.37 × 10.5 × 0.92) + (0.003 × 60) equals 13.4 ml/100 ml of blood. Thus, without any change in $PaO_2$ or $SaO_2$, a 25% decrease in hemoglobin concentration (from 14 to 10.5 g/dl) reduces the amount of oxygen in arterial blood by 24% (from 17.6 to 13.4 ml/100 ml of blood). This is an important concept for clinicians who care for patients with respiratory disease. $SaO_2$ and hemoglobin should be monitored and, if low, corrected to maintain adequate tissue oxygenation. Besides $SaO_2$ and hemoglobin, CO is the other major determinant of oxygen delivery to the tissues.

The force that loads hemoglobin with oxygen in the lungs and unloads it in the tissues is the difference in partial pressure of oxygen. In the lungs, alveolar oxygen partial pressure is higher than capillary oxygen partial pressure, so oxygen moves to the capillaries and binds to the hemoglobin. The tissue partial pressure of oxygen is lower than that of the blood, so oxygen moves from hemoglobin to the tissues. The relationship between the partial pressure of oxygen and hemoglobin is better understood with the oxyhemoglobin dissociation curve (Figure 6.1). Several factors can affect the affinity of hemoglobin for oxygen. Alkalosis, hypothermia, hypocapnia, and decreased levels of 2,3-diphosphoglycerate (2,3-DPG) increase the affinity of hemoglobin for oxygen, so less oxygen is offloaded to tissues (as shown in Figure 6.1 by a left shift of the curve). Acidosis, hyperthermia, hypercapnia, and increased 2,3-DPG have the opposite effect, decreasing the affinity of hemoglobin for oxygen so that the hemoglobin dissociation curve shifts to the right. This characteristic of hemoglobin facilitates oxygen loading in the lung and unloading in the tissue, where the pH is lower and alveolar carbon dioxide tension ($PaCO_2$) is higher. Fetal hemoglobin, which has a higher affinity for oxygen than adult hemoglobin, is more fully oxygen saturated at lower $PaO_2$ values. This is represented by a leftward shift on the hemoglobin oxygen dissociation curve.

Once loaded with oxygen, the blood should reach the tissues to transfer oxygen to the cells. Oxygen delivery to the tissue depends on cardiac output (CO) and $CaO_2$, as described in the following equation:

$$\text{Oxygen Delivery} = CO \times CaO_2$$

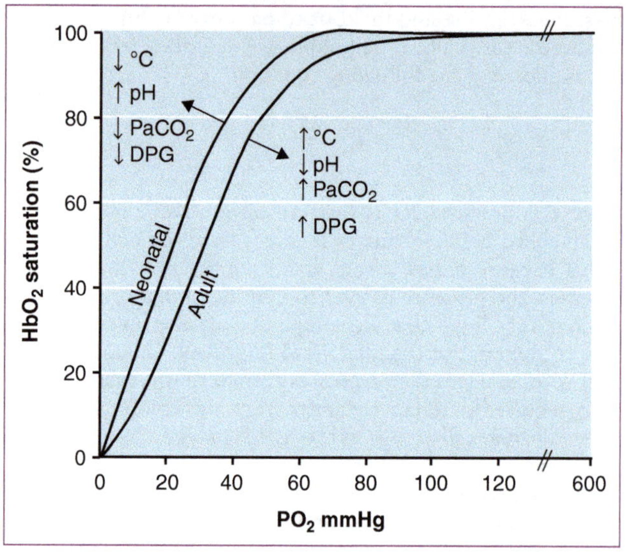


**FIGURE 6.1 Oxyhemoglobin equilibrium curves of blood from term infants at birth and from adults (at pH 7.40).**

In the case of the infant discussed previously, increased CO compensates for the decrease in $CaO_2$ that results from anemia. The key concept is that when a patient's oxygenation is assessed, more information should be considered than just $PaO_2$ and $SaO_2$. $PaO_2$ and $SaO_2$ may be normal, but oxygen delivery to the tissues is decreased if hemoglobin concentration is low or CO is decreased. With this approach, the clinician should be able to better plan the interventions needed to improve oxygenation.

As in the adult, the acid–base balance in the neonate is maintained within narrow limits by complex interactions between the pulmonary system (which eliminates carbon dioxide) and the kidneys (which conserve carbon dioxide and eliminate metabolic acids). Carbon dioxide elimination, which is more efficient than oxygenation across the alveolar-capillary membrane, is usually not as problematic as oxygenation. Carbon dioxide has a high solubility coefficient, so cellular diffusion is efficient, and no measurable partial pressure gradient exists between venous blood and the tissues unless there is severe lung disease. Therefore, elevated carbon dioxide tension ($PCO_2$) values in arterial blood samples nearly always indicate ventilatory dysfunction. Dissolved carbon dioxide moves rapidly across the cell membranes of peripheral chemoreceptors, making them sensitive to changes in ventilation. Increased intracellular $PCO_2$ elevates the cellular hydrogen ion concentration as carbon dioxide combines with water to form carbonic acid. This stimulates neural impulses to the medulla, which in turn stimulates respiration. However, excessively high $PCO_2$ levels and acidosis can depress ventilation. Acid–base balance is controlled by homeostatic mechanisms and is expressed by the Henderson–Hasselbalch equilibrium equation:

$$pH = 6.1 = \frac{\log HCO^{-}_{3}}{0.03 \times PCO_2}$$

It can be seen from this mathematical relationship that acid–base balance depends on the interplay of bicarbonate ion ($HCO_3$) and carbon dioxide ($CO_2$). Low pH (in other words, acidosis) can contribute to vasoconstriction and can result in worsening hypoxemia caused by extrapulmonary shunt across the ductus or foramen ovale. A pH of 7.20 or higher is generally considered safe in preterm infants with RDS (SUPPORT Study Group et al., 2010). A pH of less than 7.0 is not well tolerated and is associated with a poor survival rate in these patients.

If $PaCO_2$ rises above normal, as in hypoventilation, pH declines, and the patient experiences respiratory acidosis. The patient with chronic respiratory acidosis may retain bicarbonate, resulting in a compensatory metabolic alkalosis. A patient who is hyperventilated with a low $PaCO_2$ has respiratory alkalosis. Depressed bicarbonate ion concentration (less than approximately 20 mmol/L in plasma) is called *metabolic acidosis* and can be associated with any cause of anaerobic metabolism, such as poor CO from congenital heart disease—for example, hypoplastic left heart syndrome or severe aortic coarctation—or from myocardial ischemia, myocardiopathy, myocarditis, hypoxia, necrotizing enterocolitis, or septic shock. Metabolic acidosis that results from renal bicarbonate wasting commonly develops in extremely premature infants. Less common causes for prolonged and severe metabolic acidosis are the inborn errors of metabolism, including urea cycle defects and aminoacidopathies.

The clinician should become proficient at interpreting blood gas data. With knowledge of the accepted normal values and definitions of simple blood gas disorders and their compensatory mechanisms, the clinician can examine data in light of the disease process and interpret blood gas values in a fairly straightforward manner. Typically, the body does not overcompensate for a pH above or below the normal range. Therefore, when presented with an abnormal pH, the clinician should rapidly determine whether acidosis (Figure 6.2A) or alkalosis (Figure 6.2B) exists. Examining $PaCO_2$ and $HCO_3$

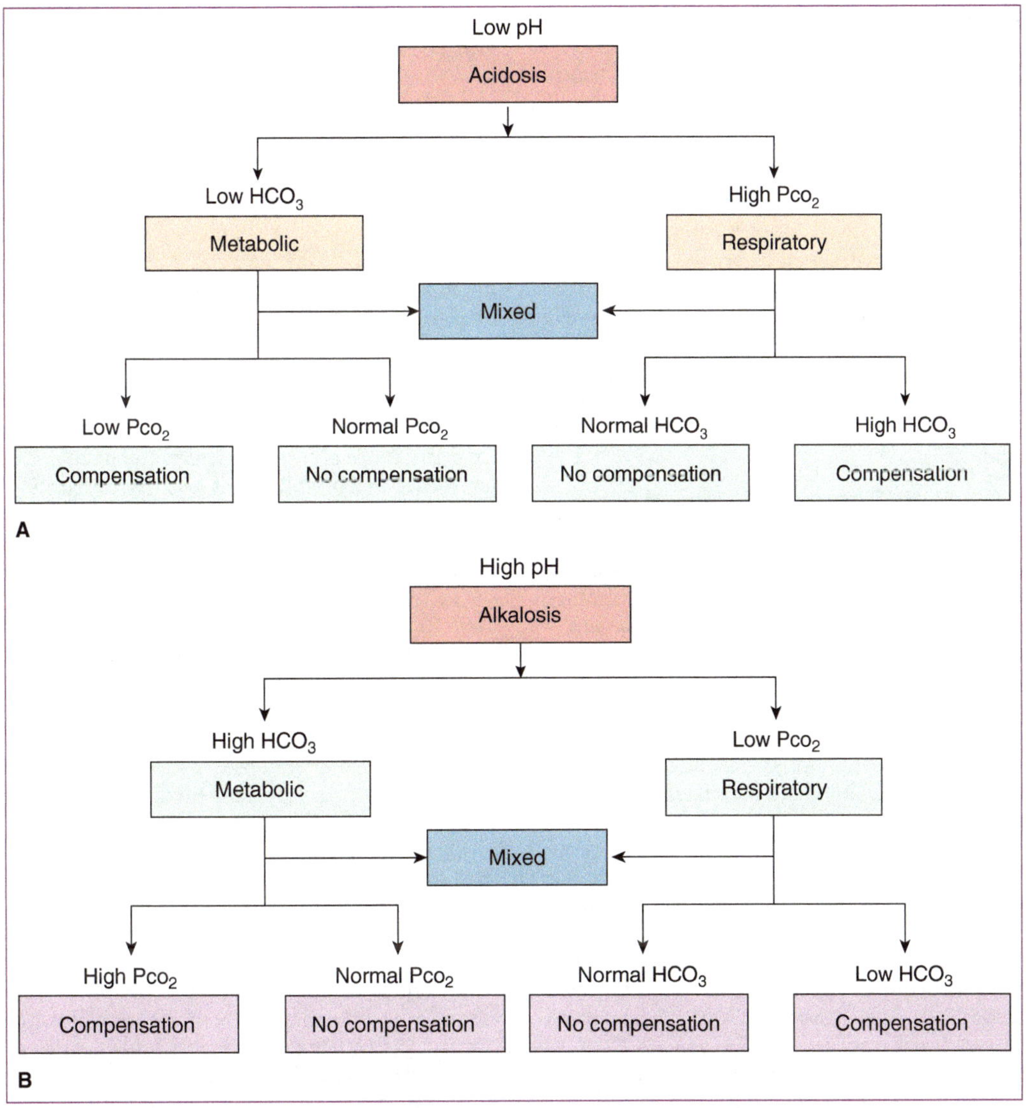


**FIGURE 6.2** **Acid–base balance: A diagnostic approach. (A) Low pH. (B) High pH.**

determines whether the process is respiratory, metabolic, or mixed. The clinician should evaluate which derangement occurred first. For example, an acidotic, acutely ill, hypoxemic infant may be experiencing a metabolic acidosis secondary to anaerobic metabolism with a subsequent high $PaCO_2$ due to hypoventilation. The infant with a low $PaCO_2$ is hyperventilating spontaneously, perhaps due to a high ammonia level, or secondary to excessive mechanical ventilation. A concomitantly low pH and low $PaCO_2$ indicate that the infant is compensating for metabolic acidosis with hyperventilation to normalize the pH. A pure metabolic alkalosis with high pH can be caused by bicarbonate administration, loop diuretics such as furosemide, or gastric losses due to pyloric stenosis or gastric suctioning. Infants with bronchopulmonary dysplasia (BPD) usually have a compensated respiratory acidosis, with an elevated $PaCO_2$ and concomitantly elevated bicarbonate. The pH may be in the normal range or slightly acidotic. A severely depressed pH usually indicates acute decompensation.

## ASSESSMENT OF THE NEONATE WITH RESPIRATORY DISTRESS

The assessment of a neonate with respiratory distress should always begin with compiling a detailed perinatal history. Every effort should be made to obtain as much pertinent information about obstetrical and fetal conditions as possible. The clinician can often gain important supplemental information from the father or visiting relatives at the bedside. A review of the maternal–prenatal history and a complete physical examination, combined with a limited laboratory and radiologic evaluation, leads to a timely diagnosis in most circumstances. Many neonatal diseases, including many with nonpulmonary origins, may manifest with signs of respiratory distress. Therefore, a comprehensive differential diagnosis must be considered (Figure 6.3).

### History

In most situations, data from a patient's history can direct the clinician to the correct diagnosis of neonatal respiratory distress. The prenatal record should be reviewed carefully for possible causes of the infant's difficulties. The mother's age, gravidity, parity, blood type, and Rh status should be recorded. The obstetrician's best estimate of gestational age should be documented as determined by first-trimester ultrasound or last menstrual period. Ultrasonography often provides information about anomalies and amniotic fluid volume, which is useful in anticipating required support at birth. Prolonged oligohydramnios may predispose to pulmonary hypoplasia and pulmonary hypertension due to poor lung growth. Polyhydramnios may indicate either poor swallowing due to a neuromuscular disorder or obstruction to swallowing from conditions that include upper airway anomalies. Historical information such as previous preterm birth is relevant because it is often associated with an increased risk of premature delivery in subsequent pregnancies. Because excessive maternal weight gain occurs with diabetes, multiple gestation, or polyhydramnios, prepregnancy weight and total gain should be noted. The clinician is often alerted to the possibility of gestational diabetes with abnormal glucose tolerance screening results, which again should be reflected in the prenatal record.

The duration of membrane rupture or oligohydramnios, the presence of maternal fever with or without accompanying chorioamnionitis, and the presence of meconium-stained amniotic fluid are important pieces of information that may help in the differential diagnosis of a newborn with respiratory distress. Additionally, antepartum and intrapartum administration of certain medications may affect respiratory outcomes. **Quality and Safety: The administration of steroids to the mother reduces the likelihood that RDS will develop in the infant; administration of narcotics to the mother close to delivery may result in poor respiratory effort by an otherwise normal infant.** The use of magnesium sulfate for either neuroprotection or for tocolysis does not result in cardiorespiratory depression or the need for increased resuscitation (De Jesus et al., 2015; Johnson et al., 2012).

### Physical Examination of the Respiratory System

General inspection is important in the initial assessment of infants with respiratory disease. Dysmorphic features may provide clues with regard to the underlying diagnosis. The presence of hydrops may suggest the presence of effusions, anemia, or associated cardiac disease. One or more of the major signs of respiratory difficulty (e.g., cyanosis, tachypnea, grunting, retractions, and nasal flaring) are usually present in neonates with both pulmonary and nonpulmonary causes of respiratory distress. Observation of the distressed infant with the unaided eye and ear is the clinician's first step in the physical assessment. Cyanosis may be central, caused by pulmonary disease and cyanotic heart disease, or peripheral, as occurs in conditions with impaired CO. However, pulse oximetry more accurately detects hypoxemia as considerable interobserver variability has been reported in clinical detection of cyanosis (O'Donnell et al., 2007). Acrocyanosis, or cyanosis noted in the extremities, is a standard normal finding in newborns during the first few days after birth.

Tachypnea typically manifests in infants with decreased lung compliance, such as RDS, whereas patients with high airway resistance (e.g., airway obstruction) usually have deep but slow breathing. Adduction of the vocal cords produces grunting during exhalation. Grunting holds gas in the lungs throughout exhalation, which helps maintain lung volume and avoid alveolar collapse. At the end of exhalation, the gas is released and rapidly propelled, causing an audible grunt. Grunting is more typical of infants with decreased functional residual capacity, such as preterm infants with RDS. Chest wall retractions may be anticipated in very premature infants because of the highly compliant chest wall (Carlo & Di Fiore, 2011). When the infant is intubated, observation of the chest gives important information. Careful observation of chest wall excursions produced by the ventilator allows the clinician to adjust the magnitude of the ventilator pressure so that optimal gas exchange is achieved while the risk of volutrauma is minimized. The chest of an intubated infant should move the same or only slightly less than that of a healthy, spontaneously breathing infant.

The clinician should assess the appropriateness of the magnitude of the chest expansion in ventilated patients. **Emergency Alert:** **A reported abrupt decrease in the chest rise may indicate atelectasis, a plugged endotracheal tube (ET), a pneumothorax, a leak in the circuit, or ventilator failure. Slow decreases in the chest rise over hours may indicate deteriorating lung compliance or gas trapping. An overinflated thorax, as determined from radiographs, is a sign of gas trapping. In the intubated infant, this observation should prompt the clinician to decrease the positive end-expiratory pressure (PEEP) or increase expiratory time to prevent gas trapping and air leakage. An anguished intubated infant with cyanosis and gasping efforts may have ET obstruction.**

Careful attention should be given to the sounds that emanate from the respiratory tract because variations in quality often aid in localizing the source of respiratory distress. Stridor is common in neonates with upper airway and laryngeal lesions. Inspiratory stridor occurs most often with upper airway and laryngeal lesions, whereas expiratory stridor suggests lower airway problems. Hoarseness is a common sign of laryngeal disorders. Forced inspiratory efforts may indicate upper airway or laryngeal involvement, whereas expiratory wheezes suggest a lower airway disease. Congenital airway disorders that may cause respiratory distress in the neonate are included in Figure 6.3.

Auscultation of the chest further aids the examiner. Infants with RDS have low lung volumes, and breath sounds are faint, usually without rales. In comparison, the infant with pneumonia may have rales indicative of alveolar filling. Auscultation allows the clinician to detect the presence of secretions in the airway and to evaluate the response to physiotherapy and suctioning. Rhonchi may be heard in neonates with airway disease, such as meconium aspiration syndrome (MAS). **Emergency Alert:** **Unequal breath sounds may be due to a pneumothorax or to one of the many causes of diminished ventilation to a lung lobe (e.g., atelectasis, mainstem bronchial intubation, and pleural effusion). A shift of the apex of the heart can occur with a pneumothorax, diaphragmatic hernia, unilateral pulmonary interstitial emphysema, pleural effusion, dextrocardia, or atelectasis, which may be differentiated by transillumination of the chest and chest imaging. Dullness to percussion may be due to a pleural effusion or solid mass. Muffled heart tones suggest a pneumopericardium or a pericardial effusion.** Respiratory distress may occur in many chest wall disorders that restrict rib cage movements. Increased oral secretions and choking with feedings are common in neonates with a tracheoesophageal fistula. Because newborns are obligate nasal breathers, those with choanal atresia typically improve with crying and have worsening respiratory distress at rest or with feeding. Characteristic Potter facies, bell-shaped chests, and other compression deformities and contractures may be present in neonates with hypoplastic lungs secondary to oligohydramnios.

Examination of the cardiovascular system and assessment of peripheral perfusion yield many clues toward a diagnosis. Pallor and poor perfusion may indicate anemia, hypotension, or hypovolemia. Polycythemia with plethora may also cause respiratory distress. Cardiovascular signs of congestive failure (e.g., hyperactive precordium, tachycardia, and hepatomegaly), poor CO, pathologic murmurs, decreased femoral pulses, and non-sinus rhythm suggest a primary cardiac cause for the respiratory distress.

When hypotonia, muscle weakness, raised hemidiaphragms, or areflexia accompanies respiratory distress, a neuromuscular cause should be considered (Box 6.1). In such cases, an accompanying history of less frequent fetal movement and polyhydramnios is often present. Sometimes, a history of muscular disease exists in the family. Brachial plexus injury or clavicle fracture may accompany phrenic nerve injury and diaphragm paralysis.

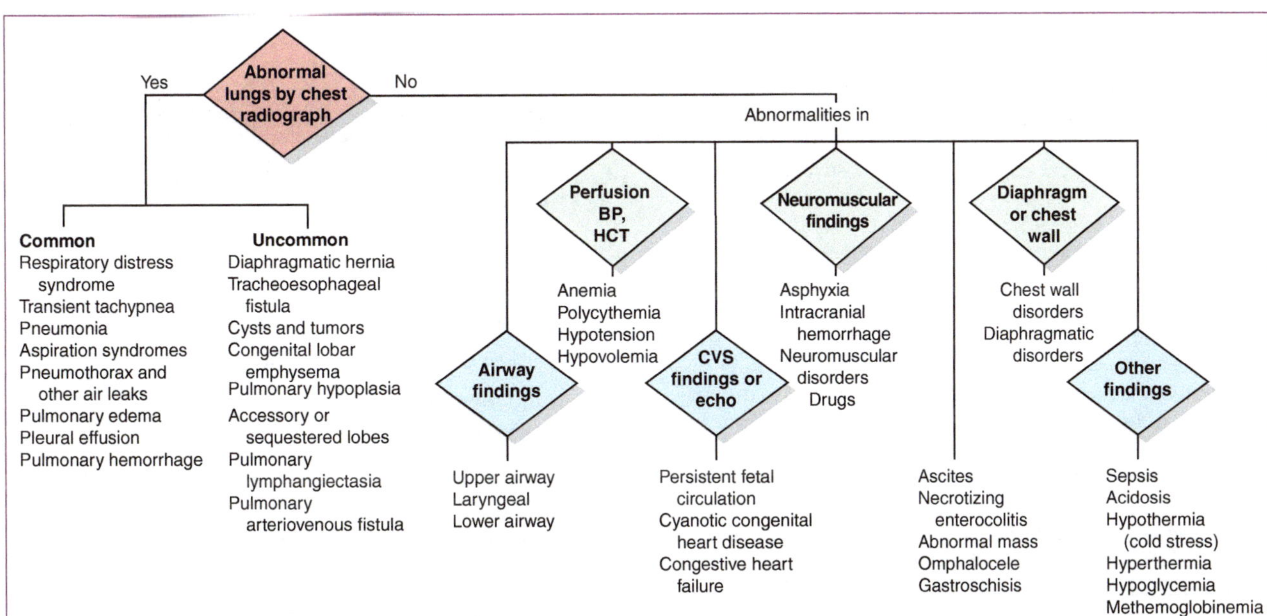


**FIGURE 6.3 Diagnostic algorithm for the neonate with acute respiratory distress.**

BP, blood pressure; HCT, hematocrit.

**BOX 6.1**

**NEUROMUSCULAR DISORDERS THAT MAY CAUSE RESPIRATORY DISTRESS IN THE NEONATE**

Myopathies

Myasthenia gravis

Werdnig–Hoffmann (spinal muscular atrophy)

Spinal cord disorder

Poliomyelitis

Others

Abnormalities found during abdominal examination enlighten the examiner about other causes of respiratory difficulty. Abdominal distention that results from causes such as ascites, necrotizing enterocolitis, abdominal mass, ileus, or tracheoesophageal fistula can cause respiratory distress, whereas a scaphoid configuration of the abdomen suggests a diaphragmatic hernia.

Other nonpulmonary disorders such as sepsis, metabolic acidosis, hypothermia, hyperthermia, hypoglycemia, and methemoglobinemia may also cause respiratory distress in the neonate.

**Radiographic and Laboratory Investigation.** Radiographic examination is often the most useful part of the laboratory evaluation and may serve to narrow the differential diagnosis. An anteroposterior view is usually sufficient, but a lateral chest radiograph may be helpful when fluid, masses, or pneumothorax is suspected. Other diagnostic imaging techniques (ultrasonography, fluoroscopy, computed tomography [CT], or magnetic resonance imaging [MRI]) may be helpful in selected patients. Thoracic ultrasound may be used at the bedside to rapidly assess the presence of effusions, pneumothorax, retained fetal fluid, consolidation, and the severity of RDS. Bronchoscopy allows direct visualization of the upper airway. This technique, albeit invasive and technically difficult, may, in selected cases, be a great aid in the differential diagnosis and treatment of patients with a suspected airway lesion.

Much can be learned from a relatively small battery of laboratory tests. In the neonatal intensive care unit (NICU) setting, the clinician is often required to collect specimens for and interpret the results of physiologic testing. Considerable skill is required in sampling venous and arterial blood from small patients at substantial risk for iatrogenic anemia and vascular damage. Ideally, the hospital laboratory is equipped to do most routine tests on microliter quantities of blood. The clinician must monitor the total amounts of blood sampled from the infant and be alert to the development of iatrogenic anemia.

Analysis of arterial blood for pH and gas tensions is one of the most common tasks of the clinicians caring for an infant with respiratory illness. Noninvasive methods to assess gas exchange, such as transcutaneous blood gas measurements or oxygen saturation, are very useful. Because oxygen delivery to the tissues so intimately depends on circulating red blood cell (RBC) volume, a hematocrit should be obtained.

## COMMON DISORDERS OF THE RESPIRATORY SYSTEM

A large variety of respiratory disorders occur in neonates, the most common of which are discussed here. Figure 6.3 lists both pulmonary and nonpulmonary disorders that cause respiratory symptoms in the newborn infant. Several diseases have their roots in the neonatal period and extend into infancy (Box 6.2). The most common is BPD, a chronic lung disease that affects newborns, mainly premature infants exposed to mechanical ventilation for RDS or other respiratory problems.

### Respiratory Distress Syndrome

RDS, formerly known as hyaline membrane disease (the term *hyaline membrane disease* originated from the histologic observation of alveolar space lined by an eosinophilic membrane formed by cellular debris), is the most common cause of respiratory distress in premature neonates (Hamvas, 2011). RDS is common in preterm infants. Most children born extremely premature have RDS, and the incidence increases as gestational age decreases. The incidence decreases from 98% at 23 weeks to 86% at 28 weeks. In rare cases, RDS develops in full-term infants born to mothers with diabetes or in full-term infants with perinatal asphyxia.

**Antenatal Steroids.** Acceleration of lung maturation with antenatal steroids is now the standard of care in women with preterm labor of up to 34 weeks. Antenatal corticosteroid therapy to the mothers of preterm fetuses of up to 34 weeks significantly reduces the incidence of RDS with odds ratios of around 0.5 and decreases mortality, with odds ratios of

**BOX 6.2**

**CAUSES OF LATE RESPIRATORY DISTRESS IN THE NEONATE**

Bronchopulmonary dysplasia

Pneumonia (bacterial, viral, or fungal)

Congestive heart failure

Recurrent pneumonitis or aspiration

Upper airway obstruction

Wilson–Mikity syndrome

Idiopathic pulmonary fibrosis (Hamman–Rich syndrome)

Pulmonary lymphangiectasia

Cystic fibrosis

Immature lungs

around 0.6 (Roberts et al., 2017). Subgroup analyses confirm that these benefits occur regardless of race and gender. No adverse effects have been reported with the usual single course of antenatal steroids. Other nonrespiratory benefits of steroid administration to mothers include reductions in intraventricular hemorrhage (IVH) and necrotizing enterocolitis (McGoldrick et al., 2020). The current guidelines recommend giving steroids to mothers between 23 and 34 weeks' gestation; however, emerging data at the limits of viability show associated benefits of giving steroids to infants as early as 22 weeks' gestation when postnatal resuscitation is planned (Carlo et al., 2011). In 2021, the American College for Obstetrics and Gynecology and the Society for Maternal-Fetal Medicine recommended considering the use of corticosteroids as early as 22 weeks' 0 days' gestation based on data suggesting that antenatal corticosteroid therapy was associated with twice the rate of survival compared to mothers not receiving antenatal corticosteroids (Backes et al., 2021). Improved survival is seen even when infants are exposed to only a partial steroid course (Carlo et al., 2011; Travers et al., 2018).

**Treatment.** The lungs of infants with RDS are deficient in pulmonary surfactant, the surface tension–reducing agent that prevents alveolar collapse and loss of lung volume at end exhalation. Surfactant-deficient lungs develop progressive atelectasis, which leads to intrapulmonary shunting, owing to perfusion of unventilated lungs and subsequent hypoxemia. The radiograph displays a characteristic ground-glass, reticulogranular appearance with air bronchograms. When lung inflation is poor due to stiff, noncompliant lungs, the arterial blood gas (ABG) analysis usually reveals respiratory acidemia and hypoxemia.

Therapy is directed toward improving oxygenation as well as maintaining optimal lung volume. Continuous positive airway pressure (CPAP) or PEEP is applied to prevent volume loss during exhalation. In severe cases, mechanical ventilation via a tracheal tube is required. Treatment with surfactant is the standard of care for preterm infants who require intubation for RDS. Exogenous surfactants (artificial and natural) are available for intratracheal instillation, improving survival and reducing some of the associated morbidities of RDS. Earlier clinical trials indicated that prophylactic surfactant administration to extremely premature infants in the delivery room was more effective than waiting for the treatment after the development of RDS (Soll & Morley, 2001). However, several subsequent trials that compared CPAP started at birth with rescue surfactant at 40% to 50% $F_IO_2$ with prophylactic surfactant at birth showed no benefit of prophylactic surfactant, though many of the infants in the early CPAP arm ultimately required surfactant administration (Finer et al., 2010; Stenson et al., 2011). The Cochrane meta-analysis showed less risk of BPD or death at 36 weeks when using early CPAP with selective surfactant administration compared to prophylactic surfactant (Rojas-Reyes et al., 2012).

Furthermore, there is limited evidence to support surfactant administration early during the clinical course of RDS. A meta-analysis attempted to identify an optimal $F_IO_2$ at which to administer surfactant 30%, 40%, and 50% but did not identify a threshold with clear benefit (Branagan et al., 2023). Moreover, a randomized trial of surfactant at a threshold of 40% compared to continuing CPAP in infants > 1,250 g did not demonstrate benefit for early surfactant (Escobedo et al., 2004). Thus, elective intubation for the administration of surfactant to preterm infants with RDS is not recommended, but individualized care based on the severity of RDS is more appropriate.

Additional methods for surfactant administration have also been evaluated. Among these, surfactant administration via a thin catheter, commonly referred to as *less invasive surfactant administration (LISA)*, has been demonstrated to reduce the risk of death or BPD compared with providing surfactant through an ET with positive-pressure ventilation (PPV) (Abdel-Latif et al., 2021).

To limit the use of invasive mechanical ventilation, noninvasive PPV is more effective for reducing the need for mechanical ventilation when compared to other forms of support, including high-flow nasal cannula and CPAP (Ramaswamy et al., 2020; Rüegger et al., 2021). In randomized trials comparing CPAP to high-flow nasal cannula, CPAP is more likely to limit the need for mechanical ventilation (Manley et al., 2019; Roberts et al., 2016).

Regarding ventilatory strategies, prophylactic high-frequency ventilation for the treatment of RDS has mixed results with limited evidence to support routine use (Cools et al., 2015), but these modes of ventilation should be considered as alternatives to conventional mechanical ventilation in specific circumstances such as in infants with air leaks including pulmonary interstitial emphysema or bronchopleural fistula. Among the conventional ventilatory strategies, the use of volume-targeted ventilation, as compared to pressure-limited ventilation, may reduce rates of death or BPD (Klingenberg et al., 2017). Infants greater than 34 weeks who have RDS and respiratory failure unresponsive to ventilatory management have responded favorably to extracorporeal membrane oxygenation (ECMO) (Thome et al., 2005).

Nursing care for infants with RDS is demanding; the most unstable infants often require a one-to-one nurse-to-patient ratio. The nurse must monitor the quality of respirations and observe the degree of difficulty the infant is experiencing. Worsening retractions may signal progressive volume loss and impending respiratory failure. **Quality and Safety: ABG tensions and pH should be measured frequently if respiratory status is changing, and continuous noninvasive monitoring of oxygenation and carbon dioxide if available, may allow early identification of gas exchange problems.** The risk of pneumothorax and right mainstem intubation is high, and the symmetry of breath sounds must be verified regularly. A crying infant loses airway pressure when the mouth is open and must be kept calm when receiving nasal CPAP. The intubated infant must be monitored for appropriate ET position and patency. Suctioning of the airway should be done carefully. The suction catheter should be passed only as far as the end of the ET because overzealous suctioning can denude the tracheal epithelium (Cordero et al., 2000). Lung volume can be lost during prolonged disconnection from the ventilator. Rapid loss of lung volume can precipitate hypoxemia, so disconnection time should be minimized. Any sudden decompensation should alert the nurse to investigate for ventilator failure, pneumothorax, or tracheal tube plugging (Figure 6.4). The infant should also be closely monitored for changes in pulmonary compliance, especially after surfactant administration.

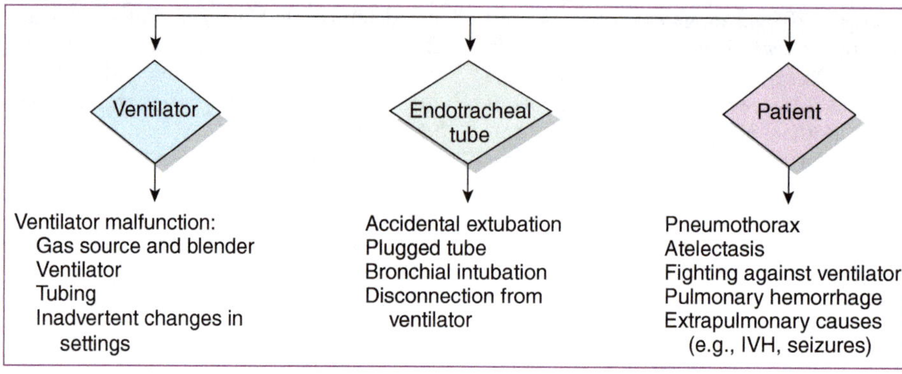


**FIGURE 6.4 Acute deterioration in a ventilated patient.**
IVH, intraventricular hemorrhage.

BPD is a common outcome in infants after RDS. BPD generally refers to chronic lung disease in preterm infants characterized by pulmonary fibrosis, bronchiolar metaplasia, emphysema, and interstitial edema. It is most commonly seen in survivors of extreme prematurity who were diagnosed with RDS, but extremely low birth weight (ELBW) infants may develop BPD without a history of RDS. According to the National Institute of Child Health and Human Development (NICHD) consensus from 2001, infants with mild BPD are those who continue to require oxygen supplementation for a total of at least 28 days, while those with moderate or severe BPD require oxygen supplementation and/or ventilatory support at 36 weeks of postmenstrual age and for more than 28 days (Jobe & Bancalari, 2001). In 2019, the NICHD proposed an alternative BPD definition in which infants with more severe forms had an increased probability of adverse long-term outcomes. In this definition, infants' disease severity is defined by the respiratory support received at 36 weeks' postmenstrual age as follows: grade 1—nasal cannula of ≤ 2 L/min; grade 2—nasal cannula > 2 L/min; grade 3—invasive mechanical ventilation (Jensen et al., 2019).

The incidence of BPD increases as gestational age decreases. Among infants less than or equal to 1,000 g at birth, 77% develop mild BPD, while 46% develop moderate BPD, and 16% develop severe BPD (Ehrenkranz et al., 2005). According to the grade definition, 39%, 23%, and 9% of infants develop grades 1, 2, and 3, respectively (Jensen et al., 2019). Of survivors to 36 weeks' corrected gestational age, 78% of infants born at 22 weeks had an oxygen requirement as opposed to 28% for infants born at 28 weeks (Bell et al., 2022). Pulmonary morbidities and adverse neurodevelopmental outcomes at 18 to 22 months were more prevalent with an increased severity of BPD. Using the evidence-based definition, the rate of death or moderate or severe neurodevelopmental impairment is 46% in infants with grade 1 BPD, 60% in infants with grade 2 BPD, and 79% in infants with grade 3 BPD (Jensen et al., 2019).

Several therapies reduce the incidence of BPD in preterm infants. A meta-analysis of the administration of vitamin A, an important mediator of pulmonary growth, showed a reduction in the incidence of BPD by 13% (Darlow & Graham, 2011). The administration of caffeine in the Caffeine for Apnea of Prematurity (CAP) trial found a reduction in BPD by 36% in infants who received caffeine compared with those receiving placebo. The administration of systemic corticosteroids after the first week of life reduces the incidence of BPD or BPD/death with available evidence not demonstrating any significant neurodevelopmental impairment (Doyle et al., 2017a), whereas giving dexamethasone earlier (before 7 days of life) reduces BPD but with an increase in the incidence of cerebral palsy (Doyle et al., 2017b).

**Air Leaks.** Air leaks frequently complicate RDS and other neonatal respiratory disorders. Air leaks are characterized by air in an ectopic location (Box 6.3). Many air-leak syndromes begin with at least some degree of pulmonary interstitial emphysema, which is the result of alveolar rupture from overdistention, usually concomitant with mechanical ventilation at lower rates and longer inspiratory times (Greenough et al., 2016) or CPAP (Morley et al., 2008). Pulmonary interstitial emphysema occurs most commonly in preterm infants but may be seen in infants of any gestational age. Lung compliance is nonuniform, and areas of poor aeration and alveolar collapse may be interspersed with alveoli of normal or near-normal compliance. The more normal lung units (those with better compliance) become overdistended and eventually rupture. Air is forced from the alveolus into the loose tissue of the interstitial space and dissects toward the hilum of the lung, where it may track into the mediastinum—causing a pneumomediastinum—or into the pericardium—causing a pneumopericardium. **Emergency Alert: The astute clinician may notice that an infant's chest becomes barrel shaped with overdistention and that breath sounds become distant on the affected side. In contrast, the infant who experiences a pneumothorax usually becomes unstable, with the development of cyanosis, oxygen desaturation, and carbon dioxide retention. The infant may become hypotensive and bradycardic because the high intrathoracic pressure impedes venous return. A tension pneumothorax, in which the free pleural air compresses the lung, is a medical emergency, and prompt relief by thoracentesis or tube thoracostomy is indicated.** Some infants are medically stable with a pneumothorax, which can be managed expectantly without decompression (**Litmanovitz & Carlo, 2008**). However, it is important to ensure that these infants are medically stable and, if they deteriorate, to be ready to intervene rapidly when needed to relieve the pneumothorax.

**BOX 6.3**

**AIR-LEAK PHENOMENA IN THE NEONATE**

Pneumothorax
Pulmonary interstitial emphysema
Pneumomediastinum
Pneumopericardium
Pneumoperitoneum
Pulmonary venous air embolism
Subcutaneous emphysema
Pseudocyst

**TABLE 6.2**

**CAUSES OF PNEUMONIA**

| Bacterial | Viral | Other |
|---|---|---|
| *Group B Streptococcus* | Cytomegalovirus | *Candida* and other fungi |
| *Escherichia coli* | Adenovirus | *Ureaplasma* |
| *Klebsiella* | Rhinovirus | *Chlamydia* |
| *Staphylococcus aureus* | Respiratory syncytial virus | Syphilis |
| *Listeria monocytogenes* | Parainfluenza | *Pneumocystis jiroveci* |
| *Enterobacter* | Enterovirus | Tuberculosis |
| *Haemophilus influenzae* | Rubella | Mycoplasma |
| *Streptococcus pneumonia* | Coronavirus | |
| *Pseudomonas* | | |
| *Bacteroides* | | |
| Others | | |

## Transient Tachypnea of the Newborn

TTN occurs typically in infants born by cesarean section, particularly in the absence of labor or in those infants born vaginally but who delivered precipitously. The cause of the disorder is thought to be transient pulmonary edema that results from decreased absorption of pulmonary alveolar fluid. The chest radiograph may show increased perihilar interstitial markings and small pleural fluid collections, especially in the minor fissure. In contrast to infants with RDS, infants with transient tachypnea tend to have a normal or low $PCO_2$. Oxygenation can usually be maintained by supplementing oxygen with a hood, although some infants benefit from a short course of positive pressure support. The infant usually recovers in 24 to 48 hours. Restricting fluid intake may also help reduce the duration of respiratory support (Stroustrup et al., 2012).

## Pneumonia

Pneumonia may be of bacterial, viral, or other infectious origin (Table 6.2). Pneumonia may be transmitted transplacentally, as has been shown with group B *Streptococcus*, or via an ascending bacterial invasion associated with maternal chorioamnionitis and prolonged rupture of the membranes. The usual causative organisms of pneumonia are group B *Streptococcus*, *Escherichia coli*, *Haemophilus influenzae*, and, less commonly, *Streptococcus viridans*, *Listeria monocytogenes*, and anaerobes.

A strong association exists between bacterial pneumonias and premature birth, which may be due to a developmental deficiency of bacteriostatic factors in the amniotic fluid. Alternatively, the infection may be a precipitating factor in preterm labor. Chorioamnionitis can occur even in the presence of intact membranes. Blood cultures and other diagnostic tests are necessary to help direct specific antimicrobial therapy. The clinician should be attuned to the labor history. Were membranes ruptured for more than 12 to 24 hours? Did the mother have a fever before delivery? Did the mother receive intrapartum antibiotics if risk factors for group B *Streptococcus* sepsis were present? Elements of the maternal history that delineate isolated maternal fever from a suspected intraamniotic infection include maternal leukocytosis, purulent cervical discharge, and fetal tachycardia (Committee on Obstetric Practice, 2017). Full-term infants with tachypnea, grunting, retractions, or temperature instability should be evaluated carefully. Although blood counts may be helpful because low white blood cell (WBC) counts, low neutrophil counts, and high immature to total neutrophil ratios are associated with higher odds of infection, these are imperfect predictors and should not solely be used to rule out infection (Hornik et al., 2012). Risk estimates based on clinical and perinatal factors may also be used in infants born at 35 weeks' gestation or later Kuzniewicz et al., 2017). Infection should be considered in any newborn with respiratory distress or more than transient oxygen requirements. Tracheal aspirates obtained within 8 hours of birth showing both bacteria and WBCs on Wright's stain are highly predictive of pneumonia.

Pending culture results, treatment usually begins with broad-spectrum antibiotics, typically penicillin and an aminoglycoside. A lumbar puncture may be undertaken or postponed until blood culture results are obtained. When cultures result in the identification of the organism, the study of antibiotic sensitivity allows the clinician to identify the most effective antibiotic or combination of antibiotics for the causative agent. Antibiotic treatment for up to 10 to 14 days may be necessary.

## Persistent Pulmonary Hypertension of the Newborn

Persistent pulmonary hypertension of the newborn (PPHN), or persistent fetal circulation, is a term applied to the combination of acute pulmonary hypertension (high pressure in the pulmonary artery), subsequent right-to-left shunting through fetal channels (the foramen ovale or ductus arteriosus) away from the pulmonary vascular bed. PPHN may be suspected when infants require high fractions of inspired oxygen and if shunting is noted with preductal oxygen saturations typically higher than postductal saturations when a patent ductus arteriosus (PDA) is present. It is important to ensure that infants have a structurally normal heart using echocardiography whenever possible because many types of congenital heart defects can present in a similar manner. The syndrome may be idiopathic or, more commonly, secondary to another disorder—such as MAS, congenital diaphragmatic hernia (CDH), RDS, asphyxia, sepsis, pneumonia, hyperviscosity of the blood, or hypoglycemia (Walsh-Sukys et al., 2000). Idiopathic causes may be related to maternal late-trimester nonsteroidal anti-inflammatory drug use or maternal use of selective serotonin reuptake inhibitors (SSRIs) (Dhillon, 2011).

The neonatal pulmonary vasculature is sensitive to changes in $PaO_2$ and pH and, during stress, can constrict to cause increased pressure against which the neonatal heart cannot force blood flow to the lungs. If the pulmonary artery pressure is higher than systemic pressure, blood flows through the path of least resistance, away from the lungs through the foramen ovale and the ductus arteriosus. The infant becomes progressively hypoxemic and acidemic, which accentuates the problem of increased pulmonary vascular resistance.

Management of infants with PPHN demands high vigilance. Because the pulmonary vasculature is unstable, almost any event can precipitate severe hypoxemia, including routine procedures such as ET suctioning, weighing, positioning, and diaper changes. Under these circumstances, minimal stimulation is usually practiced.

Occasionally, sedation and even muscle paralysis are necessary to prevent spontaneous episodes of hypoxemia or deterioration associated with procedures (e.g., suctioning and position changes). Mild alkalosis—either with bicarbonate infusion or by mild hyperventilation—often relaxes the pulmonary vascular bed and allows better pulmonary perfusion and, thus, oxygenation. The approach to respiratory therapy should be directed toward preventing hypoxemia and acidosis. The critical pH necessary for overcoming pulmonary vasoconstriction seems to be unique to the individual. High-applied ventilator pressures predispose the lung to air-leak syndromes, further increasing the risk of sudden destabilization. Since the early 1990s, inhalation of nitric oxide—alone and in association with high-frequency ventilation—is an effective therapy for PPHN (Barrington et al., 2017; Davidson et al., 1998; The Neonatal Inhaled Nitric Oxide Study Group, 1997). The use of milrinone can also be considered due to its vasodilatory effects on the pulmonary circulation. For infants with hypotension, vasopressors such as vasopressin, epinephrine, or dobutamine are often used in conjunction with targeting normal $CO_2$ values, but controlled data are not available. Vasopressors may act to improve contractility of the stressed myocardium, which improves CO, and raises systemic arterial pressure above pulmonary artery pressure to reduce right-to-left shunting.

When conventional therapies fail, high-frequency ventilation may be attempted. Approximately 30% to 60% of patients who fail conventional mechanical ventilation respond to high-frequency ventilation. However, the exact role of high-frequency ventilation in mortality or in preventing the need for ECMO needs further evaluation.

When oxygenation cannot be accomplished despite using conventional mechanical ventilation, high-frequency ventilation, or nitric oxide, ECMO has proven to be an effective therapy (UK Collaborative ECMO Trial Group, 1996). Neonatologists have differing views about the exact indications for ECMO, and some centers report impressive survival statistics without using ECMO (Mok et al., 1999). However, ECMO is often the only treatment that improves the outcome of some infants who fail less invasive therapies.

## Meconium Aspiration Syndrome

MAS is the most common aspiration syndrome that causes respiratory distress in neonates. The role of meconium in the pathophysiology of aspiration pneumonia has become controversial. It is unclear whether the material itself causes pneumonitis severe enough to lead to hypoxemia, acidosis, and pulmonary hypertension or whether the presence of meconium in the amniotic fluid is merely a marker for other events that may have predisposed the fetus to severe pulmonary disease. The severely ill infant with MAS typically comes from stressed labor and has depressed cord pH from metabolic acidosis. These infants are often postmature and exhibit classic signs of weight loss, skin peeling, and deep staining of the nails and umbilical cord. Pharyngeal suctioning at the time of birth does not reduce MAS (Vain et al., 2004). Guidelines for the resuscitation of non-vigorous infants with meconium-stained fluid were revised in 2015 and no longer include routine intubation and tracheal suctioning (Wyckoff et al., 2015). This change in clinical practice was due to concerns for the potential delay in bag-mask ventilation in these infants without any known benefit and possible harm of endotracheal suctioning because randomized controlled trials showed no benefit of routine endotracheal suctioning in non-vigorous newborns (Chettri et al., 2015; Nangia et al., 2021). Additionally, suctioning the mouth and nose provides no benefit compared to wiping the mouth as part of routine resuscitation (Kelleher et al., 2013).

Pulmonary disease in infants with MAS arises from chemical pneumonitis, interstitial edema, small airway obstruction, and concomitant persistent pulmonary hypertension. The infant may have uneven pulmonary ventilation with hyperinflation in some areas and atelectasis in others, leading to ventilation–perfusion mismatching and subsequent hypoxemia. The hypoxemia may then exacerbate pulmonary vasoconstriction, leading to deeper hypoxemia and acidosis. Infants with MAS may have evidence of lung overinflation with a barrel-chested appearance. Auscultation reveals rales and rhonchi. The radiograph shows patchy or streaky areas of atelectasis and other areas of overinflation.

As with other cases of pulmonary hypertension, nursing care of infants with MAS centers on the maintenance of adequate oxygenation and acid–base balance and on the avoidance of cold stress, which contributes to acidosis. A high incidence of air leaks exists in these infants, and PPV is best avoided if the patient can be adequately oxygenated, even at very high-inspired oxygen concentrations. Antibiotics are often used, particularly in critically ill infants, at least until a bacterial infection is ruled out, but antibiotic therapy may not be necessary. The infant is often exquisitely sensitive to environmental stimuli and should be treated in as quiet an environment as possible. Interventions should be preplanned to maximize the efficiency of handling the infant. Infants with very severe respiratory failure and MAS improve with the administration of exogenous surfactant because aspiration may lead to secondary surfactant deficiency (El Shahed et al., 2007). Inhaled nitric oxide (iNO) can be considered to treat acute pulmonary hypertension, which often complicates MAS. Some infants may require ECMO despite maximal support.

Although aspiration of meconium is most common, the neonate may become symptomatic as a result of the aspiration of blood, amniotic fluid, or gastrointestinal contents. The history is important in the differential diagnosis because radiographs are nondiagnostic.

### Pulmonary Hemorrhage

Pulmonary hemorrhage is rarely an isolated condition and usually occurs in an otherwise sick infant. RDS, asphyxia, congenital heart disease, aspiration of gastric content or maternal blood, disseminated intravascular coagulation (DIC), and other bleeding disorders may play a role in the cause of pulmonary hemorrhage. A PDA increases the risk of a clinically significant pulmonary hemorrhage that requires increased respiratory support and/or blood products. Prophylactic indomethacin reduces the risk of clinically significant pulmonary hemorrhage by 35% (Alfaleh et al., 2008). The risk for pulmonary hemorrhage is increased by approximately 5% in infants receiving either natural or artificial surfactant. Massive bleeding may also occur as a complication of airway suction secondary to direct trauma of the respiratory epithelium.

Pulmonary hemorrhage is manifested by the presence of bloody fluid from the trachea. **Emergency Alert:** **When massive, a pulmonary hemorrhage may be heralded by a sudden deterioration with pallor, shock, cyanosis, or bradycardia.** Attention must be given to the maintenance of a patent airway because an obstructed ET requires emergency replacement. However, replacing an occluded airway in the context of a massive pulmonary hemorrhage should be undertaken with caution because the bleeding can make visualization of the trachea difficult. Although studies have been reported describing the benefits of administration of surfactant in neonates after pulmonary hemorrhage due to secondary surfactant inactivation by the blood, there are no high-level-of-evidence studies to support its use (Aziz & Ohlsson, 2012). Suctioning must be done with great care to avoid precipitation of further bleeding. Clotting factors can be consumed rapidly, and the nurse should be alert to signs of generalized bleeding. Some clinicians increase the mean airway pressure (MAP) to decrease pulmonary blood flow in the context of pulmonary overcirculation, but there is limited data on this practice.

## PLEURAL EFFUSIONS

Pleural effusions may be caused by the accumulation of fluid between the parietal pleura of the chest wall and the visceral pleura enveloping the lung. A pleural effusion may also be due to chylothorax (lymphatic fluid) or hemothorax (blood). Lymphatics drain fluid that filters into the pleural space. Fluid accumulates in the pleural space due to increased filtration or decreased absorption. An increased filtration pressure, as seen with increased venous pressure in hydrops fetalis or congestive heart failure, leads to pleural effusion. The rate of filtration into the pleural space also increases if the pleural membrane becomes more permeable to water and protein, as occurs with infection.

Pleural effusion with high glucose content in an infant who is receiving parenteral nutrition via a central venous catheter should raise the suspicion of catheter perforation into the pleural space. If the infant also receives a lipid infusion, the fluid may appear milky and be confused with chylothorax.

Chylothorax may be either congenital or acquired. Congenital chylothorax frequently presents at delivery or shortly after with respiratory distress. Chylothorax can also be acquired as a surgical complication of repair of diaphragmatic hernia, tracheoesophageal fistula, or congenital heart defect. Congenital chylothorax may be suspected in the infant who is hydropic and cannot be ventilated in the delivery room. Breath sounds are difficult to hear, and chest movement with ventilation is minimal. Bilateral thoracenteses may be lifesaving. The typical pleural fluid in a chylothorax—opalescent and rich in fat—is present only if the infant has been fed. Therefore, the fluid aspirated in the delivery room or shortly after birth in a child with congenital chylothorax often has a low triglyceride level. However, the fluid will still have marked lymphocytic predominance at birth.

Pleural effusions that impede respiratory function typically require drainage by thoracentesis or tube thoracostomy. It may be necessary for chest tubes placed for chylothorax and thoracic duct injury to remain in place for extended periods while the infant is given total parenteral nutrition (TPN), receiving nothing by mouth, thus minimizing thoracic duct flow. Somatostatin administration (such as octreotide) has reduced the need for ventilator support (Yin et al., 2017). Several commercial formulas containing a higher percentage of medium-chain triglycerides (MCTs) that bypass the lymphatic system are also available for infants transitioning off parenteral nutrition. Due to the loss of lymphocytes and immunoglobulins through chylous drainage, these infants may also become immunocompromised and may benefit from immunoglobulin replacement.

## APNEA

Apnea is the typical end product of a myriad of neonatal physiologic events. Hypoxemia, infection, anemia, thermal instability, metabolic derangement, drugs, and intracranial disease can cause apnea. These causes should be considered before idiopathic apnea of prematurity is diagnosed.

Apnea is observed in more than half of surviving premature infants who weigh less than 1.5 kg at birth. The respiratory control mechanism and central responsiveness to carbon dioxide are progressively less mature at the lower gestational age, and preterm infants may require a higher carbon dioxide level to trigger respiration. In contrast to adults, infants respond to hypoxemia with only a brief hyperpneic response followed by hypoventilation or apnea. In any infant who has apnea, hypoxemia should always be ruled out before the clinician embarks on any other workup or institutes therapy.

Care of the infant experiencing apneic episodes requires close observation and careful positioning with a neutral airway position to reduce the risk of obstructive apnea. Obstructive apnea cannot be detected with the impedance respiratory monitor because normal or pronounced respiratory excursions of the chest wall exist. Prompt tactile stimulation for mild "spells" is often sufficient to abort the apnea episode, obviating further therapy. Infants with apneic episodes accompanied by profound bradycardia need prompt attention to their immediate respiratory needs as well as more aggressive diagnostic and therapeutic intervention.

Many apneic neonates respond to nasal CPAP at low pressures because the majority of apneic episodes have an obstructive component. Pressure support may also stimulate pulmonary stretch receptors, thus stimulating respiration. Use of methylxanthines, such as caffeine and aminophylline, has markedly simplified the apnea treatment in some premature infants. Xanthines appear to exert a central stimulatory effect on brainstem respiratory neurons and often markedly decrease the frequency and severity of apneic episodes. The clinician must be attuned to the toxicities of xanthines, including tachycardia, excessive diuresis, and vomiting. Caffeine may be associated with a lower risk of BPD and neurodevelopmental impairment (Schmidt et al., 2006). The timing of caffeine initiation, as well as optimal dosing in preterm infants, remains controversial. Little evidence supports the early administration of caffeine (within 36 hours of birth) with the possibility of harm (Amaro et al., 2018). Higher caffeine doses later on (i.e., in the setting of extubation) may confer neurodevelopmental benefits (Gentle et al., 2018; Gray et al., 2011). Sensory stimulation with waterbeds or other means can sometimes be used to manage these infants, particularly those with mild apnea.

Nursing care that is directed toward promoting a neutral thermal environment, normoxia, optimal airway maintenance, and prevention of aspiration is essential in the care of neonates at risk for apnea.

## CONGENITAL ANOMALIES THAT AFFECT RESPIRATORY FUNCTION

### Diaphragmatic Hernia

CDH occurs at a frequency of 1 in 2,500 live births and may be unsuspected until birth. Herniation of abdominal contents into the chest cavity early in gestation is accompanied by ipsilateral pulmonary hypoplasia. By mechanisms that are not well understood, there is often some degree of pulmonary hypoplasia on the contralateral side. Most infants are symptomatic at birth, with severe respiratory distress in the delivery room. The affected newborn's abdomen is usually scaphoid, and breath sounds are absent on the side of the defect (a left-sided defect occurs in 90% of cases). Bowel sounds may be heard in the chest, and heart sounds may be heard on the right side because the herniated abdominal contents push the mediastinum to the right.

**Quality and Safety:** **As soon as the diagnosis is suspected, bag and mask ventilation should be avoided because it fills the herniated intestinal contents with gas, leading to further lung compression and worsening ventilation.** When CDH has been diagnosed prenatally, the use of fetoscopic endoluminal tracheal occlusion may improve survival in severe left-sided defects compared to expectant care (Deprest et al., 2021). Infants receiving expectant management should be intubated, and mechanical ventilation should be initiated immediately after birth. An orogastric tube should be placed to aid in decompression of the herniated abdominal viscera. Ventilation should be attempted at a rapid rate and with low inflation pressure while tolerating hypercapnia. Symptomatic neonates often have pulmonary hypertension and progressive right-to-left shunting that may respond to the administration of iNO. Hypotension is common, and vasopressors may be helpful when adequate intravascular volume is established. Studies of iNO have shown limited evidence for effectiveness in treating diaphragmatic hernia (Barrington et al., 2017). Although evidence of surfactant deficiency in these newborns exists, surfactant administration does not appear to improve their clinical course or outcome (Colby et al., 2004).

The use of ECMO, more commonly required in infants with liver herniation or smaller lung volumes, may not lead to improvement in survival (Zalla et al., 2015). Surgery to repair the defect is indicated. Controversy regarding the urgency of the procedure exists among pediatric surgeons, and some prefer to stabilize the patient with mechanical ventilation, vasopressors, and correction of acidosis before undertaking surgical intervention; others perform surgical repair while the patient is maintained on ECMO.

### Congenital Heart Disease

Congenital heart disease commonly manifests with signs of respiratory distress. Neonates with congenital heart disease who demonstrate right-to-left shunting and decreased pulmonary blood flow (e.g., tetralogy of Fallot, pulmonary valve atresia, and tricuspid valve atresia or stenosis) usually present with profound cyanosis unresponsive to oxygen supplementation. Neonates with congenital heart disease who demonstrate increased pulmonary blood flow or obstruction to the left outflow tract (e.g., transposition of the great vessels, total anomalous pulmonary venous return, atrioventricular canal, hypoplastic left heart syndrome, and critical coarctation of the aorta) may transiently improve with oxygen supplementation. However, oxygen supplementation in some conditions, such as hypoplastic left heart syndrome, can worsen systemic flow and make the child worse. Neonates with noncyanotic lesions such as PDA and ventricular septal defect (VSD) may present later with signs of congestive heart failure (see Chapter 7, "Cardiovascular System").

## Choanal Atresia

Choanal atresia causes upper airway obstruction in the neonate. The choanae, or nasal passages, are separated from the nasopharynx by a structure known as the *bucconasal membrane*, which normally perforates during gestation. Failure of this developmental event results in an obstructed airway, occurring bilaterally in 50% of cases. Most affected infants are female, and half of the affected infants have associated anomalies such as CHARGE (coloboma, heart defects, atresia of the choanae, retardation of growth and development, genital and urinary abnormalities, and ear abnormalities and/or hearing loss) syndrome. Because newborns are obligate nasal breathers, they have chest retractions and severe cyanosis (particularly during feeding) and paradoxically turn pink when crying. This condition is suspected when a nasogastric (NG) tube fails to pass one or both nostrils. Diagnosis can be made via nasal endoscopy; however, CT imaging is also typically performed. Emergency treatment consists of tracheal intubation or placement of an oral airway. Surgical correction is indicated, though the ideal surgical intervention remains unclear (Cedin et al., 2012). In cases where atresia is bilateral, surgery usually occurs in the first week after birth.

## Cystic Hygroma

A variety of space-occupying lesions can impose on the newborn's airway (Box 6.4). Most are derived from embryonic tissues. Cystic hygroma, derived from lymphatic tissue, is the newborn's most common lateral neck mass. It is multilobular and multicystic, and, when large, obstructs the airway. Surgery or sclerotherapy is curative, although it is sometimes technically difficult. The clinician must always be mindful of the airway and its patency. Many of these lesions are of great cosmetic concern and cause great distress to the parents. A care plan should address these parental concerns. It is sometimes helpful to facilitate contact with parents of other children with similar problems who can share similar experiences.

**BOX 6.4**

**THORACIC CYSTS AND TUMORS THAT MAY CAUSE RESPIRATORY DISTRESS IN THE NEONATE**

Teratoma

Cystic hygroma

- Neurogenic tumor
- Neuroblastoma
- Ganglioneuroma
- Neurofibroma

Bronchial or bronchogenic cyst

Intrapulmonary cyst

Gastrogenic cyst

Hemangioma

Angiosarcoma

Mediastinal goiter

Thymoma

Mesenchymoma

Lipoma

Cystic adenomatous malformation

## Pierre Robin Sequence

The primary feature of Pierre Robin sequence is micrognathia (a small mandible). The tongue is posteriorly displaced into the oropharynx, thus obstructing the airway. Sixty percent of affected patients also have a cleft palate. Obstructive respiratory distress and cyanosis are common and may be severe. As with all airway obstructions (obstructive apnea), tracheal intubation should be undertaken in an emergency. Infants with Pierre Robin sequence are nursed in the prone position to prevent the tongue from falling backward. NG tube feedings are usually required in the neonatal period. With good care, the infant has a good prognosis for survival; the mandible usually grows, and the problem resolves by 6 to 12 months of age. Some infants will require surgical intervention if positioning changes do not enable an infant to successfully feed by mouth or prevent apneic symptoms. Surgical correction includes mandibular distraction or tongue-to-lip adhesion, both of which have reduced or eliminated the need for tracheostomy (Khansa et al., 2017).

# COLLABORATIVE MANAGEMENT OF INFANTS WITH RESPIRATORY DISORDERS

## Supportive Care

Supportive care of the infant in respiratory distress requires attention to detail. The clinicians' primary goals are to minimize oxygen consumption and carbon dioxide production. These goals are accomplished by maintaining a neutral thermal environment. The nurse must be skilled in physical assessment to interpret signs and symptoms, such as cyanosis, gasping, tachypnea, grunting, nasal flaring, and retractions. By understanding the pathophysiology of breathing, the nurse knows that the infant with retractions has decreased lung compliance and that the cyanotic infant has poor tissue oxygenation.

Excellent communication is needed between the neonatal nurse and the rest of the neonatal team. Acutely ill neonates with respiratory disease are often unstable, and their condition can deteriorate rapidly, so astute observation skills are necessary. Assessment is a continuous process, and effective communication among nurses, respiratory therapists, physicians, and support staff is required to properly deliver intensive care. The nurse, who is the primary bedside caregiver, is the gatekeeper for all interactions between the patient and the environment. The nurse caring for an unstable patient should be the patient's advocate, whether such a role involves regulating the timing of a physical examination by the physician or venipuncture for laboratory investigation.

Technical competence is a critical facet of the nurse's repertoire. The nurse is responsible for maintaining intravenous (IV) lines and tracheal tube patency, accurately measuring volumes of intravenous intake and urinary output, and operating advanced electronic machinery. Moreover, the nurse must also be adept at interpreting ABG and laboratory data to communicate these to the rest of the care team and develop a cogent management plan. Many functions are shared to some degree with respiratory therapists. Whether nurses or respiratory therapists make ventilator changes, the nurse should become familiar with the effects of ventilator setting changes on blood gases. $PaCO_2$ is affected by changes in ventilator rate and tidal volume. Tidal volume depends on the difference between PIP and PEEP. Thus, to decrease $PaCO_2$, either rate or inspiratory pressure should be increased. $PaO_2$ depends on the fraction of inspired oxygen concentration ($F_IO_2$) and MAP. MAP depends on PIP, PEEP, inspiratory to expiratory time ratio, and gas flow. To improve $PaO_2$, the most effective changes are to increase MAP by increasing PIP or PEEP or to increase $F_IO_2$. The nurse should also be familiar with ventilator functioning so that malfunctions can be detected promptly. The nurse should always be prepared to bag-ventilate an intubated neonate if decompensation occurs while the status of the ventilatory apparatus is checked. Nurses and respiratory therapists often share such functions as airway suctioning, monitoring and recording of inspired oxygen concentration, and delivery of chest physical therapy.

The delivery of oxygen therapy should constantly be monitored. Desired oxygenation parameters should be recorded in the nurse's notes and followed using continuous pulse oximetry and measurement of ABGs as indicated. The acutely ill infant should have $F_IO_2$ measured continuously and recorded frequently. The goal for oxygenation depends on the patient's diagnosis and condition. For example, in infants with PPHN, an acceptable saturation may occur despite marked right-to-left shunting. In preterm infants, oxygen saturation should be kept in the low 90s, thus avoiding the risks associated with hyperoxia or hypoxemia. Large randomized controlled trials (e.g., Carlo et al., 2010; Schmidt et al., 2013; Stenson et al., 2013) and meta-analyses (e.g., Askie et al., 2017, 2018) indicate that targeting lower oxygen saturations (85%–89%) versus higher saturations (91%–95%) in extremely preterm infants less than 28 weeks' gestation increases mortality and necrotizing enterocolitis without decreasing blindness. Targeting different saturations does not result in differences in neurodevelopmental impairment. Thus, targeting 91% to 95% or 90% to 95% oxygen saturations, as others have suggested, is now recommended by most experts to reduce mortality and necrotizing enterocolitis in extremely preterm infants. The use of oxygen saturation histograms may be used clinically to improve the achievement of desired oxygen saturation targets (Gentle et al., 2020).

Airway suctioning is a procedure that may be associated with cardiopulmonary derangement, hypoxemia, bradycardia, and hypertension. Various techniques to perform airway suctioning exist—including preoxygenation (increase in $F_IO_2$ before the procedure), normal saline instillation before the suctioning to improve secretion aspiration and using a closed system to avoid disconnection from the ventilator. The nurse should become familiar with the techniques used in the NICU and be aware of the associated complications. Suctioning of the airway should be done only as often as necessary to remove pulmonary secretions that could occlude the airway. The suction catheter should be passed no further than the end of the tracheal tube because the epithelium is easily damaged. There is perhaps little need to vigorously suction the intubated infant with RDS in the first days after birth because secretions are minimal, and lung volume is lost with every disconnection of the ventilator circuit.

The sudden decompensation of a ventilated infant should alert the nurse to assess disconnection of the ventilator, pulmonary air leak, ventilator failure, or obstructed tracheal tube (see Figure 6.4). The very small infant who suddenly decompensates may have experienced a severe intracranial hemorrhage.

Care of the infant who is receiving CPAP can be particularly challenging. These infants should be kept calm and swaddled if necessary. Crying releases pressure through the mouth; thus, lung volume is lost. Nasal CPAP is effective, but particular attention must be given to maintaining the patency of the nose, the nasal prongs, and the pharynx. The infant's nares and nasal septum should be guarded against pressure necrosis from inappropriately applied prongs and the use of barrier dressings as needed (Imbulana et al., 2018). The infant with respiratory disease must be constantly assessed for airway patency. If the infant cannot grunt against a closed glottis and maintain positive airway pressure, the condition may worsen if airway pressure is not maintained properly. Vibration and percussion should be used judiciously in infants with pulmonary secretions to loosen them and allow removal via suction.

## ASSESSMENT AND MONITORING

The most crucial aspect in monitoring patients with respiratory disease is the close and continuous observation of signs and symptoms. The color of the patient gives valuable clues. An infant with pink lips and oral mucosa has good oxygenation and perfusion; a cyanotic patient has poor tissue oxygenation. If the hemoglobin concentration is too low, the patient can be hypoxemic, but because the concentration of deoxyhemoglobin is low, there may be no cyanosis. An infant with tachypnea and retractions usually has decreased lung compliance. A patient with a barrel-shaped thorax, taking deep breaths, and with a normal or low respiratory rate probably has increased airway resistance and gas trapping.

Observation of the intubated patient is especially important. An anguished infant who is cyanotic and breathing deeply may have an obstructed endotracheal tube. Despite no change in ventilatory pressures, an infant with RDS and increased chest expansion over time is experiencing improvement in lung compliance. The same infant with later asymmetry in the chest and sudden deterioration of oxygenation may have a pneumothorax. Cardiac beats, easily seen through the thoracic wall, may be caused by a symptomatic PDA. A recently extubated infant, in whom increased retractions and inspiratory stridor develop, probably has upper airway obstruction. Auscultation helps diagnose increased airway resistance or the presence of secretions. It also allows the clinician to assess the response to different treatment maneuvers, such as suctioning, chest physiotherapy, and bronchodilation. Asymmetries in auscultation suggest mainstream bronchial intubation, atelectasis, pneumothorax, or pleural effusion.

Great progress has been made in noninvasive monitoring of blood gas tensions, but blood sampling is still necessary for pH determination, and arterial samples are preferable. Capillary specimens are undependable, especially for $PO_2$. If peripheral perfusion is adequate, capillary blood approximates arterial values of pH and $PCO_2$. However, capillary blood $PO_2$ values do not reflect arterial oxygenation.

Neonatal care has changed dramatically with the advent and widespread use of transcutaneous $PaO_2$, $PaCO_2$, and $SaO_2$ monitoring. The neonatal intensive care team should become familiar with the devices used in noninvasive gas monitoring. It is essential to know the basis for their functioning as well as how to interpret the information they provide and be aware of clinical situations in which the information provided is not reliable or needs to be complemented before any management decisions are made.

Transcutaneous pulse oximetry ($TcPO_2$) monitoring has been largely supplanted by continuous pulse oximetry. Arterial oxygen saturation is computed from absorption of emitted low-intensity red or infrared light. The probe is attached to a finger or toe in large infants or a hand or foot in small premature infants. Pulse oximetry offers the following advantages over transcutaneous oxygen monitoring: (a) avoidance of heating the skin and the risk of burns; (b) elimination of a delay period for transducer equilibration; (c) accurate measurement regardless of the presence of edema or patient age; (d) in vitro calibration not required; and (e) frequent position changes not required. However, the nurse should know that an $SaO_2$ higher than 97% may be associated with a $PaO_2$ higher than 100 mm Hg. This is important in premature infants who are at risk for retinopathy of prematurity. $SaO_2$ targets of 91% and 95% are probably associated with a safe range of $PaO_2$. With an $SaO_2$ over 95% to 97%, especially when it is 100%, the clinician cannot predict a patient's $PaO_2$. When the saturation is 100%, the $PaO_2$ can be approximately 100 mm Hg or much higher (see Figure 6.1). This situation is particularly important in infants with PPHN because the decision of whether to wean ventilator settings may depend on $PaO_2$. In these patients, the simultaneous use of $TcPO_2$ and pulse oximetry is a useful alternative.

A common problem of pulse oximetry is the presence of *motion artifact*, an altered signal caused by movement of the part of the body where the sensor is applied. Because the pulse waveform is not detected, this movement is recognized by the loss of correlation between the oximeter pulse rate and the electrical monitor heart rate. With current technology, the motion artifacts have been minimized (Malviya et al., 2000). Peripheral pulse oximetry may not detect pulse signals in patients with hypotension and poor perfusion. $TcPO_2$ may also give false readings in this situation. The clinician should be aware that the probe's pressure over the skin can produce skin pressure necrosis. This consideration is particularly important in premature infants. Phototherapy may interfere with accuracy of $SaO_2$ monitoring, but this problem can be avoided by covering the sensor with an opaque material (e.g., a diaper or band).

Transcutaneously measured $PCO_2$ is accomplished with a glass electrode that is pH sensitive. Transcutaneous $PCO_2$ response is slower than that of $TcPO_2$, and the value measured must be corrected for skin production of carbon dioxide. Thus, transcutaneously measured values are approximately within 5 mm Hg of arterial $PCO_2$ values (Setar et al., 2024). This modality is especially useful for monitoring chronically ventilated patients without indwelling catheters and also to reduce the number of laboratory tests in infants with indwelling catheters. Blood gas values during arterial puncture or vigorous crying during the procedure are often affected by breath-holding and shunting and thus may be misleading.

## ENVIRONMENTAL CONSIDERATIONS

Maintenance of the therapeutic environment is an important nursing function. Much attention has recently been given to the effects of sensory stimulation on infants with respiratory distress. The sick newborn often has unstable pulmonary vasculature and may be particularly prone to hypoxic vasoconstriction. Excess stimulation, such as loud noise, handling, or venipuncture, may trigger this phenomenon in some individuals. It has been shown that the agitated neonate has more difficulty with oxygenation and that a quiet, minimally stimulating environment allows for more stable oxygenation (Als, 1998). The nurse should develop a care plan that allows the baby long periods of undisturbed rest by clustering interventions into short periods whenever possible. Positioning the infant in the flexed or fetal position or "nesting" may help calm some infants. Always watch for stress cues to see how the infant tolerates the care. Clustering of care only works if the infant tolerates a more extended period of care rather than episodic care. Either way, the infant needs undisturbed periods where rest and recovery can occur.

## FAMILY CARE

Neonates with respiratory distress frequently require multiple instrumentations. They are typically in an incubator and may have endotracheal tubes, umbilical catheters, oximeter probes, chest leads, and other paraphernalia attached or applied to the skin. These interventions can give parents a feeling of increased separation from the infant. The nurse should explain the equipment surrounding the bedside and the function of invasive catheters, monitoring leads, and tracheal tubes.

Terminology appropriate to the parents' level of understanding should be used. Even the most astute parents may be bewildered, and repetition is necessary. Staff should maintain consistent terminology so that the parents do not become confused between "respirators" and "ventilators." Whenever possible, the use of frightening or inaccurate terms should be avoided. Imagine the fear engendered by the phrase, "We paralyzed your baby last night."

Parents should be involved in developing and implementing the plan of care as much as possible. The mother who plans to breastfeed can be assisted in pumping her breasts and freezing the milk, even if enteral feedings are delayed for some time. This pumping may be the only thing she can do for her baby.

Often lost in the bustle of critical care is the need for privacy. The perceptive nurse senses this need and backs away from the bedside when appropriate, allowing the parent some time with the infant. Care of the neonate requires a team—a coordinated team, and that includes the parents!

## SUMMARY

Most infants admitted to the NICU present with breathing difficulty. Nursing care of these infants requires a broad knowledge of newborn physiology and practical skills in the application of therapies that are directed toward solving the many problems that sick infants can have. The nurse often must anticipate these problems. While managing the nursing care for several patients, the neonatal nurse must also care for the sickest of infants. Parents and families of all infants in the NICU require special attention not only to achieve an understanding of the complex issues surrounding the infant's illness but also to calm fears and guilt that are often experienced. The rewards of being part of the accomplishments in the NICU may be overlooked because they are usually slowly achieved. However, when recognized, the victories surpass the greatest of expectations.

## CASE STUDY

**Identification of the Problem.** A term infant was admitted to the NICU. The infant developed respiratory distress soon after birth. Birth weight was 4,000 g. Since birth, the infant has had an increasing oxygen requirement, and because of a recent desaturation episode, the infant is now receiving 100% oxygen on a ventilator. The ventilatory settings are PIP of 25 cm $H_2O$, PEEP of 5 cm $H_2O$, ventilator rate of 60 per minute, and inspiratory time of 0.4 seconds. A recent ABG showed a pH of 7.35, $PCO_2$ of 42, $PO_2$ of 60, and bicarbonate of 22.

**Assessment: History and Physical Examination.** The infant was born by emergency C-section because of late decelerations and thick meconium-stained fluid. No signs of infection were observed. The mother had gestational diabetes and was maintained on insulin. The infant was not vigorous at birth and received bag-mask ventilation at birth because endotracheal suction is no longer recommended. Blow-by oxygen was then administered and the infant responded well, initially weaned to 40% oxygen. However, after transfer to the NICU, the infant had increasing oxygen requirements.

The physical examination is pertinent for excellent chest rise, equal breath sounds, central cyanosis with oxygen saturations in the mid-80s, good color and perfusion, and normal tone and reflexes.

**Differential Diagnosis.** Many conditions should be considered in the differential diagnosis in this patient.

1. Persistent pulmonary hypertension of the neonate. This is likely, given the severity and persistence of the very abnormal alveolar to arterial oxygen gradient ($AaDO_2$). Pulmonary hypertension may be associated with MAS. It is important to consider that right-to-left shunting can be associated with disorders such as myocardial dysfunction, sepsis, metabolic abnormalities, and others.
2. MAS. MAS with intrapulmonary (ventilation–perfusion mismatch) or extrapulmonary shunting (atrial or ductal shunting with pulmonary hypertension) may lead to desaturation despite high oxygen supplementation.
3. Pneumothorax. Infants with MAS are at high risk for pneumothorax. A pneumothorax can cause severe desaturation.
4. Gas trapping. Because this infant has a large tidal volume for the given pressure gradient (PIP–PEEP) and likely high compliance, a long-time constant of the respiratory system leading to gas trapping at a borderline high ventilator rate should be considered.
5. Other causes. There are other less frequent but important causes of the differential diagnosis. Congenital heart disease should be included in the differential diagnosis, given the $PaO_2$ is less than 100 mm Hg while on 100% oxygen. Infection should be considered in a critically ill neonate.

**Diagnostic Tests.** The chest radiograph was obtained, repeat blood gases were followed, and pre-and postductal pulse oximetry and transcutaneous measurements of gases were monitored continuously. In addition, a complete blood count (CBC) and blood culture were obtained. Four extremity blood pressures and an echocardiogram were obtained.

**Working Diagnosis.** The chest radiograph showed bilateral gas trapping. The CBC and the blood cultures were negative. The echocardiogram was consistent with persistent pulmonary hypertension.

**Development of Management Plan.** The infant was given surfactant, and initial improvement was seen. However, during the next 24 hours, there were episodes of repeated intracardiac and ductal shunting, which led to the initiation of nitric oxide.

**Implementation and Evaluation of Effectiveness.** Nitric oxide resulted in a marked reduction in the shunting episodes. The infant was gradually weaned off $F_IO_2$ and subsequently weaned off nitric oxide before extubation. The infant was entirely weaned off the ventilator and $F_IO_2$ over the subsequent 3 days.

## EVIDENCE-BASED PRACTICE

RDS is the most common cause of respiratory distress in preterm neonates (Hamvas, 2011). Most children that are born extremely premature develop RDS in the first hours after birth. The incidence of RDS is progressively more common the lower the infant's gestational age. Up to 98% of infants born at 23 weeks and 86% of infants born at 28 weeks develop RDS (Stoll et al., 2010). Many of these are treated with surfactant (Stoll et al., 2010). RDS can develop in term infants born to mothers with diabetes or in term infants who have experienced asphyxia, but it is substantially less frequent than in premature infants.

Antenatal steroids accelerate lung maturation (Roberts et al., 2017). Present recommendations are to give steroids to all mothers between 23 and 34 weeks and consider administration at 22 weeks' gestational age with threatened delivery. Antenatal steroids significantly reduce the incidence of RDS in premature infants. Antenatal steroids also decrease mortality, intraventricular hemorrhage, necrotizing enterocolitis, and neurodevelopmental impairment (Carlo et al., 2011; Schmidt et al., 2006). Adverse effects have not been reported with the usual single course of antenatal steroids (Carlo et al., 2011; Schmidt et al., 2006). Data at the limits of viability (i.e., < 25 weeks) show benefits to giving steroids to infants as early as 22 weeks with a reduction in mortality at all gestational ages between 23 and 27 weeks (Carlo et al., 2011; Travers et al., 2018).

The hallmark of RDS is deficiency of pulmonary surfactant. Surfactant reduces the alveolar surface tension, thus preventing alveolar collapse. Therapy is directed toward improving oxygenation as well as maintaining optimal lung volume. CPAP can be used to prevent volume loss during exhalation. Exogenous surfactants are also quite effective at treating RDS. Early clinical trials indicated that prophylactic surfactant administration to extremely premature infants in the delivery room is more effective than waiting for the treatment after development of RDS (Soll & Morley, 2001). However, subsequent trials indicated that early CPAP with selective surfactant for infants who require intubation reduces death/BPD when compared with prophylactic surfactant administration in extremely preterm infants (Rojas-Reyes et al., 2012). More recent trials suggest that less invasive or minimally invasive surfactant administration through a thin catheter without exposure to PPV may improve pulmonary outcomes in preterm infants.

### References

Carlo, W. A., McDonald, S. A., Fanaroff, A. A., Vohr, B. R., Stoll, B. J., Ehrenkranz, R. A., Andrews, W. W., Wallace, D., Das, A., Bell, E. F., Walsh, M. C., Laptook, A. R., Shankaran, S., Poindexter, B. B., Hale, E. C., Newman, N. S., Davis, A. S., Schibler, K., Kennedy, K. A., ... Higgins, R. D.; for the Eunice Kennedy Shriver National Institute of Child Health and Human Development Neonatal Research Network. (2011). Association of antenatal corticosteroids with mortality and neurodevelopmental outcomes among infants born at 22 to 25 weeks' gestation. *Journal of the American Medical Association*, *306*, 2348–2358. https://doi.org/10.1001/jama.2011.1752

Dunn, M. S., Kaempf, J., de Klerk, A., de Klerk, R., Reilly, M., Howard, D., Ferrelli, K., O'Conor, J., & Soll, R. F.; for the Vermont Oxford Network DRM Study Group. (2011). Randomized trial comparing 3 approaches to the initial respiratory management of preterm neonates. *Pediatrics*, *128*(5), e1069–e1076. https://doi.org/10.1542/peds.2010-3848

Finer, N. N., Carlo, W. A., Walsh, M. C., Rich, W., Gantz, M. G., Laptook, A. R., Yoder, B. A., Faix, R. G., Das, A., Poole, W. K., Donovan, E. F., Newman, N. S., Ambalavanan, N., Frantz, I. D., Buchter, S., Sánchez, P. J., Kennedy, K. A., Laroia, N., Poindexter, B. B., ... Higgins, R. D.; for the NICHD Neonatal Research Network and the SUPPORT Study Group. (2010, May 27). Early CPAP versus surfactant in extremely preterm infants. *The New England Journal of Medicine*, *362*(21), 1970–1979. https://doi.org/10.1056/NEJMoa0911783

Hamvas, A. (2011). The respiratory system: Part 3 pathophysiology and management of respiratory distress syndrome. In A. A. Fanaroff, R. J. Martin, & M. C. Walsh (Eds.), *Fanaroff & Martin's neonatal-perinatal medicine: Diseases of the fetus and infant* (9th ed., pp. 1106–1115). Mosby.

Roberts, D., Brown, J., Medley, N., &Dalziel, S. R. (2017). Antenatal corticosteroids for accelerating fetal lung maturation for women at risk of preterm birth. *Cochrane Database of Systematic Reviews*, (3), CD004454. https://doi.org/10.1002/14651858.CD004454.pub4

Rojas-Reyes, M. X., Morley, C. J., &Soll, R. (2012). Prophylactic versus selective use of surfactant in preventing morbidity and mortality in preterm infants. *Cochrane Database of Systematic Reviews*, *2012*(3), CD000510. https://doi.org/10.1002/14651858.CD000510.pub2

Schmidt, B., Roberts, R. S., Davis, P., Doyle, L. W., Barrington, K. J., Ohlsson, A., Solimano, A., & Tin, W.; for the Caffeine for Apnea of Prematurity Trial Group. (2006). Caffeine therapy for apnea of prematurity. *The New England Journal of Medicine*, *354*(20), 2179–2180. https://doi.org/10.1056/NEJMoa054065

Soll, R. F., & Morley, C. J. (2001). Prophylactic versus selective use of surfactant for preventing morbidity and mortality in preterm infants. *Cochrane Database of Systematic Reviews*, *2001*(2), CD000510. https://doi.org/10.1002/14651858.CD000510

Stoll, B. J., Hansen, N. I., Bell, E. F., Shankaran, S., Laptook, A. R., Walsh, M. C., Hale, E. C., Newman, N. S., Schibler, K., Carlo, W. A., Kennedy, K. A., Poindexter, B. B., Finer, N. N., Ehrenkranz, R. A., Duara, S., Sánchez, P. J., O'Shea, T. M., Goldberg, R. N., Van Meurs, K. P., ... Higgins, R. D.; for the Eunice Kennedy Shriver National Institute of Child Health and Human Development Neonatal Research Network. (2010). Neonatal outcomes of extremely preterm infants from the NICHD Neonatal Research Network. *Pediatrics*, *126*, 443–456. https://doi.org/10.1542/peds.2009-2959

(*continued*)

## EVIDENCE-BASED PRACTICE (*continued*)

Travers, C. P., Carlo, W. A., McDonald, S. A., Das, A., Bell, E. F., Ambalavanan, N., Jobe, A. H., Goldberg, R. N., D'Angio, C. T., Stoll, B. J., Shankaran, S., Laptook, A. R., Schmidt, B., Walsh, M. C., Sánchez, P. J., Ball, M. B., Hale, E. C., Newman, N. S., &Higgins, R. D.; for the Eunice Kennedy Shriver National Institute of Child Health and Human Development Neonatal Research Network. (2018). Mortality and pulmonary outcomes of extremely preterm infants exposed to antenatal corticosteroids. *American Journal of Obstetrics and Gynecology*, *218*(1), 130.e1–130.e13. https://doi.org/10.1016/j.ajog.2017.11.554

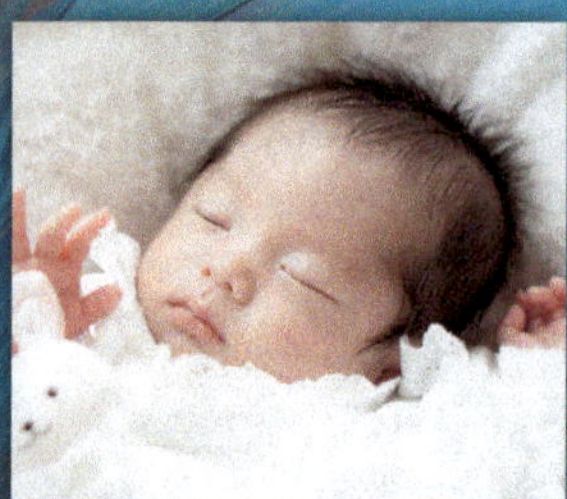

*Source:* Chihana/Adobe Stock.

## PARENT VOICES

### Heather McKinnis

Our micro-preemie was a complete surprise. My perfect pregnancy ended abruptly after just 4 hours of labor. I was given one steroid injection as they rapidly prepped me for my emergency C-section. Owen came into the world with low Apgar scores that did slightly improve as the NICU team worked on him. He was stabilized and moved to the NICU. When I first saw him, 12 hours later, he was so tiny and hooked up to so many pieces of equipment, including a vent that we would get to know well over the next week. Miraculously, my little fighter only required intubation for 8 days. He spent another week on CPAP and several weeks on high-flow cannula. We had prepared to take him home with oxygen support but a week and a half before discharge, he proved us all wrong and came off oxygen as well. Throughout this entire journey, I was incredibly grateful for the patience and kindness of our nurses. They took the time to explain everything to me, helped me wrap my mind around the fragility of my baby, and how I could best help him thrive.

### Laurel Kapferer, MS

Our son Blake was born via a scheduled C-section at 37 weeks. When he was born, everything appeared to be fine. He weighed 7 lb 1.4 oz and was breathing on his own. He was placed on my chest as soon as we left the operating room and began breastfeeding almost immediately. When he was 2 hours old, he went for a routine examination at which time everything quickly changed. During his examination, Blake went into respiratory distress and was rushed to the NICU.

The doctors told us that his respiratory distress was due to his lungs not being completely matured, the presence of fluid in his lungs, or both. Blake was hooked up to monitors and oxygen, which made holding him difficult. Anytime it was loud or Blake got excited, his oxygen saturation would drop, and eventually he had to be intubated and given two rounds of surfactant. Seeing Blake with tubes down his throat was absolutely excruciating for us. Even though we had been in the NICU before, nothing could have prepared us for that. Fortunately, the surfactant worked and all tubes and oxygen were removed. Blake was able to maintain his $O_2$ sats on room air. When he was 6 days old, he was discharged from the NICU. Today Blake is a happy, healthy 5 year old. The only complication that he has from his NICU stay are fractures in the base of his baby teeth from being intubated.

Blake's journey was made more difficult because we knew the pain of losing a child. His brother had passed away the year prior while in the NICU. We were so very fortunate to have such amazing NICU doctors and nurses caring for Blake. They all knew our story and they all did everything they could to help us through. They went above and beyond and really understood the trauma and posttraumatic stress disorder (PTSD) that we experienced. They took the time to look at the details of our past and made sure to put us in a different room from our previous NICU stay. They made sure not to discharge us on the same count of days that our other child passed on. They also met with us every day and told us what would likely happen so that we were emotionally prepared.

The compassion and understanding that our NICU team showed us had such an incredible effect on our journey and we are eternally grateful for them.

(*continued*)

## PARENT VOICES (*continued*)

### Jennifer M. Driscoll

Our daughter, Lilian Hope, was born 7 weeks premature, weighing only 2 lb 12 oz and 15 inches long. Lily's lungs were her main problem, as they are for many preemies, because the lungs are the last thing to develop. On the day she was born, she was doing well, but still needed a CPAP machine to help her breathe. As the day progressed, her condition worsened. She was given nitric oxide, put onto a ventilator to breathe for her, and needed an oscillator to vibrate the lungs to help the flow of oxygen. Due to the force of the ventilator and oscillator, an air sac in her lungs burst and she had a chest tube inserted. Additionally, she had an erratic blood pressure, jaundice, and needed multiple blood transfusions. But the miracle continued as she began to gain strength inside herself; she came off the oscillator after 7 days and took out the ventilator herself. By day 8 we were able to hold her for the first time. She ended up only needing to stay in the NICU at Lehigh Valley Hospital for 24 days and was able to come home at a mere 3 lb 11 oz.

Our son, Aidan Patrick, was also born only 4 weeks premature, weighing 4 lb 11 oz and 18 inches long. These few weeks, pounds, and inches may seem small but were huge victories for us. I was labeled high risk as soon as I found out I was pregnant and put on aspirin and bed rest much sooner because we knew what happened when Lily was born. Aidan's NICU stay was much shorter than Lily's, only a few days. Unfortunately, because of that, Aidan didn't qualify for the respiratory syncytial virus (RSV) vaccine as Lily did, and by 4 months old he was hospitalized on oxygen for over a week with RSV. This incident catapulted his asthma and subsequent allergy issues. Aidan has been hospitalized seven times since that RSV diagnosis with severe asthma flare-ups. Allergies and sickness trigger his asthma, so he is on two maintenance inhalers and daily medication and continues to see pediatric pulmonologists and allergists for his lung issues.

Both Aidan and Lily were born early because I had preeclampsia. They both had a very rough beginning, but with their strength, wonderful doctors and nurses, hope, and prayers, they have been able to rise above it all.

### Keira Sorrells

One of my daughters spent 14 months on the ventilator and had severe reflux, causing her to have extreme oral aversions and tracheomalacia. We spent the first 60 days of her 291-day NICU stay simply staring at her because we were told she was too fragile to hold. As a parent, this was absolutely devastating. NICU parents confront so many barriers in access to their children, from the locked door we have to be buzzed through to gain entry to the yellow gowns we wear over our clothing and of course the isolette, tubes, and wires encasing our babies. Parents of typical, healthy newborns obtain instantaneous and open access to their babies at birth while we are stripped of every maternal instinct we have. I wish, during those 60 days, something could have been done to allow us to be closer to her. If there was any chance of holding her before she was 2 months old, we would have cherished every minute. We spent so many hours simply sitting next to her and watching the hours pass by, hoping and praying she would be strong enough to hold.

## ONLINE RESOURCES

**CourseConnect**

Resources for this chapter are online and available at www.springerpub.com/courseconnect.

## REFERENCES

References for this chapter are online and available at www.springerpub.com/courseconnect.

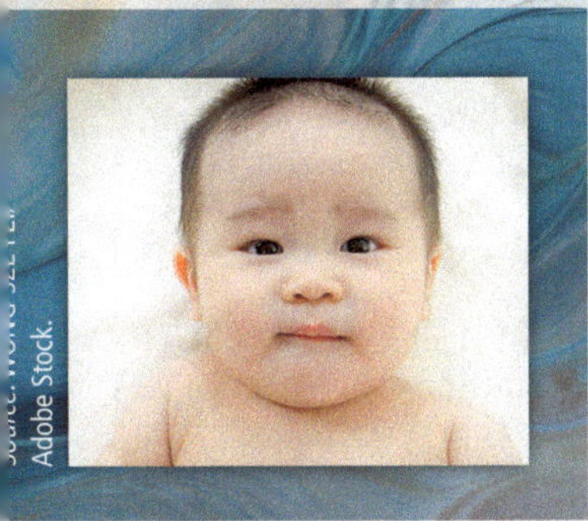

Adobe Stock.

# CHAPTER 7

# Cardiovascular System

**Gloria Johnson and Donna A. Goff**

## INTRODUCTION

This chapter presents the physiology of normal cardiac function, including fetal circulatory patterns and the changes that occur during transition to extrauterine life. The most common congenital heart defects (CHDs) and cardiac complications are described including information about the incidence, hemodynamics, manifestations, diagnosis, and medical and surgical management. The importance of prenatal detection of CHD and critical congenital heart defect (CCHD) pulse oximetry screening is discussed. Risk factors for brain injury in the neonate with CHD and age-related neurodevelopmental (ND) problems are reviewed. The chapter concludes with a discussion about the support of the family of an infant with a CHD. A case study is used to illustrate the complex care required by infants and families of infants with cardiac disorders.

## CARDIOVASCULAR ADAPTATION

### Fetal Circulation

Knowledge of the normal route of fetal blood flow is essential to understand the circulatory changes that occur in the newborn at delivery. The pattern of fetal circulation is illustrated in Figure 7.1. Fetal circulation involves four unique anatomic features.

In fetal life, the placenta serves as the exchange organ for oxygen and carbon dioxide and for nutrients and waste. Fetal circulation involves parallel circulation, which is different from series circulation—the right ventricle (RV) pumps deoxygenated blood to the lungs, which return oxygenated blood to the left ventricle (LV), which pumps blood to the body—seen postnatally. The oxygenated blood from the placenta enters the umbilical vein (UV), and the ductus venosus (DV) allows approximately one-third of this oxygenated blood to bypass the liver to stream right to left across the foramen ovale (FO), an opening in the atrial septum. This oxygenated blood enters the LV, which then pumps the well-oxygenated blood to the developing brain. Deoxygenated blood from the

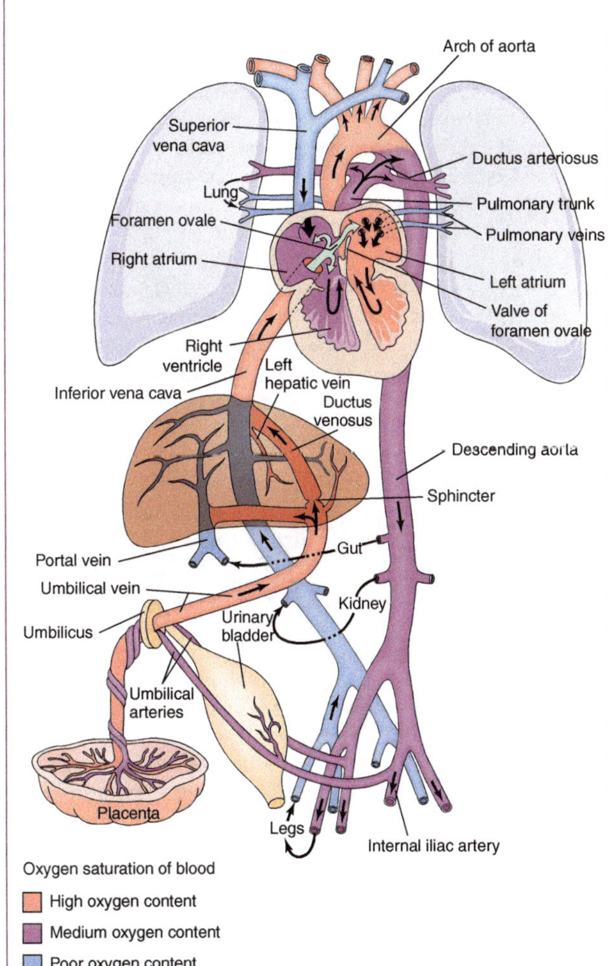


**FIGURE 7.1 Anatomic features and pattern of fetal circulation.**
*Source:* Adapted and modified from Ross Laboratories, Columbus, OH, Clinical Education Aid, 1985.

superior vena cava (SVC) and inferior vena cava (IVC) enters the right atrium (RA) to the RV, which pumps the blood into the main pulmonary artery (MPA). Because the lungs are only growing and not functioning in utero, only 5% to 10% of the blood flow in the pulmonary artery perfuses the lungs, so the majority of the blood flow shunts across the ductus arteriosus (DA) into the descending aorta and returns to the placenta via the umbilical artery (UA; Park & Salamat, 2022; Valente et al., 2022).

## Extrauterine Circulation

The cardiac and pulmonary systems undergo drastic changes at birth; these changes usually occur immediately upon onset of respiration. The most significant change is that the lungs now assume the role of primary oxygenator. Clamping of the umbilical cord removes the placenta and subsequently results in immediate circulatory changes in the newborn. With the first breath and occlusion of the umbilical cord, the newborn's systemic vascular resistance increases, decreasing the amount of blood flow through the DA. Cord occlusion causes an increase in blood pressure and a corresponding stimulation of the aortic baroreceptors and the sympathetic nervous system. The onset of respiration and consequent lung expansion causes a decrease in pulmonary vascular resistance secondary to the direct effect of oxygen and carbon dioxide on the blood vessels. Pulmonary vascular resistance decreases as arterial oxygen content increases and arterial carbon dioxide decreases (Park & Salamat, 2022; Valente et al., 2022).

Most of the RV output flows through the lungs and increases the pulmonary venous return to the left atrium (LA). This increased blood flow into the lungs that returns to the heart results in increased pressure in the LA and combined with the increased systemic vascular resistance, functionally closes the FO.

The DA functionally closes around 12 to 15 hours after birth because of constriction of the medial smooth muscle. The DA is anatomically constricted, becoming the ligamentum arteriosum by 3 weeks of age because of changes that occur in the endothelium and subintimal layers in response to oxygen, prostaglandin $E_2$ ($PGE_2$), acetylcholine, and bradykinin. Clamping of the umbilical cord causes the cessation of blood flow through the UV, DV, and UA (Park & Salamat, 2022).

*Functional closure* refers to the cessation of flow through the structure caused by changes in pressure. *Anatomic closure* refers to obliteration of the structure by constriction because of intraluminal growth of tissue.

Because anatomic closure of the fetal pathways lags behind the functional closure, the shunts may open and close intermittently before anatomic closure, resulting in transient functional murmurs.

Pulmonary artery pressure remains high for several hours after delivery. As the pulmonary vascular resistance decreases, the direction of blood flow through the DA changes. Initially, the patent ductus arteriosus (PDA) is bidirectional, the flow becomes entirely left to right typically by 24 to 48 hours of life, and the DA may be functionally insignificant by 48 hours of life. Intermittent or functional murmurs do not cause any cardiovascular compromise for the newborn and are not clinically significant. Conditions that cause transient opening of fetal shunts, allowing deoxygenated blood to shunt from the right side of the heart to the left, thereby bypassing the pulmonary circuit, produce transient cyanosis. Any murmur or cyanosis in the newborn should be carefully evaluated and monitored to detect cardiovascular abnormalities (Jones et al., 2021; Park & Salamat, 2022; Valente et al., 2022). Hypoxemia and acidosis can cause a functionally constricted DA to reopen, while the pulmonary artery and arterioles respond by constricting (Park & Salamat, 2022; Valente et al., 2022).

# NORMAL CARDIAC FUNCTION

The normal anatomy of the heart is shown in Figure 7.2.

## Cardiac Valves

Blood flow through the heart is directed through two sets of one-way valves. The *atrioventricular valves* (AVs) consist of the *tricuspid valve* and the *mitral valve*. The tricuspid valve connects the RA and the RV. The mitral valve connects the LA and the LV. The *semilunar valves* consist of the *pulmonary*

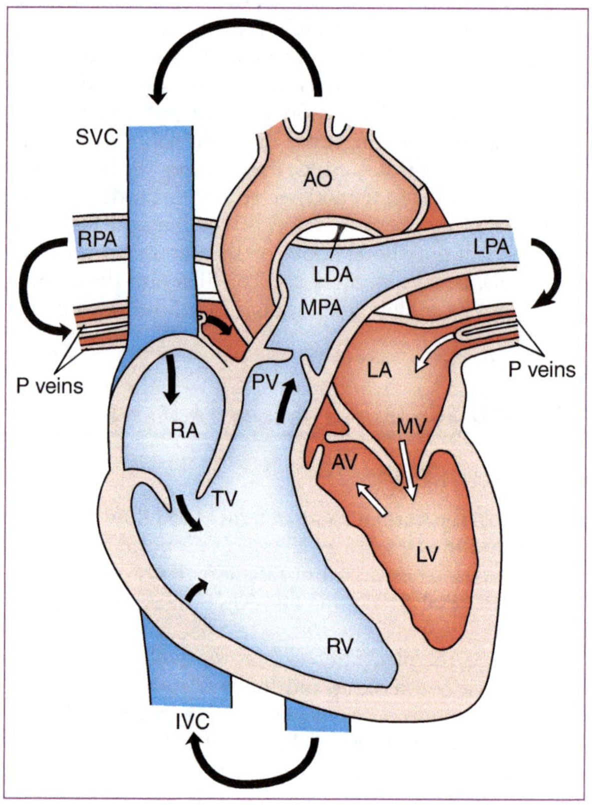


**FIGURE 7.2 Normal cardiac anatomy and circulation.**

AO, aorta; AV, aortic valve; IVC, inferior vena cava; LA, left atrium; LDA, ligamentum ductus arteriosus; LPA, left pulmonary artery; LV, left ventricle; MPA, main pulmonary artery; MV, mitral valve; PV, pulmonary valve; P veins, pulmonary veins; RA, right atrium; RPA, right pulmonary artery; RV, right ventricle; SVC, superior vena cava; TV, tricuspid valve.

*Source:* Adapted and modified from Ross Laboratories, Columbus, OH, Clinical Education Aid, 1985.

*valve* and the *aortic valve*. The pulmonary valve connects the RV and the pulmonary artery. The aortic valve connects the LV and the aorta.

## Cardiac Cycle

Normal cardiac function involves two stages: *systole* and *diastole*. During systole, contraction of the ventricle causes the pressure inside the ventricle to increase to approximately 70 mm Hg in newborns (compared with 120 mm Hg in adults). When sufficient pressure is generated, the aortic and pulmonary valves open and blood is ejected from the ventricles. As the blood flows from the ventricles, the pressure decreases, causing the aortic and pulmonary valves to close.

During diastole, the mitral and tricuspid valves open, and 70% of the blood in the atria enters the ventricles. A small portion of the aortic blood flows back into the coronary arteries to perfuse the heart. At the end of diastole, a small atrial contraction occurs (4–6 mm Hg on the right side; 7–8 mm Hg on the left side), and then the mitral and tricuspid valves close. Metabolism of the heart is decreased during diastole. The average newborn's cardiac cycle is approximately 0.4 second, with 0.2 second for diastole and 0.2 second for systole (based on a heart rate [HR] of approximately 150 beats per minute [beats/min]) (Bers & Borlaug, 2022).

## Cardiac Output

Cardiac output (CO) is the amount of blood pumped by the LV in 1 minute. Cardiac output is equal to the stroke volume (SV) times the HR (CO = SV × HR). The SV is the volume of blood pumped per beat from each ventricle; the higher the SV, the greater the volume of blood in the systemic circulation. CO is influenced by changes in HR and pulmonary and systemic vascular resistance.

CO is influenced by the amount of blood returned to the heart, as explained by the Frank-Starling law, which states that within physiologic limits, the heart pumps all the blood that enters it without allowing excessive accumulation of blood in the veins. The passive movement of blood through the veins, the thoracic pump, and the venous muscle pump determines venous return; normally, when increased volume enters the heart, contractility is increased as a response to stimulation of stretch receptors in the heart muscle. The newborn's heart has fewer muscle fibers and is unable to stretch sufficiently to accommodate increased volume; therefore, increased HR is the only effective mechanism by which the newborn can respond to increased volume (Bers & Borlaug, 2022; Hasenfuss & Mann, 2022).

Cardiac failure occurs when the volume exceeds the ability of the heart to pump. Local factors that affect venous return to the heart include hypoxia, acidosis, hypercarbia, hyperthermia, increased metabolic demand, and increased metabolites (potassium, adenosine triphosphate, and lactic acid).

Vascular pressure and resistance also influence CO. Pressure and resistance are inversely related: If pressure in the arterial bed is increased, resistance decreases, and flow improves. The size (radius) of vessels influences resistance: the greater the radius of a vessel, the lower the resistance. Vessels obstructed by thrombosis or constriction have greater resistance to vascular flow (Bers & Borlaug, 2022; Hasenfuss & Mann, 2022).

## Autonomic Cardiac Control

Cardiovascular function is modulated by the autonomic nervous system (ANS). Baroreceptors and chemoreceptors in the aorta and carotid sinus provide feedback to the ANS. Feedback from these receptors stimulates the parasympathetic (PNS) or sympathetic nervous system (SNS). Most PNS and SNS effects are on the atria, but decreased ventricular contractility may also occur.

The PNS is less powerful than the SNS. Stimulation of the PNS results in vagal nerve stimulation and decreased HR. Right vagal stimulation affects the sinoatrial (SA) node, and left vagal stimulation affects the AV node. Acetylcholine is the active neurotransmitter for the preganglionic neurons of the PNS and SNS (Bers & Borlaug, 2022).

Stimulation of the SNS through the ganglionic chain releases norepinephrine and epinephrine, which act on the SA node, the AV node, the atria, and the ventricles. Maximal stimulation of the SNS can increase HR to 250 to 300 beats/min. Contractility can be improved by approximately 100%. Alpha-adrenergic and beta-adrenergic receptors are stimulated. Alpha receptors cause increased contractility (inotropic) and increased rate (chronotropic); beta-2 receptors cause vasodilation, bronchodilation, and smooth muscle relaxation (Bakris & Sorrentino, 2022).

Term newborns have fewer receptors but are capable of normal cardiovascular system function. The preterm newborn is not able to smoothly maintain autonomic function, and energy expenditure is increased. Hence, cardiovascular signs such as color changes and bradycardia may occur because of excessive demand for ANS function.

# CARDIAC ASSESSMENT

## Prenatal Screening and Diagnosis

In many regions of the United States, less than 50% of CHD is detected prenatally (Quartermain et al., 2015). Early recognition of signs and symptoms of CHD resulting in earlier CHD diagnosis and treatment can potentially result in improved outcomes (Eckersley et al., 2016). CCHD pulse oximetry screening typically performed around 24 hours of age may contribute to earlier CHD diagnosis before ductal closure with the resultant hemodynamic collapse. Careful newborn assessment is a crucial component of newborn care. Cardiac assessment includes history taking, physical assessment, and interpretation of diagnostic tests. Review of the maternal, fetal, and neonatal history and type of prenatal screening performed is helpful in the cardiac evaluation of the newborn. Box 7.1 lists maternal and fetal conditions that are considered higher risk for fetal cardiac conditions resulting in referrals for fetal echocardiograms (Donofrio et al., 2014). Table 7.1 lists heart defects commonly associated with maternal drug use and conditions.

Typically, these pregnant mothers are considered higher risk and are screened with detailed ultrasounds and fetal

## BOX 7.1

### COMMON MATERNAL AND FETAL INDICATIONS FOR REFERRAL FOR FETAL ECHOCARDIOGRAM

**Indications With the Highest Risk Profile (Estimated > 2% Absolute Risk for Fetal Cardiac Disease)**

Maternal pregestational diabetes mellitus

Diabetes mellitus diagnosed in the first trimester

Maternal phenylketonuria (uncontrolled)

Maternal autoantibodies (SSA/SSB+)

Maternal medications (ACE inhibitors, retinoic acid, NSAIDs in third trimester)

Maternal first-trimester rubella infection

Maternal infection with suspicion of fetal myocarditis

Assisted reproductive technology

CHD in first-degree relative of fetus (maternal, paternal, or sibling)

First- or second-degree relative with disorder with Mendelian inheritance with CHD association

Fetal cardiac or extracardiac abnormality suspected on obstetric ultrasound

Fetal karyotype abnormality

Fetal tachycardia or bradycardia, or frequent or persistent irregular heart rhythm

Fetal increased NT > 95% (> 3 mm)

Monochorionic twinning

Fetal hydrops or effusions

**Indications With a Lower Risk Profile (Estimated > 1% but < 2% Absolute Risk for Fetal Cardiac Disease)**

Maternal medications (anticonvulsants, lithium, vitamin A, SSRIs [only paroxetine], NSAIDs in first or second trimester)

CHD in second-degree relative of fetus

Fetal abnormality of umbilical cord or placenta

Fetal intraabdominal venous anomaly

ACE, angiotensin-converting enzyme; CHD, congenital heart defect; NSAIDs, nonsteroidal antiinflammatory drugs; NT, nuchal translucency; SSA, Sjogren's Syndrome A; SSB, Sjogren's Syndrome B; SSRI, selective serotonin reuptake inhibitor.

*Source:* From Donofrio, M., Moon-Grady, L., Hornberger, L., Copel, J., Sklansky, M. S., Abuhamad, A., Cuneo, B. F., Huhta, J. C., Jonas, R. A., Krishnan, A., Lacey, S., Lee, W., Michelfelder, E. C., Rempel, G. R., Silverman, N. H., Spray, T. L., Strasburger, J. F., Tworetzky, W., & Rychik, J., on behalf of the American Heart Association Adults with Congenital Heart Disease Joint Committee of the Council on Cardiovascular Disease in the Young and Council on Clinical Cardiology, Council on Cardiovascular Surgery and Anesthesia, and Council on Cardiovascular and Stroke Nursing. (2014). Diagnosis and treatment of fetal cardiac disease: A scientific statement from American Heart Association. *Circulation, 129*, 2183–2242. https://doi.org/10.1161/01.cir.0000437597.44550.5d.

## TABLE 7.1

### MATERNAL CONDITIONS AND ASSOCIATED FETAL CARDIAC DISEASE

| Condition | Defect |
|---|---|
| ***Maternal Disease*** | |
| Diabetes mellitus | Cardiomyopathy, TGA, VSD, PDA |
| Systemic lupus erythematosus (SLE) | Congenital heart block |
| Collagen disease | Congenital heart block |
| Congenital heart defect (CHD) | Increased risk for congenital heart defect (3%–4%) |
| ***Viral Disease*** | |
| Rubella | |
| First trimester | PDA, pulmonary artery branch stenosis |
| Later | Various cardiac and other defects |
| Cytomegalovirus | Various cardiac and other defects |
| Herpes virus | Various cardiac and other defects |
| Coxsackie virus B | Cardiomyopathy |
| ***Drugs*** | |
| Amphetamines | VSD, PDA, ASD, TGA |
| Phenytoin | PS, AS, COA, PDA |
| Trimethadione | TGA, TOF, HLHS |
| Progesterone/estrogen | VSD, TOF, TGA |
| Alcohol | VSD, PDA, ASD, TOF |

AS, aortic stenosis; ASD, atrial septal defect; COA, coarctation of the aorta; HLHS, hypoplastic left heart syndrome; PDA, patent ductus arteriosus; PS, pulmonary stenosis; TGA, transposition of the great arteries; TOF, tetralogy of Fallot; VSD, ventricular septal defect.

*Source:* Data from Park, M. K. (2014). *Pediatric cardiology for practitioners*. Mosby.

echocardiograms resulting in prenatal detection of cardiac conditions (Donofrio et al., 2014). Sometimes, pregnant mothers who are considered higher risk may not have received adequate prenatal ultrasound screening and fetal echocardiogram screening; therefore, their newborns will require screening after birth because they are at increased risk for cardiac conditions. In addition, the fetal effects of uncontrolled diabetes during pregnancy, especially during the third trimester, may go undetected and will result in a newborn who is large for gestational age (LGA), sometimes with hypertrophic cardiomyopathy. There is a 30% risk of hypertrophic cardiomyopathy in fetuses exposed to elevated blood sugars during pregnancy (Hornberger, 2006; Rychik, 2012).

The medical team caring for women with pregnancies complicated by fetal CHD should consider referral to tertiary hospitals for specialized care. Hospital-based navigation programs with patient navigators can provide emotional support and support patients during their journey from prenatal to postnatal care in a complex healthcare system.

## Methods of Assessment

Assessment of evidence of a cardiac problem begins with a careful history, followed by a thorough physical examination. Family history of hereditary diseases, CHD, or rheumatic fever increases the risk for certain CHD lesions (Table 7.2).

The overall incidence of CHDs is approximately 1%, or eight per 1,000 live births, excluding persistent PDA in preterm newborns. Maternal history of CHD, however, increases the risk of recurrence from 3% to 7% (Donofrio et al., 2014).

A neonatal history of cyanosis, tachypnea without pulmonary disease, sweating, poor feeding, and pulmonary edema or failure to gain weight, is suggestive of CHD. Careful evaluation of the maternal, fetal, and neonatal history, in conjunction with a thorough physical assessment, helps identify infants for whom further diagnostic testing with echocardiogram is indicated.

Physical examination of the newborn with a suspected cardiac condition includes inspection, palpation, and auscultation (Park & Salamat, 2022).

Nursing documentation is a critical component of patient care. A standardized document should be utilized to ensure consistency and optimize care of the neonate with CHD.

**TABLE 7.2**

**CONGENITAL HEART DEFECTS ASSOCIATED WITH SPECIFIC GENETIC OR CHROMOSOMAL ABNORMALITIES**

| Disease or Syndrome | Defect |
|---|---|
| Trisomy 13, 18 | PDA, VSD |
| Trisomy 21 | AVC, VSD, PDA |
| Marfan syndrome | MVP, aortic dilation, and/or aneurysm |
| Noonan syndrome | PS, HCM |
| Turner syndrome | BAV, COA |
| Williams syndrome | Supravalvar AS and PS |
| 22q11 deletion syndrome<br>DiGeorge sequence<br>Velocardiofacial syndrome | Conotruncal defects (Truncus, TOF, IAA-B) conoventricular VSDs and aortic arch anomalies (DAA, RAA, and other arch anomalies |

AS, aortic stenosis; AVC, atrioventricular canal defect; BAV, bicuspid aortic valve; COA, coarctation of the aorta; DAA, double aortic arch; HCM, hypertrophic cardiomyopathy, IAA, interrupted aortic arch; MVP, mitral valve prolapse; PDA, patent ductus arteriosus; PS, pulmonic stenosis; RAA, right aortic arch; TOF, tetralogy of Fallot; VSD, ventricular septal defect.

*Sources:* Data from Park, M. K. (2014). *Pediatric cardiology for practitioners.* Mosby; Goldmuntz, E., & Crenshaw, M. L. (2016). Genetic aspects of congenital heart defects. In H. D. Allen, R. E. Shaddy, D. J. Penny, T. F. Feltes, & F. Cetta (Eds.), *Moss and Adams heart disease in infants, children and adolescents* (9th ed., Vol. 1, pp. 87–116). Lippincott Williams & Wilkins; Goldmuntz, E. (2020). 22q11.2 deletion syndrome and congenital heart disease. *American Journal of Medical Genetics Part C: Seminars in Medical Genetics, 184*(1), 64–72. https://doi.org/10.1002/ajmg.c.31774; Goldmuntz, E., Bassett, A. S., Boot, E., Marino, B., Moldenhauer, J. S., Óskarsdóttir, S., Putotto, C., Rychik, J., Schindewolf, E., McDonald-McGinn, D. M., & Blagowidow, N. (2024). Prenatal cardiac findings and 22q11.2 deletion syndrome: Fetal detection and evaluation. *Prenatal Diagnosis, 44*(6–7), 804–814. https://doi.org/10.1002/pd.6566.

## Inspection

Valuable information about the cardiovascular system of the newborn can be obtained by observation of the newborn's general appearance before examination. The following states of the newborn should be observed: sleeping or awake, alert or lethargic, anxious or relaxed. Respiratory effort, including signs of respiratory distress such as nasal flaring, expiratory grunting, stridor, retractions, or paradoxical respirations, should be noted. Tachypnea and tachycardia are early signs of LV dysfunction (Park & Salamat, 2022).

The newborn's color should be observed. Cyanosis is the bluish color of the skin, mucous membranes, and nail beds that occurs when there is at least 5 g/100 ml of deoxygenated hemoglobin in circulation. If cyanosis is present, note whether it is peripheral or central and whether it improves, stays the same, or becomes worse with crying. Cyanosis can result from pulmonary, hematologic, central nervous system, or metabolic diseases, as well as from cardiac defects. Pulmonary and cardiac defects are the two most common causes of central cyanosis in the newborn.

Pallor may indicate vasoconstriction resulting from congestive heart failure (CHF) or circulatory shock caused by severe anemia. Prolonged physiologic jaundice may occur in infants with CHF or congenital hypothyroidism, which is associated with PDA and pulmonary stenosis (PS). A ruddy or plethoric appearance is often seen in polycythemia. These infants may appear cyanotic without significant arterial desaturation.

The presence of significant diaphoresis, particularly with feeding, is very suggestive of a CHD in the newborn. The cause of sweating is sympathetic overactivity as a compensatory mechanism for decreased CO (Park & Salamat, 2022).

## Palpation

Palpation includes the palpation of the precordium and peripheral pulses. Palpation of the precordium detects a thrill, hyperdynamic activity, and the point of maximal impulse (PMI). Irregularities or inequalities of rate or volume can be detected by counting the peripheral pulse rate. Evaluation of the carotid, brachial, femoral, and pedal pulses detects differences between right and left sides and upper and lower extremities. If pulses are unequal, four extremity blood pressures should be measured. Strong arm pulses with weak leg pulses suggest coarctation of the aorta (COA) (Park & Salamat, 2022).

Heart defects that lead to "aortic runoff," or diastolic reversal of flow in the descending aorta, such as PDA, aortic insufficiency (AI), large arteriovenous malformations, or truncus arteriosus, may cause bounding pulses. Preterm newborns frequently have a bounding pulse secondary to relatively decreased subcutaneous tissue and/or PDA. Cardiac failure or circulatory shock causes weak or thready pulses (Park & Salamat, 2022).

The hyperdynamic precordium indicates a heart defect with volume overload, such as CHDs with large left-to-right shunts (e.g., PDA, ventricular septal defects [VSDs]) or valvular regurgitation (e.g., aortic regurgitation or mitral regurgitation). The location of the PMI depends on whether the RV or LV is dominant. With RV dominance, the PMI is at the lower left sternal border (LLSB). LV dominance places the PMI at the apex. A diffuse, slow-rising PMI is called a *heave* and is associated with volume overload. A sharp, fast-rising PMI is called a *tap* and is associated with pressure overload. The normal newborn has RV dominance. The LV apical impulse of the newborn is normally felt in the fourth intercostal space to the left of the midclavicular line. Lateral or downward displacement of the apical impulse may indicate cardiac enlargement (Park & Salamat, 2022).

The presence and location of a thrill provides important diagnostic information. The palms of the hands, rather than the fingertips, should be used to feel for a thrill, except in the suprasternal notch and carotid arteries. The examiner should palpate for the presence of thrills in the upper left, upper right, and LLSB, in the suprasternal notch, and over the carotid arteries. A thrill in the upper left sternal border is derived from the pulmonary valve or pulmonary artery. Thrills in the LLSB suggest PS, or occasionally PDA. A thrill felt in the upper right sternal border signifies aortic origin, usually aortic stenosis (AS), or, less frequently, PS, PDA, or COA. A thrill over the carotid arteries along with a thrill in the suprasternal notch suggest COA or AS, or other defects of the aorta or aortic valve (Park & Salamat, 2022).

Palpation of the abdomen is performed to determine the size, consistency, and location of the liver and spleen. Increased liver size is a frequent finding with CHF (Park & Salamat, 2022).

## Auscultation

Careful auscultation by a skilled evaluator is an essential component of any cardiovascular assessment. Auscultation includes HR and regularity, heart sounds, systolic and diastolic sounds, and heart murmurs. The skillful evaluation of cardiac sounds requires systematic auscultation and much practice.

## Identification of Heart Sounds

Individual heart sounds should be identified and evaluated before evaluation of cardiac murmurs is attempted. There are four individual heart sounds: $S_1$, $S_2$, $S_3$, and $S_4$. However, $S_3$ and $S_4$ are rarely heard in the newborn. $S_1$ is the sound resulting from the closure of the mitral and tricuspid valves following atrial systole and is best heard at the apex or LLSB. $S_1$ is the beginning of ventricular systole. Splitting of $S_1$ is infrequently heard in newborns. Wide splitting of $S_1$ is heard in the right bundle branch block or Ebstein anomaly (Park & Salamat, 2022).

$S_2$ is the sound created by closure of the aortic and pulmonary valves, which marks the end of systole and the beginning of ventricular diastole. $S_2$ is best heard in the upper left sternal border or pulmonic area. Evaluation of the splitting of $S_2$ is important diagnostically. The timing of the closure of the aortic and pulmonary valves is determined by the volume of blood ejected from the aorta and pulmonary artery and the resistance against which the ventricles must pump. In the immediate newborn period, there may be no appreciable splitting of $S_2$. Because the RV and LV pump similar quantities of blood and the pulmonary pressure is close to the aortic pressure, these valves close almost simultaneously. Thus, $S_2$ is heard as a single sound. As the pulmonary vascular resistance decreases, the pulmonary resistance becomes lower than the aortic pressure, causing a splitting of $S_2$ as the valve leaflets on the left side of the heart (aortic valve) close before those on the right (pulmonary valve). By 72 hours of life, $S_2$ should be split. The absence of a split $S_2$ or the presence of a widely split $S_2$ usually indicates an abnormality. A fixed, widely split $S_2$ occurs in conditions that prolong RV ejection time or shorten LV ejection time. It occurs in (1) atrial septal defect (ASD) and partial anomalous pulmonary venous return (PAPVR; the amount of blood ejected by RV is increased, resulting in volume overload); (2) PS (stenosis delays right ventricular (RV) ejection time, resulting in pressure overload); (3) right bundle branch block (delayed electrical activation of RV); and (4) mitral regurgitation (decreased forward output, decreased LV ejection time) (Park, 2014).

A narrowly split $S_2$ occurs when there is early closure of the pulmonary valve (pulmonary hypertension) or a delay in aortic closure. A single $S_2$ is significant because it could represent the presence of only one semilunar valve (e.g., aortic atresia [AA], pulmonary atresia [PA], or truncus arteriosus). A single $S_2$ may also occur with critical PS, in which the pulmonary closure is not audible. Severe AS may also cause a single $S_2$ because aortic closure is delayed. Severe pulmonary hypertension may cause early closure of the pulmonary valve, thus causing a single $S_2$.

The relative intensity of the aortic and pulmonary components of $S_2$ must be assessed. In the pulmonary area (upper left sternal border), the aortic component is usually louder than the pulmonary component. Increased intensity of the pulmonary component, compared with the aortic component, occurs with pulmonary hypertension. Conditions that cause decreased diastolic pressure of the pulmonary artery (e.g., critical PS, tetralogy of Fallot [TOF], tricuspid atresia) may cause decreased intensity of the pulmonary component. Evaluation of intensity and splitting of $S_2$ is difficult, particularly in newborns with faster hearts, and requires frequent practice listening to heart sounds (Park & Salamat, 2022).

As discussed, $S_3$ and $S_4$ are rarely heard in the neonatal period; their presence denotes pathologic origin. Likewise, a gallop rhythm, the result of the presence of $S_3$ or $S_4$ gallop, is abnormal and associated with CHF (Park & Salamat, 2022).

After evaluation of individual heart sounds, the systolic and diastolic sounds are evaluated. The ejection sound, or click, occurs after $S_1$ and may sound like splitting of $S_1$. The ejection click is best heard at the upper left or right sternal border. The pulmonary click can best be heard at the second or third left intercostal space and is louder with expiration. The aortic click, best heard at the second right intercostal space, does not change in intensity with change in respiration. Ejection clicks are associated with PS or AS or with the dilated great arteries seen in systemic or pulmonary hypertension (Park & Salamat, 2022).

## CARDIAC MURMURS

Cardiac murmurs should be evaluated for intensity (grades 1–6), timing (systolic or diastolic), location, transmission, and quality (musical, vibratory, or blowing).

The grade scale for murmurs is as follows:

Grade 1: barely audible
Grade 2: soft but easily audible
Grade 3: moderately loud, no thrill
Grade 4: loud, thrill present
Grade 5: loud, audible with stethoscope barely on chest
Grade 6: loud, audible with stethoscope near chest

The murmur grade is recorded as 1/6, 2/6, and so on. Again, practice in auscultation improves the practitioner's evaluation skills. The intensity of the murmur is affected by CO; anything that increases CO (e.g., anemia, fever, exercise) increases the intensity of the murmur (Park & Salamat, 2022).

The next step in evaluating a murmur is its classification in relation to $S_1$ and $S_2$. There are three types of murmurs: systolic, diastolic, and continuous.

### Systolic Murmurs

Most heart murmurs are systolic, occurring between $S_1$ and $S_2$. Systolic murmurs are either ejection or holosystolic murmurs. Systolic ejection murmurs (SEMs) occur after $S_1$ and end before $S_2$ and are a result of blood flow through narrowed or deformed semilunar valves or increased flow through normal semilunar valves. SEMs are best heard at the second left or right intercostal space. Regurgitant and holosystolic murmurs begin with $S_1$, with no interval between $S_1$ and the beginning of the murmur and continue throughout systole. These murmurs are caused by flow of blood from a chamber at a higher pressure than the receiving chamber throughout systole. Regurgitant and holosystolic murmurs are typically associated with mitral and tricuspid regurgitation (TR) and VSDs (Park & Salamat, 2022).

### Location

The location of the maximal intensity of the murmur is helpful in evaluation of the cardiac murmur. Figure 7.3 shows the locations at which various systolic murmurs can be heard.

Related to the location is the radiation of the murmur. Knowledge of radiation of the murmur can help determine the origin. A SEM that radiates well to the neck is usually aortic in origin, whereas one that radiates to the back is usually pulmonic

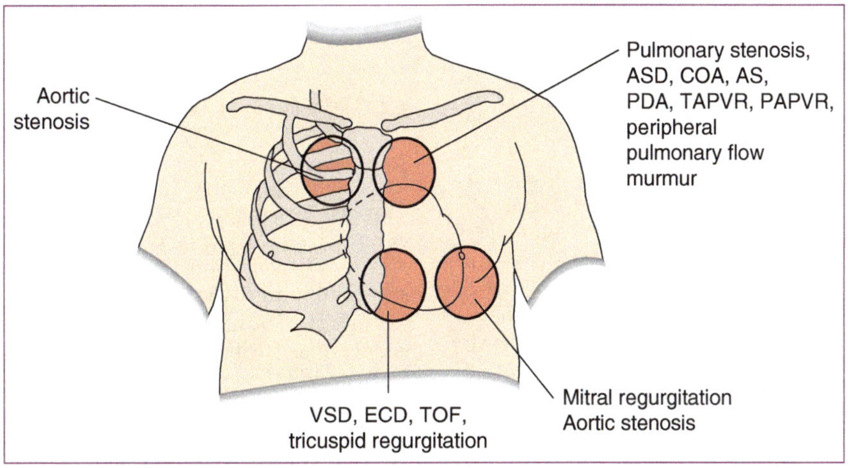


**FIGURE 7.3 Location of systolic murmurs.**

AS, aortic stenosis; ASD, atrial septal defect; COA, coarctation of the aorta; ECD, endocardial cushion defect; PAPVR, partial anomalous pulmonary venous return; PDA, patent ductus arteriosus; TAPVR, total anomalous pulmonary venous return; TOF, tetralogy of Fallot; VSD, ventricular septal defect.

in origin. An apical systolic murmur that radiates to the left axilla and lower back is characteristic of mitral regurgitation, but one that radiates to the upper right sternal border and neck is likely to be aortic in nature (Park & Salamat, 2022).

## Quality

Murmurs are described as musical, vibratory, or blowing (Park & Salamat, 2022). VSDs or mitral regurgitation murmurs have a high-pitched, blowing quality. AS and PS murmurs have a rough, grating quality. Establishing the quality of the murmur is subjective, and expertise is gained only after extensive practice and experience.

## Diastolic Murmurs

Diastolic murmurs occur between $S_1$ and $S_2$. Diastolic murmurs are classified according to their timing in relation to heart sounds as early diastolic, mid-diastolic, or presystolic.

Early diastolic (protodiastolic) murmurs occur early in diastole, right after $S_2$, and are caused by incompetence of the aortic or pulmonary valve. Aortic regurgitation murmurs are high pitched and are best heard with the diaphragm of the stethoscope at the third left intercostal space. Aortic regurgitation murmurs radiate to the apex. Bounding pulses are present with significant aortic regurgitation. Aortic regurgitation murmurs occur with the bicuspid aortic valve. Pulmonary regurgitation murmurs are medium pitched unless pulmonary hypertension is present, in which case they are high pitched. Diastolic regurgitation murmurs are heard best at the second left intercostal space, radiating along the left sternal border (LSB). Pulmonary regurgitation murmurs are common with postoperative TOF and pulmonary valvotomy for PS, or other deformities of the pulmonary valve where there is no competent pulmonary valve and severe or free pulmonary insufficiency (Park & Salamat, 2022).

Mid-diastolic murmurs result from abnormal ventricular filling. These murmurs are low pitched and can best be heard with the bell of the stethoscope placed lightly on the chest wall. The murmur results from turbulent flow caused by stenosis of the tricuspid or mitral valve. Mitral mid-diastolic murmurs are best heard at the apex and are referred to as *apical rumbles*. Mitral mid-diastolic murmurs are associated with mitral stenosis or large VSDs with a large left-to-right shunt or PDA, producing relative mitral stenosis secondary to increased flow across the normal-sized mitral valve. Tricuspid mid-diastolic murmurs can best be heard along the LLSB and are associated with moderate to large ASDs, PAPVR or total anomalous pulmonary venous return (TAPVR), or abnormal stenosis of the tricuspid valve. Presystolic or late-diastolic murmurs result from flow through AV valves during ventricular diastole because of active atrial contraction ejecting blood into the ventricle. These are low-frequency murmurs found with true mitral or tricuspid valve stenosis (Park & Salamat, 2022).

## Continuous Murmurs

Continuous murmurs begin in systole and continue throughout $S_2$ into all or part of diastole. Continuous murmurs are caused by (1) aortopulmonary or AV connection (e.g., PDA, AV fistula), (2) disturbances of flow in veins (e.g., venous hum), and (3) less commonly by disturbances of flow in arteries (e.g., severe COA or pulmonary artery stenosis) (Park & Salamat, 2022).

PDA is the most auscultated continuous murmur in the newborn. The PDA murmur is described as a machinery murmur, louder during systole, peaking at $S_2$, and decreased in diastole. PDA murmurs are loudest in the left infraclavicular area or the upper LSB (Park & Salamat, 2022).

## Other Murmurs

Functional or innocent cardiac murmurs are common in newborns and in school-age children. Innocent murmurs occur in the absence of abnormal cardiac structures. Functional murmurs are asymptomatic. The presence of any unusual or abnormal finding warrants further evaluation with cardiac consultation. Findings such as cyanosis, enlarged heart size on examination or enlarged cardiac silhouette on chest radiograph, abnormal electrocardiogram (ECG), diastolic murmur, a loud murmur (grade 3/6 systolic murmur or associated with a thrill), weak or bounding pulses, or other abnormal heart sounds have pathologic origins and must be investigated (Park & Salamat, 2022).

Peripheral PS murmur or pulmonary flow murmur of infancy is commonly auscultated in newborns. The murmur is thought to be secondary to anatomic discrepancy in size between the MPA and the branch pulmonary arteries or the angle of takeoff of the branch pulmonary arteries. In utero, the lungs only receive 5% to 10% of the RV CO, so the branch pulmonary arteries are relatively small compared to the MPA because most of the flow shunts from the PA to the ductus to return to the placenta via the UA. The increased flow after birth creates turbulence in the small vessels, which is transmitted along the smaller branches of the pulmonary arteries. This murmur is best heard at the upper LSB with grades of 1/6 to 2/6 intensity radiating to the right and left chest, both axillae, and back. There are no other significant cardiac findings. Typically, it is no longer present after 3 to 6 months of age, and persistence beyond this period should lead to further evaluation for true pathologic peripheral pulmonary artery stenosis (Park, 2014).

# CONGENITAL HEART DEFECTS

## Etiology

Cardiac development typically is completed by 8 weeks of gestation. CHDs can be multifactorial or genetic.

Many chromosomal abnormalities are associated with structural heart defects. Approximately 50% of newborns with trisomy 21 (Down syndrome) have CHD, most commonly endocardial cushion defect (ECD)/AV canal (AVC) defects, VSD, and TOF with and without an AVC defect (Goldmuntz, 2020; Goldmuntz & Crenshaw, 2016; Goldmuntz et al., 2024).

Maternal or environmental factors include maternal illness and drug ingestion. Maternal rubella during the first 7 weeks of pregnancy carries a 50% risk of congenital rubella syndrome with major defects of multiple organ systems. Heart defects include PDA and branch pulmonary artery stenosis. Other viral diseases, such as cytomegalovirus, or protozoal diseases, such as toxoplasmosis, are also associated with CHDs. The diagnosis of CHD calls for a careful maternal history to identify viral-like illnesses that may have been unrecognized or unreported at the time of occurrence and careful examination to rule out the presence of other congenital defects (Park & Salamat, 2022; Seidman et al., 2012).

Maternal drug use may also cause cardiac malformations. Fifty percent of newborns with fetal alcohol syndrome have CHD. Only a few drugs are proven teratogens (e.g., thalidomide); however, *no* drugs are known to be completely safe.

Metabolic disease of the mother increases the risk for CHDs. Infants of diabetic mothers have a 3% to 5% risk of having CHD (double outlet RV, truncus, *d*-transposition of the great arteries [TGA], hypoplastic left heart syndrome [HLHS], VSD) and 30% risk of hypertrophic cardiomyopathy (Hornberger, 2006; Rychik, 2012).

Most CHDs are of multifactorial origin; these defects are probably the result of an interaction effect of the other causes. Research into genetic causes of cardiac defects may identify specific genetic causes for some heart defects that are currently thought to have multifactorial origin. Infants with extracardiac anomalies often have associated CHDs. Multiple congenital defects affect the development of structures that are forming at the time, resulting in interference with normal fetal development.

## Incidence

CHDs occur in the US in about 1% or 40,000 births annually (Centers for Disease Control & Prevention [CDC], n.d.-a). About 4.2% of all neonatal deaths are related to heart disease (CDC, n.d.- a).

Although only 50% of CHD is detected prenatally (Quartermain et al., 2015), with the introduction of pulse oximetry screening for CHD it is expected that most CHDs will be detected earlier or at least before discharge from the newborn nursery. Some of these defects will require surgery in the neonatal period while others may be medically managed. The following discussion of CHDs extends beyond the neonatal period. Table 7.3 provides an overview of the diagnosis of CHD.

The discussion of defects is based on the common pathophysiologic features. CHDs can be classified in numerous ways. The simplest classification is based on whether the defect produces cyanosis, a method described by Dr. Helen Taussig in 1947. Cyanosis is the bluish discoloration of the

**TABLE 7.3**

**DIAGNOSIS OF CONGENITAL HEART DEFECTS**

| Defect | Chest Radiograph | Electrocardiogram | Echocardiogram | Catheterization |
|---|---|---|---|---|
| PDA | Cardiomegaly, increased pulmonary vascularity | In large PDAs: LA enlargement and LV hypertrophy | PDA size, shunt direction, LA/LV dilation, LA/Ao ratio, diastolic reversal of flow in descending aorta | Increased $O_2$ saturation in pulmonary artery; increased RV and pulmonary artery pressure (with pulmonary hypertension) |
| VSD | Cardiomegaly, increased pulmonary vascularity | Moderate VSD: LVH and LA enlargement, large VSD: BVH +/−LA enlargement | VSD type/location, size, and number, shunt direction, LA/LV dilation | Increased $O_2$ saturation in RV, evaluation for elevated pulmonary pressures |
| ASD | Cardiomegaly, increased pulmonary vascularity | Right-axis deviation; RV hypertrophy or RBBB | ASD type and size, shunt direction, RA/RV dilation | Increased $O_2$ saturation in RA; normal right side pressure; 10% PAPVR |
| ECD/AVC | Cardiomegaly, increased pulmonary vascularity | Left-axis deviation; LA enlargement; RVH; incomplete RBBB | Primum ASD and inlet VSD size, regurgitation of AV valves, RV/LV outflow tract obstruction | Increased $O_2$ saturation in RA; increased RV and/or pulmonary artery pressure; with angiography, a "goose neck" deformity of ventricular outflow area |
| PS | Normal heart size; normal pulmonary vascularity; enlarged pulmonary artery | Right-axis deviation; RA enlargement; RVH | PS gradient (mild, moderate, or severe), level of obstruction: subvalvar, valvar, supravalvar | Evaluation of level of RVOT obstruction, gradient from RV across the pulmonary artery |

(*continued*)

## TABLE 7.3

### DIAGNOSIS OF CONGENITAL HEART DEFECTS (*continued*)

| Defect | Chest Radiograph | Electrocardiogram | Echocardiogram | Catheterization |
|---|---|---|---|---|
| TOF | Normal heart size; boot-shaped contour; decreased pulmonary markings; prominent aorta; right aortic arch in 13 cases | Right-axis deviation; RVH | VSD size and number, overriding aorta, PS gradient (mild, moderate, or severe), level of obstruction: valvar, subvalvar; size of right and left pulmonary arteries, arch sidedness, coronary artery patterns | Demonstrates anatomy of RV outflow region, VSD directionality, coronary pattern |
| PA/IVS | Normal heart size or cardiomegaly; decreased pulmonary vascularity | LVH, RA enlargement, occasionally RVH | PA, size of TV, TR, RV coronary fistula, branch pulmonary artery size, PDA | RV angiogram to evaluate for presence of coronary sinusoids, RF perforation of pulmonary valve in two-ventricle approach |
| TAPVR | Cardiomegaly; increased pulmonary vascularity | RVH, RA enlargement | TAPVR connections, RA/RV dilation, pulmonary hypertension, PFO right to left | Higher $O_2$ saturation in RA; angiography reveals abnormal pulmonary venous return |
| AS | Normal heart size; slight prominence of LV and aorta in older kids | Normal in mild cases, LVH with strain in severe obstruction | Aortic valve morphology, level of obstruction in LVOT, LVH, LV function | Performed to evaluate level of LVOT obstruction and gradient, LV end diastolic pressure |
| COA | Cardiomegaly, pulmonary edema | RVH or RBBB in infants, LVH in older kids | Transverse arch size, discrete or long segment coarctation, LV function, bicuspid aortic valve, mitral valve abnormality, LVOT obstruction | In infants, performed in patients with recurrent obstruction after surgery |
| HLHS | Cardiomegaly; increased pulmonary vascularity | RVH | HLHS subtype: AS or AA, MA or MS, ascending aorta size, ASD size, RV function, TR | Balloon atrial septostomy and stenting if ASD is inadequate |
| TGA | Cardiomegaly; increased pulmonary vascularity | Right-axis deviation; RVH | Aortic outflow arises from RV, ASD size, coronary pattern, RV or LV outflow tract obstruction, presence of a VSD | Balloon atrial septostomy if ASD is inadequate; increased RV pressure; catheter can enter aorta from RV; pulmonary artery can be entered only through PDA or ASD |
| Truncus | Cardiomegaly; increased pulmonary vascularity | BVH | Truncus type, truncal stenosis or insufficiency, arch sidedness, VSD size | Left-to-right shunt at level of ventricle; pressure equal in ventricles, truncus, and pulmonary arteries |

AA, aortic atresia; AS, aortic stenosis; ASD, atrial septal defect; AV, atrioventricular; AVC, atrioventricular canal; BVH, biventricular hypertrophy; COA, coarctation of the aorta; ECD, endocardial cushion defect; HLHS, hypoplastic left heart syndrome; LA, left atrium, LA/Ao, left atrium to aortic root; LV, left ventricle; LVH, left ventricular hypertrophy; LVOT, left ventricular outflow tract; MA, mitral atresia; MS, mitral stenosis; PA/IVS, pulmonary atresia with intact ventricular septum; PAPVR, partial anomalous pulmonary venous return; PDA, patent ductus arteriosus; PFO, patent foramen ovale; PS, pulmonary stenosis; RA, right atrium; RBBB, right bundle branch block; RF, radiofrequency; RV, right ventricle; RVH, right ventricular hypertrophy; RVOT, right ventricular outflow tract; TAPVR, total anomalous pulmonary venous return; TGA, transposition of the great arteries; TOF, tetralogy of Fallot; TR, tricuspid regurgitation; TV, tricuspid valve; VSD, ventricular septal defect.

*Source:* Data from Park, M. K. (2014). *Pediatric cardiology for practitioners.* Mosby.

skin that occurs when there is approximately 5 g/100 ml of desaturated hemoglobin in the circulating volume (Taussig, 1947). Thus, the appearance of cyanosis depends on the hemoglobin concentration. An infant with low hemoglobin may be hypoxic but may not appear cyanotic; thus, low hemoglobin cannot be the sole criterion for determining pathologic origin. Cyanosis in the extremities, or acrocyanosis, is frequently seen in newborns because of reduced blood flow through the small capillaries. Oxygen is extracted from the hemoglobin in the capillaries, giving the skin a blue appearance. This blue appearance is a normal phenomenon in the newborn. Differentiation of central cyanosis from peripheral or acrocyanosis is essential because acrocyanosis is a benign condition while central cyanosis is associated with respiratory, cardiac, or metabolic conditions.

The presence or absence of cyanosis depends on whether or not deoxygenated blood is oxygenated by going through the lungs. Congenital heart defect lesions that allow the blood to go through the lungs and then shunt from the left side of the heart and back to the right side of the heart are generally acyanotic and typically result in too much pulmonary blood flow. Defects that shunt deoxygenated blood directly to the left side of the heart, bypassing the lungs, are cyanotic heart defects and are typically a result of inadequate pulmonary blood flow. Some defects have mixed anatomic or functional features and do not fit into this schema, or there is overlap between the classifications. For this discussion, the following categories are used: (1) acyanotic defects with a left-to-right shunt due to communication between the systemic and pulmonary circulations typically resulting in too much pulmonary blood flow; (2) cyanotic defects that typically are a result of inadequate pulmonary blood flow; (3) left-sided obstructive defects with inadequate systemic blood flow; and (4) defects with abnormal aortopulmonary connections.

## Defects with Left-to-Right Shunts

Typically, these defects have left-to-right shunts with increased pulmonary blood flow and volume overload on the heart. These defects typically result in too much pulmonary blood flow and include PDA, VSD, ASD, and ECD or AVC.

## Patent Ductus Arteriosus

The DA is a vascular connection between the pulmonary artery and the aorta. The DA originates from the MPA and enters the aorta distal to the left subclavian artery; it allows deoxygenated blood from the RV to bypass the lungs and enter the descending aorta. The DA functionally closes around 15 hours of life. During the first 24 hours of life, there may be some shunting of blood, but typically it is insignificant unless the ductal opening is large and remains patent.

Closure of the DA occurs in response to increased arterial oxygen concentration after the initiation of respiratory function. Other factors that contribute to closure of the DA include a decrease in prostaglandin E and an increase in acetylcholine and bradykinin (Park, 2014). Closure of the DA occurs within 48 hours in 80% of newborns and close to 100% close within 96 hours. PDA in the preterm newborn presents a different clinical problem and is discussed separately from PDA in the term newborn (Park & Salamat, 2022; Valente et al., 2022).

## Patent Ductus Arteriosus in the Term Newborn

### Incidence

PDA accounts for approximately 5% to 10% of all CHDs, excluding those in preterm newborns. There is a higher ratio of PDA in females (about 3:1). PDA is more common in infants with Down syndrome or those whose mothers had rubella during pregnancy (Park & Salamat, 2022).

### Hemodynamics

In extrauterine life, the flow of blood through the DA is reversed. In utero DA flow is right to left while after birth the PDA flow is left to right, thereby reentering the pulmonary circuit and increasing pulmonary blood flow. The amount of blood flow through the PDA and the effect of the ductal flow depends on the difference between systemic and pulmonary vascular resistance and the diameter and length of the ductus.

Over time, high pulmonary blood flow causes increased pulmonary vascular resistance, pulmonary hypertension, and RV hypertrophy. Figure 7.4 depicts the hemodynamics of PDA.

### Manifestations

A small PDA may be asymptomatic. A large PDA with significant shunting may cause signs of CHF including tachypnea and poor feeding. Frequent lower respiratory tract infections, poor feeding, and poor weight gain are common in older infants with PDA.

### Diagnosis

The diagnosis of PDA is based on history and physical examination findings, chest radiograph, and echocardiogram. Characteristic findings on physical examination include bounding

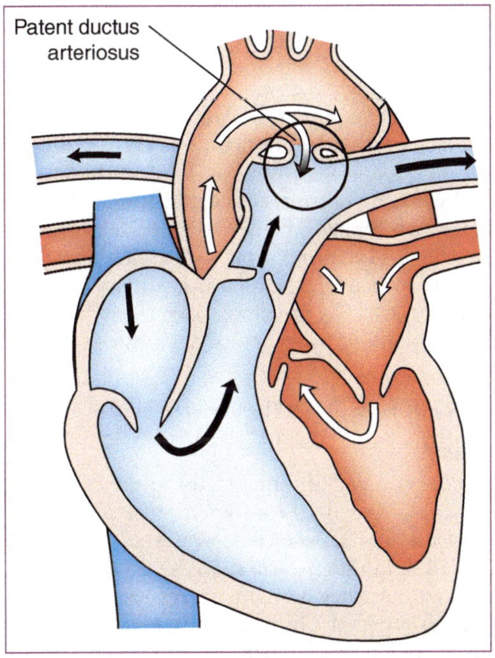


**FIGURE 7.4 Patent ductus arteriosus (PDA) is a communication between the pulmonary artery and the aorta.**

*Source:* Adapted and modified from Ross Laboratories, Columbus, OH, Clinical Education Aid, 1985.

peripheral pulses, widened pulse pressure (> 25 mm Hg), and a hyperdynamic precordium. A systolic thrill may be felt at the upper LSB. A grade 1/6 to 4/6 continuous "machinery" murmur is audible at the upper LSB or left infraclavicular area. The murmur is heard throughout the cardiac cycle because of the pressure gradient between the aorta and the pulmonary artery in both systole and diastole. In cases of a large PDA with a significant shunt, the $S_2$ may be accentuated because of pulmonary hypertension (Park & Salamat, 2022; Valente et al., 2022).

A small PDA may not be distinguishable on chest radiograph. With more significant shunting, there may be cardiomegaly and increased pulmonary vascularity. An ECG may demonstrate left atrial enlargement and left ventricular hypertrophy (LVH) and an abnormal QRS axis, more leftward, for age. The definitive diagnosis is made by echocardiogram. Echocardiogram provides diagnostic imaging of size and directionality of PDA, LA-to-aortic ratio (LA/Ao ratio), presence of LA and LV dilation, arch sidedness, diastolic flow reversal in the descending aorta, ventricular function, and pulmonary hypertension.

### Management

The treatment of the clinically significant PDA is medical or surgical closure. However, there is no absolute agreement on the criteria for determining clinical significance in the term newborn. If the term newborn's signs and symptoms are not affecting feeding and weight gain, a conservative approach to management may be used because the ductus may close over time on its own. Conservative treatment includes fluid management, diuretics, and close observation to ensure that the baby is feeding well and gaining weight. The incidence of spontaneous closure decreases as the infant becomes older. **Quality and Safety: If the newborn exhibits signs of increased pulmonary blood flow, such as respiratory distress or inability to feed, closure of the PDA is indicated.** Closure by medications is not effective in term infants; so, a clinically symptomatic PDA requires transcatheter device closure in the cardiac catheterization laboratory. Over the last decade there has been significant improvement in transcatheter devices available for PDA closure is surgical ligation through a posterolateral thoracotomy is limited to cases of large PDAs or if there are structural challenges due to anatomic variations. The mortality rate for surgical ligation is less than 1% (excluding preterm newborns). The prognosis is excellent, and complications are rare (Park & Salamat, 2022; Valente et al., 2022).

## Patent Ductus Arteriosus in the Preterm Newborn

PDA is a common complicating factor in the care of preterm newborns. As the newborn recovers from respiratory distress, pulmonary vascular resistance decreases as oxygenation improves. The DA in the preterm newborn is not as responsive (compared to term newborns) to increased oxygen content and will remain patent. Decreased pulmonary vascular resistance causes blood to shunt from left to right, resulting in increased pulmonary blood flow and pulmonary venous congestion, which decreases lung compliance. Consequences of large PDA shunts include CHF symptoms, inability to wean ventilatory support, and/or increased oxygen requirement.

Clinical findings indicative of PDA include bounding peripheral pulses, hyperdynamic precordium, widened pulse pressures (> 25 mm Hg), and a continuous murmur, best heard at the upper left and middle sternal borders. Chest radiograph findings include increased pulmonary vascularity and pulmonary edema along with cardiomegaly. (Park & Salamat, 2022; Valente et al., 2022).

Management of PDA depends on the severity of the symptoms. In asymptomatic or mildly symptomatic newborns, conservative management may be elected to allow for spontaneous closure, because one-third of extremely low birthweight (ELBW) neonates undergo spontaneous PDA closure. Conservative treatment includes strict fluid management, diuretics as needed, and close observation to assure that the baby is receiving optimal calories, tolerating feeds, and gaining weight (Park & Salamat, 2022).

In symptomatic and/or ventilator-dependent preterm newborns, closure of the DA may improve oxygenation. Two medications can be used to promote ductal closure. Indomethacin is a prostaglandin synthetase inhibitor. Prostaglandin $E_2$ is produced in the walls of the DA to prevent closure during fetal life. Indomethacin inhibits the production of $PGE_2$ and promotes ductal closure. Smaller babies may require a higher dose to obtain effective plasma levels. Indomethacin is highly nephrotoxic; so, the blood urea nitrogen (BUN) and creatinine (Cr) levels must be followed to monitor renal function. Contraindications to using indomethacin include renal failure, low platelet count, bleeding disorders, necrotizing enterocolitis (NEC), and hyperbilirubinemia (Park & Salamat, 2022; Valente et al., 2022). Ibuprofen is an effective alternative to indomethacin (Ohlsson et al., 2018). In babies who have contraindications to indomethacin/ibuprofen or have failed treatment with these medications, acetaminophen may be a treatment option to avoid transcatheter device closure or surgical intervention (Luecke et al., 2017) and may require two courses (Jasani, 2022; Kumar et al., 2020). In recent years, improvements in device availability for PDA closure in low birthweight (LBW) infants has provided options for PDA closure in the catheterization lab (Agrawal et al., 2019; Barry et al., 2023). Transcatheter device closure or surgical ligation is reserved for cases where indomethacin or ibuprofen and/or acetaminophen fails or is contraindicated. Mortality from surgical ligation is highest in the more preterm, sicker infants, especially if pulmonary hypertension has developed (Park & Salamat, 2022; Valente et al., 2022). Associated complications of short- and long-term outcomes of ligation, such as ND outcomes, must be considered in the selection of PDA management.

## Ventricular Septal Defect

A VSD is a defect or opening in the ventricular septum caused by inadequate septal formation during early fetal development. There are several types of VSDs that involve the membranous or muscular part of the ventricular septum. The location, size of the defect, and the degree of shunting are important in determining the hemodynamic effect and need for intervention. With a small defect, there is a large resistance to the left-to-right shunt at the defect, and the shunt does not depend on the pulmonary vascular resistance. With a large VSD, there is little resistance at the defect and the amount of left-to-right shunt depends on the level of pulmonary vascular resistance (Park & Salamat, 2022; Valente et al., 2022).

### Incidence

VSD is the most common CHD in children. It accounts for approximately 20% to 25% of all CHDs.

### Hemodynamics

The hemodynamic consequences of a VSD depend on its size: small, moderate, or large.

#### Small Ventricular Septal Defects

Small VSDs produce minimal shunting and may not be symptomatic. Chest radiograph and ECG are generally normal. A loud high-frequency holosystolic heart murmur may be best heard in the third and fourth left intercostal spaces at the sternal border (Park & Salamat, 2022; Valente et al. 2022). Figure 7.5 shows a VSD.

#### Moderate Ventricular Septal Defects

With moderate-sized VSDs, the blood is shunted from the LV to RV because of higher pressure in the LV and higher systemic vascular resistance. The shunt of blood occurs during systole, when the RV contracts, such that the blood enters the pulmonary artery rather than remaining in the RV.

#### Large Ventricular Septal Defects

With large VSDs, blood is shunted from the LV to RV. The volume of blood shunted is related to the size of the VSD and the pulmonary vascular resistance. The larger the VSD, the greater the volume of blood shunted, and the higher the pressure in the RV and pulmonary artery. If pulmonary artery pressure is significantly increased, thickening of the walls of the pulmonary arterioles may develop, and the increased resistance may decrease the left-to-right shunt. If left untreated, over long periods of time, pulmonary vascular disease can develop and lead to Eisenmenger syndrome with fixed right-to-left shunting resulting in significant cyanosis.

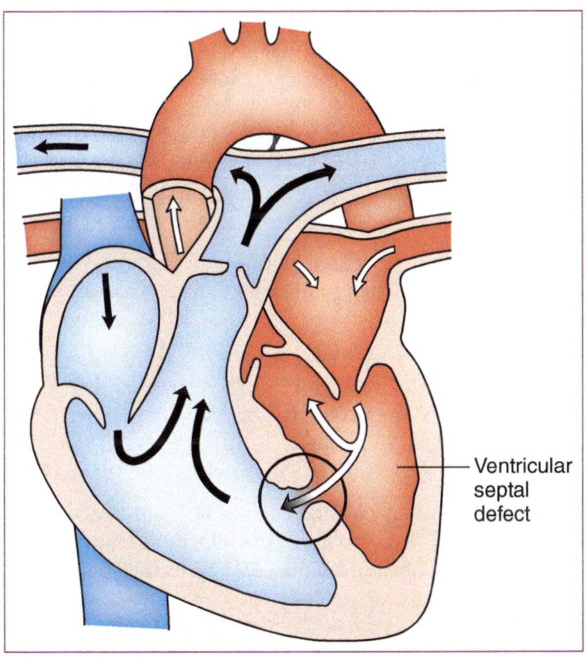


**FIGURE 7.5 Ventricular septal defect (VSD) is a communication between the right and left ventricles.**

*Source:* Adapted and modified from Ross Laboratories, Columbus, OH, Clinical Education Aid, 1985.

### Manifestations

Manifestations of VSD depend on the degree of shunting. Small VSDs may produce no hemodynamic compromise and no clinical symptoms but will typically be detected by a cardiac murmur on examination. Larger defects are associated with inadequate feeding, poor growth, symptoms of CHF, and can also be associated with recurrent pulmonary infections.

### Diagnosis

VSDs typically will have a 2/6 to 4/6 holosystolic murmur best heard at the LSB. There may also be an apical diastolic rumble, and the pulmonary heart sound may be loud.

Chest x-ray findings of moderate-to-large VSD include cardiomegaly because of LA and LV dilation and increased pulmonary vascularity and edema. ECG may reveal LV hypertrophy. RV hypertrophy may also be present in severe cases. An echocardiogram will provide information about the location and size of the VSD, directionality of the flow, and presence of LA and LV dilation along with presence of additional VSDs.

### Management

Treatment of the VSD depends upon the size of the defect and the resultant cardiovascular symptoms. Spontaneous closure of the VSD can occur; therefore, infants with hemodynamically insignificant defects may be followed clinically to allow time for spontaneous closure to occur. Small VSDs generally close spontaneously over the first few years of life.

**Quality and Safety: Initial management of the hemodynamically significant VSD includes monitoring for signs of CHF and prompt initiation of therapy.** CHF in the older infant is treated with diuretics, angiotensin-converting enzyme (ACE) inhibitors, and/or digitalis.

Surgical management involves primary suture or patch closure of the VSD. Cardiopulmonary bypass is required for surgical correction. The timing of the surgery depends on the location and size of the VSD. Large VSDs typically result in a significant left-to-right shunt with left atrial and ventricular dilation and CHF symptoms of poor feeding and inadequate weight gain. **Emergency Alert: If CHF symptoms cannot be medically managed, then this is an indication for surgical repair** (Park & Salamat, 2022).

The aggregate surgical mortality rate for VSD correction is less than 0.6%. The mortality rate is higher among small infants less than 2 months of age and those with other defects or multiple VSDs (Jacobs et al., 2018; Park & Salamat, 2022).

## Atrial Septal Defect

An ASD is a defect or opening in the atrial septum that develops because of inadequate septal formation early in fetal cardiac development.

There are three types of ASDs (Park & Salamat, 2022; Valente et al., 2022):

1. ostium secundum ASD
2. ostium primum ASD, associated with AVC
3. sinus venosus ASD, typically associated with partial anomalous pulmonary venous connection

### Incidence

Atrial septal defects account for 5% to 10% of all CHDs.

### Hemodynamics

An ASD usually does not produce symptoms until pulmonary vascular resistance begins to decrease and RV end-diastolic and RA pressures decline. All types of ASDs produce some blood flow alterations. With an ASD, blood shunts from left to right across the defect because the RV offers less resistance to filling, due to it being more compliant than the LV. Any factors that decrease RV distensibility or obstruct flow into the RV (e.g., PS or tricuspid stenosis) can reduce or reverse the shunt direction. The left-to-right shunt increases RV volume, but pulmonary vascular resistance decreases, so pulmonary artery pressure is almost normal. Over long periods of time, typically years, the increased pulmonary blood flow due to a large ASD gradually leads to increased pulmonary artery pressures and CHF in adults (Park & Salamat, 2022). Figure 7.6 illustrates an ASD.

### Manifestations

Newborns with ASDs are usually asymptomatic. In infants and children, a grade 2/6 to 3/6 SEM can best be heard at the upper LSB with a fixed, widely split $S_2$. With a large secundum ASD, there may be a mid-diastolic rumble caused by the relative tricuspid stenosis audible at the LLSB (Park & Salamat, 2022; Valente et al., 2022). On chest radiograph, the heart is enlarged with a prominent MPA segment and increased pulmonary vascularity. ECG enhances detection of ASD, showing RA deviation and RV hypertrophy. In addition, there may be incomplete right bundle branch block (Park & Salamat, 2022).

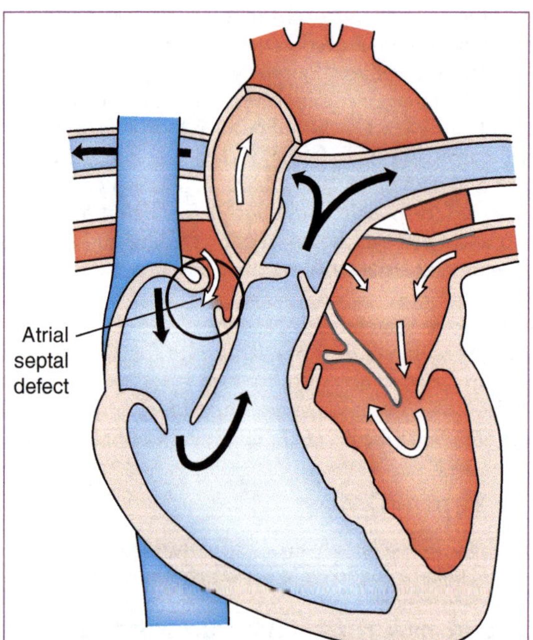


**FIGURE 7.6 Atrial septal defect (ASD) is a communication between the right and left atria.**

*Source:* Adapted and modified from Ross Laboratories, Columbus, OH, Clinical Education Aid, 1985.

Diagnosis can be made by echocardiogram, which demonstrates the ASD type, size, and associated RA and RV dilation because of a hemodynamically significant left-to-right shunt in moderate-to-large secundum ASDs.

### Management

Untreated ASDs can lead to CHF, pulmonary hypertension, and atrial dysrhythmias in adults. Spontaneous closure of ASDs occurs in the first 5 years of age in up to 40% of children (Park & Salamat, 2022). Atrial septal defects typically are asymptomatic. Large ASDs may result in right-sided dilation, and rarely CHF. Secundum ASDs that are hemodynamically significant with right-sided dilation may be closed using transcatheter device closure in the cardiac catheterization laboratory. This approach is less invasive because it involves access via femoral vein/arteries, does not require cardiopulmonary bypass, and the patient typically can be discharged the next day.

Surgical correction is reserved for infants for whom the transcatheter approach is unsuccessful due to the size of the ASD or inadequate septum attachments for the device, for primum ASDs, and sinus venosus ASDs. Surgical correction is accomplished by a simple patch or with direct closure during open-heart surgery using cardiopulmonary bypass. Timing of surgery varies depending on the ASD type, size, and presence of a significant left-to-right shunt with RA and RV dilation. The surgical mortality rate is less than 0.5% with a higher risk for mortality in small infants with CHF or increased pulmonary vascular resistance (Park, 2014; Webb et al., 2012).

## Atrioventricular Canal Defects/ Endocardial Cushion Defects

Endocardial cushions result from inadequate fusion of the ECDs during fetal development, resulting in a common AV valve with an ASD (ostium primum) and inlet VSD. There are three types of AVC defects: a complete AV canal with a primum ASD and inlet VSD, a transitional AVC with a primum ASD and a restrictive inlet VSD, and an incomplete AV canal with only a primum ASD. The type of AVC defect is important in the presentation of clinical symptoms and timing of surgery (Park, 2014).

### Incidence

AVC defects account for 2% of all CHDs. AVC defects are common in infants with Down syndrome (Park & Salamat, 2022).

### Hemodynamics

The hemodynamic consequences of AVC defects depend on the type of defect. There may be interatrial and interventricular shunts, LV to RA shunts, or AV valve regurgitation. Figure 7.7 shows an ECD.

### Manifestations

The manifestations of AVC defects result from the increased pulmonary blood flow from left-to-right flow from the VSD and regurgitation of the common AV valves if present. **Emergency Alert: The newborn may have respiratory distress, signs of CHF, tachycardia, and a cardiac murmur. The mitral regurgitation may be heard as a grade 3/6 holosystolic regurgitant murmur audible at the LLSB and may be audible at the apex.** There is also a mid-diastolic rumble at the LLSB or apex caused by the relative stenosis of tricuspid and mitral valves (Park & Salamat, 2022).

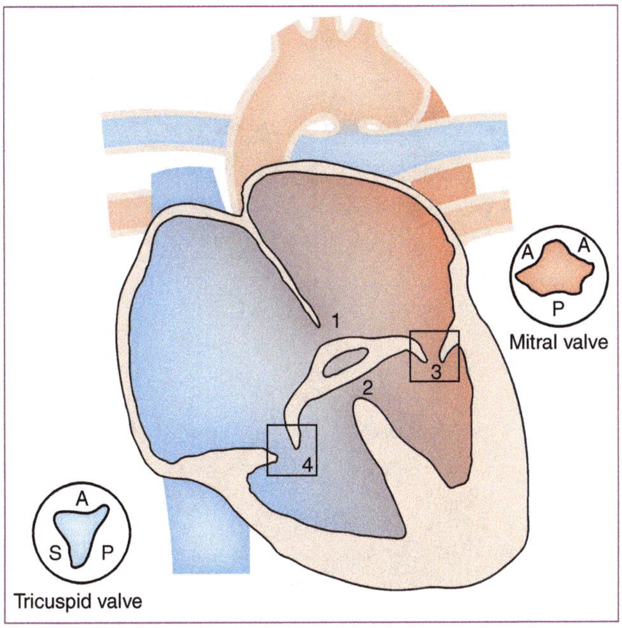


**FIGURE 7.7 Endocardial cushion defect (ECD).** (1) Ostium primum atrial septal defect; (2) a ventricular septal defect in the inlet portion of ventricular septum; (3) cleft in anterior mitral valve leaflet; (4) cleft in septal leaflet of the tricuspid valve, resulting in common anterior and posterior cusps of the atrioventricular valve.

A, anterior; P, posterior; S, septal.

Chest radiograph reveals generalized cardiomegaly with increased pulmonary vascularity and a prominent MPA segment. ECG shows left axis deviation with a prolonged P-R interval, right and left atrial enlargement, RV hypertrophy, and incomplete right bundle branch block. An infant with an AVC defect may demonstrate signs of CHF with failure to thrive due to poor feeding, inadequate weight gain, and recurrent respiratory infections. Physical examination of an untreated infant with AVC defect may show signs of a poorly nourished infant with respiratory distress and tachycardia (Park & Salamat, 2022).

### Management

Initial medical management is aimed at preventing or treating CHF with diuretics, ACE inhibitor, and/or digitalis. Definitive management consists of surgical closure of the ASD and VSD, with reconstruction of AV valves under cardiopulmonary bypass, or in rare cases, pulmonary artery banding may be performed as a temporizing palliative procedure as part of a two-staged surgical correction.

Surgery is indicated when there is CHF with failure to thrive that is unresponsive to medical therapy and/or a large shunt with development of pulmonary hypertension and increasing pulmonary vascular resistance. Timing of surgical repair depends on the type of defect. Complete AVC defects undergo repair around 2 to 4 months of age, sometimes earlier if the CHF symptoms cannot be medically managed. Transitional AVC defects typically undergo repair within the first year of life and incomplete AVC defects between 1 to 2 years of age, sometimes even older if they are asymptomatic. The aggregate mortality rate is 2.7%. Factors that increase the risks of mortality for AVC defect repair include (1) very young age, (2) severe AV valve incompetence, (3) hypoplastic LV, and (4) severe symptoms before surgery (Jacobs et al., 2018; Park & Salamat, 2022).

## CYANOTIC DEFECTS

These CHDs are defects with obstruction to RV outflow that result in reduced pulmonary blood flow or abnormality in venous return. The defects described in this section include PS, TOF, pulmonary atresia with intact ventricular septum (PA/IVS), and TAPVR.

## Pulmonary Stenosis

PS is caused by abnormal formation of the pulmonary valve leaflets during fetal cardiac development. PS can be valvular, subvalvular (infundibular), or supravalvular. Valvular PS is the most common, accounting for 90% of cases. PS is frequently seen in Noonan syndrome. It is one of the four defects found in TOF. Isolated infundibular PS is uncommon.

### Incidence

PS makes up 5% to 8% of all CHDs. It is often associated with other defects.

### Hemodynamics

Pulmonary stenosis results in obstruction to blood flow from the RV to the pulmonary artery, and there is a spectrum of disease from mild PS to critical PS (duct dependent). In cases of more severe obstruction, the RV hypertrophies in response to the increased pressure caused by the obstruction to outflow. Pulmonary blood flow volume is normal in the absence of intracardiac shunting. PS is shown in Figure 7.8.

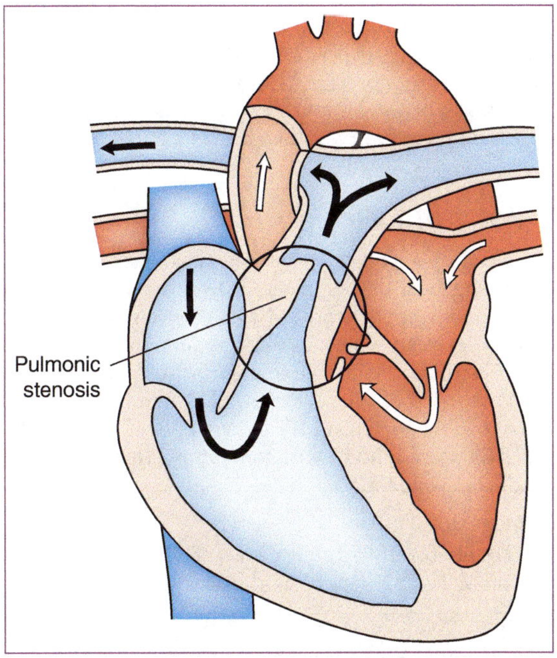


**FIGURE 7.8 Pulmonary stenosis.**

### Manifestations

PS may be asymptomatic if it is mild or moderate with normal oxygen saturations. Neonates with severe or critical PS may have saturations less than 95%.

### Diagnosis

The findings of PS depend on the severity of the defect. A pulmonary systolic ejection click may be heard at the upper LSB and $S_2$ may be widely split with the pulmonary component soft and delayed. A SEM (grade 2/6–4/6) is audible at the upper LSB and radiates to the back. The severity of the PS is directly related to the loudness and duration of the murmur. A systolic thrill can sometimes be felt at the upper LSB, which would result in a grade 4/6 SEM.

The ECG is normal in mild PS. There may be right-axis deviation and RV hypertrophy with moderate stenosis and right atrial enlargement and RV hypertrophy with strain with severe PS.

Chest radiograph demonstrates normal heart size with a prominent MPA segment. In mild-to-moderate PS, pulmonary markings are normal. The critical type of PS causes decreased pulmonary markings. Echocardiogram evaluation involves determining level of obstruction (subvalvular, valvular, and supravalvular), valve morphology, PDA patency, and associated defects. There may be a decreased motion of the pulmonary valve leaflets and poststenotic dilation of the MPA segment (Park & Salamat, 2022).

### Management

Management of PS is determined by the severity of the obstruction to flow. The mild type generally requires no therapy unless there is worsening of the PS. Moderate-to-severe PS is treated through balloon valvuloplasty during cardiac catheterization. Surgical correction is performed in children with critical PS when balloon valvuloplasty is not successful in relieving the gradient, or when the pulmonary valve fails to grow after balloon valvuloplasty. Infants with critical PS require prostaglandin E1 ($PGE_1$) infusion to maintain ductal patency until surgery is performed (Park & Salamat, 2022).

The overall prognosis for PS is excellent. The mortality rate is less than 1% in older infants. The mortality rate is higher in newborns with critical PS and CHF (Park & Salamat, 2022).

## Tetralogy of Fallot

Edward Fallot, a French physician, first described TOF in 1888. During fetal development, TOF is a result of anterior deviation of the conal septum (wall between the aortic and pulmonary valves), which causes subpulmonary/pulmonary outflow obstruction and a large anterior malalignment VSD. TOF is comprised of four defects: VSD, pulmonary valve stenosis, overriding aorta, and RV hypertrophy. There is a spectrum of TOF from mild PS with no cyanosis (pink TOF) to PA that is duct dependent.

### Incidence

TOF accounts for 10% of all CHDs. TOF is the most common cyanotic heart defect beyond infancy.

### Hemodynamics

In TOF, the large VSD causes equalization of pressure in the ventricles. Unsaturated blood flows through the VSD into the aorta because of the obstruction to blood flow from the RV into the pulmonary artery. TOF is illustrated in Figure 7.9.

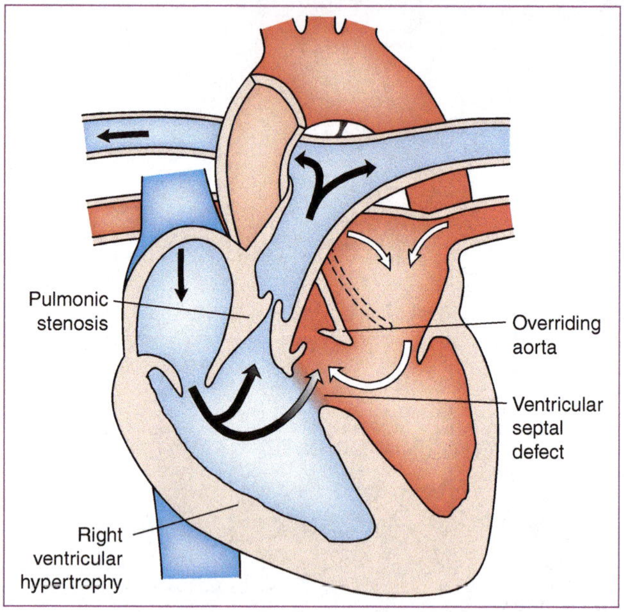


**FIGURE 7.9 Tetralogy of Fallot (TOF) consists of pulmonary stenosis, ventricular septal defect, overriding aorta, and hypertrophy of the right ventricle.**

*Source:* Adapted and modified from Ross Laboratories, Columbus, OH, Clinical Education Aid, 1985.

### Manifestations

Newborns may be asymptomatic or may present with a loud murmur and/or cyanosis. Severe decompensation or "tet" spells may occur in infants or children, but these can also occur in neonates. Children instinctively assume a squatting position, which traps venous blood in the legs, decreases systemic venous return to the heart, and increases systemic vascular resistance to increase left-to-right flow (Park & Salamat, 2022).

### Diagnosis

Neonates with TOF exhibit varying degrees of cyanosis, depending on the severity of the obstruction of blood flow through the right ventricular outflow tract (RVOT). A long, loud, grade 3/6 to 4/6 SEM is heard at the upper LSB. A PDA murmur may also be heard in TOF with critical PS or PA (Park, 2014).

Chest radiograph demonstrates decreased or normal heart size with decreased pulmonary vascularity. The contour of the heart may be boot shaped due to the concave MPA segment with upturned apex. There may also be RA enlargement and some patients may have a right aortic arch.

Echocardiogram demonstrates a large anterior malalignment VSD with overriding aorta, degree of PS and level of RVOT obstruction, coronary artery pattern, and presence of additional VSDs or right aortic arch.

### Management

The definitive therapy for TOF is surgical repair under cardiopulmonary bypass. The surgical correction can sometimes be delayed with careful medical management. **Quality and Safety: Careful follow-up is essential to detect signs of**

**clinical deterioration and worsening cyanosis.** Parents need adequate instructions on home care and self-care support (Park & Salamat, 2022).

Parents must be taught how to recognize the early signs and symptoms of decompensation. They must also be taught to recognize and treat hypercyanotic or tet spells (Table 7.4). Tet spells are precipitated by events that lower the systemic vascular resistance, producing a large right-to-left ventricular shunt. Increased activity, crying, nursing, or defecation may trigger a hypoxemic episode. The right-to-left shunt causes a decreased $PaO_2$, increased $PaCO_2$, and decreased pH, which stimulate the respiratory center, causing increased rate and depth of respirations (hyperpnea). The hyperpnea causes increased systemic venous return by increasing the efficiency of the thoracic pump. The RVOT obstruction prevents the increased blood flow from entering the pulmonary artery, so the increased flow is shunted through the VSD to the aorta, which further decreases the arterial $PO_2$. Severe, uninterrupted hypercyanotic spells lead to loss of consciousness, hypoxemia, seizures, and death.

Surgical treatment is indicated in the presence of hypercyanotic spells (tet spells) that result in increased hypoxemia, metabolic acidosis, inadequate systemic perfusion, and increased cyanosis. Systemic perfusion can be evaluated by observing peripheral pulse intensity, urine output, capillary filling time, blood pressure, or peripheral vasoconstriction.

**TABLE 7.4**

**RECOGNITION AND TREATMENT OF TETRALOGY OF FALLOT ("TET") SPELLS**

| Manifestations | Treatment | Rationale |
|---|---|---|
| Irritability, crying, hyperpnea | Knee-to-chest or squatting position | Traps blood in lower extremities to decrease systemic venous return; increases pulmonary blood flow |
| Cyanosis | Oxygen administration | Improves arterial oxygen saturation |
| Diaphoresis, loss of consciousness | Morphine sulfate (0.1–0.2 mg/kg/dose) | Suppresses respiratory center to decrease hyperpnea |
| Seizures | Bicarbonate | Corrects acidosis and eliminates stimulation of respiratory center |
| Decreased murmur | Propranolol (Inderal; 0.15–0.25 mg/kg/dose) | May decrease spasm of RVOT or may act peripherally to stabilize |

RVOT, right ventricular outflow tract.

Surgical management can be either palliative or corrective. Palliative procedures are undertaken to improve pulmonary blood flow by creating a pathway between the systemic and pulmonary circulations. In addition, these procedures allow time for the right and left pulmonary arteries to grow. Palliative procedures are indicated for newborns with TOF with PA or critical PS (duct dependent) or children with a hypoplastic pulmonary artery, in whom early corrective surgery may be difficult (Park & Salamat, 2022).

Surgical correction is performed under cardiopulmonary bypass, and the timing of surgery depends on the cardiac center. Some centers perform complete TOF repair in the neonatal period; some perform palliative surgery for TOF/PA or critical PS with a Blalock-Taussig (BT) shunt and then complete repair after 6 months of age. The defect is repaired by patch closure of the VSD with widening of the RVOT with a transannular patch if the pulmonary valve is moderate to severely hypoplastic. Postoperative care of the newborn requires careful assessment and monitoring so that complications can be prevented or ameliorated. Complications of cardiac surgery are listed in Tables 7.5 and 7.6. The mortality rate for TOF

**TABLE 7.5**

**COMPLICATIONS OF CARDIAC SURGERY**

| Low Cardiac Output | Low Cardiac Output |
|---|---|
| Hypovolemia | Pulmonary hypertension |
| Hemorrhage | Inadequate ventilatory support |
| Diuresis | Ineffective pleural drainage |
| Inadequate fluid volume | Hypoventilation secondary to pain |
| Tamponade | **Renal Dysfunction or Failure** |
| Mediastinal bleeding | Poor systemic and renal perfusion |
| Inadequate mediastinal drainage | Intravascular hemolysis |
| Decreased cardiac contractility | Thromboembolus |
| Hypervolemia | Nephrotoxic drugs |
| Electrolyte imbalance | **Electrolyte Imbalance** |
| Cardiac dysfunction | Effects of cardiopulmonary bypass |

(continued)

**TABLE 7.5**

**COMPLICATIONS OF CARDIAC SURGERY (*continued*)**

| | |
|---|---|
| **Low Cardiac Output** | **Low Cardiac Output** |
| Increased systemic vascular resistance | Diuretics |
| Increased pulmonary vascular resistance | Stress response |
| Arrhythmias | Fluid administration |
| Hypothermia | Blood administration |
| **Congestive Heart Failure** | Renal failure |
| Uncorrected CHD (after palliative procedure) | **Neurologic Abnormalities** |
| Corrected CHD, causing alterations in ventricular preload, contractility, and afterload | Hypoxia |
| Hypervolemia | Acidosis |
| Electrolyte imbalance | Poor systemic perfusion |
| Arrhythmias | Thromboembolism |
| **Respiratory Distress** | Electrolyte imbalance |
| Atelectasis | **Infection** |
| Pneumothorax | Surgery |
| Hemothorax | Prosthetic material |
| Pleural effusion | Invasive monitoring and/or procedures |
| Chylothorax | Inadequate nutrition |
| CHF | |

CHD, congenital heart defects; CHF, congestive heart failure.

varies with the severity of the circulatory compromise caused by the defect. The aggregate mortality rate is now 1.1% for uncomplicated TOF. More severe cases have a higher mortality rate, exhibit residual pulmonary outflow tract obstruction, and may require further surgery (Jacobs et al., 2018; Park & Salamat, 2022).

## Pulmonary Atresia With Intact Ventricular Septum

PA with intact ventricular septum results in the absence of communication between the RV and the pulmonary artery and is a duct-dependent lesion. Determining whether the RV is adequate based on the tricuspid valve annulus size and Z score is important to determine if the neonate will require a single ventricle palliation or two ventricle repairs. Evaluation for RV-dependent coronary circulation is important to determine the pathway of single ventricle palliation versus two ventricular repairs. If the RV is inadequate and/or there are RV-dependent coronaries, then the patient will require single ventricle palliation pathway with a modified BT shunt in the neonatal period, bidirectional Glenn (BDG), and subsequent Fontan. If the RV is adequate and there are no RV-dependent coronaries, then a two-ventricle approach with radiofrequency (RF) perforation of the pulmonary valve along with balloon dilation of the pulmonary valve in the cardiac catheterization laboratory can be undertaken. The presence of a PDA, ASD, or patent foramen ovale (PFO) to allow blood mixing of which is crucial for survival. PA with intact ventricular septum is illustrated in Figure 7.10.

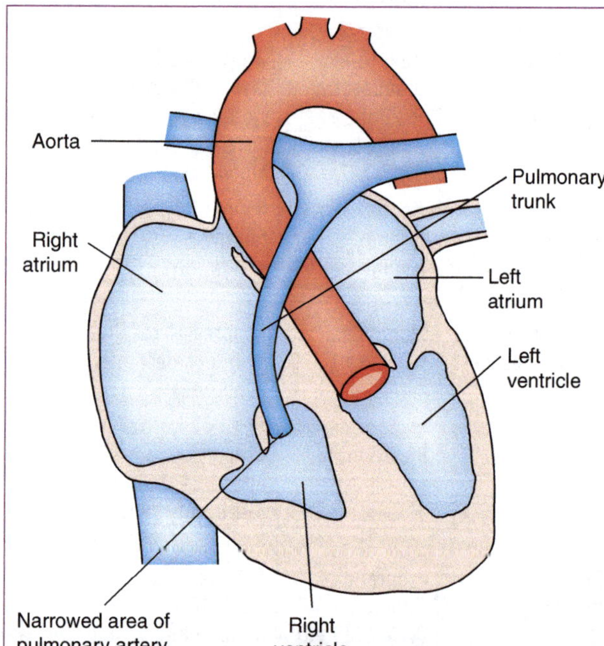


**FIGURE 7.10 Pulmonary atresia.**

**TABLE 7.6**

**COMPLICATIONS OF CARDIAC SURGERY: POSTOPERATIVE SYNDROMES**

| | Causes | Manifestations | Treatment |
|---|---|---|---|
| Postcoarctectomy syndrome | Results from changes in pressure and flow | Severe intermittent abdominal pain, fever, and leukocytosis; abdominal distention, melena, and ascites with gangrenous bowel; rebound systemic hypertension | Monitor blood pressure; prevent hypertension; delay postoperative feeding |
| Postpericardiotomy syndrome | Immunologic syndrome in response to blood in the pericardial sac | Fever, chest pain, pericardial and pleural effusions, hepatomegaly, leukocytosis, left shift, increased ESR, persistent ST and T wave changes on ECG; rare in children younger than 2 years of age | Rest, aspirin for pain, corticosteroids in severe cases, pericardiocentesis if tamponade develops, diuretics |
| Postperfusion syndrome | Cytomegalovirus | Onset 3–6 weeks after surgery; fever, splenomegaly, atypical lymphocytosis | Supportive care; self-limiting disease process |
| Hemolytic anemia syndrome | Trauma of RBCs or autoimmune action | Onset 1–2 weeks postoperatively; fever, jaundice, hepatomegaly, reticulocytosis | Iron supplementation or blood transfusions, correction of turbulent flow |

ECG, electrocardiogram; ESR, erythrocyte sedimentation rate; RBC, red blood cell.

### Incidence

PA accounts for less than 1% of all CHDs (Park, 2014).

### Hemodynamics

PA with intact ventricular septum manifests as a spectrum of tricuspid valve (TV) and RV hypoplasia. The absence of a RVOT results in high RV end-diastolic pressure, causing TR, increasing RA pressure, and causing systemic venous blood to shunt from the RA to the LA through the PFO or ASD. Mixed venous blood flows into the LV and aorta. This is a duct-dependent lesion and the PDA is the only source of pulmonary blood flow. Closure of the PDA causes severe cyanosis, hypoxemia, and acidosis.

### Manifestations

PA with intact ventricular septum results in cyanosis at birth secondary to right-to-left shunt at the atrial level. Tachypnea is present, but there is no obvious respiratory distress. $S_2$ is single, and TR may produce a harsh regurgitant holosystolic murmur along the lower right and left sternal borders (Park & Salamat, 2022).

Chest radiograph demonstrates a normal or enlarged heart with a concave MPA segment, like the appearance of tricuspid atresia. Pulmonary vascular markings are decreased and continue to decrease as the PDA closes.

ECG may reveal a normal QRS axis, LVH type I, or, less frequently, RV hypertrophy (type II), and RA enlargement is seen in approximately 70% of cases (Park, 2014). Echocardiogram demonstrates presence of an atretic pulmonary valve, degree of hypoplasia of the RV cavity and TV, amount of TR, size of ASD, and possible RV coronary fistula.

### Management

Immediate management of PA is administration of prostaglandin to maintain ductal patency. $PGE_1$ (Prostin) is given as a continuous intravenous (IV) infusion. The initial dose varies from 0.025 to 0.1 mcg/kg/min. When the desired effect is achieved, the dose is incrementally decreased to a maintenance dose of 0.01 mcg/kg/min. Careful attention to the site of the infusion is important.

Surgical correction versus cardiac catheterization is determined by the size of the TV. If the RV is inadequate in size based on a TV annulus *Z* score and/or presence of RV-dependent coronaries, then the neonate will require palliative procedures beginning with a systemic pulmonary artery shunt using Gore-Tex graft tube between the brachiocephalic artery and the pulmonary artery (modified BT shunt) in the neonatal period. The surgical mortality rate varies, depending on whether single-ventricle palliation or two-ventricle repair is required.

## Total Anomalous Pulmonary Venous Return

TAPVR is a result of the pulmonary veins draining into the RA (rather than the LA). There are four types of TAPVR (Park, 2014), based on the path of pulmonary venous return. The supracardiac type is the most common and involves drainage of the pulmonary veins via a confluence to the left vertical vein, innominate vein, and right SVC into the RA. The infracardiac type involves pulmonary veins entering a confluence, descending vertical vein that enters the portal vein in the liver to return to the RA via IVC. This TAPVR type involves drainage to the coronary sinus. The infracardiac type is the most common type to be obstructed and typically requires emergent surgery to relieve the obstruction and repair the anomalous pulmonary veins. The mixed type involves a combination of pulmonary venous drainage.

### Incidence

TAPVR accounts for 1% of all CHDs. There is a 1:1 male-to-female ratio of occurrence.

### Hemodynamics

TAPVR has an obligate right-to-left shunt at the atrial level to allow some of the oxygenated blood from the anomalous pulmonary venous return that mixes with deoxygenated blood to shunt into the LA to the LV, pumping blood into the aorta and to the systemic circulation.

Two clinical hemodynamic states exist with TAPVR. If pulmonary blood flow is not obstructed, pulmonary flow is greatly increased. The result is highly saturated blood in the RA and mild cyanosis. If there is obstruction to pulmonary blood flow, the volume of flow is decreased, cyanosis is severe, and there is associated pulmonary hypertension. Obstruction to pulmonary blood flow is a common occurrence when the TAPVR is the infracardiac type (Park & Salamat, 2022).

### Manifestations

The manifestations of TAPVR depend on the presence of pulmonary venous obstruction (PVO). TAPVR without PVO includes a history of mild cyanosis and tachypnea. TAPVR with PVO causes severe cyanosis, respiratory distress, and poor CO (Park & Salamat, 2022).

### Diagnosis

TAPVR without PVO produces a precordial bulge with hyperactive RV impulse. The PMI is at the xiphoid process or LLSB. $S_2$ is widely split and fixed; the pulmonic sound may be pronounced. A grade 2/6 to 3/6 SEM can be heard at the upper LSB, and there is always a mid-diastolic rumble at the LLSB. The rhythm is a quadruple or quintuple gallop (Park & Salamat, 2022).

TAPVR with PVO may produce minimal cardiac findings. $S_2$ is loud and single, and there is a gallop rhythm. There may be a faint SEM at the upper LSB. Pulmonary rales may be audible.

Chest radiographic findings of TAPVR without PVO include mild-to-moderate cardiomegaly and increased pulmonary markings. The characteristic "snowman" sign occurs because of the anatomic appearance of the left SVC, the left innominate vein, and the right SVC. This sign is seldom visible before the patient is 4 months of age. With TAPVR with PVO, the heart size is normal on chest radiograph, and there are signs of pulmonary edema (Park & Salamat, 2022).

On ECG, TAPVR without PVO has right axis deviation of the QRS axis and sometimes RA enlargement. TAPVR with PVO has right-axis deviation for age and RV hypertrophy in the form of tall R waves in the right precordial leads.

Echocardiography of TAPVR demonstrates right-to-left flow across the atrial septum, RA and RV dilation, pulmonary veins draining to a confluence returning to the heart via a vertical vein to the SVC or innominate vein in the supracardiac type, or descending vein to the portal system in the infracardiac type. The infracardiac type is the most common to present with obstruction secondary to obstruction of flow that occurs when the descending vein enters the portal system to return to the RA via the DV and IVC. The supracardiac type can also present with obstruction, particularly when blood flow increases to the lungs as the pulmonary vascular resistance decreases. The vertical vein typically passes between the left bronchus and left pulmonary artery and can become compressed by these two structures (Brown & Geva, 2016).

### Management

Management of TAPVR is surgical, and surgery is emergent when PVO is infracardiac. Medical management is aimed at preventing or treating CHF and preventing hypoxemia until surgical correction. Diuretics may be required to manage pulmonary edema. Balloon atrial septostomy at cardiac catheterization is performed to enlarge the interatrial communication and promote better mixing of blood. Surgery may be delayed when response to medical management is good, but it is usually performed when the patients are neonates (Park & Salamat, 2022). The surgical procedure depends on the site of the anomalous drainage. Cardiopulmonary bypass is required. Surgery involves the anastomosis of the pulmonary veins to the LA, closure of the ASD, and division of the anomalous connection. The surgical mortality rate is between 5% and 10% for infants with the unobstructed type. This rate can be as high as 20% for infants with the infracardiac type (Park & Salamat, 2022).

# DEFECTS WITH LEFT VENTRICLE OUTFLOW OBSTRUCTION

These are CHDs resulting from a defect with obstruction to LV outflow, causing reduced or inadequate systemic blood flow. The defects described in this section include AS, COA, and HLHS.

## Aortic Stenosis

AS is one of a group of defects that produces obstruction to ventricular outflow. AS may be valvular, subvalvular, or supravalvular. Valvular stenosis is the most common, and supravalvular is the least common (Park & Salamat, 2022).

In valvular stenosis, there is usually a bicuspid valve. Subvalvular stenosis can involve either a subaortic membrane or a long tunnel-like ventricular outflow tract. Idiopathic hypertrophic subaortic stenosis is a form of subvalvular stenosis that presents as a cardiomyopathy. Supravalvular stenosis is associated with Williams syndrome, or elfin facies, characterized by mental retardation, short palpebral fissures, and thick lips (Park & Salamat, 2022).

### Incidence

AS accounts for 5% of all CHDs. It is four times more common in males.

### Hemodynamics

AS causes increased pressure load on the LV, leading to LV hypertrophy. The resistance to blood flow through the stenosis gradually causes a pressure gradient between the ventricle and the aorta, and coronary blood flow decreases. AS is illustrated in Figure 7.11.

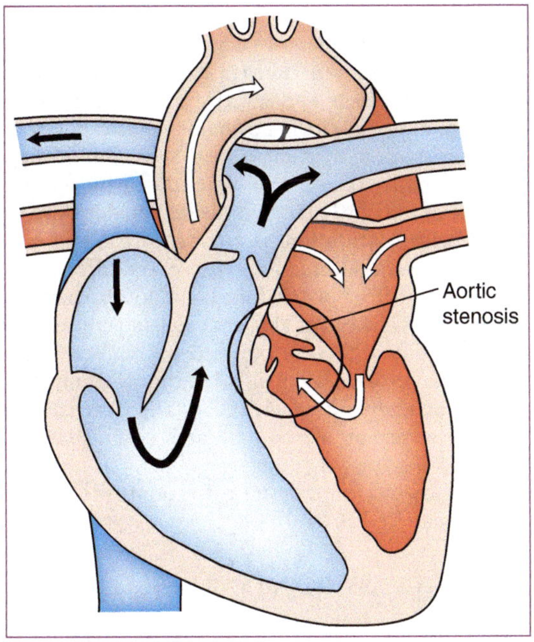


**FIGURE 7.11 Aortic stenosis is a narrowing or thickening of the aortic valvular region.**

*Source:* Adapted and modified from Ross Laboratories, Columbus, OH, Clinical Education Aid, 1985.

### Manifestations

Symptoms depend on the severity of the defect. Mild AS is typically asymptomatic; with more severe defects, there is activity intolerance, chest pain, presyncope, or syncope. With severe defects, CHF develops.

### Diagnosis

Physical examination reveals normal development without cyanosis. There may be a narrow pulse pressure and a higher systolic pressure in the right arm with severe supravalvular AS. There is a systolic murmur of approximately grade 2/6 to 4/6, best heard at the second right or left intercostal space with transmission to the neck. With valvular AS, there may be an ejection click. With severe AS, there may be paradoxical splitting of $S_2$. AI may cause a high-pitched, early diastolic, decrescendo murmur if there is bicuspid aortic valve or subvalvular stenosis (Park & Salamat, 2022).

Chest radiographs may be normal or may show a dilated ascending aorta, or, in the case of valvular stenosis, a prominent aortic "knob" caused by poststenotic dilation (Park, 2014). Cardiomegaly is present if there is CHF or severe aortic regurgitation. ECG may be normal or may show mild LVH and inverted T waves. Echocardiogram may demonstrate a bicuspid aortic valve, dysplastic thickened aortic valve, or in rare cases a unicuspid aortic valve, degree of AS, presence of AI, LVH, and subvalvular and supravalvular AS. Cardiac catheterization may be performed to identify the exact anatomy and to analyze pressure gradients.

### Management

Management is aimed at preventing or treating the CHF with fluid restriction, diuretics, and/or digitalis. In children with moderate-to-severe AS, activity is restricted to prevent increased demand on the heart. Balloon valvuloplasty is sometimes performed at the time of cardiac catheterization to improve circulation. In newborns with critical AS, maintenance of the patency of the DA with $PGE_1$ at a dose of 0.01 to 0.1 mcg/kg/min is required to prevent inadequate CO with poor perfusion and metabolic acidosis.

The type of surgical correction depends on the exact location and severity of the defect. The procedure may consist of aortic valve commissurotomy or valve replacement with a prosthetic valve or a graft. The placement of prosthetic valves is usually deferred until adult-sized prosthetic valves can be inserted. The timing of the surgery depends on the severity of the defect. Infants with severe AS without AI will require balloon valvuloplasty and potentially surgery if the gradient does not improve or there is severe AI. Surgery is typically performed on children when there is a peak systolic pressure gradient greater than 50 to 60 mm Hg (Park & Salamat, 2022).

The surgical mortality risk varies depending on the timing and surgical approach required. Surgical mortality for neonates with critical AS is 10% (Park & Salamat, 2022).

## Coarctation of the Aorta

COA is a narrowing or constriction in the aortic arch. The most common location is in the isthmus region located distal to the left subclavian artery. It may be a discrete coarctation or long-segment coarctation associated with aortic arch hypoplasia. Coarctation of the aorta may occur as a single lesion due to improper development of the aorta, or in rare instances may occur after constriction of the DA. The severity of the circulatory compromise depends on the location and degree of constriction. Many infants with COA, more than 75%, have a bicuspid aortic valve (Park & Salamat, 2022). Coarctation is illustrated in Figure 7.12.

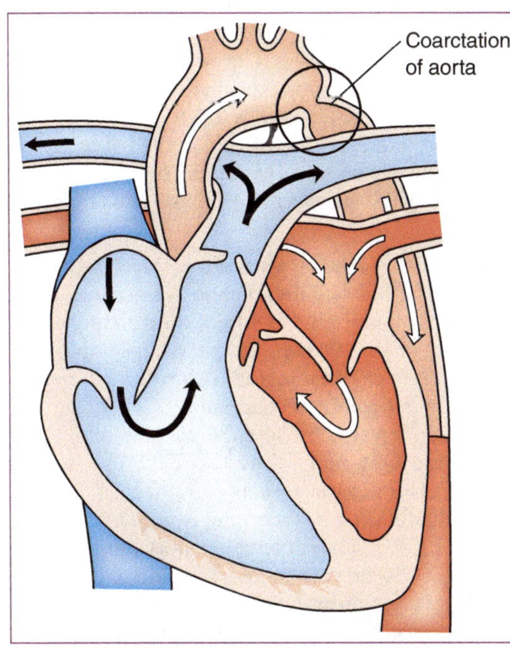


**FIGURE 7.12 Coarctation of the aorta is a narrowing or constriction of the aorta near the ductus arteriosus.**

*Source:* Adapted and modified from Ross Laboratories, Columbus, OH, Clinical Education Aid, 1985.

### Incidence

Coarctation of the aorta accounts for 8% of all CHDs. Coarctation occurs twice as often in males. Coarctation of the aorta is found in 30% of infants with Turner syndrome (Park & Salamat, 2022).

### Hemodynamics

Coarctation of the aorta causes obstruction to flow that leads to varying pressure across the aortic arch, with the portion of aorta proximal to the constriction with an elevated pressure, resulting in increased LV pressure. In newborns, RV hypertrophy is a predominant finding because the RV is the main pumping chamber in utero. In cases of delayed diagnosis, the increased LV pressure results in LV hypertrophy and dilation; over time, collateral circulation develops from the proximal to distal arteries, bypassing the constricted segment of the aorta. This is a compensatory mechanism to increase flow to the lower extremities and abdomen resulting in decreased pulses in the lower extremities. Children with delayed diagnosis of coarctation will present with elevated systolic blood pressures in the right arm and decreased femoral pulses (Park, 2014).

### Manifestations

The severity and time of appearance of symptoms of COA depend on the degree of constriction and associated aortic arch hypoplasia, as well as the presence of associated cardiac defects. Coarctation of the aorta and/or arch hypoplasia may be missed prenatally (Anuwutnavin et al., 2016). Those neonates with a murmur or who fail pulse oximetry screening for CHD will be diagnosed before becoming symptomatic. Some neonates may go undetected by CCHD pulse oximetry screening, only being diagnosed with coarctation after developing symptoms as the DA closes. In these cases, symptoms of coarctation include CHF with tachypnea, diaphoresis, poor feeding, and weak or delayed pulses in the lower extremities with bounding pulses in the upper extremities. In the presence of CHF, however, all pulses may be weak. With severe COA, $S_2$ is loud and single, a systolic thrill may be felt in the suprasternal notch, and a SEM of grade 2/6 to 3/6 can be heard at the upper right, middle, or LLSB, and at the left interscapular area on the infant's back; however, no murmur is heard in more than half of infants with COA (Park & Salamat, 2022).

### Diagnosis

Diagnosis of COA is based on history, physical findings, chest radiograph, ECG, and definitive diagnosis by echocardiogram. In asymptomatic infants and children, chest radiographs may show a normal or slightly enlarged heart. In symptomatic infants and children, chest radiographs show cardiomegaly and increased pulmonary venous congestion.

The ECG in asymptomatic children may show left-axis deviation of the QRS and LV hypertrophy. In symptomatic children, the ECG reveals normal or right-axis deviation of the QRS. Right ventricle hypertrophy is present in infants because the RV is the main pumping chamber in utero, whereas LV hypertrophy is present in older children (Park, 2014). Echocardiogram demonstrates the location and degree of the coarctation, presence of aortic arch hypoplasia, and associated defects such as VSD, bicuspid aortic valve, and LV dysfunction.

### Management

In neonates prenatally diagnosed with coarctation, a postnatal echocardiogram is performed to assess the severity of coarctation and presence and severity of arch hypoplasia. In some cases, findings from the postnatal echocardiogram will determine postnatal management, with close monitoring for detection of definitive coarctation after the ductus closes versus initiation of $PGE_1$ to maintain ductal patency until surgical repair. Oxygen saturations in the right hand and right or left foot should be monitored for a significant difference, with saturations in the right or left foot being lower than that in the right hand. The surgical approach depends on the extent of arch obstruction. If there is a discrete coarctation, then surgical repair can be performed via a left thoracotomy. If there is significant arch hypoplasia with coarctation, then a surgical approach via a median sternotomy arch augmentation will be needed.

The mortality rate for surgical corrections is less than 5% (Park & Salamat, 2022).

## Hypoplastic Left Heart Syndrome

HLHS consists of a group of cardiac defects, including a hypoplastic aortic valve and mitral valve with stenosis or atresia, and a small LA and LV. The great vessels are normally related. There are four different subtypes (mitral atresia with AA, mitral stenosis with AS, mitral atresia with AS, and mitral stenosis with AA). HLHS is illustrated in Figure 7.13.

### Incidence

HLHS occurs in about one per 3,955 babies born in the United States annually (CDC, n.d.-b).

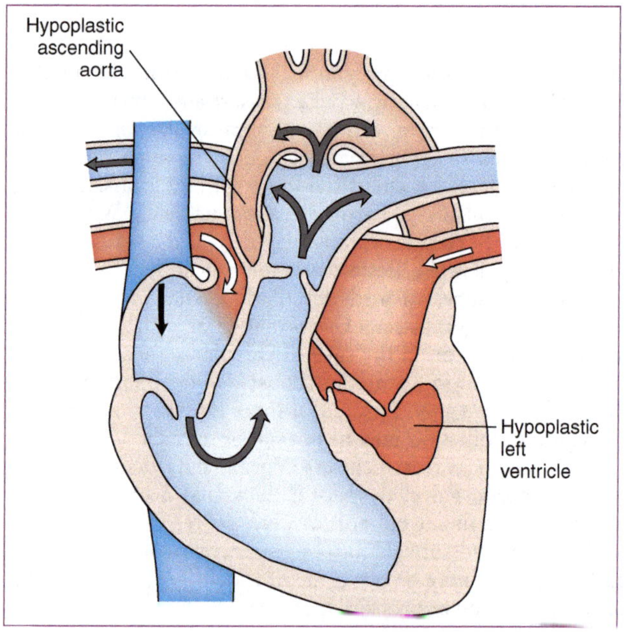


**FIGURE 7.13** Hypoplastic left heart syndrome.

### Hemodynamics

HLHS is a duct-dependent lesion requiring prostaglandin to maintain ductal patency to provide systemic blood flow. Because the LV is inadequate or absent, LV output is greatly reduced or absent. Retrograde flow through the aortic arch supplies the head, upper extremities, and coronary arteries. Left atrial and pulmonary venous pressures are elevated and may result in pulmonary edema.

Although circulation is abnormal in utero, the high pulmonary vascular resistance and the low systemic vascular resistance make survival possible. The RV maintains normal perfusion pressure in the descending aorta by a right-to-left ductal shunt. At birth, the onset of pulmonary ventilation causes decreased pulmonary vascular resistance. The systemic vascular resistance increases because the placenta is eliminated. In cases where HLHS is not prenatally detected, closure of the DA results in a decrease in systemic perfusion leading to metabolic acidosis and circulatory shock (Park & Salamat, 2022).

### Manifestations

Neonates with HLHS may be asymptomatic and have near-normal saturations if there is adequate atrial communication and mixing of blue and pink blood. Importantly, these neonates may not be detected by CCHD pulse oximetry screening typically performed at 24 hours of age because the ducts may be patent. As the ductus closes, circulatory shock develops resulting in metabolic acidosis with signs and symptoms of progressive cyanosis, tachypnea, tachycardia, and poor peripheral pulses. Typically, the $S_2$ is single, and a cardiac murmur may be absent in neonates with mitral and AA. In neonates with mitral stenosis and AS, there may be a grade 2/6 to 3/6 systolic murmur (Park & Salamat, 2022).

### Diagnosis

Chest radiograph of HLHS demonstrates mild-to-moderate heart enlargement and pulmonary venous congestion or pulmonary edema. RV hypertrophy is the characteristic finding on ECG. Echocardiography is diagnostic demonstrating hypoplastic or even absent left-sided heart structures. There may be mitral or AS, or mitral or AA associated with a hypoplastic LA, LV, and ascending aorta/aortic arch, RV dilation, and hypertrophy. The size of the ASD and presence of TR should also be documented.

### Management

Medical management of HLHS is aimed at maintaining ductal patency through continuous infusion of $PGE_1$ to prevent significant hypoxemia and metabolic acidosis. In rare cases of a restrictive atrial septum, balloon atrial septostomy and/or stenting of the atrial septum may be required if there is inadequate atrial communication.

Surgical palliation of HLHS is complex and has a high mortality rate; however, over 30 years ago, HLHS was once considered 100% fatal. The goal of surgical palliation is to separate the deoxygenated and oxygenated blood in three stages. The first-stage procedure, the modified Norwood procedure, is typically performed in the first week of life. The Stage I/Norwood procedure involves building a neoaorta utilizing the MPA and a BT shunt (Gore-Tex graft tube) or a Sano (RV-PA conduit tube) to provide stable pulmonary blood flow with an atrial septectomy to create adequate atrial communication. Infants who have undergone a Stage I/Norwood procedure typically have oxygen saturations of 75% to 80%. The second-stage procedure, the BDG, is typically performed at 4 to 6 months of age. The BDG involves dividing the SVC and anastomosing it to the RPA (right pulmonary artery) along with ligating the BT shunt. Infants with BDG have saturations of 80% to 85%. The third-stage procedure, a modified Fontan procedure, is typically performed at 2 years of age. The modified Fontan procedure involves dividing and anastomosing the IVC to the RPA. Children who have undergone a Fontan procedure have normal oxygen saturations unless they have a fenestrated Fontan. In some patients who are higher risk for a Fontan procedure or in some centers, the Fontan is fenestrated, and these patients will have lower saturations until the fenestration spontaneously closes or is closed later via transcatheter device closure (Goff et al., 2000; Marino et al., 2006).

See Table 7.7 for a description of these procedures (Park & Salamat, 2022).

The aggregate surgical mortality rate for the Stage I/Norwood palliation procedure, which includes HLHS, is 15.8%. If patients survive up to the BDG/hemi-Fontan and Fontan procedure, the aggregate surgical mortality rate decreases to 2.1% and 1.1%, respectively (Jacobs et al., 2018).

Nursing care focuses on assessment of CO, systemic perfusion, and adequate pulmonary blood flow during the immediate postoperative period. Postoperative care requires close monitoring of vital signs, chest tube output, urine output, laboratory values (hemoglobin, platelets, BUN/Cr, aspartate aminotransferase/alanine aminotransferase [AST/ALT]), and pulmonary and circulatory status. Attention to nutritional status is important for long-term recovery.

Dopamine at 5 mcg/kg/min may be needed to augment CO along with milrinone 0.5 to 1 mcg/kg/min. Diuretics and/or peritoneal dialysis may be necessary to maintain fluid balance. Fentanyl and Versed drips may be used for sedation and analgesia. In many institutions, Stage I/Norwood patients return to the cardiac intensive care unit on extracorporeal membrane oxygenation (ECMO) to maintain oxygenation and CO during the immediate postoperative period, whereas many other institutions maintain an open chest for several days to allow optimization of CO and ventilation (Marino et al., 2006).

Nutritional support is provided through total parenteral nutrition (TPN). Monitoring of daily weights, of urine for ketones, glucose, and protein, and of serum levels of electrolytes and trace minerals is necessary to adjust the parenteral fluids. Enteral feedings may be started in the first few weeks postoperatively once the neonate has been deintensified, is hemodynamically stable, and where NEC risk is somewhat decreased.

Although an alternative treatment approach for HLHS is cardiac transplantation, the wait time for heart transplant in infants is on average 4 to 6 months in many regions. Therefore, listing for heart transplant is primarily utilized for those neonates with poor RV function who are not good candidates for the Stage I/Norwood procedure. It is essential that parents be counseled and informed of all available treatment options, including risks and short- and long-term prognoses. Improvement in overall survival has led to an increased focus on

**TABLE 7.7**

**COMMON CARDIAC SURGICAL PROCEDURES**

| Procedure | Type | Defect | Description |
|---|---|---|---|
| Modified BT shunt | Palliative | Single ventricle with PA, TOF/PA, PA/IVS | Synthetic tube from the brachiocephalic artery to the pulmonary artery to provide a stable source of pulmonary blood flow |
| Stage I Procedure Norwood/ Damus-Kaye-Stansel | Palliative | HLHS/HLH variants | 1. MPA is divided, and anastomosed to the hypoplastic ascending aorta to provide unobstructed systemic and coronary blood flow<br>2. Modified BT shunt to provide a stable source of pulmonary blood flow<br>3. Atrial septectomy to allow interatrial mixing |
| Superior caval connection (bidirectional Glenn) | Palliative | Single ventricles | 1. SVC anastomosis to the RPA<br>2. Ligation and division of the BT shunt |
| Modified Fontan | Palliative | Single ventricles | Lateral tunnel (inferior baffle from IVC to SVC) or extracardiac conduit (Gore-Tex tube connection between the vena cava) |
| Rashkind | Corrective | TGA, HLHS restrictive atrial septum | Balloon atrial septostomy to enlarge the atrial communication |
| Jatene/arterial switch procedure | Corrective | TGA | Switching of TGA to their anatomically correct position along with reimplantation of coronary arteries into the neoaorta |
| Rastelli | Corrective | TGA, TOF, PA, truncus arteriosus | Commonly applied to all valved conduits from the RV to pulmonary artery |
| Pulmonary artery banding | Palliative | Multiple VSDs, single ventricles with unobstructed outflow | Placement of a band around the pulmonary artery to decrease the blood flow to the lungs |

BT, Blalock-Taussig; HLH, hypoplastic left heart; HLHS, hypoplastic left heart syndrome; IVC, inferior vena cava; IVS, intact ventricular septum; MPA, Main pulmonary artery; PA, pulmonary artery; RPA, right pulmonary artery; RV, right ventricle; SVC, superior vena cava; TGA, transposition of the great arteries; TOF, tetralogy of Fallot; VSD, ventricular septal defect.

*Sources:* Data from Marino, B. S., Ostrow, A. M., & Cohen, M. S. (2006). Surgery for congenital heart disease. In V. Vetter (Ed.), *Pediatric cardiology: The requisites in pediatrics* (pp. 277–320). Mosby Elsevier; Park, M. K. (2014). *Pediatric cardiology for practitioners.* Mosby.

long-term morbidity, particularly neurobehavioral and neurocognitive issues. Neurodevelopmental problems are common in this cohort and are further discussed in the section on age-related ND problems (Marino et al., 2012).

## DEFECTS WITH ABNORMAL AORTOPULMONARY CONNECTIONS

These CHDs result from a developmental defect of either the vascular or the valvular system, frequently with cyanosis. The defects described in this section include TGA and truncus arteriosus.

### Transposition of the Great Arteries or Vessels

Transposition of TGA is the result of abnormal rotation of the outflow tracts during fetal cardiac development. Transposition of the great arteries may be dextrotransposition of the great arteries (*d*-TGA) or levotransposition of the great arteries (*L*-TGA). In *d*-TGA, the aorta arises from the RV and the pulmonary artery arises from the LV. The aorta receives deoxygenated systemic venous blood and returns it to the systemic arterial circuit. The pulmonary artery receives oxygenated pulmonary venous blood and returns it to the pulmonary circulation. *d*-TGA is illustrated in Figure 7.14.

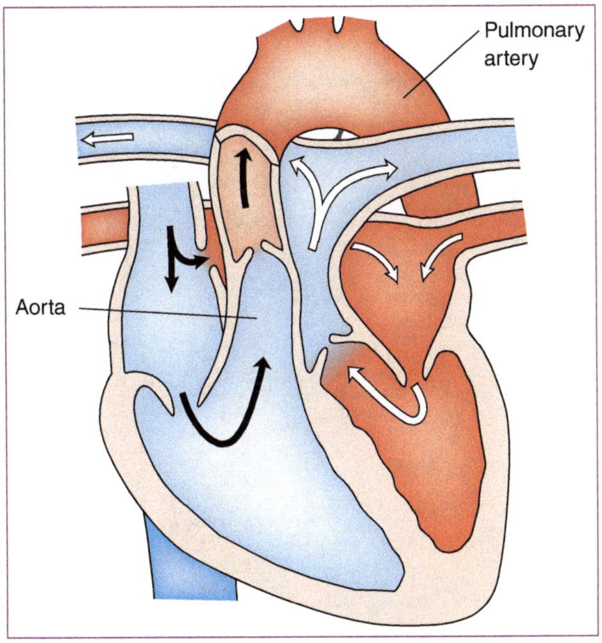


**FIGURE 7.14 Transposition of the great arteries or vessels is a condition in which the aorta arises from the right ventricle and the pulmonary artery arises from the left ventricle.** The result is two distinct circulatory (parallel) pathways.

In *L*-TGA, both the ventricles and the great vessels are transposed, with the aorta arising from the left-sided RV and the pulmonary artery arising from the right-sided LV. The aorta is to the left and anterior to the pulmonary artery. This type of transposition is called *corrected,* because physiologically the cardiac hemodynamics are normal except that the RV is the systemic pumping chamber. The oxygenated blood comes into the LA, enters the left-sided RV, and is pumped via the aorta to the systemic circulation. Frequently, there are other associated cardiac defects; but in the absence of these defects, *L*-TGA may go undetected until a patient reaches adulthood and develops right ventricular (RV) heart failure adult CHD; (Park & Salamat, 2022).

### Incidence

*d*-TGA accounts for 5% of all CHDs. It is more common in males (3:1). *d*-TGA is the most common cyanotic heart defect in newborns.

### Hemodynamics

Hemodynamically, *d*-TGA results in parallel circulation. Oxygenated blood from the lungs is returned to the LA and enters the LV, which pumps blood back to the lungs via the pulmonary artery. Deoxygenated blood from the systemic veins returns to the RA and enters the RV, which pumps blood into the systemic circulation via the aorta. The result is that the heart, brain, and other vital tissues are perfused with deoxygenated blood. **Emergency Alert: This defect is incompatible with life unless there is an adequate atrial communication to allow mixing of the oxygenated and deoxygenated blood.** Some cases of *d*-TGA have associated VSDs, which may contribute a little to mixing of oxygenated and deoxygenated blood, but the ASD is required for adequate mixing of blood (Park & Salamat, 2022).

### Manifestations

In cases detected prenatally, $PGE_1$ is initiated after birth and arterial blood gases (ABGs) are monitored for significant hypoxia. In cases not detected prenatally, cyanosis is typical and may be severe if the atrial communication is restrictive. If the atrial communication is restricted, the right upper arm saturation typically is lower than the right or left lower leg oxygen saturation.

### Diagnosis

Chest radiograph of *d*-TGA demonstrates a classical finding of an egg-shaped heart, where the heart is enlarged with a narrow base because the aorta is anterior to the pulmonary artery (Park, 2014). On ECG, there is right-axis deviation of the QRS and RV hypertrophy. Echocardiography is important to evaluate the adequacy of the atrial communication, presence, and size of VSDs, aortic or pulmonary valve abnormalities, and coarctation. The coronary pattern is important because a small percentage of coronary patterns will require an alternative surgical approach in rare cases.

### Management

*d*-TGA may be a cardiac emergency in those neonates who are not prenatally detected and have a restrictive atrial septum. Immediate medical management includes initiation of $PGE_1$; correction of acidosis, hypoglycemia, hypocalcemia; administration of oxygen; and access to emergent balloon atrial septostomy to promote mixing of oxygenated and deoxygenated blood at the atrial level (Park & Salamat, 2022).

Surgical correction involves the Jatene or arterial switch operation (ASO), which involves switching the arteries and coronaries (Jatene procedure) along with bringing the branch pulmonary arteries across the anterior aspect of the aorta (LeCompte). See Table 7.7 for a description of these procedures.

Outcomes after the ASO are quite good, with aggregate mortality rates of 2.7% for *d*-TGA without a VSD and 5.3% for *d*-TGA with VSD (Jacobs et al., 2018). In the long term, these patients may develop problems with branch pulmonary arteries and coronary problems. Children with *d*-TGA status post ASO have been one of the most widely studied groups for ND problems (Marino et al., 2012).

## Truncus Arteriosus

Early fetal development involves a single, large great vessel or trunk arising from the ventricles, which ultimately gives rise to the systemic and pulmonary circulations. During development, if there is inadequate septation of the trunk then both the pulmonary and aortic outflows will arise from one large vessel, and inadequate septation of the ventricular septum will result in a large VSD. Four types of truncus arteriosus have been described; see Table 7.8 for the classifications (Park & Salamat, 2022). Truncus arteriosus is illustrated in Figure 7.15.

### Incidence

Truncus arteriosus accounts for less than 1% of all CHDs.

### Hemodynamics

Deoxygenated blood from the RV and oxygenated blood from the LV mix via the large VSD and enter the truncal artery. The pressures of both ventricles are equal as a result of the large

**TABLE 7.8**

**FOUR MAJOR TYPES OF TRUNCUS ARTERIOSUS**

| Type | Incidence (%) | Description |
|---|---|---|
| I | 60 | MPA arises from truncus and divides into left and right pulmonary artery; results in increased pulmonary blood flow |
| II | 20 | Pulmonary artery arises from posterior portion of truncus arteriosus; pulmonary blood flow is normal or increased |
| III | 10 | Pulmonary artery arises from sides of truncus arteriosus; pulmonary blood flow is normal or increased |
| IV | 10 | Bronchial arteries arise from descending aorta to supply lungs; pulmonary blood flow may be decreased |

MPA, main pulmonary artery.

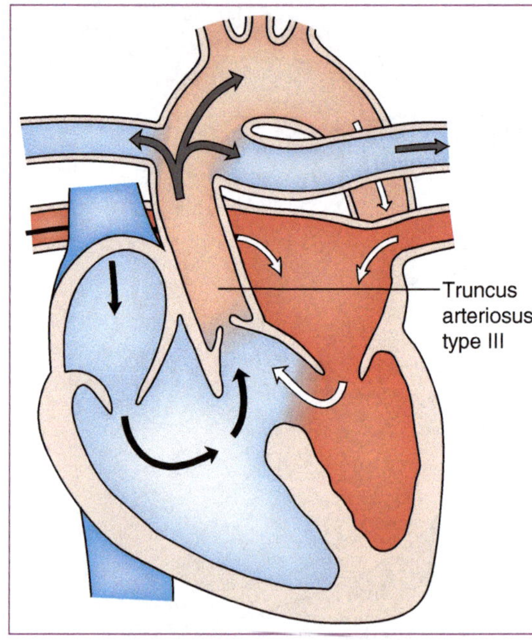


**FIGURE 7.15 The truncus arteriosus is a single arterial vessel that gives rise to the coronary arteries, pulmonary arteries, and aorta.**

*Source:* Adapted and modified from Ross Laboratories, Columbus, OH, Clinical Education Aid, 1985.

VSD. The amount of flow to the pulmonary and systemic circulations depends on the resistance of the two circulations. Pulmonary vascular resistance is high at birth, so pulmonary and systemic flows are relatively equal initially. Pulmonary resistance gradually decreases, causing increased pulmonary blood flow. CHF may develop because of increased pulmonary blood flow and there may be associated inadequate systemic perfusion. If not corrected early, over time, pulmonary vascular disease develops in response to increased pulmonary blood flow; subsequently, pulmonary blood flow decreases because of development of increased pulmonary vascular resistance. These changes, although compensatory initially, complicate the hemodynamics with increased risk for pulmonary hypertension in the postoperative period. The volume overload can also be compounded by incompetent truncal valves that allow regurgitation of blood into the ventricles.

## Manifestations

If truncus arteriosus is not prenatally diagnosed, it typically will be detected in the newborn period because of a murmur, cyanosis, symptoms of poor feeding, and signs of CHF; or it may be detected on CCHD pulse oximetry screening. The presence of cyanosis depends on the amount of pulmonary blood flow, and signs of CHF due to increased pulmonary blood flow may be the first indication of truncus arteriosus. On auscultation, $S_2$ is single and there may be a systolic click at the apex and upper LSB. A murmur may be auscultated if there is truncal stenosis or insufficiency. Truncal valve insufficiency produces a high-pitched, early diastolic decrescendo murmur. There may be bounding arterial pulses and a widened pulse pressure. The right upper oxygen saturation and lower right and left oxygen saturations will be similar and less than 95%.

## Diagnosis

On chest radiograph, the heart size is increased, and pulmonary blood flow may be increased. Thirty-five percent of cases have a right aortic arch, and this finding increases the risk of deletion of 22q11. ECG reveals a normal QRS axis and ventricular hypertrophy. Echocardiography demonstrates the presence of a single common arterial truncal valve overriding a large VSD and further details of the type of truncus with location of the pulmonary arteries, presence of truncal stenosis/insufficiency, additional VSDs, and arch sidedness (Park & Salamat, 2022).

## Management

Medical management consists primarily of treatment of CHF. Current surgical correction consists of complete primary repair, with closure of the VSD, committing the common arterial trunk to the LV, and reconstruction of the RVOT with a conduit from the RV to the branch pulmonary arteries (Park, 2014). The definitive surgical correction is the Rastelli procedure (see Table 7.7 for a description of common surgical procedures). Surgery is typically performed in the first week of life. The aggregate surgical mortality rate for truncus is 10.1%. Repeat surgery typically is required to enlarge the conduit as growth occurs (Jacobs et al., 2018; Park & Salamat, 2022).

## Congenital Arrhythmias

Cardiac arrhythmias in infants generally arise from primary cardiac lesions as a result of abnormal conduction pathways. Alternatively, cardiac arrhythmias can develop following cardiac surgical palliation or repair. It is not clear whether the arrhythmia is secondary to the cardiac lesion or the surgical procedure. Some arrhythmias are a result of electrolyte imbalances, neurologic conditions, or infections. Generally, in infants, rhythm disturbances are not the primary manifestation of a cardiac problem. CHF or cyanosis may be present before dysrhythmias occur. Some conditions present with rhythm disturbances in the newborn period. The most commonly occurring include congenital complete heart block (CCHB) and supraventricular tachycardia (SVT). These two arrhythmias are discussed in more detail.

## Congenital Complete Heart Block

The AV node and the bundle of His arise as separate structures that join. CCHB is a result of a discontinuity between the atrial conduction pathway and the AV node, or the bundle of His and the AV node. One risk factor for CCHB is exposure to SSA and SSB antibodies in utero due to maternal systemic lupus erythematosus (SLE). In most cases, the heart structure is normal and the etiology of CCHB is unknown. Congenital heart block can also be a manifestation of CHDs, including congenitally corrected TGA or *L*-TGA.

Prenatally, CCHB can be detected by fetal bradycardia (HR < 100 beats/min) on auscultation, electronic monitoring, or screening ultrasound. Fetal echocardiography is diagnostic with identification of AV dissociation with atrial rate faster and not associated with the slower ventricular rate by M-mode, and spectral Doppler techniques of the inflow and outflow of the heart (O'Connor & Shah, 2012).

### Treatment

Asymptomatic neonates do not require treatment. If the neonate has inadequate systemic perfusion due to the bradycardia, then insertion of a pacemaker may be required. Children with implanted pacemakers need close follow-up (Valente et al., 2022).

## Supraventricular Tachycardia

SVT can arise in utero or in the neonatal period. The most common arrhythmias that produce signs are paroxysmal SVT with or without ventricular preexcitation, atrial flutter, and junctional tachycardia. If the SVT occurs in utero, it can lead to heart failure and hydrops fetalis. SVT treatment depends on gestational age of the fetus, the type of SVT, whether it is intermittent or persistent, and the presence of CHF and/or hydrops. SVT treatment in the fetus depends on the presence or absence of hydrops. If the fetus is near term, then delivery with postnatal treatment may be the management strategy. If the patient is not near term, then the medication regimen depends on the type of SVT and presence or absence of hydrops. In paroxysmal SVT without hydrops, digoxin, flecainide, or sotalol may be used as first-line therapy. If first-line therapy is not successful, then combination therapy will be used (O'Connor & Shah, 2012).

In most cases of SVT, no cause is found. Ebstein anomaly of the TV can be the cause in some cases. Ten to fifty percent of infants with SVT have Wolf-Parkinson-White (WPW) syndrome, in which the atrial impulse activates the whole or some part of the ventricle, or the ventricular impulse activates the whole or some part of the atrium earlier than would be expected if the impulse traveled via the normal pathway. WPW is characterized by a normal QRS with regular rhythm and ventricular rates of 150 to 200 beats/min (Olgin & Zipes, 2012).

Symptoms produced by SVT after birth are subtle and often undetected until signs of CHF develop. Medical management typically begins with vagal maneuvers; elicitation of a diving reflex by covering the face with a cold washcloth for 4 to 5 seconds is generally successful in establishing normal sinus rhythm. If this approach is unsuccessful, then IV adenosine is attempted, typically resulting in cardioversion to sinus rhythm. A baseline 12-lead ECG is required to document presence of delta waves consistent with WPW, because it will determine the medical management and medication therapy used. Propranolol is a common medical therapy used, particularly if WPW is diagnosed. In some centers, digoxin therapy may be utilized for SVT when WPW has been ruled out. Infants are followed closely for breakthrough SVT episodes; if no further SVT is documented, then at 1 year of age medical therapy is discontinued with close follow-up to monitor for SVT recurrence. Because recurrence is more likely in WPW, these infants typically will be maintained on beta-blocker therapy.

Recurrence decreases between ages 2 and 10 years of age. Prognosis for SVT is good (Valente et al., 2022).

## Congestive Heart Failure

CHF is a condition in which the blood supply to the body is insufficient to meet the metabolic requirements of the organs. CHF is a manifestation of an underlying disease or defect, rather than a disease itself. Compensatory mechanisms are activated to maintain adequate CO before signs CHF appear (Park & Salamat, 2022). Normal mechanisms for regulation of CO are listed in Box 7.2. CHF is classified according to the cause. Box 7.3 shows common causes of CHF in newborns.

Increased volume may be caused by fluid overload or fluid retention. In the normally functioning myocardium, fluid retention does not cause CHF; however, fluid retention complicates CHF from other causes. In neonates, the most common cause of increased volume is CHD or altered hemodynamics, as in PDA.

CHF caused by obstruction to outflow occurs when the normal myocardium pumps against increased resistance. This increased resistance may be caused by structural defects, such as valvular stenosis or COA, or by pulmonary disease and/or pulmonary hypertension. CHF caused by pulmonary disease is called *cor pulmonale*. Severe systemic hypertension can also cause increased systemic vascular resistance.

CHF in the neonate usually results from abnormal stresses placed on the heart rather than from an ineffective myocardium. However, electrolyte imbalances, acidosis, and myocardial ischemia affect the ability of the heart to function effectively. Conditions such as rheumatic fever, infectious

**BOX 7.2**

**MECHANISMS OF CARDIAC OUTPUT REGULATION**

**Sympathetic Nervous System Activated By:**

Vasomotor center through peripheral sympathetic fibers

Secretion of norepinephrine from adrenal medullary "fight-or-flight" response

Symptoms

Characterized by tachycardia, increased contractility, peripheral vasoconstriction, pupil dilation.

**Parasympathetic Nervous System Activated By:**

Vagal fibers

- Atrial stimulation causes decreased heart rate.
- Ventricular stimulation causes decreased contractility.

Baroreceptor reflexes

Located in walls of carotid sinuses and in aortic arch

Pressure receptors stimulated by blood pressure

Results

Stimulation causes inhibition of the sympathetic portion of the vasomotor center and stimulation of the parasympathetic (vagal) center; decreased arterial blood pressure

**BOX 7.3**

**CAUSES OF CONGESTIVE HEART FAILURE IN THE NEWBORN**

**Noncardiac causes of congestive heart failure:**

Sepsis

Anemia

Polycythemia

Metabolic diseases (Pompe disease)

Multiple hemangiomas

Arteriovenous malformations (cranial, hepatic, abdominal)

Hyperthyroidism

Hypoglycemia

Hypocalcemia

Renal failure

Severe systemic hypertension

**Congenital heart defects:**

Hypoplastic left heart syndrome

Interrupted aortic arch

Coarctation of the aorta

Total anomalous pulmonary venous return with obstruction

Transposition of the great arteries

PDA (in preterm infants)

**Other cardiac causes:**

Myocarditis

Arrhythmias

Anomalous left coronary artery from the pulmonary artery

myocarditis, Kawasaki disease with myocarditis, and anomalous origin of the left coronary artery from the pulmonary artery may reduce the effectiveness of the heart function.

Arrhythmias that may produce CHF include complete AV block or sustained atrial or ventricular tachycardia. AVs block results in a severe bradycardia that prohibits adequate circulation of blood. Tachycardia causes insufficient time for ventricular filling, decreasing CO and leading to cardiac dysfunction over time.

Severe anemia can cause CHF because of excessive demand for CO. Because the oxygen-carrying capacity of the blood is diminished, the heart must pump more blood per minute to meet the tissue oxygenation requirements. If the heart cannot meet the excessive demand, CHF develops (Park, 2014).

Compensatory mechanisms function to meet the body's increased demand for CO. These mechanisms are regulated by the sympathetic nervous system and mechanical factors. The compensatory mechanisms can sustain adequate CO for only a short period of time. If the underlying condition is not corrected, CHF develops.

### Sympathetic Nervous System Compensatory Mechanisms

Decreased blood pressure stimulates vascular stretch receptors and baroreceptors in the aorta and carotid arteries that trigger the sympathetic nervous system. Decreased systemic blood pressure stimulates baroreceptors, causing (1) increased sympathetic stimulation, (2) increased HR, (3) increased cardiac contractility, and (4) increased arterial blood pressure. Catecholamine release and beta-receptor stimulation increase the rate and force of myocardial contraction. Catecholamines also increase venous tone, so that blood is returned to the heart more effectively. Circulation to the skin, kidneys, extremities, and splanchnic bed is decreased, allowing better circulation to the brain, heart, and lungs. Decreased renal blood flow stimulates the release of renin, angiotensin, and aldosterone. This release causes retention of sodium and fluid, resulting in increased circulating volume. The increased volume puts additional work on the heart.

### Mechanical Compensatory Mechanisms

The heart muscle thickens to increase myocardial pressure. The hypertrophy is effective in the early stages, but as soon as the muscle mass increases, compliance decreases. This change in compliance requires greater filling pressure to maintain adequate CO. The hypertrophied heart eventually becomes ischemic because it does not receive adequate oxygenation to meet its metabolic needs. Ventricular dilation occurs as myocardial fibers stretch to accommodate heart volume. Initially, this increases the force of the contraction, but it too fails after a certain threshold point.

### Effects of Congestive Heart Failure

When the RV is unable to pump blood into the pulmonary artery, the lungs oxygenate less blood, there is increased pressure in the RA and systemic venous circulation, and edema occurs in the extremities and viscera. When the LV is unable to pump blood into the systemic circulation, there is increased pressure in the LA and pulmonary veins. The lungs become congested with blood, causing elevated pulmonary pressures and pulmonary edema.

The end effects of CHF include decreased CO, decreased renal perfusion, systemic venous engorgement, and pulmonary venous engorgement and their consequent effects. Decreased CO stimulates the sympathetic nervous system, causing tachycardia, increased contractility, increased vasomotor tone, peripheral vasoconstriction, and diaphoresis. Decreased renal perfusion stimulates the renin-angiotensin-aldosterone mechanism, causing sodium and water retention. Systemic venous engorgement leads to hepatomegaly, jugular venous distention, periorbital and facial edema, and, occasionally, ascites and dependent edema. Pulmonary venous engorgement results in tachypnea, decreased tidal volume, decreased lung compliance, increased airway resistance, early closure of the small airways with air trapping, increased work of breathing, and increased respiratory effort, grunting, and rales. Stimulation of the j-receptors in the lungs causes infants to become apprehensive and irritable.

### Diagnosis

The diagnosis of CHF is based on clinical signs and symptoms, laboratory data, and chest radiography with definitive diagnosis by echocardiography. In contrast to infants with cyanotic heart disease, infants with CHF usually have significant respiratory distress with tachypnea, grunting, and retractions. They exhibit peripheral pallor, appearing to be ashen or gray in color. The precordium is hyperdynamic, and there are usually loud murmurs heard throughout systole and diastole. Pulses are usually full, but there may be a difference between the upper and the lower extremities. Hepatomegaly is common. Infants demonstrate signs of irritability because of the increased effort of breathing and air hunger.

In addition to demonstrating hypoxemia, ABG may reveal metabolic acidosis resulting from the decreased systemic blood flow. If acidosis is severe, there may be concurrent respiratory acidosis because of the pulmonary edema caused by left-sided heart failure. Pulmonary ventilation–perfusion mismatch may cause hypoxemia. Hypocalcemia is often present in infants with CHF because they have an inappropriate response to stress. In addition, infants with deletion of 22q11 may have hypocalcemia because of absent parathyroids. Conotruncal anomalies such as TOF and truncus arteriosus along with interrupted aortic arch are CHDs that are commonly associated with deletion of 22q11 (Park, 2014).

Hypoglycemia may be present in infants with severe CHF. The myocardium depends on glucose; decreased glucose levels diminish the ability of the heart to compensate for CHF. On chest radiograph, the heart is enlarged and there is increased pulmonary congestion. ECG is not generally diagnostic, unless the CHF is caused by an arrhythmia. There may be nonspecific changes in the T waves, changes in the ST segment, and an increase in the height of the P wave.

Electrolyte imbalances usually include relative hyponatremia due to increased free water. Hypochloremia and increased bicarbonate may result from respiratory acidemia and the use of loop diuretics. Hyperkalemia results from the release of intracellular cations related to poor tissue perfusion. Elevated lactic acid levels are also indicative of tissue hypoxia. Atrial natriuretic factor (ANF), a peptide hormone, may be important in the regulation of volume and blood pressure. ANF is released from the atria when they are distended. ANF release causes natriuresis, diuresis, and vasodilation. ANF acts with other volume regulators, such as renin, aldosterone, and vasopressin. An increased ANF level may be found when there is increased pulmonary blood flow, increased left atrial pressure, or pulmonary hypertension.

### Treatment

The goal of management of CHF is to improve cardiac function while identifying and correcting the underlying cause. General measures that decrease the demand on the heart are helpful; however, pharmacologic intervention is the most efficacious therapy.

### General Measures

General measures to manage CHF in infants with structurally normal hearts include the administration of oxygen to improve ventilation and perfusion at the alveolar level. Ventilation with positive end-expiratory pressure (PEEP) at 6 to 10 cm/$H_2O$ may relieve the effects of CHF by reducing pulmonary edema.

Fluid restriction may decrease the circulating volume. Careful monitoring of serum electrolytes, BUN/Cr, intake and output, and weight is essential. It is imperative that *all* fluids be counted in the total daily fluid volume. Infants with CHF do not usually feed well and may require caloric supplementation with hyperalimentation or gavage feedings (Park, 2014).

Infants with CHF are irritable and agitated, further complicating their hemodynamic status. Sedation with continuous infusions of morphine sulfate or fentanyl may improve the infant's comfort level and oxygenation by decreasing metabolic demand. Other measures that reduce metabolic oxygen demand include maintenance of a normal hematocrit, maintenance of a thermoneutral environment, and minimal stimulation (Verklan et al., 2020).

### Pharmacologic Interventions

Table 7.9 lists the medications most used in the management of cardiac conditions. Medical management of CHF *beyond* the neonatal period includes use of ACE inhibitors, diuretics, nonspecific beta blockers (carvedilol), and/or digitalis (digoxin). Digoxin slows conduction through the AV node, prolongs the refractory period, and slows the HR through vagal effects on the SA node.

The use of digoxin in preterm or term neonates is controversial. The preterm newborn is at risk for digitalis toxicity because of the narrow range between therapeutic and toxic drug levels. The preterm infant requires a lower maintenance dose because of limited renal excretion of the drug (Table 7.10).

## TABLE 7.9

### DRUGS USED IN THE MANAGEMENT OF CONGENITAL HEART DEFECTS

| Drug | Dosage | Action | Onset | Comments |
|---|---|---|---|---|
| ***Diuretics*** | | | | |
| Furosemide (Lasix) | 0.5–1 mg/kg/dose IV | Loop diuretic; inhibits sodium and chloride reabsorption in proximal tubule | 15–30 minutes | Associated with increased calcium loss |
| Furosemide (Lasix) | 1–3 mg/kg/dose PO | | 30–60 minutes | |
| Spironolactone (Aldactone) | 1.5–3.0 mg/kg/dose PO | Competitive antagonist of aldosterone | 3–5 days | Potassium sparing |
| Chlorothiazide | 20–40 mg/kg/d PO | Inhibits sodium and chloride reabsorption along the distal tubules | 1–2 hours | |
| ***Inotropic Agents*** | | | | |
| Dopamine | Low: 2–5 mcg/kg/min | Increased renal blood flow; beta-adrenergic effects | | Monitor ECG; BP |
| | Mod: 5–10 mcg/kg/min | Increased renal blood flow; HR, BP, and contractility | | |
| | High: 10–20 mcg/kg/min | Peripheral vasoconstriction, increased HR, and contractility | | |
| Dobutamine | 2–10 mcg/kg/min | Increased renal blood flow; increased contractility | Rapid | Decreased systemic vascular resistance; increased pulmonary wedge pressure |
| Isoproterenol | 0.05–0.5 mg/kg/min | Increased venous return to heart and decreased pulmonary vascular resistance | | Tachycardia, dysrhythmias, decreased renal perfusion |
| ***Prostaglandins*** | | | | |
| $PGE_1$ | 0.01–0.1 mg/kg/min | Produces vasodilation and smooth muscle relaxation of DA and pulmonary and systemic circulations; increased arterial saturation by 25%–100% | Rapid | Monitor BP; vasopressors may be required; apnea, flush, fever, seizure-like activity; decreased HR |
| ***Prostaglandin Synthetase Inhibitors*** | | | | |
| Indomethacin | 0.2 mg/kg IV (1st) q 24 h | Promotes ductal closure by inhibition of $PGE_2$ in the walls of the ductus | 12–24 hours | Monitor renal function, bilirubin, electrolytes, glucose, platelets, bleeding |
| | 0.1 mg/kg IV (2nd and 3rd) | | | |
| | > 48 hours and < 14 days: 0.3 mg/kg IV and 3 doses q 24 h | | | |
| | > 14 days and < 6 weeks: 0.2–0.3 mg/kg q 12 h | | | |

BP, blood pressure; DA, ductus arteriosus; ECG, electrocardiogram; HR, heart rate; IV, intravenously; $PGE_1$, prostaglandin $E_1$; $PGE_2$, prostaglandin $E_2$; PO, by mouth; q, every.

**TABLE 7.10**

**DIGOXIN PRESCRIPTION INFORMATION**

| | TDD (mg/kg) | Maintenance Dose (mg/kg/d) |
|---|---|---|
| Preterm | 0.025–0.05 | 0.008–0.012 |
| Term | 0.04–0.08 | 0.01–0.02 (1/8 TDD) |

To digitalize:
1. Give 1/2 TDD
2. 6–8 hours later, give 1/4 TDD
3. 6–8 hours later, get a rhythm strip; if normal, give 1/4 TDD.
4. Give maintenance dose (1/8 TDD) 12 hours after last digitalizing dose and then every 12 hours.

Slow digitalization, with decreased risk of toxicity, can be achieved by starting with the maintenance dose.

TDD, total digitalizing dose.

If digoxin is used, the neonate must be carefully monitored for signs and symptoms of digitalis toxicity. Lead II ECGs should be obtained before each dose for the first 3 days; the dose should be withheld if the PR interval is greater than 0.16 second or if there is an arrhythmia present. Digoxin levels should be monitored and should be less than 2.0 ng/ml (Park, 2014). Blood samples for digoxin levels should be drawn after the drug has achieved equilibrium in the body, approximately 6 to 8 hours after administration.

Other inotropic agents can be used to improve CO. Dopamine, a norepinephrine precursor, has direct and indirect dose-dependent beta-adrenergic effects. At low doses (2–5 mcg/kg/min), there is increased renal blood flow with minimal effect on HR, blood pressure, or contractility. Medium doses (5–10 mcg/kg/min) increase renal blood flow, HR, blood pressure, and contractility. Pulmonary artery pressure may be increased; peripheral resistance is not affected. High doses (10–20 mcg/kg/min) cause peripheral vasoconstriction, increased cardiac rate, and increased contractility (Park, 2014).

Dobutamine is a synthetic catecholamine that acts on beta- and alpha-adrenergic receptors. Dobutamine (2–10 mcg/min) has decreased effect on the HR and rhythm and causes less peripheral vasoconstriction.

**Emergency Alert: Isoproterenol (Isuprel), a synthetic epinephrine-like substance, has beta-1 and beta-2 adrenergic effects. The usefulness of Isuprel in the neonate is limited because it produces increased HR, arrhythmias, and decreased systemic vascular resistance, which may worsen the hypotension** (Park & Salamat, 2022).

### Diuretics

Diuretics are useful in the treatment of CHF to decrease sodium and water retention. The primary goal is to increase renal perfusion (with inotropic agents or vasodilators) and to increase sodium delivery to distal diluting sites of the renal tubules. Diuretic agents increase the renal excretion of sodium and other anions by inhibition of tubular reabsorption of sodium (Park & Salamat, 2022).

Furosemide, a loop diuretic, blocks sodium and chloride reabsorption in the ascending limb of the loop of Henle. Loop diuretics interfere with the formation of free water and free water reabsorption by preventing the transport of sodium, potassium, and chloride into the medullary interstitium. Loop diuretics cause increased excretion of potassium by delivering increased quantities of sodium to sites in the distal nephron where potassium can be excreted. Furosemide also increases excretion of calcium but does not affect the ability of the kidney to regulate acid–base balance.

An aldosterone antagonist such as spironolactone may be used because it is a potassium-sparing diuretic. Spironolactone works by binding to the cytoplasmic receptor sites and blocking aldosterone action, thus impairing the reabsorption of sodium and the secretion of potassium and hydrogen ion. Spironolactone has no effect on free water production and absorption. Thiazide diuretics (chlorothiazide and hydrochlorothiazide) inhibit sodium and chloride reabsorption along the distal tubules. They are not as effective as the loop diuretics and are infrequently used (Park, 2014).

### Complications of Diuretic Therapy

Diuretic therapy can cause severe electrolyte imbalances if they are not monitored carefully. The complications of diuretic therapy include (1) volume contraction, (2) hyponatremia, (3) metabolic alkalemia or acidemia, and (4) hypokalemia or hyperkalemia. When using diuretics, fluid and electrolyte balance must be maintained by the administration of water and electrolytes. The adequacy of the volume can be determined by monitoring serum electrolytes, BUN, Cr, urinary output, weight, specific gravity, and skin turgor.

The increased renal losses of sodium can lead to hyponatremia unless adequate amounts of sodium are provided. There may also be increased antidiuretic hormone (ADH) release secondary to changes in the osmoreceptors or inhibition of ADH action. Decreasing the amount of total water and improving the CO, thus increasing renal perfusion, can best manage this.

Metabolic alkalosis can result from administration of loop diuretics that interfere with sodium- and potassium-dependent chloride reabsorption. Hypochloremia results in a greater aldosterone production and an increase in bicarbonate concentration. Hypokalemia is a frequent complication of loop diuretic therapy. An increased ratio of intracellular to extracellular potassium results in the clinical signs and symptoms of hypokalemia. **Emergency Alert: Hypokalemia increases the risk for digoxin toxicity.** In contrast, hyperkalemia may result when CO is low and tissue perfusion is severely compromised. Other complications of diuretic therapy include increased calcium excretion, hyperuricemia, and glucose intolerance.

## Subacute Bacterial Infective Endocarditis

Subacute bacterial infective endocarditis (SBIE) can be a complication in certain high-risk CHD patients. Two factors are important in the development of SBIE: (1) certain structural abnormalities that create turbulent flow or pressure gradients resulting in endothelial damage and (2) bacteremia. Certain CHDs and acquired heart disease with turbulent flow or a significant pressure gradient result in trauma to the endothelial lining, predisposing the endothelium to deposition of platelets and fibrin resulting in nonbacterial thrombotic endocarditis. If certain microbial species with pathogenic potential enter the bloodstream, there is potential to cause infective endocarditis at that site. Previously, more than 90% of infective endocarditis was due to *Streptococcus viridians, Streptococcus faecalis* (enterococcus), and *Staphylococcus aureus* but these organisms now only account for 50% to 60% of the cases, while fungi and *Haemophilus influenzae, Aggregatibacter, Cardiobacterium, Eikenella,* and *Kingella spp.* organisms have increased. *Haemophilus influenzae, Aggregatibacter, Cardiobacterium, Eikenella,* and *Kingella spp.* organisms account for 17% to 30% of the cases in neonates and immunocompromised children (Park & Salamat, 2022).

### Prevention

Based on the 2007 American Heart Association guidelines, prevention of bacterial SBIE requires scrupulous daily oral care along with minimizing dental disease to decrease frequency of bacteremia in routine daily activities. SBIE prophylaxis is recommended for CHD patients considered at high risk for an adverse outcome (Box 7.4) with the following procedures: (1) all dental procedures; (2) respiratory tract procedures not including bronchoscopy; and (3) procedures involving infected skin, skin structures, or musculoskeletal tissue.

**BOX 7.4**

**CARDIAC CONDITIONS FOR WHICH SUBACUTE BACTERIAL INFECTIVE ENDOCARDITIS PROPHYLAXIS IS RECOMMENDED**

1. Prosthetic cardiac valve or prosthetic material used for cardiac valve repair
2. Previous history of infective endocarditis
3. CHD
   - Unrepaired cyanotic CHD including palliative shunts and conduits
   - Unrepaired CHD with prosthetic material or device whether placed by surgery or cardiac catheterization during the first 6 months after the procedure
   - Repaired CHD with a residual defect at the site or adjacent to a prosthetic patch or device (that inhibits endothelialization)
4. Cardiac transplant recipient who developed cardiac valvulopathy CHD, congenital heart disease.

*Source:* Adapted from Wilson, W., Taubert, K. A., Gewitz, M., Lockhart, P. B., Baddour, L. M., Levison, M., Bolger, A., Cabell, C. H., Takahashi, M., Baltimore, R. S., Newburger, J. W., Strom, B. L., Tani, L. Y., Gerber, M., Bonow, R. O., Pallasch, T., Shulman, S. T., Rowley, A. H., Burns, J. C., ... and Durack, D. T. The Council on Scientific Affairs of the American Dental Association has approved the guideline as it relates to dentistry. In addition, this guideline has been endorsed by the American Academy of Pediatrics, Infectious Diseases Society of America, the International Society of Chemotherapy for Infection and Cancer, and the Pediatric Infectious Diseases Society. (2007). Prevention of infective endocarditis: Guidelines from the American Heart Association: A guideline from the American Heart Association Rheumatic Fever, Endocarditis, and Kawasaki Disease Committee, Council on Cardiovascular Disease in the Young, and the Council on Clinical Cardiology, Council on Cardiovascular Surgery and Anesthesia, and the Quality of Care and Outcomes Research Interdisciplinary Working Group. *Circulation, 116*(15), 1736–1754. https:doi .org/10.1161/CIRCULATIONAHA.106.183095.

## NEURODEVELOPMENTAL DISABILITIES IN CONGENITAL HEART DEFECT

Over 50% of CHD patients are at risk for ND problems, including mild learning disabilities, attention deficit disorder, and speech and motor problems. Children with HLHS and *d*-TGA have been the most widely studied cohort, and at least 50% of these patients are affected by ND issues that significantly effect their academic achievement and quality of life. Several studies have demonstrated that 17% to 40% of neonates with complex CHD have evidence of periventricular leukomalacia (PVL) on preoperative MRI, whereas 50% had evidence of PVL on postoperative MRI. White matter injury or PVL has been associated with ND problems and impaired functional outcomes in very low birthweight (VLBW) and preterm neonates. By the time CHD patients reach school age, there are notable deficiencies in fine and gross motor functions, tests of intelligence and achievement, speech, language, and behavior (Marelli et al., 2016; Marino et al., 2012).

## FAMILY SUPPORT

Families of infants who are critically ill or have congenital defects generally experience confusion, guilt, anger, and fear. The family must cope with short- and long-term consequences of the CHD. Severity of the defect, availability of treatment, and prognosis influence the amount and type of support required. Parents may be overwhelmed by the knowledge of their infant's heart defect, regardless of the severity. The effect of the cardiac defect on other systems must also be included when giving parents information. Although often overlooked, neurologic prognosis is a key factor in determining the overall quality of life of a child with a CHD. Early interventions and therapies are critical to improve patient developmental outcomes, particularly when patients are at risk for ND deficiencies. Parents need frequent contact with members of the healthcare team. Caretakers should speak with parents routinely, not just when there are major changes in the infant's condition.

Although most CHDs do not have an identifiable genetic pattern, genetic counseling should be offered to all parents with a newborn with a CHD. Parents will want answers to questions about the cause of the defect and the danger of a recurrence. Although most congenital heart defects (CHDs) can be identified during the 18-to 20-week anatomy scan, nearly 90% can be detected prenatally when both the four-chamber and outflow tract views are adequately visualized (Sklansky et al., 2009) in many regions of the United States, less than 50% of CHD is detected prenatally (Quartermain et al., 2015). Healthcare professionals must be keenly aware of all options to ensure that parents receive the most up-to-date information on which to base decisions.

One of the defect diagrams and models illustrating the defect should be used. Parents need frequent reassurance and repetition of information. Parents of infants who do not require immediate surgery but who will eventually require surgical correction must be educated about all aspects of the infant's care, including signs and symptoms of deterioration, medication administration, activity limitations, and normal development. Because growth failure with a cardiac defect is common, efforts to maximize nutrition are important. Careful follow-up is important to prevent complications.

Identification of support persons for the family is extremely valuable. Parents may be encouraged to talk to other parents of newborns with the same or similar defects. Many neonatal intensive care units (NICUs) have active support groups consisting of parents of patients. Care should be taken in selection of supporters. Parents with a term newborn with a CHD may not be able to relate to parents of a preterm neonate. Other family members or friends should not be overlooked; they can become valuable support persons if they are provided appropriate guidance and education. The needs of siblings should also be assessed. Siblings need support, education, and guidance appropriate for their age and comprehension of the situation. Parents may not recognize their needs because of the overwhelming situation. Healthcare providers can facilitate the parent–child relationship during the initial period and throughout the course of the management.

Financial resources should be addressed because preoperative, operative, and postoperative care is expensive. Many parents need assistance in obtaining aid to which they are entitled. Even the most knowledgeable of parents may not be aware of resources available to them. If experimental surgery is contemplated, parents may need assistance speaking to private insurance companies regarding coverage. Referrals to appropriate local, state, federal, or private organizations that pertain to the CHD should be made for the parents. These include the Department of Family and Children Services, the March of Dimes, and Children's Medical Services. The family may qualify for the Special Supplemental Nutrition Program for Women, Infants, and Children.

Discharge planning must be comprehensive for the neonate who will receive medical management for a CHD before corrective surgery. A thorough assessment of the home may be needed before discharge. Contact with the primary care provider who will perform the routine management of the infant is imperative. Initial contact by telephone should be followed up with a copy of the complete medical record and discharge summary. If the infant requires any special equipment for home care, the equipment should be obtained before discharge so that the parents can be taught how to use it. Also, practical details such as whether there are enough electrical outlets in the infant's room must be determined. Notification of local emergency medical services, power companies, and other relevant companies should be completed before discharge.

## SUMMARY

The most common CHD lesions are reviewed along with the most common arrhythmias seen in the newborn. The diagnosis and management of the most frequent complications of CHDs, CHF, and recommendations of SBIE are included. Parental support of families with newborns and children with CHDs has been discussed.

## CASE STUDY

The NICU in a large women and children's hospital received a call for assistance from the adjacent Mother and Baby Unit to evaluate an infant for cyanosis. The nurse responded to the call and discovered that the infant was pale, cyanotic, and tachypneic. The nurse positioned the infant for optimal oxygenation and supplied oxygen via blow-by. The infant responded to the blow-by oxygen with improved color and tone. The nurse informed the infant's mother that the infant would be taken to the NICU for further evaluation and assured the mother of an update as soon as possible. In the NICU, the infant's pediatrician was called, and the birth history was obtained from the medical record supplied by the Mother and Baby Unit personnel. The infant was put in an oxyhood, and vital signs were obtained. The infant was now pink, HR was 164, respiratory rate was 76, and the mean blood pressure was 58.

The infant was born to a gravida 1, para 0 (now 1), 24-year-old mother with uncomplicated pregnancy and delivery. Birthweight was 3.3 kg, and Apgar scores were 8/9 (−1 color, −1 tone, −1 color). The infant showed no distress, and the pediatrician's examination at 3 hours postbirth was within normal limits, with some slight acrocyanosis of the hands and feet present. The infant had been in the Mother and Baby Unit and the mother was nursing. At this feeding, the mother had offered the baby a bottle following nursing. The mother called the floor nurse because the infant seemed to turn blue during the feeding.

Upon auscultation, a soft ejection-type murmur was noted at the upper LSB. Right radial ABG showed a partially compensated metabolic acidosis on 70% $F_IO_2$ per hood. The pulse oximeter registered an oxygen saturation of 58% on arms and legs. A hyperoxia test using 100% $F_IO_2$ showed no improvement in arterial oxygenation. The cardiac murmur had increased and was determined to be systolic in origin, and probably TR. Chest x-ray showed normal heart size and decreased pulmonary markings. A stat echocardiogram was ordered to determine whether a cardiac defect was present.

1. What other intervention should be initiated while the definitive diagnosis is being obtained?
2. What are the most likely cardiac defects with this presentation?
3. How does the timing of the episode influence the differential diagnosis?
4. What is the general management for PA/IVS?
5. What information should be shared with the parents regarding short- and long-term treatment and prognosis?

## EVIDENCE-BASED PRACTICE

### Screening for Critical Congenital Heart Defects with Pulse Oximetry

The overall incidence of CHD is slightly less than 1%, or eight per 1,000 live births, excluding PDA in the preterm newborn, which is the single largest factor for infant mortality due to all birth defects. CHDs that usually cause hypoxia in the newborn period and are associated with the highest mortality are classified as CCHDs. Newborns with CCHDs require immediate intervention to prevent death or disability.

Seven cardiac defects make up the CCHDs: HLHS, PA/IVS, TOF, TAPVR, TGA, tricuspid atresia, and truncus arteriosus. Approximately 4,800 babies are born each year in the United States with one of these seven CCHDs.

Delayed diagnosis of any of these defects significantly increases the risk for morbidity or mortality. Currently, diagnosis depends on prenatal ultrasound identification or physical examination of the newborn. This approach does not identify all defects, and so it leads to late diagnosis and increased morbidity and sometimes mortality. Methods that allow earlier identification of these cardiac defects would lead to quicker diagnosis, implementation of treatment, and improved outcome.

Routine screening of newborns with pulse oximetry was proposed as one method to improve early diagnosis of CCHDs. Pulse oximetry is a noninvasive, painless, relatively inexpensive, and readily available method that measures blood oxygen saturation. Most CCHDs are associated with hypoxia, and thus pulse oximetry screening could identify newborns with one of these defects. Numerous studies were conducted in the United States and in other countries, including Sweden and Germany, to determine whether routine pulse oximetry measurements on newborns improved the detection of CCHDs.

The U.S. Health and Human Services Secretary convened a group of experts to examine evidence of the effectiveness of pulse oximetry screening. The group consisted of members recommended by the Secretary's Advisory Committee on Heritable Diseases in Newborns and Children, the American Academy of Pediatrics (AAP), the American College of Cardiology Foundation, and the American Heart Association. The work group found sufficient evidence to recommend routine screening with pulse oximetry monitoring to identify low blood oxygen saturation in newborns in well-infant and intermediate nurseries. They recommended further study for screening of special populations, such as those who live in high altitudes.

Based on this review of the evidence, Secretary of Health and Human Services Kathleen Sebelius recommended the addition of pulse oximetry screening for CCHD in newborns in 2011. This recommendation was officially endorsed by the AAP. Most hospitals have adopted this screening method; however, there are differences in the screening process, in the number and type of conditions that are screened for in each state, and in the data collection to review efficacy of the program. As of 2015, most states have introduced or passed legislation to add pulse oximetry screening to the current newborn screening, but not all states have mandated pulse oximetry screening and data reporting. Many hospitals have implemented the screening process and have organized reporting voluntarily. This is an example of evidence-based practice change.

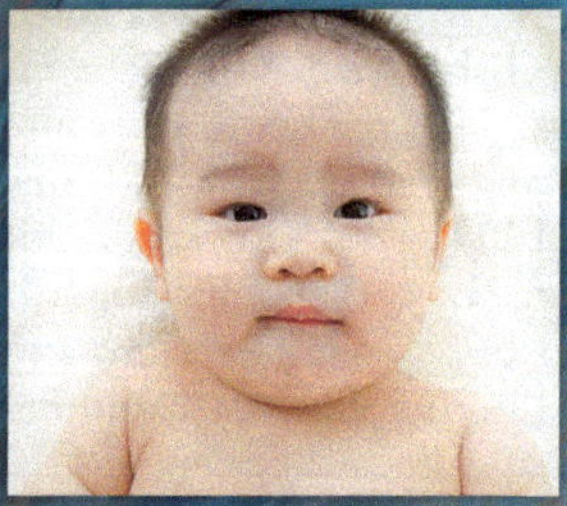

*Source:* WONG SZE FEI/Adobe Stock.

## PARENT VOICES

### Farrin Moreno

**My micropreemie was born at 25 weeks' gestational age. The doctors told me she had 0% chance of survival. In fact, while hospitalized for 6 weeks on strict bed rest leading up to her birth, my doctor tirelessly tried convincing me to terminate my pregnancy. My daughter weighed 1 lb 7 ounces and was 12 inches long. She was placed on a ventilator immediately following her birth, but on her second day of life she began breathing over it. She graduated to a nasal cannula. At 1 week of age, her breathing became harder to regulate and her weight began to drop. After several tests, we were told she had a congenital heart defect called PDA. The medical team said the PDA required a surgical closure to prevent blood from getting into her lungs. Their attempt to comfort me failed miserably as they said, "It's just a PDA, these are so common in preemies," driving me to think I was irrational for being terrified. I felt alone. The PDA ligation was performed when she was 2 weeks old. Still on a ventilator following the surgery, her progress remained slow. She developed three staph infections and remained on the ventilator nearly 2 weeks postsurgery. Almost a month later, I held my baby girl for 2 short minutes before the alarms attached to her tiny body began to sound. Nurses**

(*continued*)

## PARENT VOICES (*continued*)

**should know that every step a parent takes toward the NICU doors, they can already hear the gut-wrenching alarms echoing throughout the unit, often mentally preparing them for the worst possible news. I wish my daughter's nurses knew that though I was an unwed, 19-year-old, first-time mom, I fought every day for my child to have a chance at life, even if it meant risking mine. If only the nurses knew how much it hurt when I mustered up the courage to ask if I could change a diaper, take a temperature, or do anything that mommies do, but was told, "No, thank you" as if I were a guest. If only the nurses let me try kangaroo care. I desperately wanted to bond with her but felt completely helpless, because pumping breastmilk seemed like my only contribution. I wish they had known that every NICU interaction would be permanently engrained in my mind. Once a nurse handed me my daughter's laundry bag asking if I thought I could "handle" washing her clothing with hypoallergenic detergent. I remember feeling 2 feet tall. Another time, I rushed to the hospital to get my freshly pumped breastmilk to my daughter before her next feeding, but arrived just as her nurse began feeding her formula while looking at me saying I would need to "do better" if I expected my daughter to have an exclusive breastmilk diet. I wish her nurses knew how much their verbal and nonverbal communication affected my life well beyond the NICU, and how the trauma earned in the NICU does not go away. How you communicate matters.**

## ONLINE RESOURCES

**CourseConnect**

Resources for this chapter are online and available at www.springerpub.com/courseconnect.

## REFERENCES

References for this chapter are online and available at www.springerpub.com/courseconnect.

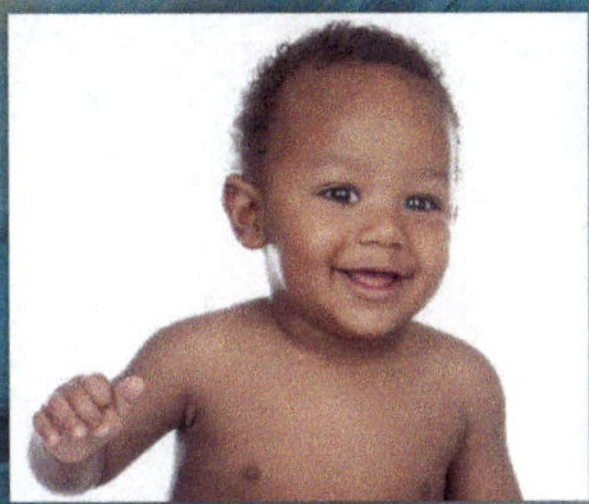

Source: Gelpi/Adobe Stock.

CHAPTER 8

# Gastrointestinal System

Khiet D. Ngo and Manoj Shah

## INTRODUCTION

The intake, digestion, and absorption of food, and the elimination of waste products are critical for normal growth, development, and long-term survival. Although many complex metabolic processes are involved, the ability to maintain adequate nutrition ultimately requires that the gastrointestinal (GI) tract be patent and structurally intact. The majority of GI diseases result from anatomic malformations, or genetic alterations leading to alterations in GI function. The diagnosis and management of GI dysfunction requires knowledge of basic embryogenesis and anatomy and physiology. External defects are immediately apparent, but many causes of dysfunction have few initial symptoms unless they are allowed to progress to serious pathophysiologic changes that result in a major threat to life. The input and support of a variety of nursing, medical, and other specialists are required for optimizing outcomes of the infant's physiologic well-being and the parents' psychosocial stability. Visible defects, especially those involving the face, appear to be particularly difficult for parents to accept. GI malformations, often associated with other congenital anomalies and prematurity, and the need for transport to a distant center for surgical and subspecialty care can place additional burdens on parental coping. The parents' and family's emotional needs and their ability to work through the grief process over the loss of the expected "perfect" child cannot be underestimated.

The GI tract is the site of the many complex transport and enzymatic mechanisms required for the digestion and absorption of nutrients. The successful intake and assimilation of these nutrients, however, rest on the ability of the gut to act as a conduit for ingestion, digestion, and elimination. Congenital malformations, particularly those involving anatomic or functional obstruction, hinder this process. Even when structurally intact, the immature supporting gastric and intestinal musculature of the newborn is relatively inefficient, increasing the tendency toward abdominal distention as a result of infrequent and irregular peristaltic movements. Transport of materials through the GI tract is further diminished in premature infants, who may have poor sucking and swallowing abilities, small gastric capacity, and an incompetent gastroesophageal sphincter. Similarly, debilitated, hypotonic infants may exhibit poor sucking and swallowing and decreased GI motility. In addition, the bowel is particularly susceptible to ischemic conditions in which blood flow is preferentially directed away from the GI tract, the kidneys, and the peripheral vascular bed toward the brain and heart.

Untoward effects of drugs commonly used in intensive care may further compromise intestinal function or integrity. Morphine, in addition to its desired analgesic effect, slows gastric emptying and reduces peristalsis. Conversely, erythromycin has been shown to accelerate gastric emptying. Ulceration of the GI tract with possible bleeding and perforation are reported side effects of tolazoline, dexamethasone, and indomethacin (Zenk et al., 2003). Mydriatics administered for ophthalmologic examination in preterm infants decrease duodenal activity and gastric emptying (James, 2002). Xanthines may cause or exacerbate gastroesophageal reflux (GER) (Jadcherla, 2002). The major purposes of this chapter are to provide a fundamental review of embryologic development and normal anatomic structure and physiology of the GI tract and to describe common causes of neonatal dysfunction and their implications for care.

## EMBRYOLOGY

Formation of the GI tract largely depends on the folding of the embryo during the first month of development (Table 8.1). At the beginning of the third week of gestation, as a result of the neural plate development, the flat, trilaminar embryonic disk begins to fold in both a cephalic-caudal and a ventral direction, invaginating the dorsal portion of the yolk sac. By the fourth week, this folding is complete, resulting in a horseshoe-shaped cylinder. This hollow tube is divided into three sections corresponding to the foregut, the midgut, and the hindgut.

### Foregut

The foregut forms part of the mouth, esophagus, stomach, proximal duodenum, pancreas, liver, and extrahepatic biliary system as well as the lower respiratory system (Sadler, 2024).

**TABLE 8.1**

**SUMMARY OF ORGAN DERIVATIVES FROM FOREGUT, MIDGUT, AND HINDGUT**

| | Foregut | Midgut | Hindgut |
|---|---|---|---|
| Organ derivative | • Pharynx<br>• Esophagus<br>• Stomach<br>• Upper duodenum (proximal to ampulla of Vater)<br>• Liver<br>• Gallbladder<br>• Pancreas<br>• Respiratory tract (trachea, bronchi, lungs) | • Lower duodenum (distal to ampulla of Vater)<br>• Jejunum<br>• Ileum<br>• Cecum<br>• Appendix<br>• Ascending colon<br>• Proximal two-thirds of transverse colon | • Distal one-third of transverse colon<br>• Descending colon<br>• Sigmoid colon<br>• Rectum<br>• Upper anal canal |
| Primary arterial supply | • Celiac artery (celiac trunk) supplies organs from esophagus to proximal duodenum (plus liver, gallbladder, pancreas)<br>• Key branches of celiac artery: Left gastric, splenic, and common hepatic arteries | • Superior mesenteric artery (SMA) supplies organs from distal duodenum to proximal two-thirds of transverse colon<br>• Key branches of SMA: Inferior pancreaticoduodenal, jejunal and ileal, ileocolic, right colic, middle colic | • Inferior mesenteric artery (IMA) supplies distal one-third of transverse colon to upper anal canal<br>• Key branches of IMA: Left colic, sigmoid arteries, superior rectal artery |

*Source:* Data from Sadler, T. W. (2024). Digestive system. In T. W. Sadler. *Langman's medical embryology* (15th ed., pp. 232–256). Wolters Kluwer.

The most cranial area of the foregut is often known as the *pharyngeal gut.* Early in the fourth week of fetal life, a depression appears on the ventral surface of the head called the *stomodeum* or primitive mouth. Oval thickenings, the nasal placodes, develop above and on either side of the primitive mouth, eventually becoming the nostrils. These nasal elevations and the area above the stomodeum merge to form the philtrum. By the eighth week, a continuous ridge forming the upper lip has developed from maxillary processes on either side of the stomodeum, fusing with the nasal pits and philtrum. The lower lip and jaw are formed when two mandibular processes below the stomodeum grow and fuse. Beginning in the fifth week, the primary palate begins to form from a wedge-shaped extension of the maxillary processes, thus separating the future nostrils from the upper lip. Lateral palatine processes also form on each side of the tongue and fuse with the nasal septum, anteriorly progressing posteriorly to form the secondary palate during the 9th to 12th week of development.

At the same time that the mouth is formed, the rest of the foregut is also developing. During the fourth and fifth weeks of gestation, an esophagotracheal septum is formed dividing the proximal foregut into the anterior trachea and posterior esophagus. Initially short, the esophagus elongates over a 2- to 3-week period to allow the development of the lungs, heart, and neck.

The stomach, first appearing as a dilation of the foregut, begins to grow with the dorsal aspect outpacing the ventral aspect, thus forming the greater curvature. As the esophagus grows, the stomach, initially in the region of the neck, descends and rotates 90° on its longitudinal axis until it reaches its final position with the greater curvature on the left and lesser curvature on the right. The duodenum develops from the caudal portion of the foregut as well as the cranial portion of the midgut. Around the 5th or 6th week, villi grow and temporarily occlude the lumen until the 9th or 10th week of gestation. Several other buds on the foregut also form the liver, gallbladder, bile ducts, and pancreas.

## Midgut

The midgut consists of the distal duodenum, jejunum, ileum, cecum, appendix, ascending colon, and the right two-thirds of the transverse colon (Sadler, 2024). Blood is supplied by the superior mesenteric artery. Although initially in tandem, the lengthening of the tubular intestine outpaces the overall elongation of the embryo.

By the sixth week of gestation, the rate of growth causes the tube to bend ventrally. Simultaneously, rapid growth of the liver quickly limits space within the abdominal cavity. Consequently, around 7 weeks' gestation, loops of the intestine begin to protrude into the umbilical cord. As the midgut herniates, it rotates in a counterclockwise fashion, approximately 90° around an axis formed by the superior mesenteric artery. At around 10 weeks, when the abdominal cavity has expanded sufficiently, and the growth of the liver has slowed, reduction of the midgut herniation occurs. As the loops of the intestine are retracted into the abdomen, they rotate another 180°, resulting in a full rotation of 270°.

This counterclockwise rotation allows the transverse colon to pass in front of the duodenum and places the cecum and appendix in the right lower quadrant of the abdomen. Once the intestine has rotated into proper placement, the mesentery attaches to the posterior abdominal wall.

### Hindgut

The GI components of the hindgut include the distal one-third of the transverse colon, the descending colon, ascending colon, sigmoid colon, rectum, and superior portion of the anal canal (Sadler, 2024). Blood is supplied from the inferior mesenteric artery. The major developmental changes occur in the terminal hindgut known as the *cloaca* and involve formation of the anus. The hindgut initially ends at the cloacal membrane, which separates it from the anal pit or proctodeum. Around the fourth week of gestation, the urorectal septum forms, and by the sixth week, divides the cloaca into a ventral urogenital sinus and a dorsal anorectal canal.

By the eighth week of gestation, the anal membrane has moved inferior and is found at the bottom of the proctodeum. In the ninth week, this membrane ruptures, completing the patency of the GI tract.

## PHYSIOLOGY OF THE GI TRACT

The GI system depends on the coordinated efforts of several organs for normal function. These organs include the oropharynx, esophagus, stomach, small intestine, liver, gallbladder, pancreas, large intestine, rectum, and anus.

The two main functions of the GI tract are digestion and absorption of nutrients and fluids and elimination. Digestion is the process by which macronutrients (carbohydrates, fats, proteins) and micronutrients are broken down to an extent such that they can be absorbed into the bloodstream. Absorption is the process by which products of digestion travel across the cells and paracellular spaces lining the GI tract and ultimately into the vascular or lymphatic circulation. Elimination is the process by which solids, liquids, and any materials that are not absorbed are expelled from the body.

Digestive, absorptive, and elimination functions are supplanted by motility and secretory functions. The layers of the GI tract, starting from the inner luminal side to the outermost layer, include mucosa, submucosa, muscularis, and serosa. The mucosa includes epithelial enterocytes that directly participate in digestion and absorption. The muscularis layer is comprised of circular and longitudinal smooth muscles that carry out motility functions of the GI tract. Myenteric and submucosal plexuses are found within the muscularis layer and submucosal layer, respectively. These plexuses are the control center of the GI nervous system that help regulate sensory, motility, and secretory functions. In addition to the network of neurons that make up the enteric nervous system, the central nervous system (CNS) can also process signals coming from the intestines as well as provide signals that affect the function of the GI tract.

There remains much to be learned about the motility functions of the GI tract. GI motility has two main functions. The first is propulsion or peristalsis, which moves liquid and solid material along different parts of the tract. Motility also contributes to the mechanical breakdown and mixing of solid materials that make food particles more accessible for digestion by digestive juices and enzymes. It is believed that the interstitial cells of Cajal, which are part of the intrinsic GI nervous system, play an essential role in regulating motility by acting as the pacemaker cells of the GI tract. The pacemaker function of the interstitial cells of Cajal is analogous to the pacemaker functions of the sinoatrial node of the heart.

The function of the GI tract is closely regulated by a complex interplay of various hormones. Some of these hormones can be classified by their endocrine, neurocrine, or paracrine functions (Barrett, 2014). Endocrine hormones include gastrin, cholecystokinin, motilin, secretin, ghrelin, and glucose-dependent insulinotropic peptide. Neurocrine hormones include acetylcholine, vasoactive intestinal polypeptide, substance P, nitric oxide, cholecystokinin, 5-hydroxytryptamine, somatostatin, and calcitonin gene–related peptide. Examples of paracrine hormones include histamine, prostaglandins, somatostatin, and 5-hydroxytryptamine (Table 8.2).

### Oral Pharynx

In children and adults, digestion begins in the mouth with the act of chewing. Enzymatic digestion of a small percentage of carbohydrates also begins in the mouth by actions of salivary amylase from the parotid glands (Hall & Hall, 2021). Because infants are edentulous and rely largely on breast milk or formula feedings, chewing does not play an important role in digestion for infants. However, the act of sucking and swallowing effectively and safely requires a complex coordination between the central and peripheral nervous systems and oropharyngeal musculature. Dysfunction of any of these structures may result in reduced or unsafe oral intake. Saliva produced by various glands serves an important role in the lubrication of the oral and esophageal mucosa, thereby facilitating the comfortable passage of materials through the oral cavity and esophagus.

Swallowing is the first step in transporting ingested fluids and solids to the rest of the GI tract. Swallowing begins when liquid or solid substances are detected by sensory nerves in the oropharynx and laryngopharynx. These sensory impulses are transmitted via the trigeminal and glossopharyngeal nerves to the swallowing center in the brainstem, where the signals are processed. The swallowing center in turn coordinates muscle function by sending motor impulses to the pharynx and upper esophagus via cranial nerves 5, 9, 10, and 12 (Hall & Hall, 2021). Breathing is temporarily inhibited during swallowing, which prevents aspiration of materials into the respiratory tract. Congenital or acquired dysfunction of the neural or muscular architecture involved in the swallowing process can lead to transient or chronic feeding problems.

### Esophagus

The esophagus serves as a conduit for liquids and solids from the mouth to the stomach. Autonomic innervation of the muscular walls of the esophagus generates esophageal peristalsis that propels solids and liquids throughout its length (Hall & Hall, 2021). Coordinated constriction and relaxation of the

**TABLE 8.2**

**SUMMARY OF SELECT HORMONES AND CHEMICALS THAT AFFECT GASTRIC FUNCTION**

| Product | Source | Functions |
|---|---|---|
| Hydrochloric acid | Parietal cell | Digestion by hydrolysis, immunologic by sterilization of meal and ingested contaminants |
| Intrinsic factor | Parietal cell | Vitamin $B_{12}$ transport and absorption |
| Pepsinogen | Chief cell | Initial protein digestion |
| Mucus, bicarbonate | Surface mucus cell; production stimulated by prostaglandin | Protection of gastric mucosa from acid injury |
| Histamine | Enterochromaffin cells | Regulate gastric secretion |
| Gastrin | G cells in gastric antrum, duodenum, and pancreas | Regulate gastric secretion |
| Gastrin-releasing peptide | Nerves | Regulate gastric secretion |
| Acetylcholine | Neurotransmitter at neural junctions | Regulates gastric secretion |
| Somatostatin | Delta cells found in pyloric antrum, duodenum, pancreatic islet cells | Multiple systemic functions including suppression of gastrointestinal hormones (gastrin, cholecystokinin, secretin, motilin, gastric inhibitory polypeptide, vasoactive intestinal peptide) |

*Source:* Adapted from Barrett, K. E. (2014). *Gastrointestinal physiology.* McGraw-Hill.

upper and lower esophageal sphincters regulate entry into the esophagus and stomach. Inappropriately low pressures generated at the lower esophageal sphincter can result in pathologic conditions such as gastroesophageal reflux disease (GERD).

## Stomach

The stomach is where a significant part of digestion begins. Gastric acid produced by parietal cells contributes to the digestive process along with gastric enzymes such as pepsinogen, which begins the breakdown of proteins. Parietal cells also produce an intrinsic factor that plays a central role in the absorption of vitamin $B_{12}$ in the terminal ileum. Even in patients who require therapy for acid-related conditions, the physiologic importance of acid in digestion and defense against infectious agents needs to be recognized.

In addition to chemical and enzymatic digestion, the intrinsic motor activity on the muscular layers of the stomach generates mechanical forces that churn, grind, and mix fluids and solids. These actions physically break down foods into smaller particles. This mechanical breakdown increases the surface area of food boluses, making it more accessible for chemical and enzymatic digestion. In addition to regulating the rate at which fluids move from the stomach into the small intestine, the pyloric sphincter muscle helps ensure that food particles exiting the stomach are small enough to be acted on by digestive enzymes and juices of the small intestine. Abnormalities in the neuromuscular function of the stomach can slow gastric motility, resulting in delayed gastric emptying. Delayed gastric emptying plays a role in other GI conditions, such as GER and feeding problems.

The lining of the stomach is normally protected from the acidic environment by a mucus layer formed by mucinous film overlying the gastric mucosa (Figure 8.1). Sandwiched in between this mucus layer and gastric mucosa is a microenvironment containing bicarbonate ions. The mucinous film serves as the first line of defense against acid injury. Any acid that is able to penetrate this layer is neutralized in the bicarbonate microenvironment. Prostaglandins, leukotrienes, and thromboxane are chemical compounds produced by the arachidonic acid pathway. Collectively, these compounds regulate numerous physiologic functions including thrombosis, inflammation, temperature regulation, and production of the mucinous layer that protects the stomach. Nonsteroidal antiinflammatory drugs (NSAIDs) such as ibuprofen are effective in treating fever, pain, and inflammation by blocking enzymes in the arachidonic acid pathway. While the antipyretic and analgesic effects are desired, the collateral reduction on prostaglandin synthesis also reduces the production of the mucosa layer, predisposing the gastric mucosa to acid injury. Devices such as nasogastric (NG) tubes used for feedings or gastric decompression can also mechanically disrupt the protective gastric lining, increasing the risk of mucosal injury.

## Small Intestine

The small intestine is the site of absorption for the majority of liquids, macronutrients, and micronutrients. Digestion continues in the small intestine as the food bolus exiting the stomach is exposed to additional digestive enzymes and secretions

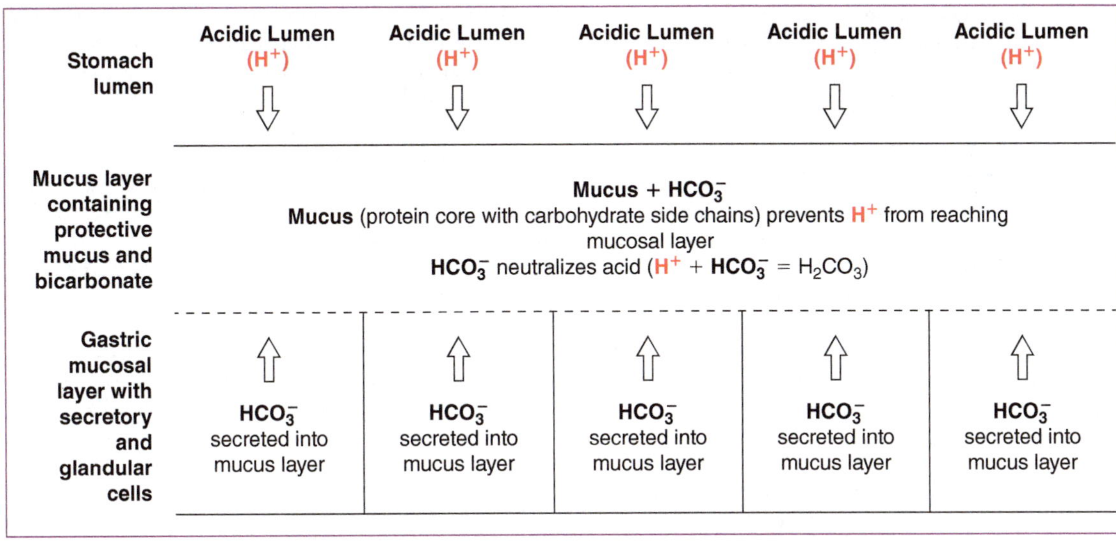


**FIGURE 8.1** Schematic of how mucus layer protects gastric mucosa from acid injury.

from the hepatobiliary system and pancreas. Food boluses are referred to as *chyme* once they enter the small intestine.

The liver performs many important metabolic functions that affect all other organ systems. Examples of these functions range from the metabolism of carbohydrate, fats, and proteins to the metabolism of medications. Another key function of the liver is the production of bile. After it is produced in hepatocytes, bile must make its way through the hepatobiliary duct system, which terminates in the first portion of the duodenum. Bile emulsifies fats, breaking them down into smaller droplets to increase their surface area for digestion by pancreatic lipases, which aids in absorption by enterocytes. Smaller fat molecules can diffuse across the enterocyte membrane, while larger fat molecules require dedicated transmembrane transporters. Congenital hepatobiliary abnormalities can result in dysfunction in the production, processing, or flow of bile (cholestasis). Hepatobiliary diseases most often present with jaundice and failure to thrive due to malabsorption. Depending on the underlying cause and severity of the condition, the size of the liver and spleen may vary. Reabsorption of bile acids in the terminal ileum, followed by hepatic recycling, accounts for over 90% of the bile pool.

The exocrine pancreas produces numerous enzymes including lipases, amylases, and peptidases that break down fats, carbohydrates, and proteins, respectively. To protect the pancreas from auto-digestion, pancreatic enzymes are secreted in an inactive form and are activated only once they reach the intestinal lumen. The pancreas also produces bicarbonate, which neutralizes acid coming from the stomach, protecting the intestinal mucosa from acid-associated injury. At the enterocyte surface, disaccharidases further break down carbohydrates into monosaccharides that can then enter the cell via dedicated transmembrane transport proteins. Amino acids, dipeptides, and tripeptides also use dedicated membrane transporters for absorption into enterocytes. Congenital or acquired causes that affect the architecture or function of these enterocyte surface enzymes can result in malabsorption.

Water absorption is mainly driven by osmotic gradients, which are initially established by the absorption of sodium and glucose. Water follows these osmotic gradients through transmembrane and paracellular pathways, moving into the enterocytes. This mechanism explains why the addition of glucose and salts in commercial rehydration solutions enhances water absorption.

## Colon

The functions of the colon are threefold: (1) maintenance of fluid and electrolyte balance, (2) formation of fecal matter, and (3) defecation. The colon provides the body's last opportunity to reabsorb water and electrolytes, a process that helps maintain fluid and electrolyte homeostasis. It also concentrates and solidifies colonic contents into stool. The main electrolytes involved in this process are sodium, potassium, chloride, hydrogen ions ($H^+$), and bicarbonate. Transmembrane proteins on the apical and basolateral surfaces of colonic cells facilitate the movement of these electrolytes. Electrolyte movement establishes electrochemical gradients, which drive water reabsorption or secretion. Disruptions in electrolyte transport mechanisms or colonic anatomy can result in profuse diarrhea and imbalances in water and electrolytes.

The process of defecation requires coordination between the local enteric nervous system, the CNS, the abdominal musculature, the internal anal sphincter, and the external anal sphincter. In healthy individuals, the urge to defecate begins after a fecal bolus in the rectum accumulates and enlarges to a threshold size that leads to the activation of mechanical stretch receptors. Activation of these mechanical receptors triggers a reflex relaxation of the internal anal sphincter. At the appropriate moment, under the individual's own volition, the external anal sphincter is relaxed. Coordination of external anal sphincter relaxation with an increase in intraabdominal pressure from contraction of abdominal muscles facilitates the expulsion of stool.

Congenital or acquired conditions affecting the neurologic or muscular processes involved in defecation can lead to disorders. Hirschsprung disease (HD) is an example of dysfunction in local neuromuscular control mechanisms, resulting in difficulty evacuating stool. The complexity of the defecation process explains the straining efforts infants often exhibit when they defecate.

## GENETIC SYNDROMES

A syndrome is a group of signs or symptoms that consistently occur together or a condition characterized by a set of associated symptoms. Many syndromes occur because of a genetic or chromosomal abnormality. Humans have 23 pairs of chromosomes, or 46 in all. Babies with chromosomal conditions have a problem with one or more of their chromosomes. Chromosomes are primarily composed of DNA, the instructions for making proteins, and genes, the building blocks of heredity. Proteins serve essential structural and functional roles throughout the body, but sometimes a mutation—a change in a gene or genes—alters the gene's instructions for making a protein such that the protein does not function properly or is missing entirely. These mutations are the basis of genetic disorders. Because one chromosome in each pair comes from the mother and the other from the father, inherited gene mutations can be from one or both parents. Abnormal genes or chromosomes may result in structural or functional abnormalities in the GI tract as well as other organ systems. Table 8.3 provides a summary of selected syndromes associated with GI abnormalities.

## DIAGNOSTIC MODALITIES

The care of neonates has vastly improved with advances in technology. However, many neonates can be evaluated using simple and noninvasive diagnostic modalities. The following spectrum of diagnostic modalities is usually available in centers with neonatal intensive care units (NICU) to manage GI problems.

### Nasogastric Tube

NG tube placement can be used for diagnostic purposes in two situations. The first is to check for patency of the nares and esophagus if anatomic anomalies are suspected. If an esophageal anatomic anomaly is present, the NG tube cannot be advanced into the stomach as seen on plain radiography. A second diagnostic application of an NG tube is the collection of a gastric aspirate sample. A gastric aspirate sample may be necessary to check for the presence of blood and to determine the blood's origin (infant or mother, via the Apt test). A gastric aspirate sample may also be used to check the gastric pH to guide acid suppression therapy; the normal gastric pH is less than 2, and effective acid suppression is achieved if the pH is greater than 4.

### Stool Studies

The stool is an excretory product of the GI tract composed of GI secretions, bile and pancreatic fluid, undigested/unabsorbed food, and microbes. Stool examination is helpful in identifying the presence and possible causes of GI pathology.

Basic clinical observations and examination of stool can yield important initial diagnostic clues. Timing of the passage of the first meconium stool should be noted, because a delayed passage of meconium (beyond 24 hours) is suggestive of a lower colonic obstruction such as Hirschsprung disease (HD) or anorectal malformation. Stool color results from bile that is altered by colonic bacteria; normal stool color is yellow to brown. Green stool is usually seen in patients with diarrhea (rapid transit). Bright red stool implies possible bleeding from the colon or anus, while dark red, maroon, or black stool suggests that the source of blood is in the small bowel or stomach. Lighter colored (acholic) or pale stool implies decreased bile in the bowel, as seen in patients with biliary obstruction (biliary atresia) or cholestasis.

Several stool tests can help as screening tests for GI tract pathology. Occult blood and white blood cells (WBCs; eosinophils) are present in patients with cow or soy milk–induced allergic colitis. A stool pH of less than 5.5 is seen in carbohydrate or fat malabsorption. Detection of reducing sugars in the stool is suggestive of carbohydrate (except sucrose) malabsorption. Stool calprotectin and lactoferrin are used as markers of inflammation in the GI tract. Their usefulness as screening markers in infants with enterocolitis (necrotizing enterocolitis [NEC] or allergic) remains unclear (Farghaly et al., 2023; Pergialiotis, et al., 2016).

Stool cultures test for bacterial pathogens in cases of diarrhea. In neonates, stool should not be routinely tested for the *Clostridium difficile* toxin, because healthy neonates can become colonized by *C. difficile* in the first few days of life (Lees et al., 2016; Shirley et al., 2023). GI stool panels are molecular-based tests that can detect a wide variety of bacteria, viruses, and parasites in stool, with results being available in less than 24 hours (Chang et al., 2021).

Fecal elastase 1 (FE1) is a useful marker of exocrine pancreatic function (Lüth et al., 2001). FE1 is usually low in meconium and reaches normal levels by day 3 in term newborns and by 2 weeks in infants born before 28 weeks of gestation. The FE1 level is a useful adjunct diagnostic test for pancreatic insufficiency in patients suspected of having cystic fibrosis (CF).

### Radiologic Studies

Radiologic studies of the GI tract are performed to look for anatomic abnormalities, obstruction, or perforation in babies presenting with vomiting, abdominal distension, constipation, or a catastrophic illness such as shock. The GI tract is filled with fluid at birth, but as the infant swallows air after delivery, air travels through the gut rapidly, filling the stomach within 30 minutes and reaching the distal small bowel by 4 hours and rectum by 6 to 8 hours. In cases of obstruction, the portion of the intestine distal to the obstruction remains airless, and the portion of the intestine proximal to the obstruction becomes dilated. As the infant continues to swallow air, the proximal intestine may become very dilated, causing a large bubblelike appearance on plain radiographs.

Plain radiographs of the chest and abdomen, taken in supine or upright positions, are valuable initial diagnostic tools for suspected GI tract obstructions. The absence of air in the stomach suggests esophageal atresia, while a dilated stomach with no air in the small intestine indicates duodenal obstruction. The absence of rectal air suggests intestinal obstruction and cross-table

**TABLE 8.3**

**COMPARISON OF GASTROINTESTINAL MANIFESTATIONS OF SELECTED GENETIC SYNDROMES**

| Syndrome | GI Problem | Cleft Lip/ Palate | Omphalocele | Malrotation | Imperforate Anus | Tracheoesophageal Fistula | Hirschsprung's Disease | Pyloric Stenosis | Duodenal Atresia | Liver Disease | Pancreatic Disease |
|---|---|---|---|---|---|---|---|---|---|---|---|
| Alagille | Cholestasis, intrahepatic biliary hypoplasia | | | | | | | | | X | |
| Apert | Cleft/narrow palate, pyloric stenosis, anterior/ ectopic anus | X | | | | | | X | | | |
| Beckwith–Wiedemann | Macroglossia, omphalocele | | X | | | | | | | | |
| Fetal hydantoin | Cleft lip and palate, pyloric stenosis, duodenal atresia, imperforate anus | X | | | X | | | X | X | | |
| Fetal valproate | Cleft lip and palate | X | | | | | | | | | |
| Meckel–Gruber | Cleft palate and/or lip, omphalocele, malrotation, imperforate anus | X | X | X | X | | | | | | |
| Sirenomelia (mermaid malformation) | Esophageal atresia, imperforate anus, tracheoesophageal fistula | | | | X | X | | | | | |
| Trisomy 13 | Cleft lip/palate, omphalocele, malrotation | X | X | X | | | | | | | |
| Trisomy 18 | Cleft lip/palate, pyloric stenosis, omphalocele, malrotation, biliary atresia | X | X | X | | | | X | | X | |

(*continued*)

**TABLE 8.3**

**COMPARISON OF GASTROINTESTINAL MANIFESTATIONS OF SELECTED GENETIC SYNDROMES (*continued*)**

| Syndrome | GI Problem | Cleft Lip/ Palate | Omphalocele | Malrotation | Imperforate Anus | Tracheoesophageal Fistula | Hirschsprung's Disease | Pyloric Stenosis | Duodenal Atresia | Liver Disease | Pancreatic Disease |
|---|---|---|---|---|---|---|---|---|---|---|---|
| Trisomy 21 | Tracheoesophageal fistula, duodenal atresia, annular pancreas, Hirschsprung disease, imperforate anus | | | | X | X | X | | X | | X |
| Waardenburg | Hirschsprung disease | | | | | | X | | | | |
| Brandt syndrome—zinc deficiency | Chronic diarrhea | | | | | | | | | | |
| Heterotaxy | Agenesis of dorsal pancreas | | | | | | | | | | X |
| Mowat–Wilson | Hirschsprung disease | | | | | | X | | | | |
| Johanson–Blizzard | Exocrine pancreatic insufficiency | | | | | | | | | | X |
| Wolf Hirschhorn | Cleft lip/palate | X | | | | | | | | | |
| Wolman disease | Liver failure, hepatomegaly | | | | | | | | | X | |
| Zellweger | Hepatomegaly | | | | | | | | | X | |
| Di George | Cleft palate | X | | | | | | | | | |
| Cornelia de Lange | Cleft palate | X | | | | | | | | | |

lateral radiographs may be helpful in visualizing air in the rectum. If perforation is suspected, a left lateral decubitus radiograph is recommended to detect free intraperitoneal air.

An upper GI series is performed using contrast (barium or Gastrografin) that is either swallowed or delivered by an NG tube before a series of radiographs are taken. An upper GI series can be considered in babies who present with vomiting, abdominal distension, or poor growth. Results of an upper GI series may be diagnostic for pyloric stenosis, intestinal malrotation, or duodenal obstruction. An upper GI series often shows reflux of gastric contents back into the esophagus; however, the study cannot distinguish between physiologic versus pathologic reflux. In addition to diagnostic purposes, the upper GI contrast study can also be used to define anatomy prior to surgical intervention such as gastrostomy tube placement or fundoplication. The study usually requires the baby to be fasting for at least one feeding (4–6 hours). In cases of suspected perforation, water-soluble contrast (Gastrografin) should be used.

A rectal contrast enema examination is performed using barium or Gastrografin to evaluate the large intestine in suspected cases of malrotation, small left colon, HD, or obstruction by meconium plug. Contrast enema examination should be done prior to the upper GI series, because a contrast from the upper GI examination may take several days to clear. If a patient already has had an upper GI series, then a gentle saline enema may help clear contrast faster; otherwise, no special preparation is needed prior to contrast enema. A saline enema may be used after a contrast enema if the contrast is not cleared.

Ultrasonography is a noninvasive test that is the modality of choice for diagnosing pyloric stenosis or intestinal duplication cyst and evaluating the gallbladder and extrahepatic biliary system. Doppler sonography may be used to diagnose portal vein thrombosis and other abnormalities in vascular flow.

A nuclear medicine scan or scintigraphy is done by performing imaging after a radioactive tracer is ingested or injected intravenously. A gastric emptying scan uses technetium-tagged formula fed to the infant and may be used to detect aspiration (with swallowing or from gastric reflux) and measure gastric emptying time in patients with feeding intolerance. A Meckel's scan is performed by intravenous (IV) injection of Tc-99m pertechnetate, which avidly accumulates in gastric mucosa, and is the study of choice in patients suspected of having a Meckel's diverticulum causing lower GI bleeding. A hepatobiliary hydroxy iminodiacetic acid (HIDA) scan, also known as hepatobiliary scintigraphy, is performed by administering radioactive tracer intravenously and obtaining images over 4 hours and then 24 hours later. The HIDA scan is used to evaluate liver, gallbladder, and bile duct pathology. At some institutions, phenobarbital is given for 5 to 7 days prior to a HIDA scan to improve accuracy (Kwatra et al., 2013; Mohamadien et al., 2021).

## Esophageal pH/Impedance Probe

An esophageal pH probe test is performed by placing a thin, flexible electrode with one or two pH sensors in the distal esophagus; data is collected by a portable recorder (Jadcherla, et al., 2021). Current pH probe catheters often include impedance monitoring, which measures intraluminal changes in electrical resistance. Impedance measurements have the advantage of being able to detect nonacidic GER episodes. After 24 to 48 hours, the probe is removed, and data are analyzed. The diagnosis of acidic GER depends on a complex scoring system based on the number of reflux episodes, the number of episodes greater than 5 minutes, the duration of the longest episode, and, most importantly, the percentage of time in reflux. It is also used to document the association of any symptom with reflux; symptoms that may be associated with reflux include apnea, bradycardia, oxygen desaturation, cough, or irritability. Because formula neutralizes acid, this test has to be done while the patient is taking bolus feedings 3 hours apart. The patient must also be off any acid-suppressive and promotility treatment for 1 to 2 days preceding and during the study period.

## Endoscopy

Diagnostic and therapeutic endoscopy is feasible even in micropremies less than 1,000 g, thanks to advances in fiber optics and digital imaging. Endoscopy can be performed at the bedside in coordination with the NICU team (Mezoff et al., 2020) (Table 8.4).

**TABLE 8.4**

**INDICATIONS FOR ENDOSCOPY**

| ***Upper Endoscopy*** | |
|---|---|
| **Diagnostic Indication** | **Entities Diagnosed** |
| Persistent vomiting without obstruction<br>Hematemesis/upper GI bleeding<br>Chronic diarrhea | Esophagitis, gastritis, gastric mucosal hypertrophy, ulcer, small bowel villous abnormalities |
| **Therapeutic Indications** | **Procedure Performed** |
| Feeding problems<br>Upper GI bleeding<br>Dysphagia<br>Esophageal stricture (after TE fistula repair) | Percutaneous endoscopic gastrostomy (PEG) tube placement<br>Control of bleeding<br>Dilation of stricture |
| ***Colonoscopy*** | |
| **Diagnostic Indications** | **Entities Diagnosed** |
| Hematochezia<br>Constipation | Colitis (allergic)<br>Hirschsprung disease (rectal biopsy) |

# TRACHEAL ESOPHAGEAL FISTULA AND ESOPHAGEAL ATRESIA

## Background

Esophageal atresia (EA) is defined as a complete interruption in continuity of the esophagus. Tracheoesophageal fistula (TEF) is a pathologic connection between the esophagus and trachea. The five major types of TEF are summarized in Figure 8.2.

Other congenital anomalies that may be associated with EA and TEF include vertebral, intestinal atresia, anorectal malformations (ARM), and cardiac, renal, and limb anomalies. VACTERL (vertebral, anorectal, cardiovascular, tracheoesophageal, renal, and limb anomalies) syndrome is diagnosed when three or more of these anomalies are present. Approximately 19% of babies with EA and TEF have VACTERL syndrome (Bruch et al., 2016). Five percent of these neonates will also have chromosomal anomalies such as trisomy 13, 18, and 21. Other conditions that may be associated with EA and TEF include CHARGE (coloboma, heart defect, atresia choanae, retarded growth and development, genital abnormality, and ear abnormality) syndrome, Potter syndrome, and pyloric stenosis (Bruch et al., 2016).

The survival rate of infants with EA with or without TEF based on birth weight (BW) and cardiac anomalies has been studied. Infants with no cardiac anomalies and a BW of greater than 2,000 g have a 100% survival rate, while infants with a BW of less than 2,000 g were found to have an 82% survival rate. Infants with a major cardiac anomaly and a BW greater than 2,000 g have a 72% survival rate, while infants with a BW of less than 2,000 g have a survival rate of 27% (Bruch et al., 2016; Okamoto et al., 2009).

## Diagnosis

Polyhydramnios and absent or small fetal gastric bubble on prenatal ultrasound should raise suspicion for esophageal atresia (Pinheiro et al., 2012). Most neonates with EA and TEF present soon after birth with difficulty swallowing even their normal production of saliva. The swallowing problems can result in choking, coughing, gagging, and/or cyanosis, particularly during feedings. Difficulty with advancing an NG tube should raise suspicion of esophageal pathology and be followed by a plain radiograph that includes views of the neck, chest, and abdomen. Coiling of the NG tube tip in the vicinity of the proximal esophagus supports the diagnosis of EA. The absence of bowel gas on a plain abdominal radiograph is suggestive of EA without a distal fistula, while the presence of gas throughout the small and large bowel suggests a distal TEF. Further mapping of a proximal fistula can be done by radiographic contrast study or rigid bronchoscopy, depending on institutional availability. Neonates who have TEF without EA (H-Type) may present beyond the newborn period (Bruch et al., 2016). In these babies, an NG tube may terminate in the stomach, but the baby will have persistent coughing and choking with feeding.

Additional findings may be associated with EA and TEF. Limb and anorectal anomalies may be observed on physical examination. Vertebral anomalies can be detected by plain radiography. Abdominal ultrasonography and echocardiogram may reveal renal abnormalities or a tethered spinal cord, and cardiac anomalies, respectively.

## Management

Management should be in collaboration with a pediatric surgery team. Prior to surgery, steps should be taken to minimize the risk of oral pulmonary aspiration. The neonate should be placed supine with the head elevated at a 30° to 45° angle. An oral or nasal esophageal tube should be placed for continuous low suction. Oral secretions can be thick and sticky, causing frequent clogging of the suction tubing. Thus, tubes may need to be routinely flushed or changed. **Quality and Safety: Patency of the tube should be checked if symptoms of increased choking, gagging, or respiratory problems arise. IV broad-spectrum antibiotics should also be started.**

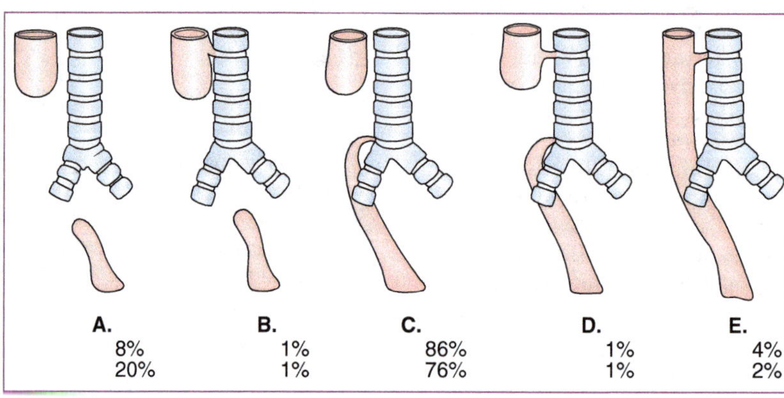


**FIGURE 8.2 Diagram of the main types of esophageal atresia (EA) with or without a tracheoesophageal fistula (TEF).** Type A is EA without a TEF and is often called pure EA. Shown are the blind upper and lower esophageal pouches next to the ringed windpipe (trachea) and the branches (bronchi) that lead to each lung. Type B has a connection (fistula) between the upper pouch and the trachea (a TEF). Type C is by far the most common form of EA and has a fistula between the lower esophagus and the trachea (one form of TEF) with a blind upper pouch. A rare form (1%) is type D with two TEFs, one between both the upper and lower esophageal segments and the trachea. Type E has only a TEF and no EA. This is usually referred to as an H- or N-shaped fistula and maybe 2% to 4% of this group. The H-fistulas are divided surgically, and nothing further needs to be done to the esophagus, which is intact and reaches normally to the stomach.

Specific details on the variations in surgical approaches have been well described (Bruch et al., 2016; van der Zee et al., 2017).

Postoperatively, the baby should be managed with parenteral nutrition (PN), antibiotics, and acid suppression. Anastomoses site leakage can be a complication after surgery and should be considered if there are acute clinical or vital sign changes. If a chest tube is in place, anastomoses site leakage may present as persistent or increased drainage. Frequent oropharyngeal suctioning and elevating the head of the bed from 30° to 45° will reduce the risk of aspiration. For oral suctioning, the catheter should be inserted to a predetermined depth that is well above the surgical site to avoid any potential trauma. The timing and initiation of gastric feedings should be determined in collaboration with the surgical team. An esophagram on postoperative days 5 to 7 can be considered to look for anastomotic leaks prior to starting oral feedings. If a leak is diagnosed, it can usually be managed conservatively by continuing IV antibiotics, parenteral nutrition, and chest tube drainage with a follow-up esophogram in about 1 week. Most leaks will seal without further surgical intervention (Dingeldein, 2025). Infants who have a gastrostomy tube or a trans-anastomotic tube ending in the stomach can be fed 2 to 3 days after surgical repair (Bruch et al., 2016).

Postoperative complications may include GER (40%–70%), anastomosis site leak (17%), anastomosis site stricture (40%–50%), fistula recurrence (5%–12%), and esophageal dysmotility (75%–100%) (Berseth & Poenaru, 2005; Kovesi & Rubin, 2004).

## GASTROESOPHAGEAL REFLUX

### Background

GER is defined as the involuntary passage of gastric contents into the esophagus with or without regurgitation and vomiting (Rosen et al., 2018). In contrast, gastroesophageal reflux disease (GERD) is when GER leads to troublesome symptoms that affect daily functioning and/or result in complications (Rosen et al., 2018). Table 8.5 lists some of the symptoms and signs that may suggest GERD. It is often a challenge to distinguish between GER and GERD in infants, because there is no consistently reliable test that has been routinely recommended to diagnose GER/GERD (Rosen et al., 2018). The diagnosis, therefore, most often relies on clinical judgment. Because the common symptoms of GER are nonspecific, conditions other than GER should also be considered in evaluating any infant (Table 8.6).

**TABLE 8.5**

**CLINICAL PRESENTATION THAT MAY SUGGEST GERD**

| Symptoms | Signs |
|---|---|
| ***General*** | |
| Persistent crying or irritability<br>Poor growth<br>Dystonic head posturing (Sandifer syndrome)<br>Sleeping problems | Anemia |
| ***Gastrointestinal*** | |
| Recurrent regurgitation<br>Hematemesis<br>Dysphagia<br>Feeding difficulties | Esophagitis |
| ***Airway*** | |
| Wheezing<br>Stridor<br>Cough<br>Hoarseness<br>Asthma refractory to therapy | Apnea<br>Brief resolved unexplained events<br>Aspiration pneumonia<br>Recurrent pneumonias |

GERD, gastroesophageal reflux disease.

*Source:* Adapted from Rosen, R., Vandenplas, Y., Singendonk, M., Cabana, M., DiLorenzo, C., Gottrand, F., Gupta, S., Langendam, M., Staiano, A., Thapar, N., Tipnis, N., & Tabbers, M. (2018). Pediatric gastroesophageal reflux clinical practice guidelines: Joint recommendations of the North American Society for Pediatric Gastroenterology, Hepatology, and Nutrition and the European Society for Pediatric Gastroenterology, Hepatology, and Nutrition. *Journal of Pediatric Gastroenterology and Nutrition, 66*(3), 516–554. https://doi.org/10.1097/MPG.0000000000001889.

Most episodes of GER are normal or physiologic and usually go unnoticed. The precise prevalence of GER and GERD in infants is unclear. Based on esophageal pH monitoring studies, healthy infants may have up to 31 episodes of gastroesophageal acid reflux a day (Vandenplas et al., 1991). The same study suggests that less than 10% of infants and children have GERD.

Three physiologic strategies limit GER and the development of GERD (Vandenplas & Hassall, 2002). First is the anatomic antireflux barrier that comprises the lower esophageal sphincter (LES), the diaphragmatic pinchcock, and the angle of His. These anatomic structures form a physical barrier that limits the frequency and severity of GER events. It is thought that inappropriate transient lower esophageal sphincter relaxation (TLESR) is the primary factor responsible for GER. The second physiologic strategy that limits the complications of GER is esophageal peristalsis and clearance, which removes any gastric content that enters the esophagus as a result of GER. Third is the epithelial layer architecture, including a protective mucous layer and tight epithelial cell junctions, which helps to reduce the esophageal injury that can result from contact with gastric contents. Compromise of one or more of these defense strategies can result in the symptoms or complications of GERD (Vandenplas & Hassall, 2002). Factors that increase intragastric pressure including increased work of breathing, mechanical ventilation, and delayed gastric emptying can contribute to GER. Risk factors for delayed gastric emptying include prematurity, feedings with increased osmolality, and certain medications.

**TABLE 8.6**

**DIFFERENTIAL DIAGNOSIS OF GERD IN NEONATES AND INFANTS**

| | |
|---|---|
| **Gastrointestinal obstruction**<br>Pyloric stenosis<br>Malrotation with volvulus<br>Hirschsprung disease<br>Antral/duodenal web<br>Abdominal tumor/mass | **Other gastrointestinal disorders**<br>Achalasia<br>Gastroparesis<br>Peptic ulcer disease<br>Eosinophilic gastroenteritis<br>Food allergy/intolerance<br>Pancreatitis<br>Cholelithiasis/cholecystitis |
| **Neurologic**<br>Hydrocephalus<br>Subdural hematoma<br>Intracranial hemorrhage<br>Intracranial mass | **Infectious**<br>Sepsis/meningitis<br>Urinary tract infection<br>Upper/lower airway infection<br>Otitis media<br>Hepatitis |
| **Cardiac**<br>Heart failure | **Renal**<br>Obstructive uropathy<br>Renal insufficiency |
| **Metabolic/endocrine**<br>Galactosemia<br>Hereditary fructose intolerance<br>Urea cycle defects<br>Amino and organic acidemias<br>Metabolic acidosis<br>Congenital adrenal hyperplasia/adrenal crisis | Pediatric condition falsification disorder by proxy<br>Child neglect or abuse<br>Vascular ring<br>Autonomic dysfunction |

GERD, gastroesophageal reflux disease.

*Source:* Adapted from Rosen, R., Vandenplas, Y., Singendonk, M., Cabana, M., DiLorenzo, C., Gottrand, F., Gupta, S., Langendam, M., Staiano, A., Thapar, N., Tipnis, N., & Tabbers, M. (2018). Pediatric gastroesophageal reflux clinical practice guidelines: Joint recommendations of the North American Society for Pediatric Gastroenterology, Hepatology, and Nutrition and the European Society for Pediatric Gastroenterology, Hepatology, and Nutrition. *Journal of Pediatric Gastroenterology and Nutrition, 66*(3), 516–554. https://doi.org/10.1097/MPG.0000000000001889.

**TABLE 8.7**

**KEY HISTORY QUESTIONS IN EVALUATING INFANT GER/GERD**

| Main Topic | Specific Data |
|---|---|
| Feeding and diet history | Duration of each feeding<br>Interval between feedings<br>Volume of each feeding<br>Current and past formula(s) used<br>Method for mixing formula<br>Maternal diet history if infant using breastmilk |
| Pattern of regurgitation, spitting up, or vomiting | Nocturnal<br>Immediately postprandial<br>Timing after meals<br>Undigested versus digested<br>Presence of red or brown material to suggest hematemesis |
| Family medical history | Food allergies/intolerance<br>Environmental allergies<br>Asthma<br>Gastrointestinal problems<br>Metabolic or neurologic conditions |
| Social history | Family psychosocial stressors<br>Mood and affect of caretakers<br>Exposure to tobacco |
| Medical history | Concurrent medical problems<br>Other symptoms and signs, including red flags<br>Growth chart parameters—weight, length, head circumference |

GER, gastroesophageal reflux; GERD, gastroesophageal reflux disease.

*Source:* Data from Rosen, R., Vandenplas, Y., Singendonk, M., Cabana, M., DiLorenzo, C., Gottrand, F., Gupta, S., Langendam, M., Staiano, A., Thapar, N., Tipnis, N., & Tabbers, M. (2018). Pediatric gastroesophageal reflux clinical practice guidelines: Joint recommendations of the North American Society for Pediatric Gastroenterology, Hepatology, and Nutrition and the European Society for Pediatric Gastroenterology, Hepatology, and Nutrition. *Journal of Pediatric Gastroenterology and Nutrition, 66*(3), 516–554. https://doi.org/10.1097/MPG.0000000000001889.

## Diagnosis

For most infants with recurrent regurgitation or spitting up, a detailed history (Table 8.7) and physical examination with attention to warning symptoms and signs (Table 8.8) that may suggest other causes is typically sufficient to make a clinical diagnosis of uncomplicated GER (Rosen et al., 2018). Neonates and infants in the hospital setting with GERD may pose a greater diagnostic challenge, because some of the symptoms and signs may be nonesophageal. Examples include apnea, bradycardia, and cyanosis during or unrelated to feedings.

Despite the frequency with which nonesophageal symptoms such as irritability and apnea trigger further investigation for or treatment of GER/GERD, a clear cause-and-effect relationship has not been well established (Abu Jawdeh & Martin, 2013; Heine et al., 2006; Ramaiah et al., 2005; Zimbric et al., 2012). Indeed, while proton pump inhibitors

## TABLE 8.8

### RED FLAG SYMPTOMS AND SIGNS THAT SUGGEST DISORDERS OTHER THAN GERD

| Symptoms and Signs | Comments |
|---|---|
| ***General***<br>Weight loss or inappropriate weight gain<br>Lethargy<br>Fever<br>Excessive irritability/pain<br>Change in character or quantity of urine | Suggesting various conditions, including systemic infections<br>May suggest urinary tract infection |
| ***Neurologic***<br>Bulging fontanel/rapidly increasing head circumference<br>Seizures<br>Macrocephaly/microcephaly<br>Lethargy | May suggest increased intracranial pressure—e.g., meningitis, brain tumor, or hydrocephalus |
| ***GI***<br>Persistent forceful vomiting<br>Vomiting not associated with feedings<br>Bilious vomiting<br>Hematemesis<br>Chronic diarrhea<br>Rectal bleeding<br>Abdominal distension | May suggest hypertrophic pyloric stenosis<br>May suggest increased intracranial pressure<br>Regarded as symptom of intestinal obstruction. Possible causes: Hirschsprung disease, intestinal atresia, or midgut volvulus or intussusception<br>Suggests a potentially serious bleed from the esophagus, stomach, or upper GI tract, possibly GERD-associated, occurring from acid peptic disease, Mallory–Weiss tear, or reflux esophagitis<br>Indicative of obstruction, dysmotility, or anatomic abnormalities |

GERD, gastroesophageal reflux disease; GI, gastrointestinal.

*Source:* Adapted from Rosen, R., Vandenplas, Y., Singendonk, M., Cabana, M., DiLorenzo, C., Gottrand, F., Gupta, S., Langendam, M., Staiano, A., Thapar, N., Tipnis, N., & Tabbers, M. (2018). Pediatric gastroesophageal reflux clinical practice guidelines: Joint recommendations of the North American Society for Pediatric Gastroenterology, Hepatology, and Nutrition and the European Society for Pediatric Gastroenterology, Hepatology, and Nutrition. *Journal of Pediatric Gastroenterology and Nutrition, 66*(3), 516–554. https://doi.org/10.1097/MPG.0000000000001889.

(PPIs) are the most effective acid suppression agents, several well-conducted studies in infants have not shown PPIs to be of benefit in reducing clinical symptoms (Davidson et al., 2013; Orenstein et al., 2009; Writing Committee for the American Lung Association Asthma Clinical Research Centers, 2012). The decision to treat with a PPI should be made only after careful deliberation benefits and potential harms because the potential risks are being increasingly recognized (Dipasquale et al., 2022; Duncan et al., 2018; Lassalle et al., 2023).

Some infants who have symptoms of GER/GERD may require additional testing. However, there are no clear indications as to when further testing may be helpful. Broad guidelines for when to consider testing may include infants who have GER before the age of 1 week, infants who have red flag signs or symptoms, and infants with unexplained extraesophageal manifestations that may be related to GER (see Table 8.8) (Rosen et al., 2018). Particular areas of ongoing controversy include the relationship of GER and respiratory disorders, and the relationship between GER and distressed behaviors in infants (Abu Jawdeh & Martin, 2013; Zimbric et al., 2012).

The current battery of tests available to evaluate for GER/GERD is outlined in Table 8.9. Routine testing beyond a thorough history and physical examination is typically not recommended unless red flag symptoms or signs are present (Rosen et al., 2018).

The 24 to 48 hours esophageal pH monitoring test with or without impedance is currently the only testing modality that enables the correlation of intraesophageal events with clinical symptoms (Salvatore & Vandenplas, 2016). The test involves inserting a nasal esophageal catheter that remains in place for 24 to 48 hours. In the case of pH monitoring, the catheter has sensors that detect changes in pH. The advantage of a dual pH/impedance catheter is that impedance sensors will also detect movement of air or liquid, regardless of pH. Thus, GER that is nonacidic will also be detected (Salvatore & Vandenplas, 2016). Because both

**TABLE 8.9**

**SELECTED STUDIES TO CONSIDER IN NEONATES AND INFANTS WITH SUSPECTED GERD**

| Study | What the Study Can Help Diagnose or Determine | Comments |
|---|---|---|
| Upper GI barium contrast | Anatomic abnormalities of the esophagus, stomach, and upper small bowel (e.g., gastric outlet obstruction, small bowel obstruction, small bowel malrotation and volvulus, pyloric stenosis, esophageal stricture, esophageal extrinsic compression, duodenal stenosis/web, hiatal hernia, tracheoesophageal fistula) | Insufficient evidence to support use of barium contrast study for the primary diagnosis of GERD |
| Ultrasound | Pyloric stenosis, hydronephrosis, ureteropelvic obstruction, gallstones | No evidence to support use of ultrasound for the diagnosis of GERD |
| EGD | Acid-related esophagitis, eosinophilic esophagitis, peptic ulcer disease, gastritis, duodenitis, *Helicobacter pylori*<br>Hiatal hernia | Insufficient evidence to support use of EGD for the diagnosis of GERD<br>Based on expert opinion, EGD with biopsies can be considered to assess complications of GERD when an underlying mucosal disease is suspected or prior to escalating therapy |
| Scintigraphy | Delayed gastric emptying, gastroparesis | Insufficient evidence to support use to establish a diagnosis of GERD |
| PPI trial | Five trials in preterm and full-term infants show reduction in symptoms | No evidence to support empiric trial of PPI for the diagnosis of GERD in infants |
| 24–48-hour esophageal pH with or without impedance monitoring | Correlation of GER episodes with clinical symptoms and signs (e.g., apnea, bradypnea, bradycardia, spitting up, cough, irritability)<br>Detection of acid- (pH) and nonacid- (impedance)-related GER episodes<br>Efficacy of acid suppression therapy | Insufficient evidence to support the routine use of pH and/or impedance monitoring for the diagnosis of GER in infants and children |

EGD, esophagogastroduodenoscopy; GERD, gastroesophageal reflux disease; PPI, proton pump inhibitor.

*Source:* Data from Rosen, R., Vandenplas, Y., Singendonk, M., Cabana, M., DiLorenzo, C., Gottrand, F., Gupta, S., Langendam, M., Staiano, A., Thapar, N., Tipnis, N., & Tabbers, M. (2018). Pediatric gastroesophageal reflux clinical practice guidelines: Joint recommendations of the North American Society for Pediatric Gastroenterology, Hepatology, and Nutrition and the European Society for Pediatric Gastroenterology, Hepatology, and Nutrition. *Journal of Pediatric Gastroenterology and Nutrition, 66*(3), 516–554. https://doi.org/10.1097/MPG.0000000000001889.

acidic and nonacidic refluxate may contribute to clinical symptoms, dual monitoring may offer additional helpful information compared to pH monitoring alone (Jadcherla et al., 2021).

## Management

Beyond regurgitation and vomiting, the symptoms often attributed to GER/GERD are nonspecific and insensitive for establishing a diagnosis. This diagnostic uncertainty makes the decision of whether to treat and how to treat GER/GERD equally challenging. Treatment options can be divided into pharmacologic and nonpharmacologic approaches.

Nonpharmacologic strategies should be considered in most infants with GER/GERD because time and maturation are the most effective treatment for GERD (Craig et al., 2004; Duncan & Rosen, 2016; Horvath et al., 2008; Vandenplas & Sacre, 1987). Nonpharmacologic approaches include thickening feedings, modifying feeding volumes, eliminating cow's milk protein, and position changes (see Table 8.10) (Bautista et al., 2004; Rosen et al., 2018). Despite the possible benefits of left lateral and prone positioning in the treatment of GER, only the supine position is recommended by the National Health Service and the American Academy of Pediatrics as the safest position to reduce the risk of sudden unexpected infant death syndrome (SUID) (Duncan & Rosen, 2016; Moon, 2011).

**TABLE 8.10**

## SUMMARY OF NONPHARMACOLOGIC OPTIONS FOR GER/GERD

| Intervention | Comments | References |
|---|---|---|
| Thickened feedings | May reduce observable regurgitation episodes, but may not affect the actual frequency of GER | Chao & Vandenplas, 2007; Corvaglia et al., 2006; Horvath et al., 2008; Iacono et al., 2002 |
| Reducing feeding volumes | Recommended based on expert opinion | No RCT has looked at effects of reduced feeding volume |
| Elimination of cow's milk protein | Some infants with cow's milk protein allergy may have regurgitation as their primary symptom<br>Trial of protein hydrolysate formula can be considered if CMPA is suspected (hematochezia, eczema, family history of allergic conditions)<br>Amino acid formulas should be reserved for infants with CMPA refractory to treatment with a protein hydrolysate formula | No RCT specifically evaluating effects of eliminating CMP on GER<br>Some studies show reduced regurgitation in infants with CMPA treated with amino acid–based formula<br>For breastfed infants, eliminating cow's milk-containing products and beef from mother's diet can be considered |
| Positioning therapy | Left lateral decubitus position may reduce total number of reflux episodes | Loots et al., 2014; Moon, 2011; Omari et al., 2004; Rosen et al., 2018 |

A minimum 2-week trial is recommended for each nonpharmacologic strategy to assess for symptom improvement before considering other therapeutic options. CMP(A), cow's milk protein (allergy); GER, gastroesophageal reflux; GERD, gastroesophageal reflux disease; RCT, randomized controlled trial.

*Source:* Data from Rosen, R., Vandenplas, Y., Singendonk, M., Cabana, M., DiLorenzo, C., Gottrand, F., Gupta, S., Langendam, M., Staiano, A., Thapar, N., Tipnis, N., & Tabbers, M. (2018). Pediatric gastroesophageal reflux clinical practice guidelines: Joint recommendations of the North American Society for Pediatric Gastroenterology, Hepatology, and Nutrition and the European Society for Pediatric Gastroenterology, Hepatology, and Nutrition. *Journal of Pediatric Gastroenterology and Nutrition, 66*(3), 516–554. https://doi.org/10.1097/MPG.0000000000001889.

Acid-suppression therapy and prokinetic agents are two common medical management options. PPIs and histamine-2 receptor antagonists ($H_2A$) are the two most prescribed acid-suppression agents. After reviewing the current evidence addressing the use of PPIs in infants, the GER guideline committee concluded that it is uncertain whether the use of PPIs or $H_2As$ reduces crying/distress, visible vomiting/regurgitation, or signs and symptoms of GERD (Rosen et al., 2018). The working group subsequently recommended against the routine use of $H_2A$ or PPI for the treatment of crying/distress or visible regurgitation in otherwise healthy infants. However, the same group determined that the current body of evidence does support the use of PPIs as the first line for treating GERD-related erosive esophagitis (Rosen et al., 2018). Considering that few infants undergo endoscopy with biopsy, which is the gold standard for diagnosing erosive esophagitis related to GERD, clinicians are left with clinical symptoms as the primary determinant of whether acid suppression treatment is warranted. An added challenge to the decision whether to use acid suppression therapy is that not all GER is acid related. It is thought that preprandial acid GER predominates while nonacid GER predominates postprandial. The benefits of acid suppression must be balanced with potential risks. As an acidic environment is one measure of defense against infection, raising gastric pH may be associated with an increased risk for infection, including sepsis.

If the decision is to proceed with treatment, a reasonable approach may be to begin with a time-limited trial with an $H_2A$ agent. If there is no improvement in targeted symptoms, then a subsequent trial with a PPI can be considered. If target symptoms fail to improve or resolve with acid suppression therapy, the treatment should be discontinued. Practitioners should also be aware that while PPIs may effectively reduce esophageal acid reflux in neonates, they may not affect the symptoms associated with GERD (Davidson et al., 2013).

Prokinetic agents are a second class of drugs available to treat GER/GERD. Metoclopramide is one of the more commonly prescribed prokinetic agents in infants, although its effectiveness is far from satisfactory (Craig et al., 2004). Coupled with its unfavorable side effects profile, including somnolence, irritability, galactorrhea, extrapyramidal reactions, and potentially permanent tardive dyskinesia, metoclopramide is not highly recommended in infants (Putnam et al., 1992).

Over the past 15 years, there has been increasing use of erythromycin as prokinetic therapy. Erythromycin is an antibiotic that is also a motilin receptor agonist. Motilin is a physiologic hormone that increases GI motility when bound to the motilin receptor located throughout the GI tract. While there have not been sufficient studies for or against its effectiveness, there have been a limited number of studies to suggest that erythromycin ethylsuccinate (EES) may be helpful in some infants at reducing GER/GERD symptoms (Rosen et al., 2018).

EES is a CYP3A inhibitor and may alter the levels of other drugs and has also been associated with arrhythmias and prolonged QT interval.

For infants with GERD symptoms refractory to medical therapy, transpyloric tube feedings may be effective at improving feeding tolerance (Malcolm et al., 2009; Misra et al., 2007). Surgical intervention can be considered in rare cases in which medical management is not effective and the benefits of surgery outweigh the risks and potential long-term side effects (Rosen et al., 2018).

## HYPERTROPHIC PYLORIC STENOSIS

### Background

Hypertrophic pyloric stenosis (HPS) is characterized by progressive thickening of the circumferential muscle layer of the pyloric sphincter that results in the narrowing and elongation of the pyloric channel that clinically manifests in a high-grade or complete gastric outlet obstruction (Seifarth & Soldes, 2016). HPS is the most common gastric surgical disorder in neonates (Seifarth & Soldes, 2016). The precise etiology and pathogenesis of HPS is unclear. Several factors are thought to play a role in the development of HPS. There seems to be a genetic predisposition with male predominance (Olivé & Endom, 2019; Seifarth & Soldes, 2016).

Regional variations in the prevalence of HPS suggest environmental factors may contribute to the development of HPS (Olivé & Endom, 2019). Other environmental factors that are thought to increase the risk for developing HPS include bottle feeding (McAteer et al., 2013), maternal smoking (Svenningsson et al., 2014), and exposure to macrolide antibiotics (Eberly et al., 2015).

### Diagnosis

Infants with HPS typically develop progressive symptoms between 3 and 6 weeks of age. The predominant symptom is nonbilious forceful ("projectile") emesis that occurs almost immediately after feeding (Olivé & Endom, 2019). If the vomiting has gone on for some time, there may be evidence of brown coloration or blood streaks from vomiting-induced gastritis or esophagitis. The infant often exhibits a robust appetite even after vomiting episodes. The inability to tolerate feedings may result in severe dehydration, lethargy, and failure to thrive. Abdominal examination may reveal the hypertrophied pylorus as an olive-shaped mass at the lateral edge of the rectus abdominis muscle in the right upper quadrant of the abdomen (Olivé & Endom, 2019). Because adrenal crisis associated with congenital adrenal hyperplasia may also present with significant vomiting, examination for evidence of ambiguous genitalia should also be part of the physical examination (Olivé & Endom, 2019).

Electrolyte losses and physiologic compensatory mechanisms result in hypochloremic, hypokalemic, and contraction metabolic alkalosis with paradoxical aciduria. Hypoglycemia may also uncommonly precipitate seizures. Bloodwork may also show a mild unconjugated hyperbilirubinemia that is thought to correlate with decreased hepatic conjugation function. The complete blood count (CBC) is typically normal in HPS, so an elevated WBC should prompt evaluation for additional causes of vomiting, including infectious causes. Abdominal ultrasound has a sensitivity and specificity greater than 95% when performed by experienced technicians or radiologists (Niedzielski et al., 2011). The diagnostic appearance on ultrasound is a target sign that represents the outer ring of low echo-density musculature and the inner ring of high echo-density mucosa (Seifarth & Soldes, 2016). Because HPS can evolve over time, a previous "normal" ultrasound should not preclude repeating the study if the infant's symptoms persist or worsen.

If ultrasonography is unavailable or inconclusive, an upper GI contrast study may be obtained. The most common signs on upper GI are an elongated and narrowed pyloric channel ("string" sign), two thin tracks of contrast along the pyloric channel from the compressed pyloric mucosa ("double-track" sign), a tapered point ending the pyloric channel ("beak" sign), and a prepyloric bulge of contrast ("shoulder" sign; Olivé & Endom, 2019).

### Management

Pyloromyotomy is the surgical treatment for HPS. Prior to surgery, dehydration and electrolyte abnormalities should be corrected (Rich & Dolgin, 2021). Multiple boluses with 10 to 20 ml/kg of 0.9% normal saline may be required to correct the hypovolemia. Maintenance fluid then can be started with 5% dextrose in 0.45% to 0.9% saline at 1.5 to 2.0 times the maintenance rate depending on the degree of dehydration (Olivé & Endom, 2019). Once urine output is established, 10 to 20 mEq/L of potassium chloride may be added to the IV fluid mixture (Seifarth & Soldes, 2016). Electrolytes should be monitored every 8 to 12 hours until normalized. Surgery may be delayed for 24 to 48 hours to correct dehydration and electrolyte abnormalities (Hackam et al., 2019). Unlike other abdominal surgical conditions associated with vomiting, continuous suction with an NG tube should be avoided so as not to exacerbate electrolyte abnormalities.

There are no guidelines on the timing and type of feedings to start after surgery. A common protocol used at some centers begins feedings within 4 to 8 hours after surgery. One-half to 1 oz of an electrolyte solution is started and progresses every 2 to 3 hours to 2 oz of breastmilk or formula (Seifarth & Soldes, 2016). Most infants can be discharged within 48 hours after surgery (Seifarth & Soldes, 2016).

## INTESTINAL ATRESIA

### Background

Intestinal atresia (IA) is defined as a congenital defect of a hollow viscus resulting in complete or partial obstruction of the bowel lumen (Wesson, 2018). Duodenal atresia make up approximately 50% of intestinal atresias (Wesson, 2018). The classification scheme for duodenal atresia is summarized in Table 8.11. Duodenal atresia is hypothesized to be caused by a failure of recanalization of the duodenal lumen during embryonic development (Schneider & Oldham, 2016). Up to 30% of infants with duodenal atresia may have associated congenital anomalies such as intestinal malrotation, esophageal atresia, imperforate anus, thoracoabdominal heterotaxia,

**TABLE 8.11**

**CLASSIFICATION OF DUODENAL ATRESIA**

| Type | Description |
|---|---|
| I | Intestinal lumen obstructed by a membrane or web<br>Membrane obstruction complete or fenestrated |
| II | Fibrous band connecting two ends of duodenum with typically dilated proximal and small distal segments |
| III | Complete discontinuity between atretic segments<br>Two blind-ending bowel loops with no mesentery in between<br>May be associated with biliary anomalies<br>Least common type |

***Classification of Jejunal Atresia***

| Type | Description |
|---|---|
| I | Intraluminal web in continuity with muscle layers of proximal and distal segments<br>Least common type |
| II | Fibrous cords connect proximal and distal bowel segments with blind ends |
| III | Significant mesenteric defects<br>Subtype IIIA—V-shaped mesenteric defect with intestinal discontinuity<br>Subtype IIIB—mesenteric defect with distal segment receiving entire blood supply in retrograde fashion via ileocolic or right colic artery; "apple peel" or "Christmas tree" deformity<br>Associated with significant bowel loss<br>Most common type |
| IV | Multiple atresias within a single length of bowel |

*Sources:* Adapted from Best, K. E., Tennant, P. W., Addor, M. C., Bianchi, F., Boyd, P., Calzolari, E., Dias, C. M., Doray, B., Draper, E., Garne, E., Gatt, M., Greenlees, R., Haeusler, M., Khoshnood, B., McDonnell, B., Mullaney, C., Nelen, V., Randrianaivo, H., Rissmann, A., & Rankin, J. (2012). Epidemiology of small intestinal atresia in Europe: A register-based study. *Archives of Disease in Childhood—Fetal and Neonatal Edition, 97*(5), F353–F358. https://doi.org/10.1136/fetalneonatal-2011-300631; Amin, R., & Oldham, K. T. (2021). Small and large bowel stenosis and atresias. In R. Wyllie, H. S. Hyams, & M. Kay (Eds.), *Pediatric gastrointestinal and liver disease* (6th ed., pp. 588–592). Elsevier; Wesson, D. E. (2018). Intestinal atresia. In J. A. Garcia-Prats & M. B. Heyman (Eds.), *UpToDate*. https://www.uptodate.com/contents/intestinal-atresia.

cardiac anomalies, gallbladder agenesis, and trisomy 21 (Best et al., 2012; Dingeldein, 2025).

Jejunal and ileal atresia each make up approximately 20% of IAs (Best et al., 2012). Unlike duodenal atresia, the pathophysiologic model for jejunal and ileal atresias begins with vascular compromise that leads to intestinal necrosis and subsequent reabsorption of the bowel tissue (Louw, 1959). Causes of vascular compromise may include intussusception, segmental compromise of the mesenteric blood supply, volvulus, internal bowel herniation, and gastroschisis (Wesson, 2018). Less than 5% of patients with jejunal or ileal atresia have associated chromosomal abnormalities (Best et al., 2012).

## Diagnosis

IA typically presents within the first 72 hours of life. These newborns may have abdominal distension, bilious or nonbilious vomiting, or fail to pass meconium (Amin & Oldham, 2021; Wesson, 2018). A supine anteroposterior plain radiograph with either upright, lateral decubitus, or cross-table lateral views should be obtained in neonates and infants with suspected intestinal obstruction. Table 8.12 summarizes the possible findings on plain radiography.

**Duodenal Atresia.** Less than 50% of IAs are diagnosed prenatally (Haeusler et al., 2002). Prenatal ultrasound of neonates with duodenal atresia may show polyhydramnios and/or dilation of the stomach and proximal duodenum (Amin & Oldham, 2021; Grosfeld & Rescorla, 1993). The vomiting-associated duodenal atresia is typically bilious. Abdominal

**TABLE 8.12**

**PLAIN RADIOGRAPH FINDINGS OF SELECTED INTESTINAL PATHOLOGIES**

| Diagnosis | Plain Radiograph Finding |
|---|---|
| Intestinal perforation | Abnormal accumulation of extraintestinal air<br>Pneumoperitoneum<br>Intraperitoneal calcification (prenatal intestinal perforation, meconium peritonitis) |
| Duodenal atresia | Double-bubble sign (dilation of stomach and duodenum)<br>Absence or paucity of air in distal bowel<br>Air-fluid level in duodenum |
| Jejunal or ileal atresia | Dilated loops of small bowel with air-fluid levels |
| Malrotation | Contrast study findings:<br>Low-lying or displaced duodenojejunal junction and coiling of bowel with partial or complete obstruction |

distension may or may not be present because vomiting may be sufficient to decompress proximal obstructions (Schneider & Oldham, 2016). Abdominal radiograph often reveals simultaneous gastric and duodenal distension (double-bubble sign) with a paucity of air in the remainder of the bowel.

**Jejunal Atresia.** Prenatal ultrasound in neonates with jejunal atresia may show polyhydramnios and dilated loops of bowel (Amin & Oldham, 2021; Phelps et al., 1997). Infants may present with bilious vomiting, abdominal distension, and/or jaundice. Plain radiographs may show moderate to severely dilated bowel loops and air-fluid levels. A rectal contrast enema may reveal a microcolon in the setting of small bowel atresia.

**Contrast Studies.** If there is no evidence of perforation on a plain radiograph, most infants should undergo an upper GI contrast study to look for malrotation or midgut volvulus. If plain radiographs and upper GI contrast studies do not provide a likely diagnosis, a contrast enema should be considered to further evaluate for IA or other causes of intestinal obstruction (Wesson, 2018).

Evaluation for other associated congenital anomalies should be considered, as summarized in Table 8.13 (Kimble et al., 1997).

## Management

Definitive treatment for IA is operative. Preoperative therapy includes electrolyte and fluid resuscitation, antibiotics, and upper GI decompression via an orogastric or NG tube (Amin & Oldham, 2021). An echocardiogram should be considered to look for associated cardiac anomalies, particularly in patients with a murmur or trisomy 21.

**TABLE 8.13**

**ADDITIONAL TESTING TO CONSIDER IN PATIENTS WITH INTESTINAL ATRESIA**

| Test | Consider in Neonates and Infants With. . . |
|---|---|
| Echocardiogram | Duodenal atresia<br>Down syndrome |
| Chest radiograph | Infants with any small bowel atresia looking for vertebral anomalies |
| Renal ultrasound | Duodenal atresia |
| CF mutation testing | Small bowel atresia and meconium plugs |

*Source:* Adapted from Kimble, R. M., Harding, J., & Kolbe, A. (1997). Additional congenital anomalies in babies with gut atresia or stenosis: When to investigate, and which investigation. *Pediatric Surgery International*, *12*, 565–570. https://doi.org/10.1007/bf01371900.

Postoperatively, GI decompression is continued. Parenteral nutrition (PN) may be required until oral feedings are started. Once the gastric aspirate appears clear and there is evidence of GI function, feedings can be started and carefully advanced until full enteral feedings are tolerated. Achieving full enteral feedings may take several weeks (Schneider & Oldham, 2016). Patients who require extensive bowel resection may take longer to tolerate enteral feedings or develop short bowel syndrome (SBS), requiring chronic PN therapy.

# INTESTINAL MALROTATION

## Background

Normal intestinal development in the fetus follows an orchestrated sequence of growth, elongation, and rotation, followed by intestinal fixation to the body wall during fetal development (Table 8.14) (Sato & Sato, 2021). Malrotation occurs when any step in this process fails to happen, resulting in abnormal intestinal rotation and fixation (Sato & Sato, 2021). The most catastrophic complication of malrotation occurs when the intestine twists along its mesenteric axis, resulting in volvulus, bowel ischemia, necrosis, and loss of bowel. Approximately 30% of infants with malrotation presenting before 1 month of age will develop volvulus (Fonkalsrud, 2003). Fifty percent of infants with malrotation are diagnosed in the first month of life, and 90% by 1 year of age (Ford et al., 1992; Nehra & Goldstein, 2011; Sato & Sato, 2021).

Other anomalies associated with intestinal malrotation include congenital diaphragmatic hernia, cardiac anomalies, abdominal wall defects (omphalocele, gastroschisis, prune belly syndrome), IA, EA, biliary atresia, Meckel diverticulum, ARM, and Cornelia de Lang syndrome (Brandt, 2019).

## Diagnosis

Because malrotation can quickly evolve into catastrophic volvulus, evaluation and treatment should be pursued emergently. Newborns and infants with malrotation typically present with one or more of the following symptoms and signs: bilious or nonbilious vomiting, abnormal abdominal examination (distension, tenderness), and hemodynamic instability. Irritability, lethargy, feeding intolerance, reduced oral intake, and/or poor growth are nonspecific findings that may also suggest malrotation. Many of these symptoms and signs overlap with those of other critical conditions, such as shock syndromes (e.g. cardiogenic, septic, hypovolemic). Therefore, a high index of suspicion coupled with a low threshold for diagnostic imaging is essential for optimizing outcomes (Sato & Sato, 2021; Yang et al., 2024).

**Emergency Alert: Late findings in babies with intestinal malrotation or volvulus include persistent bilious emesis associated with hemodynamic instability (tachycardia, hypotension, tachypnea), persistent abdominal distension, peritoneal signs, and poor vascular perfusion.** The evaluation may reveal occult blood-positive stools, metabolic acidosis, elevated serum lactate, and coagulopathy (Brandt, 2019; Nehra & Goldstein, 2011; Sato & Sato, 2021).

**TABLE 8.14**

**FETAL EVENTS LEADING TO NORMAL POSITION OF THE INTESTINES**

| Stage | Event |
|---|---|
| I | Fifth week of gestation<br>Herniation of primary intestinal midgut loop into umbilical cord base<br>Omphalomesenteric duct located at apex of midgut loop rotates 180° counterclockwise so that proximal prearterial half of loop passes posterior to SMA<br>Prearterial segment gives rise to proximal duodenum (right of midline)<br>Distal prearterial segment that passes posterior and to the left of SMA becomes third and fourth portions of duodenum<br>Distal duodenum normally fixed to left of aorta at ligament of Treitz after 270° counterclockwise rotation from original position<br>Jejunoileal segment elongates to form remainder of small bowel<br>Postarterial segment gives rise to cecum and right colon, which undergoes a 270° counterclockwise rotation to move from the initial position on the left to the right of SMA before attaching to posterior wall of right iliac fossa |
| II | 10th–12th week gestation<br>Duodenojejunal junction has passed posterior to SMA and midgut rotated 180° counterclockwise<br>Small intestine initially remains to right of midline; cecum and ascending colon still anterior to SMA on return of the intestine to the abdominal cavity |
| III | 12th week of gestation<br>Normal points of fixation: cecum in right iliac fossa, duodenojejunal junction at ligament of Treitz<br>Fixation of intestines to posterior body wall with a broad base extending from ligament of Treitz to cecum<br>Fixation prevents torsion of intestinal mesentery around its vascular supply |

SMA, superior mesenteric artery.

*Source:* Adapted from Sato, T. T., & Sato, E. H. (2021). Abnormal rotation and fixation of the intestine. In R. Wyllie, H. S. Hyams, & M. Kay (Eds.), *Pediatric gastrointestinal and liver disease* (6th ed., pp. 581–587). Elsevier.

In a patient with suspected volvulus who is hemodynamically unstable, imaging should not delay surgical exploration (Brandt, 2019). Radiographic studies can proceed in hemodynamically stable patients. Initial plain abdominal radiography may reveal gastric or proximal bowel distension with a paucity of distal bowel air on plain abdominal radiographs. Upright anteroposterior or cross-table lateral views to look for pneumoperitoneum suggestive of intestinal perforation should also be obtained.

If there is no evidence of perforation on plain radiographs, an upper GI contrast study should be performed to confirm malrotation (Applegate, 2009). Malrotation may appear as a corkscrew or coiled spiral pattern with contrast imaging. The position of the duodenojejunal junction or ligament of Treitz on the right side of the abdomen also suggests malrotation (Applegate, 2009). Upper GI contrast studies have a sensitivity of over 90% for detecting malrotation (Sizemore et al., 2008; Yang et al., 2024). For infants who undergo rectal contrast enema, the cecum may be positioned in the midline or to the left of the vertebra. However, in 20% of cases of malrotation, the cecum may appear in its normal anatomic location in the right lower quadrant (Applegate, 2009).

Ultrasound is a modality that is gaining increasing popularity. Normally, the superior mesenteric vein is to the right of the superior mesenteric artery (SMA). In the presence of malrotation, the superior mesenteric vein may be found ventral or to the left of the SMA (Sato & Sato, 2021; Weinberger et al., 1992). It should be noted that a normal ultrasound does not eliminate the possibility of malrotation (Ashley et al., 2001; Orzech et al., 2006).

## Management

Prompt consultation with pediatric surgeons is paramount in all cases of suspected malrotation or volvulus. Preoperative management includes NG tube decompression and circulatory and electrolyte resuscitation. Broad-spectrum antibiotics should be considered because signs and symptoms of malrotation/volvulus can overlap with sepsis, or there may be concomitant systemic infection. Acid suppression with an $H_2A$ blocker should be considered because vomiting or the presence of an NG tube may increase the risk of developing gastritis or esophagitis.

A general operative approach is shown in Box 8.1.

**BOX 8.1**

**GENERAL OPERATIVE STRATEGY FOR MALROTATION AND VOLVULUS**

Delivery of the entire midgut and inspection of vascular mesentery

Reduction of volvulus and evaluation of intestinal viability

Division of Ladd's bands

Broadening the base of mesenteric vascular pedicle

Appendectomy

Return of GI tract with small intestine in the right abdomen and the large intestine in the left abdomen

*Source:* Data from Abdullah, F., & Karim, O. (2018). *BMJ best practice: Intestinal malrotation*. BMJ Publishing Group.

Recovery of GI function may be delayed postoperatively, particularly in the presence of volvulus; prolonged nasogastric decompression and PN may be required (Feitz & Vos, 1997; Sato & Chang, 2016). Some infants and children may have persistent postoperative vomiting or feeding intolerance with significant intestinal dysmotility (Devane et al., 1992). Prokinetic agents such as metoclopramide or erythromycin can be considered along with continued acid suppression therapy in postoperative infants with persistent symptoms of dysmotility. Neonates who require extensive bowel resection due to a delay in diagnosis may develop short bowel syndrome (SBS), necessitating chronic PN therapy.

## ABDOMINAL WALL DEFECTS

### Background

The prevalence of omphalocele and gastroschisis is approximately 3 to 4 per 10,000 live births (Friedman et al., 2016), representing the most common types of abdominal wall defects in neonates. Table 8.15 compares key features of omphalocele and gastroschisis.

An omphalocele is a midline abdominal wall defect of variable size typically covered by a membrane of amnion and peritoneum containing abdominal contents. The defect is at the base of the umbilical cord, with the umbilical vessels inserted into the apex of the omphalocele sac. Sac contents may include the stomach, small bowel loops, colon, and liver. Larger omphaloceles may also contain the bladder, gonads, and spleen. The pathogenesis of omphaloceles begins during weeks 3 to 4 of fetal development when the embryo lengthens and folds onto itself to enclose various body cavities. Two lateral folds normally form and meet anteriorly in the midline at the umbilicus. Failure of the folds to meet in the midline results in an omphalocele (Stephenson et al., 2018). The omphalocele membrane provides a barrier that protects against potential injury from exposure to amniotic fluid.

Gastroschisis is an abdominal wall defect that is usually 5 cm or less and located to the right of the umbilical cord. The herniated abdominal contents usually include only the small bowel. The pathogenesis of gastroschisis is less clear. Several hypotheses have been proposed, including failure of differentiation of the embryonic mesenchyme, rupture of the amniotic membrane at the base of the umbilical cord at the area of the right umbilical vein, and vascular compromise (deVries, 1980). Bowel portions involved in gastroschisis can appear matted, edematous, and inflamed. Microscopic injury is characterized by serosal inflammation, submucosal fibrosis, muscular hypertrophy and hyperplasia, and villous atrophy and blunting. The gross and microscopic injury is hypothesized to be caused by exposure to amniotic fluid, and partial closure of the defect around the base of the affected intestine. The latter results in constriction around the intestinal mesentery resulting in obstruction of the intestinal lumen, lymphatic, and venous outflow. These pathologic sequelae help to explain why some neonates with gastroschisis may require long-term PN even with a relatively normal length of bowel (Dingeldein, 2025).

**TABLE 8.15**

**COMPARISON OF GASTROSCHISIS AND OMPHALOCELE**

| | Gastroschisis | Omphalocele |
|---|---|---|
| Incidence | 1.5 per 10,000 live births | 2-2.5 per 10,000 live births |
| Defect location | Right periumbilical | Umbilical ring/central |
| Covering sac | Absent | Present (amnion and peritoneum) |
| Description | Free intestinal loops | Firm mass including bowel, liver, and so on |
| Umbilical cord | Normal insertion | Inserts into sac |
| Necrotizing enterocolitis | Common | Uncommon |
| Associated anomalies | Gastrointestinal<br>Intestinal atresia<br>Malrotation<br>Cryptorchidism<br>Stenosis<br>Perforation<br>Volvulus | Trisomy syndromes<br>Gastrointestinal<br>Genitourinary<br>Cardiac defects<br>Genetic syndromes (Trisomy 13, 18, 21; Beckwith–Wiedemann Syndrome; VACTERL association; EEC syndrome (ectodermal dysplasia, ectrodactyly, cleft palate) |

*Sources:* Adapted from Chabra, S., & Gleason, C. A. (2005). Gastroschisis. *NeoReviews, 6*(11), e493–e499. https://doi.org/10.1542/neo.6-11-e493; Polites, S. F., & Nathan, J. D. (2021). Newborn abdominal wall defects. In R. Wyllie, H. S. Hyams, & M. Kay (Eds.), *Pediatric gastrointestinal and liver disease* (6th ed., pp. 593–602). Elsevier.

### Diagnosis

The diagnosis of gastroschisis and omphalocele can be made by prenatal ultrasound. Omphalocele can be differentiated from gastroschisis by the presence of a sac and a liver within the defect in most cases (Stephenson et al., 2018). Gastroschisis can be identified by free-floating loops of the bowel within the amniotic fluid. Ultrasound may also detect associated anomalies such as intestinal atresia and cardiac defects (see Table 8.15) (Hughes et al., 1989; Walther & Nathan, 2016). Both omphalocele and gastroschisis can be associated with elevated maternal serum alpha fetoprotein (Saller et al., 1994).

Omphalocele can be associated with chromosomal abnormalities such as trisomy 13, 18, or 21, Turner syndrome, and triploidy. Structural anomalies may include other GI anomalies, cardiac defects, genitourinary anomalies, orofacial clefts, neural tube defects, and diaphragmatic defects (Stephenson et al., 2018). Other syndromes associated with omphalocele include pentalogy of Cantrell, amniotic band sequence, schisis association, OEIS syndrome (omphalocele, exstrophy of the bladder, imperforate anus, spinal defects), Shprintzen syndrome, Carpenter syndrome, Goltz syndrome, Marshall–Smith syndrome, CHARGE syndrome, and Beckwith–Wiedemann syndrome (Stephenson et al., 2018).

### Management

Presurgical management of infants with gastroschisis or omphalocele presents added challenges compared to infants with other surgical conditions. Infants with respiratory distress may require supplemental oxygen or ventilator support. IV lines should preferentially be placed in the upper extremities due to possible inferior vena cava (IVC) compression during bowel reduction (Polites & Nathan, 2021). An NG or orogastric tube should be placed to decompress the stomach and help minimize small bowel distension.

The omphalocele sac should be wrapped with saline-soaked gauze and an impervious dressing to reduce fluid losses and hypothermia. In neonates who have gastroschisis with an eviscerated bowel or a ruptured omphalocele, the bowel should be wrapped in saline-soaked gauze and placed in a central position; the infant should be placed on the right side to prevent vascular compromise from mesenteric kinking. The bowel is then wrapped in an impervious dressing, such as a plastic wrap (BMJ Best Practice, 2017; Polites & Nathan, 2021).

If the gastroschisis defect is small and there is evidence of vascular compromise, the defect should be enlarged to increase blood flow (Polites & Nathan, 2021). Infants should be placed in a warm environment to maintain core body temperature. Due to ongoing fluid losses, infants may require fluid volumes greater than maintenance amounts. Electrolytes should be followed closely and corrected as needed. Repositioning the baby may be needed if there are signs of vascular compromise to the bowel such as hypotension, tachycardia, or a dusky bowel appearance.

Surgical options for gastroschisis include primary reduction and fascial closure, silo placement with serial reduction, delayed fascial closure, or primary or delayed reduction without fascial closure (BMJ Best Practice, 2017; Polites & Nathan, 2021). The main goal in managing omphalocele is the gradual reduction of the viscera into the abdominal cavity, followed by closure of the fascia and skin. Central venous access should be secured in anticipation of lengthy postoperative PN needs associated with intestinal dysmotility and decreased absorptive function that is frequently encountered.

For neonates with omphalocele, the priority for abdominal wall repair is preservation of blood flow to the intestines and eviscerated organs (Stephenson et al., 2019). Small defects (2–3 cm) can usually be closed in the first 24 to 72 hours of life (Stephenson et al., 2019). Larger and more complex defects may require initial silo placement followed by gradual reduction and definitive closure (Pacilli et al., 2005). Depending on the size of the abdominal wall defect, it may take 3 to 7 days before sufficient reduction is achieved to allow closure of the fascia and skin. Serial Doppler ultrasound may be used to ensure sufficient blood flow to the organs during the omphalocele reduction process.

During the postoperative period, infants are at risk of developing abdominal compartment syndrome after fascial closure. Repeated physical examination, ventilator settings, intraabdominal pressure measurements, heart rate, blood pressure, and urine output may provide clues indicating increased abdominal pressure (Stephenson et al., 2018). NG or orogastric decompression should continue until there is clinical evidence of bowel function and the abdominal examination is reassuring. PN should continue until a sufficient volume of enteral calories is reached. There is no clear consensus as to the optimal time for starting enteral feedings. Tolerance of full enteral feedings may take time due to the intestinal dysmotility commonly associated with gastroschisis. However, introducing even the smallest amounts of enteral feedings may help lower the risk of developing cholestasis as a result of delayed enteral feedings and PN. Oral stimulation should be provided as much as possible, even during the slow process of advancing feedings, to minimize the risk of developing feeding problems from the loss of the suck–swallow reflex (Polites & Nathan, 2021).

## NECROTIZING ENTEROCOLITIS

### Background

NEC is the most common GI emergency in neonates and carries a high rate of long-term complications (Gregory et al., 2011; Neu & Walker, 2011). NEC occurs in 1 to 3 per 1,000 live births and increases with decreasing gestational age (Llanos et al., 2002; Thompson & Bizzarro, 2008). While NEC can occur at any age, approximately 90% occur in preterm infants who have been fed enterally (Kim, 2019a; Yee et al., 2012). Characteristics inherent to premature infants that most likely contribute to their increased risk for developing NEC are circulatory instability, permeable GI mucosal barrier that is prone to bacterial translocation, undeveloped local host defense mechanisms, and immature bowel motility and function (Kim, 2019b).

NEC can be localized in the case of segmental mucosal necrosis or extensive in the case of transmural necrosis of the small and large bowels. While the pathogenesis of NEC is not well defined, characteristic features most likely include ischemic injury leading to necrosis of the intestinal mucosa, altered host epithelial defense mechanisms, dysregulated mucosal immune and inflammatory responses, abnormal bacterial colonization particularly by gas-forming organisms, and dissection of gas into the muscularis layer of the intestines and portal venous system (Kim, 2018; Neu & Walker, 2011). The convergence of these pathogenic mechanisms culminates in massive intestinal injury and multiorgan system failure (Iben & Rodriguez, 2016).

## Diagnosis

A high index of suspicion is essential because clinical evidence of NEC can be nonspecific, such as increased gastric residual with feedings, poor feeding, apnea, lethargy, temperature instability, vomiting, change in stool character, occult blood positive stools, abdominal distension or tenderness, discoloration of abdominal skin, and/or bilious output from enteral feeding tubes (Kim, 2019a). Respiratory failure and signs of septic shock may also be present. Bacteremia is also common with NEC (Kim, 2019a). Laboratory findings may include leukocytosis, neutropenia, thrombocytopenia or thrombocytosis, acute anemia, disseminated intravascular coagulation (DIC; increased prothrombin time, decreased fibrinogen, increased fibrin split products), elevated C-reactive protein, hyperglycemia, electrolyte abnormalities (hyponatremia common), elevated lactate, and acidosis (metabolic/respiratory) (Bethell et al., 2025; Kim, 2019a). Contrast enemas are contraindicated in suspected NEC due to the risk of perforation.

Successful management of NEC begins with early diagnosis, which stems from being vigilant about clinical changes (Table 8.16). When NEC is suspected, screening assessment can include plain abdominal radiography, stool for occult

**TABLE 8.16**

**MODIFIED BELL STAGING CRITERIA FOR NEC**

| Stage | Classification | Systemic Signs | Intestinal Signs | Radiographic Signs |
|---|---|---|---|---|
| IA | Suspected NEC | Temperature instability, apnea, bradycardia, lethargy | Increased gastric residuals, mild abdominal distension, vomiting, heme-positive stool | Normal or dilated bowel loops, mild ileus |
| IB | Suspected NEC | Same as IA | Bright red blood from rectum | Same as above |
| IIA | Proven NEC—mildly ill | Same as above | Same as above, plus absent bowel sounds, with or without abdominal tenderness | Intestinal dilation, ileus, pneumatosis intestinalis |
| IIB | Proven NEC—moderately ill | Same as above plus: mild metabolic acidosis, mild thrombocytopenia | Same as above, plus absent bowel sounds, abdominal tenderness, with or without abdominal cellulitis or right lower quadrant mass | Same as IIA, plus portal venous gas, with or without ascites |
| IIIA | Advanced NEC—severely ill, bowel intact | Same as IIB, plus hypotension, bradycardia, severe apnea, combined respiratory and metabolic acidosis, DIC, and neutropenia | Same as above, plus signs of generalized peritonitis, marked tenderness, and distention of abdomen | Same as IIB, plus definite ascites |
| IIIB | Advanced NEC—severely ill, bowel perforation | Same as IIIA | Same as IIIA | Same as IIB, plus pneumoperitoneum |

NEC, necrotizing enterocolitis.

*Source:* Lee, J. S., & Polin, R. A. (2003). Treatment and prevention of necrotizing enterocolitis. *Seminars in Neonatology: SN, 8*(6), 449–459. https://doi.org/10.1016/S1084-2756(03)00123-4.

blood and calprotectin, sepsis evaluation, CBC, coagulation studies, and serum chemistries (electrolytes, $CO_2$, BUN, Cr, glucose, lactate). Plain abdominal radiographs should include cross-table lateral and/or left lateral decubitus views to help detect pneumoperitoneum. Other abdominal radiographic signs can range from nonspecific findings such as a gasless abdomen, ascites, and dilated loops of the bowel to ominous signs, including pneumatosis intestinalis, portal venous air, or sentinel loops. Pneumatosis intestinalis is the result of gas dissecting into the bowel wall. Sentinel loops are bowel loops that remain in a fixed position on serial radiographs and may be evidence for necrotic bowel and/or perforation (Kim, 2019a).

Abdominal ultrasonography is playing an increasingly important complementary role in the evaluation and diagnosis of NEC (Garbi-Goutel et al., 2014; Hwang et al., 2022; Silva et al., 2007). A central echogenic focus with a hypoechoic rim may suggest necrotic bowel. Ultrasonography may also identify air in the liver parenchyma and portal venous system, fluid collections, and/or changes in bowel wall thickness and echogenicity associated with NEC. Doppler ultrasound can also detect abnormal bowel wall perfusion (Garbi-Goutel et al., 2014; Kim, 2019a; Silva et al., 2007).

### Management

Management of NEC begins with bowel rest (nil per os [NPO]), prompt initiation of broad-spectrum antibiotics, and abdominal decompression. Decompression via an NG tube set to low suction is continued until there is clinical improvement and the abdominal distension and any pneumatosis that is present resolves. Because the period of NPO can range from 10 to 14 days, PN should provide complete nutritional requirements. Inotropic support, large-volume fluid resuscitation, and ventilator support may be needed in some infants who become critically ill. Close monitoring and correction of electrolyte and metabolic abnormalities will also be required in many infants with NEC (Iben & Rodriguez, 2016; Kim, 2019a).

Because up to 30% of infants with NEC will have concomitant bacteremia (Ballance et al., 1990; Holman et al., 1997; Hunter et al., 2008; Kim, 2018; Neu & Weiss, 1999), blood cultures should be obtained prior to antibiotic therapy. There are several broad-spectrum antibiotic combination options, but any regimen should include coverage of gram-negative and anaerobic organisms (Gill et al., 2022; Kim, 2018). **Quality and Safety:** **Antifungal therapy should additionally be considered if there is suspicion for intestinal perforation or if the neonate is critically ill.** The length of antimicrobial therapy is typically 10 to 14 days. Enteral feedings can be restarted after 10 to 14 days of NPO as the clinical picture improves. Enteral feedings are advanced slowly so as to reach full feedings over 7 to 10 days (Iben & Rodriguez, 2016). Given the potential for significant bowel injury with NEC, normal GI function, including digestion, absorption, and motility, may be slow to return.

A CBC with differential, electrolytes, creatinine, BUN, and acid–base tests should be obtained every 12 to 24 hours in the acute stages of managing NEC. The frequency of monitoring serum lactate, liver enzymes, and coagulation studies should be guided by the initial results of these studies. **Emergency Alert:** **Worsening or persistent low platelet count, metabolic acidosis, or increasing serum glucose are associated with worsening or persisting NEC (Kim, 2019b).** Plain radiographs taken every 6 to 12 hours in the initial acute phase of NEC are likely a prudent strategy. Radiographs should also be obtained as needed for any clinical change or deterioration.

The timing of surgical intervention, if necessary, requires clinical judgment and evaluation of the overall clinical condition in close consultation with pediatric surgeons. Indications for surgical intervention may include lack of clinical improvement with medical management, worsening clinical picture, free intraabdominal air, or suspected bowel necrosis. **Emergency Alert:** **Worsening laboratory values (metabolic acidosis, thrombocytopenia, coagulopathy), inability to ventilate, persistent or worsening skin discoloration, protracted or refractory hypotension, escalation of inotropic support, persistent or worsening thrombocytopenia, or fixed bowel loops on plain radiography are signs that should trigger consideration of surgical management.** Surgical options include placement of peritoneal drain(s) with or without irrigation, or open laparotomy. The main aim of open laparotomy is removal of necrotic bowel, irrigation of contaminated abdominal cavity, and proximal diversion with the goal of preserving viable bowel (Iben & Rodriguez, 2016; Kim, 2018).

## INTESTINAL FAILURE AND SHORT BOWEL SYNDROME

### Background

At 27 weeks' gestation, the length of the average small bowel is 100 cm and increases to 200 cm by 40 weeks' gestation (Struijs et al., 2009). Term neonates have a small bowel length of approximately 250 cm at birth with continued substantial growth during the first year of life. Preterm infants have an even greater potential for bowel growth because their intestinal length increases substantially during the last trimester of gestation (Goulet et al., 2019; Struijs et al., 2009). By 3 years of age, the mean intestinal small bowel length is 350 cm. SBS is most commonly used to describe patients whose native bowel length or bowel function is insufficient to digest and absorb the appropriate nutrients and liquids for normal growth and hydration. However, the term *SBS* may be misleading in that the name implies a deficiency in the length of bowel, which may or may not be accurate depending on the underlying etiology. For example, infants who have a normal bowel length but depend exclusively on PN secondary to congenital villus pathology are often referred to as "SBS." A second and perhaps more accurately encompassing term is *intestinal failure* (IF).

IF is defined as the reduction of gut function below the minimum necessary for the absorption of macronutrients and/or water and electrolytes, such that IV supplementation is required to maintain health and/or growth (Pironi et al., 2015). The reduction of gut absorptive function that does not require IV supplementation to maintain health and/or growth can be considered "intestinal insufficiency" (Pironi et al., 2015). Thus, IF is a broader umbrella term that encompasses SBS.

The ultimate goal for all infants with SBS who initially require PN is to transition to full oral or enteral feedings. While there are no perfect predictors of weaning from PN, it is generally thought that longer bowel length, the presence of an intact ileum and ileocecal valve (ICV), the presence of a colon, and continuity of the GI tract represent favorable prognostic factors for weaning from PN (Andorsky et al., 2001; Goulet et al., 2005, 2019; Infantino et al., 2013; Quirós-Tejeira et al., 2004; Sondheimer et al., 1998).

Intestinal adaptation refers to the physiologic and anatomic changes that the intestine undergoes over time that enables an increase in its digestive and absorptive functions (Kaufman, 2016). The large surface area, along with its high concentration of digestive enzymes and density of transport proteins, makes the jejunum the primary site for digestion and absorption of most macronutrients, micronutrients, and fluids. Thus, a functional or anatomic loss of the jejunum results in a corresponding loss of nutrient absorption.

The ileum also plays an important role in the absorption of fluids entering from the jejunum. In addition, it is the primary site for vitamin $B_{12}$ absorption and bile acid reabsorption. Malabsorption of vitamin $B_{12}$ results in macrocytic anemia, while malabsorption of bile acids causes fat and fat-soluble vitamin malabsorption. The ICV serves at least two key physiologic functions that likely contribute to intestinal adaptation. First, the ICV serves as a barrier that blocks the translocation of colonic bacteria into the small intestine, where they can flourish and promote small intestine bacterial overgrowth (SIBO). SIBO is thought to contribute to further malabsorption of certain nutrients such as vitamin $B_{12}$ and deconjugation of bile acids that contribute to fat malabsorption and diarrhea (DiBaise et al., 2006). The ICV is also essential in its role as a physiologic brake, slowing the transit from the intestine to the colon and allowing more time for the intestine to carry out its digestive and absorptive functions. The presence of an ICV is believed to improve the chances of weaning from PN (Goulet et al., 2005; Quirós-Tejeira et al., 2004).

The causes of IF can further be classified as SBS, congenital diseases of enterocyte development, and severe motility disorders (D'Antiga & Goulet, 2013; Goulet & Ruemmele, 2006). In children, the most common cause of IF is SBS. Common causes of SBS in infants include NEC, midgut volvulus, gastroschisis, and IA (D'Antiga & Goulet, 2013; Goulet & Ruemmele, 2006).

Several factors influence the long-term prognosis of infants with SBS. These factors include: the underlying diagnosis, the type of intestinal segments that remain, the preservation of the ICV and colon, a long-term stoma versus a primary anastomosis, the number of surgical procedures, and the age at time of surgery (Belza et al., 2019; Goulet et al., 2019; Nusinovich et al., 2013).

## Diagnosis

The diagnosis of neonates with SBS is usually straightforward. These patients typically have been diagnosed with NEC, gastroschisis, omphalocele, intestinal volvulus, or IA, most often associated with surgical bowel resection. Symptoms of feeding intolerance, such as massive diarrhea, abdominal distension, and vomiting, are also common in patients with SBS.

Other causes of IF in the neonatal period, such as congenital villus abnormalities and idiopathic pseudo-obstruction syndrome, are less common. However, these causes may exhibit similar symptomatology of feeding intolerance and failure to grow in the neonatal period. Likewise, these babies will also require PN to survive.

In neonates who do require surgical intervention, it is helpful to note the quality, quantity, and location of the remaining small bowel and colon on operative reports. A precise understanding of the remaining anatomy can guide management decisions as well as facilitate discussions regarding prognosis with family members.

## Management

The mainstay of management of infants with SBS is PN. In order to provide an adequate amount of PN, a central venous catheter should be placed. The quantity of PN should be sufficient to support normal growth, normalization of electrolytes, and maintenance of euvolemia. Initially, it is common for infants with SBS to have excess fluid and electrolyte losses that will need to be accounted for in developing the PN recipe. PN is typically delivered over 24 hours initially. Once a maintenance PN program achieves appropriate growth, stable electrolytes, and euvolemia, the PN nutrition cycle can be compressed to 16 to 18 hours in most infants.

While PN may provide the majority of calories for infants with SBS, it is critical to offer and encourage oral or enteral feedings as much as tolerated. There is no standardized approach to enteral or oral feedings. Stamm and Duggan (2018) have proposed a strategy to feed infants with SBS. Breastmilk is preferred when available. In the United States, if breastmilk is not available many centers favor a protein hydrolysate or an amino acid–based formula. Hydrolysate and amino acid–based formulas have a theoretical advantage because they eliminate the need for most physiologic digestive processes that may be impaired in infants with SBS. In addition, these formulas may be less likely to trigger an immunologic response that infants with SBS may be at increased risk for developing.

Feedings are usually started at 10% to 20% of the goal. After feedings are started, advancement can be considered if stool output is less than 10 stools/day (or < 10 g/kg/d) or ostomy output is less than 2 ml/kg/hr, perianal skin irritation is manageable, and urine output is greater than 1 ml/kg/hr. The same authors recommend advancing feedings by 10 to 20 ml/kg/d to a maximum goal of 150 to 200 ml/kg/d. If stool output is 10 to 12 stools/day (or 10 to 20 g/kg/d) or ostomy output is 2 to 3 ml/kg/hr, and there is minimal or mild perineal erythema, then feedings can continue at the same rate without advancement. Intolerance to feedings is suggested by increased abdominal distension, greater than 12 stools/day or greater than 20 g/kg/d or ostomy output greater than 3 mL/kg/hr, moderate or severe perineal breakdown, or urine output less than 1 mL/kg/hr. Any of these signs of feeding intolerance should trigger a reduction in the rate of feedings or holding the feedings altogether. When feedings are restarted after being held, restart can commence at 50% to 75% of the previous rate (Stamm & Duggan, 2018). Infants who do not have NG or gastric tube feedings should be offered oral feedings as tolerated.

In general, diarrhea or increased stool output related to oral or enteral intake can be tolerated as long as electrolytes and hydration can be maintained, and the irritant effects of the diarrhea on perianal skin is manageable. Vomiting or spitting up can be managed using a combination of acid suppression and/or prokinetic therapy. As long as oral or enteral feeding does not result in complications such as respiratory symptoms or excess irritability, feedings may continue. Even the smallest amounts of oral or enteral feedings are important. First, enteral feeding is thought to be protective against intestinal failure-associated liver disease (IFALD), because oral intake and the passage of nutrients through the GI tract likely help stimulate physiologic hormones that promote hepatic bile flow. Second, infants who do not learn to suckle during infancy are more likely to develop long-term oral aversion, even once intestinal adaptation has occurred and PN is no longer needed. Trophic feedings may also help maintain intestinal mucosal integrity, lowering the risk of bacterial translocation and subsequent bacteremia.

Two complications common in infants requiring PN are IFALD and central catheter-related bloodstream infection (CRBSI). IFALD is suspected when bilirubin levels and/or liver enzymes (alanine aminotransferase [ALT], gamma glutamyl transferase [GGT], alkaline phosphatase [ALP]) are persistently high in infants receiving chronic PN. The pathophysiology of IFALD is not well understood, but the cause is likely to be multifactorial. Three likely contributing factors include the toxic effects of PN on the liver, the lack of physiologic stimulation of bile flow associated with regular oral feedings, and the toxic effects of repeated episodes of CRBSI and its associated antimicrobial treatment (Zafirovska et al., 2023).

Over the last 15 years, particular interest has been paid to the role of the lipid component of PN in contributing to IFALD. The standard lipid emulsion used in the United States is soy based and contains polyunsaturated fatty acids (PUFAs) such as omega-3 fatty acids and omega-6 fatty acids. PUFA oxidation leads to oxygen free radical production, which can bind to DNA and proteins to cause cell damage and death. PUFAs are also the precursor to a host of proinflammatory cytokines that can contribute to IFALD (Nandivada et al., 2013). Alternative lipid emulsions such as fish oil–based products contain a higher proportion of omega-3 fatty acids that are believed to have antiinflammatory effects. Omegaven® is a fish oil–based lipid emulsion that has been shown to mitigate the effects of IFALD in some infants (Gura et al., 2008; Nandivada et al., 2013; Zafirovska et al., 2023). Smoflipid® is a mixture of soy oil, medium-chain triglycerides (MCTs), olive oil, and fish oil that contains a higher proportion of omega-3 fatty acid. However, data on its effectiveness in preventing or treating IFALD is limited (Belza et al., 2017). Cycling of PN rather than continuous infusion when possible may also mitigate the effects of IFALD.

Independent of the effects of bacteremia and antimicrobial treatment on the liver, CRBSI represents a leading cause of mortality and morbidity in infants with SBS (Chan & Wu, 2014). The ideal management of CRBSI involves treatment with antibiotics and removal of the central line in cases of severe sepsis or persistent bacteremia (Mermel et al., 2009). Unfortunately, infants only have approximately four (two subclavian and two internal jugular) standard sites for central venous access (Kaufman et al., 2001). Once a central line is removed, the vessel is at risk for scarring, rendering it unsuitable for subsequent access.

Thus, recurrent CRBSI may ultimately lead to loss of vascular access for PN. For patients whose vascular access is exhausted, intestinal transplantation is an option (Kaufman et al., 2001; McNelis et al., 2023). However, the survival rate of long-term PN remains more favorable than intestinal transplantation. Therefore, management strategies aimed at preventing CRBSI are essential. There are no standard guidelines for the care and management of central lines in pediatric PN patients. At Loma Linda University Children's Pediatric Intestinal Care and home PN program, when a central line is accessed or when a central line site dressing is changed, the site or catheter is cleansed with three alcohol and three chlorhexidine pads or swabs. Each pad or swab is applied for approximately 30 seconds. Care providers are asked to wear a mask and to perform vigorous hand washing techniques recommended by the Centers for Disease Control (CDC) for 30 seconds prior to accessing the line site or catheter (CDC, 2024).

SIBO is not an uncommon problem in babies with SBS. Symptoms of SIBO include abdominal distension, nausea and vomiting, and increased stool output. SIBO may lead to lactic acidosis, which can present as altered mental status and elevated blood lactate levels (Nes et al., 2024). Usually, SIBO in infants is diagnosed based on clinical symptoms. Therapeutic options may include but are not limited to one of the following agents: metronidazole, trimethoprim-sulfamethoxazole, amoxicillin, or amoxicillin clavulanic acid.

Most infants with SBS have an increase in the production of gastric acid within the first 3 to 6 months after surgery. The increased risk for dyspepsia related to this hypersecretory state and a paucity of oral or enteral feedings can be mitigated by therapy with a $H_2A$ such as ranitidine or famotidine. The agents can be administered enterally, orally, or added to the PN mixture.

## INTUSSUSCEPTION

### Background

Intussusception is a common cause of intestinal obstruction that occurs when one segment of the intestine invaginates into an adjacent segment. Intussusception can involve any segment of the small or large intestine, but ileocolic intussusception is the most common type. In most cases, a more proximal bowel segment invaginates into an adjacent distal segment. The majority of cases are idiopathic without an identifiable lead point, which is the part of the bowel or mesentery that prevents reduction of the involved bowel segment after it has telescoped. The proximal segment is referred to as the *intussusceptum*, while the distal segment, into which it telescopes, is called the *intussuscipiens*. Ileocolic intussusception accounts for approximately 90% of cases (Mandeville et al., 2012). Ileoileocolic, jejunojejunal, jejunoileal, and colocolic intussusceptions are also possible.

The telescoping of one segment of the intestine into an adjacent part is observed periodically during GI endoscopy. These telescoping episodes are a part of normal peristalsis and typically self-reduce, returning bowel segments to their native states. Most of these episodes are transient and unlikely to cause clinical symptoms. Intussusception results when the mesentery of the intussusceptum bowel becomes "stuck" during one of these telescoping events. The consequences of intussusception are twofold: (1) partial or complete small bowel obstruction and (2) progressive vascular compromise if untreated.

The majority of intussusception is idiopathic. However, in a subset of patients, intussusception may be associated with viral or bacterial infections (Arbizu et al., 2014; Bhisitkul et al., 1992; Nylund et al., 2010). It has been proposed that infections cause hypertrophy of lymphatic tissues, which can serve as a lead point that traps bowel segments in the telescoped position, resulting in intussusception (Vo & Sato, 2019). The greater density of lymph tissue in the terminal ileum helps to explain why the majority of intussusception involves the ileum.

Up to 25% of patients with intussusception have an underlying disorder (Vo & Sato, 2019). These underlying disorders can include Meckel diverticulum (St-Vil et al., 1991), polyps (Hwang et al., 2001), small bowel lymphoma (Abbasoğlu et al., 2003), vascular malformations (Morgan et al., 2000), and vasculitis (Choong & Beasley, 1998).

## Diagnosis

Intussusception presents between 3 and 36 months of age, with over 50% presenting during infancy (Mandeville et al., 2012). Infants and toddlers with intussusception typically experience a sudden onset of colic and progressive abdominal pain that is episodic (Abdulhai & Ponsky, 2021; Ross, 2010). During episodes, the infant or toddler may cry inconsolably and draw its legs up toward the abdomen. A period of lethargy may follow the episodes of pain, which may become more frequent over time. Vomiting is commonly associated with pain episodes and may begin as nonbilious vomiting that progresses to bilious vomiting as the intussusception becomes fixed. Fever is not a typical feature of intussusception.

Between the episodes of pain, the infant or toddler can appear completely normal, which can make the diagnosis difficult to make in the early stages. The classic triad of intussusception, including colicky abdominal pain, vomiting, and red "currant jelly" stools, may not be evident until the later stages of the disease. The currant jelly stools are caused by a mixture of intestinal mucus and blood resulting from mucosal sloughing due to vascular compromise (Abdulhai & Ponsky, 2021). A mass may be palpable on physical examination, but this finding is variable (Ross, 2010).

Intussusception is an abdominal emergency that can result in acute bowel ischemia if the diagnosis is delayed (Morreale et al., 2023). Abdominal ultrasound is noninvasive, safe, and often the test of choice to screen for intussusception. The sensitivity of the technique is nearly 100% when performed by experienced ultrasonographers and interpreted by radiologists familiar with diagnosing intussusception (Mandeville et al., 2012). The classic finding of intussusception on ultrasound is a "target sign," which forms when layers of intestines are trapped within the intestine (Abdulhai & Ponsky, 2021).

Rectal enemas using air or contrast can be employed for diagnostic or therapeutic purposes in infants and children with suspected intussusception. A plain abdominal radiograph is performed prior to enemas to confirm the absence of pneumoperitoneum that may suggest intestinal perforation. The hydrostatic or pneumatic pressure from the enema relieves the intussusception in 70% to 80% of cases (Abdulhai & Ponsky, 2021). Contraindications to rectal enemas include evidence of intestinal perforation or peritonitis.

## Management

Depending on the infant or toddler's clinical status, there are nonoperative and operative management options. Patients who are hemodynamically stable and have no concerns for intestinal perforation or peritonitis are candidates for nonoperative management. Even when the nonoperative approach is tried first, the surgical team should be consulted in case operative management is required emergently.

Intravenous resuscitation and broad-spectrum antibiotics should be initiated prior to nonoperative or operative management. An NG tube for decompression can be considered if there is gastric or abdominal distension or persistent vomiting. Nonoperative management typically involves a rectal enema using air and/or hydrostatic pressure. Ideally, the pressure should separate the proximal and distal segments of the intussusception. Nonoperative management is successful in 60% to 90% of cases (Heurn et al., 2014).

Surgical management is indicated in patients who are clinically unstable, have evidence of intestinal perforation or peritonitis, or in whom nonoperative reduction has been unsuccessful. Surgical options include an open or laparoscopic approach. The goal of either approach is to first attempt to manually reduce the involved intestinal segments. If manual reduction is unsuccessful or if a lead point is identified, then resection with primary anastomosis is performed (Heurn et al., 2014).

# CONGENITAL AGANGLIONIC MEGACOLON (HIRSCHSPRUNG DISEASE)

## Background

Normal intestinal motility depends on the coordinated contraction and relaxation of the longitudinal and circular muscle layers throughout the GI tract. Control of motility relies on the function of ganglia that innervate the muscle layers. HD or congenital aganglionic megacolon is a congenital motor disorder of the colon caused by failure of neural crest cells to migrate completely to the muscular layers during fetal intestinal development (Heuckeroth, 2018). This migration failure results in missing ganglion cells in affected segments of the colon. Affected colonic segments fail to relax, resulting in a functional pseudo-obstruction (Heuckeroth, 2018).

The majority of patients with HD have short-segment disease that involves the rectum and distal sigmoid colon

(Wesson & Lopez, 2019). Twenty percent of patients have long-segment disease in which the aganglionosis extends from the rectum to the proximal sigmoid colon (Wesson & Lopez, 2019). Approximately 5% of patients have total colonic aganglionosis that involves the entire colon. The small bowel is rarely affected by HD. Short-segment HD generally carries the best prognosis.

The incidence of HD is about 1 in 5,000 live births with a male predominance (Best et al., 2014; Suita et al., 2005). The recurrence rate in siblings is between 3% and 17%, depending on whether the HD is a short or long segment. Several chromosomal abnormalities are associated with HD. These abnormalities include trisomy 21, Bardet–Biedl syndrome, cartilage-hair hypoplasia, congenital central hypoventilation syndrome, familial dysautonomia, multiple endocrine neoplasia type 2, Mowat–Wilson syndrome, Smith-Lemli-Opitz syndrome, and Waardenburg syndrome (Wesson & Lopez, 2019). Genitourinary abnormalities, visual and hearing problems, congenital heart disease, and ARM may also be found in about 20% of patients with HD (Wesson & Lopez, 2019).

## Diagnosis

Most patients with HD are diagnosed within the first 2 months of life, while up to 10% of patients may not be diagnosed until childhood (Arshad et al., 2012). Three of the more common presentations of HD are neonatal bowel obstruction, chronic constipation, and enterocolitis. Bilious or nonbilious vomiting, abdominal distension, feeding intolerance, and failure to pass meconium within 48 hours of life should raise the possibility of HD (Tabbers et al., 2014). While delayed meconium passage is a hallmark feature, a history of meconium passage within 48 hours of life does not fully exclude the possibility of HD. A forceful expulsion of stool and gas may be seen during digital rectal examination because the finger used for the examination dilates the affected rectosigmoid segment. **Emergency Alert: Infants with HD may also present with enterocolitis that can progress to toxic megacolon if untreated. Clinical evidence of enterocolitis includes fever, vomiting, diarrhea, and persistent abdominal distension even with inspiration and expiration during the respiratory cycle.**

Plain radiographs may show dilated bowel loops proximal to the aganglionic segments and an absence of gas in the rectosigmoid region. Contrast enema, anorectal manometry, and rectal biopsy are the three most common modalities for diagnosing HD. Rectal biopsy and anorectal manometry have the highest sensitivity and specificity of over 90%. Contrast enemas have sensitivities and specificities of 70% to 80% (Langer, 2021). Selection of which test(s) to use may be dictated by institutional availability of equipment and expertise to interpret the results.

Initial evaluation often involves a water-soluble contrast enema to look for a transition zone. In patients with short- or long-segment HD, the transition zone represents a change from a standard caliber or narrowed aganglionic rectum to a more dilated proximal colon (Langer, 2021). In patients with total colonic aganglionosis, the colon may appear normal in size, but dilated loops of distal small bowel may be seen. The rectosigmoid index is the ratio between the diameter of the rectum and the sigmoid colon. In children without HD, this ratio is greater than 1, while in children with HD, the ratio may be less than 1 (Garcia et al., 2007). Retained contrast for greater than 24 hours can also be suggestive of HD. A high false-negative rate for HD limits its use as a gold standard examination. Suction rectal biopsy and anorectal manometry are considered more sensitive for diagnosing HD (Heuckeroth, 2018).

Anorectal manometry involves inserting a pressure transducer with a balloon at its tip into the rectum. As the balloon is inflated, the transducer continuously measures the pressure of the anal sphincter. Usually, the inflation of the balloon should trigger a reflex relaxation of the anal sphincter. In patients with HD, this reflex anal relaxation is absent.

A rectal biopsy is performed to confirm the diagnosis of HD before surgical intervention. The procedure is performed by inserting a suction rectal biopsy instrument 2 to 3 cm into the rectum, applying negative pressure via an attached syringe to suction in intestinal mucosa into a side hole at the end of the device, and then triggering a blade within the biopsy device that excises a small piece of tissue (Noblett, 1969; Langer, 2021). Samples should contain tissue that includes submucosa to be interpretable. The procedure is convenient, can be done at the bedside, and does not require sedation or local analgesia. Uncommon complications include bacteremia, refractory bleeding, and bowel perforation (Langer, 2021; Rees et al., 1983). Histologic features of HD include absence of ganglion cells, hypertrophy of nerve fibers, and increased acetylcholinesterase staining (Langer, 2021).

## Management

Surgery is the definitive treatment for HD. Most surgery for HD is nonemergent. After fluid resuscitation, an NG or orogastric tube should be placed for intermittent or continuous suction, and broad-spectrum antibiotics should be started. Twice-daily rectal irrigations and daily digital rectal examinations are also used at some centers (Levitt & Langer, 2020). Evaluation for comorbid conditions, including cardiac, renal, and chromosomal abnormalities, should also be done prior to surgical correction. Surgery usually involves resection of the aganglionic portion of the colon and rectum, followed by the creation of a neorectum using ganglionated normal proximal bowel.

HD-associated enterocolitis is a form of severe infectious colitis unique to patients with HD that can occur before or after surgery (Levitt & Langer, 2020). Risk factors for enterocolitis include a family history of HD, trisomy 21, long-segment disease, and prior episodes of enterocolitis (Frykman & Short, 2012; Langer, 2021). Common symptoms and signs of enterocolitis include poor feeding, abdominal distension, explosive diarrhea, vomiting, fever, lethargy, rectal bleeding, and shock (Frykman & Short, 2012; Langer, 2021). Plain radiography with lateral decubitus or cross-table lateral views may show a dilated proximal bowel, absence of air in the sigmoid or rectum, and air-fluid levels. Treatment of enterocolitis generally includes broad-spectrum antibiotics that target intestinal flora, rectal irrigation with normal saline, and fluid resuscitation. The patient should be kept NPO until there is evidence of clinical improvement or resolution of signs and symptoms. The duration of antibiotic treatment ranges from 5 to 14 days, depending on the severity of the enterocolitis. Contrast enemas should be avoided in patients with enterocolitis due to the increased risk of intestinal perforation.

## SMALL LEFT COLON

### Background

The neonatal small left colon, also known as the *micro left colon*, is characterized by uniform narrowing of the left colon from the splenic flexure to the anus. Neonatal small left colon is thought to result from functional immaturity of the colon (Ngo et al., 2018). The colon is dilated proximal to the splenic flexure with a cone-shaped transitional zone between dilated and narrow areas.

Approximately 40% of patients with a small left colon are infants of mothers with diabetes (Ngo et al., 2018). The exact cause of the micro left colon is unknown but is thought to represent a colonic motility problem. Normal colonic motility is achieved at term by myenteric plexuses that innervate smooth muscles of the colon. These myenteric plexuses migrate to the colon in a cephalocaudal direction between 5 and 12 weeks' gestation; they mature to normal function as gestation progresses. Failure of migration leads to the absence of ganglion cells as observed in HD; immaturity of migrated myenteric plexuses leads to decreased motility and micro left colon. Histologic examination of the colon in such patients reveals morphologically immature plexuses.

### Diagnosis

Infants with small left colon present with signs and symptoms of a lower intestinal obstruction, including abdominal distension, bilious vomiting, and failure to pass meconium. Plain radiographs of the abdomen reveal multiple gas-filled loops of dilated small bowel and proximal colon, with decreased air in the distal colon or rectum (Ngo et al., 2018). These features are indistinguishable from HD or meconium plug syndrome. Very rarely, significant distal obstruction with marked dilation proximally may lead to cecal perforation. Contrast enema (barium or Gastrografin) reveals a uniformly small left colon, cone-shaped transition zone in the splenic flexure, and dilated proximal colon (Ngo et al., 2018). HD may have similar findings. A distinguishing feature of micro left colon in contrast to HD is that following contrast enema, infants evacuate the contrast promptly and begin passing stools spontaneously with resolution of lower intestinal obstruction. In some cases, a rectal biopsy may be needed to rule out HD. In the micro left colon, rectal biopsy reveals the presence of ganglion cells, albeit immature; ganglion cells are absent in HD.

### Management

Initial management is similar to that of any intestinal obstruction: decompression by NG tube, maintenance of hydration, and correction of electrolyte abnormalities. Contrast enema is both diagnostic and therapeutic. Oral feedings should be started as soon as the patient starts having bowel movements after an enema and gradually advance as tolerated. The baby should be diligently monitored for abdominal distension, vomiting, or decreased stool, because these may be harbingers of the recurrence of obstruction. The small left colon spontaneously resolves in the neonatal period, and the long-term outlook is good with usually normal bowel movements.

## MECONIUM ILEUS

### Background

Meconium ileus (MI) is an obstruction of the distal ileum due to an accumulation of abnormally thick meconium (Carlyle et al., 2012). In the past, a majority (almost 90%) of infants with MI were thought to have CF (Boczar et al., 2015). However, several studies have since reported that 30% to 50% of children with MI do not have CF (Paradiso et al., 2011). Non-CF causes of MI include HD, prematurity, and low birth weight.

In CF patients, MI is the result of thick meconium, which in turn is the result of exocrine pancreatic insufficiency—a lack of hydrolytic enzymes results in meconium with an abnormally high content of protein and mucus glycoprotein, resulting in very viscous meconium (Eichenwald, 2025). It is also postulated that unusually high-fat content in the distal ileum increases neurotensin secretion, which may slow intestinal motility and result in MI (Carlyle et al., 2012). The histologic hallmark of MI is distension of the goblet cells of the intestinal mucosa.

### Diagnosis

Neonates with MI typically present within the first 12 to 24 hours of life. The presentation of MI may be divided into two forms: simple or complicated. In simple MI, the distal ileum is obstructed by very viscid meconium, the proximal small bowel is dilated and thick-walled, and the colon is narrow and empty (microcolon). Complicated MI cases have additional features such as intestinal volvulus, atresia, necrosis, perforation, meconium peritonitis, and meconium pseudocyst.

Affected infants develop signs and symptoms of small bowel obstruction, including abdominal distension, bilious vomiting, and absence of stool. Physical examination of the abdomen may reveal a doughy or puttylike ball of meconium that is movable. Rectal examination reveals a normal anal sphincter tone and an empty rectal vault without meconium or stool.

Radiologic findings on plain radiographs may show a dilated proximal small bowel and a "soap bubble" or ground-glass appearance in the right lower quadrant (Ngo et al., 2018). Contrast enema shows microcolon. In complicated MI, plain radiographs may show ascites, peritoneal calcifications, or pneumoperitoneum. A sweat chloride test and DNA analysis for CF mutations should be performed in all patients suspected of having MI. Neonatal screening for CF may be helpful, although it may not provide immediate results in the first few days of life.

### Management

The initial treatment is stabilizing the patient with respect to hydration and correcting electrolytes. In simple MI, mildly hypertonic Gastrografin or Hypaque with acetylcysteine is delivered into the distal ileum via a contrast enema under fluoroscopy to break up inspissated meconium (Carlyle et al., 2012). The loosened meconium is then passed by normal peristalsis. Maintaining adequate hydration is vital, as fluid from the intravascular space is drawn into the intestinal lumen with the hyperosmolar agent. Generally, 4 ml of half-normal saline solution is given for every 1 ml of retained enema. Surgery is indicated if nonsurgical measures fail or in cases of complicated MI (Carlyle et al., 2012). Inspissated meconium is removed surgically by simple enterotomy. A temporary ileostomy may be needed in some cases.

Once intestinal function is adequate, elemental formula feedings are started. For patients with CF, pancreatic enzyme replacement should be initiated alongside feedings. Pulmonary maintenance care should begin as soon as possible, and if CF is diagnosed, parents should be referred to a genetic counselor. The long-term prognosis depends on the underlying etiology; non-CF patients have better outcomes than CF patients.

## MECONIUM PLUG

### Background

Meconium plug syndrome causes distal colonic obstruction caused by thick meconium with no associated pancreatic enzyme deficiency. Obstruction is relieved by the passage of meconium, and there are no long-term consequences. It is essential to distinguish meconium plug syndrome from HD and micro left colon.

The most likely cause of meconium plug syndrome is abnormal gut motility associated with immaturity or hypotonia. Approximately 13% of patients with meconium plug syndrome have HD (Keckler et al., 2008). Premature infants and infants with hypotonia are especially prone to developing a meconium plug. Infants of diabetic mothers (IDMs) are also at increased risk of developing a meconium plug, which is considered a variant of the micro left colon.

### Diagnosis

Meconium plug patients usually present with signs and symptoms of distal bowel/colonic obstruction; there is gradually increasing abdominal distension, bilious vomiting, and failure of meconium passage. Plain radiographs reveal multiple dilated small bowel loops. Contrast enema reveals a normal-caliber colon (as compared to the micro left colon) and dilated bowel proximal to the meconium plug.

### Management

Initial management consists of supportive care, including NG decompression and maintenance of hydration and electrolyte balance. A contrast enema is often therapeutic, resulting in the dislodgement of the plug and relief of the obstruction (Cuenca et al., 2012). Once the plug is evacuated, distension has resolved, and normal intestinal function has returned, feedings can be started and advanced as tolerated. A rectal biopsy should be considered in all patients with meconium plug syndrome, particularly if constipation persists after the initial resolution of obstruction, to rule out Hirschsprung disease. Overall, the prognosis is good, and complete recovery is expected.

## IMPERFORATE ANUS/ANORECTAL MALFORMATION

### Background

ARM includes a spectrum of congenital malformations involving the anus and rectum; many are associated with a fistula between the rectum and urogenital system or between the rectum and perineum (Herman & Teitelbaum, 2012). ARM is thought to result from abnormal development of the urorectal septum, which separates the anorectum from the urogenital system, or failure of the migration of the anus. ARM may occur in isolation, as part of the VACTERL association, or other anomalies involving the sacrum, lower spinal cord, or kidneys (Bulas, 2018).

For clinical purposes, ARM is classified according to the lesion location in relation to the internal anal sphincter or levator ani muscle complex. In low lesions, the rectal pouch ends below the internal anal sphincter and opens into the perineum as a narrow opening (anal stenosis, type I) or a fistula (type II). In high lesions, the rectal pouch ends above the internal anal sphincter and communicates externally through a fistula (type III) to the urinary bladder, urethra, or vagina; in rare cases, there may not be any external communication (type IV), causing complete obstruction. In high lesions, the internal sphincter is either absent or very malformed, with associated sacral abnormalities. In both types of lesions, the external sphincter is almost always present.

The incidence of ARM in the general population is about 1 in 5,000 live births; it increases to 1 in 100 for siblings of affected individuals (Bischoff et al., 2021). The cause of abnormal urorectal septum development or arrested migration of the anus is not known. However, both environmental and genetic factors are involved. The mildest form of low lesions presents as anal stenosis, where the anus and rectum are patent but very narrowed. The anus therefore looks very small; it may be missed, because the newborn may be able to pass pasty or loose stools. Other low lesions may be associated with a thin membrane covering the anal opening or a complete absence of an anal opening; in these cases, stool is passed through a fistula in the perineum. In high lesions, there is no anal opening, and stool is passed with urine via a fistula to the bladder, urethra, or vagina.

### Diagnosis

ARM presents with a variable degree of GI obstruction because of failed or incomplete passage of stool. Symptoms include abdominal distension, poor feeding, vomiting, and delayed or absent passage of meconium. In low lesions, perineal examination will reveal a very small anus or no discernible anal opening, ectopic anal opening, fistula, or bulge in the perineum. In high lesions, there is no anal opening or fistula externally; there may be stool mixed with urine or excreted from the vagina. A careful perineal examination is mandatory and diagnostic in identifying and categorizing ARM.

## Management

ARM may be associated with other anatomical abnormalities involving the esophagus, spine, kidneys, and heart. Because these associated conditions may also require urgent management, testing to consider in the first 24 hours after birth should include an echocardiogram, spinal ultrasound, abdominal and kidney ultrasound, and plain radiograph of the chest and abdomen (Bischoff et al., 2021).

The treatment of ARM depends on the nature of the defect; it is imperative to define low versus high lesions. As mentioned earlier, careful perineal examination is all that is needed for diagnosis. Prone cross-table lateral x-ray film at 12 to 16 hours after birth may reveal a dilated rectal pouch that ends blindly above the perineum, but it is unreliable for determining the level of the lesion; the larger the distance from the perineum (more than 1.5 cm), the more likely it is to be a high lesion. An ultrasound, computed tomography (CT), and magnetic resonance imaging (MRI) of the pelvis may better define the level of the lesion, and one or more of these modalities may be used before a surgical approach.

A pediatric surgeon needs to be involved in managing ARM as soon as the defect is identified. Anal stenosis (type I, low lesion) is treated by repeated anal dilation using Hegar dilators. The infant can be discharged once it can pass stool and there are no signs of obstruction; daily anal dilation is continued at home, because parents are trained before discharge. The other simple low lesion, where a thin membrane covers the anal opening, requires minimal surgical intervention. The membrane is ruptured or excised, and repeated anal dilation is performed as previously noted.

Low lesions with a perineal fistula are corrected by posterior sagittal anorectoplasty, in which the rectal pouch is brought down through the external sphincter (identified using a nerve stimulator) and sutured to the skin at the anal opening. Any fistulous connection is removed. Postoperatively, the infant may need gentle rectal irrigation until stool passes. Anal dilation using the Hegar dilator is usually started after 2 weeks, depending on the pediatric surgeon, and continued at home.

High lesions may require complex reconstructive surgery. These patients have significant intestinal obstruction and require stabilization before surgery. Gastric decompression is achieved with NG tube placement, and dehydration or an electrolyte imbalance is corrected. Usually, the defect is corrected in two stages. Initially, a left-sided colostomy is created as soon as possible for decompression and fecal diversion. If there is any fistula, it is excised. In the second stage, definitive repair is accomplished in 3 to 12 months by abdominal perineal pull-through surgery, where the rectal pouch is pulled through the levator ani muscle sling and the external sphincter, and the subsequent anastomosis is done at skin level. The timing of definitive surgery depends on the adequate growth and nutritional status of the patient.

Postoperative care of neonates depends on the type of surgery performed. Care of anoplasty patients requires gentle cleaning with saline and monitoring for infection at the suture site and mucosal prolapse. Parents need to be trained in the care of the wound site, as well as possible dilation as needed. Because there is a risk of recurrence of fistulas, patients should be observed for the passage of any stool mixed with urine and for any new opening in the perineum. Once the site is healed, feedings can be started. Initially, a stool softener may be required to prevent formed stool. If the patient requires a colostomy, then daily inspection of the colostomy is mandatory to ensure proper functioning and site integrity. Parents need to be trained to care for the colostomy.

The long-term outcome is measured in terms of achieving continence and a normal stool pattern. Patients with anal stenosis have a very good prognosis, and some may need stool softeners long-term. There may be late complications for all other patients, including rectocutaneous anastomosis stricture, recurrent rectourinary fistula, mucosal prolapse, constipation, and fecal incontinence. Children with low lesions (below the levator ani complex) generally achieve normal continence, while only a minority (about one-third) with high lesions achieve continence before school age. The overall mortality rate of patients with anorectal malformation is 15%; death is mainly due to complex surgical intervention and is more likely from associated anomalies. About 75% of patients have good outcomes in achieving regular bowel movements and continence.

# SUPPORT OF FAMILY OF AN INFANT WITH A GI SYSTEM DISORDER

The birth of an infant with a congenital anomaly or one who is acutely ill elicits feelings of loss, guilt, and confusion for parents. Nurses and other health professionals must expect grief reactions and be prepared to help the family cope with the crisis. Strategies to cope include support for early contact between parents and infant and open lines of communication to provide factual information about the infant's condition and care plan. Healthcare providers also need to patiently reinforce information on an ongoing basis as the family begins to process and accept the diagnosis. Understanding the disease process is essential for parents to cope with the prognosis and ongoing healthcare needs. Encourage parents to hold their infants and provide skin-to-skin (kangaroo) care as early as possible. Additionally, they should be encouraged to express their concerns before they are discharged home.

Today's parents and families have access to more information than ever. How parents and families receive and process information from social media and numerous other internet-related platforms can support coping mechanisms or exacerbate fears and concerns. Maintaining an open dialog and trust with parents and families is essential. In addition to making connections with parents, every conversation should include an invitation to share any information they have learned from social media and internet resources. Trusted resources should also be shared with parents and families.

## SUMMARY

The GI system is vital to human growth, development, and long-term survival. The vast majority of conditions that cause GI diseases in the infant result from congenital anatomic malformations or dysfunction. Additionally, any condition or situation that leads to ischemia and bacterial overgrowth places an infant at risk for certain conditions such as NEC and resultant long-term sequelae. An effective interprofessional team of nursing, medical, and other specialists is required for optimal outcomes of the infant's physiologic well-being and the family's psychosocial wellness. The primary purposes of this chapter were to present the embryologic development of the GI tract and resultant anatomic structure and to describe common causes of neonatal dysfunction with implications for care.

## CASE STUDY

### Intestinal Volvulus

**Identification of the Problem.** A 14-day-old, 36 weeks' gestation female infant presented to the emergency department with a 1-day history of vomiting consisting of golden yellow fluid, abdominal distension, and poor feeding. The infant had an unremarkable perinatal course. The mother reported that the infant had been feeding well until the past 24 hours when the infant became inconsolable and started vomiting. The infant was transferred to the NICU for further evaluation and management.

**Assessment: History and Physical Examination.** A 36-week gestation female infant, born by cesarean section to a 32-year-old, G2, P1001 mother, with a normal pregnancy and routine prenatal care. Birth weight was 2,850 g, and Apgar scores were 8 at 1 minute and 9 at 5 minutes. The infant had been feeding normally since birth and had no prior history of vomiting or feeding intolerance.

On day of life (DOL) 13, the mother noticed vomiting, irritability, and abdominal distension. The vomiting was initially clear but became yellow after a few hours. The infant was brought to the emergency department on DOL 14, where an NG tube was placed and bilious fluid was drained.

Vital signs: temperature 98.9°F (37.2°C), heart rate (HR) 158 beats/min, respiratory rate (RR) 45 breaths/min, blood pressure (BP) 85/55 mm Hg, capillary refill time (CRT) 4 seconds, weight 2,770 g.

Pediatric surgery service consulted immediately upon admission of the infant to the NICU even prior to imaging studies.

Physical examination upon arrival to the NICU:

- GENERAL: irritable, pale infant, slightly lethargic
- HEENT: anterior fontanelle soft and flat, eyes with + red reflex and no icterus
- CARDIOVASCULAR: regular rate and rhythm (RRR), no murmur, pulses 2 + and equal
- RESPIRATORY: room air, clear breath sounds bilaterally
- ABDOMEN: distended, tender, bowel sounds absent, little movement of abdominal wall with inhalation and exhalation
- GENITOURINARY: normal female genitalia
- NEUROLOGIC: lethargic, irritable, mildly hypotonic

Evaluation included laboratory work (CBC, electrolytes, blood gas), and imaging (abdominal radiograph and upper gastrointestinal [UGI] series).

#### Differential Diagnosis

- Intestinal volvulus
- NEC
- Midgut malrotation
- Intussusception
- Hirschsprung disease, enterocolitis

#### Diagnostic Tests

Laboratory Tests:

- CBC: WBC 9.8 x$10^3$/mcl, segmented neutrophils 35%, bands 15%, hematocrit 44%, platelets 250,000/$mm^3$
- Electrolytes: sodium 137 mEq/L, potassium 4.5 mEq/L, chloride 101 mEq/L, bicarbonate 19 mEq/L
- CRP: 7.0 mg/dl
- Blood cultures: pending

Imaging Tests:

- Abdominal radiograph: gaseous distension of the small bowel, no air in the rectum
- Upper GI series: evidence of malrotation with a corkscrew appearance of the midgut, consistent with volvulus

#### Working Diagnosis

- Midgut volvulus secondary to malrotation: based on UGI findings and bilious vomiting
- Early sepsis suspected due to elevated CRP and clinical presentation

#### Development of Management Plan

- Immediate discussion with pediatric surgery for potential midgut volvulus
- NPO status and NG tube to low suction for gastric decompression
- Fluid resuscitation with IV fluids (normal saline boluses followed by maintenance fluids)
- Broad-spectrum antibiotics (ampicillin, gentamicin, and metronidazole) initiated
- Continuous monitoring of vital signs and abdominal girth

#### Implementation and Evaluation of Effectiveness

Implementation of Management Plan:

- Infant was taken to the operating room for an exploratory laparotomy. A midgut volvulus was confirmed, and a Ladd procedure was performed to correct the malrotation and untwist the volvulus. No bowel resection was required.
- Gastric decompression with an NG tube was maintained postoperatively.
- IV fluids continued at 140 ml/kg/d with total parenteral nutrition (TPN) initiated after surgery.

- Antibiotics were continued for suspected sepsis.
- Postoperative pain managed with fentanyl as needed.

### Evaluation of Effectiveness

- Abdominal girth decreased within 8 hours postsurgery.
- Infant stabilized postoperatively with improvement in abdominal distension and overall activity level.
- Blood cultures remained negative, and antibiotics were discontinued on postoperative day (POD) 5.
- The infant remained NPO for the first 4 days postoperatively and was then transitioned to slow advancement of enteral feedings. TPN continued until full enteral feedings were tolerated by POD 7.
- Electrolytes and CBC remained stable throughout the postoperative course.

**Outcome.** The infant was successfully extubated on POD 2 and transitioned to room air. The infant was discharged home on full enteral feedings with weight gain on POD 10. Follow-up was arranged with pediatric surgery in 2 weeks and the primary care provider within 1 week of discharge.

## PARENT VOICES

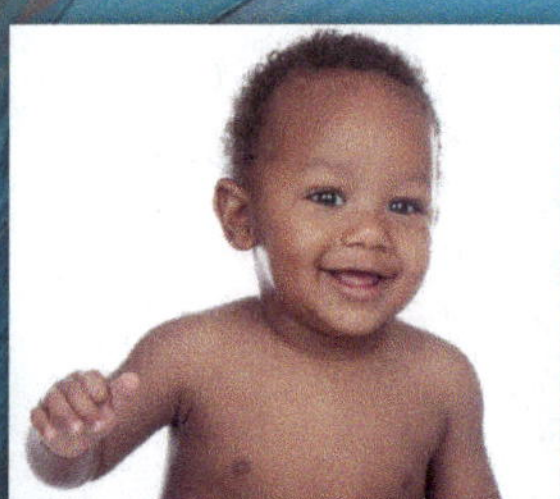

*Source:* Gelpi/Adobe Stock.

### Laurel Kapferer, MS

Our son Grayson was born via emergency C-section at 34 weeks. He had experienced IUGR, and at the time of his birth, he weighed only 2 lb 14 oz. Grayson was a very curious, aware, feisty baby with a larger-than-life personality. He would always interact with us and enjoyed skin-to-skin contact, being sung to, stories, his binky, and having his head rubbed gently.

During the first few days in the NICU, Grayson was progressing well. He was breathing on his own and regulating his own temperature. We thought for sure he would be home in no time. All that changed when Grayson was 6 days old. His color became pale and ashy, and his personality was completely different. That entire day he was crying and fussy. Nothing would comfort him. Later on in the day, Grayson developed a small pink area on his abdomen; x-rays later that day confirmed that he had developed necrotizing enterocolitis. Very quickly, his abdomen became distended and purple. He was eventually transferred to another hospital where his condition continued to worsen. His disease quickly progressed; we were told that Grayson's blood would not clot and surgery would not be possible. Eventually, Grayson's intestines were perforated, which led to sepsis.

My husband and I held our son in our arms as he took his last breaths. Less than 18 hours after Grayson was diagnosed with NEC, he lost his life. This disease progressed rapidly and before we even could understand what it was, our son was gone.

Every moment that parents have with their children is precious, especially in the NICU. Things can turn around so quickly and there is not always a happy ending. It is so critical that as nurses you do everything you can to support families bonding with their babies, and that you help them create special moments to hold onto. When we knew that Grayson was losing his battle, we were able to get hand and footprints, a lock of hair, and pictures. In the end, those items along with his blankets, hats, binkies, bracelets, and our memories are all we have left of our son. In those times where it is clear that a child may not be making it home, please be mindful not to throw anything away. Instead, hold on to it for the family. We are so grateful that the NICU nurses thought to do this for us. Having items that were Grayson's, that he touched, and in some way connected with, mean the world to us now.

### Jennifer M. Driscoll

Our daughter, Lilian Hope, was born 7 weeks premature, weighing only 2 lb 12 oz and 15 inches long. Lily's lungs were her main problem, as they are for many preemies, because the lungs are the last thing to develop. On the day she was born, she was doing well but still needed a CPAP machine to help her breathe. As the day progressed, her condition worsened. She was given nitric oxide, put onto a ventilator to breathe for her, and an oscillator to vibrate the lungs to help the flow of oxygen. Due to the force of the ventilator and oscillator, an air sac in her lungs burst and she had a chest tube inserted. Additionally, she had an erratic blood pressure and jaundice, and needed multiple blood transfusions. But the miracle continued as she began to gain strength inside herself; she came off the oscillator after 7 days and took out the ventilator herself. By day 8, we were able to hold her for the first time. She ended up only needing to stay in the NICU at Lehigh Valley Hospital for 24 days and was able to come home at a mere 3 lb 11 oz.

(*continued*)

## PARENT VOICES (*continued*)

**Aside from Lily's lung issues at birth, Lily experienced severe GI issues from the time she was discharged from the NICU until age 5. Lily was bottle-fed because my milk never came in. This was beneficial for her in some ways because we were able to monitor how much she was eating and supplement with high-calorie formula and formula that was geared toward preemies. Unfortunately for her, she would have severe vomiting and lose what seemed like an entire bottle, often during a feeding, or just after she was done, and it would literally fly from her mouth across the room with very severe force. We saw many specialists because she would experience discomfort with the reflux, but it was hard to keep giving this tiny, fragile baby so much medication. Finally, once she began some solid foods, the reflux slowed down; however, it immediately led to other motility issues for her. Over her next few years, she would experience failure to thrive, worsened motility issues, and an eventual emergency surgery at Children's Hospital in Philadelphia. It took her one full year under the care of a specialist to work through those issues and begin to stabilize, which was by age 5.**

## ONLINE RESOURCES

CourseConnect

Resources for this chapter are online and available at www.springerpub.com/courseconnect.

## REFERENCES

References for this chapter are online and available at www.springerpub.com/courseconnect.

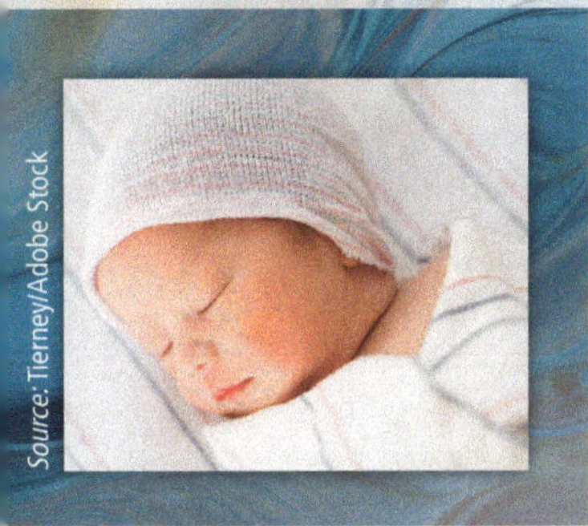

Source: Tierney/Adobe Stock

# CHAPTER 9

# Metabolic System

Susan Kau, Leilani Kahoano, Lorelei Crowder, and Carole Kenner

## INTRODUCTION

Metabolism is a sequence of chemical reactions that occurs in cells. These reactions result in a breakdown of nutrients and the generation of energy. Inborn errors of metabolism (IEMs), also known as errors of metabolism (EMs), comprise a group of disorders that cause blockages in metabolic pathways, which can lead to clinically significant consequences. Chemical compounds or enzymes are responsible for metabolic reactions. Cofactors, also known as compounds, help these enzymes react. Examples of metabolism include breaking down carbohydrates, protein, and fats in food to release energy and transforming excess nitrogen into waste products that are excreted in urine.

EMs comprise a heterogeneous group of monogenic diseases that can affect metabolic pathways. Most EMs are named for an enzyme that is not working properly. Depending on the enzyme's job, its absence means that toxic chemicals may build up, or an essential product may not be produced. A pair of genes usually contains the code or blueprint to produce an enzyme. Most people with inherited metabolic disorders inherit two defective copies of the gene—one from each parent. Both parents are carriers of the bad gene, meaning that each parent carries one normal gene copy and one defective gene copy. A mutation in the gene causes it not to function properly or not function at all. The parents can inherit these gene mutations from their parents or the mutations may occur spontaneously.

The likelihood that someone in the family has the same EM depends on several factors:

- inheritance pattern of EMs
- whether an at-risk family member is a male or female
- rest of family history (i.e., how many family members have previously been tested or diagnosed with the disorder already)

It is important to understand that everyone has two copies of most genes, with one copy inherited from the mother and one copy inherited from the father. This is not the case for genes that are on our sex chromosomes (the "X" and the "Y" chromosomes). The recommendation is for family members who may be at risk for having an EM to talk to a metabolic or genetics specialist, who may coordinate genetic testing, if deemed appropriate.

The earlier an infant develops symptoms of an EM, the more severe the disorder is. The severity of symptoms is based on several factors: the position of the defective enzyme within the metabolic pathway, whether any functional enzyme or cofactor is being produced, and other genetic or environmental factors. EM are considered multisystemic diseases; as such, infants may present with various symptoms dependent on the specific metabolic pathway. Symptoms of substrate and intermediary metabolism develop once a significant number of toxic metabolites accumulate following the initiation of feeds and may include the following: poor feeding, vomiting, diarrhea, temperature instability, tachypnea, apnea, bradycardia, poor perfusion, irritability, involuntary movements, posturing, abnormal tone, seizures, and altered level of consciousness. For EMs of energy deficiency, symptoms usually develop within 24 hours and are generally present at birth. Neonates with EM that result in defects in energy production usually have dysmorphic features, skeletal malformations, cardiopulmonary compromise, organomegaly, and severe generalized hypotonia. For those infants with errors in substrate and intermediary metabolism, physical examination findings are usually unremarkable. Acute decompensation in the neonate includes certain forms of tyrosinemia, organic acidemia, urea cycle defects, fatty acid oxidation defects, and galactosemia. An infection in an infant with an EM can result in a metabolic crisis (McGuire, 2017). This condition can result in death. Inherited metabolic disorders manifesting in the early neonatal period are this chapter's foci.

## GENERAL PRINCIPLES: THE NEONATE WITH A METABOLIC DISORDER

### Pathophysiology of Errors of Metabolism

The genetic mechanisms through which biochemical disease is inherited include autosomal dominant, autosomal recessive, sex-linked recessive, or a mutation in mitochondrial DNA (Cederbaum, 2018). The genetic mutation leads to an absent or defective gene product or enzyme, causing either an accumulation of precursors before a blocked step in a metabolic pathway, a deficiency of a critical metabolic product, or both. In disorders involving the intermediary metabolism of small molecules (such as maple syrup urine disease [MSUD]), the accumulated molecules give rise to an "intoxication syndrome" because of the profoundly toxic nature of these substances and their effect on the central nervous system (CNS). Disorders involving energy metabolism (such as pyruvate dehydrogenase [PDH] and PDH deficiency) lead to failure of energy production or utilization with a broad range of symptoms and physiologic consequences. Other disorders, such as lysosomal storage diseases, involve complex molecules, and symptoms that arise from these disorders are permanent, progressive, and independent of intercurrent events.

## Clinical Manifestations of Errors of Metabolism

Most neonates who are eventually diagnosed with EMs appear essentially normal at birth and have no history of antepartum or intrapartum complications. The placenta and maternal circulation protect the fetus from the damaging effects of toxins. The ingestion of formula, milk, or fructose unmasks some metabolic disorders. Others are unrelated to feeding or may be brought on by fasting, infection, or stress.

Metabolic disease in the newborn can be clinically silent, indolent, or acute (Cederbaum, 2018). Five common presentations have been described (Leonard & Morris, 2010):

- neurologic presentation—acute encephalopathy, seizures, lethargy
- hypoglycemia
- acid–base abnormalities—particularly metabolic acidosis and respiratory alkalosis
- cardiomyopathy and cardiac arrhythmias
- acute liver disease

A complete family history should be obtained to determine if others have an EM or have experienced sudden infant unexpected infant death (SUID).

## Diagnosis of Errors of Metabolism

The trigger for a metabolic workup varies with the situation. In infants initially suspected of having sepsis, a metabolic workup might be initiated when laboratory results to investigate infection fail to confirm infection. **Emergency Alert:** **Persistent metabolic acidosis with an increased anion gap, hypoglycemia, significant hyperammonemia, unexplained hepatic dysfunction, or ketonuria should always raise suspicion of an EM (Leonard & Morris, 2010).** Although only a minority of EMs are associated with dysmorphism, the possibility of metabolic disease should not be discounted in infants with congenital malformations or unusual features.

The initial laboratory investigation of a suspected EM includes a broad range of blood and urine tests (Box 9.1). Nonspecific screening tests do not provide a diagnosis; at best, they will support a strong suspicion of a metabolic disorder and suggest a specific category of disease (e.g., organic acidemia, fatty acid oxidation disorders [FAODs]). Interpretation of results can be tricky. Conditions of sampling can profoundly affect results. Blood and urine samples must be obtained prior to the initiation of therapy, and whenever possible, both should be collected when the infant is symptomatic (Mussa et al., 2017). Extra blood and urine samples should be obtained and frozen for later testing. Health professionals must understand the limitations of laboratory testing, which tests are appropriate under what conditions, and how the infant's symptoms relate to such testing (Rice & Steiner, 2016).

**Quality and Safety:** **Secondary metabolic derangements can interfere with test interpretation, and biochemical abnormalities might only occur during acute episodes.** Laboratory abnormalities can also be transient; a result within the reference range does not necessarily rule out a metabolic disorder. Studies may need to be repeated at specific times. Clinicians might be falsely reassured by screening tests that are

**BOX 9.1**

### GENERAL SCREENING TESTS FOR ERRORS OF METABOLISM

**Blood Tests**

- Glucose
- Complete blood count (CBC) with differential
- Blood gases
- Electrolytes (and anion gap[a])

**Liver Function Tests**

- Blood urea nitrogen and creatinine
- Total and direct bilirubin
- Prothrombin time (PT) and partial thromboplastin time (PTT)
- Uric acid
- Ammonia
- Lactate
- Pyruvate
- Amino acids
- Free fatty acids
- Ketones (3-OH-butyrate, acetoacetate)
- Creatinine phosphokinase
- Newborn metabolic screen/blood acylcarnitine analysis
- Cerebrospinal fluid glycine (to rule out nonketotic hyperglycinemia)

**Urine Tests**

- Glucose
- Ketones
- pH
- Reducing substances
- Ferric chloride reaction
- Dinitrophenylhydrazine (DNPH) reaction
- Amino acids
- Organic acids
- Odor
- Orotic acid (if blood $NH_4$ is elevated)

[a]Anion gap is (sodium – [chloride + bicarbonate]). Normal is less than 15 mEq/L.

inadequate to exclude certain conditions. Therefore, consultation with a metabolic specialist is recommended. Furthermore, the referral laboratory should provide clinical history and as much information as possible about the infant's symptoms and the suspected diagnosis to improve testing accuracy and interpretation of results.

**Postmortem Diagnosis.** If a neonate with a possible metabolic disorder dies suddenly, it is of great importance to continue to try to establish the proper diagnosis for purposes of genetic counseling and future antenatal diagnosis. In addition to standard blood and urine samples, a cerebrospinal fluid (CSF) sample should be obtained if possible, and whole blood and bile should be collected on filter paper. The routine state newborn screening card should be completed and sent. If the family declines a full autopsy, tissue biopsies should be obtained. Tissue samples of value are skin, liver, kidney, and muscle.

**Neonatal Screening.** Newborn screening was first introduced as a public health program in the United States in the early 1960s and has expanded to other countries worldwide, with different testing menus in each country. Both prenatal and newborn screenings have improved healthcare. The conditions included in newborn screening programs around the world vary greatly based on the legal requirements for screening programs, the prevalence of certain diseases within a population, political pressure, and the availability of resources for both testing and follow-up of identified patients.

The development of tandem mass spectrometry (MS/MS) has dramatically improved the presymptomatic detection of many EMs. With MS/MS, measuring 30 or 40 different metabolites in less than 2 or 3 minutes is possible using a single dried blood spot. MS/MS works by applying a charge to the compounds in solution, sending them through an electromagnetic field, sorting them out, and weighing them according to their mass-to-charge ratio. Expanded newborn screening using MS/MS is mandated in some states as part of the routine newborn screening program. It is also available to parents who wish to purchase it from a number of private laboratories at a nominal cost. Currently, MS/MS screens only for disorders of intermediary metabolism, including amino acid disorders, organic acid disorders, and FAODs. A normal neonatal screen, even an expanded newborn screen by MS/MS, does not rule out an error of metabolism in a suspicious clinical setting. **Quality and Safety:** **If newborn screening tests are still pending when a neonate manifests potential signs and symptoms of metabolic disease, clinicians should contact the screening laboratory promptly to determine whether a diagnosis can be provided or to expedite results (Yudkoff, Summar, & Haberle, 2017).**

## Management of the Infant With an Error of Metabolism

Treatment of EMs is tailored to the specific disorder once a diagnosis is made. In general, treatment goals are to maintain growth and development while minimizing or eliminating the buildup of toxic metabolites that result from the block in the metabolic pathway. This may be done by using diets, supplements, and medications.

As soon as it becomes apparent that the infant has some metabolic disorder, it is essential to consult a metabolic specialist/geneticist. In addition to general supportive measures, as indicated by the infant's symptoms, general and specific treatments should be initiated. **Quality and Safety:** **Oral feedings and amino acid solutions (all protein sources) are withheld, and 10% glucose solution with electrolytes is administered temporarily until the precise diagnosis is ascertained.** A glucose infusion rate of at least 5 mg/kg/min (and higher if tolerated, aiming for 120–150 kcal/kg/d) is administered because many metabolic disorders are exacerbated by tissue catabolism (Cederbaum, 2018). **Quality and Safety:** **Intralipids are withheld until FAODs have been ruled out. Acute hypoglycemia, metabolic acidosis, dehydration, hypovolemia, and electrolyte imbalances are corrected as part of the overall supportive management of a metabolic disorder. If the infant is to be transferred to a referral center, reliable vascular access should be secured before transport.** Hemodialysis or extracorporeal membrane oxygenation (ECMO) may be required for emergency management of some EMs. Liver transplantation can be lifesaving in some EMs. Many disorders with rapid neonatal or prenatal onset are lethal, and all that can be offered are palliative and symptomatic care.

Interactions with parents and other family members are critically important during diagnosis and throughout care (Box 9.2). EMs occur in newborns with a broad range of racial/ethnic backgrounds. The psychological distress experienced due to the diagnosis and management of their child's

**BOX 9.2**

### NURSING IMPLICATIONS FOR FAMILIES OF INFANTS WITH ERRORS OF METABOLISM

**Nurses should support the families of these infants in the following ways:**

1. Ensure that the programs are implemented safely and effectively.
2. Facilitate education of the nursing workforce and develop and contribute to programs of research focused on newborn screening.
3. Educate parents with appropriately timed discussion of results. Parental teaching should include materials providing descriptions of genetic screening and testing.
4. Emphasize the importance of keeping up with medical appointments.
5. Teach that dietary management requires lifelong dietary adherence.
6. Therapies: Follow-up with occupational/speech therapists may be needed.
7. Family planning: Inform families that having a child with an EM may affect family planning decisions.
8. Emergencies: Families may need to know how to manage metabolic emergencies.

*Source:* From Blake, S., Jnah, A., & Adkins, D. (2019). The metabolic and endocrine system. In A. Jnah & A. N. Trembath (Eds.), *Fetal and neonate physiology for the advanced practice nurse*. Springer Publishing Company.

EM can become extremely overwhelming. Care coordination is important for families with EM; many have treatment protocols developed by an EM specialist. It is important to provide culturally sensitive care, which includes access to interpreter services, exploration of the family's sociocultural background, and bidirectional communication as well as decision making in the child's best interest (Stockler et al., 2012).

## UREA CYCLE DISORDERS

Urea cycle disorders (UCDs) are caused by inherited defects in genes encoding enzymes or membrane transporters involved in ureagenesis. All are transmitted as autosomal recessive traits except ornithine transcarbamylase (OTC) deficiency, which is an X-linked defect and the most common of the primary defects. In aggregate, the prevalence of UCDs is believed to be approximately 1 per 10,000 live births if partial defects are included.

### Pathophysiology

The hepatic urea cycle is the mechanism used by the body to detoxify and eliminate ammonia generated from nitrogen waste. Five enzymatic reactions make up the urea cycle, leading to the incorporation of ammonia into urea and enabling its excretion in the urine (Figure 9.1). The first two steps, the carbamoyl phosphate synthetase (CPS) and OTC reactions, take place in the mitochondria and lead to the synthesis of citrulline. In a subsequent cytosolic reaction, citrulline is converted to argininosuccinate, which is hydrolyzed to arginine and fumarate. Arginine is then hydrolyzed to urea and ornithine is regenerated.

A block of the urea cycle can result from a deficiency of any one of the first five enzymes in the urea cycle pathway: carbamoyl phosphate synthetase I (CPSI deficiency), OTC deficiency, argininosuccinic acid synthetase (citrullinemia), argininosuccinic acid lyase (argininosuccinic aciduria), arginine, a cofactor producer, *N*-acetylglutamate synthase (NAGS) deficiency, or a transport protein (Yudkoff et al., 2017). A block in the urea cycle results in an accumulation of precursor metabolites, including ammonia, which have no effective alternate clearance pathway. The neonate, with an immature liver and a tendency toward catabolism, is poorly equipped to handle the excess metabolites and rapidly succumbs to the neurotoxic effects of high ammonia levels. Hyperammonemic encephalopathy results from osmotic swelling in the brain caused by glutamine accumulation in cerebral astrocytes, where glutamine synthesis is increased in response to high ammonia levels. The developing brain is much more susceptible to the deleterious effects of excess ammonia than the adult brain, leading to irreversible cortical atrophy, ventricular enlargement, demyelination, or gray and white matter hypodensities in survivors, the extent of which depends on the magnitude and duration of ammonia exposure and the degree of brain maturation (Braissant, 2010).

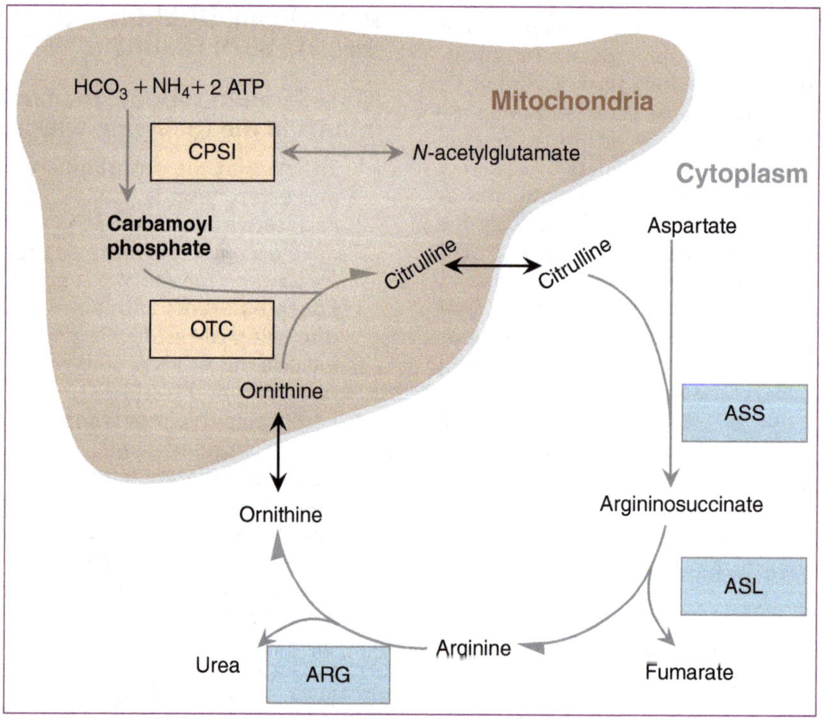


**FIGURE 9.1 The urea cycle and alternative pathways of nitrogen excretion.** Nitrogen is converted to ammonia ($NH_4$) and transported to the liver, where it is processed via the urea cycle, composed of five enzymes in the direct pathway: (1) carbamoyl phosphate synthetase I (CPSI); (2) ornithine transcarbamylase (OTC); (3) argininosuccinic acid synthetase (ASS); (4) argininosuccinic acid lyase (ASL); (5) arginase (ARG).

*Source:* Adapted from Ah Mew, N., Kimpson, K. L., Gropman, A. L., Lanpher, B. C., Chapman, K. A., & Summar, M. L. (2017). *Urea cycle disorders overview.* In M. P. Adam, H. H. Ardinger, R. A. Pagon & S. E. Wallace (Eds.), *GeneReviews®* [Internet]. University of Washington, Seattle. https://www.ncbi.nlm.nih.gov/books/NBK1217.

## Clinical Manifestations

Infants with complete urea cycle enzyme defects such as OTC and CPSI deficiency are usually born at term with no prenatal complications because the maternal circulation prevents a buildup of toxic ammonia (Yudkoff et al., 2017). Affected newborns are initially healthy, but shortly after receiving their first protein feedings, they begin to show signs of clinical decompensation and hyperammonemic encephalopathy. **Emergency Alert: The earliest signs of ammonia toxicity are irritability, hypotonia, hypothermia, lethargy, poor feeding, vomiting, and hyperventilation.** Mild respiratory alkalosis with tachypnea is a common early finding that should prompt measurement of the newborn's plasma ammonia level. Neurologic deterioration is progressive, with loss of tone and reflexes, eventually leading to respiratory failure and coma. Hepatomegaly may also be present. Without treatment, most infants will die from complications such as cerebral or pulmonary hemorrhage or neurologic or cardiac problems.

## Diagnosis

The hallmark of a UCD is an elevated blood ammonia level. A plasma ammonia level of 150 µmol/L (> 260 mcg/dl) or higher in neonates, with a normal anion gap and a normal blood glucose level, is a strong indicator of a UCD (Yudkoff et al., 2017). The exception is arginase (ARG) deficiency, which does not typically cause a rapid rise in plasma ammonia level. A normal ammonia level in a healthy infant is less than 65 µmol/L. Blood sampling and handling techniques can affect results. Blood for ammonia levels should be collected by arterial or venous sampling and kept on ice, and plasma should be separated within 15 minutes of collection. Hemolysis, delayed processing, and exposure to room air can falsely elevate ammonia levels. Because of hemolysis, blood taken by capillary puncture is inappropriate for measuring blood ammonia levels (Leonard & Morris, 2010). If the ammonia level of a newborn with a suspected UCD is only modestly elevated, it should be repeated after several hours because the level can rise rapidly.

Blood gases, electrolytes, glucose, and routine clinical laboratory tests should be obtained. Metabolic acidosis with a normal anion gap is sometimes present in UCDs but not as often as in disorders of organic acid metabolism. Blood urea nitrogen (BUN) is low, but this is not specific or sensitive for UCDs. Liver function tests are important to rule out possible causes of hyperammonemia related to liver disorders or dysfunction (Merritt & Gallagher, 2018).

Quantitative plasma and urinary amino acids are necessary for a more precise diagnosis. Plasma glutamine, alanine, and asparagine, which serve as waste storage forms of nitrogen, may all be elevated. Plasma arginine is low in all UCDs of neonatal onset. The amounts of citrulline, argininosuccinic acid, and arginine in plasma and orotic acid in urine are usually sufficient to differentiate among UCDs. Measuring enzyme activity in tissue (liver, cultured skin fibroblasts, or red blood cells) later provides a definitive diagnosis that may be desirable for genetic counseling or future prenatal testing. Molecular genetic testing using linkage analysis or mutation scanning is available for OTC and CPSI deficiencies and citrullinemia, allowing for diagnostic confirmation, carrier detection, and prenatal diagnosis. Three UCDs (citrullinemia, argininosuccinate lyase deficiency, and ARG deficiency) can also be detected by the amino acid panels of expanded newborn screening programs employing MS/MS.

**Differential Diagnosis of Hyperammonemia.** Several other EMs can cause hyperammonemia in the newborn, notably organic acidemias, propionic acidemia, methylmalonic acidemia (MMA), the FAODs, medium-chain acyl-CoA dehydrogenase deficiency (MCAD), systemic carnitine deficiency, and long-chain FAODs, although the last group is also associated with hypoglycemia. Hyperammonemia is also a feature of pyruvate carboxylase deficiency (PCD) and PDH deficiency. In transient hyperammonemia of the newborn (THAN), very high plasma ammonia levels, often matching those of UCDs, exist for which no underlying cause can be found. THAN is usually associated with prematurity and has no genetic basis, nor does it recur in infants who survive the initial episode (Merritt & Gallagher, 2018). A simple algorithm can be helpful to determine the cause of hyperammonemia (Figure 9.2).

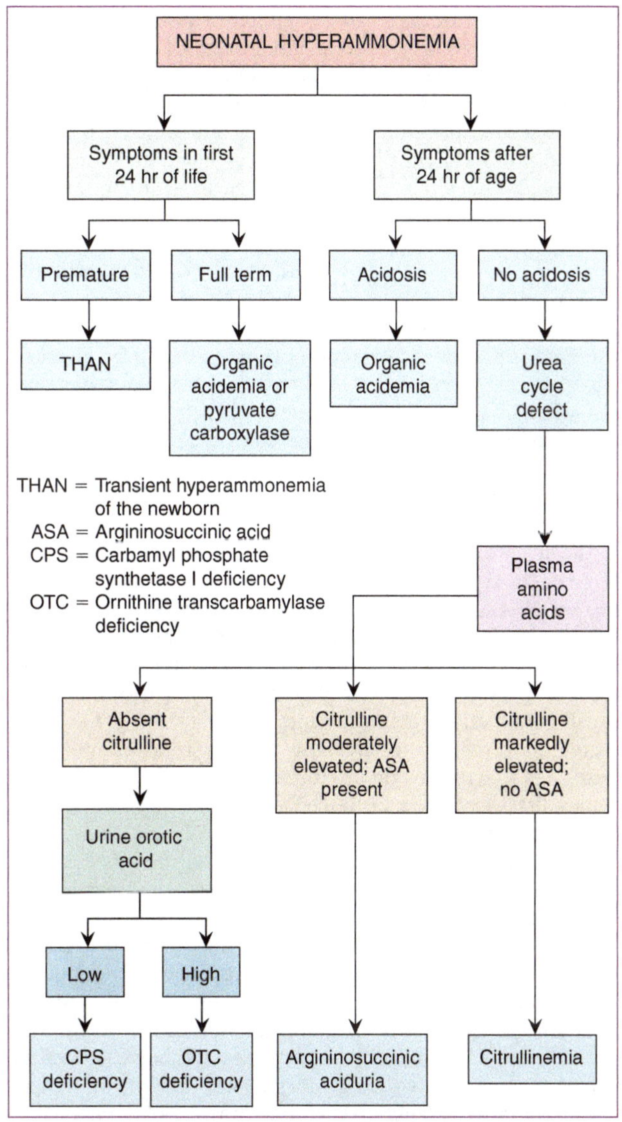


**FIGURE 9.2 Algorithm to differentiate among conditions that produce neonatal hyperammonemia.**

*Source:* Redrawn from Burton, B. K. (2000). Urea cycle disorders. *Clinics in Liver Disease, 4*, 815–830. https://doi.org/10.1016/S1089-3261(05)70143-4.

The uniform newborn screening panel was updated to include more UCDs (U.S. Department of Health and Human Services [HHS], 2018). No screening is available for OTC, CPS1, or NAGS deficiency.

## Management

Emergency treatment of an infant with a suspected UCD has three simultaneous requirements: (a) physical removal of ammonia from the circulation, (b) reversal of catabolism, and (c) scavenging of excess nitrogen (Yudkoff et al., 2017). **Quality and Safety: Dietary protein intake should cease and be replaced by high-energy intake with a protein-free formula or by intravenous (IV) glucose and lipid infusion if enteral feeding is not tolerated.** Protein intake is stopped only temporarily because failure to supply essential amino acids will eventually result in catabolism and further ammonia production. Within 48 hours, 1 to 1.5 g/kg/d of protein should be restarted, with 50% as essential amino acids. Fever, if present, must be aggressively treated. The kidneys remove ammonia poorly, so plasma ammonia levels are monitored closely, and ammonia concentrations greater than 500 µmol/L must be reduced promptly with hemodialysis or hemofiltration. Peritoneal dialysis is much less effective in clearing ammonia from the body. For this reason, it is recommended that neonates with symptomatic hyperammonemia be transferred without delay to a neonatal facility capable of providing effective toxin removal.

Compounds that conjugate to amino acids, providing an alternate route for the excretion of nitrogen, can be given to lower the nitrogen burden, and therefore the ammonia burden, of an infant with a UCD. These agents (called "scavenger drugs" or diversion therapy) include *N*-carbamylglutamate (NCG, which activates CPSI and stimulates ureagenesis), sodium benzoate (which is conjugated with glycine to form hippurate), and sodium phenylbutyrate (which is oxidized in the liver to phenylacetate and then with glutamine and excreted in the urine). *n*-Carbamylglutamate has effectively treated NAGS deficiency (Daniotti et al., 2011). Serum potassium levels must be monitored closely when these drugs are used. A preparation combining both sodium phenylbutyrate and sodium benzoate is also available. In neonates with citrullinemia and argininosuccinic aciduria, nitrogen can be excreted by increasing citrulline and argininosuccinic acid losses, respectively. Arginine supplementation enhances these metabolites' excretion by replenishing the ornithine supply. However, high doses of the IV preparation L-arginine-HCl can cause metabolic acidosis and must be administered via central line because it can cause tissue necrosis if extravasation occurs.

A neonate in acute hyperammonemic coma caused by a suspected UCD should be given loading doses followed by continuous infusions of the ammonia-scavenging drugs (L-arginine-HCl, *N*-carbamylglutamate, sodium benzoate, and sodium phenylacetate), and drug levels should be monitored to reduce the risk for toxicity. Dietary protein is reintroduced in low amounts (0.5 g/kg/d) to encourage an anabolic state, while continuing diversion therapy to control ammonia levels. Alternative therapies that have been used with variable success for neonatal UCDs include liver and hepatocyte transplantation.

**Prognosis.** Even with the most vigorous intervention, UCDs of neonatal onset are often fatal, and the few survivors have a high rate of neurologic disability (Braissant, 2010). In a recent series, a mortality rate of 32% was found in infants with UCDs who were symptomatic within the first 30 days of life (Summar et al., 2008). OTC deficiency is typically the most severe and lethal defect, particularly among males. The extent of permanent neurologic impairment in survivors is related to the duration of the hyperammonemic coma, plasma ammonia level at diagnosis, and other unidentified factors. Neonatal onset is associated with the worst prognosis (Braissant, 2010). Liver transplantation may be necessary.

# DISORDERS OF AMINO ACID METABOLISM

Amino acids play a role in literally all metabolic and cellular functions. As protein constituents, amino acids synthesize new proteins and provide a source of carbon skeletons for generating glucose and ketone bodies. Amino acids are classified as nonessential or essential, depending on whether the body can synthesize them or if they must be obtained from dietary sources.

The disorders of amino acid metabolism, also called aminoacidopathies, arise from deficiencies of enzymes required to metabolize specific amino acids or amino acid transporters. The effects of the aberrant metabolism are highly disease specific. In some aminoacidopathies, clinical symptoms are caused by the relatively rapid accumulation of toxic metabolites that are substrates for the dysfunctional enzyme (Leonard & Morris, 2006). In other amino acid disorders, the damaging effects of enzyme deficiency are more gradual and chronic in nature.

The most well-known disorder of amino acid metabolism, perhaps of all the EMs, is phenylketonuria (PKU). Clinically and biochemically heterogeneous amino acid metabolism disorders are primarily inherited as autosomal recessive traits.

## Nonketotic Hyperglycinemia

**Pathophysiology.** Nonketotic hyperglycemia (NKH) (also known as glycine encephalopathy) is a disorder of glycine metabolism that is generally fatal in its neonatal form. Glycine, a glucogenic amino acid, is typically metabolized by a complex of enzymes known as the glycine cleavage complex, consisting of four proteins encoded on four different chromosomes. A defect in any of these enzymes interferes with glycine cleavage, resulting in a steep rise in glycine concentration in the blood and CSF. The exact pathophysiology of NKH is unknown, but it is believed to be related to glycine's role as a neurotransmitter (Gibsonet al., 2017).

**Clinical Manifestations.** In classic neonatal NKH, symptoms usually start soon after birth and are not related to feedings. The clinical picture is dominated by neurologic decompensation: rapidly increasing stupor, lethargy, unresponsiveness, apnea, and sustained seizures that are difficult to control (Gibson et al., 2017). Myoclonic jerking and hiccuping (from diaphragmatic spasms) are also typical. Within 1 to 3 days, the infant becomes comatose, and death ensues. Infants who survive have intractable seizures and uniformly poor neurologic outcomes.

**Diagnosis.** Glycine is elevated in plasma, urine, and CSF. The CSF-to-plasma glycine concentration ratio of affected infants is greater than 0.09 (normal is < 0.04). The diagnostic workup fails to find evidence such as metabolic acidosis, ketosis, hyperammonemia, or abnormal organic acids in blood or urine suggestive of another EM. Electroencephalographic (EEG) tracings typically show a burst suppression pattern with hypsarrhythmia (random, high-voltage slow waves and spikes that arise from multiple foci and spread to all cortical areas). Confirmation of the exact enzyme deficiency is made by enzyme assay of a liver sample or by molecular analysis.

**Management.** No consistently effective therapy has been discovered for classic neonatal-onset NKH. Attempts to reduce plasma glycine levels with sodium benzoate and manage seizures with anticonvulsants have not changed the poor neurodevelopmental outcomes of NKH (Gibson et al., 2017).

## Hereditary Tyrosinemia

Hereditary tyrosinemia type I, also called hepatorenal tyrosinemia or fumarylacetoacetate hydrolase (FAH) deficiency, is a severe autosomal recessive metabolic disorder affecting the liver, kidneys, and nervous system.

**Pathophysiology.** Tyrosine is derived from the metabolism of dietary phenylalanine and catabolic processes. Tyrosine degradation requires a series of enzymes, the last of which is FAH. A deficiency of this enzyme characterizes tyrosinemia type I (Morris & Chakrapani, 2017). The offending compounds in tyrosinemia type I are fumarylacetoacetate and maleylacetoacetate, both of which accumulate in the cells of the liver and kidney and cause cell death by apoptosis. Although hepatocytes are quickly regenerated, liver function can deteriorate rapidly in newborns with tyrosinemia type I (Cederbaum, 2018).

**Clinical Manifestations.** Patients with hereditary tyrosinemia type I may come to clinical attention in the newborn period or within the first 3 weeks of life. Newborns present with evidence of liver dysfunction, including firm hepatomegaly, splenomegaly, bleeding from coagulation defects, jaundice, and ascites (Morris & Chakrapani, 2017). Renal tubular dysfunction and hypophosphatemic rickets are common.

**Diagnosis.** The diagnostic workup includes liver function tests, which typically show elevated transaminases and prolonged prothrombin time (PT) and partial thromboplastin time (PTT). Plasma tyrosine, phenylalanine, methionine, bilirubin, and serum alfa fetoprotein (AFP) may be elevated. The urine organic acid analysis reveals increased excretion of succinylacetone. The diagnosis can be confirmed by enzyme analysis of cultured skin fibroblasts or molecular studies. Hereditary tyrosinemia is included in the recommended uniform newborn screening panel (HHS, 2018).

**Management.** Hereditary tyrosinemia type I is now treated with nitisinone, a potent inhibitor of 4-hydroxyphenylpyruvate dioxygenase (Morris & Chakrapani, 2017). The response is monitored with urine succinylacetone, liver function tests, clotting studies, renal tubular function, and serum AFP. Most patients respond within a week with improved liver and renal function.

Dietary management involves feeding the infant a phenylalanine- and tyrosine-free formula or breastfeeding, with phenylalanine supplementation sparingly, if needed (Morris & Chakrapani, 2017). Some infants will require a liver transplant to avoid the development of hepatocellular carcinoma.

## Transient Tyrosinemia

Transient tyrosinemia in the newborn is the most common disorder of tyrosine metabolism.

**Pathophysiology.** Transient tyrosinemia is most likely caused by immaturity of 4-hydroxyphenylpyruvic acid dioxygenase (4HPPD), a vitamin C–dependent enzyme in the tyrosine degradation pathway. Risk factors include prematurity (hepatic immaturity), low vitamin C intake, and excessive protein intake. In some infants, transient tyrosinemia may be precipitated by endogenous catabolism. Tyrosinemia peaks in the first 14 days of life and resolves by 1 month of life (Morris & Chakrapani, 2017).

**Clinical Manifestations.** Lethargy and poor feeding may be seen in neonates with hypertyrosinemia, particularly in preterm infants.

**Diagnosis.** A positive newborn metabolic screen identifies transient hypertyrosinemia.

**Management.** All infants with an elevated tyrosine on the initial newborn screen should have a repeat screen, with confirmatory testing for those who remain abnormal (see Hereditary Tyrosinemia). This is usually a self-limited disorder that does not require therapy. Therapies include a low-protein diet and supplemental vitamin C as a cofactor to increase the activity of 4HPPD and accelerate the fall in tyrosine concentration.

## Phenylketonuria

Classic PKU is an autosomal recessive disorder caused by mutations in both gene alleles for phenylalanine hydroxylase, found on chromosome 12. Classic PKU occurs globally in about 1 in 23,930 live births (Hillert et. al., 2020). Although PKU rarely manifests clinically in the newborn period, it is discussed here because neonatal caregivers need to be able to provide accurate information to parents about key genetic conditions for which their newborn infants are being screened.

**Pathophysiology.** The effect of the inactive phenylalanine hydroxylase enzyme is an inability to metabolize phenylalanine, resulting in hyperphenylalaninemia. After ingesting adequate amounts of breast milk or formula, blood phenylalanine levels gradually increase. Phenylketonuric compounds are excreted in the urine, one of which (phenylacetic acid) imparts the musty odor characteristic of PKU. If dietary therapy is not implemented at birth, brain damage and CNS effects can occur (MedlinePlus, n.d.).

**Clinical Manifestations.** Biochemical manifestations of PKU are present in the newborn, but there are no outward clinical signs or symptoms. A musty odor may be detectable in the infant's urine around the end of the first week of life if plasma phenylalanine levels reach 10 to 15 mg/dl.

**Diagnosis.** **Quality and Safety:** **Early diagnosis is critical because PKU is a preventable cause of mental retardation.** Plasma phenylalanine in the normal infant is less than 2 mg/dl. In infants with PKU, the plasma phenylalanine level usually exceeds 4 mg/dl by 24 hours of age and is 20 to 40 mg/dl by the end of the first week of life. PKU is a pioneer among metabolic disorders: It was the first disorder for which a screening test was developed in 1961 (the Guthrie test, a bacterial inhibition assay), and the first disorder to be screened for using MS/MS. MS/MS has dramatically decreased the number of false-positive screening results and further clarified the prevalence of hyperphenylalaninemia variants in the population.

**Management.** PKU is currently treated with a low-phenylalanine diet; however, compliance can be a long-term problem, and dietary treatment can be associated with other nutritional deficiencies. It requires a lifetime diet with very limited intake of foods containing phenylalanine. Treatment may include taking a special nutritional supplement for life, to make sure the child gets enough essential type of protein (without phenylalanine) and nutrients for optimal growth. The U.S. Food and Drug Administration (FDA) approved the drug sepiapterin dihydrochloride, for PKU treatment. Researchers are currently investigating the use of gene therapy interventions (American Gene Technologies, n.d.).

## DISORDERS OF ORGANIC ACID METABOLISM

Organic acid disorders are disorders of intermediary metabolism resulting from a deficient enzyme or transport protein, the lack of which causes a block in a metabolic pathway. The block occurs in a step after deamination of the amino acid, and the resulting metabolites are organic acid derivatives. An organic acid is distinguished from an amino acid because it contains no nitrogen. Because these disorders lead to an accumulation of organic acids in the urine, they are often called "organic acidurias."

### Maple Syrup Urine Disease

Maple syrup urine disease (MSUD), branched-chain organic aciduria, is a disorder resulting from one or more mutations in the gene encoding the enzymes that catalyze the branched-chain amino acids (BCAA) leucine, isoleucine, and valine. MSUD refers to the intensely sweet, maple sugar odor of the cerumen, skin, and urine accompanying the disorder (Table 9.1). The U.S. incidence of MSUD is about 1 in 220,219 (Chapman et al., 2018), but in Old Order Mennonites of southeastern Pennsylvania, the frequency is 1 in 358 births (Puffenberger, 2003).

**Pathophysiology.** The second step in the degradation of a BCAA involves the enzyme branched-chain ketoacid dehydrogenase (BCKAD) complex. This enzyme catalyzes the conversion of the 3-ketoacid derivatives of the BCAA into their decarboxylated coenzyme metabolites within the mitochondria (Hoffmann et al., 2017). A deficiency of BCKAD results in an accumulation of the three BCAAs and their metabolites.

**TABLE 9.1**

**UNUSUAL ODORS ASSOCIATED WITH ERRORS OF METABOLISM**

| Disorder | Odor |
|---|---|
| Maple syrup urine disease (MSUD) | Maple syrup—burned sugar |
| Tyrosinemia type I | Cabbage or rancid butter |
| Multiple acyl-CoA dehydrogenase deficiency | Sweaty socks—rancid cheese |
| Phenylketonuria | Musty |
| Propionic acidemia | Cat urine |
| Isovaleric acidemia | Sweaty socks—rancid cheese |
| Ketoaciduria | Fruity |
| 3-Methylglutaconic aciduria | Tomcat urine |
| Trimethylaminuria | Fish |

MSUD neurotoxicity is secondary to the accumulation of the ketoacid of leucine, 2-oxoisocaproic acid, in the plasma and organs. Leucine intoxication impairs the volume-regulating mechanisms in the brain, liver, muscle, and pancreatic cells. A fall in serum sodium precipitates a redistribution of water in the intracellular spaces of the brain, causing cerebral edema. The brains of newborns with MSUD exhibit severe cytotoxic edema with the involvement of myelinated white matter on magnetic resonance imaging (MRI) (Kilicarslan et al., 2012).

**Clinical Manifestations.** The neonate with classical MSUD is usually born at term after an uncomplicated pregnancy and delivery. A short symptom-free interval occurs after birth. The usual postnatal endogenous protein catabolism causes a progressive BCAA rise with metabolic acidosis.

By about 48 hours of age, the untreated infant begins to show signs of the disorder. The earliest and most specific sign is the unique maple syrup odor of the cerumen. Other MSUD early signs and symptoms are feeding difficulties, irritability, lethargy, and dystonia. Over the ensuing hours, neurologic deterioration predominates as drowsiness and lethargy progress to coma—periods of lethargy and hypotonia alternate with muscular rigidity, hypertonia, and seizures. Opisthotonic posturing is a characteristic feature of classic MSUD (Hoffmann et al., 2017).

**Diagnosis.** Early diagnosis and management are essential to prevent permanent brain damage. MSUD is diagnosed with plasma amino acid assay. An elevated leucine level and a high leucine-to-alanine ratio are diagnostic of MSUD. A dinitrophenylhydrazine (DNPH) test of the urine, which screens for the presence of alpha-ketoacids, will be positive. Urine should also be tested for ketones, which are typically present. Ketonuria is never normal in the neonate and should always suggest the possibility of an EM. Urinary organic acid analysis should also be performed.

By the time of diagnosis on clinical grounds, many infants with MSUD are severely encephalopathic and require emergency therapy to lower the BCAA levels. Newborn screening by MS/MS allows for the detection of elevated BCAA concentrations in blood in patients with classic MSUD before the onset of severe encephalopathy. All states include MSUD on their newborn screening panels. Unfortunately, these specimens are often collected after 24 hours of age, and results are not reported until infants are 6 to 10 days of age. An infant with classic MSUD would already be seriously ill by that time.

**Management.** Treatment of MSUD aims to rapidly lower the plasma leucine level and achieve stable, long-term metabolic control with a carefully monitored low-BCAA diet. Hemodialysis, hemofiltration, or ECMO are used to remove toxins. High-energy enteral or parenteral nutrition, closely monitoring BCAA levels, is the dietary therapy used to augment toxin removal. Even after the infant is in good metabolic control, common infections and injuries can rapidly induce biochemical disturbances requiring prompt management to prevent a metabolic crisis (Cederbaum, 2018).

## ISOVALERIC ACIDEMIA

Isovaleric acidemia (IVA) is a very rare autosomal disorder of leucine metabolism caused by mutations in the gene encoding the enzyme isovaleryl-CoA dehydrogenase, mapped to chromosome 15. The disorder has both an acute and chronic form; the acute form manifests in the neonatal period as a catastrophic disease.

**Pathophysiology.** Isovaleryl-CoA dehydrogenase catalyzes the third step in the catabolism of the BCAA leucine in the inner mitochondrial matrix (Grünert et al., 2012). A deficiency of isovaleryl-CoA dehydrogenase leads to accumulations of highly toxic free isovaleric acid, 3-hydroxyvaleric acid, and N-isovalerylglycine. Excess organic acids in the bloodstream inhibit gluconeogenesis and ureagenesis, resulting in hypoglycemia, hyperammonemia, and metabolic acidosis (Khan et al., 2020). Hypoglycemia stimulates the release of free fatty acids, which are transported into the mitochondria and oxidized to produce ketones, the source of ketosis in infants with IVA, and other organic acidemias. These organic acids also arrest the maturation of hematopoietic precursors, leading to leukopenia and thrombocytopenia (Hoffmann et al., 2017; Wilcken, 2010).

**Clinical Manifestations.** Infants with IVA become extremely ill in the first week of life. Early symptoms are poor feeding, vomiting, lethargy, and hypothermia. Clinical evidence of dehydration is often present. **Emergency Alert:** **Untreated infants progress to coma, and less than half survive the initial metabolic crisis. IVA can be recognized by the unpleasant "sweaty feet" or "rancid cheese" odor of body fluids. Hepatomegaly is present in some infants.**

**Diagnosis.** The diagnosis of IVA is based on the presence of isovalerylglycine and its metabolites in urine, as well as isovalerylcarnitine in plasma. Plasma organic acid analysis also reveals markedly elevated N-isovalerylglycine and 3-hydroxyvaleric acid. A secondary carnitine deficiency can develop. Both ketosis and metabolic acidosis, with an elevated anion gap, are present. Secondary derangements include hyperammonemia, thrombocytopenia, neutropenia, and anemia. IVA can be detected by MS/MS using filter-paper blood-spot samples and is included on the recommended uniform newborn screening panel (HHS, 2018).

**Management.** Infants who are extremely ill because of the accumulation of isovaleric acid will need exogenous toxin removal with hemodialysis, hemofiltration, or ECMO (Cederbaum, 2018). Supplementation with L-glycine is also effective for IVA. Glycine promotes the formation of isovalerylglycine, which is excreted more efficiently than free isovaleric acid. L -Carnitine is given to replace lost carnitine and provide a substrate for forming isovalerylcarnitine, a nontoxic by-product that can be excreted in the urine (Cederbaum, 2018). If metabolic acidosis is severe, bicarbonate therapy is indicated. **Quality and Safety:** **Adequate fluids are mandatory to promote the excretion of isovaleric acid because the primary route of elimination is the kidney. Urine output must be carefully monitored.** Once the diagnosis is confirmed, protein is removed from the diet, and a high-energy intake of glucose and intralipid is administered. Nutritional support is subsequently provided through leucine-free amino acid mixtures, followed by a reduced leucine diet. It is important to reintroduce a balanced nutritional intake, including protein, as soon as possible to promote an anabolic state.

### Propionic Acidemia

Propionic acidemia (PA) is a severe autosomal recessive disorder caused by gene mutations that encode the propionyl-CoA carboxylase enzyme's two nonidentical subunits (alpha and beta). Its estimated incidence is less than 1 in 105,000 to 130,000 births (Gilksman, 2024).

**Pathophysiology.** Propionyl-CoA is produced by the metabolism of isoleucine, valine, threonine, methionine, odd-chain fatty acids, and cholesterol (Gilksman, 2024). A deficiency of propionyl-CoA carboxylase results in an accumulation of toxic organic acid metabolites in the mitochondria, causing severe ketoacidosis (see also Isovaleric Acidemia).

**Clinical Manifestations.** PA typically manifests shortly after birth, beginning with poor feeding, vomiting, lethargy, hypotonia, and seizures (Gilksman, 2024). Ketonuria and metabolic acidosis develop in most infants, and severe intracellular dehydration may develop. Hepatomegaly may be present. Infants with PA are susceptible to bacterial infections because of neutropenia and thrombocytopenia. The odor imparted to body fluids by propionic acid has been likened to "cat urine." Cardiomyopathy can be a presentation (Gilksman, 2024).

**Diagnosis.** Usually, a marked elevation of free propionate in the blood and urine is present. Occasionally, these findings are absent, and in those cases, significant elevations of other propionate metabolites, such as propionyl-carnitine, beta-hydroxypropionate, and methylcitrate, help establish the diagnosis. Propionyl-carnitine is not specific for PA. Plasma glycine is increased, but plasma carnitine is low. The PA diagnosis can be confirmed either by an analysis of enzyme activity in leukocytes or fibroblasts or by a specific mutation analysis. PA can be detected by MS/MS using filter-paper blood-spot samples; this test is included on the recommended uniform newborn screening panel (HHS, 2018). Molecular genetic testing for a variant in PCCA or PCCB with deficient propionyl-CoA carboxylase enzyme activity can confirm the diagnosis (Gilksman, 2024). Markers can be found in blood and urine (Children's Hospital of Philadelphia [CHOP], n.d.).

**Management.** PA is unique in that the urinary excretion of the toxin and propionic acid is negligible, and no alternate route can adequately remove the toxin from affected newborns. Emergency treatment to remove toxins using hemodialysis or hemofiltration is imperative. Initially, protein intake is stopped, and a high-calorie intake of glucose and intralipids or nonprotein formula is substituted to suppress catabolism. Protein is reintroduced in small quantities after a few days of protein restriction. A diet with low protein and some fat restrictions must be followed for life (CHOP, n.d.). Liver transplantation may be suggested in some cases (CHOP, n.d.). Discharge teaching should include the importance of seeking medical attention immediately for any sign of illness or infection because even a minor illness can lead to rapid deterioration in an infant with PA.

## Methylmalonic Acidemia

MMA comprises a group of disorders representing inherited autosomal recessive deficiencies of the activity of methylmalonyl-CoA mutase, a vitamin $B_{12}$–dependent enzyme. MMA is one of the more common organic acidemias, occurring in about 1 in 48,000 to 1 in 61,000 births in Western populations, with 1 in 4,000 to 1 in 26,000 in China (Chen et al., 2023). About half of the mutations causing MMA are in the genes encoding this enzyme; other mutations can occur in genes required to provide cobalamin cofactors. In the most severe form of MMA, enzyme activity is completely absent.

**Pathophysiology.** Methylmalonyl-CoA mutase is usually responsible for converting methylmalonyl-CoA to succinyl-CoA, a Krebs cycle intermediate. Lack of methylmalonyl-CoA mutase activity results in an intracellular accumulation of methylmalonic acid, impairing mitochondrial oxidative metabolism. A secondary inhibition of propionyl-CoA results in an accumulation of propionic acid and its metabolites. These compounds inhibit many intermediary metabolic pathways, leading to hypoglycemia, hyperammonemia, and hyperglycinemia. Mitochondrial dysfunction from metabolite accumulation results in CNS injuries (Chen et al., 2023). Conjugation with carnitine results in a relative carnitine deficiency.

**Clinical Manifestations.** Most infants with MMA begin showing symptoms before the end of the first week of life. Lethargy, hypotonia, feeding difficulties, and vomiting with signs of dehydration are followed by respiratory distress, acute encephalopathy, and eventual coma. Untreated infants develop hypoglycemia, hyperammonemia, anion gap metabolic acidosis, and ketosis. MMA is like PA in that many infants become neutropenic and thrombocytopenic.

**Diagnosis.** Plasma methylmalonic acid and propionylcarnitine are increased in MMA and can be detected by tandem mass spectrometry (MS/MS) as part of the uniform newborn screening panel (Chen et al., 2023; HHS, 2018). The presence of C4-dicarboxylic acylcarnitine distinguishes MMA from PA. Urine organic acid analysis demonstrates greatly increased methylmalonic acid and its precursors, methylcitric acid and beta-hydroxypropionate. Among the many other nonspecific laboratory findings in MMA are metabolic acidosis, hyperammonemia, hyperglycinemia, leukopenia, anemia, thrombocytopenia, and ketonuria. Molecular genetic testing is available for prenatal diagnosis. Neuroimaging can be used to examine white matter volume and other brain changes, but more research is needed in this area (Chen et al., 2023).

**Management.** The acute metabolic crisis of MMA is further managed with protein restriction and administration of IV glucose and intralipid. Some fats will be restricted (Health Resources & Services Administration [HRSA], n.d.). Adequate fluid intake will enhance the elimination of methylmalonic acid, which is relatively efficiently removed from the body by the kidneys. Blood gases should be monitored to evaluate the degree of metabolic acidosis, and sodium bicarbonate may be required to control severe metabolic acidosis. If the infant has a cofactor-responsive disease, pharmacologic doses of vitamin $B_{12}$ are given (HRSA, n.d.). Because excess propionate is also a problem in MMA, broad-spectrum antibiotics are given to inhibit anaerobic flora and reduce intestinal propionate production. Supplemental carnitine replaces carnitine depletion and promotes urinary propionylcarnitine elimination (HRSA, n.d.).

Like infants with PA, those with MMA are at high risk for infection owing to compromised immunity reflected by neutropenia and thrombocytopenia. Close monitoring of clinical and laboratory indicators of infection is warranted. These infants must also be monitored for evidence of cardiac failure related to cardiomyopathy. Discharge planning needs of infants with MMA are like those of infants with PA. Parents or other caretakers must be aware that even a minor illness or infection in their infant with MMA can represent a potential metabolic crisis and require prompt medical attention.

# FATTY ACID OXIDATION DISORDERS

FAODs comprise a subset of organic acid disorders among the most common of the known inherited disorders of metabolism. The population frequency of FAODs is estimated to be 1 in 5,000 to 10,000 births (Merritt et al., 2018). A FAOD can be caused by a deficiency of any enzymes involved in cellular uptake, transport, and mitochondrial oxidation of fatty acids. The most common is MCAD. Short, long, and very long chain forms of this enzyme deficiency also exist (SCAD,

LCAD, very long chain acyl-CoA dehydrogenase [VLCAD]), as well as carnitine transporter defects, and deficiencies of the mitochondrial trifunctional protein (MTP) complex.

## Pathophysiology

The fatty acids are the body's largest energy source and are the preferred fuel of the liver, heart, and skeletal muscles. Neonatal brown fat uses fatty acids to sustain nonshivering thermogenesis. When glucose levels are low during long periods between feedings, glucagon secreted by the pancreas stimulates adipose cell lipase to liberate free fatty acids. These fatty acids are oxidized to provide energy through the mitochondrial beta-oxidation pathway. Fatty acid oxidation also provides the substrate for hepatic ketogenesis. Fatty acids as a source of energy are particularly critical for neonates with limited glycogen stores and high metabolic rates; thus, any perturbation in the fatty acid oxidation pathway can rapidly lead to metabolic decompensation.

**Fatty Acid Oxidation.** Three subsystems are required to produce energy in the normal fat oxidation process (Figure 9.3): (a) the carnitine cycle, (b) the mitochondrial inner membrane system, and (c) the mitochondrial matrix system (Vockley et al., 2017). In the first step, L-carnitine and fatty acids are taken up by the cell, and fatty acids are conjugated to fatty acyl-CoAs in the cytoplasm by enzymes of the outer mitochondrial membrane. Medium- and short-chain fatty acids can penetrate the inner mitochondrial membrane for beta-oxidation. However, longer-chain fatty acids of dietary fat (those with carbon lengths of 14–20) must be actively transported into the matrix via the carnitine cycle. Activated acyl-CoAs are converted to carnitine esters by carnitine palmitoyltransferase I (CPT1), transported across the mitochondrial membrane by carnitine-acylcarnitine translocase, and reactivated by carnitine palmitoyltransferase II (CPT2).

Within the mitochondrion, long-chain acyl-CoAs are degraded by enzymes in the inner membrane system in a recurring cyclic sequence of four reactions (Vockley et al., 2017). These are catalyzed by VLCAD and the MTP complex encompassing the three enzymes required for a single cycle of beta-oxidation: enoyl-CoA hydratase, L to 3-hydroxy acyl-CoA dehydrogenase (LCHAD), and thiolase. In each full cycle, the fatty acid is progressively shortened by two carbons from long to medium and finally to short-chain acyl-CoAs. The final system, the mitochondrial matrix, oxidizes shorter chain-length fatty acids resulting from the enzymatic steps in the inner membrane system. L-Carnitine is not required for the latter process. The result of the beta-oxidation system is the generation of acetyl-CoA, used by the liver to produce ketone bodies and as a major source of cellular ATP.

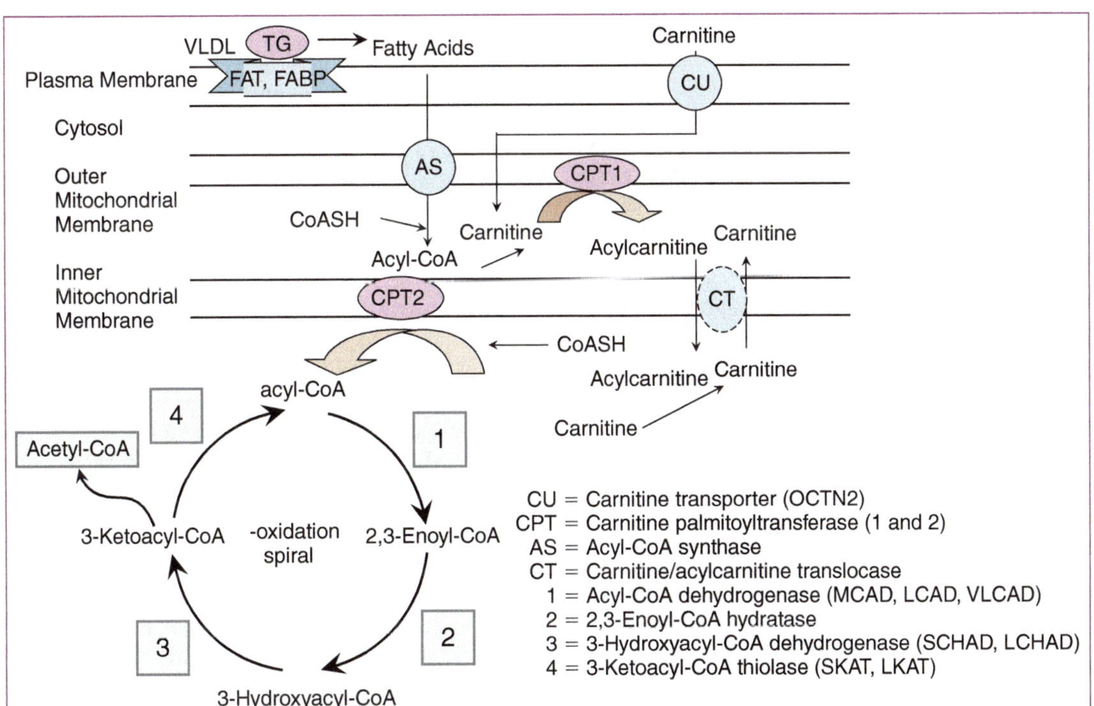


**FIGURE 9.3 The mitochondrial fatty acid oxidation pathway.** This schematic representation shows the uptake of fatty acids and carnitine into the cell, the transfer of fatty acid from the cytosol into mitochondria, and the fatty acid beta-oxidation spiral.

LCAD, long-chain acyl-CoA dehydrogenase; LCHAD, long-chain 3-Hydroxyacyl-CoA dehydrogenase; LKAT, long-chain 3-Ketoacyl-CoA thiolase; MCAD, medium-chain acyl-CoA dehydrogenase deficiency; OCTN2, an organic cation/carnitine transporter 2; SCAD, short chain acyl-CoA dehydrogenase; SCHAD, short-chain 3-Hydroxyacyl-CoA dehydrogenase; SKAT, 3-Ketoacyl-CoA thiolase; VLCAD, very long chain acyl-CoA dehydrogenase.

*Source:* Adapted from Shekhawat, P., Bennett, M. J., Sadovsky, Y., Nelson, D. M., Rakheja, D., & Strauss, A. W. (2003). Human placenta metabolizes fatty acids: Implications for fetal acid oxidation disorders and maternal liver diseases. *American Journal of Physiology, Endocrinology & Metabolism, 284*, E1098–E1105. https://doi.org/10.1152/ajpendo.00481.2002.

**Defective Fatty Acid Oxidation.** Inborn errors of fatty acid oxidation result in a buildup of toxic metabolites both proximal and distal to the block and an insufficient yield of substrate for energy production. A deficiency of any of the enzymes required for fatty acid transport or metabolism can result in a failure of fatty acid oxidation. The primary physiologic consequences are inadequate ATP, ketone body generation, and a failure of energy production. This becomes apparent during periods of increased energy demand, such as a prolonged period of fasting, fever, or other illness. Under normal circumstances, when glycogen stores are depleted in the newborn, free fatty acids are released as a source of energy. However, the neonate with a FAOD is unable to use fatty acids for fuel and rapidly becomes hypoglycemic. As a result of hypoketogenesis, the brain is without an alternate fuel source. Without early treatment, neurologic morbidity and mortality are high. A second consequence of FAODs is the accumulation of fatty acids and their derivatives, which can have toxic effects. When their oxidation is blocked, fatty acids are stored in the cytosol as triglycerides, resulting in muscular, hepatic, and cardiac lipidoses. Skeletal muscle tissue begins to break down (rhabdomyolysis), causing a skeletal myopathy characterized by muscle weakness. In defects downstream from CPT1 in the carnitine cycle, the acylcarnitine that accumulates has detergent-like properties that may disrupt the integrity of muscle membranes. In the heart muscle, accumulated long-chain fatty acyl-CoAs can produce electrophysiologic abnormalities, including arrhythmias and cardiac arrest.

## Clinical Manifestations

Affected neonates are almost always born at term. Fasting stress sufficient to reveal the disorder can result from early breastfeeding but with difficulty. Mitochondrial FAODs in the neonate present with three clinical phenotypes that, depending on the disorder, can be seen individually or in combination: hypoketotic hypoglycemia, cardiomyopathy, and skeletal myopathy (Rector & Ibdah, 2010). Neonates with MCAD, the most common of the FAODs, usually present with glucose instability, but there have been reports of acute life-threatening episodes and even sudden death (Rector & Ibdah, 2010).

Neonates with VLCAD are similarly intolerant to fasting and develop hypoglycemia without ketosis. Moreover, VLCAD can be associated with evidence of cardiomyopathy, including cardiomegaly, ventricular arrhythmias, or unexplained cardiac arrest. Other physical findings that have been reported in neonates with disorders of fatty acid oxidation include hypotonia, seizures, irritability or lethargy (mimicking acute encephalopathy), hepatomegaly, and associated congenital malformations such as cystic renal dysplasia.

## Diagnosis

A FAOD must be considered in any infant with an unexplained nonketotic hypoglycemia, hepatic dysfunction, isolated arrhythmia, or cardiomegaly. The initial screen for FAOD includes urine organic acid analysis, as well as plasma and urine-free and total carnitine collected during a period of acute decompensation. Newborn screening using tandem mass spectrometry will aid in the diagnosis (Merritt et al., 2018).

When MS/MS screening is unavailable, the most useful indirect laboratory tests in neonates with suspected FAODs are glucose, electrolytes, BUN, creatinine, lactate, ammonia, transaminases, and creatine kinase. Elevated creatine kinase and myoglobinuria reflect rhabdomyolysis. Plasma carnitine levels are markedly reduced, except in CPT1 deficiency (Vockley et al., 2017). Additional laboratory results may show hyperammonemia, metabolic acidosis, and increased uric acid and transaminases. A liver biopsy performed during the acute phase usually reveals microvesicular and macrovesicular fatty infiltration.

Family and perinatal history can be particularly important to diagnosing a FAOD. Many infants diagnosed with a FAOD have a history of a sibling who died of SUID. An association has been found between acute fatty liver of pregnancy (AFLP) or HELLP (hemolysis, elevated liver enzymes, low platelets) syndrome in the mother and fetal deficiency of LCHAD, one of the enzymes in the MTP complex. When a woman carries an affected fetus, the placenta and fetus cannot oxidize fatty acids, leading to the transfer of accumulated fatty acid intermediates to the maternal circulation. For unclear reasons, in some women, these fatty acids overwhelm the maternal liver and contribute to HELLP syndrome and maternal hepatic fat deposition (AFLP).

Newborn infants of women with AFLP or mothers who are known carriers for FAODs should be evaluated immediately after birth with blood-spot acylcarnitine profiles and treated as if they have a FAOD until test results are known.

**Neonatal Screening and Confirmatory Testing for FAOD.** The key to preventing the morbidity and mortality associated with FAOD is through presymptomatic diagnosis, allowing early treatment and avoidance of metabolic crisis. Neonatal screening for FAODs by MS/MS analyzes acylcarnitines from dried blood spots and can identify 22 different abnormalities. However, an abnormal acylcarnitine profile can represent more than one FAOD, so more specific testing is required. Using cultured skin fibroblasts (or amniocytes) incubated with deuterium-labeled fatty acid precursors and excess L-carnitine, MS/MS can rapidly detect any enzyme defect from carnitine-acylcarnitine translocase through SCAD. This method is possible because the enzymes of fatty acid oxidation are also expressed in the skin and other cells. Mutational analysis, if available, can also provide a definitive diagnosis (Vockley et al., 2017).

## Management

The primary goal is to provide nutrition to control endogenous lipolysis and prevent tissue catabolism. This involves a high-carbohydrate, low-fat diet. The newborn should be fed every 3 to 4 hours, with close monitoring of blood sugar levels. Breastfeeding mothers should receive lactation assistance to ensure successful breastfeeding with evidence of milk transfer. If hypoglycemia persists or the infant cannot tolerate enteral feeding, glucose should be administered intravenously. The nurse should closely monitor for cardiac conduction disturbances.

The nurse is in a key position to prevent stressors, such as hypothermia or pain, that could precipitate a metabolic crisis and to assess the infant for signs of intercurrent illness that might require additional therapy. Discharge teaching should emphasize the need to avoid prolonged fasting periods and seek medical attention if the infant shows signs of illness (fever, vomiting, diarrhea, refusal to eat, lethargy, or any other change in normal behavior). A consult should be made with a neonatal nutritionist or dietary specialist to arrange teaching for the family about the infant's post-discharge dietary regimen. The infant's diet will continue to be high in carbohydrates and restricted in fat.

### Multiple Acyl-CoA Dehydrogenase Deficiency (Glutaric Aciduria Type II)

**Pathophysiology.** Multiple acyl-CoA dehydrogenase deficiency (MADD), formerly known as glutaric aciduria type II, is a disorder caused by a defective electron transfer flavoprotein (ETF) or electron transfer flavoprotein dehydrogenase (ETF-QO). MADD impairs fatty acid oxidation and branched amino acids lysine and glutaric acid oxidation. The heart, liver, and kidneys become infiltrated with fat.

**Clinical Manifestations.** Two different neonatal presentations have been described for MADD; both involve overwhelming illness with rapid progression to coma and death (Vockley et al., 2017). One presentation is a neonate, often preterm, with dysmorphic facial features, polycystic kidneys, and hepatomegaly. Within the first 24 to 48 hours of life, the infant develops hypotonia, metabolic acidosis, severe nonketotic hypoglycemia, and a distinctive "sweaty feet" odor of body fluids. The alternate neonatal presentation is the infant without congenital anomalies but with similar symptoms and metabolic aberrations. Neither group lives longer than a few weeks; the few infants who survive generally succumb to cardiac failure at a few months of age.

**Diagnosis.** MS/MS rapidly detects elevated acylcarnitines (C4, C5, C8, C10, and C16). Quantitative urine organic acid analysis usually reveals a pattern of elevated organic acids: lactic, glutaric, 2-hydroxyglutaric, ethylmalonic, adipic, suberic, sebacic, and other acids, some in very high amounts. The same organic acids are increased in the plasma. Volatile acid (isovaleric, acetic, isobutyric, propionic, butyric) concentrations in plasma are excessive, accounting for the characteristic odor associated with the disorder. Plasma carnitine may be low. Mutations have been identified in the genes for flavoproteins ETF and ETF-QO.

**Management.** There is no effective treatment other than supportive care (fluids, glucose, sodium bicarbonate) for the rapid-onset, severe neonatal presentation. For the rare infant who survives the initial crisis, management involves frequent feedings with avoidance of fasting and a diet low in fat and protein and high in carbohydrates. Some patients also respond to riboflavin.

## CONGENITAL LACTIC ACIDOSIS

Congenital lactic acidosis (also called primary lactic acidosis) is a group of disorders of lactate metabolism caused by defects in the mitochondrial respiratory or electron transport chain, the tricarboxylic acid (Krebs) cycle, or in pyruvate metabolism.

Lactic acid is the major end product of anaerobic glycolysis, accumulating when pyruvate production exceeds utilization. The brain's dependence on oxidative metabolism makes it particularly susceptible to damage in disorders of oxidation that lead to lactic acidosis.

### Pyruvate Dehydrogenase Deficiency

PDH complex disorders are the most common errors of pyruvate metabolism. Most cases of PDH are caused by mutations in the X-linked *PDHA1* gene, which encodes the E1 alpha subunit of the PDH enzyme complex (Brown, 2012).

**Pathophysiology.** PDH complex efficiently and irreversibly converts pyruvate, a product of glucose metabolism, to acetyl-CoA. Acetyl-CoA is one of two essential substrates needed to generate citrate for the energy-producing tricarboxylic acid cycle (also called the citric acid cycle or Krebs cycle). Thus, PDH provides the link between glycolysis and the tricarboxylic acid cycle. PDH complex activity is regulated primarily by reversible phosphorylation (inactivation) of the enzyme's E1 alpha subunit. A deficiency in the PDH complex limits the production of acetyl-CoA and, in turn, the production of citrate, blocking the tricarboxylic acid cycle and creating an energy deficit. Persistent glycolysis without pyruvate oxidation leads to lactate accumulation because excess pyruvate is reduced to lactate in the cytoplasm. Tissues with high energy requirements, such as the CNS, are vulnerable to injury when cellular energy production is impaired.

**Clinical Manifestations.** The nonspecific early signs and symptoms of PDH deficiency develop soon after birth and are like those of other metabolic disorders. Progressive neurologic deterioration, apnea, seizures, and coma follow poor feeding, lethargy, and tachypnea. Fulminant lactic acidosis is present in infants with profound deficiencies of the PDH complex, and these patients often die early in the neonatal period. Infants with severe disease may have prenatal onset, leading to structural brain abnormalities, including microcephaly. Patients with PDH complex deficiency can also present with Leigh syndrome.

**Diagnosis.** Lactic acidosis and high pyruvate levels are important biochemical markers for mitochondrial dysfunction (Frye, 2023). Lactate and pyruvate are also often elevated in the CSF of infants with this disorder. Plasma and urine amino acid analysis reveals hyperalaninemia. A definitive enzyme activity diagnosis requires testing leukocytes, fibroblasts, tissue samples, or DNA analysis.

**Collaborative Management.** Correction of the acidosis is necessary but may not affect all of the symptoms (Frye, 2023). Cofactor supplementation with thiamine, carnitine, and lipoic acid is another facet of managing these infants (Frye, 2023).

Recently, dichloroacetate (DCA) has been used to treat PDH complex deficiency. DCA is believed to activate PDH complex activity by inhibiting PDH kinase.

### Pyruvate Carboxylase Deficiency

PCD is a disorder of energy metabolism that exists in three different forms. The most severe of these is a neonatal-onset form known as type B, a disorder with a high mortality rate. All forms of PCD have a frequency of about 1 in 250,000 live births and are recessively inherited.

**Pathophysiology.** Pyruvate carboxylase is a biotin-containing mitochondrial enzyme responsible for the ATP-dependent carboxylation of pyruvate. This enzyme catalyzes the conversion of pyruvate to oxaloacetate, thus affecting gluconeogenesis (Frye, 2023). The absence of pyruvate carboxylase activity results in the malfunction of the citric acid cycle and gluconeogenesis, disrupting energy metabolism in the brain. A deficiency of aspartic acid derived from oxaloacetate also disrupts the urea cycle, leading to a simultaneous failure of nitrogen excretion.

**Clinical Manifestations.** In PCD with neonatal onset, the earliest signs and symptoms begin at 72 hours of life and include severe truncal hypotonia and tachypnea associated with profound metabolic acidosis. Seizures, abnormal eye movements, and coma can occur. Hyperammonemia, hypoglycemia, ketosis, and ketonuria are frequent findings. Renal tubular acidosis can also accompany PCD.

**Diagnosis.** The diagnosis of PCD is based on the measurement of urinary organic acids and blood acylcarnitine profile. In type B PCD, the lactate–pyruvate ratio may be high (≥ 25). Plasma citrulline and lysine are elevated along with the ammonia level. Serum transaminases may also be elevated. The diagnosis can be confirmed by enzyme analysis of hepatic cells or leukocytes.

**Management.** PCD is a progressive disorder with no specific therapy. Some infants have biotin-responsive disease, so pharmacologic doses of biotin are administered, and the response is evaluated. Therapeutic options with citrate or aspartic acid supplements can reduce acidosis and lower ammonia levels (Frye, 2023).

## DISORDERS OF CARBOHYDRATE METABOLISM

### Galactosemia

Galactosemia is an inherited disorder of carbohydrate metabolism caused by a deficiency in one of the three enzymes of the galactose metabolic pathway: galactose-L-phosphate uridyl transferase (GALT), galactokinase (GALK), or UDP-galactose-4-epimerase (GALE). GALT deficiency, affecting the second step in galactose metabolism, accounts for more than 95% of galactosemias; thus, it has become synonymous with classic galactosemia.

Galactosemia has an estimated prevalence of 1 in 16,000 and 1 in 44,000 live births (Tisa et al., 2022). At least 24 mutations have been identified in the human GALT gene, located on chromosome 9.

**Pathophysiology.** Infants with galactosemia cannot metabolize the sugar galactose, derived from the disaccharide lactose, the major carbohydrate of mammalian milk. In normal galactose metabolism, galactose is first converted to galactose-L-phosphate by GALK, which is, in turn, converted by the GALT enzyme to uridyl diphosphate (UDP) glucose. The severe form of galactosemia features near-total deficiency of GALT enzyme activity in all body cells. In the absence of GALT, ingesting lactose-containing substances produces toxic levels of galactose-L-phosphate within cells. Surplus galactose is reduced to galactitol or oxidized to galactonate, metabolites that also have a direct toxic effect on the liver and other organs.

**Clinical Manifestations.** Most patients present in the neonatal period or the first week or two of life. After ingestion of galactose (either cow's milk-based formula or breast milk), vomiting, diarrhea, poor weight gain, jaundice, hepatomegaly, and hypoglycemia become evident. In some infants, CNS symptoms, such as lethargy and hypotonia, predominate. Untreated infants will go on to develop cataracts secondary to the accumulation of galactitol. Sepsis, usually caused by *Escherichia coli (E. coli)*, is often the presenting problem owing to low neutrophil bactericidal activity. Liver dysfunction is progressive, and many infants die during the first week of life from liver failure. In those who do survive, neurologic complications are frequent.

Two related disorders of galactose metabolism are GALK and GALE deficiencies. In GALK deficiency, galactose cannot be phosphorylated into galactose-L-phosphate. The chief clinical finding in GALK deficiency is cataract formation. In GALE deficiency, most patients are asymptomatic and have normal growth and development.

**Diagnosis.** A galactose assay, measuring blood galactose, red blood cell (RBC) galactose-L-phosphate, and GALT enzyme activity, is used to diagnose classic galactosemia. GALT activity is low or absent. Galactose and galactose-L-phosphate are elevated. DNA analysis for the common mutations associated with GALT deficiency can also be done. Urine is positive for reducing substances. Galactosemia is included on all routine state newborn screening panels, allowing presymptomatic diagnosis.

**Management.** Galactosemia is treated by feeding a soy-based formula containing no galactose. **Quality and Safety: Breastfeeding is not permitted. Other sources of galactose, including medications containing galactose, must also be avoided. Dietary restriction of galactose in the newborn will reverse the hepatic, renal, brain, and immune dysfunction and reduce the accumulated galactose metabolites. Additional measures include monitoring for and treating sepsis and coagulopathy. Despite dietary treatment, long-term neurodevelopmental outcomes have not been uniformly favorable. An essential part of discharge education is dietary teaching, which assists the family in maintaining dietary control as the infant grows and develops and helps them identify occult sources of galactose in foods and other substances.**

### Hereditary Fructose Intolerance

Hereditary fructose intolerance (HFI) is an inherited inability to digest fructose (fruit sugar) or its precursors (sugar, sorbitol, and brown sugar). This autosomal recessive disorder has a frequency of approximately 1 in 22,000 births.

**Pathophysiology.** Fructose is a naturally occurring sugar used as a sweetener in many foods, including many baby foods. A deficiency of the enzyme fructose-L-phosphate aldolase activity impairs the body's ability to convert fructose-L-phosphate to glyceraldehyde and dihydroxyacetone phosphate. The outcome is an accumulation of fructose-L-phosphate in the liver, kidney, and small intestine, which inhibits glycogen breakdown and glucose synthesis and causes severe hypoglycemia following fructose ingestion. This disorder can be life threatening to infants.

**Clinical Manifestations.** In the neonate, the onset of clinical symptoms follows ingestion of cow's milk formula and resembles that of galactosemia. Signs and symptoms include pallor, lethargy, poor feeding, irritability, vomiting, and hypoglycemia. Jaundice, hepatomegaly, and evidence of progressive liver disease may follow. In exclusively breastfed infants, symptoms will be delayed until weaning to fruits and vegetables.

**Diagnosis.** The diagnosis of HFI is usually done by molecular analysis rather than enzyme analysis or fructose tolerance testing (Merritt & Gallagher, 2018). Urine is positive for reducing substances.

**Management.** Management of HFI centers on removing all sources of fructose and sucrose from the diet. All IV solutions and other medications must also be free of fructose, corn syrup, and sorbitol. Supportive care includes management of liver failure, kidney dysfunction, and coagulopathy, if present. The infant's parents will benefit from consultation with a dietary specialist to learn about long-term dietary management.

## Fructose 1,6-Bisphosphatase Deficiency

Fructose 1,6-biphosphatase deficiency is a rare disorder of carbohydrate metabolism.

**Pathophysiology.** Fructose 1,6-bisphosphatase catalyzes the irreversible splitting of fructose 1,6-biphosphate into fructose 6-phosphate and inorganic phosphate. The enzyme's activity is highest in gluconeogenic tissues such as the liver and kidney. Fructose 1,6-biphosphatase deficiency is, therefore, a disorder of gluconeogenesis, resulting in glucose deprivation to the CNS.

**Clinical Manifestations.** In fructose 1,6-biphosphatase deficiency, hypoglycemia is precipitated by fasting, not by fructose ingestion (Merritt & Gallagher, 2018). Lactic acidosis and ketosis result from accumulating lactic, 3-hydroxybutyric, and acetoacetic acids. Hyperventilation followed by apnea may result from profound acidosis. Although the acidosis and hypoglycemia may be treated and the infant recovers from the acute attack, if the underlying disorder is not recognized, the infant can have many acute metabolic attacks and develop hepatomegaly and failure to thrive before the diagnosis is made.

**Diagnosis.** Definitive diagnosis is made by liver biopsy and assay of hepatic enzymes. Mutational analysis is available and can be used instead of biopsy.

**Management.** Acute management involves administering glucose intravenous solutions and correcting acidosis with sodium bicarbonate. Frequent feedings, avoidance of fasting, and limiting fructose and sucrose in the diet prevent further episodes. Dietary restriction includes the many prescription and over-the-counter medications with a syrup base containing sucrose. Stress management (e.g., during times of fever, infection, or vomiting) is critical because illness can induce a metabolic attack.

## Glycogen Storage Disease

Glycogen storage disease (GSD) is a group of inherited enzyme defects that affects the glycogen synthesis and degradation cycle mainly involving the liver. More than 10 different types of GSD have been identified with a collective incidence of about 1 in 20,000 to 43, 000 live births (Stone et al., 2023). Glycogen storage disease type I (GSD-I, also known as von Gierke disease), the disorder most likely to have neonatal onset, occurs in about 1 in 100,000 births and has two main subtypes (Ia, Ib). GSD-II, known as Pompe disease, is classified as a lysosomal storage disease.

**Pathophysiology.** GSD-Ia, the most common subtype, is the result of a deficiency of the hepatic enzyme glucose-6-phosphatase (G6Pase), an enzyme situated in the endoplasmic reticulum of the cell. Normally, G6Pase hydrolyzes glucose-6-phosphate to glucose and phosphate. An accumulation of glycogen in the liver, kidney, and intestines results from a deficiency of G6Pase. In the normal neonate, blood glucose falls during the first postnatal hours as the neonate uses circulating glucose obtained from the mother, but then rises as endogenous glucose production begins. In the neonate with GSD-I, blood glucose continues to decline because endogenous glucose production is severely compromised. Instead, the phosphorylated intermediate compounds of glycolysis produce an excess of lactate, resulting in hyperlactacidemia. Secondary metabolic derangements typical of GSD-I include hyperuricemia and hyperlipidemia.

**Clinical Manifestations.** The neonate with GSD-I cannot cope with the normal postnatal drop in blood sugar. Despite a plentiful supply of glycogen, the neonate is unable to mobilize free glucose and becomes hypoglycemic. The abdomen may appear distended from birth because of an enlarged liver. Acute, nonspecific clinical deterioration is related to the buildup of lactic acid in the body.

**Diagnosis.** Definitive diagnosis of GSD-I is accomplished with molecular genetic testing. Typical laboratory findings in GSD-I include increased plasma lactate and metabolic acidosis with an increased anion gap. Ketosis and ketonuria will be found during hypoglycemia. Other routine tests that should be obtained are liver function tests, plasma uric acid, triglycerides, creatinine, coagulation studies, and complete blood count (CBC) with differential. Abdominal ultrasonography is performed to determine liver and kidney size. A liver or muscle biopsy may be indicated (Stone et al., 2023).

**Management.** The goals of treatment of GSD-I are to prevent hypoglycemia and correct secondary biochemical abnormalities. Frequent feedings or continuous gastric feedings may be necessary to maintain normoglycemia and supply the brain with a steady source of glucose, even at night. Blood glucose levels must be monitored closely. Pharmacologic therapy to address hyperuricemia and prevent the development of gout may be necessary. Very severely affected infants will require a liver transplant. Parent teaching about long-term nutritional management, prevention of hypoglycemia, and special considerations during stress or other illnesses is critically important.

## PEROXISOMAL DISORDERS

Peroxisomal disorders are complex developmental and metabolic disorders caused by defects in peroxisome biosynthesis. Two of the better-known disorders, Zellweger syndrome (ZS) and neonatal adrenoleukodystrophy (NALD), are now recognized as belonging to a continuous spectrum of disorders, of which ZS is the most severe. ZS has a reported incidence of about 1 in 25,000 to 50,000 births.

### Pathophysiology

Peroxisomes are subcellular organelles that synthesize bile acids, cholesterol, and plasmalogens (a type of phospholipid found in myelin sheaths of nerve fibers). Peroxisomes are also critical in the beta-oxidation of very long-chain fatty acids. Peroxisomal disorders arise from a defect in peroxisomal biosynthesis or a single peroxisomal enzyme or protein (Scott & Olpin, 2010). Individuals with peroxisome biogenesis defects, such as ZS and NALD, synthesize peroxisomes normally but display defects in the import of peroxisomal enzymes into the lumen of the organelle (Merritt & Gallagher, 2018). Biochemical abnormalities include impaired degradation of peroxide, very long-chain fatty acids, pipecolic acid, and phytanic acid and impaired synthesis of plasmalogens, bile acids, cholesterol, and docosahexaenoic acid. In ZS, the extent of progressive multisystemic disease is profound; in NALD, the systemic involvement is milder, but the cerebral demyelination is more pronounced.

### Clinical Manifestations

Infants with ZS present with characteristic facial dysmorphism, including a high forehead, hypoplastic supraorbital ridges, flat occiput, low and broad nasal bridge, epicanthal folds, high arched palate, small nose with anteverted nares, micrognathia, large fontanelles, wide sutures, and eye abnormalities (Scott & Olpin, 2010). Typically, they have profound hypotonia, an absence of neonatal reflexes, and seizures. The disease affects every organ of the body, particularly the liver, kidney, and brain, resulting in hepatomegaly, renal cysts, white-matter abnormalities, and neuronal migration defects.

### Diagnosis

Diagnosis of peroxisomal biosynthesis defects is based on indirect evidence of the defect. Initial tests for an infant with a suspected peroxisomal disorder include plasma, very long-chain fatty acids, and plasmalogens in erythrocytes. Affected infants have elevated transaminases, bile acid intermediates, hypercholesterolemia, and increased iron and transferrin concentrations and are often hypoglycemic. A suspected peroxisomal disorder is confirmed by molecular studies, if possible (Scott & Olpin, 2010).

### Management

Currently, no successful treatment for the peroxisomal disorders is available. Management is supportive care and symptomatic therapy. The median life expectancy of ZS patients is less than 1 year. Milder forms of peroxisomal disorders may respond to dietary treatment.

## LYSOSOMAL DISORDERS

Lysosomal disorders comprise a diverse group of inherited conditions caused by dysfunctions in enzymes (called hydrolases) responsible for the degradation of complex macromolecules. Z complex substrate, normally degraded by a series of lysosomal enzymes, fails to undergo degradation owing to a deficiency or malfunction of one of these enzymes. Catabolism of the substrate into soluble end products is incomplete, and the cell cannot effectively covert or expel the waste products. More than 50 lysosomal disorders are recognized, with a collective incidence of 1 in 7,000 to 10,000 births.

**Pathophysiology.** Niemann–Pick type C (NP-C) is a disorder of intracellular cholesterol transport that accumulates unesterified cholesterol in lysosomes (Thomas et al., 2018). Unesterified cholesterol, sphingomyelin, phospholipids, and glycolipids are stored in excess in the liver and spleen, and glycolipids are increased in the brain.

**Clinical Manifestations.** Neonatal-onset NP-C is characterized by conjugated hyperbilirubinemia, ascites, hepatosplenomegaly, and hypotonia (Thomas et al., 2018). Hydrops fetalis is a rare presentation. Respiratory failure can occur.

**Diagnosis.** The diagnosis of NP-C requires specialized testing that must be coordinated with a metabolic laboratory. Mass spectrometry can be used to test for some of these diseases. Biliary atresia and congenital viral infection are the chief differential diagnoses.

**Management.** There is no definitive or consistently effective therapy for NP-C to date. Splenectomy is sometimes necessary if anemia and thrombocytopenia are severe. Liver transplantation corrects the hepatic dysfunction but not the neurodegenerative disease.

### Gaucher Disease

**Pathophysiology.** Gaucher disease, the most common of the lysosomal storage diseases, is an inborn error of glycosphingolipid metabolism caused by the deficient activity of the lysosomal enzyme acid beta-glucosidase. Widespread accumulation of glucosylceramide-laden macrophages results from enzyme deficiency. These accumulated compounds are toxic to various tissues in the body. There are three types of Gaucher disease. Type I is the most common (95%). A subset of type II, a neuronopathic form of Gaucher disease, is the only one with neonatal onset.

**Clinical Manifestations.** Neonates with type II Gaucher disease can present with congenital ichthyosis or a collodion membrane (hyperkeratotic scale), hepatosplenomegaly, and/or nonimmune hydrops fetalis, hypertonicity, seizures, and other evidence of neurologic deterioration.

**Diagnosis.** Diagnosis is made by analysis of acid beta-glucosidase activity in white blood cells (WBCs) or DNA analysis. Characteristic Gaucher cells (large, lipid-laden macrophages with foamy cytoplasm) can be seen in a bone marrow aspirate.

**Management.** Enzyme replacement therapy for Gaucher disease is available but has not been very effective for patients with type II disease. Splenectomy may be necessary to manage severe anemia and thrombocytopenia. Death from respiratory insufficiency or severe neurologic disease usually occurs shortly after birth or within the first year of life.

## GM1 Gangliosidosis

**Pathophysiology.** Gangliosides are normal components of cell membranes, particularly neurons. GM1 gangliosidosis is a devastating lysosomal storage disease caused by a deficiency of the enzyme acid beta-galactosidase, resulting in a generalized accumulation of GM1 gangliosides, oligosaccharides, and the mucopolysaccharide keratan sulfate in both the brain and viscera.

**Clinical Manifestations.** Affected infants may have coarse facial features known as a "Hurler phenotype" (frontal bossing, depressed nasal bridge, maxillary hyperplasia, large ears, wide upper lip, macroglossia, and gingival hyperplasia), hirsutism of forehead and neck, macular cherry-red spots, and corneal clouding (Figure 9.4). The dysmorphic features might not be obvious in neonates (Thomas et al., 2018). Facial edema, pitting edema of the extremities, or ascites may also be apparent, and the neonate may present with hydrops fetalis and placental evidence of vacuolated cells. Neurologic examination reveals hypotonia and hypoactivity. The liver and spleen are both enlarged upon palpation.

**Diagnosis.** Diagnosis is made by demonstrating a lack of beta-galactosidase activity in WBCs. Galactose-containing oligosaccharides can also be measured in the urine.

**Management.** Currently, there is no effective therapy for infants with GM1 gangliosidosis. Enzyme and gene therapies are being studied as potential treatments for this lethal disorder.

## Mucopolysaccharidoses

**Pathophysiology.** The mucopolysaccharidoses (MPS) are a family of seven disorders caused by deficiency of lysosomal enzymes required for the stepwise degradation of glycosaminoglycans (polysaccharides that make up an essential component of connective tissue). The undegraded glycosaminoglycans are stored in lysosomes, causing cell, tissue, and organ dysfunction. MPS VII, the type with the most prominent neonatal presentation, is caused by a deficiency of the enzyme beta-glucuronidase.

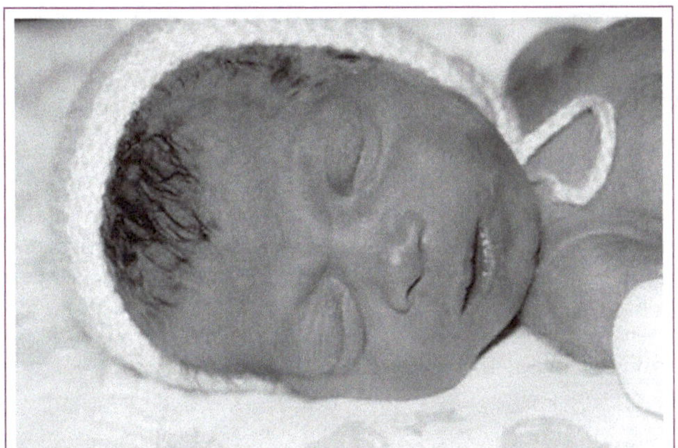

**FIGURE 9.4 The "Hurler phenotype" seen in some neonates with lysosomal storage disorders.**

*Source:* From Wraith, J. E. (2002). Lysosomal disorders. *Seminars in Neonatology, 7,* 75–83. https://doi.org/10.1053/siny.2001.0088.

**Clinical Manifestations.** MPS VII (Sly disease) has a well-recognized neonatal presentation with nonimmune hydrops fetalis, hepatosplenomegaly, ascites, pitting edema, hernias, skeletal abnormalities (dysostosis multiplex), and corneal clouding. In the most severely affected patients, MPS I (Hurler syndrome) can present in the neonatal period with an umbilical or inguinal hernia or an excess of Mongolian spots. Hearing loss is common. Clinical evidence of heart disease is present in most patients with MPS.

**Diagnosis.** MPS VII is diagnosed by evaluating beta-glucuronidase activity in WBCs. Urine glycosaminoglycans can also be quantitated.

**Management.** Management is primarily supportive care and treatment of complications. Range-of-motion (ROM) exercises are essential to preserve joint function and prevent joint stiffness. Recurrent pneumonia is a frequent complication of MPS VII. Development of hydrocephalus often necessitates the insertion of a ventriculoperitoneal shunt. An ophthalmologic examination should be performed to evaluate for corneal clouding and the development of glaucoma.

## Glycogen Storage Disease Type II (Pompe Disease)

**Pathophysiology.** Glycogen storage disease type II (GSD-II), also called acid maltase deficiency or Pompe disease, is an inherited disorder of glycogen metabolism resulting from defects in the activity of the lysosomal hydrolase acid alpha-glucosidase in all tissues of the body. This enzyme is required to degrade a portion of the body's glycogen. Without it, excessive glycogen accumulates within the lysosomes, eventually causing cellular injury and enlarging and hindering the function of the entire organ, such as the heart. Energy production is not affected, and hypoglycemia does not occur. Pompe disease has an incidence of about 1 in 40,000 U.S. births (Leslie & Bailey, 2023).

**Clinical Manifestations.** Prominent findings in infants are cardiomyopathy, progressive cardiomegaly, and left ventricular thickening that eventually leads to outflow tract obstruction. Characteristic findings on electrocardiogram (ECG) are large QRS complexes coupled with abnormally short PR intervals. The QRS complex combines the Q, R, and S waves and represents ventricular depolarization. The PR interval is the interval between the beginning of the P wave and the beginning of the QRS complex of an ECG that represents the time between the start of the contraction of the atria and the beginning of the contraction of the ventricles. Other manifestations are hepatomegaly, striking hypotonia, macroglossia, feeding difficulties, and respiratory distress complicated by pulmonary infection.

**Diagnosis.** Definitive diagnosis requires the measurement of acid alpha-glucosidase activity in cultured skin fibroblasts or WBCs. Serum creatinine kinase (CK) is elevated (up to 10 times normal). Hepatic enzymes may also be elevated. Molecular genetic testing is available (Leslie & Bailey, 2023).

**Management.** Treatment must be individualized for cardiomyopathy with special consideration of how any drug therapy may result in a life-threatening condition (Leslie & Bailey, 2023). Physical therapy for muscle weakness and respiratory support may be necessary (Leslie & Bailey, 2023). Enzyme replacement therapy (ERT) is used (Leslie & Bailey, 2023). A recombinant version of human alpha-glucosidase, a glycoprotein enzyme needed for the breakdown of glycogen in cell lysosomes, has now been developed to treat Pompe disease.

## DISORDERS OF CHOLESTEROL SYNTHESIS

### Smith–Lemli–Opitz Syndrome

Smith–Lemli–Opitz (SLO) syndrome is comprised of multiple congenital anomalies/mental retardation and is caused by an inherited defect in cholesterol biosynthesis. SLO syndrome has an estimated incidence of 1 in 10,000 to 60,000 births (Haas et al., 2017).

**Pathophysiology.** The underlying biochemical defect in SLO syndrome is a lack of the microsomal enzyme 3 beta-hydroxysteroid-delta 7 reductases (DHCR7), the final enzyme in the sterol biosynthetic pathway that converts 7-dehydrocholesterol (7DHC) to cholesterol. Without DHCR7, the precursor 7DHC accumulates to potentially toxic levels, producing insufficient cholesterol. Because cholesterol is required to develop cell membranes and myelin and produce steroid hormones and bile acids, a severe deficiency of cholesterol during morphogenesis is believed to contribute to the abnormalities associated with SLO syndrome. SLO syndrome is different from other disorders of intermediary metabolism, from which the fetus is protected until after birth. Without endogenous cholesterol, the growing embryo depends on maternal cholesterol, which may not be transported across the placenta in sufficient amounts. Thus, the fetus with SLO syndrome may have facial dysmorphia, cardiac defects, poly- or syndactyly of the toes, and underdeveloped male genitalia (Nowaczyk & Wassif, 2020).

**Clinical Manifestations.** Common findings at birth are intrauterine growth restriction (IUGR), microcephaly, and hypotonia. Facial dysmorphism may feature epicanthic folds, ptosis, anteverted nares, broad nasal tip, micrognathia, and low-set ears. Associated anomalies include syndactyly of the second and third toes (> 98%), postaxial polydactyly, small abnormally positioned thumbs, Hirschsprung disease, cataracts, and in males, hypospadias, cryptorchidism, and hypoplastic scrotum. Common clinical manifestations in the newborn include severe hypotonia, feeding difficulties with poor suck and vomiting, and excessive sleepiness with poor responsiveness (Haas et al., 2017). A severe form of SLO syndrome can result in death during the first week of life due to multisystem organ failure.

**Diagnosis.** SLO syndrome is often recognized by its distinctive clinical features. Confirmation is made by finding elevated blood levels of its direct precursor, 7DHC. Plasma cholesterol may be normal or low. Some fetuses with SLO syndrome are identified by anomalies detected prior to birth by ultrasonography, and confirmation can be made by amniotic fluid or chorionic villus sample analysis.

**Management.** Immediate management is directed toward raising body cholesterol and removing toxic precursors. Providing exogenous cholesterol not only restores low cholesterol levels but also suppresses the infant's endogenous cholesterol synthesis, decreasing the production of 7DHC (Haas et al., 2017).

## DISORDERS OF METAL METABOLISM

Errors of metal metabolism are genetic biochemical disorders in how the body processes metals: their synthesis, transport, absorption, storage, or utilization.

### Molybdenum Cofactor Deficiency

**Pathophysiology.** The molybdenum cofactor is an essential component of a large family of enzymes involved in necessary carbon, nitrogen, and sulfur metabolism transformations. Molybdenum cofactor deficiency is an autosomal recessive, fatal neurologic disorder characterized by the combined deficiency of sulfite oxidase, xanthine dehydrogenase, and aldehyde oxidase.

**Clinical Manifestations.** Affected neonates are usually born after an uneventful pregnancy and a normal delivery. Soon after birth, feeding difficulties and neurologic symptoms develop. The neurologic picture includes intractable tonic–clonic seizures, axial hypotonia, and peripheral hypertonicity (Koeller & Kaler, 2017). Typical facial features include puffy cheeks, a long philtrum, and a small nose. The neuropathologic findings are consistent with a toxic insult to the brain that causes severe neuronal loss, demyelination of white matter, reactive astrogliosis, and spongiosis. Ectopia lentis (displacement of the lens) may be noted on ophthalmologic examination.

**Diagnosis.** Molybdenum cofactor deficiency can be challenging to diagnose because there are no clues on routine laboratory studies. A positive sulfite dipstick of fresh urine is suggestive of the disorder; however, a negative test does not rule it out. Urinary S-sulfocysteine, thiosulfate, urothion, xanthine, and hypoxanthine levels aid in the diagnosis of molybdenum cofactor deficiency (Koeller & Kaler, 2017). Plasma uric acid is typically low.

**Management.** Treatment is aimed at targeting the specific deficiency. A cysteine-restrictive diet is helpful (Misko et al., 2023). Feeding may require a gastrostomy tube. Supplementation with thiamine, magnesium, and seizure treatment may be necessary (Misko et al., 2023). Surveillance for neurologic deterioration is important (Misko et al., 2023). Valproate use should be avoided (Misko et al., 2023).

## SUMMARY

The number of known inherited disorders of metabolism has risen steadily in recent years and is likely to continue. Although not all will manifest in the neonatal period, many disorders with neonatal onset are rapidly lethal if not recognized and treated without delay. Expanded newborn screening programs have saved many lives through presymptomatic diagnosis, but these programs currently screen for only a fraction of the hundreds of possible metabolic disorders. Neonatal health professionals must be vigilant and consider the diagnosis of an inborn EM in a neonate presenting with clinical manifestations resembling sepsis or in an infant becoming ill after one or more days of normal health, particularly when the laboratory data do not fit the clinical picture. Although many neonatal metabolic disorders are not yet amenable to therapy, an exact diagnosis is important for genetic counseling and prenatal diagnostic procedures that the family may desire for future pregnancies.

## CASE STUDY

**Identification of the Problem.** A newborn infant, just over 48 hours of age, was rooming with his mother, who noted him to be jaundiced and unusually sleepy. His mother could not awaken him to breastfeed, and she notified the nurse, who took him to the nursery to check his bilirubin level. His total serum bilirubin was 10.4 mg/dL. However, the infant did not respond to having his heel lanced for the blood draw, and the nurse could not awaken him to feed. She called the infant's pediatrician, who ordered a CBC with differential and a blood culture. The infant was then transferred to the neonatal intensive care unit (NICU) for further evaluation. An intravenous drip of D10W at 100 ml/kg/d was begun, and ampicillin and gentamicin were given. However, the CBC, differential, and C-reactive protein (CRP) were all within normal limits; subsequently, the blood culture was also negative.

**Assessment: History and Physical Examination.** The infant, a boy, was born by Cesarean section to a 33-year-old G3 mother who was P2 group B streptococcus (GBS)–negative and has insulin-dependent gestational diabetes that was in satisfactory glucose control during the last trimester of pregnancy. Family history was significant for a maternal brother who died on the third day of life from unknown causes. The siblings of this infant were two healthy girls. This infant's Apgar scores were 8 and 9. The birth weight was 3,790 g. The infant's blood sugar levels on day 1 were within normal limits; he appeared healthy and roomed in with his mother, breastfeeding on demand with occasional formula supplementation. He was voiding and stooling normally.

On examination, his color was pale pink with mild jaundice on room air. Respirations were regular and rapid, but there were no retractions, grunting, or flaring. His axillary temperature was 97°F (36.1°C), heart rate 122, respiratory rate 80, and blood pressure 60/36 mm Hg (mean 44). The glucose screen (point of care) was 52. An arterial blood gas (ABG) was obtained; the results were pH 7.32, $PO_2$ 71, $PCO_2$ 30, and base deficit –2. Capillary refill was 2 to 3 seconds, pulses were equal, and there was no murmur. His abdomen was rounded with mild hepatomegaly. He did not react to stimulation of any type and could not be aroused. His overall tone was decreased, he did not suck, and no Moro reflex was noted. Within 24 hours, he began having seizures, requiring treatment with phenobarbital. Severe apnea and respiratory failure led to intubation and mechanical ventilation.

**Differential Diagnosis.** The chief differential diagnosis for a full-term infant becoming ill at about 48 hours of age is neonatal sepsis. However, this mother was GBS-negative, and the infant's laboratory data did not support this diagnosis. His serum bilirubin was not high enough to explain his somnolence and lethargy as stemming from bilirubin encephalopathy. Transient tachypnea of the newborn was unlikely because he did not appear to be in any significant respiratory distress other than his rapid respiratory rate, and the clinical picture was more consistent with a neurologic insult. The history did not suggest an etiology for neonatal encephalopathy. The following most likely diagnostic possibilities would be inborn errors of intermediary metabolism that present with an "intoxication" syndrome and without hypoglycemia, following a symptom-free interval: organic acid disorders, amino acid disorders, and UCDs.

**Diagnostic Tests.** A blood ammonia level is needed to differentiate between the most likely categories of metabolic disorders. Depending on this result, other critical diagnostic tests might include electrolytes, BUN, creatinine, quantitative plasma, urine amino acids, urine organic acids, and urine orotic acid.

**Working Diagnosis.** The infant's blood ammonia level was 1,901 µmol/L. This suggests a working diagnosis of a urea cycle defect. Additional testing revealed the following:

Plasma amino acids: Glutamine 1,632 µmol/L (reference range 376–709 µmol/L)

Citrulline trace (reference range 10–45 µmol/L)

Urine orotic acid: 852 mmol/mol creatinine (reference range 0.12–3.07 mmol/mol creatinine)

Following the algorithm for neonatal hyperammonemia (see Figure 9.2), these findings point to a working diagnosis of OTC deficiency. In support of this diagnosis, the infant's symptoms began after 24 hours of age, and he had no significant acidosis.

**Development of Management Plan.** The most urgent priority was a reduction of the infant's toxic blood ammonia level. In addition, protein intake had to be stopped temporarily until the blood ammonia level was normalized; the infant was made NPO (nothing by mouth), and no amino acids were added to the IV solution. Protein would be reintroduced within 48 hours and would be small enough to prevent catabolism. While preparations were being made for hemodialysis, an umbilical venous catheter was inserted to administer "scavenger drugs," or agents that supply alternatives to urea to eliminate waste nitrogen.

**Implementation and Evaluation of Effectiveness.** A loading dose of sodium phenylacetate plus sodium benzoate 2.5 ml/kg was given via central catheter over 90 minutes (Ammonul, Ucyclyd Pharma, Scottsdale, AZ). In addition, a dose of arginine HCl 10% (2.0 ml/kg) was administered. Hemodialysis was initiated, and after about 36 hours, the infant's ammonia level was successfully reduced to less than 70 µmol/L. He showed rapid improvement in neurologic status and was extubated. Amino acids were reintroduced to the IV solution after another 24 hours, and feedings were restarted shortly after that with citrulline supplementation. Following discharge, he was maintained on this regimen, plus pharmacologic diversion therapy, and he had two metabolic crises requiring hospitalization before receiving a liver transplant. An MRI of his brain at 1 year of age revealed that the neurologic prognosis remains guarded. The family also underwent genetic counseling regarding recurrence risks and prenatal genetic diagnosis for future pregnancies.

## EVIDENCE-BASED PRACTICE

### Hyperammonemia

Hyperammonemia (plasma ammonium level > 150 µmol/L or > 260 mcg/dl) is a metabolic disturbance that is a characteristic feature of many different EMs, including disorders of organic acids, fatty acid oxidation, and the urea cycle. Ammonia, a product of protein metabolism, is a neurotoxin that can accumulate in the brain along with glutamine, resulting in osmotic swelling, brain edema, and permanent brain damage. Many areas of the developing brain are vulnerable to the effects of excess ammonia, and the neurologic sequelae are correlated with the duration and magnitude of hyperammonemia (Braissant, 2010). Therefore, the prevention or reversal of hyperammonemic coma is of prime concern in a suspected metabolic disorder. The initial management of ammonia encephalopathy must often proceed in the absence of a definitive diagnosis (Westrope et al., 2010). The kidneys clear ammonia poorly, so removal of ammonia from the body must be expedited by another method. Two means of accomplishing this are diversion therapy using ammonia-scavenging drugs, and physical removal of ammonia from the circulation with dialysis or hemofiltration.

Although the efficacy of dialysis or hemofiltration in the clearance of serum ammonia has been established, the optimal treatment modality has not. Few published studies have shown associations between specific dialysis modalities and survival rates. Owing to the rarity of the EMs, randomized controlled trials to compare these therapies do not exist. The evidence is largely retrospective and observational, from single case reports and case series.

Expert consensus suggests that first-line treatment of hyperammonemia should involve stopping protein intake, suppressing protein catabolism, and administering agents that combine with ammonia to form compounds with high renal clearance. Many case reports describe successful medical treatment of newborns with various EMs using *N*-carbamylglutamate (Filippi et al., 2010; Gessler et al., 2010; Kasapkara et al., 2011), sodium benzoate, and sodium phenylbutyrate. When plasma ammonia levels decline within 4 hours of treatment, the need for dialysis may be averted (Picca et al., 2001). During this 4-hour window, however, preparations should be underway to institute a more aggressive route of ammonia clearance in neonates who do not respond to medical treatment (Picca et al., 2008).

If detoxification with ammonia-scavenging drugs fails to reduce the plasma ammonia level within a few hours, another method of clearance must be initiated without delay. Options include hemodialysis, continuous venovenous hemofiltration (CVVHF), continuous venovenous hemodialysis (CVVHD), and peritoneal dialysis. Methods that provide continuous renal replacement (hemodialysis or hemofiltration) are preferred over peritoneal dialysis, although evidence is scant. Picca et al. (2001) reported their experience using three different extracorporeal methods of clearing ammonia (continuous arteriovenous hemodialysis, CVVHD, and hemodialysis). They found that CVVHD was the most effective method to promptly lower ammonia levels. However, they also found that the most relevant indicator of prognosis was not how quickly the plasma ammonia level was reduced, but the duration of hyperammonemic coma before the initiation of dialysis (Picca et al., 2001). Coma duration longer than 30 hours before dialysis initiation negatively affects the outcome (Picca et al., 2001). Therefore, they recommend that infants with rising ammonia levels should be transferred without delay to a facility capable of providing extracorporeal dialysis if medical therapy fails.

In a 10-year experience with CVVHF to treat hyperammonemia, Westrope et al. (2010) found this method to be safe, effective, and efficient in lowering plasma ammonia levels. However, neither the pretreatment ammonia level nor the speed of ammonia removal was associated with outcome (Westrope et al., 2010). This study suggests that the pretreatment status of the neonate may be the main determinant of outcome, reinforcing the need to initiate medical treatment and to proceed with continuous renal replacement therapy without delay.

In another study of 21 children (15 neonates), investigators retrospectively analyzed outcomes for patients receiving CVVHD or peritoneal dialysis (Arbeiter et al., 2010). A 50% reduction in serum ammonia levels was achieved significantly faster with CVVHD than with peritoneal dialysis. In neonatal patients, survival and survival without mental retardation were both better following CVVHD, although the sample sizes were small, and the duration of pretreatment encephalopathy was not known. Of interest, these investigators documented the best outcomes in patients with neonatal-onset citrullinemia.

Although it would be desirable to have randomized, controlled trial evidence of the superiority of one method of treating hyperammonemia over another, the trend toward presymptomatic detection of metabolic disorders could, in the future, lead to preventive treatments that will obviate the need for such aggressive approaches to hyperammonemia. In the meantime, clinicians should continue to collect data on the few patients encountered with these disorders to inform best practice and improve outcomes.

(*continued*)

## EVIDENCE-BASED PRACTICE (*continued*)

### References


Arbeiter, A. K., Dranz, B., Wingen, A. M., Bonzel, K. E., Dohna-Schwake, C., Hanssle, L., Neudorf, U., Hoyer, P. F., & Büscher, R. (2010). Continuous venovenous haemodialysis (CVVHD) and continuous peritoneal dialysis (CPD) in the acute management of 21 children with inborn errors of metabolism. *Nephrology Dialysis and Transplantation*, *25*, 1257–1265. https://doi.org/10.1093/ndt/gfp595

Braissant, O. (2010). Current concepts in the pathogenesis of urea cycle disorders. *Molecular Genetics and Metabolism*, *100*, S3–S12. https://doi.org/10.1016/j.ymgme.2010.02.010

Filippi, L., Gozini, E., Fiorini, P., Malvagia, S., la Marca, G., & Donati, M. A. (2010). N-carbamylglutamate in emergency management of hyperammonemia in neonatal acute onset propionic and methylmalonic aciduria. *Neonatology*, *97*, 286–290. https://doi.org/10.1159/000255168

Gessler, P., Buchal, P., Schwenk, H. U., & Wermuth, B. (2010). Favourable long-term outcome after immediate treatment of neonatal hyperammonemia due to N-acetyl glutamate synthase deficiency. *European Journal of Pediatrics*, *169*, 197–199. https://doi.org/10.1007/s00431-009-1006-0

Kasapkara, C. S., Ezgu, F. S., Okur, I., Tumer, L., Biberoglu, G., & Hasanoglu, A. (2011). *N*-Carbamylglutamate treatment for acute neonatal hyperammonemia in isovaleric acidemia. *European Journal of Pediatrics*, *270*, 799–801. https://doi.org/10.1007/s00431-010-1362-9

Picca, S., Bartuli, A., & Dionisi-Vici, C. (2008). Medical management and dialysis therapy for the infant with an inborn error of metabolism. *Seminars in Nephrology*, *28*, 477–480. https://doi.org/10.1016/j.semnephrol.2008.05.007

Picca, S., Dionisi-Vici, C., Abeni, D., Pastore, A., Rizzo, C., Orzalesi, M., Sabetta, G., Rizzoni, G., & Bartuli, A. (2001). Extracorporeal dialysis in neonatal hyperammonemia: Modalities and prognostic indicators. *Pediatric Nephrology*, *16*, 862–867. https://doi.org/10.1007/s004670100702

Westrope, C., Morris, K., Burford, D., & Morrison, G. (2010). Continuous hemofiltration in the control of neonatal hyperammonemia: A 10-year experience. *Pediatric Nephrology*, *25*, 1725–1730. https://doi.org/10.1007/s00467-010-1549-3


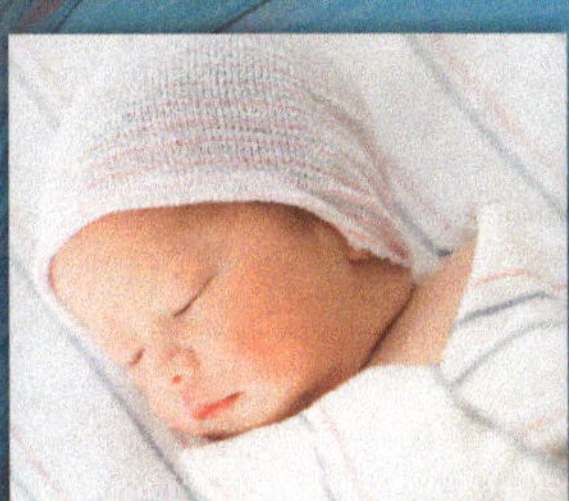
Source: Tierney/Adobe Stock

## PARENT VOICES

### Jimena Guild

**The simple act of feeding my child seems ordinary to most parents, but for us whose child experienced feeding issues, it was huge. My son Kai was born premature at 28 weeks and developed acute oral aversion among other issues during his 4-month stay in the NICU. To ensure he received the necessary nutrition, my son was fed through a tube that from his nose fed right into his stomach called a nasogastric (NG) tube. In the NICU, he fought the bottle so much I was not even going to try him on the breast. He continued to struggle with drinking from a bottle for the first 6 months of his life. He was labeled "failure to thrive" and needed assistance from nursing services and an occupational therapist (OT) who would come to help him develop the skills he needed to eat orally. Kai was tube-fed for the first 2 years of his life. Most parents whose children have feeding tubes do not know for how long their child will need the tube. We were lucky that he only had it for 2 years; he will never remember the awful nights we would struggle to get the tube put back in when he would pull it out; the screams, the cries, from both of us, were not something I wish on any parent; having to hold him down while my husband fished the tube down into his stomach, sometimes having to redo it multiple times if it went down the wrong tube (into his lungs) or came out of his mouth as he coughed. Those are days I will never forget, but it's also important to know that feeding tubes offer hope. Sure, it's an alternative way of eating by mouth, but it is one that gives children—and all people—with no other alternative, a way to thrive. Nowadays, Kai is a healthy little 7-year-old boy who, you wouldn't believe, has an insatiable hunger; he is the most non-picky child you will meet and is willing to try anything and everything once.**

## ONLINE RESOURCES

**CourseConnect**

Resources for this chapter are online and available at www.springerpub.com/courseconnect.

## REFERENCES

References for this chapter are online and available at www.springerpub.com/courseconnect.

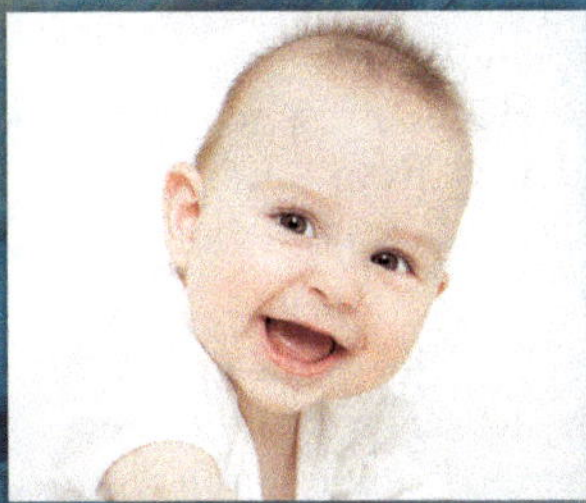
Adobe Stock.

CHAPTER 10

# Endocrine System

**Susan Kau and Carole Kenner**

## INTRODUCTION

Our understanding of endocrine disorders in the neonate advances to the molecular level in parallel with discoveries in genetics and cell biology. Endocrine processes are fundamental to the growth and development of the fetus and newborn. Prompt recognition of endocrine disorders in the neonate is the chief prerequisite in our ability to institute lifesaving treatment and minimize long-term morbidity. This chapter provides an overview of the clinical endocrine disorders that may be seen in the neonatal period.

## THE ENDOCRINE SYSTEM

The word *endocrine*, from the Greek words *endo* (within) and *krinein* (to separate), describes a diverse group of ductless organs that secrete hormones directly into the bloodstream. The classic endocrine glands are the hypothalamus, pineal, pituitary, thyroid, parathyroid, thymus, pancreatic islet cells, adrenals, ovaries, and testes, although the heart, kidneys, and intestines also secrete and regulate hormones. Among the many functions of the endocrine system are coordination and regulation of metabolism and energy, the internal environment, growth and development, and sexual differentiation and reproduction. The endocrine system provides homeostasis for the body.

The endocrine glands synthesize, store, and secrete hormones, which are the chemical messengers, or signals, of the endocrine system, that are responsible for tight regulation of diverse physiologic functions. Regulatory or effector hormones are peptides, amines, or steroids. Secreted into the blood or extracellular fluid, hormones exert their actions on specific cells, either locally or in distant tissues called *target cells*. Target cells respond to hormones that contain receptors for those precise hormones. Hormones must first bind to these receptor sites before exerting physiologic actions. Some hormones, such as insulin, are fully active on release into the circulatory system, whereas others, such as $T_4$, require activation to produce their biologic effects. Hormones that must be modified to active hormone after synthesis are known as Preprohomrones and prohormones.

Many hormones are insoluble in water and must be bound to carrier proteins to be transported in the circulatory system. Protein-bound hormones exist in rapid equilibrium with minute quantities in the aqueous plasma. The cell takes up this "free" fraction of the circulating hormone and represents the active hormone concentration that provides feedback to regulate the synthesis of the new hormone.

Target hormone levels also serve as powerful negative feedback regulators of their own production via suppression of trophic hormones and hypothalamic-releasing hormones. As the target hormone level rises, a message is sent to the anterior pituitary to reduce the production of the respective trophic hormone and to the hypothalamus to slow the production of the respective releasing hormone. Endocrine disease is classified as hormone excess, hormone deficiency, or altered tissue responses to hormones (e.g., hormone resistance). Clinical endocrine abnormalities can result from deviations in the feedback systems that control hormone levels. Genetic mutations or expression alterations are the basis of endocrine problems.

Development of the fetal endocrine system is independent of maternal endocrine influences (Divall & Merjaneh, 2018). The placenta blocks the entry of most maternal hormones into the fetal circulation, but the minute quantities that achieve transplacental passage can have profound effects. Some prenatal exposures are essential to fetal growth; others may contribute to fetal and neonatal endocrine dysfunction.

## FETAL ORIGINS OF ADULT DISEASE

When exposed to a variety of different stressors (maternal undernutrition, uteroplacental insufficiency, or psychological stress), the fetus releases glucocorticoids and catecholamines that, during critical periods of development, affect the development of the fetal hypothalamic–pituitary–adrenal (HPA) axis. Chronic stress can also induce intrauterine growth restriction, or the so-called thrifty phenotype, in the fetus, an adaptation to the limited supply of nutrients (Divall & Merjaneh, 2018).

How the fetus adapts, a concept known as *programming*, is believed to permanently alter physiology and metabolism, affecting endocrine, metabolic, and cardiac functions throughout life.

## NEONATAL ENDOCRINE DISORDERS

Endocrinopathy in the newborn can be caused by a mutation in a single gene or by genomic imprinting, when the expression of the gene depends on which parent passed on that particular gene (Divall & Merjaneh, 2018). In addition to well-described neonatal endocrine disorders such as hypothyroidism and congenital adrenal hyperplasia (CAH), endocrine dysfunction can affect the preterm infant in a variety of ways. Exposure to various exogenous agents in the environment, known as *endocrine disruptors,* can have deleterious effects on the development of the endocrine system. Numerous chemicals have known estrogenic or antiandrogenic properties and have been shown to disturb sexual differentiation in animals (Divall & Merjaneh, 2018). The extent to which endocrine disruptors are responsible for increases in hypospadias and testicular dysgenesis syndrome is unknown.

## PITUITARY GLAND AND HYPOTHALAMUS

The pituitary gland is the master gland; it produces and secretes hormones and sends signals to the other glands. The pituitary gland has two distinct structures, the anterior and posterior pituitary, with different embryologic origins. The anterior pituitary develops from oral ectoderm, a diverticulum called Rathke's pouch, and its cells differentiate into specific hormone-secreting cells. The posterior pituitary gland develops from neuroectoderm evaginating ventrally from the developing brain. The two tissues grow together into a single gland but remain functionally separate.

The hypothalamus, located just above the pituitary gland, secretes the releasing and inhibiting hormones that, in turn, influence the production of anterior pituitary hormones. Hypothalamic hormones are carried to the anterior pituitary via hypothalamic–hypophyseal portal veins, where they bind to receptors on the anterior pituitary cells. The anterior pituitary regulates growth, differentiation, and homeostasis and produces growth hormone, prolactin, adrenocorticotropic hormone (ACTH), thyroid-stimulating hormone (TSH), follicle-stimulating hormone (FSH), and luteinizing hormone (LH). Hormones secreted by the posterior pituitary include oxytocin and hypothalamic-produced vasopressin (antidiuretic hormone, ADH). The hypothalamus is the interface between the endocrine and autonomic nervous systems.

## ANTERIOR PITUITARY DISORDERS

### Congenital Hypopituitarism

Congenital hypopituitarism, rare in the newborn, has several possible etiologies. Congenital hypopituitarism can be an isolated defect or associated with malformations, including holoprosencephaly, septooptic dysplasia, and other midline cerebral anomalies, the same developmental defects of the embryonic brain that lead to hypothalamic dysfunction. Infection and hypovolemic shock stemming from birth-related complications such as placenta previa and abruptio placentae are additional etiologies.

**Pathophysiology.** Complete absence of the pituitary gland (pituitary agenesis) and other pituitary lesions can produce deficiencies of one or all pituitary hormones. Panhypopituitarism is a deficiency of all pituitary hormones. The foremost neonatal effect of congenital hypopituitarism is hypoglycemia. Owing to the absence of growth hormone and possibly cortisol, insulin is unopposed, placing the neonate at risk for hypoglycemia. Growth hormone deficiency, and often gonadotropin, combine to stunt penile growth in utero, usually referred to as *hypogonadotropic hypogonadism.* Although fetal pituitary growth hormone is not the primary stimulus for fetal growth, growth hormome does make an important contribution to birth size.

**Clinical Manifestations.** Neonates with congenital hypopituitarism can initially be asymptomatic. Pituitary hormone deficiencies develop over time. Neonates with hypopituitary syndromes can present with midline craniofacial defects such as cleft lip, cleft palate, or bifid uvula. Males may have a micropenis, defined as a normally formed and proportioned penis with a stretched penile length more than two standard deviations below the mean for age. The average penile length for preterm infants 30 weeks of age or older is 2.5 + 0.4 cm, and for term infants, 3.5 + 0.4 cm. The formula can be used for preterm infants 24 to 26 weeks' gestation: penile length in centimeters = 2.27 + 0.16 × (gestational age in weeks) (Tuladhar et al., 1998). Hypoglycemia can be mild or severe and persistent. Later in the neonatal period, infants may present with prolonged jaundice and direct hyperbilirubinemia, or evidence of other endocrinopathy, such as diabetes insipidus (DI; high urine output, dehydration, hypernatremia).

**Diagnosis.** A pediatric endocrinologist usually coordinates the diagnostic testing and interpretation. Laboratory testing is used to determine which hormone deficiencies are present. Measurement of growth hormone, thyroid hormone, and cortisol is essential. Magnetic resonance imaging (MRI) of the brain defines the anatomy and looks for a structural cause of hypopituitarism. For infants with suspected septooptic dysplasia, an ophthalmologic examination is indicated.

**Management.** The immediate goals of management are to stabilize the neonate's blood sugar and ensure that the neonate is not at risk for life-threatening cortisol insufficiency. Hypoglycemia might not resolve without growth hormone replacement. Further treatment is geared toward correcting specific hormonal deficiencies. The infant will require follow-up by the pediatric endocrinologist throughout hospitalization and after discharge.

## POSTERIOR PITUITARY DISORDERS

### Diabetes Insipidus

DI is a deficiency of ADH (vasopressin). In neonates, central or neurogenic DI can be associated with congenital midline anatomic defects (septooptic dysplasia, holoprosencephaly), central nervous system (CNS) injury such as intracranial hemorrhage or hypoxia, neoplasms, or it can be idiopathic. Ninety percent of neonates with inherited nephrogenic DI are boys with an X-linked form caused by mutations in the *arginine vasopressin receptor* 2 (*AVP2R*) gene, a condition that can be diagnosed prenatally (Richardson & Yonekawa, 2018).

**Pathophysiology.** Typically, ADH secretion is triggered by changes in osmolality detected by supraoptic and paraventricular osmosensors in the brain. Increased osmolality stimulates the posterior pituitary to release ADH, increasing the permeability of the renal collecting tubules to water-reducing urinary water loss. Damage to the osmosensors, the posterior pituitary gland, or the hypothalamic–hypophyseal axis results in a deficiency of ADH and increased urinary free water loss.

**Clinical Manifestations.** Neonates with DI may suck vigorously during feeding but vomit immediately afterward, resulting in poor growth. **Emergency Alert: Urine output in DI is high, more than 5 ml/kg/hr, with low specific gravity (<1.010). Irritability and fever may accompany evidence of dehydration (poor skin turgor, depressed anterior fontanel, sunken eyes, mottled skin, weak pulses, low blood pressure, and constipation).**

**Diagnosis.** Serum electrolytes, osmolality, and plasma ADH levels are the primary laboratory tests used to diagnose DI. Plasma ADH is normally elevated in the newborn following delivery, playing a role in the low urine output typical on the first day of life. In neonates with DI, hypernatremia may result in levels as high as 180 mEq/L with elevated serum osmolality. Urinalysis reveals inappropriately dilute urine (low urine osmolality and low specific gravity). MRI is used to visualize the pituitary gland and stalk to delineate the possible cause of DI.

**Management.** DI in neonates requires very careful fluid management. Severe dehydration and hypernatremia are corrected primarily with intravenous (IV) fluids. Insensible water losses should be minimized. **Quality and Safety: Serum electrolytes and osmolality, blood glucose, accurate intake and output, and the evidence of dehydration (weight loss, blood pressure, pulses, skin turgor, etc.) should be closely monitored during treatment of DI. Emergency Alert: Infants with severe hypernatremia must be observed for possible seizure activity.** Although serum sodium is expected to decline, very rapid shifts in serum sodium should be avoided. During therapy to correct serum sodium, the infant's neurologic status must be monitored closely for signs and symptoms of cerebral edema. **Quality and Safety: Hyperglycemia must be avoided; it may lead to glycosuria and exaggerate the diuresis.** If possible, neonatal DI should be managed with fluid therapy alone (Bin-Abbas et al., 2023). If it is impossible to manage DI with fluids alone, the agent of choice for pharmacologic treatment is desmopressin (DDAVP), a long-acting synthetic analog of pituitary ADH. Intranasal DDAVP can be diluted with normal saline for administration to the neonate. Subcutaneous and oral formulations of DDAVP are also available, as well as short-acting IV aqueous vasopressin (Pitressin) for emergency treatment of severe dehydration. **Emergency Alert: Observe the infant for hyponatremia because fluid management and drug therapies may decrease sodium levels.**

### Syndrome of Inappropriate Antidiuretic Hormone

Syndrome of inappropriate antidiuretic hormone (SIADH) is an impairment of free water clearance associated with inappropriately raised secretion of ADH.

**Pathophysiology.** An uncontrolled release of ADH can occur in sick preterm and term infants, resulting in renal free water retention that is inappropriate to the level of serum osmolality. The infant becomes hyponatremic, not because of actual sodium depletion, but because of a dilutional effect from the retained fluid. ADH levels can become elevated in infants born after fetal distress or those with severe pulmonary disease, undergoing surgery or experiencing pain.

**Clinical Manifestations.** Signs and symptoms of SIADH are oliguria, hyponatremia, low serum osmolality (< 275 mOsm/L), weight gain, and edema. Patients with SIADH are euvolemic or hypervolemic.

**Diagnosis.** The diagnosis of SIADH should be made only when hyponatremia exists with no other apparent causes (Bardanzellu et al., 2022). True SIADH, fulfilling all diagnostic criteria, is probably uncommon in the neonate. Apparent SIADH may be due to hypovolemia-induced baroreceptor-driven ADH secretion.

**Collaborative Management.** The essentials of management are fluid restriction, close monitoring of intake, output, serum electrolytes, blood glucose, accurate daily weights, evidence of increasing edema, and hydration measures. Restricting fluids can be difficult because infants receive all of their nutrition in liquid form. Diuretics are sometimes used to promote free water excretion. Comparing intake and output is essential. **Quality and Safety: A careful neurologic assessment should be performed, noting changes to fluid or sodium balance.**

## THYROID GLAND

The thyroid gland is a butterfly-shaped structure made up of two lateral lobes connected by a thin band of tissue called the *isthmus*. Composed of densely packed follicular cells containing colloid, the thyroid gland also contains parafollicular cells (C-cells) that produce the calcium-lowering hormone calcitonin.

Thyroid hormones thyroxine ($T_4$) and triiodothyronine ($T_3$) are produced from the amino acid tyrosine. This process is essential to trapping and storing iodide, a trace element required for thyroid hormone synthesis. Thyroglobulin (Tg), a thyroid hormone precursor, is synthesized in the follicular cell. Iodine is taken up by the Tg molecule, incorporated into its tyrosine residues, and returned to the colloid, where a coupling reaction occurs. This step, called *organification*, is catalyzed by the enzyme thyroid peroxidase (TPO). The coupling of two tyrosine residues produces $T_4$, whereas the coupling of diiodotyrosine (DIT) with monoiodotyrosine (MIT) produces $T_3$. These are stored in the follicular lumens until TSH stimulates their release.

The thyroid gland produces primarily $T_4$, which serves as a storage pool for $T_3$. $T_3$ is the most biologically active thyroid hormone, with a greater affinity for the thyroid receptor.

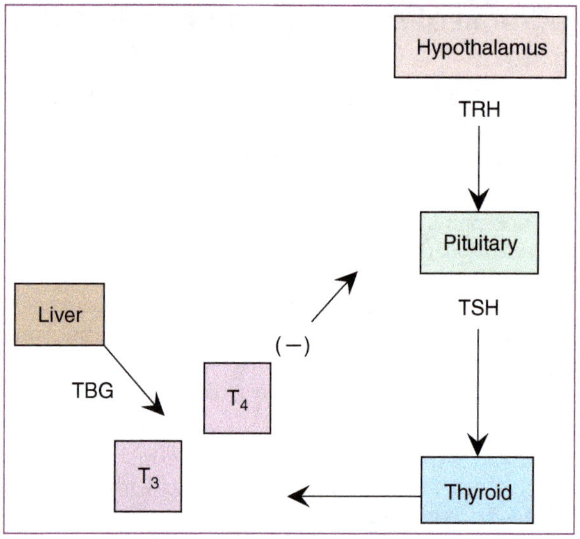


**FIGURE 10.1 The hypothalamic–pituitary–thyroid (HPT) axis.** Thyroid hormone levels are regulated by a feedback inhibition system operating along the HPT axis. The hypothalamus secretes thyrotropin-releasing hormone (TRH), which stimulates the pituitary to secrete thyroid-stimulating hormone (TSH). TSH, in turn, stimulates the thyroid gland to produce and secrete thyroid hormones ($T_4$ and $T_3$) into the circulation, which circulate bound to thyroid-binding globulin (TBG) synthesized by the liver. Once levels of $T_4$ and $T_3$ are adequate, further production of TSH is suppressed.

Circulating $T_4$ is metabolized by outer ring 5' monodeiodination to $T_3$ in the peripheral tissues. Inner ring 5' monodeiodination of $T_4$ produces reverse $T_3$ ($rT_3$), an inactive metabolite. $T_4$ and $T_3$ circulate in plasma bound to thyroid-binding globulin (TBG), leaving just a small fraction in equilibrium as a free hormone. It is possible for TBG, which is synthesized in the liver, to be deficient even though the free hormone levels are normal. The free hormone is available to the tissues, with the bound hormone acting as a circulating reservoir. The concentration of free hormones determines the individual's metabolic state.

The hypothalamic–pituitary–thyroid (HPT) axis controls thyroid hormone secretion (Figure 10.1). The hypothalamus synthesizes thyrotropin, stimulating the release of TSH from the anterior pituitary. In turn, TSH stimulates the uptake of iodine by the thyroid, thyroid hormone synthesis, and release, and increases the size and vascularity of the thyroid gland itself. The feedback loop is responsive to changes in free hormone concentration, and TSH secretion adjusts accordingly.

## FETAL AND NEONATAL THYROID DEVELOPMENT

The thyroid gland is the first endocrine organ to develop in the human embryo. Concurrent with fetal thyroid development is the growth and maturation of the hypothalamus and pituitary glands, which are required for thyroid function. At about 10 to 12 weeks' gestation, the hypothalamus begins synthesizing thyrotropin-releasing hormone (TRH), the pituitary gland starts secreting TSH, and TBG is detectable in fetal serum. Maternal thyroxine is measurable in amniotic fluid before the onset of fetal thyroid function. Before 20 weeks' gestation, transplacental passage of maternal $T_4$ largely provides for fetal thyroidal needs and is critical for normal development. Maternal hypothyroidism during early gestation can impair CNS development in the fetus. However, by the start of the second trimester, the fetal contribution to circulating thyroid hormones is significant. The capacity of the fetal thyroid gland to trap and store iodide and synthesize thyroid hormones begins at about 11 weeks' gestation. Still, hormone production is limited until 18 to 20 weeks, when iodine uptake increases markedly. The only source of iodide for the fetus is a transplacental passage from the maternal circulation and placenta.

As pregnancy progresses, the placenta becomes less permeable to maternal thyroid hormone. Permeability is likely to be highest during the first trimester because thyroid hormone is critical to fetal neurodevelopment, and no other source is available to the fetus. The fetal HPT axis develops from mid-gestation through 4 weeks postbirth, so it is not fully developed in preterm infants. In the last trimester, the fetus is less dependent on maternally derived thyroid hormone. Although thyroid hormone is required for CNS maturation, it is not needed for metabolism, growth, or heat generation. An excess of bioactive $T_3$ could be harmful to fetal development. Tissue concentration of $T_3$ must be controlled in the tissues by preferential conversion of excess fetal $T_4$ to the bioinactive reverse $T_3$ by type III deiodinase. In the event of $T_4$ deficiency, as in fetal hypothyroidism, $T_4$ is shunted to the brain where it is deiodinated to $T_3$ to provide a critical source of intracellular $T_3$.

Birth represents a temporary state of hyperthyroidism for the newborn. In response to sudden exposure to a cold environment, the pituitary releases a surge of TSH that peaks at 70 to 100 mU/ml at 30 minutes after birth. This cold-stimulated TSH surge provokes rises in serum $T_4$, $T_3$, and free $T_4$, all of which peak at about 48 hours. $T_4$ increases in most infants to 6.5 mcg/dl or higher. The rise in $T_4$ causes the TSH to decline to 20 mU/ml or less (the cutoff used in most screening programs for congenital hypothyroidism [CH]) because of feedback inhibition. Free and total $T_4$ and $T_3$ gradually decrease over the next 1 to 2 months.

## CONGENITAL HYPOTHYROIDISM

CH is a deficiency of thyroid function present at the time of birth. With an incidence of 1 in 3,000 to 4,000 births (Tuli et al., 2020), it is the most common congenital endocrine disorder (Polak et al., 2017). Depending on the underlying etiology, CH is classified as either permanent or transient. Early diagnosis and appropriate treatment are essential to prevent permanent neurologic damage. Because most affected infants are asymptomatic at birth, neonatal screening for hypothyroidism is now mandated so that infants with CH are promptly identified and treated.

## Causes of Congenital Hypothyroidism

**Thyroid Dysgenesis.** The most common cause (85%) of permanent CH is thyroid dysgenesis, which includes thyroidal ectopy, hypoplasia, and complete thyroid agenesis. The severity of thyroid dysfunction varies, depending on the amount of functional thyroid tissue present. Thyroidal ectopy accounts for two-thirds of neonates with thyroid dysgenesis. Ectopic thyroid tissue (lingual, sublingual, subhyoid) provides adequate amounts of thyroid hormone in some infants. Occasionally, ectopias are associated with thyroglossal duct cysts. Most of these infants have a thyroid remnant, found midline at the base of the tongue, because of failure of the gland to descend normally during embryologic development.

Thyroid dysgenesis occurs in 1 in 4,000 live births; however, the incidence in Black infants is 1 in 32,000 live births, and in Hispanic infants, 1 in 2,000. The disorder has a female-to-male ratio of 2 to 1. Trisomy 21, or Down syndrome, is associated with an increased prevalence of thyroid dysgenesis, and extrathyroidal abnormalities (cardiac, gastrointestinal [GI], CNS, and eyes) are also more common. No serum Tg is measurable in thyroid agenesis, distinguishing it from functional thyroid tissue associated with measurable serum Tg concentrations.

**Thyroid Dyshormonogenesis.** About 10% to 20% of infants with CH have inborn defects of thyroid hormone metabolism. Mutations in genes coding for proteins involved in thyroid hormone synthesis, secretion, or transport result in the failure of one of the steps in this process, leading to thyroid insufficiency. These biochemical defects are usually inherited as autosomal recessive traits, including TSH hormone resistance, iodide organification defects, iodide transport defects, iodotyrosine deiodinase defects, and thyroglobulin deficiency. Deficient activity of the enzyme TPO is one of the most common disorders of thyroid synthesis caused by mutations of *THOX1* or *THOX2* (Kim et al., 2018). Although dyshormonogenesis eventually results in a compensatory goiter, it is not typically apparent during the neonatal period.

**Thyroid-Binding Globulin Deficiency.** Infants born with congenital TBG deficiency have low TBG and total $T_4$ but normal TSH concentrations and are normal with respect to thyroid function. Familial congenital TBG deficiency is an X-linked trait that can be complete or partial and is frequently an incidental finding on neonatal screening. A TBG level can confirm the diagnosis for parental counseling, but no treatment is recommended.

**Hypothalamic–Pituitary Hypothyroidism.** Between 5% and 10% of infants with CH can be accounted for by what is called secondary–tertiary or central hypothyroidism. A deficiency of hypothalamic TRH or pituitary TSH can occur because of a pituitary or hypothalamus developmental defect. Central hypothyroidism is generally associated with other anomalies of the midbrain (such as the absence of the septum pellucidum or other midline defects), hypopituitarism, pituitary stalk interruption, or empty sella syndrome, all of which lead to low serum $T_4$ and low or inappropriately normal serum TSH.

**Thyroid Hormone Resistance.** Increasing numbers of patients are being found with resistance to the actions of endogenous and exogenous $T_4$ and triiodothyronine ($T_3$), a form of "peripheral hypothyroidism." Most involve a genetic mutation for the gene encoding for thyroid hormone receptor-beta. Most patients have goiter, and $T_4$, $T_3$, free $T_4$, and free $T_3$ levels are elevated. These findings have often led to the erroneous diagnosis of Graves' disease, although most affected patients are clinically euthyroid. The unresponsiveness to thyroid hormone may vary among tissues.

## Clinical Manifestations of Congenital Hypothyroidism

Few neonates are diagnosed with CH solely on clinical grounds. Signs and symptoms of CH can be slow to develop owing to the persistence of the maternal thyroid hormone. When present, signs and symptoms of CH in the neonate are subtle and nonspecific; thus, they are not immediately linked with hypothyroidism. **Quality and Safety: Early diagnosis of CH is critical, however, to ensure prompt treatment that will reduce the risk of intellectual disability.** The signs and symptoms of hypothyroidism in the neonate reflect the wide-ranging actions of thyroid hormones on metabolism, intestinal motility, cardiac function, temperature regulation, neurologic function, and skeletal maturation (Box 10.1). CH must be considered with a birth weight more than the 90th percentile, prolonged jaundice, hypothermia, cold mottled skin, an enlarged (> 1 cm) posterior fontanel, umbilical hernia, and feeding difficulties.

Other features traditionally associated with hypothyroidism (macroglossia, dry skin, lethargy, hypotonia, hoarse cry, coarse hair, and constipation) evolve over the first weeks of life. A palpable, enlarged thyroid gland (a goiter) can be associated with impaired thyroid hormone synthesis and hypothyroidism. The thyroid glands' hyperplasia results from TSH hypersecretion in response to low $T_3$ and $T_4$ levels. Infants with suspected central hypothyroidism may present with midline or cranial defects or other signs of pituitary deficiency. Central hypothyroidism should be suspected in infants presenting with septooptic dysplasia, hypoglycemia, micropenis, or cleft lip/palate.

**BOX 10.1**

**SIGNS AND SYMPTOMS OF HYPOTHYROIDISM IN THE NEONATE**

- Birth weight > 4,000 g, gestation longer than 42 weeks
- Large, open posterior fontanel (> 1 cm)
- Umbilical hernia
- Abdominal distension
- Poor feeding
- Hypothermia, cool extremities
- Prolonged jaundice
- Bradycardia
- Poor muscle tone
- Mottled skin
- Delayed skeletal maturation

## Diagnosis of Congenital Hypothyroidism

**Neonatal Screening.** Because even severe CH can be clinically silent, universal newborn screening for CH is widely practiced. Routine screening of all newborn infants for CH has greatly improved early detection and treatment of the disorder, preventing much of the mental retardation that was previously associated with CH.

The incidence of CH, as detected through newborn screening, is approximately 1 per 3,000 to 4,000. Screening all newborns for CH is mandated in all U.S. states and Canada.

Some screening programs in North America measure the TSH directly from blood samples collected on filter paper. Other programs initially measure $T_4$ on all specimens, followed by TSH measurement only if $T_4$ is low. Owing to the physiologic surge in TSH in the first hours of life as the newborn adapts to the extrauterine environment, the screening specimen must be collected when the infant is at least 24 hours of age, preferably between 2 and 4 days of age. If blood is collected earlier, a false-positive result can occur. In those instances, a repeat specimen must be collected within the first 7 days of life, regardless of prior test results. Protein intake is not required before screening.

False negatives can also occur with screening. When only $T_4$ testing is done, as many as 8% of infants with central CH can be missed (Kim et al., 2018). Their initial $T_4$ levels are normal (Kim et al., 2018). Infants who have hypothyroxinemia with delayed TSH elevation and those with residual thyroid tissue (such as an ectopic thyroid gland) have initial $T_4$ levels in the normal range. All these infants would be detected by repeat screening at 2 to 6 weeks of age.

Certain infants are at risk for a missed or delayed diagnosis, including those born at home, those who are extremely ill in the neonatal period, and those who are transferred between hospitals at an early age. Screening errors, including incorrect specimen collection or improper storage and transport, can result in a false-negative test. Thyroid medications taken by the mother during pregnancy can also produce false-negative results. Blood transfusions can alter test results. Preservatives (ethylenediaminetetraacetic acid [EDTA] or citrate) in blood-collection containers can result in false-negative or false-positive screening results.

When a low $T_4$ and elevated TSH level (> 40 mU/L) are encountered, the neonate should be presumed to have primary hypothyroidism until proven otherwise. A thorough examination for signs and symptoms of CH is indicated, along with confirmatory serum testing. Treatment with L-thyroxine should be initiated while awaiting the results of further testing.

**Laboratory Testing.** Low serum total, free $T_4$ and $T_3$, and elevated TSH levels confirm CH in the neonate. Permanent congenital CH is highly likely in a full-term neonate with a serum $T_4$ less than 6 mcg/dl and a serum TSH greater than 50 mU/L. A normal $T_4$ (e.g., > 10 mcg/dl) in combination with elevated TSH suggests that the infant has enough functional thyroid tissue to respond to excess TSH stimulation, the pattern seen in a subgroup of infants with compensated or subclinical hypothyroidism. Age-related reference norms for both gestational age and hours of age should be used when interpreting all thyroid test results. If maternal antibody-mediated hypothyroidism is suspected, maternal antithyroid (TSH receptor–blocking, TRBAb) antibody testing should be done. Other thyroid autoantibodies that can produce hypothyroidism include thyroglobulin (TGAb) and thyroid peroxidase antibodies (TPOAb). TBG levels can be measured to rule out TBG deficiency. Thyroglobulin levels in infants with possible CH can help to differentiate between thyroid agenesis and dyshormonogenesis, as an adjunct to thyroid imaging. Genetic studies have already helped identify the etiology of CH in some infants.

**Imaging Studies.** Infants with biochemical evidence of CH usually undergo scintigraphy with iodine-123 ($^{123}I$) or pertechnetate ($^{99m}TcO_4$), which is trapped by the thyroid gland and, like iodine (Polak et al., 2017), aids in the detection of an ectopic (lingual or sublingual) or missing gland. A normal or enlarged gland suggests a defect in thyroxine synthesis as the source of CH. Thyroid ultrasound can also be useful initially to demonstrate the presence or absence of a gland. Lateral radiographs of the knee and foot reveal bone age, indicating the degree of intrauterine hypothyroidism experienced by the fetus. Ossification of the distal femoral epiphysis usually appears at 36 weeks' gestation; its absence in a term or postterm infant suggests delayed bone maturation from long-standing hypothyroidism.

## Management of Hypothyroidism

Early, adequate treatment of permanent CH is critical for optimal neurologic development. The goal of hormone replacement therapy is to rapidly normalize the infant's serum $T_4$ level and maintain it in the upper half of the normal range, which should result in a TSH of 0.5 to 4 mU/L (Kim et al., 2018). The agent of choice is sodium-L-thyroxine ($NaT_4$) because it is substantially converted to $T_3$ within the brain. Tablets are crushed and given in a small amount of liquid. One method is instructing parents to crush the tablet and place it on the baby's tongue just before feeding (Polak et al., 2017). The tablet should not be diluted in the entire volume of the baby's bottle because if the bottle is not finished, the baby will not receive the full dose. Parents should be counseled about the importance of consistent medication administration and instructed on actions to take if a dose is missed or vomited.

Infants receiving thyroid replacement therapy must be monitored closely for treatment adequacy and evidence of thyrotoxicosis (irritability, tachycardia, poor weight gain). Serum $T_4$ should normalize in 1 to 2 weeks; serum TSH can take longer to normalize.

# TRANSIENT DISORDERS OF THYROID FUNCTION

## Transient Hypothyroxinemia of Prematurity

About 50% of infants born at less than 30 weeks' gestation exhibit transiently low thyroxine levels compared to their full-term counterparts. This relative hypothyroxinemia is primarily a function of HPT axis immaturity, a physiologically normal stage of thyroid system development. Other factors may affect thyroid function, especially in the very preterm infant. The abrupt cessation of maternal $T_4$ supply at birth contributes to low thyroid hormone levels. Other factors include the immature ability to concentrate iodine, synthesize, and iodinate thyroglobulin. Preterm infants may also experience insufficient iodine intake during the early weeks after birth before full enteral feeding is established. Iodine excess related to using iodine-containing antiseptics and radiopaque agents can block thyroid hormone release from the thyroid gland.

**Pathophysiology.** The postnatal TSH surge of the preterm infant is similar yet quantitatively lower than that of the more mature infant. Likewise, the corresponding rise in $T_4$ in preterm infants is blunted compared to term infants. It takes approximately 4 to 8 weeks, depending on the gestational age at birth, for normal-term hormone levels to be reached. The more premature the infant, the more severe the hypothyroxinemia is. Infants with transiently low thyroxine need follow-up testing to ensure the low $T_4$ levels rise into the normal range over time.

Extremely preterm infants (24–27 weeks' gestation) are at an even greater disadvantage, having a distinct and more ineffective pattern of postnatal thyroid function. The TSH surge of these very immature infants is significantly attenuated, and TSH levels continue to fall after birth to less than cord blood values by 7 hours of age. Such very low TSH levels fail to stimulate a postnatal rise in $T_4$. $T_4$ levels in extremely immature infants remain quite low and are even slightly lower than cord blood values at 24 hours of age.

**Clinical Manifestations.** Hypothyroxinemia of prematurity is a subtle condition with no overt signs or symptoms of hypothyroidism. Many classic signs and symptoms of hypothyroidism are common clinical findings in preterm infants (slow intestinal motility, distension, prolonged jaundice, low muscle tone, mottled skin, etc.). **Quality and Safety: Thyroid hormones are critical to brain development, so prolonged low thyroxine levels while the brain is still developing could contribute to poor neurocognitive outcomes in these infants.**

**Diagnosis.** Hypothyroxinemia of prematurity is identified by routine newborn screening. $T_4$ and free $T_4$ are low, but TSH is not elevated above the cutoff of 20 mU/L. This is the critical difference between transient hypothyroxinemia of prematurity and CH. A repeat test is conducted after several weeks to recheck $T_4$ and monitor for a possible delayed rise in TSH.

**Management.** The bothersome fact about hypothyroxinemia of prematurity is that it is associated with higher mortality and neurodevelopmental deficits. Yet, cumulative evidence has not demonstrated the clear benefits of routinely supplementing these infants with thyroxine during early life. Thyroid function tests should be followed carefully in preterm infants at risk for hypothyroxinemia, and treatment should be instituted promptly if indicated by elevated TSH. Flag or highlight the low thyroid results from the initial newborn screen to ensure that repeat thyroid testing is not overlooked.

## Nonthyroidal Illness

In some ill preterm infants, $T_4$ is preferentially converted to $rT_3$ instead of $T_3$, possibly as an adaptive response to lower the metabolic rate during severe illness. The outcome is low serum concentrations of both $T_4$ and $T_3$. Reverse $T_3$ is elevated, and TSH is normal. This condition, also known as "low $T_3$ syndrome" or "euthyroid sick syndrome," occurs in infants who have immature lungs or infections. Cytokines are produced that inhibit thyroid function and metabolism. The low $T_4$ from nonthyroidal illness reverses spontaneously when the infant's condition improves. No treatment is required. Similar effects are seen in infants who are receiving dopamine or glucocorticoids.

## Transient Primary Hypothyroidism

Hypothyroidism is defined as transient when a low $T_4$ and elevated TSH in apparently healthy full-term infants revert to normal spontaneously or after several months of thyroxine supplementation. About 5% to 10% of the cases identified by newborn screening with CH are transient. Initial management is the same as for CH.

## Transplacental Passage of Drugs or Antibodies

Transient hypothyroidism in the newborn can be precipitated by transplacental passage of antithyroid agents taken during pregnancy for the treatment of maternal Graves' disease. Medications such as propylthiouracil (PTU), methimazole, radioiodine, and amiodarone can inhibit fetal thyroid production. A similar inhibitory effect can occur if the fetus is exposed to excess iodine in utero. If the mother has a history of autoimmune thyroid disease, maternal TSH receptor–blocking antibodies (TRBAb, also termed thyrotropin-binding inhibitor immunoglobulin, or TBII) readily cross the placenta and block the fetal thyroid, producing hypothyroidism. These TRBAbs can persist in the infant's circulation for 2 to 3 months after birth before they are entirely metabolized and disappear. It can be challenging to predict the effects of these antibodies because some mothers will simultaneously produce TSH receptor–stimulating antibodies that will offset the effect of the TRBAbs.

**Clinical Manifestations.** Like CH, transient hypothyroidism is usually asymptomatic in the newborn. If present, the signs and symptoms are the same as for CH. Transient hypothyroidism caused by antithyroid drugs (goitrogens) can cause a goiter in the neonate. Iodine deficiency or excess has a similar effect.

**Diagnosis.** Transient hypothyroidism is typically detected by routine neonatal screening or is based on maternal history. The neonate displays the thyroid profile of low $T_4$ and elevated TSH that is characteristic of hypothyroidism. When the maternal history is positive for autoimmune thyroid disease, thyroid-stimulating hormone antibodies (TRSAb) and TRSAb levels (as indicated) are also obtained for baseline purposes. Thyroid imaging tests may also be conducted.

**Management.** Transient hypothyroidism caused by maternal antithyroid medication will resolve spontaneously when the medication is cleared from the infant's circulation, usually within a day or two after birth. The infant's serum $T_4$ and TSH levels should be monitored to ensure they return to normal. Supplementation with L-thyroxine is not usually necessary. Transplacentally acquired TSH receptor–blocking antibodies can slowly degrade completely; therefore, most infants will require supplementation for several months. TRBAb levels in the infant can be monitored to determine when to discontinue therapy. Breastfeeding is not contraindicated in neonates whose mothers continue their antithyroid medication in the postpartum period because very little passes into the breast milk.

## Hyperthyroidism (Neonatal Graves' Disease)

**Pathophysiology.** The transient condition neonatal Graves' disease occurs in infants born to mothers with active or inactive Graves' disease, to those who have undergone thyroidectomy or radioiodine ablation of the thyroid gland, and to women taking antithyroid drugs. Maternal TRSAbs cross the placenta readily and stimulate the fetal thyroid gland, causing an overproduction of thyroid hormone and, in some cases, the development of a goiter. The higher the TRSAb level in the mother, the more severely affected the infant will be. Hyperthyroidism in the neonate is typically transient, lasting approximately 3 to 12 weeks. The clinical course varies depending on the maternal disease and treatment. Onset may be delayed for a week or longer in neonates whose mothers produce TRSAb and TSH receptor–blocking antibodies. Suppose the mother took antithyroid medication during pregnancy. In that case, the neonate might not exhibit evidence of hyperthyroidism for several days until the drugs are metabolized (and, in fact, some infants are hypothyroid during that time). Occasionally, the hyperthyroidism persists beyond the expected recovery period and becomes true, permanent Graves' disease.

**Clinical Manifestations.** Neonates may be born preterm, often with evidence of intrauterine growth restriction (IUGR). Common clinical signs of thyrotoxicosis include tachycardia, arrhythmias, hypertension, tachypnea, poor feeding, vomiting, sweating, hyperthermia, flushing, diarrhea, restlessness, tremors, irritability, and hyperalertness. In severe cases of untreated maternal Graves' disease, advanced bone age, craniosynostosis, and microcephaly are evident in both the fetus and newborn. The infant should be examined for a goiter, which can be very small or large enough to compress the trachea and cause respiratory distress in the newborn. A goiter is a symmetrical, smooth enlargement of the gland and can be recognized as a swelling in the anterior neck of the neonate (Figure 10.2). To examine the neonate for goiter, place the infant supine and elevate the trunk while allowing the head to fall back gently (Escobar et al., 2018). A goiter can increase in size during the early neonatal period.

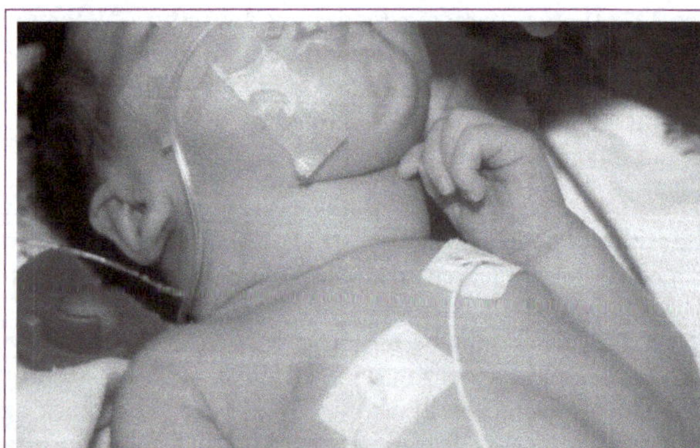

**FIGURE 10.2** Newborn infant presenting at birth with goiter.

**Diagnosis.** Serum $T_4$, free $T_4$, and $T_3$ are elevated, and serum TSH is low, all relative to age-appropriate norms. A TRSAb titer in the neonate will indicate the expected severity of the disease course. **Emergency Alert: Infants at risk (e.g., high maternal titer of TRSAb) for severe thyrotoxicosis require frequent monitoring of free $T_4$ and TSH.** A good maternal history is essential (e.g., history of radioablation therapy, antithyroid drugs taken during pregnancy and when they were taken, and maternal symptoms, if any).

**Management.** The mainstays of treatment of hyperthyroidism in the neonate are iodine, antithyroid medication, sedation, and beta-adrenergic blockers, if needed. Treatment is tailored to the severity of the infant's symptoms. Lugol's iodine solution (potassium iodide), given in a single drop three times daily, acutely inhibits the release of thyroxine from the thyroid gland. Other preparations include iodine-based contrast agents (ipodate), PTU, and methimazole. Propranolol can be used to manage cardiovascular symptoms. The infant's serum $T_4$ must be followed closely during treatment for possible iatrogenic hypothyroidism. TRSAb levels are also observed to monitor the infant's recovery and determine the appropriate time for weaning antithyroid medication.

# ADRENAL GLAND

The highly vascular adrenal glands are located at the superior poles of the kidneys. Each gland comprises two distinct, independently functioning organs: the outer cortex, which produces steroid hormones (mineralocorticoids, glucocorticoids, and androgens), and the inner medulla, which produces catecholamines. Adrenal steroid production and regulation require a functional HPA axis. Cortisol is released in response to stress, hypoglycemia, surgery, extreme heat or cold, hypoxia, infection, or injury.

Aldosterone, the most important mineralocorticoid, regulates renal sodium, water retention, and potassium excretion. Aldosterone influences not only electrolyte balance but blood pressure and intravascular volume as well. Aldosterone is regulated by the plasma renin-angiotensin system.

Adrenal androgens include dehydroepiandrosterone (DHEA), DHEA sulfate, and androstenedione and are regulated by ACTH. These steroids have minimal androgenic activity but are converted in peripheral tissues to potent androgens: testosterone and dihydrotestosterone (DHT), which are required for normal sexual differentiation.

# FETAL ADRENAL GLAND

The fetal adrenal gland is evident from 6 to 8 weeks' gestation and rapidly increases in size. Fetal cortisol is secreted at 8 weeks' gestation. Early in gestation, the fetal adrenal cortex differentiates into three regions: an inner prominent fetal zone, an outer definitive zone, and a transitional zone. After birth, the fetal zone involutes, and the definitive zone is transformed into the mature gland. Cortisol maintains intrauterine homeostasis and influences the development of various fetal tissues. Cortisol is essential for the prenatal maturation of organ systems, including the lungs, GI tract, liver, and CNS, which are vital for neonatal survival.

The fetal adrenal gland and the placenta are an integrated endocrine system known as the *fetoplacental unit*. The fetal zone of the developing adrenal gland produces DHEA and DHEA sulfate, precursors for placental estrogen, which is critical to maintaining the pregnancy and fetal well-being. In turn, the placenta regulates fetal exposure to maternal cortisol by oxidizing cortisol to the biologically inactive cortisone, protecting the fetus from excessive cortisol levels. The placenta also releases corticotropin-releasing hormone (CRH), which heightens the activity of the fetal HPA axis and stimulates fetal cortisol production. All of this contributes to the prenatal cortisol surge that prepares the fetus for the stress of birth and adaptation to the extrauterine environment.

## NEONATAL ADRENOCORTICAL FUNCTION

Plasma cortisol levels are elevated at birth but decline in the first few days of life. In term infants, a nadir is seen on day 4 of life. Likewise, levels of cortisol precursors such as 17-hydroxyprogesterone (17-OHP) are high at birth but decrease to normal neonatal levels by 12 to 24 hours of age. Cortisol is regulated by pituitary ACTH, which hypothalamic CRH controls via a negative feedback loop. Cortisol in the newborn plays a key role in the response to stress and illness. It also helps to maintain blood pressure.

Aldosterone and plasma renin activity (PRA) are elevated in neonates compared with values for older infants, allowing for positive sodium balance until the kidneys fully mature. Hyponatremia and urinary sodium losses often seen in preterm infants during the early postnatal weeks are due to a relative mineralocorticoid deficiency because of the immaturity of both the kidneys and the adrenal glands.

## ADRENAL DISORDERS IN THE NEONATE

### Transient Adrenocortical Insufficiency of Prematurity

A limited ability of the adrenal glands to maintain cortisol homeostasis in the early days of life has been observed in some preterm newborns. Manifestations are a low serum cortisol, normal or exaggerated pituitary response, and good recovery of adrenal function occurs by the end of 2 weeks of life. Whether a relative adrenal insufficiency contributes to hemodynamic instability and hypotension in critically ill infants is still under debate (Fechner, 2018).

### Neonatal Adrenal Hemorrhage (NAH)

Adrenal hemorrhage in the neonate can be precipitated by traumatic delivery, breech presentation, macrosomia, or disseminated intravascular coagulation (DIC). The large size and vascularity of the fetal adrenal gland predispose the gland to injury and rupture during the birth process. NAH is a newborn's most common adrenal mass (Lee et al., 2024). Although it is often asymptomatic, classic findings include jaundice, pallor, or a flank mass on either side (although hemorrhage is more common on the right), abdominal mass, poor feeding, vomiting, lethargy, hypotonia, hypertension, and scrotal edema (Lee et al., 2024). In severe cases, the infant may exhibit signs of adrenal insufficiency. Small hemorrhages can be initially undetected but eventually manifest in anemia and persistent jaundice (Askenazi et al., 2018). Abdominal ultrasound confirms the diagnosis and treatment depending on the clinical picture (Lee et al., 2024).

### Congenital Adrenal Hyperplasia

CAH is a spectrum of autosomal recessive disorders resulting from a deficiency of one of the five enzymes required to synthesize cortisol from cholesterol in the adrenal cortex. Each enzyme is encoded by its gene, and mutations in the 21-hydroxylase (21-OHD) gene, *CYP21A2*, are the most frequent.

**Pathophysiology.** A lack of 21-OHD prevents the conversion of progesterone to its two end products: cortisol and aldosterone (Figure 10.3). By reduced negative feedback regulation, the absence of cortisol causes oversecretion of ACTH, which chronically stimulates the adrenal cortex, resulting in hyperplasia of the gland. The precursor steroids proximal to the blocked step accumulate and are shunted into other metabolic pathways, such as androgen biosynthesis. In a female fetus, these superfluous yet potent systemic androgens cause virilization of the developing external genitalia. Also, the effects of this androgen exposure on the developing CNS may be important. Internal reproductive organs (ovaries, fallopian tubes, and uterus) are not affected by androgen exposure and develop normally.

Classic 21-OHD has a worldwide incidence of about 1 in 15,000 live births (Merke & Auchus, 2024). Two-thirds of those have a severe form known as either salt-wasting or salt-losing, in which there is a concurrent inability to produce aldosterone. High sodium excretion leads to profound hyponatremia, dehydration, and hyperkalemia. Glucocorticoid deficiency impairs carbohydrate metabolism, resulting in hypoglycemia and leading to hypotension, shock, and cardiovascular collapse from adrenal insufficiency. The remaining one-third of those with classic 21-OHD have a simple virilizing form. These infants have an incomplete enzymatic block, with enough aldosterone biosynthesis to maintain fluid and electrolyte homeostasis.

**Clinical Manifestations.** Affected female infants are usually recognized at birth by their nontypical genitals, a cardinal feature of CAH. Clitoromegaly, posterior fusion of the labia majora with rugae, and a single perineal orifice instead of separate urethral and vaginal openings may be present. In the last instance, the vagina joins the urethra above the perineum, forming a single urogenital orifice. In severe cases, clitoral hypertrophy is so marked that it resembles a penile urethra (Figure 10.4). These infants can be mistaken for boys with bilateral cryptorchidism and hypospadias. There may also be hyperpigmentation of the genital skin resulting from excessive pituitary ACTH secretion. Male infants with 21-OHD are phenotypically normal and may not be identified in the immediate neonatal period because the onset of adrenal symptoms is delayed until 7 to 14 days of life. Undetected

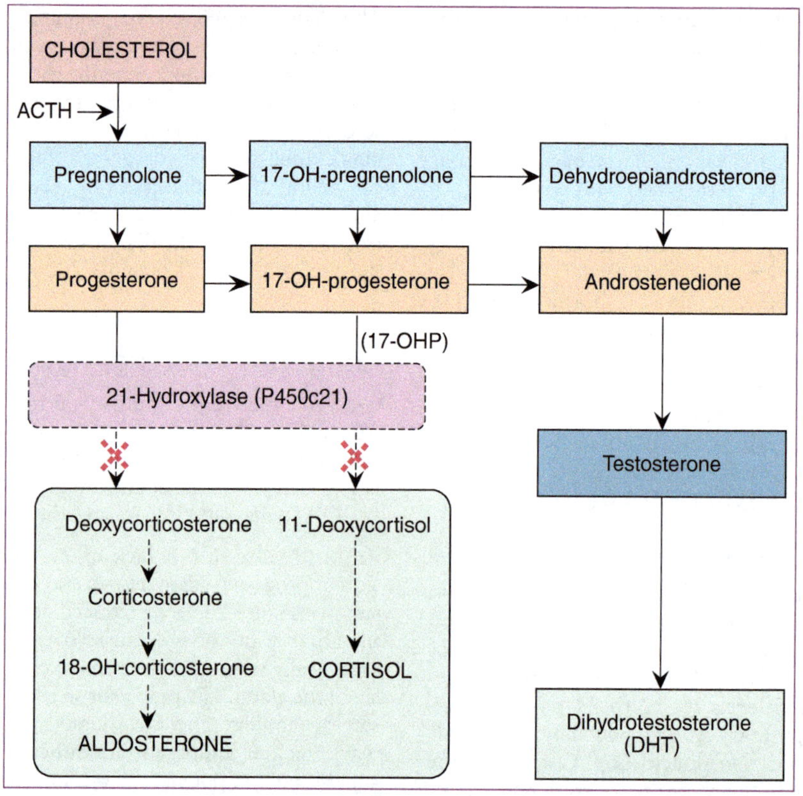


**FIGURE 10.3 Pathophysiology of congenital adrenal hyperplasia caused by 21-hydroxylase (21-OHD) deficiency.** A deficiency of the enzyme 21-OHD prevents the normal conversion of cholesterol to aldosterone and cortisol. Precursor steroids, including 17-hydroxyprogesterone (17-OHP) proximal to the blocked step, are shunted into the androgen synthesis pathway, resulting in excess production of androgens.

ACTH, adrenocorticotropic hormone.

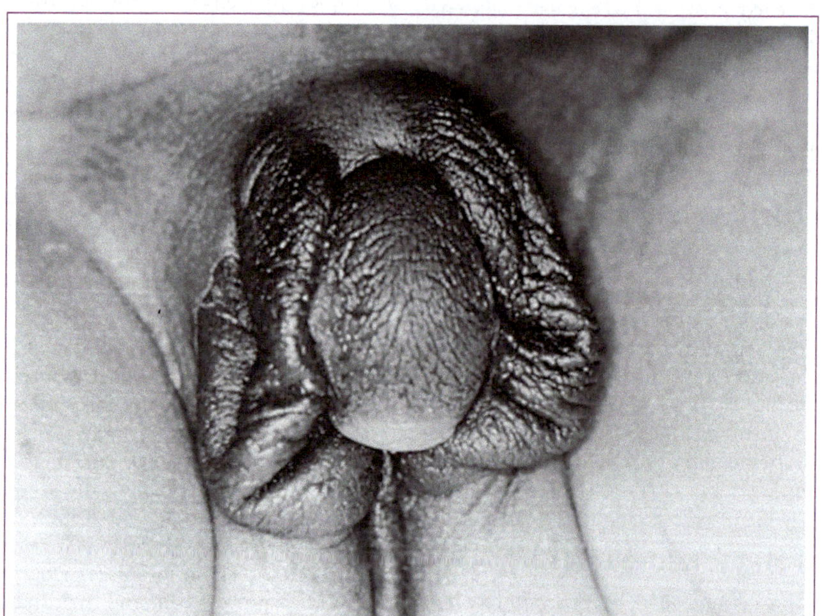

**FIGURE 10.4 External genitalia of 46,XX neonate with congenital adrenal hyperplasia.** Note clitoromegaly with rugosed, hyperpigmented, and partly fused labioscrotal folds.

*Source:* From Stokowski, L. (2015). Endocrine disorders. In M. T. Verklan & M. Walden (Eds.), *Core curriculum for neonatal intensive care nursing* (5th ed., pp. 632–661). Elsevier.

infants may present with impending adrenal collapse: vomiting, weight loss, lethargy, dehydration, hyponatremia, hyperkalemia, hypoglycemia, hypovolemia, and shock. Untreated infants of either sex will undergo rapid postnatal growth and sexual precocity. Salt loss can result in death.

**Diagnosis.** A markedly elevated 17-OHP level is diagnostic for classic 21-OHD deficiency. Random 17-OHP levels in affected infants can reach 10,000 ng/dl (normal is < 100 ng/dl). However, such high 17-OHP levels may not be reached until the second or third day of life, so a specimen drawn too early could lead to false reassurance that the infant does not have CAH. Prenatal or postnatal steroids can suppress the 17-OHP level and produce a false-negative result as well. Biochemical support for diagnosing CAH also includes elevated serum DHEA and androstenedione levels in males and females and elevated serum testosterone in females. Molecular genetic analysis is not usually essential for the diagnosis but may help confirm the exact defect type and aid in genetic counseling.

Part of the evaluation of every newborn with ambiguous genitalia is a karyotype or fluorescence In Situ hybridization (FISH) test for sex chromosome material, and this is also true when the suspected diagnosis is CAH. Imaging studies, including pelvic and abdominal ultrasound, will determine the presence or absence of a uterus, evaluate adrenal size, and more rapidly identify the infant's sex.

The increased serum 17-OHP levels in affected infants permit screening for the disorder using blood filter specimens on routine newborn screening panels. **Quality and Safety: The major objectives of newborn screening for CAH are the presymptomatic identification of infants at risk for the development of life-threatening adrenal crises and the prevention of incorrect sex assignment of affected female infants with ambiguous genitalia.** The former is particularly important for affected boys whose initial manifestation may be an adrenal crisis. All 50 states now screen newborns for CAH. False positives occur in about 1% of all tests.

**Management.** CAH requires urgent expert medical attention. When the diagnosis is confirmed, physiologic replacement dosing of cortisol is initiated. Aldosterone replacement maintains fluid and electrolyte homeostasis. Agents of choice in the newborn are hydrocortisone, a glucocorticoid, plus fludrocortisone, a mineralocorticoid. Daily checking weight, adrenal steroid concentration, PRA, electrolytes, blood glucose, and other data guide further clinical management. PRA should be compared against age-specific norms, because basal PRA is higher in newborns than older infants. Dietary sodium chloride supplementation is often necessary.

Hypertrophy of the clitoris will gradually abate with medical therapy; however, severe virilization will not be reversed. Parents of virilized female infants may have many questions about possible genital surgery. Although such surgery is not usually performed until the infant is 2 to 6 months of age, it is helpful for the parents to meet with the pediatric endocrinologist and pediatric urologic surgeon well before the surgery is planned. The goals of genital surgery for virilized girls with CAH are to achieve genital appearance compatible with gender, unobstructed urinary emptying without incontinence or infections, and good adult sexual and reproductive function. The surgery has good outcomes and low complications (Ibrahim et al., 2024). After discharge, a pediatric endocrinologist must closely follow infants with CAH to assess hormone levels, blood sugar, blood pressure, growth, skeletal maturation, and other parameters necessary to guard against over- or undertreatment.

Some authorities now use the term *disorder of sex development* or *DSD related to physical changes in genitalia,* or the older term, *ambiguous genitalia,* discussed in the next section (Houk et al., 2019). Whether to force a specific sexual identification early is still hotly debated and often results in ethical considerations—especially the wishes of the family.

## GENITALIA

### Sexual Development in the Fetus

Sexual differentiation is a sequential process with three stages: (a) fertilization (determination of chromosomal sex), (b) gonadal differentiation, and (c) differentiation of phenotypic sex (internal ductal system and external genitalia (Shnorhavorian & Fechner, 2018). At conception, the sex chromosome complement of the fertilizing sperm determines the chromosomal sex.

Genes direct the following events. During the early weeks of development, all embryos have bipotential gonads and structures for both male and female internal and external genitalia. Male-specific development requires the expression of the testis-determining gene (*SRY*) located on the short arm of the *Y* chromosome. This directs the gonad to differentiate to a testis.

Numerous other genes are required for normal gonadal development. Mutations in many of these genes (such as *SRY, WT1, SOX9, DAX-1, DMRT1,* and *SF1*) are the source of identified syndromes of gonadal dysgenesis, such as Swyer syndrome, Denys–Drash syndrome, campomelic dysplasia, dosage-sensitive sex reversal, and gonadal dysgenesis. It was formerly believed that the ovary developed as a "default" gonad (in the absence of genes for testis development). Still, we now know that specific genes are necessary for normal ovarian differentiation (Shnorhavorian & Fechner, 2018).

### Internal Genitalia

The following events in sexual development are hormonally mediated and predicated on the established gonadal sex (Shnorhavorian & Fechner, 2018). By 7 weeks' gestation, the fetus has two sets of primitive ducts that will become the internal reproductive tracts: the Müllerian (female) and Wolffian (male). In the XY fetus, the testis differentiates by the end of week 7. The embryonic testis develops two types of hormone-producing cells: the Sertoli and the Leydig cells. The Sertoli cells begin secreting Müllerian-inhibiting factor (MIF), causing the Müllerian ducts to regress. By the ninth week, testicular Leydig cells are secreting the androgens necessary for further virilization of the male fetus.

Testosterone, the major androgen produced by the testes, acts locally in high concentrations to induce the development of the Wolffian ducts into the epididymis, vas deferens, and seminal vesicles. Without testosterone, the Wolffian ducts regress at 11 weeks' gestation. Müllerian ducts require no ovarian hormonal inducement to develop into fallopian tubes, uterus, and upper vagina. This occurs in fetuses with a normal ovary or on any side lacking a gonad.

## External Genitalia

The primitive external genital structures are identical in both sexes (Figure 10.5). In this indifferent stage, a genital tubercle forms and elongates to form a phallus and urogenital sinus, surrounded by inner urogenital folds and labioscrotal swellings. Between the 8th and 14th weeks of gestation, male differentiation of the external genitalia occurs. Central to this development is the availability of DHT, a potent metabolite produced from testosterone by the enzyme 5 alpha-reductase-2 (5-ARD-2). With 10 times the binding affinity of testosterone, DHT binds to androgen receptors in the genital tissues, stimulating the fusion of the urethral folds to form the penile shaft and the labioscrotal swellings to form the scrotum. The urogenital sinus becomes the urethra. Penile growth continues throughout gestation, and migration of the testes from the abdominal cavity to the scrotum is a late event at 25 to 35 weeks' gestation. Androgen exposure after about 14 weeks contributes to further phallic enlargement (Shnorhavorian & Fechner, 2018).

In the absence of DHT, feminization of the external genitalia occurs. The phallus becomes a clitoris, and the labioscrotal swellings remain unfused to form the labia majora and minora. The urogenital sinus develops into the lower vagina and urethra. Feminine external genital development is complete by 11 weeks of gestation. Androgen exposure after this critical period can promote growth of the clitoris but does not cause labial fusion or the development of a penile urethra (Shnorhavorian & Fechner, 2018).

## General Principles of Management of Disorders of Sexual Development

The fact that doctors and nurses are not quite sure if one's long-awaited newborn baby is a male or a female must surely be one of the most incomprehensible things that parents can

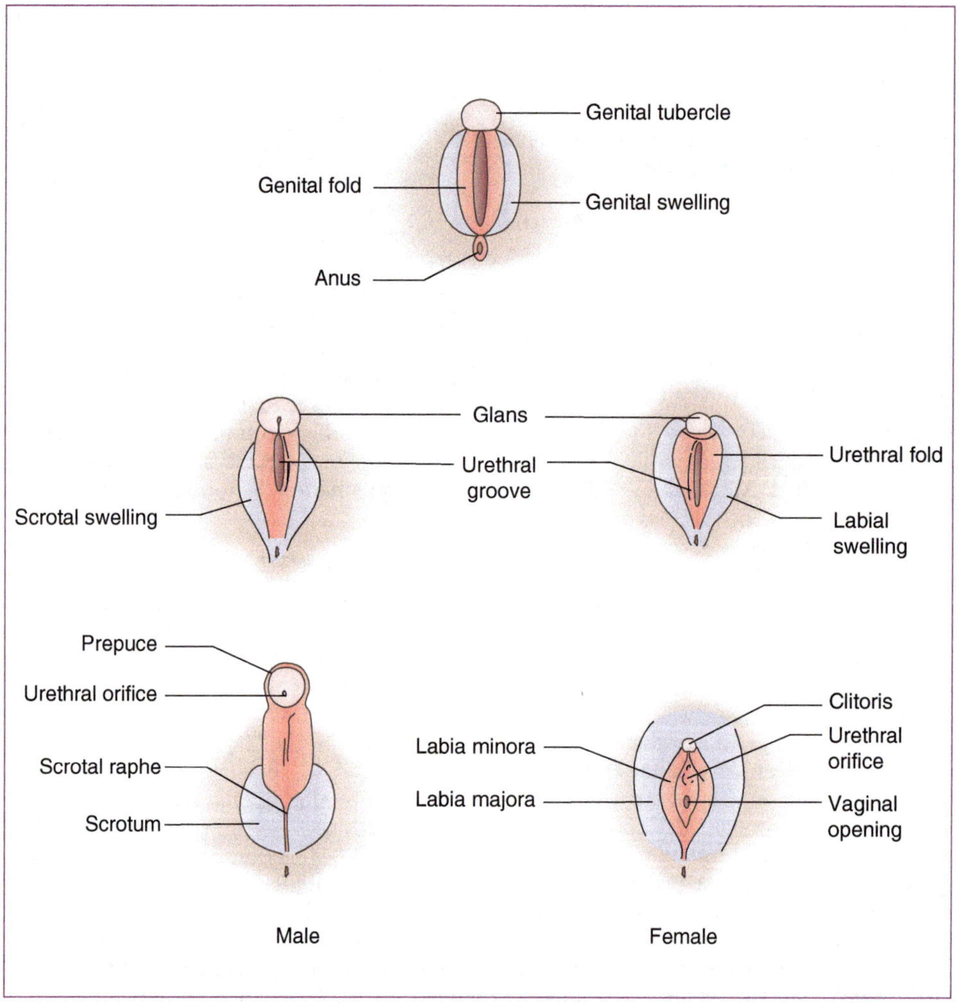


**FIGURE 10.5 Development of the external genitalia.**

*Source:* Adapted from Griffin, J. E., & Ojeda, S. R. (1988). *Textbook of Endocrine Physiology.* Oxford University Press, USA.

hear in the delivery room. This situation requires a high degree of sensitivity and tact. Many infants are identified prenatally following ultrasound recognition of genital ambiguity or a karyotype/phenotype discordance, and these families will be prepared, to some degree, for the experience of having a baby of uncertain sex. Others will be taken entirely by surprise. Despite the family's desire for a quick answer, the baby's assignment should not be done at birth. Neonates who do not have health concerns requiring intensive care monitoring or treatment should not be transferred to the NICU.

**Clinical Manifestations.** Essential to the evaluation of the neonate with genital ambiguity is obtaining a detailed family history. Any of the following could indicated a congenital or inherited DSD: maternal virilization or ingestion of hormones or oral contraceptives during pregnancy; consanguinity; history of urologic abnormalities, infertility, or genital ambiguity in other family members; or previous neonatal deaths that may suggest an undiagnosed adrenal crisis. Dysmorphic features raise suspicion of a syndrome.

A detailed assessment of the genitalia should be conducted. Examinations should respect the privacy of the infant and the family. Because of the considerable overlap in the genital anatomy among DSDs, the physical assessment alone does not permit a firm diagnosis (Shnorhavorian & Fechner, 2018). Some findings can provide clues to the underlying pathophysiology and guide the diagnosis. A precise description of the anatomy is more useful than simply staging classifications. If preferred, however, the degree of virilization can be documented by Prader staging from a phenotypic female with mild clitoromegaly (Prader stage II) to a phenotypic male with glandular hypospadias (Prader stage V; Figure 10.6). Look for symmetry or asymmetry of the genitalia, which provides an important clue. The presence of a uterus can be determined by digital rectal examination as an anterior midline cordlike structure.

**Gonads.** Determine whether gonads are palpable. The presence or absence of palpable gonads helps to differentiate the major categories of DSDs. An apparent male infant with bilateral or a single impalpable testis with hypospadias should be considered as having a potential DSD until proven otherwise. A palpable gonad excludes the diagnosis of a virilized genetic female (46,XX) with CAH. A gonad palpated below the external inguinal ring is presumed to contain testicular tissue. Because ovaries are rarely palpable, a unilateral gonad is usually a testis or occasionally an ovotestis. To palpate testes, place fingers flat from the internal ring and milk down into the labioscrotal folds. Gonads may be situated high in the inguinal canal, requiring a careful examination. Sweep the fingers down along the line of the inguinal canal on each side, beginning well above the site of the internal inguinal ring. A gonad milked down by this maneuver is gently grasped by the other hand, and its size and consistency are noted. Ovotestes will feel softer than testes. Bilateral absence of the testes is known as *cryptorchidism*.

**Phallus.** Phallic size should be measured with a straight-edge ruler, depressing the fat pad, and measuring the stretched length from the pubic tubercle to the tip of the penis, not including the foreskin. Both the length and mid-shaft diameter of the penis should be noted. Chordee, ventral curvature of the penis caused by residual urethral tissue that tethers the phallus to the perineum, should be emphasized because it can reduce the apparent length of the penis (Shnorhavorian & Fechner, 2018). If present, the actual position of the urethral meatus and the severity of hypospadias should be determined.

Clitoral size should also be measured when clitoromegaly is present. A clitoral length greater than 9 mm in term infants is considered excessive. Clitoral size often appears large in preterm infants because breadth remains constant from 27 weeks onward. A prominent, but not truly enlarged, clitoris or a normally sized penis concealed by an abundance of prepubic fat are two normal assessment findings.

**Labioscrotal Folds.** Labial fullness, a benign finding, is another feature occasionally mistaken for genital ambiguity. The labioscrotal folds are examined for fusion, which starts posteriorly and moves anteriorly, increasing the anogenital distance. The perineum is inspected by gently separating the labia and using an exam light to confirm the presence of separate urethral and vaginal openings or a single urogenital orifice (an opening connected to both urinary and genital systems). Visualization of voiding is helpful. If skin tags with a slightly bluish hue are seen, a hymen and vagina are present. Note rugosity or hyperpigmentation of the labioscrotal fold, signifying hypersecretion of ACTH associated with CAH. Other variations include a bifid scrotum (a deep

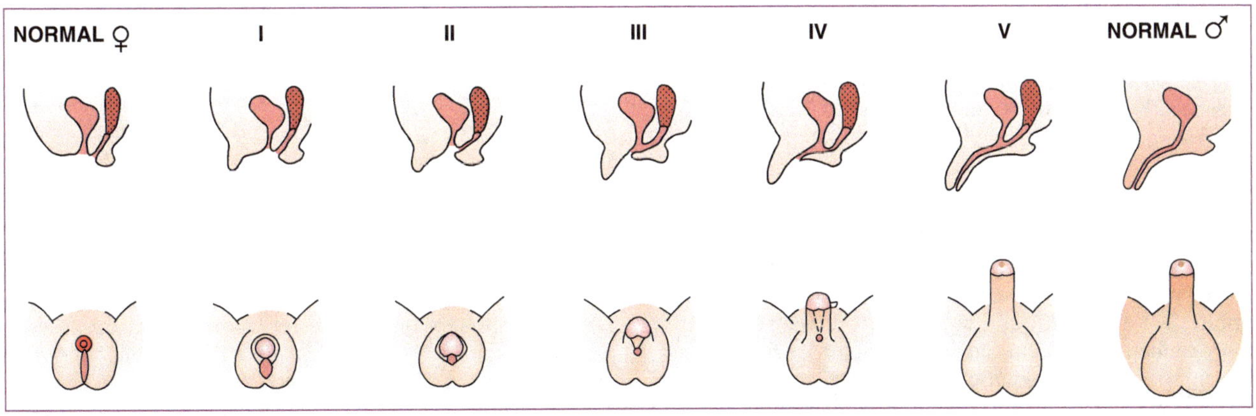


**FIGURE 10.6 Degrees of genital virilization according to the stages of Prader.** The upper panel shows a sagittal view, and the lower panel shows a perineal view.

midline cleft) or a shawl scrotum (the scrotum surrounds the penis like a shawl).

**Diagnostic Studies.** DSDs are diagnosed with biochemical, hormonal, imaging, and molecular testing. The principal aim of an initial investigation is to rule out a life-threatening illness such as CAH, which can precipitate an adrenal crisis. Such testing includes serum 17-OHP level (after 24–48 hours of age), electrolytes, glucose, baseline levels of testosterone, DHT, and other steroid precursors (progesterone, DHEA, delta 4-androstenedione, and 17 alpha-hydroxypregnenolone). A karyotype with X- and Y-specific probe detection is obtained from all infants.

A urinary steroid profile is helpful in the diagnosis of disorders of steroid biosynthesis. Other investigations that may be warranted include ACTH stimulation test, PRA, and serum MIF, LH, and FSH. An hCG stimulation test is undertaken to delineate a block in testosterone biosynthesis from androstenedione (17 beta-hydroxysteroid dehydrogenase deficiency) or conversion of testosterone to DHT (5 alpha-reductase deficiency). A human chorionic gonadotropin (hCG) test involves measuring baselinc lcvels of testosterone and its precursors, DHEA or DHEA sulfate, and androstenedione and its metabolite DHT. One to three intramuscular injections of high-dose hCG are given at 24-hour intervals. Repeat testosterone at least 24 hours after last injection.

Imaging studies include abdominopelvic ultrasound (to determine the presence or absence of a uterus, to visualize the presence or absence of gonads in the inguinal region, and to assess the Müllerian anatomy), genitourethrogram (to delineate the anatomy of the vagina and urethra, and where the vagina opens into the urogenital sinus), and pelvic MRI. Laparoscopic exploration with gonadal biopsy may be necessary to evaluate gonadal histology. Finally, molecular analysis may be required to arrive at a definitive diagnosis.

**Interpretation of Findings.** The most common cause of genital ambiguity in the newborn is 21-OHD deficiency. This form of CAH, responsible for over 90% of cases of ambiguous genitalia, presents with a virilized XX (female) with a uterus but gonads unpalpable.

Among the remainder of cases of ambiguous genitalia, the most common diagnoses are gonadal dysgenesis, followed by partial androgen insensitivity syndrome (PAIS) and testosterone biosynthetic disorders. An undervirilized male will exhibit external genitalia, with or without palpable gonads, and no uterus. A micropenis should prompt investigation for hypopituitarism or growth hormone deficiency, particularly in the presence of hypoglycemia (Shnorhavorian & Fechner, 2018).

A diagnosis in the undervirilized male infant is not always possible. Provisional diagnostic groupings can be determined based on the presence or absence of a uterus, symmetry of the external genitalia, and presence of gonads (Table 10.1).

## TABLE 10.1

### DIAGNOSTIC GROUPING SUGGESTED BY ASSESSMENT FINDINGS

| Diagnostic Grouping | Assessment Finding | | |
|---|---|---|---|
| | **Uterus** | **Gonads** | **External Genitalia** |
| CAH (21-OHD) virilized female | Present | Not palpable | Symmetrical hyperpigmented |
| Undervirilized male (PAIS or testosterone biosynthetic defect) | Absent | Palpable | Symmetrical |
| Gonadal dysgenesis (with Y chromosome) ovotesticular DSD | Present | Palpable | Asymmetrical |

21-OHD, 21-hydroxylase; CAH, congenital adrenal hyperplasia; DSD, disorder of sex development; PAIS, partial androgen insensitivity syndrome.

**Talking With Families.** Optimal care of the infant with a DSD involves a well-coordinated team approach. The team comprises, at minimum, the attending neonatologist, neonatal nurse, endocrinologist, pediatric surgeon/pediatric urologic surgeon, social worker, counselor or other mental health professional, and, in some instances, geneticist. The initial contact with parents of a newborn with a DSD is extremely important. This interaction should emphasize that a DSD is not a shameful condition. A single person should be identified to communicate diagnostic findings and plans with the family. When discussing possible diagnoses with the family, language must be carefully chosen. The role of the healthcare team is to provide information, share and explain all diagnostic findings, inform parents of all available options, and support the parents in the decision-making process. A relationship of trust is paramount, and this requires open and honest communication and full disclosure of available information (Shnorhavorian & Fechner, 2018), including candid discussion of the controversies and dilemmas concerning gender assignment and early genital surgery. Professionals must also recognize and respect the cultural and psychosocial influences on parents' decisions about care (Shnorhavorian & Fechner, 2018).

**Sex Assignment.** Parents are naturally anxious to find out their baby's sex so that they can name the baby and announce the birth to family and friends. Nevertheless, it must be sensitively communicated that although their distress is acknowledged, when sex is in doubt, a sex-of-rearing decision is one with lifelong implications and cannot be made in haste. Sex assignment must be deferred until an expert evaluation of the newborn takes place (Shnorhavorian & Fechner, 2018).

Unfortunately, some tests required for evaluation of a DSD must be sent out to referral laboratories, and the long wait for results can be frustrating for the parents. Questions about the infant's future management and treatment needs, gender identity/gender role development, and potential long-term outcomes should be addressed by clinicians who have extensive experience with DSDs.

## DISORDERS OF SEXUAL DEVELOPMENT

Most DSDs result from one of two events: either a failure in one of the steps of the male sexual developmental pathway or the exposure of an XX fetus to androgens during a sensitive period of development. Less frequent are DSDs resulting from gonadal differentiation, chromosomal disorders, and syndromes associated with ambiguous genitalia (Shnorhavorian & Fechner, 2018). The genes and multigenic factors responsible for DSDs are just beginning to be understood, but this information has yet to prove beneficial in terms of clinical management.

### 46,XX DSD Trimester

The most frequently encountered DSD in the neonate is the virilized female or the 46,XX infant with ambiguous external genitalia but normal female internal structures. The most common etiology is CAH, caused by 21-OHD deficiency. This enzyme deficiency results in an overproduction of androgens at a critical stage of development, causing masculinization of the external, but not the internal (ovaries, uterus, fallopian tubes), and genitalia. In the most severe cases, the excess androgens also prevent the vagina from fully descending into the perineum, leaving a common urogenital canal (see the section Adrenal Disorders in the Neonate).

Other possible, yet rare, causes of virilization of external genitalia in the 46,XX infant are placental aromatase deficiency, maternal androgen-producing or adrenal tumors, and maternal medications with androgenic action taken during pregnancy.

### 46,XY DSD

The combination of a 46,XY karyotype with ambiguous genitalia results from a failure in one of the steps involved in the synthesis or response to testosterone during sexual differentiation and penile growth. These infants have bilateral testicular development but incomplete virilization of the internal or external genitalia. An external phenotype result ranging from completely female to isolated hypospadias or cryptorchidism. Another condition associated with incomplete virilization in the XY male is cloacal exstrophy, a defect of embryogenesis involving bladder exstrophy. Although not a DSD, significant ambiguity of external genitalia may be present. In most cases of 46,XY DSD, a genetic mutation cannot be determined.

### Androgen Insensitivity Syndrome

**Pathophysiology.** Androgen insensitivity syndrome (AIS) is caused by a loss-of-function mutation in the androgen receptor gene located on the long arm of the X chromosome. More than 300 mutations have been identified (Shnorhavorian & Fechner, 2018). Both testosterone and its target tissue metabolite, DHT, must bind to androgen receptors to masculinize the genital tissues. When androgen receptor activity is impaired, androgen binding is insufficient. One variant of AIS is receptor negative: Cytosol receptors are incapable of binding DHT. Another variant is receptor-positive: Receptors can bind DHT, but this does not result in normal differentiation. Both internal Wolffian structures and external genitalia fail to respond to high levels of testosterone and DHT. The disorder has partial and complete forms, resulting in different degrees of undervirilization. In PAIS, the clinical phenotype varies and often parallels the severity of androgen resistance, but genotype-phenotype correlations have not been found.

**Clinical Manifestations.** Infants with PAIS have undervirilization ranging from simple hypospadias to microphallus with a labia majora–like bifid scrotum, undescended testes, and a urogenital sinus. No visible features distinguish PAIS from other causes of incomplete masculinization. Infants with complete androgen insensitivity (CAIS) are born with apparently female genitalia. However, these neonates may have palpable inguinal or labial masses, which further testing will reveal to be testes. Some may also have a short, blind-ending vagina.

**Diagnosis.** The diagnosis of CAIS is missed in the newborn period unless the infant presents with bilateral masses in the labia or inguinal canals, or a male was expected based on a prenatal karyotype. CAIS might also be discovered during inguinal hernia repair, or there may be a history of similarly affected family members. Important investigations include a karyotype and levels of testosterone, DHT, and LH. In PAIS, the ratio of androstenedione to testosterone is normal. Testosterone, estradiol, and LH levels are normal or high; the FSH level is usually normal.

Androgen receptor (AR) binding assays are not always helpful because normal ligand binding does not rule out androgen insensitivity caused by mutations in other domains of the androgen receptor (Shnorhavorian & Fechner, 2018). A test for direct sequencing of the AR for mutational analysis is commercially available, but AR mutations are not always found in PAIS (Shnorhavorian & Fechner, 2018). Imaging studies reveal the absence of female internal reproductive structures (uterus, fallopian tubes). Two normal testes are present.

**Management.** Infants with CAIS have unambiguously female external anatomy and are raised in the female sex. Testes are removed (usually after puberty) to prevent later malignancy. When the phenotype is predominantly male, male sex rearing is recommended. However, no consensus exists for the management of infants with severe perineoscrotal hypospadias and microphallus. When it is contemplated to rear as male sex, a therapeutic trial with pharmacologic doses of androgen, especially in those with an identified AR mutation, is often used to predict potential androgen responsiveness at puberty. If the phallus does not grow in response to testosterone, some experts would recommend consideration of a female sex assignment. However, many experts now believe that, given the putative influence of prenatal androgen exposure on the developing CNS, and the possibility that the child will develop a male gender identity.

### Testosterone Biosynthetic Defects

**Pathophysiology.** Defects in the chain of steroidogenic enzymes involved in the testosterone biosynthesis pathway result in insufficient androgen concentrations during fetal development. Disorders include congenital lipoid adrenal hyperplasia

(CLAH), 3 beta-HDD, 17 alpha-hydroxylase/17,20 lyase deficiency, and 17 beta-hydroxysteroid dehydrogenase deficiency (17 beta-HSD). CLAH is caused by a defect in the steroidogenic acute regulatory (StAR) protein, which is responsible for transporting cholesterol to the inner membrane of the mitochondria. Insufficient testosterone in affected males leads to underdeveloped Wolffian duct structures and external male anatomy. Müllerian structures are absent because there is normal testicular MIF production.

**Clinical Manifestations.** Male infants with CLAH present with complete adrenal insufficiency: vomiting, weight loss, and hypotension. Genital appearance is primarily female. Infants with 3 beta-HDD can present with varying degrees of genital ambiguity and evidence of salt-losing crisis (see 21-OHD). Infants with 17 alpha-hydroxylase/17,20 lyase deficiency have genital ambiguity, whereas patients with primary 17 alpha-hydroxylase deficiency also have hypertension. Male infants with 17 beta-HSD present with what appears to be external female genitalia that may include mild clitoral enlargement. An inguinal hernia may be present, possibly the only finding that will bring the infant to medical attention.

**Diagnosis.** General laboratory investigations in suspected testosterone biosynthetic defects include chromosomes, baseline levels of testosterone, androgen precursors and DHT, and levels of steroids and steroid precursors. An hCG stimulation test can measure the ratio of androstenedione to testosterone; an elevated ratio suggests 17 beta-HSD deficiency. In CLAH, ultrasound, computed tomography (CT), or MRI may show enlarged, lipid-laden adrenal glands (Shnorhavorian & Fechner, 2018).

**Management.** Acute management of these disorders requires complete steroid replacement with both glucocorticoids and mineralocorticoids. Genetic XY infants with CLAH are raised in the female gender. Children with 17 beta-HSD often virilize significantly at puberty owing to increased peripheral conversion of androstenedione to testosterone by 17 beta-HSD isoenzymes, making sex assignment of those diagnosed as neonates a less straightforward decision.

## 5-Alpha-Reductase-2 Deficiency

**Pathophysiology.** 5-ARD-2 deficiency is an autosomal recessive disorder caused by more than 20 different mutations of the *5-ARD* gene. 5-ARD-2 is an enzyme found in the genital skin and fibroblasts of the developing fetus, without which testosterone is not converted to DHT, and fetal external genitalia does not virilize. Development of the internal structures is unaffected because DHT is not required, so the Wolffian ducts generally differentiate in response to testosterone, and the Müllerian ducts regress. At puberty, the external genitalia become virilized, and fertility is possible (Misra & Lee, 2005).

**Clinical Manifestations.** The spectrum of findings ranges from mild (isolated micropenis or hypospadias) to severe (a female phenotype with clitoromegaly, mild rugation, or pigmentation) undervirilization (Figure 10.7). Testes are intact and are found in the inguinal canals or labioscrotal folds or are retained in the abdomen. The uterus and fallopian tubes

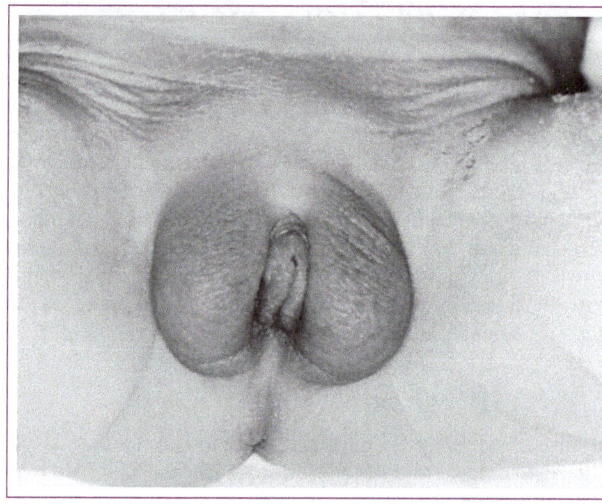

**FIGURE 10.7 External genitalia of 46,XY neonate with 5 alpha-reductase deficiency.** Undervirilization is so severe in this infant that the phenotype is almost completely female, with labia majora–like bifid scrotum and severe microphallus.

*Source:* From Stokowski, L. (2015). Endocrine disorders. In M. T. Verklan & M. Walden (Eds.), *Core curriculum for neonatal intensive care nursing* (5th ed., pp. 632–661). Elsevier.

regress because of the normal secretion of Müllerian inhibiting substance (MIS). Wolffian duct differentiation is not affected because DHT is not required. Male internal ducts terminate in a blind pseudovaginal pouch or on the perineum.

**Diagnosis.** Diagnosis is made by assessing the ratio of testosterone to DHT following an hCG stimulation test. A normal T/DHT ratio is less than 4 to 1. In 5-ARD-2 deficiency, this ratio is higher than 14 to 1 (Shnorhavorian & Fechner, 2018). The hCG stimulation test also rules out other causes of undervirilization, such as Leydig cell hypoplasia and testosterone biosynthetic defects. Analysis of 5-ARD-2 activity in genital skin fibroblasts provides a definitive diagnosis.

**Management.** Males with 5-ARD-2 respond to endogenous testosterone and undergo virilization and penile growth at puberty. The mechanism behind this late virilization may be extraglandular DHT formation due to peripheral conversion of increased testicular testosterone by unaffected isoenzymes. For this reason, it is recommended that when the diagnosis is made in the newborn period, a male sex assignment is usually made.

## Gonadal Dysgenesis

This group of disorders is usually associated with chromosomal anomalies or mutations or deletions of genes responsible for sexual differentiation. Karyotypes producing gonadal dysgenesis include 46,XY; 46,XX; 46,XY/46X; and mosaic forms, including the Y chromosome.

**Pathophysiology.** Dysgenetic gonads are characterized by variable degrees of immaturity or dysfunction, which can manifest in a variety of genital ambiguities. Gonadal dysgenesis is considered partial or incomplete when testes are dysgenic or incompletely formed and complete when the gonads are streaks containing only stromal tissue. Mixed gonadal dysgenesis occurs when one gonad is a streak and the other is a well-formed testis. Internal ducts correlate with the ipsilateral gonad. On the side of a streak gonad, a fallopian tube and hemiuterus develop, and on the side of a normal testis, the vas deferens and epididymis form.

**Clinical Manifestations.** External genitalia are highly variable depending on how much testosterone is produced. In mixed gonadal dysgenesis, the external genitalia are asymmetric, appearing male on one side and female on the other. A vagina and uterine cavity may be present. Complete (or pure) gonadal dysgenesis is a form of sex reversal that results in unambiguously female genitalia with features of Turner syndrome. These infants might not be identified in the newborn period unless a discrepancy is noted between a prenatal karyotype (46,XY) and the appearance of the genitals.

**Diagnosis.** Determining the sex chromosome complement by FISH testing is the most important diagnostic test. Imaging studies, genitography, or laparoscopy define the internal anatomy. Gonadal histologic analysis is necessary to differentiate gonadal dysgenesis from ovotesticular DSD, wherein elements of both testes and ovaries are present in the same individual (see Ovotesticular DSD in this chapter).

**Management.** Determining the sex of rearing for the infant with partial or mixed gonadal dysgenesis can be a difficult decision, one that is typically based on the degree of virilization and details of the internal anatomy. When a uterus is present, the female sex assignment may be preferred. Most infants with complete gonadal dysgenesis are raised as females.

### Ovotesticular DSD

In ovotesticular DSDs, both ovarian and testicular components are present in the same individual. Possible combinations include an ovary on one side and a testis on the other, an ovary or testis with an ovotestis, or two ovotestes. More than half the affected babies will have an XX karyotype. This condition was formerly known as true hermaphroditism, a label that is considered outdated.

**Pathophysiology.** The amount of testosterone produced by the testicular tissue that is present determines the degree of differentiation of Wolffian ducts, regression of Müllerian ducts, and virilization of external genitalia. Internal ducts usually parallel the ipsilateral gonadal histology. Ovarian tissue can be normal.

**Clinical Manifestations.** Asymmetry of the external genitalia is a hallmark of ovotesticular DSD. Genital ambiguity ranges from a female phenotype with slight clitoromegaly to a mildly undervirilized male phenotype.

**Diagnosis.** FISH testing is used to determine the sex chromosome complement. Imaging studies are used to define the internal anatomy. A diagnosis is based on the presence of functional ovarian and testicular tissue. Laparoscopy with gonadal biopsy is necessary at some point to confirm the diagnosis.

**Management.** Management for true ovotesticular DSD are like those of gonadal dysgenesis.

## PANCREAS

The pancreas is both an exocrine and endocrine gland. The endocrine pancreas is responsible for the hormonal regulation of blood glucose levels. The endocrine functions are performed by clusters of cells called *islets of Langerhans*, which include alpha, beta, and delta cells. Hormones secreted by the endocrine pancreas include glucagon, insulin, amylin, and somatostatin.

Fetal insulin, present by 8 to 10 weeks' gestation, is secreted in response to glucose and amino acids. The fetus is critically dependent for growth on its own supply of insulin, which does not cross the placenta. Insulin stimulates the uptake of glucose by muscle and adipose tissue. The fetal pancreas becomes progressively more responsive to glucose in late gestation, and beta-cell mass increases markedly. When the maternal glucose supply ceases at birth, the neonate's blood glucose level declines, along with plasma insulin. A concomitant surge in the counter-regulatory hormones epinephrine and glucagon sets in motion the production of glucose that will sustain the neonate until milk feeding is established.

The exocrine portion of the pancreas constitutes 80% of the total gland. Acinar cells secrete digestive enzymes, including trypsin, lipase, and amylase, into the duodenum. Epithelial cells along the pancreatic ducts secrete bicarbonate and water that neutralize gastric acid.

## DISORDERS OF THE PANCREAS

Rare pancreatic disorders in the newborn include congenital anomalies such as pancreatic agenesis, pancreatic hypoplasia, and annular pancreas. Disorders of the endocrine pancreas include neonatal diabetes mellitus (NDM) and hyperinsulinism, as well as the developmental disorder of the pancreas seen in the infant of the diabetic mother (IDM). The most common newborn disorder of the exocrine pancreas is cystic fibrosis (CF).

### Infant of a Diabetic Mother

Diabetes in pregnancy affects about 14% of women globally (Eades et al., 2024). Macrosomia or higher birthweight is linked to gestational diabetes mellitus (GDM) (Leth-Moller et al., 2024). Newborns will be at risk for problems associated with glucose intolerance and abnormal glucose regulation and childhood obesity (Leth-Moller et al., 2024).

**Pathophysiology.** If maternal glycemic control is poor in the third trimester, high circulating maternal glucose levels chronically stimulate the fetal pancreas to release insulin, leading to fetal fat deposition. Fetal macrosomia is more likely to occur in women whose hyperglycemia occurs episodically. At birth, the neonatal beta-cells adjust to the lower circulating glucose level and continue to secrete insulin, preventing the mobilization of glycogen and fat as sources of glucose. This failure of normal metabolic adaptation places the baby at risk of hypoglycemia. Hyperinsulinemia, regardless of whether the mother has type 1 or type 2 diabetes, can result in increased glucose utilization, decreased glucose production, and reduced availability of alternate substrates.

Excess fetal insulin may also cause delayed maturation of type II alveolar cells and pulmonary surfactant deficiency seen in some IDMs. Transient functional anomalies of the heart, including cardiomyopathy and intraventricular septal hypertrophy, begin in utero with glycogen loading of the septum. A delayed adaptation in parathyroid regulation after birth is the source of hypocalcemia and hypomagnesemia of the IDM. An increase in fetal erythropoiesis leading to polycythemia in the IDM is common, but its etiology is unknown. Hyperbilirubinemia results from the presence of excess hemoglobin (Hb), which, in turn, results in a larger-than-normal bilirubin load.

The higher rate of congenital anomalies associated with diabetic pregnancy is related to maternal glycemic control at the time of conception and during early gestation, when organogenesis is taking place. Congenital malformations associated with maternal diabetes include those of the CNS (anencephaly, meningomyelocele, encephalocele, caudal dysplasia), the heart (transposition of the great vessels, coarctation of the aorta, ventricular septal defects, atrial septal defects), the kidneys (hydronephrosis, renal agenesis), and the gastrointestinal tract (duodenal atresia, small left colon syndrome).

**Clinical Manifestations.** As a result of fat accumulation in late gestation, affected fetuses can develop macrosomia, with birth weights that are not in proportion with their length and head circumference measurements. Intrauterine growth restriction is a less common presentation seen in advanced maternal diabetic vascular disease. Skin tones may be ruddy with a sluggish capillary refill. The neonate may present in respiratory distress. If there is a history of a difficult vaginal delivery with shoulder dystocia, the infant may present with musculoskeletal or peripheral nerve findings, suggesting fractured clavicle or humerus or brachial plexus palsy. With the latter condition, the affected arm is held limply at the side, and movements, including Moro responses, are asymmetric. Deep tendon reflexes (DTRs) are absent. Crepitus may be palpated along the clavicle if a fracture is present.

**Diagnosis.** Macrosomia at birth is a good marker for detecting the infant at risk for neonatal morbidities related to maternal diabetes. Despite the IDM's size, it is also important to determine gestational age to assess the risk of prematurity-related problems. **Quality and Safety: The IDM must be monitored for hypoglycemia, usually within an hour or two of birth. Objective measurements of blood and plasma glucose should be used rather than relying on symptoms of hypoglycemia, because the latter are nonspecific and unreliable.** Point-of-care blood glucose test results indicating hypoglycemia (< 40 mg/dl in the newborn) should be verified with serum laboratory glucose; however, treatment should not be delayed while awaiting the laboratory test results. If no treatment is initiated and the serum glucose confirms hypoglycemia, valuable time is wasted, but if treatment is begun and the serum glucose is higher than the point-of-care glucose, the treatment is relatively benign.

Additional testing required for the IDM is a serum calcium concentration, and if this is low, serum magnesium is done. Hemoglobin level should be measured with a venous, rather than a capillary, blood sample. Additional diagnostic tests will depend on the findings of the initial physical examination.

**Management.** Unless life-threatening complications, such as perinatal asphyxia, are present, prevention of hypoglycemia is typically the primary concern in the early management of the IDM. Early, frequent milk feedings in stable infants are ideal if tolerated. Infants born preterm may display immature feeding skills despite their large size and require gavage feedings. **Quality and Safety: Severe or persistent hypoglycemia is managed with IV glucose boluses, followed by continuous glucose infusion starting at 6 to 8 mg/kg/min.** Glucose infusions must be weaned slowly, with close monitoring of blood glucose levels, as the neonate begins to sustain a normal blood sugar level between feedings.

## Neonatal Diabetes Mellitus

NDM is a rare disorder manifested by persistent, insulin-sensitive hyperglycemia occurring as early as the first week of life and lasting more than 2 weeks. About half of all cases of NDM are of the transient form (TNDM) and half of the permanent form (PNDM).

**Pathophysiology.** The fundamental problem in NDM is the failure of the pancreas to release sufficient insulin in response to high blood glucose levels. NDM is unrelated to the presence of anti-insulin or anti-islet cell antibodies. In TNDM, diabetes develops within days of birth and resolves again within weeks or months before recurring, in a milder form, in late childhood. PNDM develops within days to months after birth and persists throughout life. Most cases of PNDM are caused by transcription factors involved in beta-cell development and in insulin secretion, the glucose-sensing enzyme glucokinase, and a gene-regulating immune response.

**Clinical Manifestations.** A common feature of NDM is IUGR, a result of insufficient insulin secretion and subsequent failure to thrive in utero. IUGR in infants with deficient insulin secretion in utero highlights the importance of insulin as a growth hormone. In addition to being small for gestational age, infants with NDM exhibit hyperglycemia, glycosuria, osmotic polyuria, dehydration, and minimal ketoacidosis.

**Diagnosis.** The diagnosis is made by demonstrating hyperglycemia with low levels of insulin, insulin-like growth factor-1, and C-peptide. The hyperglycemia responds to insulin infusion. Antibodies to insulin or islet cells are absent. If there are signs and symptoms of malabsorption, pancreatic agenesis should be ruled out by abdominal ultrasound. Based on clinical course, TNDM and PNDM cannot be differentiated in the neonatal period; genetic testing for chromosome 6 anomalies is required. If the neonate is shown to have a mutation of the adenosine triphosphate-sensitive postassium channels (KATP) channel, treatment with oral sulfonylureas rather than insulin is possible, tremendously beneficial to the child's glucose control and quality of life.

**Management.** Insulin therapy is necessary for some affected infants to manage hyperglycemia and achieve adequate growth, initially by continuous drip and transitioning to subcutaneous injection of an intermediate-acting insulin preparation when the condition permits. A high caloric intake can be challenging to maintain. In some infants, insulin therapy can be withdrawn after a period when it is observed that exogenous insulin induces hypoglycemia. The disease course in NDM is highly variable. Some infants with TNDM will have spontaneous recovery with no recurrence, whereas others will have apparent remission with a recurrence of permanent disease in late childhood. Infants with PNDM have no remission.

The opportunity for parents to speak with the pediatric endocrinologist and geneticist should be provided for information and guidance about the cause of NDM and the plans for continuing care for their infant. Close follow-up is essential even if the diabetes has resolved because of the high rate of recurrence later in childhood.

## Congenital Hyperinsulinism

Congenital hyperinsulinism is not a single disorder but a group of disorders with the common feature of hyperinsulinemic hypoglycemia. It is the most frequent cause of severe, persistent hypoglycemia in the newborn, with an incidence of 1 in 30,000 to 50,000 live births (Werny et al., 2018). Several different genetic forms have been described. Between 10% and 15% of congenital hyperinsulinism is transient and will spontaneously resolve at 1 month of age. Beckwith–Wiedemann syndrome is a congenital overgrowth syndrome with hyperinsulinism caused by beta-cell hyperplasia.

**Pathophysiology.** Hyperinsulinism is caused by unregulated insulin release from the entire pancreas (diffuse beta-cell hyperfunction) or confined areas of the pancreas (focal adenomatous islet-cell hyperplasia). Insulin lowers circulating glucose, suppressing lipolysis and ketogenesis and decreasing the availability of free fatty acids and ketone bodies. Because these are alternative energy substrates for the brain during hypoglycemia, hyperinsulinemia puts the infant at risk of severe neurologic dysfunction and seizures as consequences of neuroglycopenia.

**Clinical Manifestations.** Most infants with congenital hyperinsulinism present within the first postnatal days. Generally, they are born at term and are normal or large for gestational age. Many are macrosomic with a characteristic facial appearance. Neonates with Beckwith–Wiedemann syndrome present with a constellation of findings, including macroglossia, abdominal wall defects, Wilms' tumors, renal abnormalities, and facial nevus.

**Diagnosis.** Congenital hyperinsulinism is recognized by severe hypoglycemia with an insulin level that is inappropriate to the level of blood glucose that is present (e.g., insulin level > 5 U/ml with a plasma glucose level < 50 mg/dl).

Diagnostic criteria are a high glucose requirement (> 6–8 mg/kg/min) needed to maintain normoglycemia, low serum blood glucose by laboratory analysis, measurable insulin, raised C-peptide, low free fatty acids, and low ketone body concentrations. Blood sampling must occur during hypoglycemia to be of diagnostic value (Werny et al., 2018). The administration of glucagon during hypoglycemia results in a glycemic response.

**Management.** The cornerstones of management are a high caloric intake and pharmacologic therapy to inhibit insulin secretion by the pancreas. A central venous catheter is required to administer high glucose infusates during the acute phase safely. **Quality and Safety: Hypoglycemia must be avoided at all costs to decrease the chances of neurologic complications (Gillespie, 2022).** Drugs include diazoxide, which inhibits insulin secretion by blocking the sulfonylurea receptor of the beta-cell, and octreotide, a somatostatin analog. Diazoxide must be used cautiously in hyperbilirubinemia because it is highly protein bound and will displace bilirubin from albumin-binding sites.

Unfortunately, the responsiveness of infants with hyperinsulinism to these agents is inconsistent and variable. Babies who do not show an adequate and immediate response may require pancreatectomy to prevent recurrent neuroglycopenia. Preoperative localization procedures and intraoperative biopsies will determine the exact nature of the lesion and how much of the pancreas must be removed. Focal disease may require only a partial pancreatectomy, but a near-total (> 95%) removal of the pancreas is indicated for diffuse congenital hyperinsulinism. Loss of the pancreas can pose additional risks, such as pancreatic insufficiency and diabetes mellitus.

## Cystic Fibrosis

CF is an autosomal recessive disorder caused by mutations in the CF transmembrane conductance regulator (CFTR) gene that regulates the DFTR protein (NIH, NHLBI, n.d.). The incidence rate is decreasing, and survival is increasing to the fifth decade of life (Scotet et al., 2020). In the population of European descent, the incidence is 1 in 3,000 to 6,000 (Scotet et al., 2020).

**Pathophysiology.** Mutations in the *CFTR* gene affect the cyclic adenosine-5'-monophosphate (AMP)-mediated signals that stimulate chloride conductance in the epithelial cells of the exocrine ducts. Deficient chloride transport and the associated water transport abnormalities result in the production of abnormally viscid mucus. Nearly all organs and systems of the body are affected, including the lungs and upper respiratory tract, GI tract, pancreas, liver, sweat glands, and genitourinary (GU) tract. In the neonate, hyperviscous secretions in the intestines and a deficiency of pancreatic enzymes can create a sticky plug of meconium, a condition known as *meconium ileus*. The meconium has a higher protein and lower carbohydrate concentration, making it more viscid than normal meconium.

**Clinical Manifestations.** Without a family history or prenatal screening, CF is not recognized at the time of birth in most affected neonates unless a meconium ileus is present. A simple meconium ileus is usually identified at 24 to 48 hours of age (occasionally earlier) when there are signs of intestinal obstruction: abdominal distension, bilious vomiting, and either failure to pass meconium or passage of gray-colored stools. On examination, the dilated bowel loops have a doughy character that indents on palpation. A complicated meconium ileus has a more dramatic presentation with severe abdominal distension and signs of peritonitis such as tenderness, erythema, and clinical evidence of sepsis. The neonate may be acutely ill and require urgent surgical attention. Although not always present in the neonatal period, most patients with CF have pancreatic enzyme insufficiency and present with digestive symptoms or failure to thrive early in life.

**Diagnosis.** The possibility of CF is raised in the neonate with meconium ileus, and the diagnosis can be confirmed with DNA testing. A sweat test can also be performed after the first 48 hours of life if the infant is not edematous. A sweat test uses electrical-chemical stimulation of the skin to induce sweat, which is collected and analyzed for chloride content. Prenatal or carrier screening and newborn screening have impacted the declining incidence (Scotet et al., 2020). A meconium ileus is sometimes identified on prenatal ultrasound as a hyperechoic mass in the terminal ileum, representing thickened or dried meconium and dilated bowel loops. Postnatal abdominal radiographs show an unevenly dilated bowel and, occasionally, a characteristic "soap bubble" pattern, or small bubbles of gas caused by air mixing with the tenacious meconium.

**Management.** A meconium ileus requires prompt attention to prevent complications such as volvulus, bowel necrosis, or intestinal perforation. Treatment for simple meconium ileus is a therapeutic Gastrografin (diatrizoate meglumine) enema performed under fluoroscopy. Gastrografin is a hyperosmolar, radiopaque solution that evacuates the dried or thickened meconium from the intestine. Gastrografin is not used in infants with evidence of volvulus, gangrene, perforation, peritonitis, or atresia of the small bowel. The risks of the procedure are ischemia, hypovolemic shock, and perforation. It is essential to provide adequate hydration to compensate for the rapid fluid losses that can occur with the Gastrografin enema. It usually takes 24 to 48 hours to evacuate the softened meconium, and serial radiographs are typically ordered to monitor the evacuation. Feedings are started when signs of obstruction have subsided. **Quality and Safety: An infant who has undergone a Gastrografin enema should be observed closely for at least 48 hours for signs and symptoms of bowel perforation; late perforation is a rare but possible complication that can occur as long as 48 hours after the procedure.**

CF is also managed with a diet high in energy and fat to compensate for malabsorption and the increased energy demand of chronic inflammation. In addition to vitamin and mineral supplementation, a hydrolyzed protein formula containing medium-chain triglycerides (MCTs) is used. MCTs do not require digestion by pancreatic enzymes for absorption, but pancreatic enzyme supplements are also needed to improve fat absorption. Meticulous care of the perianal area must be taken because these enzymes can cause severe perianal dermatitis. Breastfeeding has been shown to have significant benefits for infants with CF.

Preventing pulmonary infections is important, as is removing mucus that can become trapped in the lungs. Targeted gene therapies called CFTR modulators, antibiotics, antiinflammatory agents, mucus-thinning agents such as hypertonic saline, bronchodilators to open the airways, pancreatic enzymes, stool softeners, and antacids are usual treatments (Chalmers, n.d.). CFTR modulators include ivacaftor, elexacaftor, and tezacaftor are used depending on the gene type of CF that is present (Chalmers, n.d.)

Finally, of utmost importance, the care of the neonate with CF requires a team approach.

## SUMMARY

Some neonatal endocrine disorders are rare; recognizing them requires a high index of suspicion. Neonatal screening programs have permitted the presymptomatic diagnosis of some of these disorders, which has led to earlier treatment and reduced morbidity. However, most endocrine disorders still require lifelong therapy for the affected infant.

## CASE STUDY

**Identification of the Problem.** A 34-week-gestation, 1.33-kg male infant was admitted to the NICU for small size and prematurity. Admission vital signs were heart rate (HR) 128, respiratory rate (RR) 72, blood pressure (BP) 42/23 (mean 30), and axillary temperature 97.4°F (36.3°C). The blood glucose screen (point of care) was 104.

A peripheral IV was started with $D_{10}W$ at 80 ml/kg/d (GIR 5.5 mg/kg/min), and the infant was made nothing by mouth (NPO). A repeat blood glucose screen on $D_{10}W$ showed a result of 545. Because this was believed to be an error, it was repeated, resulting in 550. A serum glucose level was drawn, and the IV fluids were changed to $D_5W$. The serum glucose was 535. The initial $D_{10}W$ fluid bag was sent to the laboratory for analysis.

The repeat blood glucose screen on $D_5W$ was 550 (serum 632). After IV fluids were changed to normal saline, the repeat blood glucose was 443 (serum 635). An insulin drip was started at 0.05 U/kg/hr and titrated to maintain a blood glucose level of less than 250.

**Assessment: History and Physical Examination.** The infant was born by cesarean section to a 25-year-old G1 P0 mother following a pregnancy complicated by oligohydramnios. Apgar scores were 7 and 9, and the arterial cord pH was 7.27. The infant's length was 38.5 cm, and the head circumference was 28 cm, placing the infant below the 10th percentile for all growth parameters.

Arterial blood gas (ABG) is taken in room air: pH 7.30, $PCO_2$ 35, $PO_2$ 128, base excess −7.7

Following this, 10 ml/kg of normal saline was given for metabolic acidosis.

Examination revealed a tiny but healthy-appearing male infant without evidence of respiratory distress.

**Differential Diagnosis.** The initial suspected "diagnosis" for the highly elevated blood glucose, in this case, was operator error; when the same result was obtained with a repeat specimen and confirmed by serum glucose, it was still viewed with a high degree of suspicion, and the IV fluids were sent to the laboratory for analysis. The differential diagnosis of hyperglycemia in neonates includes iatrogenic causes, poor insulin sensitivity of the very-low-birthweight or growth-restricted infant, sepsis, pancreatic agenesis, insulin resistance, TNDM or PNDM, and side effects of medications such as glucocorticoids and theophylline. Several of these were ruled out because they did not apply (the infant was not extremely premature, nor had the infant received any medications known to cause blood glucose elevation). Furthermore, the problem persisted after changing the IV fluids, ruling out an iatrogenic cause. Insulin resistance was ruled out because the infant responded promptly to an insulin infusion. The infant showed evidence of IUGR, but it was believed more likely that this was a consequence of the infant's primary problem rather than a cause of the primary problem.

**Diagnostic Tests.** The following tests were ordered to research the cause of hyperglycemia further:

- Complete blood count (CBC): hematocrit (Hct) 42%; white blood cells (WBCs) 4.4; segments (Segs) 20; bands 8; platelets 274,000
- Blood cultures were negative at 24 and 48 hours.
- Abdominal ultrasound (to rule out pancreatic agenesis): The organ appeared normal.
- Insulin autoantibodies were negative; the insulin drip was stopped for 2 hours, and insulin and C-peptide levels were drawn.
- RESULTS: Insulin level less than 2 mIU/ml
- C-peptide less than 0.5 ng/ml (reference range 0.8–3.1 ng/ml)
- Concurrent plasma glucose was 412

**Working Diagnosis.** The infant's presentation at birth and clinical course were most consistent with a diagnosis of NDM. The infant was IUGR, indicating a prenatal onset of the condition, and had mild metabolic acidosis. The infant had no evidence of autoimmune or structural pancreatic disease. The infant did not have septicemia or evidence of other infections. Furthermore, the laboratory studies revealed severe insulinopenia. The low level of C-peptide, a single-chain amino acid typically released with insulin in equal amounts, supports this diagnosis. It was not known whether the infant's NDM was transient or permanent; this would require molecular genetic analysis, a test that was not done during the initial hospitalization.

**Development of Management Plan.** The management plan was to reintroduce glucose while continuing the insulin infusion, advancing to total parental nutrition as tolerated. Glucose levels would be monitored at least every 2 hours to keep the blood glucose under 250. The plan included the introduction of feedings as early as feasible to improve control of blood glucose. Continuous insulin would be weaned as tolerated. If the diabetes showed no signs of resolution, subcutaneous insulin would be started for long-term management. The infant would continue to be followed by the pediatric endocrinologist.

**Implementation and Evaluation of Effectiveness.** Stabilizing the blood glucose level over the first few days proved difficult. On total parenteral nutrition (TPN), the infant fluctuated between hyperglycemia and hypoglycemia. Feedings were introduced, providing stability, although weight gain remained slow. The infant was eventually successfully managed with and discharged on subcutaneous insulin.

## ONLINE RESOURCES

CourseConnect

Resources for this chapter are online and available at www.springerpub.com/courseconnect.

## REFERENCES

References for this chapter are online and available at www.springerpub.com/courseconnect.

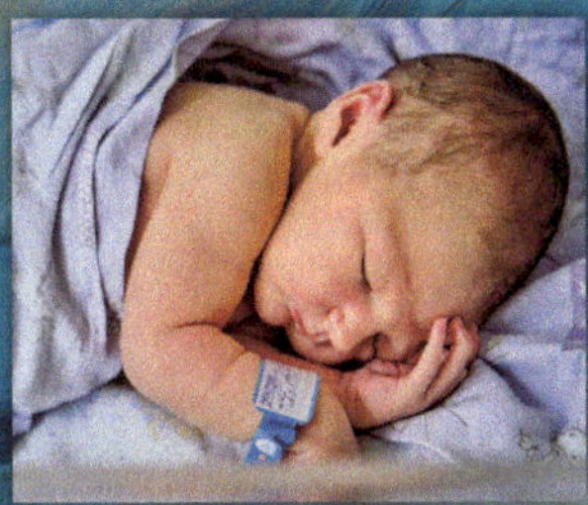

Adobe Stock.

CHAPTER 11

# Immune System

**Jacqueline Hoffman and Mike Kurz**

## INTRODUCTION

Despite all the lessons we have learned, neonatal sepsis continues to be a leading cause of neonatal and infant morbidity and mortality. The intact uterine environment helps to protect the fetus from a variety of pathogens including bacteria, viruses, fungi, protozoa, and parasites. Although there is protection, it is not absolute: Breaches do occur. The birth canal may not be a sterile environment, as once thought. New evidence has shown the presence of pathogens in the placenta and amniotic fluid in asymptomatic term pregnancies. However, the role of transfer of the placental microbiome from birthing parent to fetus, and whether this influences the infant gut is less clear (Gil et al., 2020). The newborn is exposed to a wide variety of microorganisms during labor and delivery. The level of exposure is increased in the event of ruptured membranes. The extrauterine environment exposes the infant to even more potential pathogens.

To understand and appreciate the challenges infants face in the first few days and weeks of life, it is necessary to review the basics of innate and adaptive immunity and potential alterations to the neonatal immune system. This chapter will discuss the development of the immune system and will describe assessment parameters for evaluating the infant with suspected and culture-proven infection as well as diagnostic measures and treatment for the most common causes of newborn infection. Due to the importance of a broader approach to combating mortality from neonatal sepsis, a global perspective will be presented. The emergence of resistant organisms and the possible detrimental effects of prolonged antibiotic usage are becoming more influential in the treatment choices in individual units; therefore, the importance of antibiotic stewardship will be introduced.

## DEVELOPMENT OF THE IMMUNE SYSTEM

The overall goal of the immune system is to recognize foreign substances and activate subsystems to inactivate, destroy, and eliminate this material from the body. Immaturity of the immune system, especially in preterm infants, contributes to increased susceptibility to bacterial, viral, and fungal infections. The immune system consists of two separate immune responses: the innate immune response and the adaptive immune response. The innate immune system is what you are born with and is the first line of defense. It consists of external barriers such as the skin and mucous membranes, leukocytes and other defense cells, enzymes, and proteins in the blood. Natural killer cells are an important part of the innate immune system. These cells destroy invasive cells with cytotoxins (Benjamin et al., 2025). It is easy to see why this system is considered the first line of defense. The adaptive system takes over when the innate system fails to destroy the foreign substance. It may be delayed, but it is more accurate and efficient. This system produces memory cells, which are responsible for immunologic memory. The adaptive immune system is composed of T lymphocytes, B lymphocytes, and antibodies (Simon et al., 2015).

### Innate Immune System

The innate or natural immune system is the first line of defense, acting within minutes of initial exposure. This system does not require prior exposure to the pathogen to mount a response (Lewis et al., 2025). This system consists of granulocytes (mainly neutrophils), antigen-presenting cells (monocytes), and natural killer cells. Neutrophils are the first phagocytic cells to reach the site of infection; sensing the foreign pathogen, neutrophils adhere to the vascular endothelium and, when pathogens invade, are the first to migrate toward the site of infection to engulf and kill the pathogen. The response to the infectious process is to release more neutrophils from the storage pool. When the immune system is overtaxed or immature, the result is a release of both mature and immature neutrophils, resulting in what is known as a left shift (Box 11.1).

The innate immune system utilizes toll-like receptors (expressed on monocytes), nucleotide-binding oligomerization domain (NOD)–like receptors, and retinoic acid-inducible gene (RIG)–like receptors to identify and respond to pathogen-associated molecular patterns leading to the production of

**BOX 11.1**

**CALCULATING THE I:T RATIO FOR NEONATAL SEPSIS**

Clinical application: The immature-to-total (I:T) ratio is a common tool used when there is a concern for neonatal sepsis. To calculate:

**Total number of immature neutrophils** (promyelocytes, myelocytes, metamyelocytes, and banded neutrophils) divided by the **total number of immature + mature neutrophils**

A shift to the left of > 0.2, or 20%, is concerning for potential infection

cytokines, resulting in proinflammatory responses, and activation of the adaptive immune system (Santacroce et al., 2024). Neonates have a decreased ability to produce proinflammatory cytokines, in particular tumor necrosis factor (TNF) and interleukin (IL)-6. Neonates also have decreased neutrophil and dendritic cell functions, decreased adhesion ability, and decreased response to chemotactic factors affecting the ability to deform and penetrate the vascular endothelial lining (Basha et al., 2014; Camacho-Gonzalez et al., 2013). Additionally, there is reduced cytokine production, resulting in decreased activation of natural killer cells. All of these conditions in the neonate place the neonate at increased susceptibility to bacterial and viral infections (Camacho-Gonzalez et al., 2013).

## Adaptive Immune System

The adaptive or acquired immune system relies on exposure and memory; this antigen-specific response is guided by recognition from prior exposure to pathogens. The adaptive immune system relies on T lymphocytes and B lymphocytes. T lymphocytes provide cell-mediated immunity. They develop in the thymus and then circulate to the periphery (Lewis et al., 2025). There are two different types of T lymphocytes: CD4 T cells and CD8 T cells. The CD4 T cells are "helper" cells that stimulate antibody production, whereas CD8 T cells act as cytotoxic killer cells. B lymphocytes provide humoral immunity. They develop in the bone marrow and circulate to the peripheral lymphatic system, where they differentiate into plasma cells that secrete five types of immunoglobulins: immunoglobulin A (IgA), immunoglobulin D (IgD), immunoglobulin E (IgE), immunoglobulin G (IgG), and immunoglobulin M (IgM). The only immunoglobulin transplacentally transferred is IgG. Active transplacental transfer of IgG is noted in the fetus beginning at 13 weeks and approximates 50% of birthing-parent levels by 32 weeks' gestation; levels begin to fall rapidly after birth. The presence of IgM in the neonate at birth reflects a response to intraamniotic infection exposure (Lewis et al., 2025).

To minimize the overwhelming inflammatory response that would otherwise occur at the time of delivery from a relatively sterile environment, the adaptive immune system function increases slowly in the newborn. Skin and mucosal barriers in preterm infants are less effective than those in term and older neonates (Collins et al., 2018). The neonate has decreased cytotoxic function and decreased cell memory, impacting the ability to respond effectively to infections (Camacho-Gonzalez et al., 2013).

The development of the immune system in the fetus and newborn cannot be studied in isolation from influences provided by the birthing parent. The ability of the birthing parent's body to tolerate the fetus during pregnancy, rather than rejecting it as a foreign body, is not thoroughly understood. It is well documented that birthing-parent blood with immunocompetent T lymphocytes circulates in contact with fetal cells, that both fetal and birthing-parent cells are exchanged through the placenta, and that humoral and cellular immunity to fetal antigens develop in the birthing parent. Recent studies have focused on birthing-parent antibody transfer because it protects the newborn from infection prior to childhood immunizations and the infant's natural responses to infection. Secretory IgA in breast milk may also interfere with successful immunization, particularly with live poliovirus, by neutralizing the virus by antibodies in the gastrointestinal (GI) tract (Jennewein et al., 2017; Remington et al., 2025).

Birthing-parent placental transfer of IgG is inversely related to gestational age; there is minimal birthing-parent IgG transfer in the first trimester but increases occur throughout gestation with the most significant increases occurring during the third trimester. This late transfer leaves premature infants with a relative IgG deficiency (only 50% transfer by 32 weeks' gestation). Such immunity is transient; nevertheless, it may provide protection during a vulnerable time of life (Camacho-Gonzalez et al., 2013; Lewis et al., 2025). An exciting area of study is the use of prenatal immunization provided to the birthing parent as a promising strategy to enhance the transfer of pathogen-specific IgG to the fetus, providing newborns with crucial early immunity (Wessel & Dolatshahi, 2023). After birth, levels of IgG fall to their nadir between 2 and 4 months of age, which is referred to as *physiologic* or *transient hypogammaglobulinemia*. Infants do not begin producing their own IgG in response to exposure to pathogens until around 6 months of age.

New and exciting evidence is available concerning the effect of birthing-parent microbiota on neonatal immune development. It is now recognized that the birthing parent's diet, including micronutrients and the birthing parent's microbiome, significantly influences the neonatal innate and adaptive immune systems. It is known that the birthing parent's gut and genital microbiota are transferred to the infant at birth and through the placental pathway (Jennewein et al., 2017).

## Global Perspective on Neonatal Infection

The incidence of infection varies according to the level of perinatal care available, economic standards, and other perinatal risk factors in newborns, such as prematurity. Because the world is becoming smaller in terms of travel and cross-cultural engagement, it is no longer sufficient to concern ourselves with what is relevant to the North American continent. Our greatest concern is the challenge to eliminate the gaps in healthcare access and, therefore, to improve health outcomes worldwide. One of the barriers to understanding the overall burden of neonatal infection globally is the general paucity of data from low- and middle-income countries (Fleischmann-Struzek et al., 2018). Although child and infant mortality is declining globally, infant morbidity is not. Over the past three decades, there has been a significant decrease in mortality from neonatal infection, with Global Burden of Disease 2021 data showing that neonatal sepsis and infection make up only 5% of deaths in children under 5 years of age (Institute for Health Metrics and Evaluation, 2021). During the same time period, however, there has been a 46% increase in the global incidence of neonatal sepsis and infection (Li et al., 2023). In the United States, the incidence of culture-proven early-onset sepsis (EOS) is estimated to be 0.77 to 1 per 1,000 live births. The incidence and mortality in very low birth weight (VLBW) infants are significantly higher. In the United States, there is a large disparity in rates of infection and mortality, with Black infants, preterm especially, having the highest rates of sepsis and mortality at 5.14 per 1,000 live births (Gollehon, 2019; Simonsen et al., 2014). In those settings with the highest mortality (low- and middle-income countries), neonatal infections may account for up to 40% of all neonatal deaths (Imam et al., 2025). Improved knowledge and technology to care for premature and growth-restricted newborns have led to an increased population of newborns at higher risk for bacterial infection. Understanding the importance of optimizing nutritional support, thermoregulation, and acid–base status of the infant at risk for being compromised as a result of infection is important to maximize the benefit of management. Major complications of infection include respiratory distress, septic shock, acidosis, disseminated intravascular coagulation (DIC), and meningitis. Long-term morbidity remains a concerning consequence of neonatal infections.

## ASSESSMENT AND MANAGEMENT OF THE INFANT WITH SUSPECTED OR PROVEN INFECTION

Host defense mechanisms begin to develop early in gestation; however, they remain immature and often do not function efficiently even in the term newborn. Although the neonate's immune system is not fully developed, the newborn is able to respond to the environment, resulting in specific markers that can be detected in lab studies, such as the complete blood count (CBC) and the C-reactive protein (CRP). Even so, the infant's immature immune system is easily overwhelmed. The immaturity of the immune system is responsible for the relatively high prevalence of infectious disease during the neonatal period and the occurrence of neonatal infection from microorganisms that do not generally cause infection in older individuals. The susceptibility to infectious processes and the associated high morbidity and mortality make early identification and treatment of newborn infection a critical component of care (Gollehon, 2019).

### Clinical Signs of Infection

Identifying and caring for a newborn with an infection can be one of the greatest challenges in nursing. Bedside caregivers are often the first to recognize that there is something "wrong" with an infant, and this often leads to investigation of the signs. Generally, treatment is begun once a presumptive diagnosis of infection is made because the benefits of early treatment most often outweigh the risks of unnecessary treatment. Signs and symptoms of neonatal sepsis are nonspecific and are often related to the specific organism responsible. The presentation and differential diagnosis may also be attributed to other diseases or conditions such as respiratory distress syndrome (RDS), metabolic disorders, or stress from a difficult delivery. These other diagnoses must be ruled out while maintaining a high index of suspicion for sepsis. The most commonly recognized signs and symptoms of infection are listed in Box 11.2. Temperature instability, hypothermia in particular, and the inability of the neonate to maintain temperature in the normal range with core temperature less than or equal to 95°F (35°C) is a strong predictor for infection. Newborns traditionally do not have well-developed febrile mechanisms;

**BOX 11.2**

**SIGNS AND SYMPTOMS OF NEONATAL INFECTION**

**Clinical**

- General appearance
- Poor feeding
- Irritability
- Lethargy
- Temperature instability

**Skin**

- Petechiae
- Pustulosis
- Sclerema
- Edema
- Jaundice

**Respiratory**

- Grunting
- Nasal flaring
- Intercostal retractions
- Tachypnea/apnea

**Gastrointestinal**

- Diarrhea
- Hematochezia
- Abdominal distention
- Emesis
- Aspirates

**Central Nervous System**

- Hypotonia
- Seizures
- Poor spontaneous movement

**Circulatory**

- Bradycardia/tachycardia
- Hypotension
- Cyanosis
- Decreased perfusion

(*continued*)

**BOX 11.2**

**SIGNS AND SYMPTOMS OF NEONATAL INFECTION (*continued*)**

**Laboratory Values**

WBC count

- Neutrophils
- < 5,000 cells/mm³, neutropenia
- > 25,000 cells/mm³, neutrophilia
- Absolute neutrophil count (neutrophil and bands)
- < 1,800 cells/mm³ (during first week)
- Immature: total neutrophil ratio
- > 0:2
- Platelet count
- < 100,000, thrombocytopenia
- Cerebrospinal fluid (results outside the normal ranges below suggest CNS infection)
- Protein (normal values)
- 150 to 200 mg/L (term)
- 300 mg/L (preterm)
- Glucose (normal values)
- 50% to 60% or more of blood glucose level

*Note:* Symptoms and values are based on over 30 years of practice and observation by the authors. Individual practices must rely on current literature for diagnosis and treatment plans.

therefore, the absence of fever does not indicate the absence of infection. More often, premature infants present with a low body temperature. Hyperthermia may occur in both bacterial and viral infections in term newborns, with core temperatures greater than 100.4°F (38°C), but this is relatively rare in preterm infants. An infected infant may present with lethargy, poor feeding, decreased reflexes, abdominal distention, delayed gastric emptying time, and perhaps diarrhea or loose green or brown stools. Hypoglycemia or hyperglycemia, as well as glycosuria, may result from impaired glucose metabolism and the inability to maintain normal metabolic processes (Gordon et al., 2025).

Vascular perfusion is typically decreased; the infected neonate may appear gray, mottled, or ashen in color with poor perfusion, prolonged capillary refill time, and hypotension (the hallmark of septic shock). Skin changes may also include cyanosis and petechiae. Thrombocytopenia is often present. Infections can cause DIC, resulting in altered prothrombin time (PT), partial thromboplastin time (PTT), and fibrin split product laboratory values. Hemolytic anemia may occur as a part of the inflammatory process, and this can significantly decrease oxygen-carrying capacity, especially in preterm infants. Cardiovascular shock and hypotension can be a sudden clinical sign of fulminant infection that requires immediate and aggressive intervention to restore adequate circulation. Unexplained bradycardia, sclerema, sudden purpura, rash, or petechiae are other signs of systemic infection (Weinberg & D'Angio, 2025).

Apnea in a term (nonsedated) newborn in the first few hours of life should be considered a serious sign of inability to regulate the brain's respiratory center. Apnea in the first 24 hours of life in a preterm newborn is a common sign of infection. Respiratory distress can be an early sign of pneumonia and must be considered carefully. Jaundice, hepatosplenomegaly, and irritability may also be found in infants with infection. The wide variability of signs of infection warrants the inclusion of infection as part of the differential diagnosis in any ill-appearing infant.

## Risk Factors

Prematurity is the most prevalent risk factor for infection because premature infants are far more susceptible to the invasion of foreign microorganisms and far less capable of mounting an immune response. Preterm infants have decreased birthing-parent antibodies (passive immunity). The birthing-parent antibodies, developed by exposure to antigens and subsequent creation of an antibody defense system, provide temporary protection to the newborn. Still, preterm newborns are born before the majority of birthing-parent antibodies are transferred from the birthing parent's circulation. Also, the cellular immune system is not well developed in the preterm newborn; thus, there are decreased phagocytic cellular defenses.

Prolonged rupture of the fetal membranes (PROM) is a well-known risk factor for the development of infection. The fetus is at increased risk because a break in the amniotic sac provides a pathway for the migration of microorganisms up the vaginal vault to the fetus. Delaying delivery in pregnancy in a birthing parent with PROM and a preterm fetus before pulmonary maturity is achieved creates the potential environment for bacterial proliferation and subsequent newborn infection. In this case, the benefit of promoting the maturity of the immature lungs is weighed against the risk of overwhelming infection in the baby. The development of pulmonary hypoplasia is another serious concern when delivery is delayed after premature PROM (Riley & Swamy, 2025). PROM, a rupture of membranes lasting longer than 18 hours, is considered a risk factor in evaluating infants for potential infections (Jefferies, 2017; Shah & Padbury, 2014).

Although the most common cause of birthing-parent fever in labor is dehydration, a fever may indicate birthing-parent intraamniotic or systemic infection and warrants further assessment. A birthing parent with an infection before or during delivery may transmit it to the infant. If the birthing parent's temperature is greater than or equal to 100.4°F (38°C) during labor, evaluation for infection in he newborn is warranted (Riley & Swamy, 2025). Birthing parent cervical or amniotic fluid cultures may identify the causative microorganism. If the birthing parent's illness suggests viral infection, newborn viral cultures should be obtained. Early identification of causative agents in the birthing parent may help in the management of the newborn by allowing faster identification of the microorganism and initiation of appropriate antimicrobial therapy.

Foul-smelling amniotic fluid is an indication for newborn antimicrobial therapy in symptomatic infants. Routine blood cultures and a CBC with differential are indicated as a screen for newborn infection. Under these circumstances, the placenta should be sent for pathologic evaluation. Other risk factors associated with newborn infection are antenatal or intrapartum asphyxia, iatrogenic complications of treatment, and invasive procedures.

Stress inhibits the ability to fight infection by increasing the metabolic rate, which requires more oxygen and energy. A severely compromised, hypoxemic newborn may have regional tissue damage. Ischemic or necrotic areas in the lungs, heart, brain, or GI system promote colonization and overgrowth of normal bacterial flora. This overgrowth of bacteria is one of the most common sources of newborn infection. Tissue damage can be prevented or repaired only if the infectious process is reversed and adequate tissue perfusion is restored.

Several known birthing parent factors are associated with newborn infection: low socioeconomic status, malnutrition, inadequate prenatal care, substance abuse, premature or prolonged rupture of membranes, presence of a urinary tract infection (UTI) at delivery, peripartum infection, clinical intraamniotic infection, and general bacterial colonization. Newborn risk factors include antenatal stress, intrapartum stress (perinatal asphyxia), congenital anomalies, male sex, multiple gestations, concurrent neonatal disease processes, prematurity immaturity of the immune system, invasive admission procedures, and antimicrobial therapies.

## Diagnostic Workup

A high index of suspicion for infection, early identification of the microorganism, and institution of appropriate therapy provide the best outcome. The index of suspicion is directly proportional to the birthing parent's history and risk factors. Early and accurate diagnosis of infection in the newborn is a difficult task and is often complicated by the nonspecific signs associated with sepsis exhibited by the newborn. The evaluation for infection in the newborn often depends on whether EOS or late-onset sepsis (LOS) is suspected. EOS is most often defined as sepsis that presents within the first 72 hours of life; however, many definitions include sepsis that occurs within the first 6 days of life. LOS is, therefore, sepsis that presents after the first week of life. Very LOS may occur up to 3 months of age, usually from group B streptococcus (GBS; Gordon et al., 2025).

The perfect screen for neonatal sepsis has not been determined, although some laboratory aids have been found to be very helpful in diagnosing neonatal sepsis. A CBC is often the first step in evaluating for infection. The CBC of an infected infant may reveal leukopenia (low white blood cell [WBC] count < 5,000 cells/mm$^3$), elevated WBC (WBC count > 25,000 cells/mm$^3$), or a preponderance of immature neutrophils with the immature-to-total cell ratio (I:T) greater than 0.2. The I:T ratio is the most studied ratio of neutrophil counts and adds a level of confidence that is not appreciated with a banded neutrophil count alone. More importantly may be the negative predictive value of the I:T ratio. If I:T ratios are normal, it is unlikely that the infant is septic. Keep in mind that if the CBC is obtained early in the infectious process, it may not reflect abnormalities. A follow-up CBC in 12 to 24 hours should be considered for the infant with an initially normal CBC but who is symptomatic for sepsis; this CBC may reflect abnormalities at that time. The use of the CRP has added another level of confidence in excluding serious infection, in evaluating the infant's response to treatment, and in determining the length of therapy. Serial CRPs have been found to be more reliable than a single level. In the presence of EOS, CRP levels may be normal at the onset of symptoms but are typically elevated by 24 hours of age and remain elevated during the acute phase of infection or inflammation.

If signs of central nervous system (CNS) involvement are present, a lumbar puncture (LP) for cerebrospinal fluid (CSF) cultures is indicated, whether EOS or LOS is suspected. Because UTIs are extremely uncommon during the first few days of life, a urine culture is not indicated for EOS (Shane et al., 2017). Gram stain of the CSF or urine can give an early indication of the type of microorganism responsible for the infection. Evaluation of the WBC count, protein, and glucose levels of the CSF may also indicate the presence of infection. A chest radiograph in an infant with respiratory distress can identify the presence of pneumonia. Other tests that may be useful include latex agglutination (LA) or counter-immunoelectrophoresis (CIE) of urine or CSF or other body cavity fluids and erythrocyte sedimentation rate (ESR). Serum procalcitonin (PCT) is a test that is gaining favor in the diagnostic evaluation of possible bacterial sepsis in older infants and adults but is not commonly used to diagnose bacterial infection in newborns. The known fluctuations seen in the newborn during the first 48 hours complicate its usefulness. Traditionally, culture-positive sepsis from blood, CSF, urine, and other body fluids is the most valid diagnostic sign.

## Differential Diagnosis

The microorganisms responsible for newborn infection have changed over the past 60 years, and there are marked regional variations. Organisms responsible for EOS differ from those responsible for LOS; therefore, the antimicrobial agents of choice differ based on the timing of symptoms. Even with the implementation of prophylactic use of intrapartum antibiotics, GBS remains the leading cause of EOS followed by *Escherichia coli* (*E. coli*). Some microorganisms, including *E. coli*, groups A and B treptococci, and *Listeria monocytogenes*, are often implicated in EOS and LOS. Other organisms, including *Staphylococcus aureus*, coagulase-negative staphylococci (CoNS), and *Pseudomonas aeruginosa*, are typically associated with LOS (Gordon et al., 2025). After day 7, nosocomial microorganisms should be considered. CoNS is the most frequently identified organism in newborn infants with nosocomial infection, particularly when invasive medical devices have been used, with gram-negative organisms and fungi following. Hospitalized preterm newborns are often affected by repeated episodes of infection. Many of these episodes are termed presumed, suspected, or clinical infection because no microorganism is recovered and cultured, despite clinical evidence of infection that responds to antimicrobial therapy (Shane et al., 2017).

## Prognosis

The introduction of broad-spectrum antimicrobial agents dramatically improved the prognosis for infection and resulted in a decline in infection-associated neonatal and infant deaths in the United States. However, infection still accounts for significant morbidity and mortality in the neonatal period.

Consequences of bacterial infection include prolonged hospitalization, increased hospital costs, and increased mortality. Term infants who are promptly and adequately treated for sepsis rarely have long-term, sepsis-associated health problems; however, neurologic sequelae are seen in 15% to 30% of infants with septic meningitis. Preterm infants with sepsis are more likely to experience long-term neurologic damage, especially if shock is present (Gollehon, 2019).

## Management

Management of a newborn with an infection is aimed at the traditional "ABCs": airway (including oxygen, ventilation, and correction of acidosis), breathing, and circulation, with the addition of volume expansion, antimicrobial agents, and consideration of immune therapy. The exact management plan is based on an assessment of clinical signs, careful history, and appropriate laboratory findings with consideration of the most likely microorganisms. Treatment should begin as soon as sepsis is suspected due to the newborn's state of immuno-immaturity. Antimicrobial agents should be started as soon as relevant diagnostic tests have been completed (Gollehon, 2019).

## Antimicrobial Agents

The selection of antimicrobial agents is based on the identification of the microorganism and the infant's response to therapy. Treatment decisions are divided into empirical (suspected sepsis) or definitive (known pathogen). The prudent use of empiric therapy is necessary in this age of increasingly resistant organisms in our hospitals and communities. Infectious microorganisms are divided into two broad classes based on Gram-stain results: gram-positive and gram-negative (Shane et al., 2017). The shape of the microorganism categorizes it as either a coccus or a rod. Generally, gram-positive organisms respond to broad-spectrum antibiotics, such as penicillin analogues and first-generation cephalosporins (beta-lactamases), and the beta-lactamase penicillins. The gram-negative microorganisms are most often susceptible to aminoglycosides and cephalosporins. Tests must be run to determine the specific sensitivity of a microorganism to the antimicrobial agent selected to ensure that the appropriate agent is prescribed (Shane et al., 2017). In the United States and Canada, empiric therapy for EOS sepsis is generally treated with a combined approach such as intravenous (IV) ampicillin and an aminoglycoside (usually gentamicin); a third-generation cephalosporin should be considered if there is concern for meningitis (Gollehon, 2019). This approach provides coverage for the most likely organisms, which include gram-positive organisms such as GBS and gram-negative bacteria such as *E. coli*. If LOS is suspected, antibiotic choices should be based on the site of infection and those that are effective against known hospital-acquired infections, such as *S. aureus, S. epidermidis,* and *Pseudomonas* species (Simonsen et al., 2014).

Generally speaking, antimicrobial choices are based on organisms known to be present in the local nursery. Gram-positive cocci generally respond to penicillin, unless the microorganism produces beta-lactamase (or penicillinase). The beta-lactamase destroys the penicillin. *Staphylococcus aureus* is a beta-lactamase–producing microorganism and is, therefore, not responsive to penicillin. A group of semisynthetic penicillins with added side chains are used for the treatment of *S. aureus* infection. Of this group, nafcillin and oxacillin are most often used. Other similar drugs are methicillin, dicloxacillin, and cloxacillin. First-generation cephalosporins, such as cefazolin, cephalexin, and cephalothin, are also resistant to beta-lactamase. *Staphylococcus epidermidis* and *S. aureus* strains may be resistant to penicillin, semisynthetic penicillins, and cephalosporins. Methicillin-resistant *S. aureus* (MRSA) is unresponsive to the semisynthetic penicillins. In this case, vancomycin is the drug of choice (Simonsen et al., 2014). It may also be used for *S. epidermidis* and infection related to foreign bodies or invasive procedures. The emergence of resistant strains to available antimicrobial agents is an increasing concern due to the lack of other safe and effective antimicrobial agents to treat the infection (Shane et al., 2017).

Third-generation cephalosporins are used to treat gram-negative cocci that are penicillin and methicillin resistant. Carbapenems, such as meropenem, may also be considered for extended-spectrum beta-lactamase–producing gram-negative bacilli infections. *Listeria monocytogenes*, a gram-positive rod, generally responds to ampicillin therapy. Aminoglycosides or third-generation cephalosporins are the drugs of choice for gram-negative enteric rods (Shane et al., 2017). Some gram-negative rods are classified according to their lactose fermentation ability. The lactose fermenters, *E. coli* and *Klebsiella*, are sensitive to aminoglycosides and third-generation cephalosporins. *Shigella* and *Salmonella* are non–lactose fermenters that respond well to ampicillin and third-generation cephalosporins. *Haemophilus influenzae* is usually sensitive to ampicillin and third-generation cephalosporins, although some strains are ampicillin resistant. *Pseudomonas* requires the following combination therapy: aminoglycoside and an antipseudomonal penicillin such as azlocillin, carbenicillin, imipenem, mezlocillin, piperacillin, or ticarcillin (Simonsen et al., 2014).

Two anaerobic microorganisms, *Bacteroides fragilis* (gram-negative) and *Clostridium* (gram-positive), are sometimes the cause of newborn infections. *Bacteroides fragilis* is susceptible to metronidazole (Flagyl), clindamycin, chloramphenicol, and some of the newer beta-lactamases, such as imipenem and ampicillin with sulbactam. *Clostridium* is usually susceptible to penicillin. A combination of ampicillin or penicillin and gentamicin is useful for antibacterial action against *Streptococcus*, *L. monocytogenes*, and gram-negative enteric rods. This combination of antimicrobial agents has a synergistic effect (in vitro), increasing the efficacy of either drug therapy used alone. Additional therapy or selection of other agents is necessary if staphylococcal infection is suspected, if *Pseudomonas* or *Bacteroides* (most often iatrogenic) is present, if there is an outbreak of resistant organisms, or if prolonged ampicillin and gentamicin therapy has been used (Simonsen et al., 2014). Antimicrobial agents must be reevaluated after completion of cultures and sensitivity testing. Tables 11.1 and 11.2 show generally recommended antimicrobial choices for infections caused by gram-positive and gram-negative microorganisms.

**TABLE 11.1**

**GENERAL ANTIMICROBIAL SELECTION GUIDELINES FOR GRAM-POSITIVE MICROORGANISMS**

| Microorganism | Antimicrobial |
|---|---|
| *Streptococcus* | Penicillin or ampicillin |
| *Staphylococcus aureus* | Semisynthetic penicillins, such as methicillin (or methicillin-type), nafcillin, oxacillin, dicloxacillin, cephalin, cephalothin |
| MRSA | Vancomycin |
| *Staphylococcus epidermidis* | Vancomycin |
| *Listeria monocytogenes* | Ampicillin |
| *Clostridium difficile* | Penicillin |

MRSA, methicillin-resistant *S. aureus.*

**TABLE 11.2**

**GENERAL ANTIMICROBIAL SELECTION GUIDELINES FOR GRAM-NEGATIVE MICROORGANISMS**

| Microorganism | Antimicrobial |
|---|---|
| *Escherichia coli* | Aminoglycosides or third-generation cephalosporins |
| *Klebsiella* | Aminoglycosides or third-generation cephalosporins |
| *Shigella* | Ampicillin and third-generation cephalosporins |
| *Salmonella* | Ampicillin and third-generation cephalosporins |
| *Haemophilus influenzae* | Ampicillin and third-generation cephalosporins; some strains are ampicillin resistant |
| *Pseudomonas* | Aminoglycoside plus an antipseudomonal penicillin |
| *Serratia* | Aminoglycoside plus an antipseudomonal penicillin |
| *Bacteroides fragilis* | Metronidazole, clindamycin, some beta-lactamases such as imipenem, and ampicillin with sulbactam; and chloramphenicol |

## TYPES OF NEONATAL INFECTION

This section briefly describes the types of microorganisms that typically cause neonatal infection and their clinical manifestations, diagnosis, and collaborative management. The discussion includes both congenitally acquired and nosocomially acquired infections caused by bacterial, viral, fungal, and protozoal organisms.

### Bacterial Infections

#### Group B Streptococcus

Group B beta-hemolytic streptococci were unknown to the perinatal scene until the early 1970s when they replaced *E. coli* as the single most common pathogen associated with bacterial meningitis during the first 2 months of life. Since the implementation of intrapartum antibiotic prophylaxis (IAP) for the prevention of neonatal GBS disease, rates of EOS with GBS have declined to 0.23 to 0.25 cases per 1,000 live births in the United States; however, GBS sepsis continues to be the most common pathogen in term infants (CDC, 2024b; Ratner et al., 2025).

**Epidemiology.** The number of newborn deaths associated with either early-onset or late-onset GBS infections continues to be high, particularly in high-risk urban centers. The potential for permanent neurologic sequelae for infant survivors of meningeal infections is significantly high (32%–46% with some degree of long-term neurologic effects). The mortality rate of infected newborns varies according to time of onset. Early-onset infection (within the first week of life) has a mortality rate of 2% to 10%, which has decreased from 50% in the 1970s; late-onset (after the first week of life) mortality is approximately 3% (Ratner et al., 2025). Although the incidence of GBS EOS has declined, universal screening and IAP has not resulted in a decline in the incidence or morbidity of LOS;

the incidence of late-onset GBS now exceeds that of early-onset GBS at 0.29 cases per 1,000 live births in the United States in 2020 (AAP, 2024f). More research is needed related to disparity and the burden of prenatal GBS (AAP, 2024f; Puopolo et al., 2019).

GBS is a gram-positive diplococcus with an ultrastructure similar to that of other gram-positive cocci. It was classified as hemolytic because of its double zone of hemolysis surrounding colonies on blood agar plates. Culture of body fluids, such as blood, urine, CSF, and other secretions, is the most common method of identifying group B streptococci. More rapid techniques, DNA probe assays, LA assays, and nucleic acid amplification assays, such as polymerase chain reaction (PCR), enable a presumptive diagnosis before cultures are returned. Rapid identification of the GBS organism is important in treating the colonized pregnant birthing parent and in the early diagnosis and treatment of infection in the sick, unstable septic infant. To accurately predict birthing parent colonization with group B streptococci, both vaginal and rectal areas should be cultured on more than one occasion (AAP, 2024f; Puopolo et al., 2019).

**Clinical Manifestations.** GBS has been identified as a relatively common cause of midgestational fetal loss in birthing parents who experience vaginal hemorrhage, PROM, fetal membrane infection, and spontaneous abortion. The rate of stillbirth is reported to be as high as 61% in association with these bacteria. Early-onset neonatal infections with GBS can be asymptomatic or can manifest with severe symptoms of respiratory distress and shock, which can rapidly progress to death (Gordon et al., 2025).

**Early-Onset Group B Streptococcus.** Early-onset GBS infection usually appears within the first 24 hours of life, with approximately 95% of all cases occurring within 48 hours. Although early-onset GBS infection is a higher risk in preterm and low birth weight (LBW) infants, *E. coli* is now the most common pathogen in this group (Ratner et al., 2025). Common presentations are bacteremia (80%–85%), pneumonia (~10%), and meningitis (5%–10%) (Ratner et al., 2025). Congenital pneumonia is a more common presenting sign in infants who weigh 1,000 g or less. Signs of respiratory distress (apnea, grunting, tachypnea, and cyanosis) are common with early-onset GBS. Hypotension and metabolic acidosis are found in up to one-third of newborns with GBS infection; these infants are at risk for cardiopulmonary collapse. Nonspecific signs of infection include lethargy, poor feeding, temperature instability, abdominal distention, pallor, tachycardia, and jaundice (Ratner et al., 2025). Experienced nurses may observe that the neonate "just doesn't look right," which is sometimes a critical point for early detection and implementation of therapy. Overwhelming GBS septicemia is often compounded by meningitis. LP and examination of the CSF are the only ways to exclude meningeal involvement and, therefore, represent an important part of the workup. Seizures may occur in infants with GBS meningitis.

**Late-Onset GBS Infection.** Late-onset infection with GBS can present in term newborns from 7 days to 89 days of age, with a typical presentation at 3 to 4 weeks of age (AAP, 2024f; Ratner et al., 2025). The incidence in the United States has not changed over the past 20 years and remains at 0.3 to 0.4 cases per 1,000 live births, with a higher risk in infants born < 37 weeks' gestation (Ratner et al., 2025). Bacteremia without a focus accounts for approximately 60% of cases, with meningitis complicating a third of the cases. The mortality rate for LOS GBS meningitis in term newborns, based on findings from two U.S. centers was 10%. The study parameters included death during acute hospitalization combined with later death due to complications of GBS meningitis; of significance was that 44% of survivors in this study had neurodevelopmental impairment ranging from mild to severe. The effect on VLBW infants is even greater, with a 1.6-fold increased odds risk of neurologic impairment compared to the VLBW infant without meningitis (Gordon et al., 2025).

Complications include global or profound intellectual disability, spastic quadriplegia, cortical blindness, deafness, uncontrolled seizures, hydrocephalus, and diabetes insipidus. Thus, early treatment is a critical part of preventing long-term serious sequelae. Initially, an infant with a positive blood culture can be asymptomatic. The diagnosis of GBS infection is complicated because signs and symptoms of neonatal infection are not specific, and symptoms may represent other conditions of the neonate. For example, apnea may be a symptom of CNS immaturity in the preterm neonate, but it is also associated with infection. The caregiver must have a high index of suspicion for infection in all conditions involving the neonate. Infection should be considered in the differential diagnosis of most newborn illnesses. Screening tests, such as CBC with differential, are often used to identify the need for further evaluation for infection. Abnormal results indicate the necessity for definitive testing and implementation of empiric antimicrobial therapy. Definitive diagnosis is made by positive culture from normal sterile sites such as blood, urine, or CSF. The use of PCR-assay can result in decreased time to detection, and in cases where culture is obtained after antibiotic therapy has already started, it may enhance bacterial yield for diagnosis (Ratner et al., 2025).

**Treatment.** Regional and hospital differences in infectious agents must be considered when selecting antimicrobial therapy. Before culture results are returned, administration of a broad-spectrum penicillin and an aminoglycoside provides coverage for the most prevalent microorganisms. Generally, ampicillin and gentamicin are selected until culture results and sensitivities are available. Although most strains of GBS are resistant to aminoglycosides, a synergistic effect is observed when gentamicin and ampicillin are used in combination until these results are known. GBS is generally very sensitive to penicillin G, and, in many institutions, penicillin G is substituted for ampicillin once the diagnosis is made. It is acceptable practice to discontinue gentamicin when cultures confirm GBS infection. Therapy is maintained for a minimum of 10 days for uncomplicated bacteremia or pneumonia and a minimum of 14 days for meningitis (Ratner et al., 2025; Simonsen et al., 2014). The LP may be repeated midway or at the end of therapy in infants with complicated meningitis to ensure that there are no microorganisms remaining in the CSF (AAP, 2024f). Fluid management, volume expansion, and appropriate antimicrobial therapy are the key components of nursing care. Infants with GBS infection are often very labile and do not tolerate frequent interventions. Minimal handling is often required for their care.

**Prevention.** The most potentially lasting method for prevention of early- and late-onset infections, as well as birthing-parent morbidity associated with GBS, appears to be active immunization of all women of childbearing age, either before pregnancy or late in pregnancy (at ~7 months gestation). Passive transmission of antibodies to the newborn occurs via the placenta; however, women often deliver infants prematurely before the successful transmission of appropriate protective antibodies. Because 65% to 85% of all infants with GBS disease are born at term, vaccines given to women early in the third trimester could prevent up to 95% of these infections. The cost of developing a suitable vaccine would probably be less than the cost of the care required by the critically ill newborn and the chronically ill, debilitated, severely handicapped newborn. To date, there are no licensed birthing parent vaccines for neonatal GBS prevention, although much research has been done and development is progressing (Ratner et al., 2025).

### Staphylococcus

Staphylococcus is another gram-positive bacterium. From the 1950s to the 1970s, coagulase-positive *S. aureus* was the main organism identified as a hospital pathogen. In the 1980s, coagulase-negative organisms, in particular *S. epidermidis*, were discovered to be equally important.

**Epidemiology.** These organisms have caused many serious and even fatal infections in newborns. Critically ill and preterm newborns are already immunocompromised and, therefore, are especially vulnerable to infections. Open skin lesions, surgical incisions, or puncture wounds caused by diagnostic tests or procedures are conducive to bacterial growth, especially *S. aureus* or *S. epidermidis*. Nosocomial infections may also be transmitted to the neonate through contaminated articles or from the hands of healthcare providers. Overgrowth of *S. epidermidis* may occur in nurseries where an attempt has been made to reduce colonization of *S. aureus*. The development of resistant organisms is a risk for critically ill or preterm infants who require extensive invasive treatments. CoNS or methicillin-resistant *Staphylococcus aureus* (MRSA) can potentially cause a wide variety of significant clinical syndromes, including those with high mortality. Staphylococci release endotoxins that have systemic effects, including alterations in the skin's protective layer. Scalded skin syndrome is one of the most common examples of this effect (Liu & Bradley, 2025).

**Treatment.** Management and supportive therapy for staphylococcal infection are initially the same as for infection with group B streptococci. Antimicrobial therapy begins with ampicillin and gentamicin. Once definitive cultures and sensitivities are available, and if the organism is ampicillin resistant, the drug of choice is one of the synthetic penicillins: oxacillin, methicillin, cloxacillin, dicloxacillin, or nafcillin. If the organism is methicillin resistant, the best available drug is vancomycin. The choice of antimicrobial agent must be carefully made and reconsidered when culture results are available.

### Escherichia coli

*E. coli* is second to GBS as the most common cause of EOS in the term newborn and is the most common cause of early-onset gram-negative infection in preterm infants (Lawrence et al., 2025).

**Epidemiology.** *E. coli* is associated with preterm delivery, LBW, prolonged ROM, intrapartum fever, and birthing-parent intraamniotic infection (Mendoza-Palomar et al., 2017). As with other organisms associated with the birthing parent GI tract, coliform organisms are common in the birthing parent's birth canal, causing a high incidence of colonization in newborns' lower GI or respiratory tract during labor or at delivery (Gordon et al., 2025).

**Treatment.** Uncomplicated bacteremia due to susceptible organisms should be treated for 14 days following the first negative culture; culture-positive meningitis should be treated for a minimum of 21 days. Although there appears to be increasing resistance to ampicillin and gentamicin in the United States, this combination remains the best choice for empiric therapy until sensitivities are available (Lawrence et al., 2025; Simonsen et al., 2014). The use of third-generation cephalosporins for empiric therapy is not recommended due to increasing resistance unless gram-negative meningitis is highly suspected (Mukherjee & Ryan, 2025). **Emergency Alert: Due to increasing ampicillin resistance patterns, it is important to follow blood culture sensitivities when treating organisms with ampicillin.**

### Listeria Monocytogenes

**Epidemiology.** *L. monocytogenes*, a gram-positive rod, has been recognized as a cause of perinatal complications since the early 1900s. From 2009 to 2011 in the United States, 1,651 cases were reported to surveillance systems with a case-fatality rate of 21%. Those at greatest risk are older adults, pregnant women (10–20 times increased risk), and immunocompromised individuals. *Listeria* is found in birds and mammals, including domestic and farm animals, and in unpasteurized milk, soil, and fecal material (McKinney & Freitag, 2025).

**Clinical Manifestations.** A birthing parent infected with *Listeria* commonly has flu-like symptoms, including malaise, fever, chills, diarrhea, and back pain. It is also possible to contract the infection and remain asymptomatic or have only minor symptoms (AAP, 2024j). If contracted between 17 and 28 weeks' gestation, *Listeria* can cause fetal death or premature birth of an acutely ill newborn who may develop EOS, LOS, or meningitis. However, early birthing-parent treatment with IV ampicillin and gentamicin has been associated with a normal newborn outcome. Infection late in pregnancy may cause the infant to be born with a congenital infection, usually pneumonia. Mortality rates are high but are usually related to the degree of prematurity. Late-onset listeriosis, which can occur up to 4 weeks after delivery, can easily result in meningitis (AAP, 2024j). A term newborn with listeriosis has a lower chance of dying but often experiences complications of hydrocephalus and cognitive disability. However, in either preterm or term neonates in whom meningitis develops, there is a 70% mortality rate if treatment is delayed. Newborns infected with *Listeria* may be meconium stained (or have brown-colored amniotic fluid); exhibit apnea and flaccidity; have a papular, erythematous skin rash; have hepatosplenomegaly; and be poor feeders. Preterm birth associated with the appearance of meconium staining of amniotic fluid should always be considered suspicious for listeriosis (AAP, 2024j; McKinney & Freitag, 2025).

**Treatment.** Intrapartum administration of antibiotics may decrease fetal morbidity and mortality rates. Ampicillin, in combination with an aminoglycoside, is the most common treatment. Investigators have shown that newborn survival rates are significantly different if the birthing parent as well as the infant receives treatment (71% versus 29%) (McKinney & Freitag, 2025). Treatment for bacteremia is typically 14 days, whereas meningitis is treated for 21 days. It is recommended that diagnostic imaging of the brain be performed near the end of the anticipated treatment course to determine if prolonged therapy is needed for parenchymal involvement of the brain (AAP, 2024j). Careful handwashing is a very important aspect of caring for an infant infected with *Listeria*. Institutional policy may require that the infant be isolated for the first 24 hours of life until the antibiotics are initiated. The birthing parent's urine, stool, and lochia should be cultured, and if positive, she should be given ampicillin. Listeriosis often presents suddenly in the last trimester of pregnancy, precipitating an unexpected preterm delivery. Extensive emotional support may be necessary for the birthing parent and family. In the United States, listeriosis is a nationally reportable disease for state and local health departments (AAP, 2024j).

**Neonatal Meningitis Epidemiology.** Meningitis is commonly associated with newborn infection. The single most important factor in the enhanced risk for sepsis or meningitis in the newborn is LBW (Gordon et al., 2025). Mortality rates have decreased over the past decades but remain estimated at 10% to 20% in high-income countries; rates in low- and middle-income countries are significantly higher, ranging from 40% to 58% (Mathias et al., 2024). Meningitis can be associated with both early- and late-onset infection but is more common as a complication of late-onset infection (Gordon et al., 2025). In up to two-thirds of cases, meningitis with bacteremia was present. Thus, an inoculation of organisms may pass the blood–brain barrier and infect the CSF.

Although the overall incidence of neonatal bacterial meningitis in developed countries is less than 1%, the incidence is much higher in preterm and VLBW infants (Mathias et al., 2024). Male infants are more vulnerable to infection and, consequently, meningitis. Female infants have lower rates of RDS and lower rates of most congenital infections. Geography and socioeconomic factors are influential in patterns of neonatal disease. These differences most likely reflect populations served, including unique cultural activities and sexual practices, as well as local customs. Differences also likely reflect different treatment patterns in local nurseries and variations of antimicrobial selections (Gupta et al., 2024).

**Clinical Manifestations and Diagnosis.** Initially, the infant with meningitis presents with signs and symptoms of generalized infection. In addition, the meningeal irritation results in increased irritability, alterations in consciousness, lethargy, tremors or twitching, seizure activity, and decreased muscle tone. Focal signs include hemiparesis, horizontal deviation of the eyes, and some cranial nerve involvement. Bulging fontanelles may or may not be a presenting finding due to the flexibility of the cranial sutures (Gordon et al., 2025). The most common organisms responsible for bacterial meningitis are GBS, *E. coli*, and staphylococcus, followed by other gram-negative organisms (Gordon et al., 2024). Herpes simplex virus (HSV) is a significant cause of neonatal viral meningitis and carries a 50% risk for neurologic sequela (Gupta et al., 2024). Obtaining CSF for culture before initiating antibiotics is the gold standard for diagnosing meningitis. Broad-range PCR assays offer a quick and reliable method of identifying pathogens in the CSF; however, large-scale, randomized controlled trials are lacking in the neonatal population (Gordon et al., 2024). Cytologic tests on the CSF can identify the presence of an inflammatory response. A Gram stain of the CSF fluid should be prepared, and other appropriate cultures should be obtained. High CSF protein and low glucose levels are also indicators of meningitis, although parameters may overlap between those with and without meningitis. As with all procedures in the neonate, the LP is not without risks, which must be weighed against the benefit of obtaining a CSF culture. Often, the preterm infant may be so critically unstable that the LP is deferred; in these cases, the infant should be assumed to have meningitis and, therefore, require a longer antibiotic duration (Gordon et al., 2024).

**Treatment.** The selection of antimicrobial therapy for meningitis is based on the causative microorganism. Supportive therapy is necessary for the newborn with meningitis. Acute observation and monitoring of vital signs and activity levels are crucial. Infants who become critically ill with meningitis may deteriorate quickly and need rapid, acute interventions. Infants often require long-term antibiotic therapy, and peripheral venous access can be problematic due to poor perfusion. Placement of a percutaneous central line for antibiotic therapy and parenteral nutrition may be necessary. Families need education and emotional support during long-term hospitalizations, particularly if complications develop. Because signs and symptoms of neonatal infection are nonspecific and are often the same, with or without meningitis, it is imperative to begin empiric therapy once suspicion is established. Empiric therapy for sepsis of unknown etiology includes initiation of broad-spectrum antibiotics, generally ampicillin and gentamicin for EOS; nafcillin or vancomycin with gentamicin are most commonly used for LOS but are driven by local pathogen patterns. When meningitis is highly suspected, cefotaxime or cefepime is used due to better blood–brain barrier penetration (Mathias et al., 2024; Saleh et al., 2024). It is important to realize that cephalosporin-resistant strains of many gram-negative bacteria are emerging. Resistance of *E. coli* and *Klebsiella* species to ampicillin, gentamicin, and cephalosporins continues to make treatment choices more difficult (Gupta et al., 2024). Due to the risk of recurrence or relapse of CNS disease seen in some studies, especially in neonates/infants with *E. coli* meningitis, it is recommended to repeat the LP prior to discontinuation of antibiotic therapy to document bacterial clearance (Saleh et al., 2024).

**Prevention.** Preventive measures are in place for the most common causes of neonatal meningitis. GBS prophylaxis and IAP for birthing parents who test positive for GBS or have certain risk factors has led to a steady decrease in EOS GBS sepsis and meningitis. Control measures for *Listeria* and *E. coli* include avoiding certain foods by pregnant birthing parents and those who may become pregnant. Foods that have a known risk for being contaminated with listeria include soft cheeses made with unpasteurized milk; uncanned, smoked seafood; and unpasteurized milk. The food industry must be strict with the handling of foods to prevent the growth of *Listeria* and *E. coli*. The most likely foods for contamination are raw sprouts, melons, and meats such as hot dogs, deli meats, and cold cuts (Gordon et al., 2024; Gupta et al., 2024).

**Prognosis.** Mortality from neonatal meningitis has decreased dramatically, with higher rates among preterm infants; substantial neurologic morbidity continues to be seen among survivors. Complications of neonatal meningitis include mental and motor problems, seizure disorders, hydrocephalus, hearing loss, blindness, and abnormal speech patterns. It is estimated that 35% will have mild deficits, and 20% will have moderate or severe neurologic sequelae (Valentine & Wallen, 2024).

## Congenital TORCH Infections

Historically, the microorganisms most often responsible for congenitally acquired infections were grouped together as TORCH infections. Torch stands for toxoplasmosis, others, rubella, cytomegalovirus (CMV), and herpes. The "others" category included additional microorganisms responsible for congenital infections. However, the list of microorganisms implicated in congenital infections has grown, and the acronym is no longer inclusive. A more appropriate acronym, ToRCHES CLAP, is suggested by Remington et al. (2025). This new acronym includes: **To**, *Toxoplasma gondii* (*T. gondii*); **R**, rubella; **C**, CMV; **H**, HSV; **E**, enteroviruses; **S**, syphilis (*Treponema pallidum*); **C**, chickenpox (varicella-zoster virus [VZV]); **L**, Lyme disease (*Borrelia burgdorferi*); **A**, acquired immunodeficiency syndrome (AIDS/HIV); and **P**, Parvovirus B19 (Remington et al., 2025).

### Toxoplasmosis

Initially thought to be an animal disease, the clinical importance of the parasite *T. gondii* in humans gained importance throughout the 1900s. Toxoplasma is a pathogen ever present in the natural environment worldwide (Wallon et al., 2025). The life cycle of toxoplasma is complicated. The predominant host of this organism is the ordinary house cat that has ingested contaminated meat or fomites excreted by other infected cats; however, other animals, such as farm animals (cows, pigs, and sheep), can become infected if they ingest food or water containing cat feces with oocytes present (Kaufman et al., 2025). The oocyte form of the parasite persists in soil contaminated by cat feces.

**Epidemiology.** Congenital toxoplasmosis is transmitted from the birthing parent to the fetus after ingestion of undercooked meat or food or from fomites in cat feces. The risk of infection by the pregnant birthing parent is related to certain activities such as changing litter boxes, playing with children in sandboxes, and gardening in soil used by cats. Congenital toxoplasmosis is almost exclusively the result of a primary infection in the birthing parent. The transmission rate during pregnancy is directly related to the gestational age of the fetus when the birthing parent's infection occurs (lowest during the first trimester, increasing up to as high as 70% transmission during the third trimester) (Wallon et al., 2025). On the other hand, there is an inverse relationship between the timing of infection and fetal damage (first-trimester infection will have more devastating fetal effects compared with third-trimester acquisition) (McAuley, 2014). The risk of infection when the birthing parent was infected prior to pregnancy is extremely low, except in the immunocompromised woman (McLeod & Boyer, 2025). After infection in the birthing parent, the microorganisms invade and multiply within the placenta, eventually entering fetal circulation. The greatest risk is when a nonimmune birthing parent is exposed to *T. gondii* during fetal organogenesis (weeks 4–8 of gestation), when the risk for congenital anomalies is high. In the United States, approximately 40 million people (11% of the population over the age of 6) are seropositive for this protozoan (CDC, 2024d). There is wide variability in the prevalence of seropositive birthing parents of childbearing age among countries, geographic regions of the same country, and ethnic origin; different cultural practices regarding food are probably the primary cause of this difference. Because meat is the main vector for transmission, areas where there is less *T. gondii* present in meat because of improved methods for processing or cooking meat have lower prevalence rates (Wallon et al., 2025).

**Clinical Manifestations and Diagnosis.** Acute toxoplasmosis in a pregnant birthing parent often goes undetected and undiagnosed because the signs and symptoms are not severe. Clinical questioning after the identification of an infected newborn or infant often leads to reflection and memories of a period of enlarged lymph nodes and fatigue without fever. Birthing parents sometimes report a mononucleosis-like or flu-like syndrome that may have a febrile course, with malaise, headache, fatigue, sore throat, and sore muscles. These symptoms may persist for several months. Newborns with congenital toxoplasmosis most often lack symptoms at birth. However, a small number can present with the classic triad of hydrocephalus, chorioretinitis, and intracranial calcifications (Wallon et al., 2025). This is especially true in infants of birthing parents who were not treated during pregnancy. There are a wide variety of clinical signs in the scope of the disease, and many of these closely mimic congenital CMV. The newborn can appear clinically well at birth or exhibit severe erythroblastosis, hydrops fetalis, purpura, and other clinical signs. Neurologic signs similar to encephalitis (e.g., convulsions, bulging fontanelles, nystagmus, and increased head circumference) may be the only significant presentation of this clinical problem. If the newborn receives treatment and there is no permanent neurologic damage, signs may disappear, allowing for normal cerebral growth and development (McLeod & Boyer, 2025; Wallon et al., 2025).

Mild cases of the disease may not be recognized in the newborn period. Signs of delayed onset of disease in premature newborns include severe CNS or eye lesions appearing at 3 months of age. In term newborns, delayed disease may occur in the first 2 months of life and is usually mild. Clinical signs include generalized infection, enlarged liver and spleen, late-onset jaundice, enlarged lymph nodes, or late-onset CNS problems, including hydrocephalus and chorioretinitis. Infants with congenital toxoplasmosis may have new lesions appearing until age 5 years (Wallon et al., 2025). When congenital toxoplasmosis is suspected, neonatal peripheral blood for toxoplasma IgG and IgM immunosorbent agglutination assay should be sent to a reference laboratory. Serum transaminase tests and a CBC with differential should also be obtained (AAP, 2024n).

**Treatment.** Treatment for congenital toxoplasmosis is pyrimethamine plus sulfonamides. The suggested dosing of pyrimethamine is 2 mg/kg/d in two divided doses orally for 2 days followed by 1 mg/kg/d for 2 or 6 months, then 1 mg/kg/d every Monday, Wednesday, and Friday for a 12-month total duration of treatment. Sulfadiazine is given in doses of 100 mg/kg/d in two divided doses orally for 12 months. Leucovorin (folic acid) is given in doses of 10 mg per dose three times weekly during and up to 1 week after pyrimethamine therapy to minimize toxicity (AAP, 2024n). Close monitoring is necessary during therapy due to the possibility of toxicity. Corticosteroids are given in the form of prednisone at 1 mg/kg/d in two divided doses until there is resolution of elevated protein in CSF or active chorioretinitis (AAP, 2024n). As expected, it is evident that the outcome for infants with congenital toxoplasmosis is much better when treatment is given than for those without treatment (AAP, 2024n; Wallon et al., 2025). Nursing management is supportive and dependent on the severity of the infection. Neurologic impairment at birth can be significant, requiring mechanical ventilation and seizure control.

**Prevention.** The best and most effective treatments are prevention and early recognition. The cost effectiveness of pregnancy serology screening depends on the costs of the tests and the estimated cost of treating the infection if identified early. Presently, in the United States, screening is done erratically, and there are no particular screening standards. Counseling education for the prevention of toxoplasmosis in seronegative birthing parents should focus on avoiding raw meat and using gloves during feline litter box cleaning and gardening in what may be contaminated soil. Toxoplasmosis cannot be contracted by merely handling or being around a cat, so the family cat does not need to be banished. It is imperative for pregnant birthing parents to inform their healthcare provider if they experience any signs that could be attributed to *T. gondii* infection. Transmission of toxoplasmosis in humans occurs only from birthing parent to child; therefore, the risk to healthcare personnel is negligible. There is a theoretical risk from contaminated urine, however (AAP, 2024n).

### Rubella

Rubella (German measles) is usually a mild disease of infants and children involving a variable rash and fever; it is more severe and associated with more complications in adults. The clinical significance for infants is transplacental infection leading to congenital rubella syndrome (CRS). CRS is commonly recognized as a constellation of defects seen in a newborn with congenital rubella infection. These include a combination of ophthalmologic defects, congenital heart defects, and hearing loss, with or without CNS complications (Gans, 2025; Reef & Plotkin, 2025).

**Epidemiology.** The spread of endemic rubella, and consequently CRS, has been eliminated in the United States. The only reported cases of rubella appear to have been imported from countries where the disease remains endemic. Before introducing the rubella vaccine in 1996, the incidence of rubella was 78% higher, and the incidence of CRS was 69% higher than after 1996. A two-dose regimen was implemented following a resurgence of both rubella and CRS between 1989 and 1991. This new schedule has been successful in controlling the disease in the United States, but elimination of rubella has not been achieved nationally; this may partly be related to vaccine hesitancy. Due to this, high levels of immunity must be maintained in the United States (Gans, 2025; Reef & Plotkin, 2025).

Most cases of CRS occur after a primary infection in the birthing parent with subsequent viremia and intrauterine transmission. Effects on the fetus are related to the timing of the infection during the pregnancy. First-trimester perinatal infection carries the highest morbidity. There may be fetal death, stillbirth, or CRS. Some fetuses are unaffected, and not all affected fetuses develop CRS. The placenta is an effective barrier during the 12th to 28th weeks; however, the fetus is very vulnerable in the first and third trimesters (Desai et al., 2025).

**Clinical Manifestations and Diagnosis.** A presumptive diagnosis of CRS should be high on the differential diagnosis list for any infant born to a birthing parent with documented or suspected rubella during pregnancy. The diagnosis should also be considered for any infant with presenting signs known to be associated with CRS. The abnormalities most commonly associated with CRS are auditory (e.g., sensorineural deafness), ophthalmic (e.g., cataracts, microphthalmia, glaucoma, chorioretinitis), cardiac (e.g., patent ductus arteriosus [PDA], peripheral pulmonary artery stenosis, atrial or ventricular septal defects [ASD/VSD]), and neurologic (e.g., microcephaly, meningoencephalitis, intellectual disability). In addition, infants with CRS frequently exhibit both intrauterine and postnatal growth restriction. Other conditions sometimes observed among babies with CRS include radiolucent bone defects, hepatosplenomegaly, thrombocytopenia, and purpuric skin lesions ("blueberry-muffin spots"). Newborns who are moderately or severely affected by CRS are readily recognizable at birth. Still, mild CRS (e.g., slight cardiac involvement or deafness) may be detected months or years after birth or not at all (Desai et al., 2025; Gans, 2025; Reef & Plotkin, 2025).

The possibility of subclinical infection with rubella highlights the need for laboratory confirmation. Attempting to isolate the rubella virus in tissue culture is very valuable in the diagnosis of CRS. The virus is readily obtainable from the posterior pharynx, but it is less reliable in specimens obtained from the conjunctivae, spinal fluid, or urine. Specimens should be obtained when CRS is suspected because viral shedding decreases during infancy. The detection of rubella antibodies confirms the presence of the infection. Cord serum is a reliable source of assay for the presence of rubella-specific IgM because IgM is derived from the fetus. Rubella-specific IgG persists for life and can be detected by enzyme immunoassay (EIA). Demonstration of rubella-specific IgM in fetal blood obtained by cordocentesis has been used to establish diagnosis in utero. Chorionic villus sampling has also demonstrated recovery of the virus during the first trimester (Desai et al., 2025; Reef & Plotkin, 2025).

**Treatment.** Unfortunately, there are no specific treatment modalities available for either rubella or CRS. Treatment is supportive and related to the associated complications. CRS is not a static disease, and the primary physician must take time to define the extent of the associated problems and coordinate efforts to maintain a broad, multidisciplinary approach to infant care. Ongoing care of an infant with CRS involves coordinated follow-up and evaluation by pediatricians, cardiologists, audiologists, ophthalmologists, and neurologists. Hearing screens are particularly important because intervention is known to improve outcome in hearing (Gans, 2025).

**Prevention.** The primary goal in the United States is to eliminate rubella with vaccination, because active immunization is the only practical means to prevent CRS. Control techniques include isolation of those infected with rubella. Patients are considered infectious from the seventh day before the onset of symptoms to the fifth to seventh day after the onset of the rash. Children with CRS are considered infectious for the first year unless repeated pharyngeal or urine cultures are negative (Reef & Plotkin, 2025). Reports of rubella epidemics in Japan, Poland, and Romania, with cases of CRS, are mostly attributed to cost, lack of public awareness, and public health commitments (Lambert et al., 2015). These recent epidemics highlight resurgence as a result of misunderstandings, misinformation, and parents' refusal of vaccinations during childhood. There is much speculation that the incidence of many preventable infections will increase as a result of parent refusal of childhood immunizations. It will be prudent to follow trends.

### Cytomegalovirus

CMV, a member of the herpes family, is the most common congenital viral infection in developed countries and is the leading cause of infectious birth defects in the United States. CMV is a DNA virus covered with a glycoprotein coat that closely resembles the herpes virus and VZV.

**Epidemiology.** CMV infection is endemic, and although it has been identified in the great apes, it is believed that humans are the only host. By adulthood, most people have been exposed to CMV, and antibodies have developed to it. CMV infection is more prevalent in lower socioeconomic groups and is especially common in developing countries. In the United States, nearly one-third of children under the age of 5 years are infected, and well over half of the adult population have been infected by the age of 40; the rate continues to increase with age. Racial differences are also noted, with African American and Hispanic populations showing higher seroprevalence than White populations (CDC, 2024a; Permar & Gantt, 2025). The virus is usually transmitted from person to person through body fluids and secretions. Blood, urine, breast milk, cervical mucus, semen, and saliva harbor CMV. The virus can cause an infectious mononucleosis-like syndrome, with general malaise, liver complications, fever, and general fatigue (Desai et al., 2025; Permar & Gantt, 2025). Transplacental transmission is directly related to advancing gestational age with up to 75% risk during the third trimester. Congenital infection is associated with more severe sequelae when acquired during the first half of pregnancy (AAP, 2024c). Although infection of the fetus can occur at any time during pregnancy, the risk of malformations and developmental delays is most common during the period of organogenesis (Desai et al., 2025). Perinatal transmission can occur within 2 to 3 days of infection by transplacental crossing of the organism. The fetus can also contract the virus during the intrapartum period from infected cervical secretions while descending through the birth canal. CMV can be transmitted through infected breastmilk. CMV infection may occur at any stage of gestation and is not always the result of a primary infection in the birthing parent. In the United States, congenital CMV occurs in approximately 0.2% to 2% of all newborn infants (Desai et al., 2025; Permar & Gantt, 2025).

**Clinical Manifestations and Diagnosis.** Congenital CMV is divided into two categories, symptomatic congenital CMV and asymptomatic congenital CMV. The majority of infants identified with congenital CMV will not present with symptoms at birth (asymptomatic). Infants who do not present with symptoms at birth generally have a better prognosis; however, approximately 10% will develop sensorineural hearing loss (SNHL). Congenital CMV infection is the leading nongenetic cause of SNHL in the United States, occurring in up to 50% of children with symptomatic illness at birth (AAP, 2024c). These infants require close follow-up for neurologic and motor defects as well as chorioretinitis. Symptomatic disease is most often accompanied by intrauterine growth restriction (IUGR), microcephaly, periventricular calcifications, SNHL, chorioretinitis, congenital cataracts, profound intellectual disability, hepatosplenomegaly, and jaundice (Boppana et al., 2013; Permar & Gantt, 2025; Swanson & Schleiss, 2013).

Suspicious clinical findings or obstetric history warrant further investigation for CMV infection. Diagnosis in the neonate can be confirmed by viral detection in bodily fluids or PCR, culture, or antigen testing. Preferred specimens include urine and saliva due to the high viral load found in these specimens. After the first 3 weeks of life, congenital infection cannot be distinguished from postnatally acquired disease. IgG and IgM antibody titers cannot reliably be used in diagnosis. Elevated IgM in the first 2 weeks of life reflects fetal antibody response to CMV; however, after 2 weeks, elevated titers may be related to postnatal acquisition of the virus. Elevated neonatal IgG titers may reflect the seropositive status of birthing parents, with the IgG antibodies becoming undetectable between 4 and 9 months in the uninfected infant; in the infected infant, these antibodies persist for a much longer interval (AAP, 2024c; Permar & Gantt, 2025; Swanson & Schleiss, 2013).

**Treatment.** Newborns infected with CMV display a wide range of signs and symptoms. General supportive therapy is based on the presence of these clinical manifestations. Treatment with antivirals offers the best outcome for infants with symptomatic CMV. The most beneficial treatment is oral valganciclovir, although ganciclovir can be used for initial therapy if GI absorption in the newborn is compromised. These drugs are generally safe and well tolerated by newborns. It is important to involve an infectious disease specialist, who can follow the infant after discharge and recommend a length of needed therapy (AAP, 2024c; Permar & Gantt, 2025; Swanson & Schleiss, 2013). IV immunoglobulin therapy provides passive immunity to at-risk infants but not to those already infected. Two live attenuated vaccines for CMV have been developed and are being tested on renal transplant patients and healthy volunteers. Theoretically, these vaccines would be useful preconceptionally or perinatally to prevent vertical transmission; however, only limited research has been done, and efficacy has been inconsistent. Chemotherapy offers the most promise for the treatment of neonatal CMV infection; however, clinically, it has not been shown to be effective in improving long-term outcomes (Permar & Gantt, 2025; Swanson & Schleiss, 2013).

**Prevention.** CMV is a common and often undiagnosed infection. Prevention of the spread of the virus is virtually impossible due to the lack of symptoms in most hosts. Careful surveillance of childbearing women will assist in recognizing the risk of infection in the newborn. Hospital workers who are of childbearing age are often concerned about their risk of contracting CMV from their virus-shedding patients. Generally, this risk is dependent on the prevalence of CMV secretion, the susceptibility of the worker, and the degree of exposure. Since the implementation of universal precautions, the risk of nosocomial transmission of the virus has been very low. It is considered lower than the risk of acquiring the infection in the community (Permar & Gantt, 2025). Transmission of CMV via infected blood products has been significantly decreased through the use of CMV-negative donors or irradiation of blood products. Premature and LBW infants are especially vulnerable to the infusion of this virus in blood products. The best method of prevention is the institution of universal precautions, including good handwashing techniques.

### Herpes Simplex Virus

HSV types 1 and 2 are family members of large DNA viruses. Common sites of infection include the skin, oral mucosa, eyes, and genital tract. Although these two types are capable of causing primary infection at any site, type 1 is more likely to cause recurrence at oral mucosal sites, and type 2 has a greater propensity for recurrence at genital sites (Stanberry, 2006).

**Epidemiology.** Neonatal infection can result from either type, with a worldwide estimate of 75% of cases caused by HSV type 2 and 25% of cases of type 1 (Allen & Robinson, 2014). HSV possesses the quality of "latency," whereby the virus can persist in a latent state for a period of time and then be reactivated by certain stimuli. A strand of the viral DNA persists in an infected individual for a lifetime; thus, the virus maintains a "foothold" in its host. Clinical experiences demonstrate that, after primary HSV infection, at the site of the infection (perhaps an oral or genital site), the microorganism invades the sensory nerve endings and remains there (Scott & Kimberlin, 2025). Primary infections appear to be more severe as the host is seronegative. Potential stimuli for HSV reactivation include periods of stress, emotional trauma, and prolonged exposure to the sun (Desai et al., 2025). Maintenance of the latency state and recurrence of the virus are topics of intense current research. There are many unanswered questions about what triggers latency and about the cofactors for reactivation of the virus.

Greater than 90% of neonatal HSV infection is the result of birthing parent–fetal transmission, with up to two-thirds of cases occurring in birthing parents with an asymptomatic primary infection. Transmission of the infection to the fetus can be caused by passage through infected genital secretions in the intrapartum period or by ascending infection from the vaginal vault via ruptured (or not) membranes. Many birthing parents can be asymptomatic and still be shedding HSV. Recurrent infections are the most common problem in pregnancy. The risk is greater with primary or nonprimary first infection than with exposure from a recurrent infection. Although primary infection is less common, it causes the most severe neonatal disease, most likely including CNS problems, disseminated disease into other organ systems, and probable death. During a primary genital infection, there is a higher viral load, prolonged viral shedding, and little or no passive antibodies from the birthing parent, resulting in a higher incidence of fetal or neonatal infection. The incidence of intrapartum transmission with a primary infection or nonprimary first infection is approximately 25% to 60%. Many neonatal complications, such as prematurity, intrauterine restriction, and RDS, can potentiate the neonate's illness, limiting the ability to fight off HSV. There is a broad range of severity of neonatal infection, from severe to benign and asymptomatic. HSV is the most reported cause of fatal encephalitis in both children and adults (Stanberry, 2006).

Intrapartum transmission is more likely to occur in the presence of ruptured membranes. Other risk factors include intrauterine fetal monitoring, fetal scalp sampling, and other instrumentation such as forceps or vacuum-assisted delivery. It is recommended that women infected with HSV not be monitored by these methods (Desai et al., 2025). Transmission from birthing parent to infant from an infected breast lesion has been reported. Transmission has also been documented from oral lesions.

**Clinical Manifestations and Diagnosis.** Acquisition of HSV in utero can result in spontaneous abortion, preterm birth, or a normal baby. Clinical manifestations of the disease are broad and are related to the initial site of infection or category. The clinical presentation of the congenital acquisition of the infection includes skin vesicles or scarring, hypopigmentation, chorioretinitis, microcephaly, and hydranencephaly. There are three categories of neonatal HSV disease. These categories may occur in isolation or there can be overlap of presentation. The most common category (~45%) includes patients with localized infections of the skin, eyes, or mouth (SEM disease). The typical skin finding is a cluster of discrete vesicles on an erythematous base.

The second category (~30%) includes patients with encephalitis (CNS disease). In this group, neurologic sequelae occur in approximately 50%, and mortality is high in untreated HSV encephalitis. Approximately one-third of these patients do not have skin vesicles and are identified by history alone. CSF is positive for the virus in 25% to 40% of these cases. The presence of cells and increased protein are very common in the CSF of patients with encephalitis. The third category of neonatal patients (~25%) includes those with disseminated disease characterized by irritability, seizures, respiratory distress, jaundice, DIC, shock, and other symptoms of viral and bacterial infection. All major neonatal organs may be involved. The liver, lungs, and adrenal glands are the most common reservoirs for the virus. The CNS is involved in 60% to 75% of affected neonates. In greater than 40% of newborns with disseminated disease, skin vesicles do not develop or develop late, making identification of infected infants more difficult. The mortality rate for untreated disseminated disease is greater than 80%, making early and accurate diagnosis a priority in the ill newborn (Desai et al., 2025; Scott & Kimberlin, 2025). **Emergency Alert: HSV infection should be considered in any clinically ill, septic-appearing neonate with negative bacterial cultures. Fever is also highly suggestive, especially within the first 3 weeks of life.**

Expert consultation is important in the early stages of identification and evaluation. Laboratory tests are available to differentiate HSV infection from other bacterial and viral infections but must be interpreted considering the clinical context (Allen & Robinson, 2014). Routine surface cultures of the newborn from oral mucous membranes, rectum, nasopharynx, and conjunctivae should be delayed to 24 to 48 hours after birth to differentiate viral replication from transient colonization of the newborn at birth. Earlier testing from these sites may confound the results (Desai et al., 2025; Scott & Kimberlin, 2025). The clinical diagnosis of neonatal HSV is necessary for proper treatment and continuing management. Standard diagnostic tests include nucleic acid amplification test (NAAT) of CSF, swabs of any vesicular lesions, and specimen collection from the conjunctivae, mouth, nasopharynx, and anus. Serum for HSV NAAT and alanine aminotransferase (ALT) level should also be obtained. Positive HSV cultures from non-CNS sites are diagnostic for neonatal HSV infection and remain the gold standard. Viral DNA detection by PCR assay is the gold standard diagnostic method for CNS disease (Scott & Kimberlin, 2025).

**Treatment.** Early and consistent therapy with IV acyclovir (ACV) has been determined to be the standard of care for all three presentation types of neonatal HSV infection. Because definitive results may take days to obtain, treatment must begin when HSV infection has been suspected. There is convincing evidence that early therapy has the potential to decrease mortality and morbidity and improve long-term outcomes for infants with neonatal HSV infection (Allen & Robinson, 2014; Desai et al., 2025; Scott & Kimberlin, 2025). The recommended dose of ACV for neonates is 60 mg/kg/d in three divided doses given every 8 hours; if renal function is normal for SEM disease, treatment is continued for 14 days. For disseminated or CNS disease, treatment should be continued for a minimum of 21 days, with CSF sampling at the end of 21 days. ACV may be discontinued for suspected SEM disease when it is determined that the infant is not infected and after 21 days of treatment for the infant with CNS involvement who is shown to have negative CSF studies (Allen & Robinson, 2014; Stanberry, 2006). A topical agent should be administered along with ACV in neonates with eye disease (AAP, 2024h).

**Prevention.** Great progress has been made in surveillance for and treatment of neonatal HSV infection. However, the ideal approach to prevention is eliminating exposure of the fetus to the virus or the newborn to active infection in the birthing parent at the time of delivery. There is growing concern about the transmission of the virus to unborn children with the concomitant increase in genital herpes as a sexually transmitted infection (STI). Increases in risky sexual practices and the high incidence of HSV type 2 in the United States lead to increasing numbers of women of childbearing age who are at risk for newly acquired infection (Scott & Kimberlin, 2025). The presence of active HSV genital lesions or prodromal symptoms in the birthing parent is a contraindication to vaginal delivery. If the membranes have been ruptured 4 hours or longer, cesarean section may or may not prevent transmission to the neonate. Daily use of oral antiviral prophylaxis with valganciclovir or ACV in the last trimester of pregnancy may reduce the risk to the infant and may reduce the number of elective cesarean sections (Desai et al., 2025; Scott & Kimberlin, 2025).

**Quality and Safety: Postnatal nosocomial transmission is greatly reduced with good handwashing techniques and universal precautions.** Hospitalized infected infants must be isolated because viral shedding provides a reservoir for infecting other infants in the nursery. HSV continues to be a life-threatening neonatal infection in the United States. It is important for all healthcare providers in the perinatal areas to maintain a high index of suspicion in infants whose symptoms may be compatible with HSV infection. Early identification allows prompt treatment, necessary continued observation, or both. Ongoing research may produce a more rapid method of virus identification and a safe and effective vaccine. Prevention of neonatal HSV depends on improved knowledge regarding the factors of virus transmission between birthing parents and infants (Scott & Kimberlin, 2025).

Primary nursing responsibilities in the management of a family with HSV infection are education and support. Birthing parents should be educated about the mode, methods, and possible origins of the HSV infection, and concerns should be addressed regarding potential transmission to newborns. Nurses are often the first to document a birthing parent's comment that the parent "had a small bump or blister and fever" right before their infant was born. **Quality and Safety: Careful history taking and thorough questioning can often identify potentially infected patients early.** With the diagnosis of genital herpes and subsequent monitoring procedures, families often feel stigmatized as well as anxious. Parents and responsible family members need education and support. Birthing parents with a history of genital HSV should be investigated for findings of active infection during the peripartum period. Breastfeeding is contraindicated if the birthing parent has a lesion on their breast. Infants are not isolated unless they are infected. Many nurseries have guidelines regarding a 24- to 48-hour observation period to check cultures on an infant who was delivered vaginally through an infected genital area. An uninfected neonate does not require prolonged hospitalization, and on discharge, the family needs information and education. Families should be informed that immediate medical consultation should be obtained with the development of major findings, including malaise, irritability, fever, temperature instability, respiratory distress, apnea, large abdomen or liver, sudden changes in skin color, new skin vesicles, lesions on the mucous membranes, or conjunctivitis. The sudden onset of systemic disease in a small, recovering preterm infant can include DIC and shock. Skin lesions are often absent in these severe cases, which may delay diagnosis (Scott & Kimberlin, 2025).

All family members with active lesions anywhere on the body should be taught careful handwashing techniques to use before handling the baby. Any person with an oral HSV infection who handles the infant must wash well, wear a mask, and not kiss the infant anywhere until the lesions are completely crusted over and healed (Scott & Kimberlin, 2025). The implementation of contact isolation provides healthcare workers and other patients with excellent protection against HSV infection in the workplace. Healthcare workers with active oral–facial lesions (cold sores) should take precautions, particularly when caring for high-risk patients such as newborns, immunocompromised individuals, and patients with chronic skin conditions (Stanberry, 2006).

### Nonpolio Enteroviruses

The genus *Enterovirus* (EV) consists of a broad range of viruses belonging to the family *Picornaviride*. The original classification system divided the EV into three main groups based on their replication patterns known at the time: polioviruses, coxsackieviruses (A & B), and echoviruses (Abzug, 2014; Krogstad & Cherry, 2025). This section will focus on the nonpolio neonatal diseases caused by coxsackievirus A, coxsackievirus B, and echovirus.

**Epidemiology.** As the genus name implies, the GI tract is the main site for replication and source of transmission (Abzug, 2014). The EVs have a worldwide distribution with seasonal prevalence in the more temperate regions (summer and fall). In tropical climates, there is year-wide prevalence (AAP, 2024d). The overall prevalence is difficult to estimate because the nonpolio viruses are not reportable, and unrecognized infections mask the known numbers. Experts estimate EV disease incidence to be equal to or exceed that of GBS, HSV, and CMV (Abzug, 2014). Because of the seasonal occurrence, swimming pools may be a threat to children, who are the main susceptible group (AAP, 2024d). Oral transmission is also possible through the air, by ingesting contaminated materials, or by contamination from environmental objects. The incidence of infection and antibodies in general, does not differ between males and females (Krogstad & Cherry, 2025). The human neonate is particularly susceptible in the first 2 weeks of life when associated with birthing-parent illness and prematurity, with this unique group demonstrating a higher incidence in males. Prenatal and perinatal infection is also possible, leading to infection of the neonate. The infant may present with typical signs of sepsis, although a wide variety of more serious findings may accompany EV infections (AAP, 2024d; Modlin, 2015). The incubation period is typically 3 to 6 days, except for acute hemorrhagic conjunctivitis, with an incubation period of 1 to 3 days (AAP, 2024d). Infected, symptomatic, and asymptomatic children frequently shed the virus from the respiratory tract for up to 3 weeks, whereas fecal shedding may continue for almost 3 months (AAP, 2024d).

**Clinical Manifestations and Diagnosis.** Although the majority of infants infected with EV may remain asymptomatic, those with severe disease have devastating disease with death or long-term sequelae resulting. It is important to emphasize that fatal infections account for only a small fraction of all congenital and neonatal EV infections. The most serious infections present with myocarditis, hepatitis, and encephalitis, with pneumonitis being seen less frequently (AAP, 2024d; Modlin, 2015). Unfortunately, pathology reports are only available from postmortem examinations. Because of the similarity of the presentation of EV infection with other viral, bacterial, and fungal infections, diagnosis cannot be made based on clinical findings alone, although suspicion may be increased based on time of year, exposure, incubation period, and certain clinical symptoms (Krogstad & Cherry, 2025).

Definitive diagnosis is made by detecting the virus from various sources, including stool, rectal swab, CSF fluid, oral swabs, serum, and urine. PCR assays have a higher sensitivity than viral cultures and provide a quicker turnaround time (AAP, 2024d; Krogstad & Cherry, 2025).

**Treatment.** There are no approved definitive treatments for EV infections in the United States. Human immune globulin may be offered to infected infants in an effort to boost antibodies, although efficacy for acute illness has not been established (AAP, 2024d). Pleconaril, an antiviral drug, shows promise in neonatal EV infection; however, it has not gained approval from the U.S. Food and Drug Administration (FDA). Supportive therapy is the mainstay of current treatment modalities. Infants who require intensive care may require respiratory support, cardiovascular agents, and eventually heart or liver transplants. Family support and involvement are needed, with breastfeeding encouraged (Krogstad & Cherry, 2025; Modlin, 2015).

**Prevention.** As with any congenital or neonatal disease, eliminating the agent is the only way to eradicate EV diseases. Vaccine development may be the best direction to follow globally. There has been a 99% reduction in infection with poliomyelitis, primarily because of vaccination, but the disease still exists. Infection control practices are in place and, with careful attention, should be effective in preventing outbreaks in hospital nurseries. When illness is detected, isolation and use of the cohort system is paramount (Krogstad & Cherry, 2025; Nikonov et al., 2017).

### Congenital Syphilis

Syphilis is an STI caused by the bacterium *T. pallidum*. This bacterium is a gram-negative spirochete and is one of the few bacteria that can readily cross the placenta, resulting in fetal infection. Although most cases are the result of transplacental transmission, a few cases may result from contact with genital lesions during the delivery process (Desai et al., 2025; Lawrence, 2025).

**Epidemiology.** The World Health Organization (WHO) reports that more than two million pregnancies are complicated by syphilis annually, and approximately two-thirds of those pregnancies end in poor outcomes (Lawrence, 2025). After reaching a historic low in the United States between 2000 and 2001, the national rate of syphilis has increased by 52% from 8.6 to 12.7 cases per 100,000 population from 2016 to 2020 (AAP, 2024m). This increase is mostly attributable to sexual practices, particularly among gay and bisexual men (AAP, 2024m).

**Clinical Manifestations and Diagnosis.** Untreated syphilis adversely affects pregnancy outcomes. Vertical transmission of treponemas can occur at any time during pregnancy, with the likelihood increasing with advanced gestational age. The microorganisms can cause preterm labor, stillbirth, hydrops fetalis, congenital infection, or neonatal death (AAP, 2024m). The incidence of congenital infection where the birthing parent was untreated or inadequately treated is highest during the 4 years following acquisition of primary infection, secondary infection, and early latent disease. When newborns acquire syphilis from hematogenous spread across the placenta, the effects are on the major organ systems of the fetus, especially the CNS. Common early presentation of the infant with congenital syphilis are hepatosplenomegaly, jaundice, LBW, IUGR, snuffles (copious nasal secretions), mucocutaneous lesions, anemia, and osteochondritis. There is often a bilateral superficial peeling of the skin (desquamation) on the neonatal palms and soles. Some findings may not be apparent until years after birth but can be prevented by treatment of early infection (AAP, 2024m). Nonimmune hydrops is a common presentation in congenital syphilis. The symptoms of perinatal syphilis are similar to those of any other viral infection that spreads hematogenously from the birthing parent to the placenta and on to the developing fetus (AAP, 2024m; Lawrence, 2025).

The serologic status of all birthing parents who deliver in a hospital should be determined before the newborn is discharged (AAP, 2024m). All infants born to seropositive birthing parent require, at a minimum, careful physical examination and a nontreponemal test such as the Venereal Disease Research Laboratory (VDRL) slide test or the rapid plasma regain (RPR) test. In the event of a positive nontreponemal test in the infant or abnormal neonatal physical examination, further testing, such as chest radiograph, eye examination, liver function tests, neuroimaging, and auditory brainstem response, is required. Because an infant's RPR/VDRL will be positive if born to a RPR/VDRL-positive birthing parent, the titers are more diagnostic than the positive result. The infant's quantitative nontreponemal test is considered significant if the titers are fourfold (or greater) higher than the birthing parents. A test positive at two dilutions is the same as a fourfold increase. An LP for CSF analysis (including quantitative VDRL) and radiographs of the long bones can further the definitive diagnosis of syphilis in the neonate and should be performed in all cases of probable congenital syphilis. Radiologic changes such as osteochondritis (a blurring of the epiphyseal borders) demonstrate recent fetal infection, and periostitis represents prolonged involvement, probably within 16 weeks or second-trimester infection (AAP, 2024m; Lawrence, 2025).

**Treatment.** The recommended treatment for a newborn presumed to be infected with congenital syphilis is aqueous penicillin G. Treatment plans are based on whether the infant is suspected to have or is proven to have congenital syphilis. Treatment guidelines are available on the CDC website (https://www.cdc.gov/std/treatment-guidelines/congenital-syphilis.htm) and in the 2024 to 2027 AAP Red Book (AAP, 2024m). A newborn with an antibody titer four or more times higher than the birthing parent level should be treated as if a definitive diagnosis has been obtained. For proven or highly probable congenital syphilis, aqueous crystalline penicillin G, 50,000 U/kg, given intravenously every 12 hours for the first week and then every 8 hours after the first week for a total of 10 days, is the preferred treatment. When the IV route is not feasible, procaine penicillin G, 50,000 U/kg, intramuscularly (IM) as a single daily dose for 10 days is acceptable. For asymptomatic infants whose birthing parent was treated adequately during pregnancy, treatment is not necessary unless follow-up cannot be ensured. Some clinicians recommend a single dose of benzathine penicillin, 50,000 U/kg IM, if the infant is not likely to be followed up. If birthing parent treatment does not include penicillin and if neonatal follow-up is likely to be unreliable, the neonate is given a full 10-day course (AAP, 2024m; Lawrence, 2025).

**Emergency Alert:** **It is imperative for the physician or nurse practitioner (NP) writing the order for penicillin to be clear on the form of penicillin to use. Aqueous crystalline penicillin G is approved for IV usage. Benzathine penicillin G and procaine penicillin G can only be administered IM; IV administration may cause life-threatening side effects or death.**

Standard precautions are recommended for infants with suspicious symptoms until appropriate treatment is given (AAP, 2024m). There is a definite role for nursing education and support in the treatment of an infant exposed to syphilis. The 10-day course of penicillin treatment may lead to the establishment of a trusting relationship between the nurse and family, thus providing an opportunity to give more information regarding sexual risk factors. Families often need encouragement and support to get treatment for other sexual partners and to obtain other necessary medical evaluations (such as HIV screening or drug counseling).

**Prevention.** Prevention of congenital syphilis is accomplished by prevention of syphilis in childbearing birthing parents. Identification and adequate treatment of pregnant birthing parents is necessary. Infants with confirmed congenital syphilis should receive careful follow-up evaluations. Regular childhood well-child visits should be ensured. Serologic nontreponemal measurements can be made at follow-up visits with their primary care physician (AAP, 2024m). In infants with congenital neurosyphilis, CSF examinations should be done every 6 months, with retreatment as needed, until the studies are normal. The infection can be effectively treated, but the physiologic and developmental prognosis depends on the degree of organ damage sustained during fetal development.

### Other Sexually Transmitted Diseases

**Gonorrheal Ophthalmia.** Ophthalmia neonatorum is the result of infection of the mucous membranes by *Neisseria gonorrhoeae* or *Chlamydia trachomatis;* these infections may be found simultaneously. Neonatal conjunctivitis caused by *N. gonorrhoeae* is the primary concern when birthing-parent gonorrhea has been diagnosed. Although infection of mucosal surfaces is more common in infants born to an infected birthing parent, scalp abscesses and systemic infection can occur (Embree, 2025).

**Epidemiology.** *Neisseria gonorrhoeae* is a species of small gram-negative diploid bacteria. *Neisseria gonorrhoeae* is the second most reported of STIs, exceeded only by *C. trachomatis* (CDC, 2024d). There were 194.1 cases per 100,000 population in the United States in 2022 (CDC, 2024d; Embree, 2025). Rates are higher in the non-White communities as a result of social disparities. Infection with this organism is seen most frequently in young adults 20 to 24 years of age (Embree, 2025). Other risk factors include unprotected sex, multiple sex partners, drug and alcohol abuse, and low-income status. In females, the infection may be asymptomatic, compromising the disease's detection. Neonatal gonococcal conjunctivitis occurs in up to one-third of cases where the birthing parent cervical infection is present (Embree, 2025). The incubation period is typically 2 to 7 days; however, gonococcal infection should be considered in any infant with conjunctivitis present 24 hours after birth (Embree, 2025).

**Clinical Manifestations and Diagnosis.** Gonococcal conjunctivitis in the newborn has historically been a risk from transmission via the birth canal. Although asymptomatic colonization has been reported, typically, the infected infant presents with acute purulent conjunctivitis and edema of the eyelids. Other possible neonatal findings include scalp infection or systemic manifestations, including pneumonia, sepsis, osteomyelitis, or meningitis. Untreated, the illness may spread to the connective tissues and cornea (Embree, 2025).

Although conjunctivitis may be obvious based on clinical signs, a definitive diagnosis is necessary for planning the management and treatment. Ophthalmia neonatorum from other organisms must be differentiated from conjunctivitis from different organisms. Gram stain of the drainage will reveal the gram-negative diplococcic typical of *N. gonorrhoeae*. This provides a presumptive diagnosis. If Gram stain is positive, cultures should be obtained of the eye drainage as well as from additional mucosal sites in the infant. Testing of the birthing parent and their sexual partner is essential. Specifics for testing of adults are beyond the scope of this chapter on neonatal illnesses but are a prerequisite for the management and treatment of the newborn (Darville, 2025; Embree, 2025).

**Treatment.** Globally, *N. gonorrhoeae* is increasingly resistant to penicillin; therefore, this antibiotic is no longer recommended unless the specific isolate has been proven to be sensitive. Infants who are delivered to a birthing parent who is infected and untreated are usually given a complete infection workup, including an LP, and given a single dose of ceftriaxone or cefotaxime IV or IM. If cultures confirm the presence of the microorganism, the infant with scalp abscess or disseminated gonococcal infection should be treated with ceftriaxone, 25 to 50 mg/kg/d (maximum of 125 mg) IV or IM in a single dose for 7 days (10–14 days if meningitis is confirmed) (AAP, 2024e). Cefotaxime is recommended for infants with hyperbilirubinemia, especially if born prematurely, because ceftriaxone competes for bilirubin binding sites on albumin (Darville, 2025; Embree, 2025). For gonococcal ophthalmia neonatorum, a one-time single dose of ceftriaxone is recommended to prevent progression to corneal ulceration and/or perforation (AAP, 2024e). An important addition to the management plan is irrigation of the eyes with a normal saline solution frequently until drainage is no longer seen. This practice has been shown to decrease long-term consequences. The addition of ophthalmic antibiotic drops has not been shown to improve outcomes and is not deemed necessary. Education and support regarding the origin of the infectious agent are important in the treatment of gonorrhea. Sexual partners of infected persons should be encouraged to seek testing and appropriate antibiotic treatment for gonorrhea (AAP, 2024e; Embree, 2025).

**Prevention.** Targeting the treatment of pregnant birthing parents is the best strategy for the prevention of fetal and neonatal infection. The use of silver nitrate solution or erythromycin for the prevention of gonococcal ophthalmia neonatorum is one of the early achievements in preventive medicine. Silver nitrate was discontinued due to the universal development of chemical conjunctivitis. Routine prophylaxis is mandated by law in most states and has significantly improved treating ocular disease if administered within 1 hour of birth. Erythromycin ointment in both eyes is a well-established and efficacious prophylactic practice for preventing gonococcal ophthalmia (Embree, 2025). Chlamydia conjunctivitis has become far more common than gonococcal conjunctivitis in the neonate because of the continual screening for gonorrhea.

**Chlamydia Conjunctivitis.** *Chlamydia* is a genus of intracellular bacteria that may affect virtually all animal species. Although the genus *Chlamydia* is divided into at least four groups, this chapter will focus on the organism *Chlamydia Trachomatis* (*C. trachomatis*). *C. trachomatis* infection is the most commonly reported and notifiable STI in the United States (Darville, 2025). Birthing-parent infection may lead to neonatal conjunctivitis and chlamydia pneumonia. Neonatal conjunctivitis can be expected in 20% to 50% of infants born to infected but untreated birthing parents. Pneumonia caused by C. trachomatis will develop in 5% to 20% of newborns of birthing parents with active, untreated chlamydia infection (Darville, 2025). Conjunctivitis will be the focus of this section.

**Epidemiology.** *C. trachomatis* is the most common STI in Western industrialized nations. Most infected individuals are asymptomatic, leading to underestimation of the prevalence. This is a worrisome fact because this could theoretically support a large reservoir within our societies that can sustain the pathogen. Risk factors are the same as for other STIs—young age (< 20 years), socioeconomically disadvantaged, geography, and number of sexual partners. The infection can present in birthing parents as cervicitis, salpingitis, urethritis, or pelvic inflammatory disease (PID). *C. trachomatis* infection has been identified as causing a significant increase in the incidence of PROM, the number of LBW babies, and the rate of infant mortality (Darville, 2025). Thus, screening pregnant birthing parents for chlamydia is an essential part of prenatal care.

**Clinical Manifestations and Diagnosis.** Chlamydia conjunctivitis can present in the newborn with a very watery discharge that may progress to purulent exudate. The incubation period is anywhere from 5 to 14 days but may be shorter in cases of prematurely ruptured membranes. Prior to treatment, the eyelids may swell, and a "pseudomembrane" consisting of inflammatory exudate may form and stick to the conjunctiva (Darville, 2025).

Diagnosis of chlamydial infections is based on physical and laboratory examination. In cases of conjunctivitis, Giemsa-stained conjunctival scrapings (not exudate alone) provide a method of direct fluorescent antibody (DFA) testing. This method is the only FDA-approved culture-independent method for detecting chlamydia from conjunctival swabs. The organism is not detectable on routine Gram stains. Cell culture demonstrates high specificity but is expensive. NAATs are **not** FDA approved but exhibit higher sensitivity and can also test for both *C. trachomatis* and *N. gonorrhoeae* simultaneously. The definitive diagnosis for chlamydial pneumonia is made by culture of the respiratory tract or identification of high levels of IgM antibodies to chlamydia; however, serologic testing is not widely available (AAP, 2024b; Darville, 2025). Two NAAT tests were FDA approved in 2019, suggesting utility when the nasopharyngeal specimen is obtained in the newborn (Darville, 2025).

**Treatment.** Universal eye prophylaxis with antibiotics is required by law in most states for every newborn. Application of erythromycin ointment at birth for ocular prophylaxis successfully treats gonococcal conjunctivitis but has not been as successful in treating chlamydial conjunctivitis. Even for infants born to birthing parents known to have untreated chlamydial infection, prophylactic antimicrobial treatment is not indicated due to the unknown efficacy of such treatment. In these cases, the infants should be monitored clinically with appropriate diagnostic workup and appropriate treatment if the infant becomes symptomatic (AAP, 2024b; Darville, 2025). The treatment of highly suspected chlamydia infection in the newborn usually begins with ampicillin and gentamicin if the infant's workup is for generic infection. Once the chlamydia organism is identified, treatment with oral erythromycin base or ethylsuccinate (50 mg/kg/d in four divided doses daily) for 14 days for chlamydial ophthalmia neonatorum or chlamydial pneumonia is recommended. An alternative treatment for both types of infection is azithromycin (20 mg/kg as a single daily dose for 3 days; however, data on effectiveness is limited (AAP, 2024b; Darville, 2025). In the case of neonatal conjunctivitis, topical therapy, in addition to systemic treatment, is indicated. Follow-up of infants treated for chlamydial conjunctivitis is recommended to determine if treatment was effective (AAP, 2024b).

**Prevention.** Prevention of STIs is the same regardless of the organism in question. The only definitive method of prevention is screening and treating the infected pregnant birthing parent. Education and counseling regarding the method of transmission of chlamydia are important. This organism may be present for many years in the birthing parent's genital tract and produce no symptoms. The organism does not respond to partial treatment; sexual partners must receive full treatment immediately. A condom should be used during sexual relations to prevent transmission. Without treatment, the severe complications for the birthing parent include PID, ectopic pregnancy, and endometritis (Darville, 2025).

### Varicella-Zoster

Varicella is a member of the human DNA herpes viruses. Primary infection with the VZV causes chickenpox. This primary infection is followed by a lifelong period of latent infection of the sensory ganglion neurons. Herpes zoster (shingles) may develop later in life in those who had varicella, especially the elderly and those with immune deficiency. Chickenpox is extremely contagious and commonly occurs in childhood. Varicella is known as the most communicable of all diseases and is only found in humans (AAP, 2024o; Shah et al., 2025; Moss, 2025). Because of the devastating effects of congenital varicella syndrome (CVS), varicella will be the focus of this section.

**Epidemiology.** The incidence of this virus in pregnant birthing parents is very low, approximately in the range of 0.5 in 10,000 pregnancies, primarily due to the success of the varicella vaccine. The virus is transmitted by direct contact with the virus in vesicular lesions or by airborne droplets spread via the respiratory tract. Symptoms of varicella are usually present 10 to 21 days after exposure and include fever, malaise, and an itchy rash. Administration of varicella-zoster immune globulin (VZIG) may delay onset for up to 28 days. An infected individual is considered contagious from 1 to 2 days before the onset of symptoms until all lesions have crusted. The maculopapular rash eventually forms vesicles and crusts around 6 days after onset (AAP, 2024o; Desai et al., 2025; Moss, 2025). In utero, infection occurs as a result of transplacental passage of the virus during gestation in the infected birthing parent. The severity of the effect on the fetus or newborn is related to the timing during gestation. The lowest risk of CVS occurs when the birthing parent is infected during the first trimester and rises slightly during weeks 13 through 20. CVS rarely occurs after the 20th week of gestation. There is a higher case-fatality rate in offspring when illness develops in the birthing parent from 5 days before to 2 days after birth of the infant. The severity of CVS is decreased when varicella develops in the birthing parent more than 5 days before delivery and after 28 weeks' gestation. It is thought that the birthing parent's transfer of varicella-zoster–specific IgG is responsible (AAP, 2024o).

**Clinical Manifestations and Diagnosis.** CVS is characterized by cicatricial skin lesions with scarring, limb hypoplasia, CNS involvement, and abnormalities of the eye, renal system, and autonomic nervous system. Neonatal death is most often the result of pneumonia (Desai et al., 2025; Shah et al., 2025).

In the neonate, identified infection in the birthing parent will easily lead to a diagnosis of CVS when clinical manifestations are obvious, such as a widespread vesicular exanthema. A similar presentation is more difficult to identify when there is no known birthing parent infection. The definitive diagnosis of varicella is made by the identification of VZV from vesicular fluid using a PCR test. Other methods are available, but the PCR assay is the diagnostic method of choice. Culture and DFA testing are less sensitive and, therefore, unreliable. The presence of specific IgM may only indicate recent exposure or infection and is not a reliable indicator for CVS (AAP, 2024o; Desai et al., 2025).

**Treatment.** Although some believe that the consequences of CVS do not progress in severity after birth, there is limited data that the use of acyclovir for the treatment of severe disease in newborns, whether congenital or postnatally acquired, may be beneficial. The recommended dose is 30 mg/kg/d divided in three doses for 7 to 10 days or until no new lesions have appeared for 48 hours in the neonate with varicella infection progressing beyond mild infection (Shah et al., 2025). There is a limited window for the best outcome of antiviral therapy for varicella (Moss, 2025; Shah et al., 2025). Early therapy maximizes benefit. VZIG can be given to newborns to decrease the severity of infection in those exposed and should be administered as soon as possible after birth (AAP, 2024o;

Desai et al., 2025). **Emergency Alert: Children with varicella should not be given salicylate or salicylate-containing products (aspirin, bismuth subsalicylate). These products are known to increase the risk of Reye syndrome.**

**Prevention.** The primary approach to prevention of CVS is vaccination of birthing parents of childbearing age before pregnancy. Although not 100% effective, vaccination could protect 85% of birthing parents and their infants. Strict isolation of identified infants or those whose symptoms are highly suspicious of infection is necessary. Infants should be vaccinated according to established vaccination schedules. Hospitals should initiate and strictly enforce guidelines for maintaining the immunity of hospital personnel. Isolation for airborne and contact illnesses should be followed. Typically, if a birthing parent has contracted varicella infection late in pregnancy, other persons, such as healthcare workers, family members, or other newborns, may have been exposed (Moss, 2025). In cases where the birthing parent was infected during pregnancy, and the infant does not show evidence of disease at birth, the birthing parent and infant should be isolated separately until the birthing parent's lesions have crusted over. If the infant develops clinical evidence of disease, the birthing parent may care for the infant if they are well enough. Isolation should continue during hospitalization and after discharge for a total of 21 days (28 days if intravenous immunoglobulins (IVIG) was given; AAP, 2024o).

VZIG can be given to newborns to decrease the severity of infection in those exposed; it does not prevent infection. If exposure occurs within a neonatal intensive care unit (NICU), it is recommended that if there is a risk of significant exposure (such as in an open-bed environment as opposed to a single-room environment), all premature infants less than 28 weeks or less than 1 kg receive VZIG regardless of the birthing parent's immunity status, because there has been inadequate transfer of birthing parent antibodies. VZIG should also be given in the NICU when there is significant exposure in the 28th week of gestation or more and in neonates with birthing parent seronegative immunity status (AAP, 2024o; Moss, 2025; Shah et al., 2025).

## Lyme Disease

Lyme disease is the most common vector-borne disease in the United States. It is caused by the spirochete *B. burgdorferi*. Lyme disease is transmitted to humans by the bite of the blacklegged tick, commonly known as the deer tick. Because other spirochetes are known to cause significant and often devastating outcomes when transplacental infections occur, the risk of disease in the newborn from Lyme disease is of considerable interest (Sood & Shapiro, 2025).

**Epidemiology.** Lyme disease has been identified in more than 50 countries. In the United States, more than 63,000 cases were reported by state health departments to the CDC in 2022 (CDC, 2024c). It is known that this is only a proportion of the actual cases. The most recent estimate based on a commercial insurance claims database is that the number of people diagnosed may be around 476,000. There is a concentration of cases in the Northeast, Mid-Atlantic, and Upper Midwest, with 14 states accounting for over 95% of reported cases (AAP, 2024k; CDC, 2024c; Sood & Shapiro, 2025). Tick larvae become infected by feeding on animals that are infected. Ticks in the nymphal stage are the most likely to infect humans with the spirochete. This stage emerges in the spring to early fall, when deer activity is greatest, making this season the most likely time for humans to become infected. Evidence indicates that the risk of Lyme disease after a deer tick bite is only 1% to 3%. Late disease, mainly arthritis, occurs at any time. Although infection can occur at any age, the reported incidence is greater in children from 5 to 9 years of age and adults 55 through 69 years (AAP, 2024k; CDC, 2024c; Sood & Shapiro, 2025; Swami, 2025).

**Clinical Manifestations and Diagnosis.** In adults, clinical manifestations can be divided into early (early localized or early disseminated) disease or late disease. Early-localized disease is characterized by a distinct lesion at the site of a recent tick bite, although the person may not be aware of having been bitten by a tick. There is a classic "bull's eye" appearance in some, but not all, cases. There may be an accompanying clinical presentation of extreme tiredness, headache, mild neck stiffness, muscle pain, and maybe fever. In early-disseminated disease, multiple lesions of erythema migrans may appear 3 to 5 weeks after the tick bite. These lesions are smaller but similar to the primary lesion. There may be palsies of the cranial nerves, lymphocytic meningitis, and rarely carditis. The signs of early-localized disease can be expected as well. Late Lyme disease occurs in people who were not treated early and most commonly presents in Lyme arthritis in children who were not treated (AAP, 2024k; Swami, 2025).

In areas where Lyme disease is endemic, transplacental infection is known to occur, although congenital infection is rare. There are case reports of fetal loss and newborns with anomalies. Although skin anomalies and cardiac defects have been noted in infants born to birthing parents with Lyme disease, the inconsistency in findings suggests that there is no recognized syndrome associated with fetal infection. Attempts to investigate the significance of congenital Lyme disease on the newborn have been limited. First, the prevalence is low, and second, diagnosis based on current methods of seropositivity, history of tick bite, and reports of clinical symptoms in the birthing parent is unreliable. Because of increased awareness of the problems associated with Lyme disease, most childbearing women are being identified and treated, especially if pregnancy is suspected. *Borrelia burgdorferi* has been identified from several abortuses and a few live-born children with congenital anomalies.

Furthermore, evidence suggests no difference in the prevalence of congenital malformations in infants born to women with serum antibodies against *B. burgdorferi* and the offspring of those without such antibodies (Sood & Shapiro, 2025; Swami, 2025). The CDC currently recommends a two-step process in the testing for evidence of Lyme disease. These steps can be done together using the same blood sample. The first step uses an EIA or enzyme-linked immunosorbent assay (ELISA). Rarely is an indirect immunofluorescence assay (IFA) used. If this first step is negative, no further specimen testing is recommended. If the first step is positive or equivocal, the second step should be performed. The second step consists of the Western immunoblot (Western blot). Results are considered positive only if both steps render a positive result. The two steps of Lyme disease testing are designed to be done together. Skipping the first step is not recommended due to many false-positive reports (CDC, 2024c). Keep in mind that serologic testing may be falsely negative during the first 4 to 6 weeks after infection, so diagnosis and treatment should be started based on the characteristic appearance of erythema multiforme (EM) lesion plus likely exposure in geographic areas of known incidence (AAP, 2024k; CDC, 2024c).

**Treatment.** Current treatment protocols include an oral regimen of doxycycline, amoxicillin, or cefuroxime axetil. Doxycycline previously was not recommended for use in young children under the age of 2 years due to reports of permanent teeth staining; these findings, although present in older tetracyclines, have not been documented with the use of doxycycline. Therefore, the AAP now accepts the safety of doxycycline use regardless of age (Sood & Shapiro, 2025). All persons receiving doxycycline should be warned of the side effects of photosensitivity in sun-exposed areas. Early use of appropriate antibiotics is associated with rapid and complete recovery. People with certain neurologic or cardiac forms of illness with neurologic or cardiac involvement may require IV treatment with ceftriaxone or amoxicillin (AAP, 2024k; CDC, 2024c; Swami, 2025).

**Prevention.** Reducing the risk of tick bites is the only definitive preventive measure. Methods to reduce the risk involve decreasing the known habitat of the deer tick. Keeping yards clear of brush and lawns frequently mowed may reduce exposure in endemic areas. Pesticides may effectively reduce the tick population, but many unwanted and undesirable side effects are inherent in their usage. In infants 2 months of age and older, a tick and insect repellent that contains *N,N* -diethyl-meta-toluamide (DEET) applied to the skin may provide additional protection (Sood & Shapiro, 2025).

### Human Immunodeficiency Virus

HIV is one of the greatest public health concerns of the past five decades. HIV-1 and HIV-2 are RNA-containing retroviruses of the *Retroviridae* family and belong to the *Lentivirus* genus (AAP, 2024i). Retroviruses are characterized by the presence of a viral reverse transcriptase enzyme that converts single-stranded viral RNA into double-stranded DNA. This double-stranded DNA copy integrates into the host cell genome. Because HIV-1 is more prevalent in the United States, HIV-1 will be the focus of this section, especially as it affects the newborn.

**Epidemiology.** Although a virus very closely related to HIV was originally identified in chimpanzees and monkeys in Africa, it has long been known that HIV affects humans, attacking cells containing the surface molecule, $CD4^+$, particularly T lymphocytes and macrophages. Originally thought to be a disease mainly affecting men involved in homosexual relationships, HIV is now known to occur in both men and women and children. HIV has no regard for socioeconomic status, gender, age, or nationality; however, disparities still exist. Of the roughly 38.4 million individuals infected with the HIV virus, 67% live in Sub-Saharan Africa (SSA) (Moyo et al., 2023). China follows SSA, with 4 million infected, and then the Americas (including the Caribbean), with 3 million people who are HIV infected. HIV often leads to AIDS in the untreated patient and may advance to AIDS despite treatment. Chronic immune activation, with the depletion of $CD4^+$ cells via the adaptive and innate immune systems, plays an important role in the immunopathogenesis of HIV/AIDS. The good news is that rates are declining, with the most significant declines noted in the Caribbean and SSA (AAP, 2024i; Shetty & Maldonado, 2013). The only epidemiologically implicated ways of transmission are through contact with blood, semen, cervicovaginal secretions, and human milk (AAP, 2024i). Transmission from the birthing parent to the child has declined dramatically due to early recognition and treatment of birthing parents of childbearing age; therefore, there is a relatively stable incidence of infection. Although rates are declining, the incidence is still unacceptable. The vast majority of children living with HIV are infected as a result of vertical transmission from a birthing parent who is HIV infected. In utero infection occurs through transplacental infection or fetal exposure to infected amniotic fluid. Current data suggest that in utero infection occurs during the last few weeks of gestation, when placental vasculature is proliferative. Intrapartum infection may be the result of direct exposure of the fetus or infant to infected secretions from the birthing parent or exposure to the birthing parent's blood during labor (Shetty & Maldonado, 2013). Although transmission from the birthing parent to the child occurs across a large range of viral loads, the birthing parent's viral load is the most critical determinant of vertical transmission of the virus. The risk increases with ROM and directly relates to the time of ROM. Cesarean delivery before ROM is known to reduce transmission from the birthing parent to the child. Postnatal transmission is most likely the result of transmission through human milk, especially where the provision of human milk is a common practice in low-to-middle-income families because safe alternatives to feeding the infant may not be available or may be unsafe (AAP, 2024i; Shetty & Maldonado, 2013).

**Clinical Manifestations and Diagnosis.** Perinatal HIV infection results in a wide variety of manifestations and depends on the stage at diagnosis. Most HIV-infected newborns are asymptomatic at birth because infection most likely occurs during the peripartum period. Clinical signs typically begin to manifest around 1 to 2 years of age. For some poorly understood reason, some infants, termed *rapid progressors*, may become symptomatic in the first 2 months (Desai et al., 2025). In the untreated pediatric population, early clinical signs of HIV type 1 include fevers of unknown cause, lymphadenopathy, enlargement of the liver and spleen, failure to thrive, persistent candidiasis, diarrhea, encephalopathy, either hyporeflexia/floppiness or hyperreflexia/hypertonia, and developmental delays. Recurrent opportunistic infections are common and may increase the risk of death (AAP, 2024i). The prognosis of survival for the neonate, infant, or child infected with HIV is based on the timing of infection and treatment modality. Death in untreated infants is invariable.

Unless assay results are negative, antibody assays are not helpful in the diagnosis of HIV in children under the age of 24 months because these infants and toddlers will have passive antibodies acquired from the birthing parent. These antibodies from the birthing parent make the EIA and Western blot inappropriate in infants up to 18 to 24 months of age. Currently, in the United States, the most sensitive and, therefore, the preferred test is the HIV DNA PCR or RNA assay, referred to as HIV NAAT. If the test is positive within 48 hours of birth, in-utero transmission is assumed (AAP, 2024i; Shetty & Maldonado, 2013). Some experts recommend viral testing in the first 2 days of life for all infants suspected of in-utero infection to increase the chance of early identification and treatment. Umbilical cord testing is not acceptable due to the possibility of contamination with birthing parent blood. Refer to the AAP Report of the Committee on Infectious Diseases, 2024–2027, Redbook, for a link to an algorithm for interpreting the test results and a technical update published in 2023 following FDA approval of HIV nucleic acid tests with a diagnostic claim (AAP, 2024i).

**Treatment.** It is important to know that treatment with antiviral therapy does not cure HIV; instead, it suppresses the virus with the goal of converting the active disease to a chronic disease. Because of the options available for the treatment of HIV-infected infants and children, consultation with an expert in pediatric HIV infection is the standard of care for these individuals (AAP, 2024i). The most important factors in the outcome for infants exposed to or infected with HIV are whether the birthing parent received antepartum/intrapartum antiretroviral therapy (ART) and the viral load at the time of delivery. Treatment of the birthing parent is not the purpose of this section, but if and when the birthing parent received treatment, it is paramount in the decisions around the treatment of the infant. ART resistance is becoming more evident, and therapeutic management protocols have changed with the current findings. The newborn infant, exposed to HIV in utero, should be bathed as soon as possible after birth to remove all blood and secretions from the birthing parent. Antiretroviral (ARV) prophylaxis should be started as early as possible, preferably within 6 hours after birth. Current treatment guidelines may be found online at: https://clinicalinfo.hiv.gov/en/guidelines. Enrollment of HIV-infected infants in clinical trials may provide opportunities for exposure to the newest treatment modalities (AAP, 2024i).

**Prevention.** Theoretically, prevention of HIV in adults and adolescents can be accomplished by safe sexual practices, limiting exposure to HIV-infected blood, and education to all sexually active individuals about the risk factors and ways to avoid them. Prevention of HIV transmission to the infant has been the focus of research since the first recognition of transmission from the birthing parent to the infant. The result has been the use of ART for the birthing parent with known HIV infection. Current recommendations are that all birthing parents are tested early in pregnancy and ARV therapy begins. Compliant birthing parents who desire to provide their own human milk should be supported in doing so and meet with a lactation consultant. However, ongoing birthing-parent ARV therapy compliance, antiretroviral prophylaxis for the infant, maternal viral load monitoring, and HIV infection testing in the infant should be encouraged (AAP, 2024i). Increased research efforts on adherence to recommendations and how they affect youth are needed.

### Parvovirus

The parvoviruses are a family of small, single-stranded DNA viruses of the family *Parvoviridae*. The parvoviruses are animal viruses and seem to be species specific. Parvovirus B19 and human bocavirus (HBoV) are the only two parvoviruses with proven pathogenicity in humans (Koch, 2025). Parvovirus B19 typically presents in children as an erythematous rash (erythema infectiosum), whereas HBoV manifests as a respiratory illness indistinguishable from other common viral respiratory infections. Parvovirus B19 will be the focus of this section because it is the most well studied and clinically significant in humans (Desai et al., 2025).

**Epidemiology.** The human parvovirus, B19, presenting as erythema infectiosum (fifth disease) is a common and highly contagious pathogen worldwide. In the United States, 40% to 60% of adults are seropositive, indicating a previous infection during childhood. The incidence is twice as high in Whites as in Blacks. The virus is transmitted mainly by droplets from oral or nasal secretions but can also occur from percutaneous exposure to blood or blood products (AAP, 2024l). Rapid transmission occurs due to close contact between family members or school classmates (Koch, 2025).

**Clinical Manifestations and Diagnosis.** The focus of this chapter is on the effects of disease on the neonate; therefore, this section will discuss the clinical manifestations and diagnostic tests necessary when an infant is suspected of having parvovirus B19V. There have been reports of serious, and often devastating, outcomes for the fetus and newborn when the birthing parent has a primary infection of parvovirus B19. Adverse outcomes include hydrops fetalis, isolated pleural or pericardial effusions, IUGR, fetal anemia, and intrauterine fetal demise. Although fetal infections may lead to poor outcomes, the infected neonate will likely be asymptomatic at birth. The risk of transmission from the birthing parent to the infant is low (≤ 10%); the greatest risk occurs with birthing parent infection during the first 20 weeks of gestation. Meconium ileus and peritonitis have also been reported in neonates following birthing-parent infection during pregnancy (Desai et al., 2025; Koch, 2025).

The diagnosis of parvovirus B19 in the newborn infant is based on identifying the infection in the birthing parent. Most infants are asymptomatic at birth and rarely require virologic confirmation. The preferred diagnostic test for acute or recent parvovirus B19 is the detection of serum-specific IgM antibodies. Prenatal diagnosis, when fetal hydrops is suspected, can be verified by the detection of viral DNA in fetal blood or amniotic fluid by these methods (AAP, 2024l; Koch, 2025).

**Treatment.** Treatment for the prenatally infected infant is based on clinical manifestations, if present. Fetal transfusion may be indicated in cases of hydrops fetalis with significant fetal anemia. Intrauterine transfusions may be necessary for resolution of the hydrops and associated anemia. Each transfusion is associated with increased risk to the fetus, and the birthing parent should be referred to a maternal–fetal specialist for ongoing management of the pregnancy (Koch, 2025).

**Prevention.** Pregnant healthcare providers should be informed of the potential risks to their fetus from parvovirus B19 infections. The best strategy to decrease the risk of infection is to pay attention to strict infection control procedures, including standard and droplet precautions, if hydrops has not resolved in the neonate at the time of birth (AAP, 2024l).

### Hepatitis B Virus

The hepatitis B virus (HBV) is a large, double-stranded DNA–containing virus in the family *Hepadnaviridae*. Hepatitis B surface antigen (HBsAg) is present in the chronic carrier state. A chronic carrier state is defined as the persistence of the HBsAg in serum for at least 6 months (AAP, 2024g).

**Epidemiology.** HBV has been detected worldwide, with an estimated 350,000 persons known to be chronic carriers. In the United States, the prevalence of HBV infection in pregnant birthing parents shows a distinct disparity by race and ethnicity, with the highest rates reported in Asian birthing parents; rates in Black, White, and Hispanic birthing parents are similar, with the lowest rates in Hispanic birthing parents. Chronic HBV infection is endemic in SSA, China, parts of the Middle East, the Amazon basin, and the Pacific Islands. Carrier rates are estimated to be as high as 35% in these areas. In the United States, where a successful vaccination program exists, there is still an estimated 1.25 million chronic HBV carriers (Rogers & Balistreri, 2025; Karnsakul & Schwarz, 2025). However, in Alaska, where the Alaska Native population experienced near-epidemic HBV infection rates, symptomatic HBV has been nearly eradicated by universal newborn vaccination, mass screening, and vigilant immunization of susceptible individuals (Rogers & Balistreri, 2025). The primary route of transmission is through infected blood or bodily fluids. The surface antigen, HBsAg, has also been noted in human milk, saliva, and tears. Blood, semen, vaginal secretions, CSF, and other bodily fluids, such as synovial, pleural, pericardial, peritoneal, and amniotic fluid, present the most potential for transmission of the virus. Transmission by blood or blood products in the United States has been virtually eliminated due to routine screening of donors (AAP, 2018g). HBV infection in a pregnant birthing parent does not appear to have teratogenic abilities, although there are reports of a higher incidence of LBW and prematurity. Acute HBV infection in the birthing parent early in pregnancy has a 10% transmission rate, with a higher incidence when acute infection occurs in the third trimester. Chronic infection in pregnant birthing parents does not appear to affect pregnancy outcomes (Karnsakul & Schwarz, 2025). HBV is most often the result of IV drug use, but transmission also occurs through sexual contact with an infected partner and via transmission from the birthing parent to the infant. The majority of infections transmitted from the birthing parent to the infant occur at birth or in the postpartum period. A large percentage of infants born to birthing parents with a high viral load develop chronic HBV infection (Desai et al., 2025).

**Clinical Manifestations and Diagnosis.** Clinical manifestations of HBV infection are age dependent. In adults, HBsAg is detected 1 to 3 months after exposure to the virus. Elevation of liver enzymes occurs between 2 weeks and 2 months after detection of HBsAg. The symptoms most often reported are nausea, vomiting, headache, and lethargy. This period progresses to the development of jaundice. Most adults with HBV infection have a self-limited course. A few will develop hepatic failure, and many of these will die. A chronic carrier state, or persistent HBV infection, is also possible. In the United States, 25% to 50% of all cases of chronic infection are in children. Chronic liver disease and hepatocarcinoma may result from a chronic carrier state (Rogers & Balistreri, 2025).

Ninety percent of infants born to birthing parents who are positive for both HBsAg and hepatitis B e antigen (HBeAg) are at risk for the development of chronic HBV infection by their first birthday if they are not given treatment. Infants born to birthing parents who are positive for HBsAg but negative for HBeAg have lower rates of perinatal infection (20%). Infants who do not receive treatment are likely to become carriers, which may eventually lead to cirrhosis or primary hepatocellular carcinoma. A few (6%) may develop acute hepatitis at around 2 months of age. Symptoms most reported for infants are fever, jaundice, and hepatic tenderness. Serum aminotransferases are elevated (Karnsakul & Schwarz, 2025).

The serologic diagnosis of HBV is complex and is different depending on whether the disease is acute or chronic. HBsAg is used to detect acutely or chronically infected people. HBsAg is an important test in assessing a birthing parent's risk of transmitting HBV to their unborn child. HBeAg is used to identify people who are at the greatest risk of transmitting the virus. The presence of HBsAg and HBeAg is the best indication of infectiousness. It is currently recommended that all pregnant birthing parents be screened at their first prenatal visit for HBsAg and HBeAg to prevent prenatal transmission; for high-risk populations, this should be repeated in the third trimester (Rogers & Balistreri, 2025).

**Treatment.** Hepatitis B vaccine is the gold standard for prevention of HBV. All infants should receive the first vaccine before discharge from the birth hospital, preferably within 24 hours of birth. Infants born to birthing parents who are at risk of transmitting the virus should receive the HBV vaccine along with hepatitis B immunoglobulin. An algorithm exists to determine the timing and dosage for infants according to birth weight as well as for prophylaxis according to birthing parent HBV status (AAP, 2018g). Vaccination is recommended for individuals who are at risk for exposure to HBV, including healthcare workers, family members of chronic carriers, persons with large numbers of heterosexual partners, and IV drug users. Hepatitis B vaccine is administered to the deltoid muscle once and again 1 and 6 months later (AAP, 2018g).

**Prevention.** Proper and prompt identification of birthing parents in high-risk groups and knowledge of HBV status is vital in the delivery room to determine whether the infant is at risk for infection. Following universal infection control measures, appropriate barriers protect healthcare workers from blood and body secretions. Delivery room and nursery personnel should always wear gloves when handling new infants. The infant of a birthing parent with confirmed HBV infection should be bathed with soap and water immediately, with special attention to removing all blood and secretions present on the skin and hair. The infant may be fed at the breast (unless the birthing parent's nipples are cracked) and cared for routinely. Family clustering of HBV has been identified, and spread via household contact is common (AAP, 2024g).

## Fungal Agents

### Candida albicans

*Candida* species are a group of fungi frequently found in humans; *Candida albicans* is the most prevalent form in neonates, followed by *Candida parapsilosis*. *Candida* organisms are oval, yeastlike cells that can bud to reproduce (AAP, 2024a).

**Epidemiology.** *Candida* bloodstream infections are a major cause of LOS in newborns, especially in extremely LBW infants or medically complex larger infants. The incidence of late-onset candidemia is reported to range from 4% to 15% in VLBW infants; mortality and neurodevelopmental impairment may be as high as 75% of affected extremely low-birth weight (ELBW) infants (AAP, 2024a; Bendel & Swanson, 2025). Outcomes, such as blindness, severe neurologic impairment, renal failure, and endocarditis, have been reported related to dissemination. Early recognition and treatment of fungal infections are imperative to prevent severe CNS complications and death. Besides birthing parent colonization, other risk factors include prolonged broad-spectrum antibiotic treatment for small, premature infants, which may predispose infants to *Candida* overgrowth in the GI tract. Studies have shown that up to 75% of neonates admitted to the NICU are colonized in the GI tract with Candida by the end of the first month of life. This overgrowth may predispose the infant to disseminated or systemic fungemia in the preterm infant (Bendel & Swanson, 2025). Administration of hyperalimentation, frequent use of indwelling venous lines, invasive procedures, and GI disease, especially necrotizing enterocolitis (NEC), may also predispose the infant to *C. albicans* infection. Congenital candidiasis may present at birth and results from a birthing parent's intrauterine infection or exposure to extensive vaginal infection. Chorioamnionitis is associated with intrauterine fetal death and preterm delivery (Bendel & Swanson, 2025).

**Clinical Manifestations and Diagnosis.** *Candida* species are responsible for a variety of clinical presentations in the newborn. Mild candida diaper dermatitis and oral thrush are potential findings in infants who have been on antibiotics. Systemic candidemia can be life threatening, especially in extremely premature infants. The newborn with disseminated *C. albicans* infection presents a picture similar to that of any septic infant. Early cultures reported as negative in clinically ill infants with risk factors for fungal infection should alert the caregiver to the possibility of candidemia. In the NICU, the median age at onset of symptoms varies depending on the type of candida infection, with clinical symptoms of congenital candidiasis present at birth or within 24 hours of life to systemic infections presenting after 7 days of age. An infant with candidemia often presents similar to an infant with generalized infection and may develop respiratory distress, abdominal distention, guaiac-positive stools, carbohydrate intolerance (evidenced by new-onset hyperglycemia), thrombocytopenia, candiduria, temperature instability, and hypotension as infection progresses. Candida species have a high affinity for other organs (brain, eyes, heart, kidneys, liver, and spleen), and dissemination is a concerning risk. Infants with congenital candidiasis most likely present with diffuse cutaneous disease, with widespread erythematous maculopapular rash. More severe disease presents with manifestations of systemic viral or bacterial infection (Bendel & Swanson, 2025).

Mucocutaneous disease can be tentatively diagnosed based on clinical characteristics. It is rarely necessary to obtain cultures of skin or mucous membranes. A potassium hydroxide (KOH) test for budding yeast can be used to distinguish oral thrush from other causes of white coating of the tongue and mucous membranes; KOH is also a rapid screening technique for candiduria (AAP, 2024a; Bendel & Swanson, 2025; Ericson & Benjamin, 2025). A positive *Candida* blood culture should never be considered a contaminated specimen. Intermittently positive cultures may reflect transient candidemia, and, usually, removal of any indwelling catheters and lines and changing of antibiotic therapy may be indicated. Blood, urine, and spinal fluid cultures should be obtained in fulminant disease. Brain imaging, echocardiogram, abdominal ultrasound, and dilated retinal examination are warranted for any neonate/infant with candidemia due to the higher risk for dissemination in the preterm population.

**Treatment.** For mucocutaneous disease, topical agents are indicated. Nystatin is the most commonly used therapy. Oral nystatin should be applied directly to the lesions to improve efficacy. Nystatin ointment or powder effectively treats skin lesions, including diaper dermatitis. Some clinicians prescribe oral nystatin when severe diaper dermatitis is present. This regimen is not recommended, however, because the reservoir is usually the lower GI tract. Gentian violet was extensively used in the past and is still prescribed when nystatin is ineffective in the short term. Because of the inconvenience of staining and some local irritation, most clinicians choose systemic therapy when topical treatment is ineffective (Bendel & Swanson, 2025). Amphotericin B is the drug of choice for infants with systemic *C. albicans* infection. This toxic, potent antifungal agent must be used cautiously. The recommended treatment is 1 mg/kg given every 24 hours IV; if there are concerns about renal failure, dosing should be adjusted. Therapy should continue for 2 weeks after the first negative blood culture and clearance of clinical signs of the disease (AAP, 2024a; Bendel & Swanson, 2025). Therapy for CNS involvement should include the addition of 5-fluorouracil (5-FU) because amphotericin B does not cross the blood–brain barrier well (Bendel & Swanson, 2025). Therapy should be continued for at least 3 weeks until all signs and symptoms of CNS infection have cleared, including negative CSF cultures. Prompt central line removal is advised (AAP, 2024a; Bendel & Swanson, 2025).

Kidney toxicity is a major side effect of amphotericin B therapy because it causes renal vasoconstriction and decreases both renal blood flow and glomerular filtration rate. This damage can result in hyponatremia, hypokalemia, increased blood urea nitrogen (BUN), and increased creatinine, as well as acidosis. If the medication makes the patient oliguric, most providers recommend stopping the drug until the next day. Thrombocytopenia, granulocytopenia, fever, nausea, and vomiting are the common side effects of amphotericin B (Bendel & Swanson, 2025).

**Prevention.** NICUs with a high incidence of invasive candidiasis are advised to implement a prophylaxis protocol. Antifungal drug prophylaxis is the only regimen shown to be efficacious in randomized controlled trials. Most units use an IV fluconazole prevention protocol (AAP, 2024a; Bendel & Swanson, 2025). Some use an oral nystatin protocol. A small retrospective, descriptive study in one hospital demonstrated that a topical nystatin cream protocol was associated with a very low rate of *Candida* species in extremely LBW infants with central catheters in that NICU (Bodin et al., 2015). More evidence is needed to determine when prophylaxis is needed, what agents are most efficacious, and which agents are considered safe for use in newborn infants of all gestational ages and birthweights.

## NOSOCOMIAL INFECTIONS

Both colonization and infection are nosocomial events, meaning "of or related to a hospital." In the neonate, LOS is mostly the result of nosocomial transmission, with the exception of late-onset GBS and HSV infection. Rates of nosocomial infections have declined over the past decade as efforts have been put in place for surveillance and prevention. Risk factors are prematurity, LBW, underlying medical conditions, and extended hospitalization, where many invasive procedures are required. Incidence is indirectly related to birthweight and gestational age, where the highest incidence is found in extremely premature infants. There is considerable variability between nosocomial infection rates among NICUs with reported rates ranging from 10.3% to 31.7% after adjusting for birthweight, gestational age, race, and sex (Ramasethu, 2017). Hospitals in low- to middle-income countries have higher (3–20 times higher) nosocomial infection rates, mostly due to being poorly equipped to provide aseptic techniques for procedures involving sick neonates (Remington et al., 2025).

Gram-positive organisms, gram-negative organisms, and yeast predominantly cause nosocomial infections. CoNS has been identified as a major cause of nosocomial infections in the United States since the early 1980s and remains so. Yeast infections often occur if previous antibiotic therapy has been given. This infection is also associated with colonization of vascular catheters, assisted ventilation, and necrotizing enterocolitis. The most common device-related infections are central line-associated bloodstream infections (CLABSIs), ventilator-associated pneumonia (VAP), urinary catheter-associated urinary tract infections (CAUTI), and ventricular shunt–associated infections (Mathew et al., 2025; Ramasethu, 2017).

Gram-negative and gram-positive viral organisms can cause nursery epidemics because they have (a) the ability to colonize or infect human skin or the GI tract, (b) the ability to be carried from person to person by hand contact, and (c) characteristics that allow existence on hands of personnel or in fluids or on inanimate objects, including IV fluids, respiratory support equipment, solutions used for medications, disinfectants, and banked breastmilk (Mathew et al., 2025).

Resistance to antibiotics is a serious problem in many NICUs, particularly with gram-negative enteric pathogens such as ampicillin-resistant *E. coli*. Aminoglycoside resistance is a problem in many nurseries, as are colonization and infection with MRSA and vancomycin-resistant Enterococcus. Respiratory infections with respiratory syncytial virus (RSV), influenza, parainfluenza, rhinovirus, and echovirus occur in many nurseries. These are more difficult to identify and, thus, more difficult to report. CMV infection has been reported as a transfusion-related problem in LBW infants, hence prompting the current policy of using CMV-screened blood donors, resulting in a decreased incidence (Mathew et al., 2025).

## INFECTION CONTROL POLICIES

The hospital infection control committee should set up policies and procedures in nurseries based on the recommendations of the AAP and the CDC. The significance of these policies to newborns should be detailed in a hospital policy book. The following topics should be covered: (a) ocular prophylaxis, (b) skin and cord care, (c) nursery staff ratios, (d) nursery design and environment, (e) handwashing, (f) staff apparel, (g) isolation, (h) visitors, (i) employee health, and (j) epidemic control (Mathew et al., 2025). Appropriate handwashing with soap and water is the simplest, most effective weapon for preventing infection!

## SUMMARY

Many factors place the neonate at high risk for infection and the premature newborn at even higher risk. The nurse is in a unique role in implementing methods for infection prevention in nurseries, detecting early signs and symptoms of infection, and participating in infection control. A better understanding of the neonatal immune system, methods of perinatal acquisition of organisms, common microorganisms, signs and symptoms of infections, and appropriate therapy provide the nurse with a sound basis for the management of care, as well as the development and implementation of hospital infection control policies for the NICU. Antibiotic stewardship remains one of the best practices for decreasing resistance organisms and, therefore, decreasing neonatal morbidity and mortality (McPherson et al., 2018).

## CASE STUDY

■ **Identification of the Problem.** Term, female infant is admitted to the well-baby nursery (WBN) following a repeat C-section. Presented with grunting respirations, nasal flaring, and retractions (GFR) by 15 minutes of age.

■ **Assessment: History and Physical Examination.** The infant was delivered via repeat C-section under spinal anesthesia to a G2P1001 female with an estimated gestational age (EGA) of 39 weeks. Birthing parent labs: Blood type A+, GBS negative at 35 weeks. RPR nonreactive, hepatitis B negative, HIV negative, and Rubella immune. The birthing parent reports a UTI at 36 weeks' gestation, which was treated with nitrofurantoin macrocrystals (Macrodantin). No other complications were noted. Other than this treatment, only prenatal vitamins were taken during pregnancy. Membranes ruptured at delivery with clear amniotic fluid. Apgar scores: 8 at 1 minute and 9 at 5 minutes. The infant only required drying and stimulation at delivery. The infant was admitted to the WBN at 10 minutes of age for normal newborn care. The neonatal nurse practitioner (NNP) was called to evaluate the infant at 15 minutes of age for GFR. An arterial blood gas (ABG), CBC with differential, and CRP were obtained. The ABG results were: pH 7.223, $PaCO_2$ 66, $PaO_2$ 44. CBC and CRP results are pending. The infant was transferred to the NICU with blow-by $O_2$ for further evaluation and treatment.

Physical examination of the infant on admission to the NICU was as follows:

- GENERAL: Term female infant with marked acrocyanosis. Resting supine with marked grunting, nasal flaring, and subcostal retractions; $SpO_2$ 91% with blow-by $O_2$ at 5 L/min
- Head, eyes, ears, nose, and throat (HEENT): Normocephalic, anterior fontanelle (AF) soft and slightly concave; bilateral red reflexes and pupils equally reactive to light; ears normally placed; nares patent
- RESPIRATORY: Bilateral breath sounds clear to auscultation; marked GFR; respiratory rate (RR) 40 breaths/min
- CARDIOVASCULAR: Heart rate (HR) regular with normal sinus rhythm; HR 170 beats/min; no murmur noted; brachial and femoral pulses 2+; capillary refill 4 seconds; blood pressure (BP): 76/35 mm Hg; mean BP: 37 mm Hg
- ABDOMEN: Abdomen soft and nontender with no hepatosplenomegaly or masses palpable; three-vessel cord
- GASTROINTESTINAL/GENITOURINARY: Normal female infant genitalia; patent anus; anal wink present
- NEUROLOGIC: Decreased responses, with eyes open and unblinking; muscle tone markedly decreased
- SKIN: Pale pink with mottling; no bruises or "birthmarks" noted
- EXTREMITIES: Good passive range of movement (ROM) with 10 fingers and toes in each extremity; no hip clunks noted

## Differential Diagnosis

- Transient tachypnea of the newborn
- Pneumothorax
- Sepsis
- Pneumonia
- Shock

## Diagnostic Tests

Laboratory tests:

- CBC/differential: WBC: 4.7; hemoglobin (Hb): 14.2; hematocrit (Hct): 45.2; platelet count: 105,000; segments: 35; bands: 21; metas: 2; myelos: 1
- C-reactive protein (CRP): 6.8
- Repeat ABG: pH 7.12; $PaCO_2$ 71; $PaO_2$ 49
- Blood cultures X 2: Endotracheal secretion culture. Blood cultures positive at 12 hours for gram-positive cocci; minimal inhibitory concentration (MIC) pending

Imaging tests:

- Chest x-ray: Good expansion with mild reticulogranular appearance; no pneumothorax
- Working diagnosis. GBS sepsis with possible GBS pneumonia (based on preliminary BC report and chest x-ray appearance).

## Development of Management Plan

- Respiratory support with mechanical ventilation as needed
- Umbilical arterial catheter (UAC) and umbilical venous catheter (UVC) placement for monitoring, sampling, and fluid management
- Continuous monitoring of arterial blood pressure, vital signs, and neurologic status, every 2 to 4 hours
- CBC/diff and CRP every a.m.
- BMP at 12 hours of life and every a.m.
- ABG every 3 to 4 hours as needed for ventilator management
- Maintenance fluid support; fluid boluses to support intravascular volume
- Vasopressors to maintain adequate blood pressure and cerebral blood flow
- Ampicillin and gentamicin IV
- CSF cultures when stable

## Implementation and Evaluation of Effectiveness

Implementation of management plan (immediately after initial assessment in the NICU):

- Infant intubated within the first 30 minutes of life and placed on mechanical ventilation with the following settings: SIMV: 40; PIP: 24; PEEP: 4; PSV: 12; $F_IO_2$ 50% (adjusted to keep $SpO_2$ 90%–97%)
- Chest x-ray to verify endotracheal tube (ETT) placement
- UAC and UVC placed; abdominal x-ray to verify umbilical line placement
- Dopamine 10 mcg/kg/min initiated by 1 hour of life; weaned to 5 mcg/kg/min by 36 hours

Effectiveness of management plan:

- Despite maximum ventilatory support, the infant developed severe persistent pulmonary hypertension of the newborn (PPHN) and was transferred to a children's hospital for possible extracorporeal membrane oxygenation (ECMO) on day 3 of life
- Blood cultures and ETT cultures were positive for group B streptococcus
- CSF cultures were negative
- GBS sepsis and GBS pneumonia were successfully treated with antibiotics

**Outcome.** The infant did well at the receiving hospital and did not require ECMO. The infant was treated with iNO for 3 days and was extubated by day 9 of life. Follow-up blood cultures were negative after 14 days of IV antibiotics. The infant was discharged home at 3 weeks of age and is developmentally appropriate at 3 years of age.

Although the incidence of GBS sepsis is decreasing, it remains the number-one cause of EOS in the newborn. In the case presented, a high level of suspicion for sepsis was based on the history of the UTI in the birthing parent. Although a birthing parent's GBS screen is negative when it is tested, the parent may become positive later, or the test may reveal a false negative, depending on the timing and technique used. Early recognition and rapid treatment can mean the difference between a poor outcome and a good outcome for the neonate (AAP, 2024).

## Reference

American Academy of Pediatrics. (2024). Group B streptococcal infections. In D. W. Kimberlin, R. Banerjee, E. D. Barnett, R. Lynfield, & M. H. Sawyer (Eds.), *Red book: 2024 report of the committee on infectious diseases* (33rd ed., pp. 799–806). American Academy of Pediatrics.

## EVIDENCE-BASED PRACTICE

One of the most successful evidence-based practice changes in recent history has been the implementation of a group B beta-hemolytic streptococcus (GBS) prophylaxis protocol for the prevention of GBS sepsis in the newborn. During the 1970s, GBS sepsis exceeded *Escherichia coli* as the leading cause of sepsis and meningitis in newborns (Ratner et al., 2025). Cases of GBS sepsis continued to increase over the next two decades. In 1996, the Centers for Disease Control and Prevention (CDC) published the first guidelines for the prevention of perinatal group B streptococcal disease, which were based on case reports and clinical trials demonstrating the effectiveness of intrapartum administration of antibiotics to birthing parents who were considered at risk for transmitting GBS to their newborns. These guidelines offered two prevention methods: a risk-based approach or a culture-based approach. Although there was a decrease in cases, GBS disease remained a leading cause of neonatal sepsis. Further studies comparing the two strategies revealed data that supported the culture-based method as the most effective strategy in preventing neonatal GBS disease. Therefore, in 2002, the CDC replaced the 1996 guidelines with recommendations that all pregnant birthing parents be screened for GBS between 35 and 37 weeks' gestation with the use of intrapartum antibiotic administration during labor for culture-positive birthing parents.

Significant declines in the incidence of GBS disease occurred after the implementation of the 1996 guidelines, but a more dramatic decrease occurred after the updated guidelines in 2002. The CDC and other organizations continued to collect data and the guidelines were updated again in 2010. Few changes were made except for information related to testing methods and recommendations for antibiotics for birthing parents with penicillin allergy (Puopolo et al., 2019). Since the implementation of IAP for prevention of neonatal GBS disease, rates of EOS with GBS have declined; however, GBS sepsis continues to be the most common pathogen in term infants and remains the leading cause of disease-related morbidity and mortality among newborns. It is important that we continue to evaluate our practices and make changes that are based on current evidence (Ratner et al., 2025).

### References

Puopolo, K. M., Lynfield, R., Cummings, J. J., Committee of Fetus and Newborn, Committee on Infectious Diseases, Hand, I., Adams-Chapman, I., Poindexter, B., Stewart, D. L., Aucott, S. W., Goldsmith, J. P., Mowitz, M., Watterberg, K., Maldonado, Y. A., Zaoutis, T. E., Banerjee, R., Barnett, E. D., Campbell, J. D., Gerber, J. S., & Kourtis, A. P. (2019). Management of infants at risk for group B streptococcal disease. *Pediatrics, 144*(2), e20191881. https://doi.org/10.1542/peds.2019-1881

Ratner, A. J., Nizet, V., & Puopolo, K. (2025). Group B streptococcal infections. In Y. A. Maldonado, V. Nizet, E. D. Barnett, K. M. Edwards, R. Malley, J. S. Remington, & J. O. Klein (Eds.), *Remington and Klein's infectious diseases of the fetus and newborn infant* (9th ed., pp. 348–387). Elsevier.

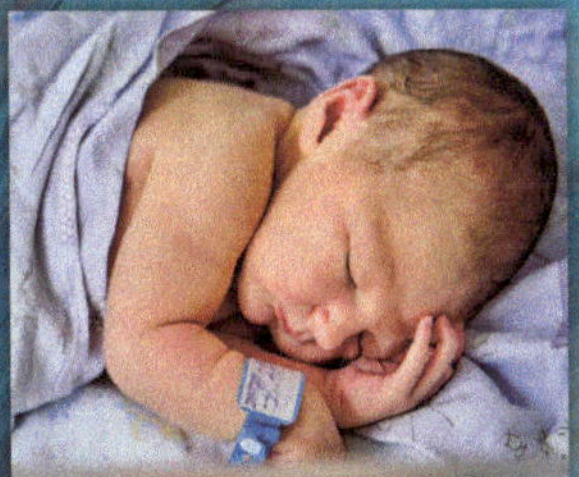

*Source:* Андрей Журавлев/ Adobe Stock.

## PARENT VOICES

### Deborah A. Discenza

**We were about 3 weeks into my daughter's stay in the NICU and had just started doing Kangaroo Care at my request. I was so excited to see how I personally could help my daughter thrive in the NICU environment. Well, one day I walked in, eager to hold her and kangaroo her when the nurse came up to us immediately and said my daughter was not well. Sure enough, we looked into her incubator and she was totally still and very sick. We were told not to touch our daughter nor to stimulate her in any way. They never told us what was wrong and I sat there by her bedside staring at her with a sense of dread. But the nurses said not to touch her, not to comfort her. There was nothing I could do. I felt completely powerless to help my daughter and I had no idea what lay ahead for her. Later we learned it was sepsis and we felt grateful for the care and the antibiotics that helped her through it. The experience left its mark on our daughter but also on us, her parents. Things can change in a second.**

## ONLINE RESOURCES

**CourseConnect**

Resources for this chapter are online and available at www.springerpub.com/courseconnect.

## REFERENCES

References for this chapter are online and available at www.springerpub.com/courseconnect.

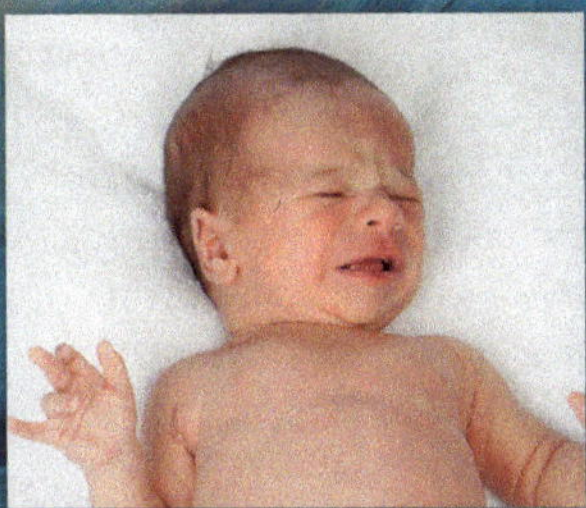

Source: Gelpi/Adobe Stock.

CHAPTER 12

# Integumentary System

Carolyn Houska Lund

## INTRODUCTION

Skin phenomena, along with other examination findings, are used to assess the maturity, duration of pregnancy, and neonatal vitality. The skin of a preterm infant makes up 13% of the body weight, compared to 3% in adults. This large organ provides a barrier against infection, protects internal organs, assists in acid mantle development, contributes to temperature regulation and prevention of insensible water loss (ISWL), stores fats, excretes electrolytes and water, and provides tactile sensory input. The sensations of touch, pressure, temperature, pain, and itch are received by millions of microscopic dermal nerve endings. The skin is instrumental in the early establishment of the mother–infant relationship in that the quality of touch and stimulation that an infant receives is responsible for the infant's later responses to other people and the environment. Thus, the skin fulfills a task of vital importance, particularly in maternal–child nursing.

Care practices that affect the fragile, underdeveloped skin of premature infants present major concerns as well as dilemmas for care providers. Life support and monitoring equipment must be securely attached and frequently removed or replaced; this practice can cause trauma to the skin. Necessary invasive procedures, such as vascular access, blood sampling, and chest tube insertion, invade the skin's barrier. Trauma to the skin can result in the diversion of an excessive proportion of caloric intake to tissue repair. Other effects of trauma to premature skin include the energy demands of electrolyte imbalances, increased evaporative heat loss through damaged or immature skin, and the risk of toxicity when substances are applied to the skin surface.

Trauma to the skin creates portals of entry for bacteria and fungi in an already immune-compromised host. Significant morbidity and mortality can be attributed to practices that cause either trauma to the skin or alterations in normal skin function. Iatrogenic skin problems—including burns and caustic lesions from isopropyl alcohol and erythema and skin craters from transcutaneous oxygen monitoring—have been reported. Increased skin permeability and percutaneous toxicity from drugs and chemicals have also been documented in neonates.

This chapter covers the development and structure of the skin, the normal physiologic variations in newborn skin, and dermatologic diseases. This information is then incorporated into the management of neonatal skin.

## SKIN STRUCTURE AND FUNCTION

Skin consists of three anatomically distinct layers: the epidermis, the dermis, and the subcutaneous tissue. The uppermost layer of the epidermis is the *stratum corneum*, primarily composed of nonliving cells made of protein with layers of lipids that bind them; this has been described as similar to the "bricks and mortar of a wall." Once exfoliated in utero, these cells form part of the *vernix caseosa*, the cheese-like substance that covers and protects fetal skin. The bottom, living basal layer contains keratinocytes, which constantly replace the keratin cells in the stratum corneum; it takes approximately 26 days for keratinocytes to migrate up to the stratum corneum. Approximately 20% of an adult's protein requirement is needed for this purpose. Keratin-forming cells—which cornify the outer layer of the epidermis—and melanocytes are contained in the lower levels of the epidermis. Melanocytes begin producing melanin, or pigment, before birth and distribute it to the epidermal cells. Active pigmentary activity can be observed before birth in the epidermis of infants of dark-skinned races, but little evidence of such activity exists in White fetuses (Torchia & Persaud, 2025).

The dermis lies directly under the epidermis and is 2 to 4 mm thick at birth. It is a closely woven layer of collagen, a fibrous protein, and elastin fibers. This fibrous complex provides mechanical strength and elasticity, allowing the skin to withstand frictional stress while extending easily over joints. At term, the dermis is well organized but is thinner and has higher water content compared to the adult dermis (Loomis et al., 2008). Many nerves and a rich supply of blood vessels are contained there. They nourish the skin cells and act as carriers of the sensations of heat, touch, pressure, and pain from the skin to the brain.

Hair originates from deep in the dermis. Down-growths, called *epidermal ridges*, which extend into the developing dermis, result from a proliferation of cells in the basal layer. These ridges are permanently established by 17 weeks' gestation and produce ridges and grooves on the surface of the palms, including the fingers, and on the soles of the feet, including the toes.

Determined genetically, this type of pattern constitutes the basis for using fingerprints in criminal investigations and medical genetics. Dermatoglyphics is the study of the pattern of these epidermal ridges. The presence of abnormal chromosome complements affects the development of the ridge patterns. For example, infants with Down syndrome exhibit distinctive hand and foot patterns that are of diagnostic value (Torchia & Persaud, 2025).

The major component of the subcutaneous layer is fatty connective tissue. The subcutaneous fat functions as a heat insulator, a shock absorber, and a calorie reserve area. Fat accumulation occurs predominantly in the last trimester. Sebaceous glands are found in both the dermis and the subcutaneous layer. Well-developed and potentially functional at birth, these glands have minimal function until puberty. Sweat glands are also found in the dermis and the subcutaneous layer and are affected directly by external environmental temperature. In premature infants, sweat gland maturation occurs between 21 and 33 days of age. In term infants, this maturation occurs at about 5 days of age. Poor sweat production in the premature infant is caused by sweat gland immaturity. However, adult function is not achieved until the second or third year of life.

Term-infant skin is soft, wrinkled, velvety, and covered with vernix caseosa (Visscher et al., 2005). Transformation of the fetal circulation is evident soon after the cord is cut, because the skin develops the intense red coloration characteristic of the newborn. This color may remain for hours. A blue, blotchy appearance may occur if the infant is exposed to a cool environment.

The insulating layer of vernix is usually lost during the first few days of life through traditional newborn skin care (Dyer, 2013). This results in a loss of insulation for the stratum corneum, which then peels off, thus resulting in skin with a grayish-white or yellowish hue. Visible desquamation of newborn skin comes to an end after about 7 days. The vernix protects the fetus from maceration by the amniotic fluid, facilitates the development of the *stratum corneum*, assists in the development of the acid mantle, provides bactericidal protection, and contributes to the development of epidermal barrier function (Visscher et al., 2015, 2021).

Compared to the skin of the term infant, the premature infant's skin is more transparent, gelatinous, and unwrinkled. Lanugo, which has been lost in the full-term infant, may be present in varying degrees and is one criterion used to estimate gestational age. Additionally, subcutaneous edema may be present and is clinical evidence of a cutaneous excess of water and sodium. This edema decreases within the first few days of life, and the skin then lies loosely over the infant's entire body. The immaturity of the infant's skin is linked to the premature newborn's difficulty maintaining body temperature. A poorly developed fat supply and a large body surface area in relation to body weight add to temperature instability.

The premature infant has been shown to have a less well-developed stratum corneum; at less than 30 weeks' gestation, there may be only two to three layers of stratum corneum. This immaturity results in the premature infant's decreased capacity to resist particles, viruses, parasites, and bacteria in the external environment, leaving the infant readily susceptible to skin infection and irritation (Lawton, 2013).

Transferring from the intrauterine aquatic environment to the external atmospheric environment stimulates and accelerates the maturation of skin functions. Embryologic skin development is described in Exhibit 12.1.

## Developmental Variations

Several factors are responsible for the functional differences between premature and term infants' skins. These differences subside with increasing gestational and postnatal ages (Table 12.1).

### EXHIBIT 12.1

**Embryologic Development of Skin**

The skin consists of two morphologically different layers derived from two different germ layers. The epithelial structures (epidermis, pilosebaceous-apocrine unit, eccrine unit, and nails) are ectodermal derivatives. The ectoderm also gives rise to the hair, the teeth, and the sense organs of smell, taste, hearing, vision, and touch—everything involved with events that occur outside the organism. Mesenchymal structures (collagen, reticular, and elastic fibers; blood vessels; muscles; and fat) originate from the mesoderm. These developments are outlined in Table 12.2.

The epidermis, which develops from the surface ectoderm, consists of one layer of undifferentiated cells in a 3-week-old embryo. By 4 weeks' gestational age, it has an inner germinative layer of cuboidal cells with dark, compact nuclei and an outer layer of slightly flatter cells covered by microvilli. By about the middle of the second month of gestation, some of the cells begin to be crowded to the surface and form a thin, protective layer of flattened cells known as the periderm. The cells of this layer continually undergo keratinization and desquamation and are replaced by cells arising from the basal layer. The periderm is often called the *epitrichial* ("upon the hair") layer of the epidermis because the hairs that later grow up from the deeper layers are said not to penetrate this thin surface layer but to push it up on their growing tips, thus causing it to be cast off if it has not already disappeared. These exfoliated cells form part of the vernix caseosa.

During the latter part of the second month, the epithelium tends to become thicker. This occurs (at first) by a staggering of the nuclei and the beginning of cell rearrangement, which leads rapidly to the formation of an intermediate layer between the flattened cells of the epitrichial layer and the basal layer adjacent to the underlying dermis. The cells of this intermediate layer tend to become enlarged and show a high degree of vacuolation. The basal layer of the

(*continued*)

## EXHIBIT 12.1 (*continued*)

epidermis is later called the *stratum germinativum* (Torchia & Persaud, 2025).

At the end of the second month of gestation, the cutaneous nerves, detectable in the embryonic dermis by about the fifth week of gestation, appear to be functional, although the skin is primitive by comparison with that of an adult.

At about 10 weeks' gestation, fingernail development begins at the tips of the digits. A thickened area of epithelium on the dorsum of each digit is the first sign of nail formation. Our nails are adaptations of the epidermis, homologous to the claws and hooves of lower mammals, and are formed by a modified process of keratinization. Development of the fingernails is begun and completed (30–34 weeks) before that of the toenails (35–38 weeks).

By about 11 weeks' gestation, collagen and elastic connective tissue fibers begin to develop in the dermis. The epidermal–dermal junction, which has been smooth up to this time, now becomes wavy as epidermal thickenings grow down into the dermis of the palm and the soles of the feet. Dermal papillae develop in these dermal projections. Capillary loops develop in some dermal papillae and Meissner corpuscles, which are the sensory nerve endings of touch, form in others (Torchia & Persaud, 2025). These epidermal ridges produce ridges and grooves in a genetically determined pattern and are the basis for fingerprinting and footprinting. The development of these ridges can be distinctly affected by the presence of abnormal chromosome complements (e.g., as occurs in Down syndrome-trisomy 21). These ridges are permanently established by about 17 weeks of gestation.

During the third to fourth month of gestation, the stratum germinativum differentiates from the rest of the epithelium. These cells are termed the germinative layer because they undergo the repeated cell divisions that are responsible for the growth of the epidermis.

During the fourth month of gestation, the epithelium starts to become many cells thick and keratin begins to accumulate in the cells above the stratum germinativum layer. Daughter cells from the basal layer are crowded upward and undergo progressive changes in each layer and finalize in cornification. The thin stratum granulosum epidermidis, which contains keratohyalin granules, is the layer directly above the stratum germinativum. The next higher layer is the thin and clear stratum lucidum epidermidis, the content of which is a fluid—eleidin—that replaces the granules. Above that is the keratinized multilayered stratum corneum epidermidis (Torchia & Persaud, 2025). As the keratin accumulates in these cells, they become more and more sluggish and finally die, so that the surface layer of the epidermis is made up of tough, scalelike, dead cells that form a relatively impermeable membrane.

In areas such as the soles of the feet and the palms of the hands, where the skin is subjected to more than ordinary wear, the keratinization of the outer layer is much heavier than in the general body surface. Of interest, however, is that the greater thickness of palmar and plantar epidermis becomes evident in the embryo long before it is possible for these areas to have been subjected to any more wear than other parts of the skin. When the layers are all completely differentiated, the structure of fetal epidermis resembles that of adult epidermis.

During the early fetal period, neural crest cells migrate into the dermis and differentiate into melanoblasts. At about 17 to 20 weeks of gestation, these melanoblasts differentiate into melanocytes, migrate to the epidermal–dermal border, and begin to produce melanin. Fetal melanocytes in White races contain little or no pigment, whereas in dark-skinned races, they produce melanin granules. The skin of Black newborns is only a little darker than that of White newborns. Skin at the bases of the fingernails and toenails is often noticeably darker, however.

The skin of Black infants continues to darken after birth as increased melanin production occurs in response to light. When melanocytes remain behind in the dermis, they appear bluish through the overlying cutaneous tissue and are called CDM. Some believe that it is not the number of melanocytes present that is important but rather their activity level. The hormone secreted by the pituitary gland that controls the clumping or dispersion of the melanin granules is a melanocyte-stimulating hormone.

At around 20 weeks' gestation, the eyebrows, upper lip, and chin hair are first recognizable. On the general body surface, the hair makes its appearance about a month later. These fine hairs are called *lanugo*. The emergence of this hair breaks off the periderm and the periderm becomes one component of the vernix caseosa. The other components of vernix are sebum from the sebaceous glands, fetal hair, and desquamated cells from the amnion (Torchia & Persaud, 2025). The vernix protects the epidermis against a macerating influence that would be exerted by the amniotic fluid and acts as a lubricant to prevent chafing injuries from the amnion as the growing fetus becomes progressively confined in its fluid-filled sac.

Between 21 and 24 weeks' gestation, the fetal skin is wrinkled, translucent, and pinkish-red because blood in the capillaries has become visible. Head and lanugo hair are well developed in a 26- to 29-week fetus. At this same time, eccrine sweat glands are anatomically developed and are found over the entire body. Their function is somewhat immature in the perinatal period.

Brown adipose tissue cells begin to differentiate in the seventh month of gestation, and the accumulation of subcutaneous fat begins to smooth out the many skin wrinkles. Between the 30th and 34th week of gestation, the skin is pink and smooth and the lanugo is beginning to shed. The fingernails reach the fingertips but the distal part of the nail is still thin and soft (Torchia & Persaud, 2025). During the last trimester of pregnancy, subcutaneous fat accumulates and the fetus acquires a plump appearance. Composition of amniotic fluid tested reflects skin function. The number of anucleated cells and keratinized lipid-containing skin flakes increases.

**TABLE 12.1**

**STRUCTURAL DIFFERENCES BETWEEN INFANT AND ADULT SKIN**

| | Premature | Full Term | Adult |
|---|---|---|---|
| Epidermis | Thinner cells compressed | Stratum corneum appears as adherent cell layers | Good resistance to penetration |
| | Fewer desmosomes | Melanin production low | |
| | Fewer layers of stratum corneum | | |
| | Melanin production low | | |
| Dermoepidermal junction | Fewer hemidesmosomes | | |
| | Less cohesion between layers | | |
| Dermis | Fewer elastin fibers | Fewer elastin fibers | Full complement of elastin fibers |
| | Thinner than in the adult | Thinner than in the adult | |
| Eccrine glands | May be more typical of fetus than adult | Equivalent in structure to adult | Distribution less dense than in infant |
| | Ducts patent | Denser distribution | |
| | Secretory cells undifferentiated | | |
| Hair | Lanugo hair may be present | Vellus hair characteristic | Both vellus and terminal hairs |
| | Hair growth synchronous | Hair growth synchronous | Hair growth dyssynchronous |
| Sebaceous glands | Large and active | Large and active but diminishing rapidly in both size and activity for several weeks after birth | Large and active |
| Nerve and vascular system | Not fully organized | Vascular system not fully organized until 3 months | Adult pattern |
| | Most nerves are small in diameter, unmyelinated, sensory, and autonomic | Cutaneous nerve network not fully developed; may continue to develop until puberty | |
| | Unmyelinated nerves are typically fetal in structure | Most nerves are small in diameter, unmyelinated, sensory, and autonomic | |
| | Meissner touch receptors not fully formed | Meissner touch receptors not fully formed | |
| | | Good resistance to penetration | |

(continued)

**TABLE 12.1**

**STRUCTURAL DIFFERENCES BETWEEN INFANT AND ADULT SKIN (*continued*)**

| | Premature | Full Term | Adult |
|---|---|---|---|
| Permeability | Highly permeable | Good resistance to penetration | |
| | Higher penetrability of fat-soluble substances | Higher penetrability of fat-soluble substances | |
| | Greater absorption because of higher skin surface: body weight ratio | Greater absorption because of higher skin surface: body weight ratio | |
| Eccrine sweating | Reduced sweating capability, especially for first 13–24 days | Reduced sweating capability, especially for first 2–5 days | Full sweating capability |
| Photosensitivity | Melanin production low; will sunburn readily | Melanin production low; will sunburn readily | Sensitivity to sun depends on skin type |
| Related conditions | Reduced ability to ward off infection because of deficient immune system | Reduced ability to ward off infection | Readily sensitized to allergens |
| | Low reactivity to allergens | Low reactivity to allergens | |

*Source:* Adapted from Shalita, A. (1981). *Principles of infant skin care.* Johnson & Johnson Baby Products.

**TABLE 12.2**

**EMBRYONIC AND FETAL DEVELOPMENT OF SKIN**

| Weeks of Gestation | Development |
|---|---|
| 3 | Epidermis, which develops from surface ectoderm, consists of one layer of cells. |
| 5 | Cutaneous nerves are detectable in embryonic dermis. |
| 6–7 | Periderm, a thin, protective layer of flattened cells, is formed. |
| 11 | Collagen and elastic fibers are developing in the dermis.<br>Epidermal ridges (fingerprints) are forming.<br>Nails begin to develop at the tips of the digits. |
| 13–16 | Scalp hair patterning is determined. |
| 17–20 | Melanocytes migrate to the epidermal–dermal junction and begin to produce melanin.<br>Skin is covered with vernix caseosa and lanugo.<br>Keratin is accumulating in the epidermis. |

(*continued*)

**TABLE 12.2**

**EMBRYONIC AND FETAL DEVELOPMENT OF SKIN (*continued*)**

| Weeks of Gestation | Development |
|---|---|
| 21–25 | Skin is wrinkled, translucent, and pink to red because blood in the capillaries has become visible. |
| 26–29 | Subcutaneous fat begins to be deposited and starts to smooth out the many wrinkles in the skin.<br>Eccrine sweat glands are anatomically developed and found over the entire body; their function, however, is somewhat immature in the perinatal period. |
| 30–34 | Skin is pink and smooth.<br>Fingernails reach fingertips.<br>Lanugo begins to shed. |
| 35–38 | Fetuses are usually plump.<br>Skin is usually white or bluish-pink.<br>Toenails reach toe tips. |

The embryonic period is undoubtedly the most important period of human development because the beginnings of all major external and internal structures develop. The fetal period (ninth week to birth): primarily concerned with the growth and differentiation of tissue and organs that started to develop during the embryonic period.

*Source:* Adapted from Ackerman, A. (1985). Structure and function of the skin. In S. Moschella & H. Hurley (Eds.), *Dermatology* (2nd ed., Vol. 2). Saunders.

## Thickness of the Stratum Corneum and Permeability

The *stratum corneum* layer provides the barrier properties of the skin. This barrier is composed of keratinocytes coated by intercellular lipids. The stratum corneum begins to develop in the fetus after 21 weeks estimated gestational age (EGA). The stratum corneum in infants of 28 weeks' gestation consists of only a few cell layers and is markedly thinner than that of term infants. These findings correlate with the immaturity of barrier function of the stratum corneum and are characterized by increased permeability and increased transepidermal water loss (TEWL) (Bhatia, 2006). By 34 to 35 weeks EGA, the stratum corneum has developed sufficiently to offer some protection (Visscher et al., 2015).

The full-term infant has a fully functional stratum corneum. The stratum corneum, the nonliving layer of the epidermis, contains 10 to 20 layers in adults and term infants. The stratum corneum of term newborns has been shown to have lower TEWL and stratum corneum (SCH) than that of adult skin, with the lowest levels seen on the first day of life. This suggests that the barrier is relatively impermeable to water to protect from maceration in utero and that a gradual drying process occurs over the first few days of life. In addition, the TEWL in different areas—such as the forehead, palms, and soles—is lower in newborns, whereas levels are higher on the forearm region (Yosipovitch et al., 2000).

Despite reports of normal barrier function at birth, studies indicate that infant skin is prone to higher percutaneous absorption and exhibits a greater tendency to irritant and allergic contact dermatitis, prompting some to say that barrier function is not fully developed at birth (Hoeger & Enzmann, 2002). In addition, infant stratum corneum is 30% thinner than adult, with the overall epidermis 20% to 30% smaller. Keratinocyte cells are smaller; with a higher cell turnover rate that may explain observations of faster wound healing in infant skin (Rahma & Lane, 2022; Stamatas et al., 2011).

The stratum corneum of premature infants was once thought to rapidly mature and reach adult barrier function within approximately 2 weeks after birth. However, this is a slower process in premature infants less than 27 weeks' gestation; rates of TEWL are nearly double adult levels, even at 28 days of life (Hammarlund & Sedin, 1979). In infants of 23 to 25 weeks' gestation, skin barrier function reaches mature levels much more slowly (Agren et al., 1998), as long as 8 weeks after birth in a 23-week-gestation infant (Kalia et al., 1998). The undeveloped stratum corneum of the premature infant's skin results in increased TEWL and evaporative heat loss and contributes to the difficulty the premature newborn experiences in maintaining fluid balance and body temperature.

Neonatal skin is 40% to 60% thinner than adult skin, and the body surface/weight ratio is nearly five times greater, placing the newborn at risk for toxicity from topically applied substances (Mancini, 2004; Siegfried, 2008). The skin of a premature infant is remarkably permeable; permeability correlates inversely with gestational age. Sekkat et al. (2004) have developed an in vitro model to examine the biophysical characteristics of TEWL in premature infants. This model will help clinicians understand how procedures coupled with gestational age can affect skin integrity, permeability, and TEWL.

Toxicity due to topically applied substances secondary to the increased permeability of both preterm and term infants' skin has been reported in numerous cases (Siegfried, 2008). All topical solutions during the first month of life should be carefully evaluated in relation to potential benefits, risks, and effectiveness.

## Dermal Instability

Collagen in the dermis increases with gestational age as the tendency toward water fixation and edema decreases. The other component of the dermis, the elastin fibers, is formed mostly after birth and may not fully mature until 3 years of age. **Quality and Safety: Protection from pressure and ischemic injury includes routine turning and repositioning on surfaces such as gelled pads or water mattresses** (Association of Women's Health, Obstetric, and Neonatal Nurses [AWHONN], 2018).

## Diminished Cohesion

Another variation in the premature infant's skin structure and function is the diminished cohesion between the dermis and the epidermis. The junction of the epidermis and the dermis, normally connected by numerous fibrils, has fewer and more widely spaced fibrils in premature infants than in term infants or adults. These fibrils become stronger with increasing gestational and postnatal age (Holbrook, 1982). Because the care of premature infants in the NICU often requires intravenous (IV) lines, cardiorespiratory electrodes, endotracheal tubes, and umbilical artery catheters, the premature infant is at higher risk of blistering and stripping of the epidermis when adhesives are used to secure these devices and monitors are removed (Cousins, 2014). **Emergency Alert: The cohesion between many of the currently used adhesives and the stratum corneum may be stronger than the bond between the dermis and the epidermis.**

## Skin pH

Another developmental variation of infant skin resides in the functional capacity of the skin to form a surface pH of less than 5.0, which is the acid mantle. A skin surface pH of less than 5.0 is ordinarily seen in both children and adults.

Full-term newborns' skin was found to have a mean pH of 6.34 immediately after birth. Within 4 days, the pH decreased to a mean of 4.95; between 7 and 30 days, it further decreased to 4.7 (Behrendt & Green, 1971). In a later study of 127 low birth weight (LBW) infants, these authors documented that the mean pH decreased from 6.7 (day 1) to 5.04 (day 9). However, a different technique for measuring pH was used than in the previous study; thus, the absolute values for pH may not be comparable. They concluded that acidification of the skin is independent of gestational age (Fox et al., 1998).

An acidic skin surface is credited with having bactericidal qualities against some pathogens and serves in the defense against microorganisms. This acid mantle contributes to the stratum corneum's innate immune function by inhibiting the growth of pathogenic bacteria (Larson & Dinulos, 2005; Visscher et al., 2011). The retention of vernix caseosa has been shown to assist in earlier acidification of the newborn skin and may help to facilitate colonization by normal flora after birth (Tollin et al., 2005), while an increased pH may reduce stratum corneum integrity and enhance susceptibility to mechanical damage (Visscher et al., 2011).

## Melanin Production

One of the primary functions of melanin is to screen the skin from the sun's harmful rays by absorbing their radiant energy. Although melanin production—and therefore pigmentation—is lower during the neonatal period than later in life, certain areas—such as the linea alba, the areola, and the scrotum—are often deeply pigmented because of high circulating levels of maternal and placental hormones. Melanin production in premature infants is even less than in term infants, thus placing them at greater risk for damage from sunlight and ultraviolet light (Williams, 2008).

## Assessment and Physiologic Variations

Acrocyanosis, or peripheral cyanosis involving the hands, feet, and circumoral area, is a common finding in the newborn. It occurs because of sluggish blood flow in the feet and hands that results from limited development of the peripheral capillary circulation. Acrocyanosis usually resolves within the first few days of life but may reappear with cold stress (Lucky, 2015). It occurs more often in premature infants.

Pallor is most commonly a sign of anemia, hypoxia, or poor peripheral perfusion that results from hypotension or infection. Meconium staining is caused by the passage of meconium in utero and usually requires at least 6 hours of meconium contact to stain the skin.

Jaundice, which occurs in 50% to 70% of newborns, is a yellowing of the skin and develops because of indirect bilirubin in the blood formed from the body's normal breakdown of red blood cells. Bilirubin is normally processed by the liver and is eliminated in the urine and feces. In newborns, the body cannot eliminate bilirubin as fast as it is produced.

A bilirubin level of at least 5 mg/100 mL is required for visible staining of the skin and sclera. The predictable head-to-toe progression of jaundice over the body gives a crude estimate of the bilirubin level. The bilirubin level is typically highest at 3 to 5 days (Bromiker et al., 2012).

Risk factors for high bilirubin levels or kernicterus, a neurologically damaging condition caused by hyperbilirubinemia, are bruising at birth, prematurity, breastfeeding and poor feeding, glucose-6-phosphate dehydrogenase deficiency (G6PD), East Asian or Mediterranean descent, jaundice prior to 24 hours, and a prior sibling with jaundice. Jaundice fades after the bilirubin level returns to normal. *Linea nigra* is a line of increased pigmentation from the umbilicus to the genitals. This area of benign pigmentation may become less noticeable as the infant's skin darkens. Congenital dermal melanocytosis are collections of melanocytes in the dermis most frequently seen at birth. They are slate blue, gray, or black, shaped as irregular, bruise-like spots seen primarily over the sacrum and the buttocks but may extend over the back and shoulders.

Most commonly seen in newborns with darkly pigmented skin, they are found in 96% of African American, 86% of Asian, and 13% of Caucasian infants (Lucky, 2008). Although they look like bruises, they are harmless and resolve over several years.

Lanugo is the fine, downy hair that is most commonly seen over the back, shoulders, and facial areas of a premature newborn. It is shed at the seventh to eighth month of gestation and is one criterion used to estimate gestational age.

Milia are common papules that occur primarily on the face but may also occur in other locations. They are seen as small, white, pinhead-sized bumps scattered over the chins, cheeks, noses, and foreheads of 25% to 40% of full-term babies (Dinulos & Darmstadt, 2005). They spontaneously resolve within the first month of life. Mothers should be instructed not to squeeze or prick these pimple-like spots. Milia can develop on the foreskins of infant boys; these are called epidermal inclusion cysts. When they occur on the palate, they are called Epstein's pearls.

Miliaria (prickly heat) is a general term for describing obstructions of the eccrine duct. The cause is sweat retention due to of edema of the stratum corneum; this edema blocks eccrine pores, thus resulting in four types of miliaria: rubra, crystallina, pustulosa, and profunda. The most common locations are the forehead and upper trunk (Howard & Frieden, 2015).

*Miliaria pustulosa* and *miliaria profunda* are rarely seen in temperate climates. *Miliaria rubra* is commonly observed in infants exposed to excessive environmental temperatures with humidity. It appears as pink or white pimples with a bit of redness around them. They resolve when the infant is moved to cooler temperatures. *Miliaria crystallina* presents as clear, 1- to 2-mm superficial water blisters without inflammation. The distribution and grouping of vesicles that contain no eosinophils, help to differentiate them from *erythema toxicum neonatorum*.

Harlequin color change is a dramatic but benign phenomenon in which the color on the dependent half of an infant in a side-lying position turns deep red while the upper half is pale. The face and genitalia may be spared, and the color will reverse when the infant is turned. Attributed to a temporary imbalance in the autonomic regulatory mechanism of the cutaneous vessels, this phenomenon is more common in LBW infants—whether well or sick—but can affect up to 10% of full-term babies (Lucky, 2015).

Vernix caseosa is a grayish-white cheesy substance that is a mixture of 80% water, protein, lipids, and desquamating cells (Visscher et al., 2015). This covering protects the fetal skin while the fetus is in utero and helps the infant slide through the birth canal. Vernix production begins at the end of the second trimester and accumulates in a cephalocaudal manner (Haubrich, 2003). The vernix covering diminishes as pulmonary surfactant rises and the fetus reaches term (Moraille, et al., 2005). Surface distribution depends on gestational age, type of delivery, birth weight, race, gender, and the presence of meconium. The World Health Organization (WHO, 2015) recommends leaving residual vernix in place after initial drying to wear off with normal care and handling for at least 6 hours before bathing. **Quality and Safety:** ***The AWHONN Neonatal Skin Care Evidence-Based Practice Guideline,*** **Fourth Edition, recommends leaving vernix on the skin and delaying the first bath until between 6 and 24 hours of age (AWHONN, 2018).** In clinical care, vernix has been thought of as an unwanted soil from the intrauterine life, but recent research has revealed that vernix has many functions and potential benefits for newborns. These functions and potential benefits include protection against infection (Tollin et al., 2005), decreased skin permeability and TEWL (Visscher & Narendran, 2014; Yoshio et al., 2004), skin cleansing (Moraille et al., 2005), moisturization of the skin surface (Visscher & Narendran, 2014), development of the epidermal barrier (Tansirikongkol et al., 2007), pH development (Colwell, 2015), and temperature regulation.

*Cutis marmorata*, or mottling, is a normal physiologic vascular response to cool air. This generalized mottling reflects the infant's vasomotor instability. The marbling disappears with rewarming and is uncommon after several months of age. Mottling is often prominent in infants with Cornelia de Lange syndrome and Down syndrome (trisomy 21).

## TERMINOLOGY

Ecchymoses appear as black and blue bruises of varying sizes anywhere on the body. Primarily seen over the presenting part in a difficult vertex delivery or a vaginal breech delivery, ecchymosis is most frequently due to trauma associated with labor and delivery. It occurs more commonly in fragile, premature infants. However, this bruising can indicate serious infections or bleeding disorders. Large areas of bruising may require phototherapy as a result of hyperbilirubinemia (Jensen & Galbraith, 2015).

Petechiae are pinpoint hemorrhagic areas, less than 1 mm in diameter, scattered over the upper trunk and face due to pressure during the descent and rotation of birth. Their incidence increases when the umbilical cord has been around the neck or when the cervix clamps down after delivery of the head. They do not disappear with blanching because the blood is contained in the tissues. They usually fade within 24 to 48 hours. If they continue to develop or are unusually numerous, a complete workup for infection or bleeding disorders should be performed.

Thrombocytopenia should be suspected when the infant presents with general cutaneous petechiae. It frequently accompanies neonatal infections and is most commonly associated with the TORCH diseases (toxoplasmosis, others, rubella, cytomegalovirus [CMV], and herpes simplex).

Macules are nonpalpable, nonraised lesions less than 1 cm in diameter identified only by color change. They are seen in measles, rubella, scarlet fever, roseola, typhoid fever, and drug reactions.

Papules are superficial elevated solid lesions less than 1 cm in diameter. They are firm and not fluid filled. They may follow the macular stage in many eruptive diseases. Vesicles are skin elevations that contain serous fluid (blisters). They are commonly seen with herpes simplex, insect bites, and poison ivy.

Pustules are localized accumulations of pus in, or just beneath, the epidermis. They are often centered around appendageal structures (e.g., hair follicles) and are usually caused by bacterial infections or skin abscesses. When a pustule breaks, the degree of crusting is more marked than occurs with the rupture of a vesicle.

Nodules are deep, solid lesions larger than 1 cm in diameter. Nodules are similar to papules but are larger. Because of their size, they are more likely to have a dermal component than are papules.

## Lesions Related to the Birth Process

Caput succedaneum is a diffuse, generalized edema of the presenting part of the scalp. It is the result of venous congestion caused by the pressure of the uterus, cervix, and vaginal wall on the infant's head during prolonged labor. The borders are not well defined, and the swelling crosses suture lines because the fluid accumulates outside the periosteum. Cephalohematoma is a subperiosteal hemorrhage caused by the rupture of the emissary or diploic veins of the skull during prolonged labor and delivery. The margins of the suture lines are clearly demarcated, almost always unilateral, and the swelling never crosses suture lines. It is seen more commonly in vacuum-assisted vaginal deliveries. Estimates of underlying skull fractures range from 5% to 25% (Jensen & Galbraith, 2015).

Forceps marks are identified by their rounded contours and position. The bruised area should be checked for underlying tissue and nerve damage. Scalp lacerations can occur in many ways. The placement of an internal fetal monitoring lead or the artificial rupture of membranes (ROM) can cause a laceration.

Using a vacuum extractor may cause a circular red or ecchymotic area. Any abraded area may be a portal of entry for infection; therefore, a scalp laceration should be carefully and continuously assessed.

Lacerations can also occur to other body surfaces from scalpel injuries during cesarean birth; an incidence of 1.9% was noted in a series of 896 cesarean section deliveries. Usually, the laceration or abscess remains confined to the skin; however, reported complications include osteomyelitis.

Internal fetal monitoring sites are at risk for infection, owing to the introduction of the maternal vaginal flora directly into the subcutaneous tissue of the fetus. Scalp abscesses caused by implantation of a fetal electrode are generally benign, self-limited occurrences. Rare instances of major complications have been reported, however, including significant areas of cellulitis, osteomyelitis, and sepsis (Jensen & Galbraith, 2015).

Subcutaneous fat necrosis is an uncommon subcutaneous tissue disorder that occurs primarily in full-term and postterm infants. It has been associated with birth trauma, shock, asphyxia, and hypothermia, including therapeutic hypothermia, seizures, and peripheral circulatory collapse. One or several indurated, violet, or red plaques or sharply defined subcutaneous nodules on the buttocks, thighs, back, cheek, or arms may appear (Hoath & Narendran, 2015). Hypercalcemia has been associated with subcutaneous fat necrosis; serum calcium levels should be monitored. Most areas of subcutaneous fat necrosis gradually reabsorb over weeks to months if left alone. Residual atrophy or scarring is unusual.

*Sclerema neonatorum* may have the same cause and adipose tissue abnormality in the subcutaneous tissues as those noted in fat necrosis. However, sclerema more commonly affects premature or debilitated infants. It is a diffuse hardening of the subcutaneous tissue that results in cold, nonpitting skin. The extremities may be involved initially, but generalized involvement occurs within 3 to 4 days. Infants with this disorder are usually critically ill, and there is a high mortality rate. If the infant survives, the sclerodermatous changes rarely last beyond 2 weeks. Treatment is based on therapy for the underlying systemic disease, restoration of body temperature, and adequate nutrition. Exchange transfusions and systemic administration of steroids have been used with unconfirmed efficacy (Hoath & Narendran, 2015).

# TRANSIENT SKIN LESIONS

Erythema toxicum neonatorum, the most common rash of newborns, usually occurs within 5 days of birth and affects approximately half of term infants. However, it is rarely seen in premature infants or those weighing less than 2,500 g. It appears as small, firm, white, or pale-yellow pustules with an erythematous margin. Lesions may first appear on the face and spread to the trunk and extremities but may appear anywhere on the body except the soles and palms (Howard & Frieden, 2015). Macules, papules, and pustules are seen in varying combinations. A smear and Wright stain of the pustules reveal numerous infiltrates of eosinophils devoid of bacteria. Differential diagnosis includes transient neonatal pustular melanosis, candidiasis, staphylococcal pyoderma, and miliaria. No treatment is necessary.

Neonatal and infantile acne are two distinct conditions distinguished by the time of onset and clinical features. Neonatal acne (neonatal cephalic pustulosis) involves inflammatory, erythematous papules and pustules located primarily on the cheeks, often scattered over the face and extending into the scalp. The usual age of onset is days to weeks. Treatment with low-potency topical corticosteroids such as hydrocortisone or imidazole creams such as ketoconazole can result in quicker resolution (Howard & Frieden, 2015). Infantile acne is considered to result in hyperplasia of sebaceous activity. It is found primarily on the face and presents after 1 month of age. Infantile acne can persist for months to years but generally resolves without treatment. Infantile acne may be more persistent and even cause scarring. Some experts suggest that neonatal acne is related to sebum excretion rate while the infantile form is linked to high androgen levels, but both have genetic influences (Herane & Ando, 2003).

Transient neonatal pustular melanosis is a lesion that is like miliaria but is present at birth, usually causing the infant to be unnecessarily isolated. It occurs most commonly on the forehead, behind the ears, and on the palms of the hands and the soles of the feet of term infants. It is most commonly seen in Black infants. The differential diagnosis includes *erythema toxicum neonatorum*, staphylococcal impetigo, congenital candidiasis, *miliaria crystallina* or rubra, and acropustulosis of infancy. If the lesions are ruptured, smeared on a slide, and stained, the contents are found to be amorphous debris. The lesion is neither infectious nor contagious. It is self-limiting and requires no treatment.

Sucking blisters that contain sterile, serous fluid may be seen on the thumb, index finger, wrist, or lip. Presumably the result of vigorous sucking in utero, they are seen in approximately 1 in every 250 live births and resolve without treatment (Howard & Frieden, 2015).

## Pigmentary Lesions

Hyperpigmented lesions may be present at birth or during the first weeks of life. Some pigmentary problems are benign, such as congenital dermal melanocytosis (CDM), whereas others can be signs of a systemic or genetic disorder. Some of the more common ones are included in this section.

Café au lait spots are irregularly shaped, flat, oval lesions. Their color resembles coffee to which milk has been added. They are present in up to 20% of infants, usually over the buttocks. They should be noted on the newborn's initial physical examination; if they are larger than 4 to 6 cm or if more than six are present, a diagnosis of neurofibromatosis should be considered (Hoath & Narendran, 2015). Pigmented lesion lasers can provide a safe and effective therapy for removing café au lait spots (Mavropoulos & Cohen, 2013).

CDM is a collection of melanocytes deep in the dermis. Commonly located over the buttocks and sacrum, CDM is gray, slate blue, or black in color. It appears in 13% of Caucasians, 65% of Latinos, 86% of Asians, and 96% of African American infants (Lucky, 2015).

Hyperpigmentation that presents in a diffuse pattern is unusual in the newborn. When present, congenital Addison disease, hepatic or biliary atresia, metabolic disease (Hartnup disease, porphyria), nutritional disorders (pellagra, sprue), hereditary disorders (lentiginosis, melanism), or unknown causes (the bronze discoloration seen in Niemann–Pick disease) may be the cause. Hyperpigmentation of the labial folds with clitoral hypertrophy may result from the transplacental passage of androgens (Dinulos & Darmstadt, 2005).

Neonatal/infantile hypopigmentation results from a diverse group of conditions. It can occur due to any defect in melanocyte development, melanin synthesis and transport, or distribution of melanosomes to keratinocytes. Hypopigmentation can present as a generalized, diffuse, or localized loss of pigment in the neonate, which may stem from metabolic (phenylketonuria), endocrine (Addison disease), genetic (vitiligo, piebaldism, tuberous sclerosis, albinism), traumatic, or postinflammatory causes (Dinulos & Darmstadt, 2005).

Albinism refers to a group of genetic disorders involving abnormal melanin synthesis during embryogenesis (Chan & Tay, 2015). It may occur in any race, with an incidence of approximately 1 in 20,000, with a slightly higher rate in African Americans (Sethi et al., 1996). An autosomal recessive gene usually causes it, but rare cases of autosomal dominant inheritance have occurred (Dinulos & Darmstadt, 2005).

Partial albinism (piebaldism) is a localized, autosomal dominant disorder present at birth and easily detected in dark-skinned infants. Off-white macules are seen on the scalp, widow's peak, and forehead, extending to the base of the nose, trunk, and extremities. A white forelock, a tuft of white hair over the midfrontal scalp, is present in 80% to 90% of patients and is associated with depigmentation of the underlying scalp (Chan & Tay, 2015). When illuminated with a Wood light, the amelanotic areas of piebaldism exhibit a brilliant whiteness. Differential diagnoses are Waardenburg syndrome, vitiligo, nevus anemicus, Addison disease, and white macules of tuberous sclerosis. Photoprotection of the depigmented areas beginning early in infancy is important to protect from sunburn and to avoid skin cancers later in life.

White leaf macules are the earliest cutaneous manifestations of tuberous sclerosis, an autosomal dominant neurocutaneous syndrome with both cutaneous and neurologic abnormalities (Chan & Tay, 2015). The macules vary in size and shape but most often resemble a mountain ash leaflet. They may be difficult to see in a newborn infant and more readily observed by examination with a Wood lamp, heightening the contrast between the macule and normal skin. Normal infants occasionally have a single lesion, but the presence of one or more of these macules in an infant with neurologic problems strongly suggests the diagnosis of tuberous sclerosis. Retinal hamartomas, cardiac rhabdomyomas, and benign renal tumors are some of the other possible findings. A careful family history, detailed physical examination, and multidisciplinary management are indicated in infants with these lesions.

Waardenburg syndrome is a rare autosomal disorder characterized by depigmented patches of skin and hair, congenital nerve deafness, craniofacial anomalies, and heterochromia iris.

## Dermatologic Diseases

Diseases of the skin in newborns often present patterns different from the presentation of the same disease in adults. Therefore, a careful physical examination of the skin is necessary for an accurate dermatologic diagnosis. All lesions should be described, and their locations and patterns should be noted.

Lesions can be classified as either primary or secondary. Primary lesions are described as the initial or principal lesions identified when the disease begins. Primary lesions are classified as macule, patch, papule, plaque, nodule, tumor, vesicle, bulla, wheal, pustule, or abscess. Some conditions that present with blisters and pustules can be life threatening (Howard & Frieden, 2015). Secondary lesions are brought about by the modification of a primary lesion, resulting in a crust, scale, erosion, ulcer, fissure, lichenification, atrophy, or scar.

## Developmental Vascular Abnormalities

The following two major groups of vascular birthmarks are seen:

1. Vascular malformations composed of dysplastic vessels
2. Vascular tumors that demonstrate cellular hyperplasia

Vascular malformations have various subcategories determined by the anomalous vessels involved—including capillary, venous, arteriovenous, or lymphatic. They remain relatively stable in size; any growth is commensurate with the child's growth.

**Port-Wine Stain.** A port-wine stain is a capillary malformation consisting of dilated and congested capillaries lying directly beneath the epidermis. It appears in approximately 3 out of 1,000 newborns. This birthmark appears pink at birth but gradually darkens to purple. Port-wine stains are most commonly found on the face and neck and are permanent developmental defects. They are most sharply demarcated and flat in infancy but, over time, develop a thickened or pebbly surface. Although a port-wine stain is primarily a cosmetic problem, it is occasionally an indicator of a multisystem disorder, such as Sturge–Weber syndrome or Klippel–Trenaunay–Weber syndrome. The presence of seizures, mental retardation, hemiplegia, or intracortical calcification suggests the presence of Sturge–Weber syndrome (Hoath & Narendran, 2015). An ophthalmologic examination is extremely important in these infants. Gradual thickening and nodule formation can occur with port-wine stain, thus supporting the need for early treatment in infancy and childhood. Although the timing of intervention is somewhat controversial, many dermatologists now advise laser treatment as early as possible in infancy to decrease the stigma associated with this lesion and to prevent skin thickening (Enjolras & Garzon, 2008). The pulsed dye laser is the gold standard for treating port-wine stain birthmarks, but multiple treatments are required. While the laser effectively fades these lesions, complete resolution is achieved in only 15% to 20% of cases (Hoath & Narendan, 2015; Tremaine et al., 2012).

**Pigmented Nevus.** Congenital melanocytic nevi are benign nested clumps of melanocytes. In contrast to melanocytes, they tend to lie in groups or nests. Congenital pigmented nevi are different from pigmented nevi, which arise later because they are usually larger and more extensive. As the infant grows, the area becomes thicker and darker (Dinulos & Darmstadt, 2005).

Flat, junctional nevi are seen in about 1% of newborns. They are brown or black, and their size varies from one to several centimeters. Conservative management consists of serial observations because there is no evidence that they are premalignant lesions. Surgical excision may be considered based on the location and appearance of the lesion (Hoath & Narendran, 2015).

**Large Congenital Melanocytic Nevi.** A pigmented and softly infiltrated area characterizes a giant hairy nevus (>20 cm). The color varies from pale brown to black. When the nevi are large, they tend to have a dermatomic distribution, and their location and size give them their name (e.g., bathing trunk nevus, vest nevus, shoulder stole nevus) (Figure 12.1). On histologic examination of a biopsy specimen, the nevus cells penetrate deeply into the dermis and subcutaneous tissue.

When a giant nevus is situated on the head or neck, it may be associated with mental retardation, epilepsy, or hydrocephalus. *Spina bifida* or meningocele may occur when this nevus is present over the spine (Dinulos & Darmstadt, 2005). Other abnormalities sometimes associated with a giant pigmented nevus are clubfoot, hypertrophy or hypotrophy of the affected limb, and von Recklinghausen disease (neurofibromatosis). Besides being a cosmetic problem, the giant nevus is associated with a higher incidence of malignancy. Malignant melanomas develop in as many as 8% of these patients. Management involves surgical excision of the entire lesion to prevent the development of skin cancer in the lesion. Dermabrasion, lasers, and tissue expansion techniques have been used in conjunction with surgery. Plastic surgical reconstruction may be needed if the excision is extensive.

**Hemangiomas.** Infantile hemangiomas (IH) are the most common vascular tumors seen during early infancy and are

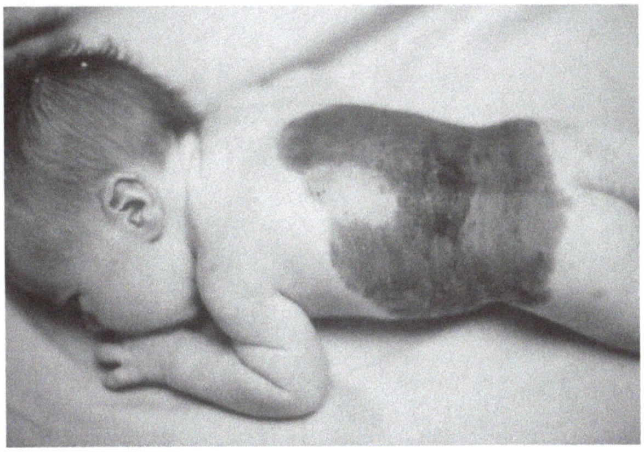

**FIGURE 12.1 The giant pigmented hairy nevus of this infant involves the thorax, abdomen, and back and is commonly called a "bathing trunk" nevus.** It is raised with fleshy elements and has a somewhat leathery texture.

*Source:* From Arya, S., & Jain, M. (2016). Giant congenital melanocytic nevus with limb hypoplasia and lipomatosis: A rare association. *Journal of Pigmentary Disorders, 3*(2). https://doi.org/10.4172/2376-0427.1000238.

characterized by the proliferation of capillary endothelium cells. These cells also possess histochemical markers present in placental vessels (Chen et al., 2013). Hypoxia has been identified as the main factor for vascular proliferation in IH (Laken, 2016). Hemangiomas appear in 1% to 3% of infants at birth and develop in another 10%, usually within the first 3 to 4 weeks of life. Females are two to three times more likely to be affected than males (Haggstrom & Chamlin, 2014). Besides gender, the other infants at highest risk are non-Hispanic Whites, premature infants, and multiple-gestation infants. The incidence is 22% in preterm babies who weigh less than 1,000 g and 15% in infants with birth weights of 1,000 to 1,500 g.

Classified by their depth, hemangioma types include superficial, deep, and compound. The treatment for most hemangiomas is "active" nonintervention. Up to 40% will develop complications requiring intervention (Hoath & Narendran, 2015). Congenital hemangiomas that resolve rapidly often leave pronounced atrophic changes in their place. They frequently appear in the skin as a single lesion, but multiple cutaneous lesions also occur, usually involving other organ systems.

The natural history of the hemangioma is characterized by its appearance during the first few weeks of life, rapid postnatal growth for 3 to 18 months (proliferative phase), a phase of stabilization for 12 to 18 months, which is followed by very slow but inevitable regression for the next 5 to 8 years (involutive phase) (Droitcourt et al., 2018). IH resolve entirely in more than 80% of children by 4 years of age, and continued improvement occurs in the remaining children. The regression rate does not seem to be related to the sex or age of the infant, the site, size, or appearance of the hemangioma, or the duration of the proliferative phase.

Strawberry or superficial hemangiomas consist of a dilated mass of capillaries in the dermal and subdermal layers that protrude above the skin's surface. They are bright red, soft, compressible tumors that can appear anywhere on the body (Figure 12.2). They generally increase in size for

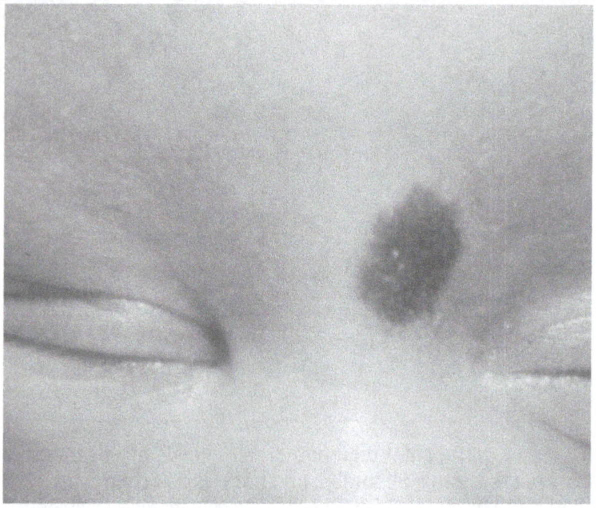

**FIGURE 12.2 This photograph shows the early hemangioma in a 28-week-gestation premature infant.** Approximately 5 weeks after birth, the first area of discoloration appeared. The irregular surface with sharp demarcation is typical of strawberry hemangioma, which eventually enlarges to twice the size that it appears in this photograph before involution.

*Source:* From Gstk. (2017, June 2). *Infantile hemangioma* [Image]. Wikimedia Commons. https://commons.wikimedia.org/wiki/File%3AInfantile_hemangioma.jpg.

approximately 6 months and then gradually begin to regress or involute spontaneously. Complete involution may take several years to occur. These marks require no treatment, but 20% to 40% of patients may have residual skin changes. Intervention is necessary when these lesions interfere with vital functions such as vision, feeding, and respiration (Enjolras & Garzon, 2008).

Cavernous or deep hemangiomas are more deeply situated in the skin than superficial strawberry hemangiomas. They are bluish-red, feel spongy when touched, and may not appear until 1 to 3 months after birth. Most hemangiomas are small, harmless birthmarks that involute to leave either normal or slightly blemished skin. However, even a small hemangioma can obstruct the airway or impair vision. A large hemangioma in the liver or an extensive cutaneous hemangioma can divert a considerable volume of blood through its extensive labyrinth of capillaries and produce high-output heart failure. The increased capillary endothelial surface that characterizes a giant hemangioma can also trap platelets and may cause thrombocytopenic coagulopathy, as seen in the Kasabach–Merritt syndrome. This syndrome carries significant mortality and requires aggressive treatment, such as transcutaneous arterial embolization (Hoath & Narendran, 2015).

A few hemangiomas grow to an alarming size or proliferate simultaneously in several organs and cause life-endangering conditions, such as soft-tissue destruction, deformation or obstruction of vital structures, serious bleeding, ulceration, and sepsis. Large lesions can expand the skin and, even after they regress, result in excess slack skin, pigment changes, and a fibro-fatty residuum.

Visceral hemangiomas may arise in many organs, most commonly in the liver and larynx, with or without cutaneous involvement; a single lesion or multiple hemangiomas may occur. Having five or more lesions puts the infant at a higher risk of hepatic hemangioma (Laken, 2016). Flow through extensive hemangiomas increases the total blood volume, causes hemodeviation, and disturbs the hemodynamic equilibrium. The hyperdynamic cardiovascular state of the hemangiomas decreases or shunts blood away from other tissues, thus resulting in hypoperfusion of other tissues. This hypoperfusion may cause brain hypoxia, acidosis, and predisposition to seizures, as seen in some cases. Close surveillance of the cardiovascular system is necessary to determine the proper time to begin digitalization.

Large, complex, or segmental lesions around the head, neck, lumbosacral, perineal, and lower extremities have been associated with congenital anomalies. Large segmental lesions on the face can indicate PHACE syndrome. This neurocutaneous syndrome includes Posterior fossa brain formations, Hemangioma greater than 5 cm, Arterial anomalies of the head or neck, Cardiac abnormalities, and Eye abnormalities. Chest wall abnormalities may also exist (Drolet et al., 2013).

**Management.** Management of both superficial and deep hemangiomas consists of a detailed history, scrutiny of the lesion or lesions, including three-dimensional measurements, and evaluation of the growth pattern of the hemangioma. Ulceration, the most common complication that occurs in about 15% to 25% of all infants, can be very painful and result in infection, hemorrhage, scarring, and functional impairment (Hoath & Narendran, 2015). As involution progresses, the color gradually changes from grayish-pink to white or pink, and the tension of the lesion decreases. Ulcerated hemangiomas should be treated with topical antibiotics to prevent infection.

While the cutaneous lesions are being monitored, the infant's clinical course and physical development must be closely observed for poor growth, altered cry, stridor, dyspnea, cyanosis, feeding difficulties, or swallowing impairment. **Emergency Alert: If any abnormal signs or symptoms appear—such as tachycardia, heart murmur, hepatomegaly, or bruit that can be heard over the liver—the infant should be examined for evidence of heart failure.** Ultrasonography, echocardiography, and computed tomography may be needed.

Management generally consists of planned neglect, which is essential in avoiding disfiguring scars. Complications of therapy may be significant, but residual scarring after complete involution is uncommon. Hemangiomas located in exposed areas often cause great parental anxiety, which increases as the hemangioma grows. This anxiety often puts pressure on the physician to do something. However, the hemangioma should be left to regress spontaneously, and preconceived notions about birthmarks should be discussed with the family.

In some cases, treatment of hemangiomas may be needed. The following indications for treatment have been proposed: life-threatening or function-threatening hemangiomas, including those that cause impairment of vision, respiratory compromise, or congestive heart failure; hemangiomas occurring in certain anatomic locations such as the nose, lip, glabellar areas, and ear that may cause permanent deformity or scars; large facial hemangiomas, especially those with a large dermal component; and ulcerated hemangiomas.

Systemic propranolol is now the standard treatment for high-risk hemangiomas, replacing high-dose corticosteroid therapy in most cases (Harter & Mancini, 2019; Pahl & McLean, 2022). Adverse effects of propranolol treatment include sleep disturbances and agitation; these are the most common. More serious side effects include hypoglycemia, hypotension, bradycardia, bronchospasm, peripheral vasoconstriction, and diarrhea. Topical management options for IH involve timolol 0.5% gel. Timolol maleate is a topical beta blocker that may have a particular role in treating superficial lesions. The recommendation is to apply one drop twice a day to affected lesions.

Surgical therapy involving either laser removal or surgical excision is also a treatment option. Excision is usually done once the hemangioma has involuted to remove residual tissue and redundant skin. Early excision is generally not recommended.

**Emergency Alert: Propranolol had the most significant response when it was started with infants younger than 4 months of age. Potentially harmful effects include hypoglycemia, hyperkalemia, bronchiolitis, bronchospasm, conduction disorders (bradycardia), and hypotension** (Droitcourt et al., 2018). The dose should be divided into three daily doses with a minimum of 6 hours between doses. Giving the dose with or right after feeding reduces the risk of hypoglycemia.

## Blistering Diseases

**Epidermolysis Bullosa.** Epidermolysis bullosa (EB) is a group of rare, congenital blistering disorders, all of which are inherited. They are considered mechanobullous diseases, meaning that trauma to or friction on the skin induces blister formation. EB is caused by defects in the complex meshwork of proteins in the epidermis, dermis, and dermoepidermal junction that allow the skin to adhere in the presence of frictional stress. The underlying defect appears to be a lack of cellular glue in the squamous epithelium, which is responsible for maintaining cellular integrity. Diagnostic studies should include a skin biopsy for light and electron microscopy and immunofluorescence mapping. In all forms of EB, gentle rubbing will result in blister formation, the Nikolsky sign (Polra et al., 2024).

The classification of EB was updated in 2020. The diagnosis of EB is now more heavily based on genetic rather than clinical or histologic features (Lucky et al., 2021). EB is classified into three major subtypes by the clinical extent and ultrastructural level of blistering, inheritance pattern, and specific genetic mutations (Hoath & Narendran, 2015; Püttgen & Cohen, 2013). Although some subtypes of EB are severe in the neonatal period and milder later, others can be fatal in the first weeks as a result of severe generalized blistering and complications that arise from this. EB can be nonscarring or scarring. Inheritance may be either autosomal dominant or autosomal recessive.

EB simplex is the mildest form of EB. Most cases are autosomal dominant. The lesions occur at the basal layer of the epidermis and do not lead to scarring and hyperkeratosis. Usually present at birth, the vesicles and bullae appear over the joints and the bony protuberances and at sites subjected to repeated trauma.

Junctional EB is a very severe but the least common type of EB with autosomal recessive inheritance. In junctional EB, severe generalized blistering is present at birth, with subsequent extensive denudation. Marked mucosal blistering occurs, and erosions of the larynx, respiratory, gastrointestinal (GI), and urinary tract may also be present. It may be fatal in a few days to a couple of years because of significant loss of electrolytes and protein or sepsis. Histopathologically, a separation occurs between the plasma membrane of the basal cells and the basal lamina at the dermal–epidermal junction (Püttgen & Cohen, 2013). In junctional EB, healing is poor, and scarring is extensive.

Dystrophic or scarring EB results in blistering that occurs below the dermal–epidermal junction and has either dominant or recessive inheritance. In the recessive form, blistering, infection, and scar formation can be severe, begin before birth, and lead to severe deformities and joint contractures. Milia may mark the healed blister sites. Complications include infections and hemolytic, nutritional, orthopedic, GI, and psychiatric sequelae. Squamous cell cancer is also associated with this life-limiting type of EB.

The dominant form of dystrophic EB is milder, with less severe blisters or red plaques seen on the distal extremities and bony protuberances (Figure 12.3). Some scar formation occurs, and the nails may be mildly dystrophic, but deforming scars and contractures occur infrequently. The external skin layer can be easily rubbed off by slight friction or injury. Milia, due to a functional disorder of the sweat glands, are found on the rims of the ears, the dorsa of the hands, and the extensor surfaces of the arms and legs. The oral, anal, and esophageal mucosa are frequently involved but not severely.

**Management.** EB can be a significant challenge in the newborn period, particularly with the more severe forms. Nursing care centers around three main issues: (a) skin breakdown,

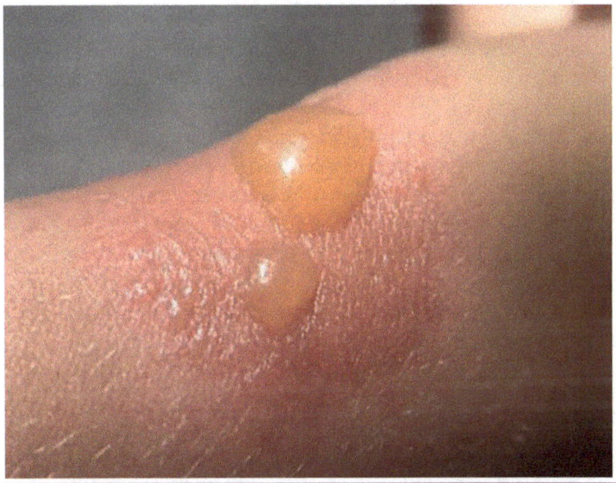

**FIGURE 12.3 This photograph of epidermolysis bullosa shows the scaling, broken bullae with underlying erythroderma.**
*Source:* OlegMalyshev/iStockphoto.

(b) prevention of secondary infection, and (c) dysphagia. Many techniques used to protect the skin of very premature infants are helpful with EB patients. Avoiding the use of tape and preventing traumatic injuries is essential. Clean, soft dressings may be helpful over bony pressure points. Wound care involves providing a moist healing environment by covering open lesions with a thick coating of petrolatum-based emollients, combined with topical antibiotic ointments, and covering with nonstick dressings.

Many dermatologists will rotate topical antibiotics every few months to prevent resistance and may use wound cultures to guide the selection of agents. Nonstick dressings include petrolatum gauze, Vigilon, EXU-DRY, or silicone-based products such as Mepitel (Direct Medical Inc., Houston, TX). After this layer, wrapping with nonadhesive cotton gauze further protects the wound; some practitioners prefer cotton mesh, and others use Coban™ (3M, Indianapolis, IN), a wrap that adheres to itself without adhesives. When blisters are tense and fluid filled, they should be "unroofed" to prevent extension. This procedure is done with sharp, clean scissors, leaving the blister roof in place. Dressings are changed daily and removed gently; some prefer to remove dressings during immersion bathing.

From birth to 6 months of age, the environment is easy to control through the use of sheepskin, loose-fitting clothes, and mittens for the infant's hands and feet. Cloth diapers softened with fabric softener are preferred over rougher, disposable diapers. Any person handling the infant should avoid wearing jewelry.

Protection of the infant becomes more difficult once the infant is mobile. The infant should always wear long pants; foam rubber pads sewn into the knees help avoid trauma during crawling. Contractures may form quickly as scarring begins to occur. The pathologic increase in elastic skin fiber adds to this process. Gentle range-of-motion exercises lessen contracture formation.

Dysphagia can occur from facial and pharyngeal scarring secondary to erosions on the buccal mucosa, tongue, palate, esophagus, and pharynx. Feedings should be performed slowly and carefully to avoid aspiration and to maintain adequate nutrition. The metabolic needs of these infants are high because of the continuous skin healing and sloughing of epithelium, which results in large protein, fluid, and electrolyte losses. Additional iron may be required to replace chronic blood loss from the skin (Püttgen & Cohen, 2013). Adding more puncture holes to a nipple may help prevent oral mucosal trauma. If oral ulcerations do occur, several weeks of hyperalimentation and high-dose steroid therapy are instituted. Gavage feedings are discouraged because of the possibility of trauma. It is essential that the family receives genetic counseling regarding the inheritance pattern associated with EB; a negative family history does not exclude its occurrence.

## Infections of the Skin

Previously, it was thought that after vaginal birth, the skin colonization with microorganisms reflected the mother's vaginal flora, and after cesarean section birth without rupture of the amniotic membranes, the skin was sterile. Recent research using DNA sequencing has begun to reveal that the skin microbiome begins in utero (Gregory, 2011). The skin microbiome of vaginally born infants does appear similar to the mother's vaginal flora, but the skin of cesarean section births resembles the mother's and caregiver's skin flora (Dominguez-Bello et al., 2010). It is now known that the skin and its normal flora are natural defense mechanisms against invading pathogens. Maintenance of the skin microbiome is essential to the immunologic functioning of the skin (Coughlin et al., 2014). A skin surface pH of between 4.0 and 4.5 facilitates the attachment of the "good" commensal bacteria (Telofski et al., 2012).

In the newborn, an immature immune system, prematurity, stress, and medical and surgical problems contribute to vulnerability and infection. Additionally, most infants in the NICU require a variety of invasive monitoring and diagnostic procedures that allow for breaks in the normally intact physical barrier of the skin, providing direct access to blood and deep tissues (Dinulos & Pace, 2008). The origin of skin infections and skin manifestations of systemic infection can be bacterial, viral, or fungal.

**Bacterial.** Bacterial skin infections can vary in initial clinical findings and potential for systemic symptoms and sequelae. The pathogen involved and the route of inoculation are two factors that affect the course of bacterial cutaneous infection (Dinulos & Pace, 2008). Types of bacterial skin infections include bullous and nonbullous impetigo, omphalitis, abscesses, and cellulitis. Severe dermatologic findings are also seen when endotoxins are released from bacteria, as in the case of staphylococcal scalded skin syndrome.

**Staphylococcus Aureus.** Infections resulting from *Staphylococcus aureus* (*S. aureus*) are seen in newborns and can result in bullous, crusted, or pustular types of skin lesions. Nonbullous impetigo is a superficial infection localized to the epidermis and is characterized by erythematous, honey-colored, crusted plaques. Bullous impetigo of the newborn involves blisters that originate in the subcorneal portion of the epidermis and are filled with clear or straw-colored fluid. Bullous impetigo often presents during the first 2 weeks of life. Few or many blisters may be dispersed widely over all areas of the body and may rupture easily, thus leaving denuded areas of skin. Bullous impetigo commonly appears on the diaper area, axilla, and periumbilical skin and is predominantly caused by *S. aureus* (Hoath & Narendran, 2015). If the bacteria are later spread via the bloodstream, the infection may result in osteomyelitis, septic arthritis, or septicemia in neonates (Dinulos & Pace, 2008). Isolation of hospitalized neonates is initiated and IV antibiotics are generally recommended in neonates after initial blood, blister fluid, and skin cultures are obtained. Treatment is then tailored to the specific organism when the antibiotic susceptibility profile is known.

**Management.** Medical and nursing management is focused on the treatment of the affected infant and on the prevention of the spread of infection to other infants because this condition is highly contagious. Blood cultures should always be obtained before initiating IV antibiotics (Hoath & Narendran, 2015). Systemic antibiotics are administered parenterally initially due to the release of an epidermolytic toxin by *S. aureus* in bullous impetigo. They may be followed by oral treatment once the infection begins to subside. Antibiotics include oxacillin, nafcillin, or methicillin; vancomycin is used if the culture indicates methicillin-resistant *S. aureus* (MRSA). Topical antibiotics are not indicated for the treatment of bullous impetigo. Additionally, mupirocin intranasally is recommended to prevent recurrent impetigo from nasal colonization. Topical antibiotics can be effectively used for nonbullous impetigo if the lesions are not extensive or involve the mouth area. Fluid and electrolyte monitoring is necessary if the denuded areas cover a large surface or if the infant is of low birth weight (LBW) (Hoath & Narendran, 2015). Compresses of warm saline can be applied to the affected sites. Isolation of the affected infant is necessary to prevent the spread of the infection throughout the nursery.

**Scalded Skin Syndrome.** Staphylococcal ("staph") scalded skin syndrome is a severe endotoxin-mediated disease with superficial, widespread blistering, often leading to desquamation (Figure 12.4). The bright erythema of this bullous eruption resembles a scald. The erythema usually begins on the face and spreads downward. Multiple sites are cultured when this disease is suspected, including any bullous lesions, blood, cerebrospinal fluid, nasopharynx, urine, conjunctival sac, and umbilicus to recover an organism. Staph scalded skin syndrome is rarely seen at birth, with most cases appearing between 3 and 7 days of life (Hoath & Narendran, 2015).

Skin will appear bright red, like a burn, followed by the development of large, loose blisters that quickly progress to sheets of skin being shed. During the course of this disease, the entire epidermis may be shed. Emollients, together with semi-occlusive dressings, provide gentle lubrication and pain relief.

**Management.** Medical and nursing management also involves the administration of the appropriate systemic antibiotic regimen and supportive measures in terms of fluid and electrolytic replacement, prevention of secondary infection through the damaged epidermis, and pain management. Applying local antibiotic solutions or ointments is not recommended; cleansing open skin areas with gentle irrigation using normal saline followed by the application of a nonadherent dressing that promotes healing and prevents secondary infection is better (King et al., 2014). The infant may be more comfortable in an incubator than in a radiant warmer because the incubator is a convective heat source that does not have a direct cutaneous effect. In contrast, the radiant heat source heats directly through the skin. In addition, the radiant heat source may further increase the degree of ISWL through the damaged epidermis. Usually, a flaking process is observed on the skin during the healing process. Emollients may help treat dry skin at this point.

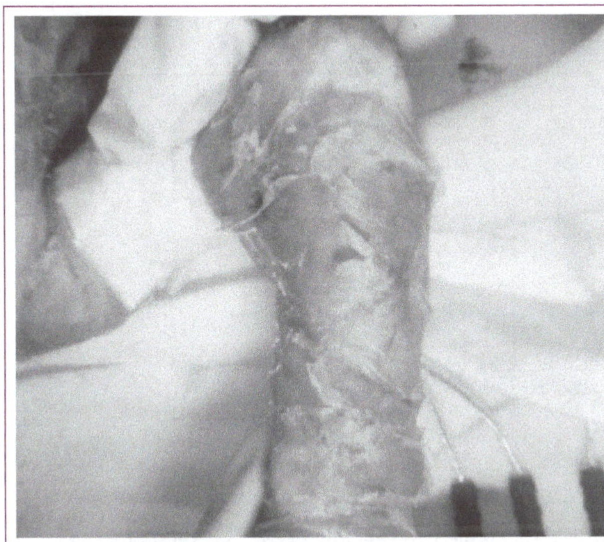

**FIGURE 12.4 The peeling, scaling skin of this premature infant had an acute onset at approximately 2 weeks of age.** This is the scalded skin syndrome that results from *Staphylococcus aureus*.

*Source:* Reprinted with permission from Clark, D., & Thompson, J. (1986). Dermatology of the newborn, Parts 1 and 2. In *Pathology of the neonate slide series* (Vol. 3, No. 4). Wyeth-Ayerst Laboratories.

**Listeria Monocytogenes.** Another bacterial skin disease is listeriosis, caused by *Listeria monocytogenes*. This organism, which can cause severe systemic disease, can also result in disseminated miliary granulomatosis in neonates (Hoath & Narendran, 2015). In some cases, miliary abscesses can occur, and occasionally, more generalized erythema or petechiae may be present. Systemic listeriosis is a severe infection that causes blood hemolysis and a high mortality rate. Prompt recognition and treatment with intravenous penicillin or ampicillin are indicated for the best prognosis. No direct skin therapy has been described as being necessary for this disease.

**Syphilis.** Congenital syphilis is another bacterial infection that has skin manifestations. Sixty percent of infants born with congenital syphilis are asymptomatic at birth (Püttgen & Cohen, 2013). If the infant with congenital syphilis is not treated after birth, a maculopapular or bullous skin eruption develops between 2 and 6 weeks of age. Sometimes, the bullous lesions may be observed at birth on the palms or the soles, signifying the presence of more severe disease (Hoath & Narendran, 2015). The fluid contained in the blisters contains spirochetes.

The lesions most commonly seen in congenital syphilis are copper-colored and maculopapular and are located on the soles and palms. In addition, open lesions may be present around the mouth, anus, or genitals, and a highly contagious nasal discharge is occasionally seen. If the syphilis remains untreated, the lesions regress in 1 to 3 months, leaving areas on the skin with either hyperpigmentation or hypopigmentation.

**Management.** Medical and nursing management for infants with congenital syphilis involves prompt, consistent administration of penicillin. Titers are obtained over the next year at 3-month intervals, and a negative serologic finding is expected at 1 year. Care of the skin lesions is primarily directed toward preventing the spread of infection during the active phase of the illness, especially when bullous lesions or open areas are apparent. No direct topical therapies have been advocated in the literature.

**Viral.** Viral infections can display a broad range of cutaneous manifestations in the neonate and can occur in utero, perinatally, or postnatally. Congenital infections are known by the acronym TORCH (Örge & Grigorian, 2015). Skin manifestations can directly result from skin infection or be a consequence of viral infection in other tissues. Viral infections that result in cutaneous manifestations include herpes simplex virus, CMV, rubella, varicella, enterovirus, parvovirus, and human immunodeficiency virus (HIV). Some of these have very specific cutaneous presentations (such as the classic "blueberry muffin" appearance of infants infected with rubella and cytomegalic virus), vesicles (as with herpes simplex), or nonspecific lesions. Toxoplasmosis, which has cutaneous manifestations and is caused by a parasite, is also discussed in this section.

**Herpes Simplex.** Herpes simplex virus (HSV) types 1 and 2 are serious pathogens in newborns. Intrauterine herpes infection typically presents with vesicles at birth or within the first 24 hours of life. The majority of newborns acquire infections from infectious vaginal secretions at the time of delivery. The 1- to 3-mm vesicles on the skin with this disease usually develop at 6 to 13 days of life. They can vary; a few faint scars may be present, or actual vesicle formations may be present with either one large swelling or discrete groups of vesicles. Frequently, an inconspicuous cutaneous lesion is a sign of systemic infection (Hoath & Narendran, 2015). Vesicles may recede and then recur over months.

HSV, types 1 and 2, is one of the most serious viral infections to affect the newborn and can appear as a disseminated infection, central nervous system (CNS) infection and infection localized to the skin, eyes, or mouth. Disseminated infection is the most devastating presentation, with a mortality rate of up to 75% without antiviral therapy and about 50% if antiviral therapy is used (Friedlander & Bradley, 2008). Vesicle formations may present with either one large swelling or smaller groups of vesicles that crust over rapidly and then recede. The absence of vesicles does not rule out the disease. Management consists of early recognition and treatment with antiviral agents, such as acyclovir, and isolation from other infants. If encephalitis develops, the prognosis is extremely poor, with either a high risk of death or severe mental retardation.

**Management.** Medical and nursing management is centered primarily on early recognition and treatment with the antiviral medication acyclovir. A definitive diagnosis is made by scraping the base of a fresh vesicle and staining with Giemsa or Wright stain, direct fluorescent antibody staining, or enzyme immunoassay detection of HSV antigens (Püttgen & Cohen, 2013).

The prognosis of systemic herpes simplex is extremely poor if encephalitis develops, with a high risk of either death or severe mental retardation. An important consideration in caring for infants with known or suspected herpes simplex infection is isolation from other patients to prevent transmission.

**Varicella.** Another viral infection that manifests in the skin is varicella. Varicella infection is rare, but when it occurs in the first 10 days of life, it is generally thought to have been acquired in the last 3 weeks of pregnancy. The vesicular eruptions are the same as those in chickenpox acquired at any age. A mortality rate of 20% is associated with varicella infection in newborns, and this infection poses a significant risk for immunocompromised infants in premature and intensive care nurseries. No systemic medication or topical treatment is required for these lesions. Occasionally, scarring can occur. Strict isolation is essential to protect other infants from exposure because this virus is airborne.

**Toxoplasmosis.** Toxoplasmosis, which is caused by an intracellular parasite (*Toxoplasma gondii*), can be transmitted transplacentally and can result in systemic infection. Some infants may have a generalized maculopapular rash, hepatosplenomegaly, jaundice, fever, and anemia. The rash may progress to desquamation and hypopigmentation in very severe cases. Direct topical therapy is not reported to be necessary or efficacious; systemic therapy may be considered.

**Cytomegalovirus and Rubella.** Both CMV and rubella have symptoms manifested in the skin. Petechial lesions can occur with both infections. These result from thrombocytopenia and dermal erythropoiesis and usually disappear in 2 to 6 weeks. In severe rubella infection, and very rarely in CMV, bluish-red papules that are 2 to 8 mm in diameter can occur on the head, trunk, and extremities (Figure 12.5), resulting in the description "blueberry muffin" syndrome. Ocular involvement in congenital rubella is common. The characteristic "salt and pepper" retinopathy is the most common finding, but cataracts are responsible for the greatest vision loss (Örge & Grigorian, 2015). Neither of these lesions requires topical therapy.

**Fungal.** *Candida albicans* infection is the primary fungal infection with cutaneous manifestations. However, other species—such as *Candida parapsilosis*, *Candida tropicalis*, *Candida lusitaniae*, *Candida glabrata*, and *Malassezia furfur*—can also potentially colonize the skin of term and preterm newborns, particularly those who are hospitalized in an intensive care nursery. During routine screening, roughly one-third of healthcare workers in the NICU test positive for *Candida* (Hoath & Narendran, 2015). Clinical symptoms of this type of infection can range from diaper dermatitis to other mucous membranes or localized skin eruptions to systemic candidiasis, resulting in significant morbidity and mortality. *Candida* is not generally found on the skin of the newborn. The primary reservoir for this organism is the GI

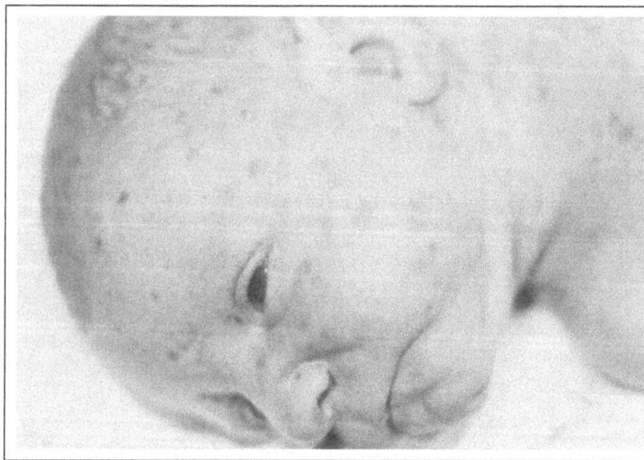

**FIGURE 12.5 This is an example of the "blueberry muffin" syndrome, seen in an infant with congenital cytomegalovirus infection.** The infant has multiple petechiae and purpura from thrombocytopenia in this systemic infection.

*Source:* From Benmiloud, S., Elhaddou, G., Belghiti, Z. A., Hida, M., & Bouharrou, A. (2012). Blueberry muffin syndrome. *Pan African Medical Journal, 13*(1), Article 23. https://doi.org/10.11604/pamj.2012.13.23.1790.

and female genital tracts so that the skin can be colonized at birth during passage through the birth canal. The incidence of *Candida* colonization also increases with the frequent use of broad-spectrum antibiotics that alter normal skin flora in infants after delivery. Nursing assessment of the LBW infant should include the observation of a monilial diaper rash or a diffuse burnlike dermatitis affecting large areas of the lower back, buttocks, chest, and abdomen (Baley & Silverman, 1988). *Candida* dermatitis is recognized as an early presentation of invasive fungal disease in the extremely low birth weight (ELBW) infant (Benjamin et al., 2010).

Premature neonates with systemic candidiasis may demonstrate cutaneous involvement. This cutaneous pattern may be a diffuse, burnlike dermatitis that affects large areas on the lower back, buttocks, chest, and abdomen. Lesions also typically appear in skin creases (Püttgen & Cohen, 2013). In a few infants, the axilla and groin are affected. Scaling follows the erythematous macular patches, and in severe cases, desquamation develops like that seen in staphylococcal scalded skin syndrome. These infants do not always have the satellite papules and pustules commonly seen with *Candida* diaper dermatitis. The onset of the generalized rash often occurs within the first 3 days to 4 weeks of life but can appear later. Skin biopsies performed on patients with this condition revealed fungal invasion that extended beyond the epidermis into the dermis. Associated factors included maternal colonization with vaginal birth, steroid administration, hyperglycemia, and skin trauma from adhesive removal. Infants who weigh less than 1,500 g are especially at risk for systemic infection. In addition to a birth weight of less than 1,500 g, risk factors for disseminated candidiasis include respiratory therapy, central line placement, antibiotic use, and parenteral nutrition (Hoath & Narendran, 2015).

Another important cause of necrotic and purpuric lesions in neonates with ecchymoses and crustlike plaques is cutaneous infection with mold species, such as *Aspergillus*, *Fusarium*, *Rhizopus*, and *Mucor* (Hook & Eichenfield, 2011). A biopsy is often part of the evaluation, particularly if surface cultures are inconclusive; cutaneous debridement and systemic antifungal agents may improve outcomes for these rare cases.

**Management.** Medical and nursing management of infants with systemic or local *Candida* infection involves therapy with systemic antifungal medications and antifungal ointments and creams. Cutaneous *Candida* in extremely premature infants less than 1 week of age requires aggressive monitoring for systemic infection and may warrant parenteral antifungal agents to prevent dissemination of the fungal infection. Yeast is sometimes challenging to culture; techniques include obtaining urine to look for hyphae or budding yeast, blood cultures, and skin scrapings prepared with potassium hydroxide (KOH) obtained from the margins of the affected areas because this is the area of active growth, and examined for pseudohyphae (Cunningham & Wagner, 2008). Nursing observation in LBW infants for evidence of diffuse, burnlike dermatitis or a spreading monilial diaper rash is essential and may expedite the initiation of parenteral antifungal therapy for systemic candidiasis. Most *Candida* species found in the NICU are sensitive to fluconazole and amphotericin (Lin et al., 2013).

Treatment for *Candida* diaper dermatitis consists of keeping the area clean and dry and applying an antifungal ointment or cream several times a day. Thrush, an oral fungal infection, appears as patches of white material scattered over the tongue that cannot be scraped off. It is treated with an oral form of nystatin.

## Scaling Disorders

A scaly appearance in the skin of a newborn can have a range of causes, from relatively benign to long-term and potentially life threatening. In this section, scaly skin due to postmaturity, essential fatty acid (EFA) deficiency, congenital ichthyosis, and eczema are discussed, and areas of nursing management are determined.

**Postmaturity.** Many term infants born between 40 and 42 weeks' gestation experience a period of shedding or desquamation considered a normal physiologic process. Postmature infants born after 42 weeks' gestation may also have this appearance, but other characteristics differ. The postmature infant may have a lean appearance and little subcutaneous fat; the weight is low in relation to length. The skin resembles parchment paper and may literally peel off in sheets, peaking near the eighth day of life (Hoath & Narendran, 2015). Fingernails may be stained with meconium and may be long. Long hair may also be present.

Skin care is not the primary problem nor the focus of medical or nursing management. Eventually, the skin underneath the peeling layers predominates; even during the period of desquamation, the skin functions well as a barrier because these infants have all the layers of stratum corneum of a term infant or adult. Aside from initially bathing with a mild baby wash, moisturizing with a petrolatum-based ointment may be appropriate. More careful attention is paid to the more compelling problems associated with postmaturity, such as hypoglycemia and meconium aspiration.

**Essential Fatty Acid Deficiency.** Newborns frequently do not receive an adequate diet because of other illnesses or surgical conditions; scaly, dry skin may signify the development of EFA deficiency syndrome. Infants may be more prone to developing this syndrome, especially if premature or postmature, because of the decreased fat stores available. It may also occur in infants with severe fat malabsorption, such as those with cystic fibrosis.

The skin appearance in EFA deficiency includes a superficial scaling and, in some cases, desquamation. Later presentation may involve oozing and irritation in the neck, groin, or perianal region.

This syndrome is sometimes confused with other conditions that cause scaling or other skin disruptions, including ichthyosis, acrodermatitis enteropathica, and candidal infection. Laboratory findings that confirm this diagnosis are decreased serum EFA levels, possibly in conjunction with thrombocytopenia and impaired platelet aggregation, because EFAs are necessary to ensure platelet function.

**Management.** Medical and nursing management consists of replacing EFAs through administering IV lipid solutions or diet. Human breastmilk and most infant formulas contain more than adequate EFAs. However, IV therapy is required if the GI system is not functioning well in digestion and absorption of nutrients.

Once skin symptoms are present, administration of an IV lipid solution can reverse the process in 1 to 2 weeks. Dietary replacement takes longer and is effective only in the presence of healthy GI function.

Prevention of EFA deficiency is possible and should be the goal. The development of EFA deficiency can be prevented by the early administration of IV lipid solutions in the first weeks of life in a dose as low as 0.5 g/kg/d.

**Ichthyosis.** The most serious cause of dry, scaly skin in the newborn is ichthyosis dermatosis, a genetically inherited disorder of cornification (Ivich, 2015). Four major types of ichthyosis exist: (1) X-linked ichthyosis; (2) lamellar ichthyosis; (3) bullous congenital ichthyosiform erythroderma, which is present at birth; and (4) *ichthyosis vulgaris*, which usually appears after the third month of life. Terms commonly used to describe infants with ichthyosis may include harlequin fetus and collodion baby, but these terms do not define which form of ichthyosis is present.

Males are primarily affected by the X-linked type of ichthyosis. Some female heterozygotes may exhibit mild scaling of the arms and lower extremities. Affected male newborns have large yellow or brown plaques that cover the whole body, except the palms, soles, midface, and over joints. At birth, some affected males may appear scaly, whereas others are often called collodion babies.

Lamellar ichthyosis, formerly called nonbullous congenital ichthyosiform erythroderma, is an autosomal recessive disorder. Initially, affected newborns may have a bright red appearance that rapidly progresses to desquamation; rarely is a collodion-baby appearance present at birth. Later, scales develop that are yellow to brown, and that may eventually become thick, horny plates. Although the prognosis is usually good, infants who are severely affected with the most severe form—harlequin ichthyosis—may die of sepsis or require extensive plastic surgery (Figure 12.6). Among them, difficulties faced are eye disease, heat intolerance, finger contractures, chronic skin infections, and hearing problems (Ivich, 2015).

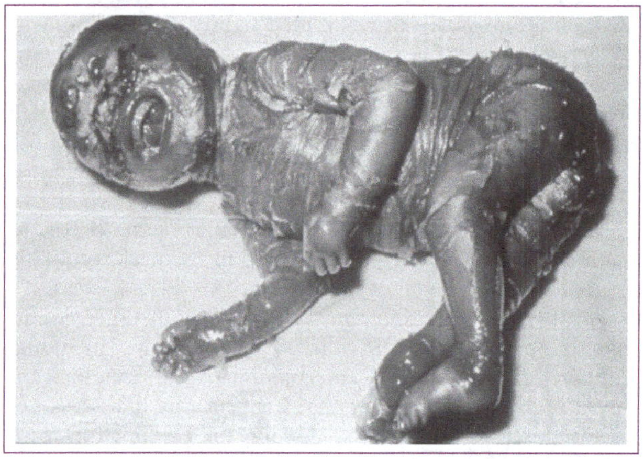

**FIGURE 12.6 This harlequin infant is an example of the most severely affected ichthyotic infant.** The skin is hard and thick, with deep crevices. The lack of elasticity of the skin results in fleshy deformities of joints and limbs.

*Source:* From Fouad, A., Bennaoui, F., Slitine, N. E. I., Soraa, N., & Maoulainine, F. (2018). Vibrio cholerae septicemia and Harlequin ichthyosis: Outstanding association. *The Open Infectious Diseases Journal, 10*(1), 76–78. https://doi.org/10.2174/1874279301810010076.

In bullous congenital ichthyosiform erythroderma, autosomal dominance is the mode of heredity; thus, several family members may be affected. Large bullae are initially seen, as are erythema and dry scaly skin; the blistering that recurs throughout childhood differentiates this form from the lamellar type. Extensive denuded areas of the skin can present a problem in the newborn as the blisters burst, and secondary life-threatening infections with *Streptococcus* or *Staphylococcus* can occur.

**Management.** Medical and nursing management of X-linked and lamellar forms of ichthyosis involves the continual use of topical emollients, prescription bathing techniques, and infection prevention. **Quality and Safety: Emollients increase hydration and help restore barrier function; keratolytics, used after the newborn period, assist in scale shedding.** Bathing is performed with water-dispersible bath oil, and soaps that are excessively drying or irritating should be avoided. Collodion babies should be placed in a high-humidity incubator to increase hydration. Emollients that preserve moisturization, such as Aquaphor ointment (Beiersdorf, Inc., Wilton, CT), should be applied several times daily.

Infants with severe skin involvement from ichthyosis may require protective isolation if they receive care in an intensive care nursery because of the higher risk of contact with nosocomial infections. Incubators provide a barrier to infection. Sterile linen, sterile gloves, and other measures are needed if large areas of denuded skin are present. Nutrition management is essential due to the infant's high metabolic demands from inflammation, evaporative calorie losses, and cutaneous hyperplasia.

Multidisciplinary involvement of genetics, ophthalmology, dermatology, and physical therapy is essential to care. Comfort is another key nursing concern in the care of an infant who is significantly affected by ichthyosis. Fussy, irritable agitation may be seen and is related to pruritus or inflammation. Some form of analgesia may help, although the topical therapies prescribed have the most direct effect. Some authors describe the use of diphenhydramine (Benadryl) if severe pruritus exists. However, this would be hard to determine in a neonate who lacks verbal or fine motor skills to communicate this symptom. A trial of this medication with careful observation might be helpful for a frantic or irritable infant when other measures (e.g., topical treatment, pacifiers, feeding) are unsuccessful.

Working with the parents of an infant with ichthyosis has many facets. The appearance of the infant, especially if he or she is severely affected, could be shocking and traumatic to the parents and could require careful interventions. As with parents of infants with other congenital abnormalities, a period of shock, denial, and grief occurs over the loss of a perfect baby. In addition, the genetic nature of this disorder and the implications for future children must be comprehended. Parents of these infants need genetic counseling, support, and education as they come to terms with this disease.

**Eczema.** Atopic eczema (AE) or atopic dermatitis (AD) is a skin disorder that causes several degrees of skin irritation. It has multiple causes but is rarely seen in the newborn period. It is more commonly seen within 3 months of age and involves an eruption that proceeds to the development of microvesicles and oozing, which later turns into the scaling of the epidermis (Blume-Peytavi & Wahn, 2011). Scaling is due to the body's attempt to regenerate the skin layer rapidly. Lichenification, or skin thickening, occurs in adult skin with eczema and is not seen in infants.

Epidermal barrier dysfunction is a contributing factor in AD. Studies have shown that maternal AD (and, to a lesser extent, paternal and sibling history) was a risk factor for the development of AD in infants (Deckers et al., 2012). Prevalence of food allergy has been reported to be between 20% and 80% in infants who develop AD (Newland et al., 2013).

Several pilot studies focused on improving skin barrier function early in life through the daily application of topical emollients suggested that AD might be preventable, along with food allergies and asthma (Horimukai et al., 2014; Simpson et al., 2014). However, two subsequent larger trials did not confirm this finding (Chalmers et al., 2020; Skjerven et al., 2020). A Cochrane systematic review concluded that the routine use of skin moisturizers during the first year of life probably does not prevent AD and may lead to increases in food allergies and skin infections, although these conclusions are not strongly made (Kelleher et al., 2022).

**Management.** Bathing infants with AD should be carried out in lukewarm water with a synthetic surfactant-based cleanser with a pH of 5.5 to 6.0; irritating or drying soaps should be avoided (Telofski et al., 2012). This is followed by applying an emollient to all skin surfaces, which is the cornerstone of treatment for AD (Chu et al., 2024). The effectiveness of any emollient increases if it is applied directly after bathing to seal in the humidity (Fernandes et al., 2011). If large areas of skin are involved, thermoregulation may be a concern, especially in dry climates. Humidification may be desirable in some climates, especially during the summer months. Air conditioning may also be necessary during the summer months. Discomfort is a significant concern because infants with eczema may experience considerable pruritus. Topical therapy is generally the first consideration, followed by the judicious use of diphenhydramine in severe cases.

## SKIN CARE PRACTICES

The most basic aspects of skin care for newborns include bathing, moisturizing with emollients, skin preparation with disinfectant solutions, use of medical adhesives for life-support devices, monitoring of vital signs, and oxygenation if the newborns are hospitalized. During all these practices, the newborn's skin has the potential for trauma or alterations in normal barrier function and pH. The literature is reviewed to determine what is currently known about these and other common nursing practices and their impact on the skin of newborns.

### Bathing

#### First Bath

The purpose of bathing newborns includes providing overall hygiene, aesthetics, and protection of healthcare workers by removing blood and body fluids. However, bathing is not an innocuous procedure, and during the immediate postbirth period, it can result in hypothermia, increased oxygen consumption, and respiratory distress. There is ongoing debate about when the first bath should be given and even whether to bathe the newborn at all (Colwell, 2015). The Neonatal Skin Care Evidence-Based Clinical Practice Guideline, developed by the AWHONN, recommends giving the first bath when thermal and cardiorespiratory stability has been achieved, between 6 and 24 hours of age (AWHONN, 2018). The WHO recommends delaying the bath for 24 hours, or, if this is not possible due to cultural reasons, waiting at least 6 hours to prevent hypothermia, especially in developing countries (WHO, 2015). However, infants born to a mother who is HIV positive should be bathed as soon as possible after delivery once their temperatures have stabilized (Kilpatrick et al., 2017).

Techniques for giving the first bath include sponge bathing with a small tub, such as those provided in the hospital, or an immersion bath in a larger tub. Immersion bathing places the infant's entire body, except the head and neck, into warm water 100°F to 101.8°F (37.8°C–38.8°C), deep enough to cover the shoulders. Studies involving over 1,000 newborns report that tub or immersion bathing, compared to sponge bathing, maintains temperature better, causes less crying and distress for the infant, and does not result in increased infection, even with the umbilical cord in place (Anderson et al., 1995; Bryanton et al., 2004; Cole et al., 1999; Hennigsson et al., 1981). In a study of 100 late preterm infants (35–36 6/7 weeks' gestation) randomized to immersion tub bathing or sponge bathing after 24 hours of life, infants had overall higher temperatures and less variability in body temperature when immersion bathed (Loring et al., 2012).

Using a swaddle cloth during bathing adds additional comfort for the newborn. A randomized controlled trial (RCT) of providing this support for full-term newborns during their first bath found that swaddled bathing was more effective in maintaining temperature and other physiologic parameters such as heart rate and oxygen saturation (Çaka & Gözen, 2017). A systematic review and meta-analysis of different bathing methods confirms the benefits of swaddle bathing for newborns (Sun et al., 2023).

The Neonatal Skin Care Guideline recommends using warm tap water with or without a mild cleansing bar or liquid cleanser that has a neutral or slightly acidic pH to assist in the removal of blood and meconium, because water alone may not easily remove some lipid-soluble substances such as meconium. An RCT using a mild cleanser or water only for the first bath showed no difference in skin pH, hydration, or barrier function with either method (Lund et al., 2019).

For premature infants less than 32 weeks, warm water only during the first week of life is the recommendation (AWHONN, 2018),

Leaving residual vernix caseosa on the skin is important, because vernix facilitates skin adaptation, including skin hydration and the formation of the acid mantle of the skin surface (Visscher et al., 2005). WHO guidelines for newborn care recommend leaving vernix intact for at least 6 hours (Visscher & Narendran, 2014; Visscher et al., 2020; WHO, 2015).

#### Routine Bathing in NICU Patients

There are many issues in determining the optimal frequency of bathing and the best techniques for administering the bath in hospitalized neonates. The NICU population can range from full-term infants with illness, infection, or the need for surgical interventions to ELBW premature infants.

Knowledge about the effect of bathing on neonatal skin barrier function as measured by parameters such as skin surface pH, TEWL, and hydration of the SCH is important to inform practice. Bathing can alter the development of the skin's acid mantle. On the first day of life, the skin surface pH is greater than 6.0, falling to less than 5.0 during the first weeks of life (Behrendt & Green, 1971; Hoeger & Enzmann, 2002; Yosipovitch et al., 2000). Premature infants' skin develops an acidic surface, reaching a pH of 5.5 at the end of the first week and 5.0 by the end of the first month (Fox et al., 1998). Once the acid mantle of the skin surface is established, bathing can transiently alter the skin pH, even with water alone, in older infants (Gfatter et al., 1997). Bathing two to three times per week with cleansing products compared to water alone has been shown to have little or no difference in skin pH, TEWL, and SCH in the neonatal period in full-term healthy infants (Dizon et al., 2010; Garcia Bartels et al., 2010; Lavender et al., 2012). Similar studies measuring skin parameters have not been performed in hospitalized neonates or premature infants.

Sponge and tub bathing in premature infants can negatively affect physiologic parameters such as heart rate, oxygenation, and behavioral cues indicating distress with bathing (Liaw et al., 2006; Peters, 1998). Because of the concern about the stress on premature infants during bathing, researchers evaluated the effect of bathing with a mild cleanser every 2 versus 4 days on normal skin colonization and pathogenic bacteria (Quinn et al., 2005). Although an initial decrease in bacterial skin colonization was noted, bacterial colonization was restored at 48 hours and remained stable between 48 and 96 hours after bathing. Another study reported a transient decrease in skin colonization in premature infants of 28 to 35 weeks' gestation with coagulase-negative staphylococcus at 30 minutes following the bath, regardless of whether the bath was given with water alone or water and liquid soap (da Cunha & Procianoy, 2005). It does not appear that decreased bathing frequency from every 2 days to 4 days in premature infants leads to an increase in skin colonization, and the use of bathing products or water also does not increase skin colonization with coagulase-negative staphylococcus. Therefore, less frequent bathing will subject premature infants to less physiologic and behavioral stress. Swaddling the premature infant during routine bathing reduced temperature loss and crying (Edraki et al., 2014). Hand containment and postural support reduces stress as well (Liaw et al., 2010).

## Emollients

The skin surface of term newborns is drier than that of adults but becomes gradually better hydrated as the eccrine sweat glands mature during the first year of life. Maintaining the hydration of the stratum corneum is necessary for an intact skin surface and normal barrier function. Skin that is dry, scaly, or cracking is uncomfortable and can be a portal of entry for microorganisms.

Treatment for dry skin includes moisturizers or emollients. Emollients are oil-in-water (ointments) or water-in-oil emulsions (creams, lotions). Ointments do not require a preservative, whereas creams and lotions require preservatives due to the higher water content (Hoath & Narendran, 2000).

Several studies have evaluated emollient use in premature infants. Premature infants of 29 to 36 weeks' gestation were treated with a cream moisturizer twice daily and had less visible dermatitis but no change in skin barrier function (Lane & Drost, 1993). An RCT of younger gestation premature infants receiving twice-daily applications of a petrolatum ointment versus routine skin care reported improved skin barrier function, measured as a lower TEWL and less visible dermatitis. No increases in skin temperature or redness were seen if the infants received phototherapy or were cared for under radiant warmers, and no increase in bacterial or fungal cultures was reported. In addition, although there were not enough subjects to verify this outcome, the treated infants had fewer positive blood or cerebrospinal fluid cultures (Nopper et al., 1996).

A large RCT of 1,191 ELBW infants (510–1,000 g) was undertaken to determine if the twice-daily prophylactic application of petrolatum-based ointment would reduce the combined outcomes of mortality and sepsis (Edwards et al., 2004). No effect was seen in these combined outcomes, although skin integrity appeared to improve in the treated infants. It is important to note that in infants less than 750 g, the incidence of bloodstream infections with coagulase-negative staphylococcus was increased in the group with prophylactic use of the emollient. However, the mechanism and relationship to twice-daily emollient use are unclear. The control infants in this study also received emollients on an "as-needed" basis for skin dryness.

A Cochrane review evaluated RCTs of emollient use in the NICU. It concluded that the prophylactic application of topical ointment increases the risk of coagulase-negative staphylococcus infection and other nosocomial infections. The routine use of emollients in preterm infants is not recommended (Conner et al., 2004).

The benefits of emollient use in premature infants must be carefully weighed against the risk of infection. In general, emollients can be safely used in this population to treat skin with excessive drying, skin cracking, and fissures. They may also be beneficial in reducing TEWL and evaporative heat loss, although methods such as using a high-humidity environment are also available for this purpose. Small tubes or jars for single-patient use are recommended to prevent contamination with microorganisms.

There is little consensus to date about the routine use of emollients for full-term newborns (Irvin & Miller, 2015). One study reports improved skin parameters in healthy full-term infants when the skin care regime included a "baby cream" emollient after bathing and did not adversely affect bacterial skin colonization (Garcia Bartels et al., 2010).

## Skin Disinfectants

Using skin disinfectants before invasive procedures such as inserting IV lines, venipuncture, arterial puncture, umbilical catheter placement, and chest tube placement is common practice in neonatal nurseries. Concerns with disinfection practices include the effects of absorption of disinfectants and skin injury resulting from topical skin preparation with these agents, which must be weighed against their effectiveness in preventing infection.

Disinfectants that are used in newborns include 70% isopropyl alcohol (IA), 10% povidone-iodine (PI), and chlorhexidine gluconate (CHG), in varying concentrations as both an aqueous solution and one combined with 70% isopropyl alcohol (CHG/IA). It is widely accepted that CHG-containing formulations are the most effective for skin disinfection in children and adults for central venous catheter insertion and dressing changes, and their use is recommended as best practice in several guidelines (Chaiyakunapruk et al., 2002; Loveday et al., 2014; Marschall et al., 2014). However, there are no studies in neonates that have confirmed the superior efficacy of CHG preparations over other disinfectants, such as PI, in the prevention of bloodstream infection (Ponnusamy et al., 2014; Sathiyamurthy et al., 2016). Therefore, the Centers for Disease Control and Prevention (CDC) guidelines have maintained that there is insufficient evidence to make a recommendation about the safety or efficacy of CHG products in infants younger than 2 months of age (O'Grady et al., 2011).

The use of 0.5% CHG in IA reduces peripheral IV catheter colonization in premature and term newborns compared with using PI (Garland et al., 1995). An RCT of 344 infants admitted to the NICU and SCN settings showed significantly fewer blood-culture contaminants in infants having skin disinfection with 1% aqueous CHG compared with those using 10% PI (Nuntnarumit & Sangsuksawang, 2013).

A sequential study reported that the rate of positive blood cultures (the number of true infections or contaminated cultures when 10% PI was used in this NICU) was not statistically different from a subsequent period when 0.5% CHG/IA was used (Linder et al., 1997). A pilot trial of 47 infants who weighed more than 1,500 g and were older than 7 days of age evaluated cutaneous tolerance of 2% CHG/IA compared with 10% PI for peripherally inserted central catheter (PICC) placement. The two groups had no differences in the number of bloodstream infections or sepsis evaluations; however, this pilot study was not powered to look at bloodstream infection rates (Garland et al., 2009). An RCT of 304 preterm infants compared 2% CHG/IA to 10% PI for insertion of 815 central venous catheters and reported no difference between the proportion of catheter-related bloodstream infections between the two disinfectants, although more infants in the PI group had thyroid dysfunction. The authors acknowledged that the study was not adequately powered to detect differences in actual numbers of catheter-related bloodstream infections and that a larger study is needed (Kieran et al., 2018). A feasibility study comparing aqueous 2% CHG to 2% CHG in 70% IA found similarly low rates of catheter colonization in both groups (Clarke et al., 2024).

**Toxicity From Skin Disinfectants.** If absorbed through the skin, PI has been shown to alter thyroid function in premature newborns. A systematic review of 15 articles reported evidence of thyroid dysfunction in premature infants exposed to iodine-containing disinfectants, with incidence ranging from 12 to 33 cases per 100 infants. The review also found no long-term neurodevelopmental studies that cited harm from exposure to iodine-containing solutions; although the researchers recommended restricting iodine-containing solutions in premature infants, more research is needed (Aitken & Williams, 2014).

Systemic toxicity from percutaneous absorption of CHG in neonates has been raised as a concern. A small study of CHG antisepsis for PICC placement and subsequent dressing changes in premature infants who weighed more than 1,500 g found measurable concentrations of CHG, ranging from 13 to 100 mcg/ml, in 7 of the 10 infants who had levels drawn. However, there were no reported systemic side effects. The role of IA in combination with CHG may be a possible contributing factor to cutaneous absorption of CHG (Garland et al., 2009). Another study involving 20 premature infants with a median gestational age of 28 weeks had an extremity disinfected with 2% aqueous CHG prior to insertion of a PICC. Ten infants had detectable serum CHG levels ranging from 1.6 to 206 mcg/ml, with the highest levels occurring 2 to 3 days after initial exposure (Chapman et al., 2013).

Past reports of neurotoxicity from exposure to hexachlorophene bathing (Anderson et al., 1981; CDC, 1973) have prompted research on the potential neurotoxicity from systemic absorption of CHG. An in vitro model of neurite cells was exposed to CHG levels comparable to the highest levels reported in premature infants. CHG inhibited L1-mediated neurite growth, and researchers concluded that it is important to determine whether the blood–brain barrier is permeable to CHG in premature infants (Milestone et al., 2014).

There is interest in using CHG to decrease infection in adult and pediatric ICU patients and patients with central venous catheters with daily wiping of skin surfaces with CHG (Milstone et al., 2013). A study was undertaken in a NICU population using 2% CHG–CHG-impregnated wipes in a quasiexperimental design, comparing the treated infants to a historical cohort. The algorithm for wiping the skin with CHG determined the frequency based on postnatal age and weight. A decrease in central line–associated bloodstream infections was reported; however, infants weighing less than 1,000 g and younger than 28 days were excluded from CHG bathing. Serum CHG levels were not obtained (Quach et al., 2014). In a study of NICU patients with CVCs receiving CHG bathing twice weekly, skin bacterial burden was reduced but returned to baseline after 72 hours, and the authors acknowledge that this frequency may be inadequate to suppress skin bacterial growth (Johnson et al., 2019).

Several case reports document chemical burns in premature infants from disinfectants containing CHG; these include various concentrations of CHG, both aqueous and alcohol preparations (Andersen et al., 2005; Bringué Espuny et al., 2010; Kutsch & Ottinger, 2014; Lashkari et al., 2012; Mannan et al., 2007; Neri et al., 2017; Reynolds et al., 2005). There have also been reports of chemical burns from IA and PI solutions in ELBW infants (Figure 12.7) (Sardesai et al., 2011).

The UK Medicines and Healthcare Products Regulatory Agency published a review of 44 case reports of chemical burns after the application of aqueous or alcohol-based CHG solutions. Most burns occurred in premature infants younger than 26 weeks' gestation or those who weighed less than 1,000 g, with long-term sequelae in some infants, including scarring, discoloration, and keloid formation (Beresford, 2015). Because of these concerns, safety labeling in the United

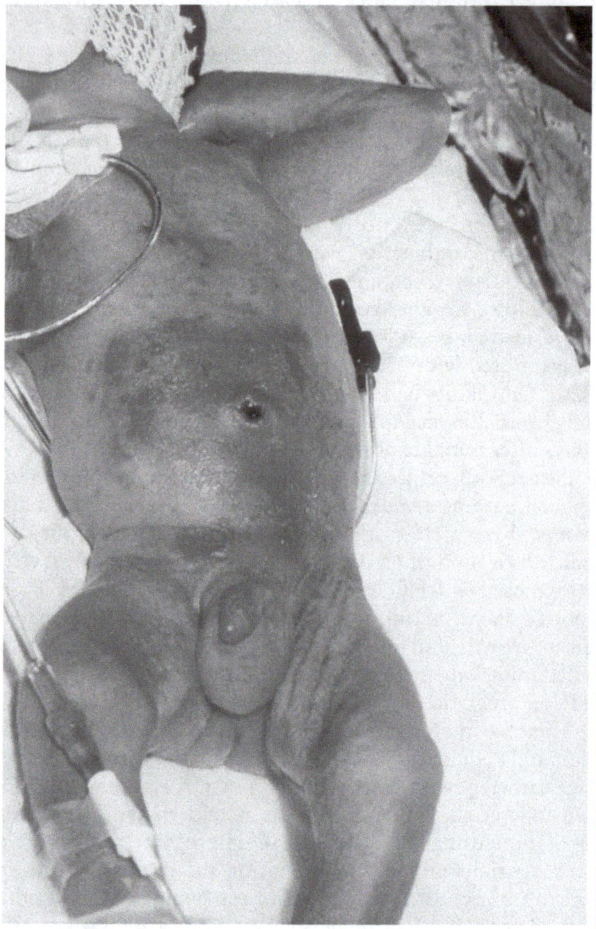

**FIGURE 12.7 Skin injury resulting from skin disinfectant.**

States and Europe continues to state the potential for chemical burns from CHG solutions used for skin disinfection in premature infants (Paternoster et al., 2017).

Several studies have been undertaken to determine how CHG affects skin integrity. A prospective study of 40 infants with a mean gestational age of 32 weeks (range 23–39 weeks) found that the use of 2% CHG/IA for PICC insertion and weekly dressing changes compromised skin-barrier function, which was measured by elevated TEWL, an increase in erythema, and dryness (Visscher, deCastro, et al., 2009). A pilot trial comparing 2% CHG/IA in 47 premature infants weighing more than 1,500 g and older than 7 days of age found no increase in skin redness or breakdown when CHG was used for PICC insertion and weekly dressing changes and only one incidence of erythema in a newborn treated with PI (Garland et al., 2009) (Figure 12.8).

The selection of appropriate disinfectants in neonates remains a dilemma, particularly for extremely premature infants during the first weeks of life. CHG products in the United States are limited to a 2% aqueous surgical scrub solution available only in 4-oz bottles and a 2% and 3.15% chlorhexidine solution in 70% IA available in single-use packaging. The U.S. Food and Drug Administration (FDA) states that chlorhexidine-containing disinfectants should be used with care in premature infants or infants less than 2 months of age because these may cause skin irritation and chemical burns. PI continues to be used in many nurseries to avoid previous complications, although the issues of thyroid toxicity remain a concern.

Although removal of disinfectants with sterile water or saline after the procedure is complete is advocated (AWHONN, 2018), the manufacturer of the 2% CHG/IA product advises that removal not be attempted because the residual effect of the disinfectant on the skin may be beneficial. However, it is not known whether this feature may contribute to skin irritancy and absorption of CHG in newborns and premature infants.

CHG should not be used as preoperative skin disinfection on the face or head because misuse has been reported to result in injury if it remains in contact with the eye or ear during surgical procedures. However, careful use before scalp intravenous or central-line insertion is acceptable, so splashing or using excessive chlorhexidine is avoided. In addition, there is no clinical data to discourage the use of chlorhexidine gluconate products prior to lumbar puncture or epidural catheter placement because this is considered skin antisepsis (Milstone et al., 2008).

## Umbilical Cord Care

Using antibiotic ointments and skin antiseptics on the umbilical cord can prolong the time to cord separation and has no beneficial effect on the frequency of infection (Zupan & Garner, 2000). Although the umbilicus is a possible route for infection by invasive pathogenic microorganisms until healed, the evidence suggests that dry cord care, defined as keeping the cord clean and leaving it exposed to air or loosely covered by a clean cloth, is effective for infants born in high-resource countries (Stewart et al., 2016).

Dry cord care is recommended for newborns born in health facilities because several studies support this practice. A cluster RCT in France involving over 8,000 near-term and term newborns found that dry cord care was not inferior to antiseptic cord care in preventing omphalitis (Gras-Le Guen et al., 2017). A group of 150 consecutively born, healthy, late preterm, and term infants born in a hospital setting in Taiwan (high-humidity, subtropical country) was randomized to alcohol or dry cord care. Cord separation time was significantly decreased for infants with dry cord care compared with those cleansed with 95% IA and the incidence of cord infection was not increased (Hsu et al., 2010). A meta-analysis showed that topical IA was not superior to dry cord care in reducing the incidence of omphalitis (Imdad et al., 2013).

## Medical Adhesives

Hospitalized full-term and premature newborns require the routine use of adhesives to secure life support and monitoring equipment such as endotracheal tubes, IV devices, oxygen saturation sensors, and electrodes. The types of medical adhesives used in the NICU are categorized as acrylates, hydrocolloids, hydrogels, and silicone-based adhesives (Lund, 2014).

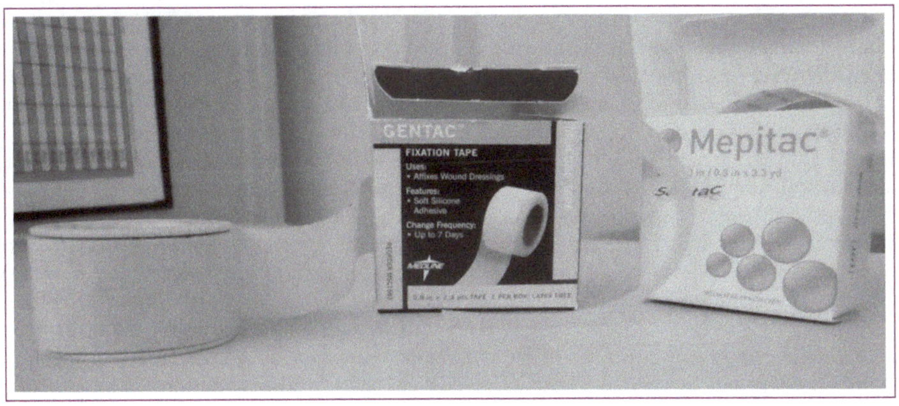


**FIGURE 12.8 Silicone-based adhesives developed for use in wound care products are now available as silicone tapes and have been shown to improve adherence to wounds and reduce discomfort when removed.**

Acrylate-based adhesives include paper, plastic, and soft cloth tape. These adhesives have increased adherence over time and may leave a residue on the skin after removal (McNichol et al., 2013). However, acrylate adhesives adhere effectively to skin and medical devices and are commonly used in intensive care settings. Polyurethane films with acrylate adhesives, such as transparent adhesive dressings, allow visualization of catheter insertion sites and are permeable to water vapor, oxygen, and carbon dioxide, allowing the skin to breathe (Darmstadt & Dinulos, 2000).

Hydrocolloid adhesives were initially used to protect peristomal skin for ostomy patients and later became a wound dressing. They are sometimes used as a platform between skin and tape and are sometimes integrated into products such as an endotracheal tube securement device. Initially, it was hoped to be gentler on the skin when removed, but hydrocolloids have been shown to cause skin trauma equal to acrylate tape when removed at 24 hours (Lund et al., 1997). Other studies have also reported decreased skin-barrier function, measured by increased TEWL and erythema, under hydrocolloids (Zillmer et al., 2006). However, these barriers are still used because they absorb moisture, mold well to skin surfaces, and, as noted previously, serve as a platform between skin and acrylate tapes and transparent dressings (Boswell & Waker, 2016; Cheng & Kroshinsky, 2011; O'Neil & Schumacher, 2014). One study found no statistically significant quantitative difference between a transparent dressing placed over a hydrocolloid base or a transparent dressing placed directly on the skin. Despite this lack of support for one method over the other, they found a theme of comments from nurses that they preferred transparent dressings placed over a hydrocolloid base as a more effective adhesive and a belief that it was gentle for the skin (Boswell & Waker, 2016).

Hydrogels are a low-trauma and highly breathable adhesive with high water content. Hydrogels are found in some adhesive products, such as ECG electrodes and temperature probe covers; they are also available as tapes to secure tubes. Hydrogels are also available as a wound dressing and may have a cooling or analgesic effect on wounds. Hydrogel adhesives have been shown to reduce the trauma associated with electrode removal (Darmstadt & Dinulos, 2000; Lund et al., 1997; Webster & McCosker, 1994). However, they do not adhere well enough to secure critical lines and tubes and do not function well in high-humidity environments such as humidified incubators.

Silicone-based adhesive products have been shown to improve adherence to skin and reduce discomfort to patients with adhesive removal. This technology holds promise for developing products that adhere and cause minimal trauma, such as erythema, skin stripping, and keratin loss, compared with acrylate-based paper tapes when removed from the skin of pediatric patients (Grove et al., 2014). Although the first generation of silicone adhesives did not adhere well to plastic devices, newer products are more adherent and have been integrated into securement devices for nasogastric tubes and cannulas (Turnbull et al., 2024). A beneficial use of silicone adhesives is as a border for dressings, which can be lifted and replaced for wound assessment. Another application for silicone adhesives is securing brain-monitoring electrodes, which adhere well to hair and can be removed with minimal discomfort.

Newborns are at high risk for medical adhesive-related skin injury (MARSI), a term first used in a consensus paper involving a number of different health providers representing several specialties, including pediatrics, gerontology, orthopedics, and dermatology and wound care experts (McNichol et al., 2013). Types of MARSI include skin stripping, skin tears, contact, and allergic dermatitis. MARSI consensus was updated in 2024 (Barton et al., 2024).

Newborns are particularly vulnerable to MARSI; the evidence-based practice project for the Neonatal Skin Care Guideline, which included skin and environment assessments for 2,820 premature and full-term newborns, found that adhesives were the primary cause of skin breakdown (Lund et al., 2001). It is known that functional changes in adult skin, including altered skin barrier function (measured as increases in TEWL), are seen after 10 consecutive applications and removals of adhesive tape (Lo et al., 1990), and after one application/removal in premature infants (Harpin & Rutter, 1983; Lund et al., 1997).

Liquid skin-barrier films are skin protectants wiped on the skin before attaching adhesives and have been shown to protect the skin from adhesives, fecal and ostomy output, and urine (Black, 2007). Silicone-based skin barrier films do not sting when applied, rapidly evaporate, and do not leave a residue, which is another benefit of silicone-based skin protectants in neonates (Irving, 2001). A study of premature infants (< 33 weeks) showed both skin protection and the additional benefit of reduced TEWL (Brandon et al., 2010).Although this study found efficacy without any safety concerns, further research is warranted in a larger ELBW population.

Removal of medical adhesives can cause trauma, such as skin stripping and pain. **Quality and Safety: A technique involving slowly pulling adhesives at a very low angle, parallel to the skin surface, while holding the surrounding skin in place may reduce epidermal stripping (Barton et al., 2024; Lund & Tucker, 2003; McNichol et al., 2013).** Adhesive removers help to aid in the atraumatic removal of adhesives. There are three categories of adhesive removers: alcohol–organic-based solvents, oil-based solvents, and silicone-based removers (Black, 2007; Cooper, 2010). Solvents contain hydrocarbon derivatives, petrolatum distillates, or IA and carry the potential for systemic and topical toxicities. A case report of a premature infant developing a severe dermatologic reaction to an adhesive remover, including blistering and hemorrhage, suggests the lack of safety with these products in a NICU (Ittmann & Bozynski, 1993). Oil-based solvents release the bond between skin and adhesive and are based on paraffin or citrus oil extracts. These do not evaporate and leave a residue that prevents adherence during the reapplication of adhesives to the site where they were previously applied.

Silicone-based removers form an interposing layer between adhesive and skin, allowing easier removal. These evaporate readily after application without drying the skin and are less likely to leave a residue. They do not cause stinging, even on broken skin. Also, they are inert, reducing the risk of toxicity. Silicone-based removers are available in spray, liquid, lotion, or wipe formulations (Cooper, 2010). Researchers have demonstrated the safety and effectiveness of silicone-based removers in the neonatal population, including infants with EB (Cooper et al., 2011; Denyer, 2011).

## Transepidermal Water Loss

Because of the poorly keratinized stratum corneum that provides minimal resistance to the diffusion of water, the preterm infant is at risk for TEWL through the skin and heat loss via evaporation. Characteristic skin factors predisposing premature infants to excessive water loss include reduced skin barrier function from fewer layers of stratum corneum and thinner epidermis, larger surface area concerning body weight, increased water content, increased permeability, and increased blood supply closer to the skin surface. Mature keratin, a major component of the tough, nonliving outer layer of the epidermis, is relatively impermeable to water. Because keratin formation is directly related to gestational age, a premature infant less than 30 weeks' gestation is at increased risk for increased TEWL and evaporative heat loss.

Premature infants of 23 to 25 weeks' gestation have TEWL 10 times higher than full-term newborns (Agren et al., 1998; Visscher et al., 2015). Mature barrier function—at one time thought to advance rapidly over a 2-week period in premature infants less than 30 weeks' gestation—has been shown to take longer in extremely premature infants of 23 to 24 weeks' gestation and occurs when the infant reaches approximately 30 to 31 weeks postconceptional age (Kalia et al., 1998).

In the delivery room, premature infants less than 28 weeks' gestation are placed in a polyethylene bag or wrap without drying the skin to reduce the degree of evaporative heat loss and hypothermia/cold stress during initial stabilization (Bissinger & Annibale, 2010; Knobel et al. 2005; Vohra et al. 2004). This technique is so effective that studies have reported hyperthermia in some infants; thus, careful temperature monitoring is needed.

High humidity, a relative humidity (RH) greater than 70%, added to an incubator has been shown to reduce evaporative heat loss and TEWL effectively; the rate of TEWL has been shown to decrease by half when the RH increases from 20% to 60% (Hammarlund & Sedin, 1979; Harpin & Rutter, 1983). The use of humidified "hybrid" incubators in premature infants less than 1,000 g are capable of providing high humidity in a convectively heated incubator and also radiant heat for procedures and emergencies. A study reported positive effects on fluid balance, electrolyte stability, and growth velocity after the hybrid humidity devices were implemented, compared to a historical control group. This study utilized high humidity levels (70%–80%) for the first week, with reduced humidity levels to 50% to 60% for the second week until the infant reached 30 to 32 weeks postconceptional age (Kim et al., 2010). In this fashion, the rationale for reducing the humidity level was based on an earlier RCT that demonstrated improved skin barrier function and maturity when humidity levels were reduced to 50% compared to 75% in the second week of life (Agren et al., 2006). Despite the widespread use of high humidity for very preterm infants in the first week of life, several recent reviews acknowledge the substantial variability among NICUs about which level of added humidity is optimal and recommend further research be done in this area (Glass & Valdez, 2021; Rizk et al., 2022).

The application of petrolatum-based emollients every 6 to 12 hours also reduces TEWL and can be used on infants on radiant warmers or under phototherapy without temperature increases or burns (Nopper et al., 1996). A novel use of a protective barrier film was also shown to reduce TEWL compared to petrolatum ointment in premature infants less than 33 weeks' gestation (Brandon et al., 2010). However, due to the concerns raised in a large RCT of infants less than 1,000 g regarding increased coagulase-negative staphylococcus infections with prophylactic use of this petrolatum ointment. These approaches are not recommended without further study.

Because of the numerous benefits of skin-to-skin holding (kangaroo care), a study was undertaken to measure evaporative loss while out of the high humidity environment. Five premature infants of 22 to 26 weeks' gestation were held skin to skin by their mothers at 3 to 9 days of age; covering with a single layer of cotton fabric resulted in decreased evaporative heat loss (Kjällström et al., 2011).

Thus, addressing the vital area of reducing excessive heat loss and TEWL is necessary in caring for extremely premature neonates to maintain adequate hydration without excessive fluid intake. The goal of maintaining hydration and normal serum sodium levels on an intake of less than 150 ml/kg/d is optimal and achievable using preventive strategies.

## MANAGEMENT OF SKIN CARE PROBLEMS

The stratum corneum can be traumatized by a variety of insults, including epidermal stripping from the removal of adhesives; chemical burns from disinfectants; pressure injuries, especially from medical devices; infection; nutritional inadequacies, such as zinc and EFA deficiency; extravasation of IV fluids; and diaper dermatitis. The goal of all skin care for neonates should be the maintenance of skin integrity; however, even with meticulous care, skin breakdown can occur.

### Skin Assessment

A thorough daily examination of all skin surfaces will reveal the state of skin integrity in critically ill or extremely premature infants in the NICU. Early signs of skin abrasions or small excoriations may call for either diagnostic or treatment procedures. A skin assessment tool such as the Neonatal Skin Condition Score (NSCS) (Box 12.1 and Figure 12.9), used in the AWHONN/National Association of Neonatal Nurses (NANN) research-based practice project, may be beneficial when assessing skin conditions (Lund et al., 2001). The NSCS was found to have both interrater and intrarater reliability, and validity was confirmed by the relationship of the skin scores with birth weight, number of observations over time, and prevalence of infection (Lund & Osborne, 2004). Identifying risk factors for skin injury in individual patients may include gestational age less than 32 weeks, use of paralytic medications and vasopressors, multiple tubes and lines, numerous monitors and probes, surgical wounds, ostomies, and technologies that limit patient movements such as high-frequency ventilation and extracorporeal membrane oxygenation.

Other scoring tools such as the Braden Q and Starkid Scale that assess risk for pressure injuries have been suggested (Curley et al., 2003; Suddaby et al., 2005). However, in these studies, the number of neonates is not indicated; patients from ages 0 to 12 months are evaluated as a single group, and

**BOX 12.1**

**NEONATAL SKIN CONDITION SCORE**

**Dryness**

1 = Normal, no sign of dry skin

2 = Dry skin, visible scaling

3 = Very dry skin, cracking/fissures

**Erythema**

1 = No evidence of erythema

2 = Visible erythema over < 50% of the body's surface

3 = Visible erythema on > 50% of the body's surface

**Breakdown/Excoriation**

1 = None evident

2 = Small localized areas

3 = Extensive

*Note:* Perfect score = 3; worst score = 9.

*Source:* Adapted from Lund, C. H., Osborne, J. W., Kuller, J., Lane, A. T., Lott, J. W., & Raines, D. A. (2001). Neonatal skin care: Clinical outcomes of the AWHONN/NANN evidence-based clinical practice guideline. Association of Women's Health, Obstetric and Neonatal Nurses and the National Association of Neonatal Nurses. *Journal of Obstetrics, Gynecology, and Neonatal Nursing, 30*(1), 41–51. https://doi.org/10.1111/j.1552-6909.2001.tb01520.x. Copyright © 2001, AWHONN.

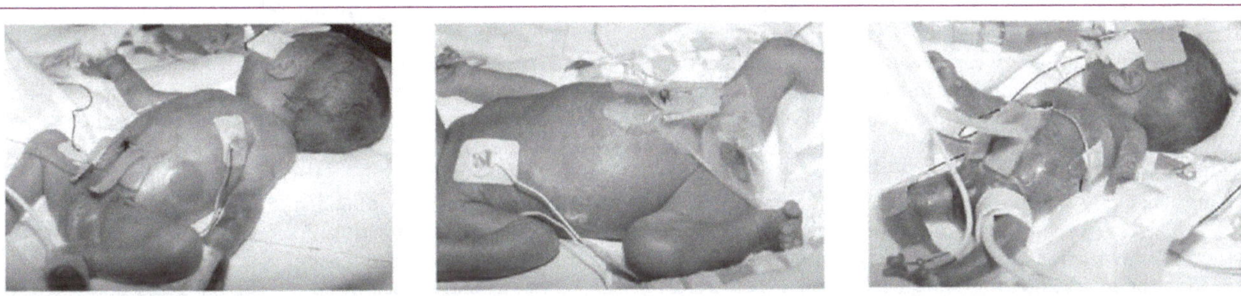

Dryness: 1 = normal, no sign of dry skin
Erythema: 2 = visible erythema < 50% body surface
Breakdown: 3 = extensive

Dryness: 2 = dry skin, visible scaling
Erythema: 1 = no evidence of erythema
Breakdown: 1 = none evident

Dryness: 2 = dry skin, visible scaling
Erythema: 3 = visible erythema > 50% body surface
Breakdown: 3 = extensive

**FIGURE 12.9** Examples of skin assessments in three infants using the Neonatal Skin Condition Score (NSCS).

no premature infants were included, so the applicability of these tools to a NICU population has not been demonstrated.

The Braden QD was developed to predict hospital-acquired pressure injuries (HAPI) in pediatric patients, including those caused by both immobility and medical devices. Their study involved 625 patients, 17% of whom were less than 1 month of age. The overall HAPI rate was lower than expected, with 86 HAPI found in 49 patients; 75% were device related (Curley et al., 2018).

The Braden QD evaluates the intensity and duration of pressure regarding the patient's mobility and sensory perception. It also evaluates skin tolerance regarding friction, shear, nutrition, tissue perfusion, and oxygenation. In addition, the number of medical devices and the ability to reposition devices and sensors is quantified. However, there is no scoring for prematurity or gestational age, both important aspects of skin tolerance in NICU patients, so the helpfulness of the use of the Braden QD in NICU patients remains questionable. It is also essential to recognize that risk assessment is not the same as skin assessment, and careful observation and documentation of the skin condition are essential components of skin care in NICU patients. A skin risk assessment and management tool developed in Australia called the SRAMT combines assessing risk, including scoring for gestational age and offering management strategies (Broom et al., 2017). This may be a better tool that deserves further study.

## Skin Injuries

Although little clinical research is available to guide the selection of topical agents and products to treat skin injuries in neonates, several principles help inform practitioners. These include moist wound healing, gentle cleansing, and understanding the proper application of appropriate dressings (Cousins, 2014; Fox, 2011). In addition, although the injury may be due to mechanical trauma, the role of microorganisms can further complicate the management of skin injury, especially in very low birth weight (VLBW) premature infants. In these cases, a skin culture may be helpful.

If the culture is positive for a candidiasis species, antifungal ointment and systemic treatment with fluconazole or amphotericin may prevent devastating, disseminated disease (Benjamin et al., 2010; Darmstadt et al., 2000). Although fungal causes are sometimes suspected, other microorganisms such as *S. aureus* species, *Escherichia coli*, and other gram-negative bacteria have also been cultured in extremely premature infants. The knowledge of their skin colonization may be useful in guiding systemic treatment should their clinical condition worsen, suggesting systemic disease, including sepsis.

Ointments are sometimes used on skin injuries because of their antibacterial or antifungal properties and because covering the wound with a semiocclusive layer promotes healing by facilitating the migration of epithelial cells across the surface. Petrolatum-based emollients and ointments cover wounds and provide a semiocclusive layer that facilitates the migration of epithelial cells across the surface and may become part of the stratum corneum layer during the healing process. Antibacterial ointments such as Polysporin, Bacitracin, or Bactroban help treat gram-positive colonized surfaces and promote the growth of gram-negative organisms (Smack et al., 1996). Many dermatologists recommend against using Neosporin because of the potential for developing later sensitization to this ointment, although sensitization to Bacitracin is being reported with increasing frequency (Marks et al., 1995). If a fungal infection is suspected, nystatin ointment is used and can also be applied to surrounding intact skin to prevent extension of the infection. Ointments are generally preferable to creams in this application because of better adherence and healing properties.

Gentle cleansing of the skin injury or wound can remove debris and exudate and promote a clean wound bed. These materials and other necrotic tissue impede wound healing, and removing them reduces bacterial contamination (Cousins, 2014). Wound cleansing is best accomplished by gentle irrigation with normal saline, either diluted or undiluted, using a 20- to 60-ml syringe and a blunt IV catheter (AWHONN, 2018). Antiseptic solutions and cleansers are to be avoided because these can cause further injury to delicate healing tissue and may delay healing (Lineaweaver et al., 1985; Rolstad & Ovington, 2007; Wilson et al., 2005).

Dressings for wound care and skin injury should be occlusive and nonadherent to promote moist healing and facilitate the migration of epithelial cells. These include silicone dressings, hydrocolloid dressings, hydrogel dressings, and transparent dressings made of foam or other composite materials. In addition, some may be impregnated with silver ions, with potential benefit due to antiinfective properties (Fox, 2011). Although silver-containing creams and dressings were initially avoided due to toxicity concerns, more recent articles demonstrate safe uses of silver-containing agents in neonates (August et al., 2015; Tenenhaus et al., 2014).

Medical-grade honey, either as an ointment or in a dressing, has also been described for use in neonates and may be used to facilitate debridement (Amaya, 2015). Benefits include antiinfective properties and facilitating moist healing cascade (Alvarez-Suarez et al., 2014). Several case studies report positive results using medical-grade honey in premature infants (Boyar et al., 2014; Esser, 2017; Mohr et al., 2014).

## Intravenous Extravasations

The extravasation of IV fluids and medications can result in skin injury and, in some cases, deep-tissue injury to muscles and nerves (Figure 12.10). Neonates are at high risk for developing extravasation injuries because of their immature skin, lack of subcutaneous tissue, and the small size of their blood vessels (Amjad et al., 2011; Casanova et al., 2001). The most severe extravasation injuries are iatrogenic complications that can lead to pain, prolonged hospitalization, and increased morbidity, such as infection. Extravasation injuries can also increase hospital costs and the potential for legal action.

Nursing actions such as monitoring IV sites and other preventive strategies, as well as immediate interventions that reduce the extent of tissue injury, are important considerations for all nurseries that care for newborns with IV devices for fluid administration and medications. Some of the risk factors for tissue injury from IV extravasations in NICU patients are listed in Box 12.2.

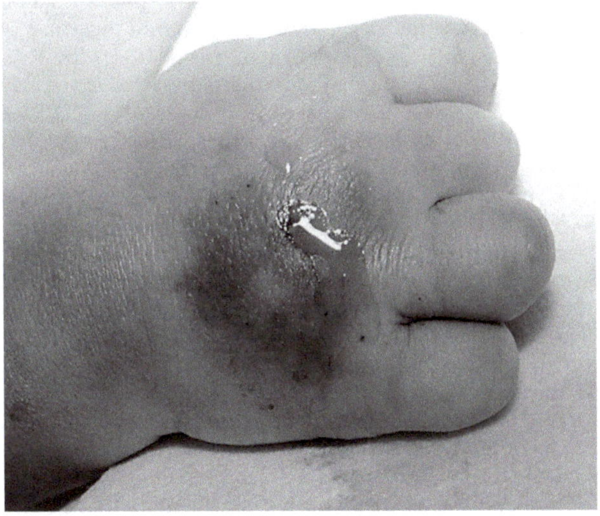

**FIGURE 12.10 Intravenous extravasation injury with swelling, discoloration, and leaking of fluid.**

**BOX 12.2**

**RISKS FOR TISSUE INJURY FROM INTRAVENOUS EXTRAVASATIONS**

Some of the factors known to increase the risk of tissue injury include:

- The length of exposure after extravasation occurs, especially when the patients are unable to verbalize the discomfort of pain or pressure
- The nature of the drug or solution; hypertonic solutions with high concentrations of calcium, potassium, glucose, or amino acids; and medications such as nafcillin have been identified as high risk for causing injury
- The mechanical compression caused by electronic infusion pumps

Hourly assessments of the insertion site, with more frequent assessments during the administration of certain medications, are recommended, as well as not relying on the infusion pump to detect infiltration of fluid into the tissue (Amjad et al., 2011; Simona, 2012; Tofani et al., 2012). Quality improvement efforts involving standardizing assessment strategies have been described and are beneficial, such as "Touch, Look, Compare" and "Assess, Compare, Touch" (Tofani et al., 2012; Wilder et al., 2014). One center included these aspects of assessment, along with the review of factors such as catheter type, securement method, and daily review of catheter necessity; these efforts resulted in a reduction in infiltration rates over a 6-month period (Watterson et al., 2018).

Prevention of skin injury after infiltration is an important consideration. Strategies include ensuring the insertion site is visible using transparent adhesive dressing or clear tape to secure the device and observing the site with appropriate documentation every hour. In addition, the tape should be carefully placed on the extremity to avoid obstructing venous return. Tape placed loosely over a bony prominence, such as the knee or elbow, permits extravasated fluids and medications to disperse over a larger surface area and thus reduce the risk of injury, compared with extravasation limited to a small surface area. Avoiding extremities with poor perfusion in favor of better-perfused scalp veins (except those on the forehead) may also be prudent; in some cases, the wiser choice may be placing central venous lines for access.

The fluid being infused is a known factor that can lead to a greater risk of extravasation. The risk relates to the fluid's chemical properties, osmolality, and pH (Gorski et al., 2017). Normal serum osmolality is 280 to 295 mOsm/kg, and solutions that exceed this are considered hypertonic. Solutions infusing through a peripheral vein in a neonate should stay within this range (Thigpen, 2007). Glucose concentrations above 12.5% risk extravasation injuries in neonates (Weinstein, 2007).

Medications can be both hyperosmolar and irritating due to pH extremes. In particular, irritating medications, and solutions, called *vesicants*, should be avoided or carefully watched during infusions. A chart showing various degrees of vesicants can be a helpful guide for neonatal patients and may also identify patients who would benefit from central venous access (Gorski et al., 2017).

Once an IV extravasation has been identified, immediate measures to reduce injury are instituted (Thigpen, 2007). The device should be carefully removed and the extremity elevated (if it is an arm or leg). Treatment with heat or moisture is not recommended because the delicate tissue could be further injured by a burn or the effects of maceration. Making multiple puncture holes over the area of greatest swelling and squeezing to allow the fluid to leak out of the tissue releases the infiltrated fluid and can potentially prevent skin injury (Chandavasu et al., 1986; Sawatzky-Dickson & Bodnaryk, 2006). Saline washout has also been described (Casanova et al., 2001; Davies et al., 1994; Kostogloudis et al., 2015), although no randomized trial has been published to compare efficacy (Gopalakrishnan et al., 2017).

Hyaluronidase is an enzyme that facilitates diffusion of the extravasated fluids by temporarily dissolving normal interstitial barriers, reducing tissue damage; also, it has been reported to reduce tissue injury following extravasation in neonates (Banta, 1992; Laurie et al., 1984; Raszka et al., 1990). A dose of 15 to 20 units is administered in five subcutaneous injections around the periphery of the extravasation (Treadwell, 2012), and this dose may be repeated. The addition of multiple punctures may also facilitate the flow of fluid from the tissues, as well as keeping the site moist for several hours using hydrogel products or moist compresses.

Topical wound care treatments are necessary if tissue damage results despite immediate care measures. In the most severe cases of deep-tissue necrosis after extravasation injury, a surgical or plastic surgery consultation may be necessary (Figure 12.11).

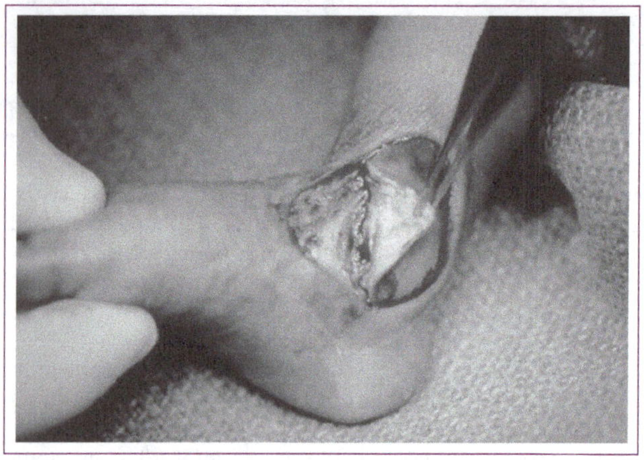

**FIGURE 12.11 This intravenous extravasation injury will require plastic surgery.**

## Diaper Dermatitis

A common skin disruption in neonates and infants is diaper dermatitis (diaper rash). This term encompasses a range of processes that affect the perineum, groin, thighs, buttocks, and anal area of infants who wear some covering to collect urine and feces. Many different mechanisms can cause diaper dermatitis, but the skin condition has a direct role in the progression of skin injury. Clinical characteristics of diaper dermatitis have been outlined in an integrative review and include age of the infant, stooling frequency, type of feeding, antibiotic exposure, previous episodes of diaper dermatitis, mode of delivery, and exposure to phototherapy (Esser & Johnson, 2020). Review articles provide an excellent background for evidence-based care in the prevention and treatment for diaper dermatitis (Adam, 2008; Heimall et al., 2012).

The pathogenesis of diaper dermatitis is partly related to the degree of wetness of the skin. Moist and macerated skin becomes more permeable and susceptible to injury because wetness increases friction. In addition, moisture-laden skin is more likely to contain microorganisms than dry skin.

Another component in skin injury from diaper dermatitis is the effect of an alkaline pH. The normal skin pH is acidic—ranging between 4.0 and 5.5—but can become alkaline when it is diapered (Visscher et al., 2000, 2002). The resulting increased pH of the skin increases its vulnerability to injury and penetration by microorganisms. Another problem associated with increased skin pH is that it stimulates fecal enzyme activity. Specifically, both protease and lipase, found in stools, can injure the skin, which is made up of protein and fat components. These enzymes can cause significant epidermal injury fairly quickly and are responsible for the contact irritant diaper dermatitis that is commonly seen.

Once the epidermis has been impaired or becomes a less efficient barrier because of one of the aforementioned mechanisms, invasion by bacteria or fungus can occur. Thus, a contact irritant diaper dermatitis can turn into a staphylococcal or fungal rash if this progression happens. *S. aureus* can be found in large numbers on the skin surface, especially if inflamed or impaired, and can result in secondary infection. The classic presentation for *S. aureus* is pustule formation at the site of hair follicles, although the overall incidence of *S. aureus*–complicated diaper dermatitis is relatively low.

Fungal rashes, primarily those caused by *C. albicans*, may have different invasion mechanisms. Many researchers have identified *C. albicans* as a secondary invader of skin that has been injured by other mechanisms, whereas, others suggest that *C. albicans* is a primary causative factor in diaper dermatitis. This theory is based on the ability of *C. albicans* to penetrate the stratum corneum, especially in a warm and moist environment, such as that found under an occlusive diaper. The resulting intense inflammation is significant and appears as brightly erythematous, sharply marginated dermatitis that involves the inguinal folds as well as the buttocks, thighs, abdomen, and genitalia, characteristically with satellite lesions that may extend the rash over the trunk (Figure 12.12). The GI tract is often the reservoir for *C. albicans*, and it can frequently be recovered in stools. Oral therapy may be indicated, especially if evidence of oral infection, such as thrush, is apparent.

Diaper dermatitis can result from a primary dermatologic condition, such as psoriasis, eczema, and seborrheic dermatitis. A significant family history of these skin conditions may identify infants especially vulnerable to developing severe reactions to inflammation in the diaper area. The role of allergens has also been implicated in some cases of diaper dermatitis and should be considered when treatment strategies fail (Smith & Jacob, 2009).

## Management

Prevention is the first goal of intervention and is paramount in breaking the cycle of diaper dermatitis. Frequent diaper changes result in drier skin with a more normal pH and a more normal functional barrier of the skin. Strategies to keep the skin dry also include using highly absorbent gelled diapers that "wick" moisture away from the skin. The use of baby powders is discouraged because of the risk of inhalation of particles into the respiratory tract.

The use of commercially available diaper wipes, although in widespread use, has variable support in the literature with

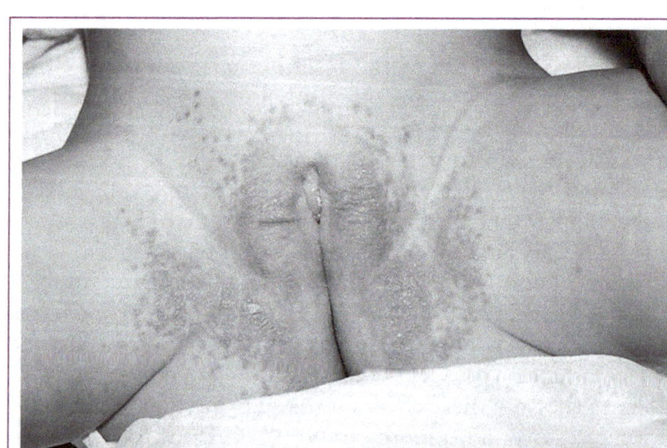

**FIGURE 12.12 Candida diaper dermatitis involving labia and inguinal folds with characteristic satellite lesions.**

reports of contact allergens and concerns with product ingredients (Ehretsmann et al., 2001; Fields et al., 2006; Smith & Jacob, 2009). A carefully controlled study of one brand of wipes compared to cloth and water for skin cleansing in the diaper area of premature infants showed improved skin pH and TEWL with the diaper wipe (Visscher, Odio et al., 2009). An RCT comparing the use of diaper wipes to cotton balls and warm water found no difference in skin barrier function and changes in skin pH between the two techniques (Lavender et al., 2013). However, these findings are not generalizable to other products with different formulations.

Once diaper dermatitis occurs—and it is not entirely avoidable in most infants—protecting injured skin during healing is the primary goal. A generous layer of protective skin barriers containing petrolatum ointment and/or zinc oxide prevents further trauma and allows impaired skin to heal (Figure 12.13). Although various amounts of zinc are found in different products, there is no evidence that one is better than the other (Stamatas & Tierney, 2014). Other beneficial ingredients include carboxymethylcellulose products that adhere exceptionally well to excoriated skin (Esser, 2016). The ingredient cyanoacrylate, found in "liquid bandages," is now found in some products for incontinence-associated dermatitis in adults and holds promise for the most severe cases of diaper dermatitis in infants and children (Brennan et al., 2017).

Opening the skin to light and air is ineffective if the fecal contents are allowed direct contact with already injured areas. Because protective skin barriers tend to adhere well to the skin, it is neither necessary nor desirable to remove them altogether during diaper changes before more cream is applied because the generated friction will injure healing tissue. It is best to generously apply more cream to the site to protect the area from further injury.

Multiple products are used in diaper dermatitis—topical emollients, diaper rash balms, and wipes—but product selection is often affected by myth and tradition rather than science. A damp diaper covered with a plastic coating enhances the risk of irritation and percutaneous absorption. The risk of absorption is even greater in newborns and premature infants because of their large surface-area-to-body-weight ratio and immature skin. The various compounds and chemicals used have been described extensively (Gilliam & Williams, 2008; Siegfried & Shah, 1999), concerning potential toxicity, irritancy, and later sensitization. Simple, inexpensive products such as zinc oxide ointment are recommended over more complex compounds.

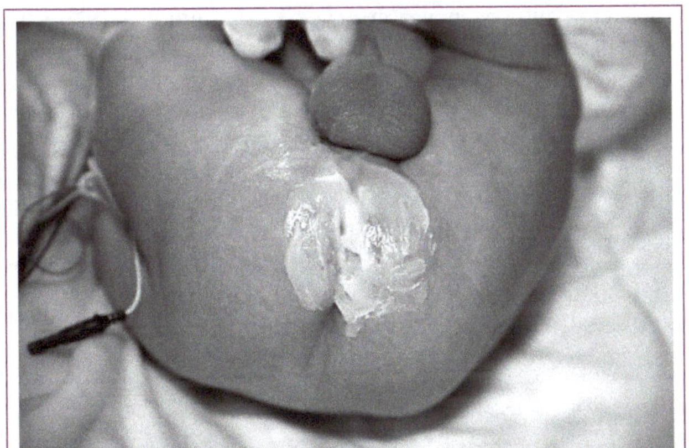

**FIGURE 12.13 A thick layer of a skin barrier, such as zinc oxide or pectin paste, will prevent reinjury of skin damage in diaper dermatitis.**

Treatment of diaper dermatitis that is solely due to invasion with *C. albicans* requires the use of antifungal creams or ointments. Some of the antifungal preparations include nystatin, miconazole, and clotrimazole. If the diaper dermatitis involves both fungus and a contact irritant component, alternating applications of the topical creams or ointments is effective.

Severe diaper dermatitis with deep excoriations can be seen in infants with malabsorption syndrome secondary to intestinal resection or mucosal injury. In these cases, the stool is highly caustic and contains a higher level of enzyme activity, a lower pH due to rapid transit through the intestine, and significant amounts of undigested carbohydrates. In the case of opiate withdrawal, stool frequency is often significantly increased. Other infants at risk for severe diaper dermatitis include those with spina bifida, exstrophy of the bladder, and infants with decreased anal sphincter tone due to early pull-through procedures for Hirschsprung disease. In cases of loss of sphincter tone, fecal material constantly dribbles to the perianal area.

Although skin disruption frequently becomes the focus of nursing interventions, this symptom may indicate more serious physiologic concerns. These infants' stools should be carefully monitored by documentation of number and volume. Infants must be observed for dehydration caused by extensive water loss and diarrhea. Once dietary manipulations and hydration have stabilized the general physiologic status, a skin protection program is imperative because some levels of chronic diarrhea may be ongoing for many weeks or months. Products such as pectin-based powders or pectin-containing pastes without alcohol may be better barriers to the caustic, constant fecal irritation if traditional zinc oxide creams do not work adequately. Antifungal creams may be applied in conjunction with protective barriers if yeast is present.

## EVIDENCE-BASED SKIN CARE GUIDELINE

Many intensive care and newborn nurseries have written protocols for various aspects of neonatal skin care. The AWHONN and the NANN collaborated to develop a comprehensive, evidence-based neonatal skin care guideline. An extensive review of the scientific basis for neonatal skin care was undertaken by a team, including advanced practice nurses and a pediatric dermatologist (Lund et al., 1999), and a neonatal skin guideline was written to address 13 aspects of skin care (Box 12.3). An evaluation project involving 51 nurseries was undertaken to evaluate the effect of using this guideline. The project involved identifying coordinators at each site willing to collect baseline information about the skin condition of infants in their units, implement the practice guideline in their respective units, and then collect skin condition information

**BOX 12.3**

**ELEMENTS OF THE AWHONN/NANN EVIDENCE-BASED PRACTICE GUIDELINE: NEONATAL SKIN CARE**

1. Newborn skin assessment
2. Neonatal skin injury
3. Bathing
4. Vernix caseosa
5. Umbilical cord care
6. Diaper dermatitis and diaper wipes
7. Circumcision care
8. Emollient use for dry skin and atopic dermatitis
9. Skin disinfectants
10. Medical adhesives
11. IV extravasation
12. Transepidermal water loss in premature infants
13. Parent education

*Source:* Adapted from the Association of Women's Health, Obstetric, and Neonatal Nurses. (2018). *Evidence-based clinical practice guideline: Neonatal skin care* (4th ed.). Author. Copyright © 2018.

again once the guideline had been introduced. Safety and feasibility were important, as was the evaluation of the effect of evidence-based practice on skin conditions.

More than 11,000 skin observations using the NSCS were performed on 2,820 newborns of varying gestational ages and weights. An improvement in skin condition was observed after implementation of the guideline, as evidenced by overall lower scores on the NSCS during the observation period. Initial scores were similar in both the preguideline and postguideline groups but improved more rapidly after the guideline had been implemented. The results were more dramatic in LBW infants, but improvement was also seen in the "well-baby" sample.

The Neonatal Skin Care Guideline was revised in 2007, with the addition of a section on vernix caseosa due to the availability of numerous studies published on this topic. A third revision was released in 2013, and a fourth in 2018.

## SUMMARY

Neonatal skin management is a complex problem that requires a collaborative approach. Some research has been conducted in this area, but a lot remains to be done regarding the use of routine NICU equipment and its effect on neonatal skin, the use of skin barriers for protection, and the effect of a consistent approach to skincare on the integrity of neonatal skin. This chapter has outlined the development and structure of the skin. It has addressed differences in the skin based on gestational age variations. Normal physiologic and common dermatologic abnormalities have been presented. Evidence-based neonatal skin care is recommended and has proven feasible and safe to improve skin conditions in the newborn.

## CASE STUDY

**Identification of the Problem.** An extremely premature infant was admitted to the NICU 3 days ago with respiratory distress syndrome; birth weight 650 g, gestational age 24 0/7 weeks. The infant has an endotracheal tube and receives assisted ventilation; catheters are inserted in both the umbilical artery and vein for blood sampling, blood pressure monitoring, and administration of IV fluids. An area of skin breakdown is noted on the abdomen where a temperature probe had been placed and removed on the first day of life. By day 3, the area is erythematous and oozing a yellow-tinged fluid. Surrounding areas are also quite red.

**Assessment: History and Physical Examination.** The infant, a baby boy, was born via vaginal delivery to a 30-year-old G1 P1 mother. The pregnancy was complicated by preterm labor starting at 20 weeks, and a cervical cerclage was performed. A month later, the mother was again hospitalized with prolonged rupture of membrane (PROM) and preterm labor. This time the efforts to stop labor were unsuccessful, and the infant was delivered vaginally 48 hours after a single course of betamethasone was administered.

The infant's Apgar scores were 4 and 7. The infant was intubated in the delivery room due to poor respiratory effort, and an initial dose of surfactant was administered. The infant was placed immediately into a polyurethane bag for reduction of evaporative heat and fluid loss in the delivery room. Upon arrival in the NICU, the infant was placed on a combination radiant warmer/incubator to insert umbilical catheters. The skin was prepared with a disinfectant (2% chlorhexidine in 70% IA) before placing umbilical catheters. After placing catheters and confirming the position with a radiograph, the disinfectant was wiped away using normal saline. The top of the heating device was lowered and converted to a convectively heated incubator with RH set at 80%.

The infant's skin was very moist and fragile in appearance. After placement of the umbilical catheters, although the periumbilical skin was cleansed with sterile water to remove the skin disinfectant, the skin was noted to be more erythematous than prior to insertion. A temperature probe with a hydrogel probe cover was attached to the infant's abdomen, which promptly slid off due to the high humidity in the environment. A silicone adhesive tape was used to secure the temperature probe, which was then covered with a reflective foil probe cover.

**Differential Diagnosis.** The chief differential diagnoses for an extremely premature infant with skin breakdown include trauma from adhesive removal, chemical burn from disinfectant used for periumbilical skin preparation, and infection. Although the original problem may be trauma, microorganisms on the skin surface can also infect the wound.

**Diagnostic Tests.** A skin culture with Gram stain and KOH prep is obtained from the area of breakdown. A complete blood count (CBC) and a blood culture are obtained. Although a catheter urine culture is requested, this is not obtained due to the extremely small size of the infant's penis and urethra; a "clean" bag specimen is collected instead.

**Working Diagnosis.** The Gram stain and KOH prep show budding yeast within 24 hours. The skin culture later shows a heavy growth of *C. albicans*. The blood and urine show no growth of microorganisms after 72 hours. The white blood cell (WBC) count remains unchanged from the first sample sent on the day of admission, but the platelet count has dropped from 100,000 to 60,000.

**Development of Management Plan.** After the Gram stain and KOH prep report, the area of breakdown appeared more extensive, and the skin over the abdomen was erythematous. The excoriated skin was gently debrided using a 30-ml syringe with warmed, one-half normal saline gently squirted through a 20-gauge Teflon catheter. Antifungal ointment, rather than cream or powder, was selected for topical treatment because of the potential healing benefits of ointments.

Because of the proximity of the excoriation to the umbilical catheter insertions, a decision was made to place a PICC line and peripheral arterial line so that the umbilical catheters could be discontinued.

**Implementation and Evaluation of Effectiveness.** After receiving the preliminary culture report and noting the drop in platelet count, it was determined that further evaluation for systemic illness would be necessary. A subsequent platelet count was 45,000, and this, coupled with the need for dopamine infusion for hypotension, prompted the medical decision to initiate systemic antifungal treatment. Fluconazole infusion was begun and a platelet transfusion was also administered.

After a second platelet transfusion, the platelet count had stabilized at 90,000 by the fifth day of treatment with fluconazole.

Despite having no growth of *C. albicans* from blood or urine samples, fungal infections in extremely premature infants can initially be cutaneous infections. If not treated early, this can quickly progress to disseminated *Candida* infections involving the blood, urinary tract, cerebrospinal fluid, or other organs.

Factors associated with cutaneous fungal infections in the first week of life are instrumentation procedures, such as cerclage placement and PROM. The infant can be colonized from maternal fungal or bacterial flora. Additional risk factors are skin breakdown from trauma or irritation and glucosuria. Several authors recommend early, aggressive management of cutaneous manifestations of fungal infection to prevent further dissemination and systemic complications.

## ONLINE RESOURCES

**CourseConnect**

Resources for this chapter are online and available at www.springerpub.com/courseconnect.

## REFERENCES

References for this chapter are online and available at www.springerpub.com/courseconnect.

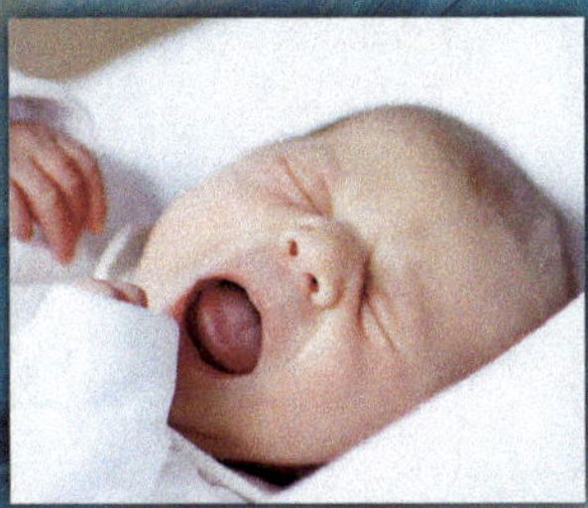
Source: Irina Schmidt/Adobe Stock.

CHAPTER 13

# Hematologic System

Wakako Eklund

## INTRODUCTION

To support the care of the prematurely born, or ill infants, it is critically important to understand the complexity of fetal development, which affects the premature infants' physiology. Infants who present with hematologic conditions, or infants who are born with premature hematologic systems, rely on the healthcare team to anticipate potential problems or to intervene in a timely manner to minimize complications. The hematologic system offers a broad range of topics, and it is beyond the scope of this chapter to address all in a complete manner. This chapter will discuss a brief historic overview of hematology, development of the hematologic system, the concept of *hematopoiesis*, and it common hematologic conditions in the neonatal period and the general descriptions of the management for these conditions.

## HISTORY AND OVERVIEW OF THE HEMATOLOGIC SYSTEM

### Historic Backdrop

More than 20 centuries ago, Hippocrates and Galen believed that the human body consisted of four elements: blood, phlegm, black bile, and yellow bile. Loss of balance among the four elements was believed to be the cause of illnesses. The study of hematology development paralleled with the advancement of various technologies, such as the invention of an early-model microscope by Leeuwenhoek in Holland and further development of complex instruments/devices and scientific methods such as staining. Leeuwenhoek published the first description of red blood cells (RBCs) using his simple microscope (Leeuwenhoek, 1674). Much later, in 1773, after the compound microscope was developed, white blood cells (WBCs) were described for the first time (Hewson, 1773). Many researchers described platelets much later; however, Bizzozero published his seminal work, which affected future work regarding platelets as distinct elements different from RBCs and WBCs (Bizzozero, 1882). Some who identified and described platelets (PLTs) early suspected PLTs as possible infectious agents, like bacteria (Osler & Burdon-Sanderson, 1874). The advancement toward cellular and molecular biology enhanced the knowledge of hematology, not only in the morphology of cells but also in blood cell development and the cells' specific functions. Newborn hematology is relatively recent knowledge. Nineteenth-century textbooks on pediatric diseases do not offer the word "hematology" and only briefly describe what was known about the state of blood circulation in infants in a few short paragraphs (Francis, 1844). It was not until 1897 when the original author, Holt, published *The Diseases of Infancy and Childhood*, which contained a 17-page section addressing blood-related diseases (Holt & McIntosh, 1937). Advanced research later explained the differences between fetal and adult hemoglobin, the various types and functions of WBCs, and the hematopoiesis mechanism. Textbooks containing normal hematologic values or newborn-specific hematologic conditions began in the mid-1900s and now provide healthcare professionals with tools that earlier periods did not offer (Pearson, 2021).

### Hematopoiesis

Hematologic cells critical to human life—such as RBCs, WBCs, or PLTs—originate from pluripotent stem cells, which later differentiate into specific types to serve human physiologic needs. Pluripotent stem cells give rise to RBC, WBCs, and PLTs, as well as lymphoid stem cells, which lead to immune cells (B or T lymphocytes). This chapter will not discuss the lymphoid cells. Progenitor cells are descendants of stem cells and possess the ability to proliferate, self-renew, and differentiate; these cells contribute to regeneration or repairs in addition to producing new blood cells (D'Souza et al., 2021). When healthy and mature, the human body produces upwards of 200 billion RBCs, 10 billion WBCs, and 400 billion PLTs a day, ensuring that needs are met for the human body to maintain homeostasis and health (D'Souza et al., 2021). The rate of production changes in times of need, such as if someone is placed in a hypoxic state, infected, or experienced injury. In these instances, additional RBCs, WBCs, and PLTs are deployed; thus, the rate of production increases (Figure 13.1).

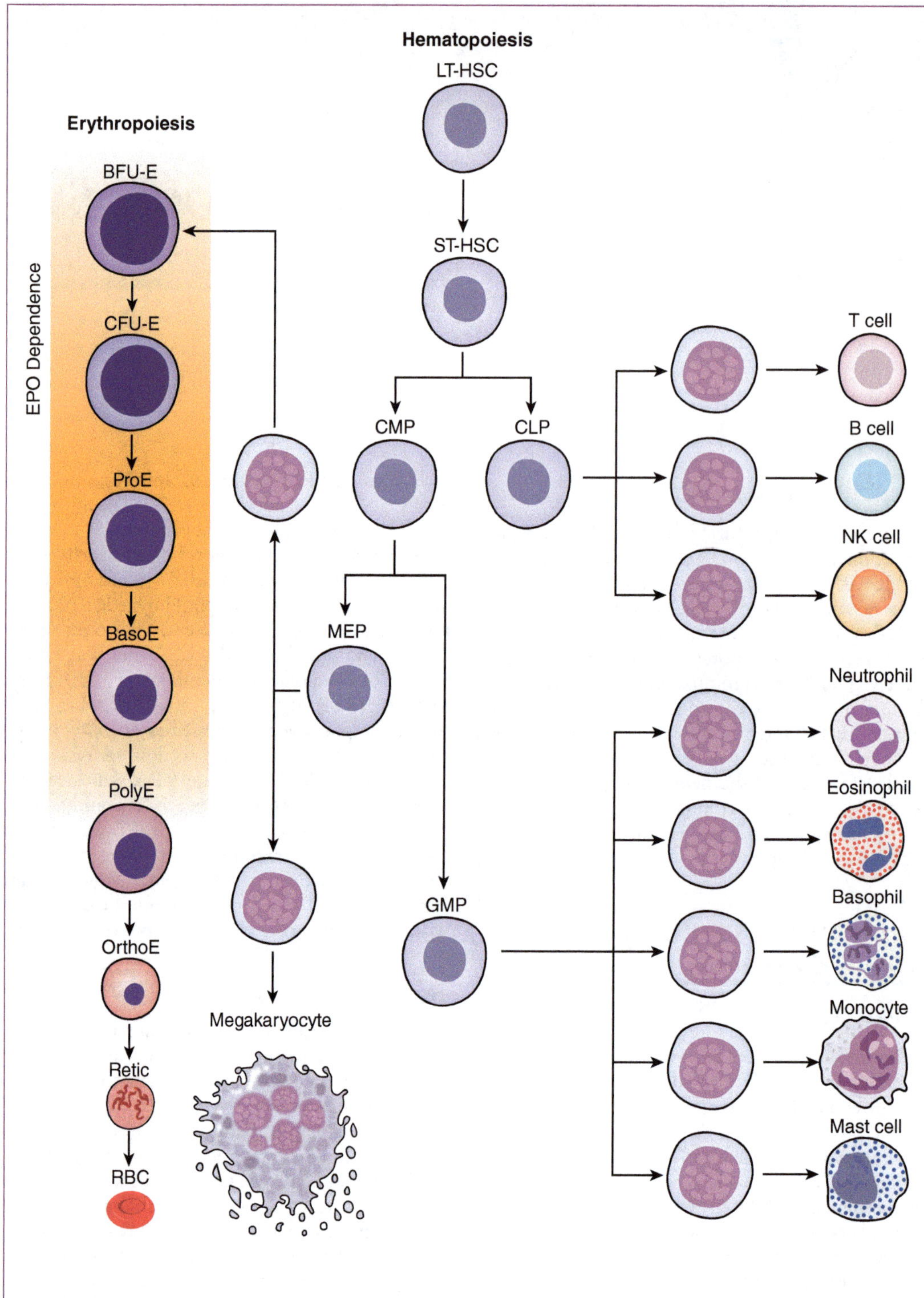


**FIGURE 13.1 Hierarchy of hematopoiesis/erythropoietin activity and erythropoiesis.**

NK, natural killer. Multipotent hematopoietic progenitors include the following: CLP, common lymphoid progenitor; CMP, common myeloid progenitor; LT-HSC, long-term engrafting hematopoietic stem cell; MEP, megakaryocytic-erythroid progenitor; ST-HSC, short-term hematopoietic stem cell. Committed erythroid progenitors include the following: BFU-E, burst-forming unit-erythroid; CFU-E, colony-forming unit-erythroid. Erythroid precursors include the following: BasoE, basophilic erythroblast; OrthoE, orthochromatic erythroblast; PolyE, polychromatic erythroblast; ProE, proerythroblast; Retic, reticulocyte.

*Source:* From Bhoopalan, S. V., Huang, L. J., & Weiss, M. J. (2020). Erythropoietin regulation of red blood cell production: From bench to bedside and back. *F1000Research*, *9*, F1000 Faculty Rev-1153. https://doi.org/10.12688/f1000research.26648.1.

Hematopoiesis describes a process of blood cell production and development from the embryonic stage of life to the entire adult life on a continuum. Hematopoiesis manufactures blood cells and makes them available by releasing them into the blood circulation. Hematopoiesis was not understood or studied until the mid-20th century due to complexities that required more than microscopes (D'Souza et al., 2021). As blood cells become old or are self-destructed or injured, hematopoietic stem cells are constantly called to action by producing numerous new blood cells to replace the damaged or injured cells by differentiating into the necessary final products, including RBCs, WBCs, or PLTs.

The initial site of hematopoiesis is in the embryonic yolk sac, and it begins as early as 7 days of embryonic life. The blood cells produced appear in the yolk sac by days 16 to 19. Then, the fetal liver begins hematopoiesis and produces blood cells from 5 to 6 weeks' gestation to 22 weeks' gestation. The liver hematopoiesis gradually diminishes from 18 to 21 weeks. Most long bones become actively engaged with hematopoiesis by weeks 11 and 12. However, it is not the primary site for hematopoiesis because the bones are still very small. The liver remains the main site for hematopoiesis from weeks 6 to 22 during fetal life (D'Souza et al., 2021). As it begins hematopoiesis, the liver becomes bright red in appearance, enriched by the presence of blood cells, which continue to mature (Torchia & Persaud, 2025). RBCs are vital for carrying oxygen to developing tissues and the vascular system. Systemic circulation is established by weeks 4 to 5, and the cardiac structure critical to the continued development of the systemic circulation is almost completed by 8 weeks' gestation. This highlights the importance of early and active hematopoiesis for optimal and continued fetal development (Torchia & Persaud, 2025).

While the long bones are small, extramedullary sites of the spleen, lymph nodes, thymus, and kidneys help with hematopoiesis. Changes in the primary location of hematopoiesis throughout fetal life and the transition from fetal to adult hemoglobin are shown in Figure 13.2.

## Red Blood Cells and Hemoglobin

The most abundant cell type is the RBCs (erythrocytes), with the critical role of transporting oxygen to the cells to remove carbon dioxide as a waste product. RBC production

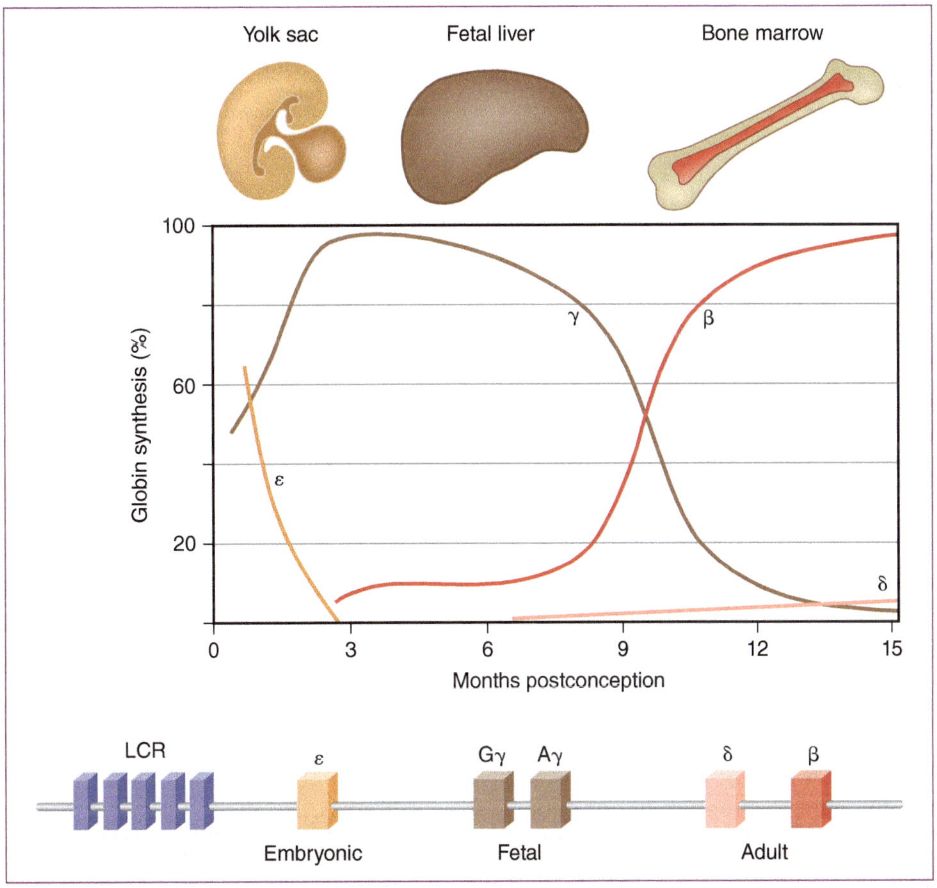


**FIGURE 13.2 There are two developmental switches in expression from the cluster, from embryonic to fetal during the first trimester of conception, and from fetal to adult around the time of birth.**

*Source:* From Bauer, D. E., Kamran, S. C., & Orkin, S. H. (2012). Reawakening fetal hemoglobin: Prospects for new therapies for the β-globin disorders. *Blood, 120*(15), 2945–2953. https://doi.org/10.1182/blood-2012-06-292078.

(erythropoiesis) is essential for the first functional organ system, the cardiovascular system (Palis, 2024). In the early 1900s, two erythroid cell population groups were discovered during embryonic and fetal life. However, the period of existence for the two types of erythroid cells overlap. The earliest type recognized in embryonic life was the primitive erythroblasts for their large and nucleated form. Another was called the definitive erythroblasts for their smaller enucleated form (Palis, 2014).

Erythropoiesis, the production of RBCs, begins in the first few weeks of gestation in the yolk sac. On the mesodermal layers of the yolk sac, primitive erythroid progenitor cells congregate, forming blood islands. Primitive progenitor cells then differentiate further to become primitive erythroblasts, which are large and nucleated. Primitive erythroblasts begin producing embryonic hemoglobin. In contrast to the primitive erythroblasts that are larger and nucleated, the definitive erythroblasts start to emerge later. The initial definitive erythroblast productions have two distinct origins that lead to further development. The definitive erythroblast progenitors (burst-forming units erythroid [BFU-E]) are formed in the yolk sac early, and they migrate and seed the fetal liver, where they mature to become the first line of definitive erythroblasts, which are smaller than the primitive erythroblasts. Secondly, hematopoietic stem cell--derived BFU-E begin to mature at the colonization site, such as the fetal liver, initially to the enucleated mature stage. The production site later moves more predominantly to the bone marrow to continue the process (Palis, 2014, 2024). Definitive erythroblast production increases from 11 to 14 weeks' gestation, and the presence of primitive erythroblasts declines sharply (D'Souza et al., 2021).

Approximately 1 to 2 days after enucleation of the erythrocytes, this reticulocyte becomes a mature RBC and enters the bloodstream. In erythropoiesis, the maturation of RBC development takes approximately 14 days from the beginning. The body can produce upward of 200 billion erythrocytes a day (D'Souza et al., 2021). Erythropoiesis is shown in Figure 13.3. Also, please refer to the earlier hematopoiesis hierarchy (Figure 13.1 in the far-left column).

The lifespan of fetal and newborn RBCs is much shorter than the 120-day life of adult RBCs. The full-term infant's erythrocytes can last 60 to 80 to 90 days, while a preterm infant's is 30 to 35 to 50 days (Driscoll, 2016; Pearson, 1967). With advancing gestation, erythrocytes become smaller in size and volume. Because of their larger size and cylindrical shape, compared to adult or older children's erythrocytes, neonatal erythrocytes are more prone to earlier destruction in the narrow splenic sinusoids (Tang & Wang, 2023).

Today, in high-resource settings, infants ranging from 22 weeks to term/postterm are admitted to the neonatal intensive care units (NICUs). Hematocrit/hemoglobin (Hct/Hb) levels increase as the gestational age increases, especially after reaching 25 to 27 weeks' gestation. Before that, the Hct/Hb is approximately 38% per 12.4 g/dl; however, after 24 to 25 weeks, Hct and Hb reach 62% per 19 g/dl. Those numbers remain relatively stable until full term, except that the hematocrit levels may rise to the mid-60s by 36 to 37 weeks and level off by 40 weeks (Stark et al., 2019).

The embryonic hemoglobin is built of a pair of alpha and a pair of epsilon globin chains (epsilon is the first to appear in the embryonic stage); however, soon afterward by 4 to 5 weeks' gestation, fetal hemoglobin with a pair of alpha and a pair of gamma-globin chains (fetal hemoglobin) appear. Embryonic and fetal hemoglobin have a stronger affinity to oxygen molecules than adult hemoglobin, allowing the embryo/fetus to attract oxygen molecules from maternal hemoglobin much easier (Figure 13.4). This is critical because the fetus is in a hypoxemic environment with the fetal partial pressure of oxygen ($PO_2$) averaging between 25 and 35 mm Hg. Adult hemoglobin with a pair of alpha and a pair of beta globin chains begins production and is detectable early in fetal life. However, the level remains very low during fetal life. Adult hemoglobin has much less affinity to oxygen molecules, which allows it to readily release oxygen molecules to tissues once extrauterine life is established with respiratory/circulatory

**FIGURE 13.3 Hematopoietic stem cells stimulated to become erythrocytes initially develop into multipotent colony-forming cells (multi-CFCs).** A portion of the multi-CFC becomes erythroid progenitor cells, the early and late erythroid burst-forming units (BFU-E), which eventually differentiate into erythroid colony-forming units (CFU-E). These progenitor cells progress to form the normoblast, the erythrocyte precursor. Multiple divisions and alterations of the normoblast lead to the development of the reticulocyte. When the reticulocyte extrudes its nucleus, it usually moves out of the predominant production sites (i.e., the liver or bone marrow) and into the blood.

*Source:* Adapted from Diab, Y., & Luchtman-Jones, L. (2015). Hematologic and oncologic problems in the fetus and neonate. In R. J. Martin, A. A. Fanaroff, & M. C. Walsh (Eds.), *Fanaroff and Martin's neonatal-perinatal medicine: Diseases of the fetus and infant* (10th ed., pp. 1294–1343). Elsevier.

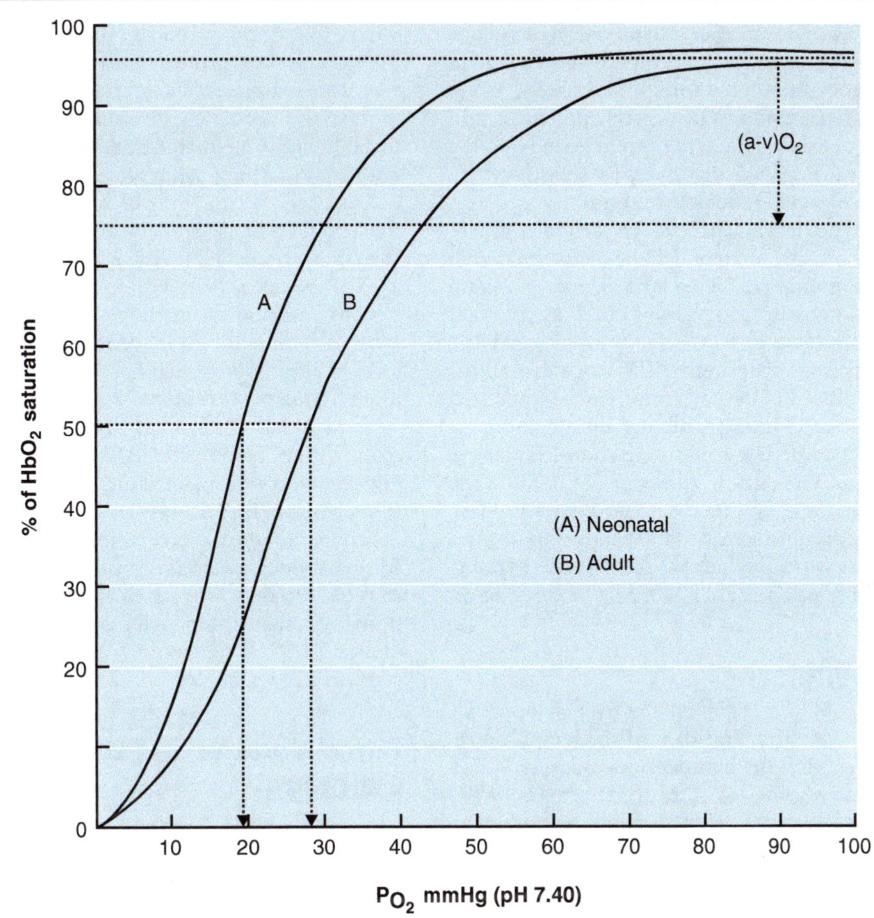


**FIGURE 13.4 The affinity for oxygen (i.e., the ability of the hemoglobin molecule to bind and hold the oxygen molecule) is markedly different between fetal and adult hemoglobin.** Fetal hemoglobin has a greater affinity for oxygen. It can bind to oxygen more readily at the intervillous spaces of the placenta, a property useful in the fetus's low partial pressure of oxygen ($PO_2$) environment. Adult hemoglobin has a diminished affinity for oxygen, allowing easier oxygen release to the tissue when metabolic needs are higher than those that arise in the fetus.

*Source:* Adapted from Sacks, L., & Delivoria-Papadopoulos, M. (1984). Hemoglobin–oxygen interactions. *Seminars in Perinatology, 8,* 168–183.

function. Fetal hemoglobin makes up 50% to 85% of the entire hemoglobin at term, and it completely disappears in healthy children by 3 to 4 years of age (D'Souza et al., 2021; Stark et al., 2019).

## Erythropoietin

A complex system or mechanism sensing the oxygen in the body regulates the production of erythropoietin (EPO). Maternal EPO does not cross the placenta. EPO is produced in the fetal liver. In the early 1900s, an observation was made by Carnot and Deafandre that the infusion of blood from anemic animals into nonanemic/healthy animals increased the RBC counts in the nonanemic/healthy animals, suggesting that there is a substance circulating in the serum of the anemic animal stimulated by anemia. Therefore, the anemic animal's blood increased the erythropoiesis in the healthy donor (Bhoopalan et al., 2020; Bunn, 2013). During the following years, extensive research continued, leading to the discovery that EPO is primarily produced in the kidneys. Further isolation of pure EPO occurred in 1977, the cloning of the EPO gene occurred in 1985, the successful manufacturing of recombinant human EPO for clinical use was approved by FDA in 1989, and the findings of a complex system that regulates EPO in the 1990s followed (Bhoopalan et al., 2020; Bunn, 2013; Jelkmann, 1986).

This circulating glycoprotein hormone EPO, the gene of which is located on the seventh chromosome, is an obligate growth factor that stimulates stem cells to become committed progenitors of the erythrocyte. The erythropoietin-dependent process of erythropoiesis is shown in Figure 13.1 to the left of the figure.

In the absence of erythropoietin, hypoxia does not increase RBC production. However, if erythropoietin production is intact, hypoxia stimulates a rapid increase in erythropoietin levels, which remain elevated until hypoxia is resolved.

The production of erythropoietin in the fetus and newborn increases within minutes to hours after a hypoxia event occurs. Although erythropoietin levels increase rapidly, no change in the number of erythrocytes is noted for approximately 5 days after a hypoxic stress encounter. When erythropoietin stimulates the production of excess RBCs, they are released into the circulation before reaching maturity (i.e., as reticulocytes); this is reflected in an elevated reticulocyte count.

Factors besides hypoxia that increase erythropoietin production in the newborn are maternal hypoxemia, maternal anemia, small for gestational age (SGA) infants, poor placental functioning, maternal smoking, and possibly other diseases that affect the integrity of maternal RBCs, for example, malaria, acquired immunodeficiency syndrome (AIDS), or tuberculosis (TB). Cord-blood levels of EPO usually are elevated compared with adult values but drop dramatically to almost undetectable levels in the newborn. The healthy newborn, therefore, produces few RBCs in the first few weeks of life because the hypoxic stimuli of low fetal $PO_2$ levels are no longer present. Erythropoietin levels do not increase in the term infant until 8 to 10 weeks of age, when the kidneys sense tissue hypoxia caused by anemia (Bhoopalan et al., 2020; Migliaccio, 2024).

## White Blood Cells

The formation of the WBCs begins in the liver at approximately 5 to 7 weeks' gestation and then in the lymph nodes at 12 weeks' gestation, with the number of circulating WBCs increasing dramatically during the third trimester. The WBC aims to work against foreign proteins found in the body. The production and function of WBCs are also affected by gestational age; this subject is covered in more detail in Chapter 11, "Immune System."

## Platelets

The hemostatic system provides a series of processes that are interlinked with complex mechanisms to achieve the cessation of bleeding by forming a "plug" to restore and maintain the circulatory network. Platelets are developed from the hemopoietic stem cells, which gives rise to common myeloid progenitor (CMP) cells and megakaryocyte/erythrocyte progenitors (MEPs). MEP develops into megakaryocytes, at which point the megakaryocytes produce the final product, the platelets, which are 2 to 4 µm in diameter (Josefsson et al., 2020). Platelets are more short-lived than WBCs or RBCs, and the daily production in healthy adults is as many as 400 billion a day (Bhoopalan et al., 2020). Once produced, platelets only live 7 to 10 days compared to RBCs, which live 80 to 100 days (Josefsson et al., 2020).

Neonatal platelet counts remain relatively the same across gestation, unlike the RBCs and hemoglobin, which increase with gestational age. Even if the structure and number of platelets (normal range is 150,000–450,000/mcL) are like that of the adults, neonatal platelets do not respond to signals as adult platelets when needed. Agonists, such as adenosine diphosphate, epinephrine, collagen, thrombin, or thromboxane, do not initiate the same responses in platelet function, and this immature response is more prominent in preterm infants (Ferrer-Marín & Sola-Visner, 2022).

Basic functions of platelets begin with the initial adhesion, which relies heavily on the blood flow; therefore, poor perfusion may compromise this mechanism. Various adhesive receptors expressed on the surface of platelets are in play to initiate the adhesion. Certain receptors, not all, are found to be lower in neonatal platelets than that of older children and adults. Along with the adhesion process, a simultaneous process occurs in which endothelial damage activates the production of some thrombin, leading to aggregation (Ferrer-Marín & Sola-Visner, 2022).

The platelets level is not the only factor in bleeding or clotting, making the pathogenesis of bleeding in preterm infants very difficult to manage. When infants have the same level of thrombocytopenia, severe bleeding appears to occur more frequently for infants with other underlining conditions, such as sepsis, necrotizing enterocolitis (NEC), or alloimmune thrombocytopenia (AIT) than infants who present with low platelets due to intrauterine growth restriction (IUGR) (Ferrer-Marín & Sola-Visner, 2022). Bleeding risk is not solely dependent on the platelet count, as evidenced by a multicenter study in which infants with platelet counts $< 60 \times 10^9$/L were studied. Bleeding was associated more with the lower gestational age than the platelet counts (bleeding in 63% for infants < 28 weeks versus 14% for 28 weeks and older) (de Vos et al., 2022; Katheria et al., 2023; Stanworth et al., 2009).

## Blood Volume and Delayed Cord Clamping

After extensive studies, the American College of Obstetricians and Gynecologists (ACOG) Committee of Obstetric Practice recommended delayed cord clamping (DCC) in 2017, and it was updated and reaffirmed in 2023. DCC directly adds to the blood volume in neonates by allowing the transfer of remaining blood in the placenta to the newborn. Benefits of DCC for term infants include: (a) increased hemoglobin, (b) increased iron stores for several months postnatally, and (c) potentially favorable effect on developmental outcomes. For preterm infants, the benefits are more significant. The benefits for preterm infants include: (a) improved transitional circulation, (b) increased RBC volume, (c) decreased need for packed RBC (PRBC) transfusions, and (d) decreased incidences of NEC and intraventricular hemorrhage (IVH). The current recommendation from ACOG is to perform DCC for 30 to 60 seconds for vigorous term and preterm infants. A minor increase in jaundice from increased RBC transfer has been recognized, and healthcare systems must have a set protocol in place to capture neonatal jaundice for timely treatment (ACOG, 2020). In term infants, DCC for 1 minute transfers 80 ml of blood volume, reaching nearly 100 ml by 3 minutes of age. The neonates' blood volume is approximately 80 to 100 ml/kg of weight and less for more preterm infants, so DCC adds significant blood volume (Koperska, 2024; Lopriore, 2023). With the additional transfer of blood volume, blood cells, immunoglobulins, and stem cells are also transferred, adding to the extensive hematologic benefits (Sanberg et al., 2010). Current recommendations differ based on the professional organizations. However, a range of 30 seconds to 2 minutes is commonly recommended for vigorous infants who do not require resuscitation (ACOG, 2020;

Hainstock & Raval, 2020; World Health Organization, 2023). When placental integrity is in question, such as in placental abruption, maternal hemorrhage, an infant needing immediate resuscitation, IUGR infants with abnormal Doppler evaluation, or any other situations where placental circulation is not intact, immediate cord clamping should be considered (ACOG, 2020).

When time is highly limited, umbilical cord milking (UCM) or stripping has been considered a potential method to improve placental blood transfusion to infants when 30 to 60 seconds of DCC causes potential delay to care, especially when immediate resuscitation is indicated. A 2019 study on UCM for preterm infants (23–27 weeks) stopped early due to the cord milking arm of infants developing IVH more frequently than the group receiving DCC (Katheria et al., 2019). IVH incidence appears to be similar for infants at 28 to 32 weeks' gestation when cord milking was performed (Katheria et al., 2023). Currently, there is insufficient evidence to support or refute UCM per the most recent ACOG recommendation, which was reaffirmed in 2023 (ACOG, 2020). Clinically, in situations of tight nuchal cord, respiratory depression, or maternal placental abruption requiring immediate resuscitation, obstetricians use clinical judgment for the individual patient in each situation.

## Reference Range

The hemoglobin concentration and hematocrit levels for adults are well established. The references for normal ranges for neonatal population is limited, due to the ethical issues related to the potential danger and risks of withdrawing blood samples across the course of the neonatal life, especially for those preterm. Hematocrit and hemoglobin values must be carefully evaluated based on the gestational age as well as the postnatal age with ongoing, thorough assessment. Gestational age and postnatal age each represent independent factors that determine the hemoglobin and hematocrit, which shows an increase of hemoglobin and hematocrit with an increase in gestational age, while there is a decrease as the postnatal age advances in days of life (Henry & Christensen, 2015; Scholkmann et al., 2019). Figure 13.5 depicts this trend.

Mean hemoglobin values in postmature infants are higher than in the term infant, possibly because of progressive placental dysfunction and oxygen deficit, which stimulates the release of erythropoietin. Table 13.1 summarizes the differences in hematologic values as a function of increasing gestational and postnatal age.

It is important to consider the sampling site and the quality of blood flow when interpreting laboratory values. The hemoglobin levels of capillary blood are 10% to 20% higher than those of venous and arterial blood. This discrepancy can be minimized by warming the extremity before drawing blood to enhance peripheral perfusion, allowing better spontaneous blood flow. Discarding the first few drops obtained on a capillary draw also improves the accuracy of the sample. Sampling by the venous route also requires care; poor blood flow through small-bore needles increases the chance of hemolysis, leading to sampling errors. Greater accuracy

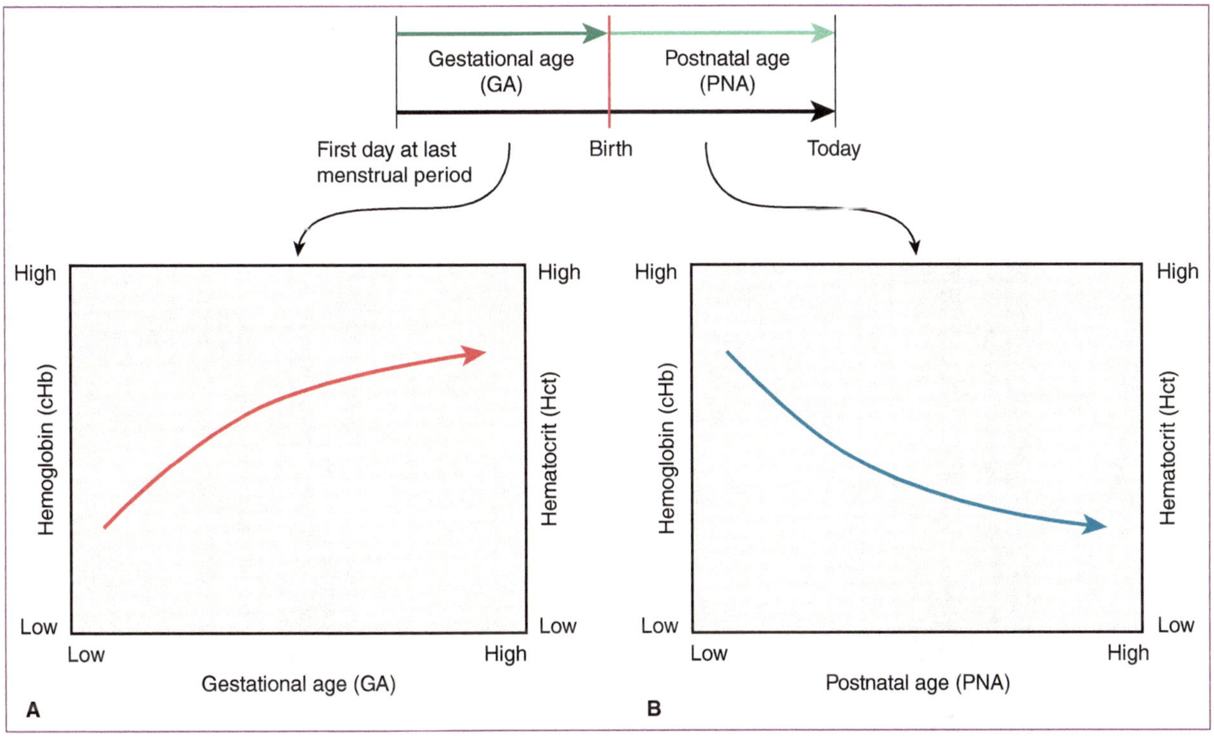


**FIGURE 13.5 Hemoglobin and hematocrit trend in neonates based on GA (A) and PNA (B) according to the findings of Henry and Christensen (2015) by Scholkmann et al. (2019).**

*Source:* From Scholkmann, F., Ostojic, D., Isler, H., Bassler, D., Wolf, M., & Karen, T. (2019). Reference ranges for hemoglobin and hematocrit levels in neonates as a function of gestational age (22–42 weeks) and postnatal age (0–29 days): Mathematical modeling. *Children (Basel, Switzerland)*, *6*(3), 38. https://doi.org/10.3390/children6030038.

## TABLE 13.1

### AGE-SPECIFIC NORMAL BLOOD CELL VALUES IN FETAL SAMPLES (26–30 WEEKS' GESTATION) AND NEONATAL SAMPLES (28–44 WEEKS' GESTATION)

| Age | Hb (g/dl)[a] | Hct (%)[a] | MCV (fL)[a] | MCHC (g/dl RBC)[a] | Reticulocytes | WBCs (× $10^3$/ml)[b] | Platelets ($10^3$/ml)[b] |
|---|---|---|---|---|---|---|---|
| 26–30 weeks' gestation[c] | 13.4 (11) | 41.5 (34.9) | 118.2 (106.7) | 37.9 (30.6) | – | 4.4 (2.7) | 254 (180–327) |
| 28 weeks | 14.5 | 45 | 120 | 31.0 | (5–10) | – | 275 |
| 32 weeks | 15.0 | 47 | 118 | 32.0 | (3–10) | – | 290 |
| Term[d] (cord) | 16.5 (13.5) | 51 (42) | 108 (98) | 33.0 (30.0) | (3–7) | 18.1 (9–30)d | 290 |
| 1–3 days | 18.5 (14.5) | 56 (45) | 108 (95) | 33.0 (29.0) | (1.8–4.6) | 18.9 (9.4–34) | 192 |
| 2 weeks | 16.6 (13.4) | 53 (41) | 105 (88) | 31.4 (28.1) | – | 11.4 (5–20) | 252 |
| 1 month | 13.9 (10.7) | 44 (33) | 101 (91) | 31.8 (28.1) | (0.1–1.7) | 10.8 (4–19.5) | – |

[a]Data are mean (number in parenthesis is –2 standard deviations [SD]).
[b]Data are mean (number in parenthesis is –2 SD).
[c]In infants younger than 1 month, capillary Hb exceeds venous Hb: at 1 hour old, the difference is 3.6 g; at 5 days, 2.2 g; at 3 weeks, 1.1 g.
[d]Mean (95% confidence limits).

Hb, hemoglobin; Hct, hematocrit; MCV, mean corpuscular volume; MCHC, mean corpuscular hemoglobin concentration; WBCs, white blood cells.

*Source:* Modified from Costa, K. (2018). Hematology. In *The Harriet Lane handbook* (pp. 364–394). Elsevier.

can be obtained by using a needle with the largest possible bore and removing the needle from the syringe before placing the sample in the specimen container. Gestational age also affects the discrepancy between reported capillary and venous results: the younger the gestational age, the more significant the discrepancy. The key to accuracy in hematology laboratory values lies in using a consistent sampling site (Bagwell & Steward, 2020).

## Blood Group Type

The RBCs have antigens on the cell membranes' surface that can cause antigen–antibody reactions. Blood is classified by groups and types based on the antigens found in the RBCs. The four major blood types are A, B, O, and AB. Antibodies to the antigens of different blood types occur naturally in the plasma (Table 13.2). For example, type A blood has A antigens on the cell surface but has circulating anti-B antibodies in the plasma. Type B blood has the opposite: B antigens on the cell surface and anti-A antibodies in the plasma. Type AB blood has A and B antigens on the cell surface and neither antibody in the plasma; type O blood has neither antigen on the cell surface but has both anti-A and anti-B antibodies in the plasma. Antigens are usually polypeptides and complex proteins; antibodies are immunoglobulins (mostly IgG and IgM).

Globally, approximately 42% of the population has type O+ blood, 31% has A+, 15% has B+, 5% has AB+, and 3% of the population has type O (Figure 13.6). Some of the blood types, however, are more commonly seen in certain population groups. It is estimated that among the Latin American population, 53% has type O+, and among the Black population, 47% has type O+. However, among the Asian population and Whites, 39% versus 37% are reported to have type O+ blood, respectively. Type B+ is more common in Asians (25%), while it is known to be around 9% for both Latin Americans and Whites (Fleck, 2023; WorldAtlas, 2024).

**TABLE 13.2**

**BLOOD GROUPS AND THEIR ANTIGENS AND ANTIBODIES**

| Blood Group Type | Antigens | Antibodies |
|---|---|---|
| O | None | Anti-A, Anti-B |
| A | A | Anti-B |
| B | B | Anti-A |
| AB | A and B | None |

*Source:* Adapted from Hall, J. E. (2016). *Guyton and Hall textbook of medical physiology* (13th ed.). Elsevier.

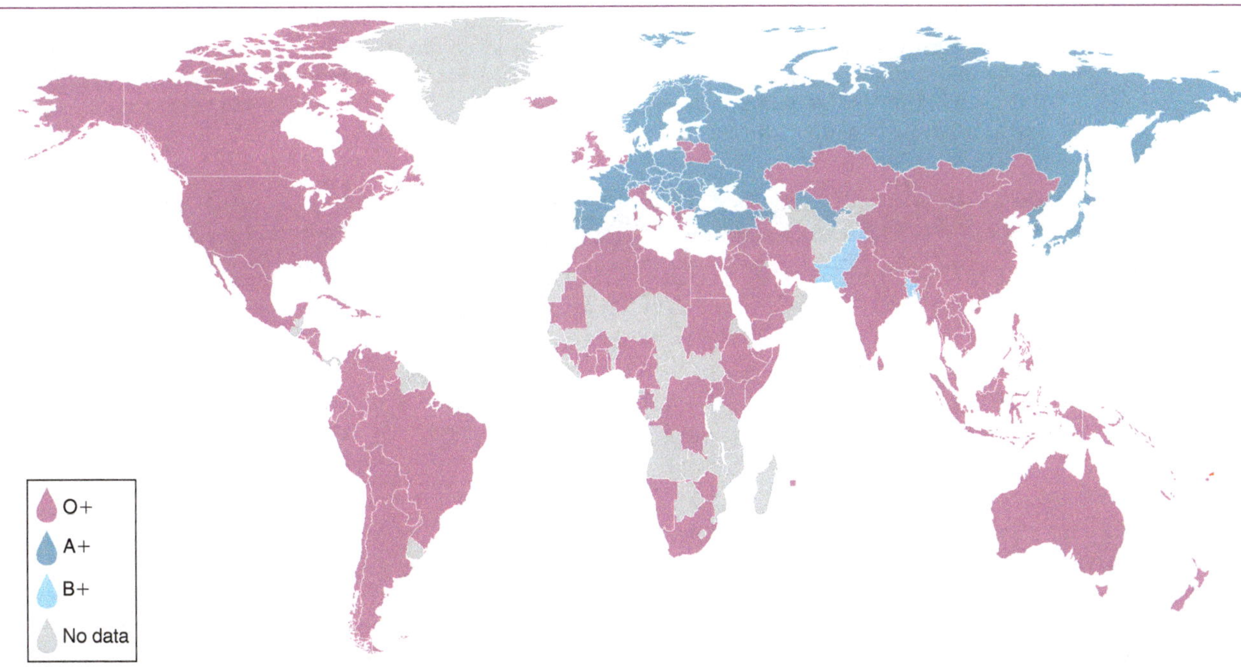


Depending on the country, the majority blood group represents between 30 percent and 75 percent of the population.

**FIGURE 13.6 The most common blood types around the world.**

*Source:* From World Population Review. Statista. https://www.statista.com/chart/28156/blood-type-by-region/.

The other type of antigen is Rh antigens. The Rh system has been known to be a very complex group system. The Rh system was discovered as the cause of severe jaundice and fetal demise by erythroblastosis fetalis in 1941 (Levine et al., 1941).

There are three presumed Rh gene loci capable of producing recognized antigens in the Rh complex: C, D, E, c, d, and e. Everyone has a paired set of these factors, having inherited a single set of C or c, D or d, and E or e from each parent. Three potential combinations are possible: two Rh positive (CDe and cDE) and one Rh negative (cde). The factors involved in Rh determination are D (most prevalent, and its presence on RBC indicates a Rh-positive cell) and d, or lack of D, which indicates Rh negative. Approximately 15% of Whites are Rh negative, 8% of the Black population, and 1% in Asians (Dean, 2005). Because of single-set inheritance from each parent, the potential exists for three different combinations of paired antigens: one pair being both d (dd: Rh negative, homozygous), another pair being both D (DD: Rh positive, homozygous) and the third pair being a combination of d and D (Dd: Rh positive, heterozygous). The end product is the presence or absence of Rh antigen on the RBC cell membrane. The Rh antigen can be detected as early as 38 days' gestation on the fetal RBCs and attains complete development during fetal life. This antigen is critically essential to the membrane structure of the RBCs (Bagwell & Steward, 2020; Fung-Kee-Fung, et al., 2024; Westhoff, 2007).

## Hemostatic System

The components involved in blood coagulation and fibrinolysis are produced in the liver, vascular wall, and tissue during early fetal life. Many of the clotting factors (procoagulants) and anticoagulants (inhibitors) are synthesized in the fetus starting around 10 weeks' gestation. At term, all the factors for coagulation and fibrinolytic system are not only present but also measurable in the laboratory. However, procoagulants, anticoagulants, and the substances in the fibrinolytic system (responsible for dissolution of a clot) do not increase in number and function to reach adult levels at the same rate, as presented in Tables 13.3 to 13.5 (Andrew et al., 1987, 1988, 1990). Some components increase with increasing gestational age, whereas others achieve normal adult levels several weeks to months before the fetus reaches term. Still, other components do not achieve normal adult levels until several weeks to months or years after birth. For example, in the coagulation system, K-dependent coagulation factors (Factors II, VII, IX, X, protein C, and S) or how the system generates thrombin are less equipped in newborns compared to adults. At the same time, some factors (fibrinogen, Factors, V, VIII, XIII) are already increased at the level of older children and adults at birth. For the fibrinolytic system, significantly decreased levels are seen in newborns for plasminogen, tissue-plasminogen activator, antiplasmin, and plasminogen activator inhibitors. Some inhibitors, such as heparin cofactor II, protein C, or antithrombin levels, are at 50% level at birth compared to older children. However, other components, such as alpha 2-macroglobulin, are elevated twice the level of adult. Although the function of coagulation factors and anticoagulants in the fetus are not identical to that in an older child or adult, initial vascular response to injury by release of tissue thromboplastin is functional in the fetus as early as 8 to 10 weeks (Albisetti & Monagle, 2021; Andrew et al., 1990). Age-dependent range of plasma concentration of various components must be used to interpret the laboratory values for newborns who present with clinical symptoms related to bleeding. Hemostasis consists of a delicate and dynamic balance between factors that prevent bleeding and those that keep the blood in a fluid form. The balanced interrelationship ensures orderly hemostasis and fibrinolysis when vascular integrity is destroyed or interrupted. The four constituents involved are vascular spasm, platelets and their activating substances, coagulation or plasma factors, and the fibrinolytic pathway (Bagwell & Steward, 2020)

**TABLE 13.3**

**NORMAL COAGULATION TEST RESULTS AND BLOOD LEVELS OF COAGULATION FACTORS IN THE FETUS (19–27 WEEKS' GESTATION) AND NEWBORN (28 WEEKS' GESTATION TO TERM)**

| Test/Factor | 19–27 Weeks Mean ± SD | 28–31 Weeks Mean (boundary) | 30–36 Weeks, Day 1 Mean (boundary) | 30–36 Weeks, Day 5 Mean (boundary) | Full Term, Day 1 Mean (boundary) | Full Term, Day 5 Mean (boundary) |
|---|---|---|---|---|---|---|
| ***Test*** | | | | | | |
| Prothrombin time (seconds) | – | 15.4 (14.6–16.9) | 13 (10.6–16.2) | 12.5 (10–15.3) | 13 (10.1–15.9) | 12.4 (10–15.3) |
| Activated partial thromboplastin time (seconds) | – | 108 (80–168) | 53.6 (27.5–79.4) | 50.5 (26.9–74.1) | 42.9 (31.3–54.5) | 42.6 (25.4–59.8) |

*(continued)*

**TABLE 13.3**

**NORMAL COAGULATION TEST RESULTS AND BLOOD LEVELS OF COAGULATION FACTORS IN THE FETUS (19–27 WEEKS' GESTATION) AND NEWBORN (28 WEEKS' GESTATION TO TERM) (*continued*)**

| Test/Factor | 19–27 Weeks Mean ± SD | 28–31 Weeks Mean (boundary) | 30–36 Weeks, Day 1 Mean (boundary) | 30–36 Weeks, Day 5 Mean (boundary) | Full Term, Day 1 Mean (boundary) | Full Term, Day 5 Mean (boundary) |
|---|---|---|---|---|---|---|
| Thrombin clotting time (seconds) | – | – | 24.8 (19.2–30.4) | 24.1 (18.8–29.4) | 23.5 (19–28.3) | 23.1 (18–29.2) |
| ***Factor*** | | | | | | |
| Fibrinogen (g/L) | 1 ± 0.4 | 2.56 (1.6–5.5) | 2.43 (1.5–3.73) | 2.8 (1.6–4.18) | 2.83 (1.67–3.99) | 3.12 (1.62–4.62) |
| Factor II (U/ml) | 0.12 ± 0.02 | 0.31 (0.19–0.54) | 0.45 (0.2–0.77) | 0.57 (0.29–0.85) | 0.48 (0.26–0.7) | 0.63 (0.33–0.93) |
| Factor V (U/ml) | 0.41 ± 0.1 | 0.65 (0.43–0.8) | 0.88 (0.41–1.44) | 1 (0.46–1.54) | 0.72 (0.34–1.08) | 0.95 (0.45–1.45) |
| Factor VII (U/ml) | 0.28 ± 0.04 | 0.37 (0.24–0.76) | 0.67 (0.21–1.13) | 0.84 (0.3–1.38) | 0.66 (0.28–1.04) | 0.89 (0.35–1.43) |
| Factor VIII (U/ml) | 0.39 ± 0.14 | 0.79 (0.37–1.26) | 1.11 (0.5–2.13) | 1.15 (0.53–2.05) | 1 (0.5–1.78) | 0.88 (0.5–1.54) |
| von Willebrand factor (U/ml) | 0.64 ± 0.13 | 1.41 (0.83–2.23) | 1.36 (0.78–2.1) | 1.33 (0.72–2.19) | 1.53 (0.5–2.87) | 1.4 (0.5–2.54) |
| Factor IX (U/ml) | 0.1 ± 0.01 | 0.18 (0.17–0.2) | 0.35 (0.19–0.65) | 0.42 (0.14–0.74) | 0.53 (0.15–0.91) | 0.53 (0.15–0.91) |
| Factor X (U/ml) | 0.21 ± 0.03 | 0.36 (0.25–0.64) | 0.41 (0.11–0.71) | 0.51 (0.19–0.83) | 0.4 (0.12–0.68) | 0.49 (0.19–0.79) |
| Factor XI (U/ml) | – | 0.23 (0.11–0.33) | 0.3 (0.08–0.52) | 0.41 (0.13–0.69) | 0.38 (0.1–0.66) | 0.55 (0.23–0.87) |
| Factor XII (U/ml) | 0.22 ± 0.03 | 0.25 (0.05–0.35) | 0.38 (0.1–0.66) | 0.39 (0.09–0.69) | 0.53 (0.13–0.93) | 0.47 (0.11–0.83) |
| Prekallikrein (U/ml) | – | 0.26 (0.15–0.32) | 0.33 (0.09–0.57) | 0.45 (0.26–0.75) | 0.37 (0.18–0.69) | 0.48 (0.2–0.76) |
| High-molecular-weight kininogen (U/ml) | – | 0.32 (0.19–0.52) | 0.49 (0.09–0.89) | 0.62 (0.24–1) | 0.54 (0.06–1.02) | 0.74 (0.16–1.32) |
| Factor XIIIa (U/ml) | – | – | 0.7 (0.32–1.08) | 1.01 (0.57–1.45) | 0.79 (0.27–1.31) | 0.94 (0.44–1.44) |
| Factor XIIIb (U/ml) | – | – | 0.81 (0.35–1.27) | 1.1 (0.68–1.58) | 0.76 (0.3–1.22) | 1.06 (0.32–1.8) |
| Plasminogen (U/ml) | – | – | 1.7 (1.12–2.48) | 1.91 (1.21–2.61) | 1.95 0.35 (44) | 2.17 ± 0.38 (60) |

SD, standard deviation.

*Source:* Modified from Andrew, M., Paes, B., & Johnston, M. (1990). Development of the hemostatic system in the neonate and young infant. *American Journal of Pediatric Hematology/Oncology*, *12*, 95–104. https://doi.org/10.1097/00043426-199021000-00019.

**TABLE 13.4**

## NORMAL BLOOD LEVELS OF COAGULATION INHIBITORS IN NEWBORNS (30 WEEKS' GESTATION TO TERM)

| Coagulation Inhibitors | 30–36 Weeks' Gestation | | Full Term | |
|---|---|---|---|---|
| | Day 1 Mean (boundary) | Day 5 Mean (boundary) | Day 1 Mean (boundary) | Day 5 Mean (boundary) |
| Antithrombin III (U/ml) | 0.38 (0.14–0.62) | 0.56 (0.3–0.82) | 0.63 (0.39–0.87) | 0.67 (0.41–0.93) |
| Alpha2-macroglobulin (U/ml) | 1.1 (0.56–1.82) | 1.25 (0.71–1.77) | 1.39 (0.95–1.83) | 1.48 (0.98–1.98) |
| C1 esterase inhibitor (U/ml) | 0.65 (0.31–0.99) | 0.83 (0.45–1.21) | 0.72 (0.36–1.08) | 0.90 (0.6–1.2) |
| Alpha1-antitrypsin (U/ml) | 0.9 (0.36–1.44) | 0.94 (0.42–1.46) | 0.93 (0.49–1.37) | 0.89 (0.49–1.29) |
| Heparin cofactor II (U/ml) | 0.32 (0.1–0.6) | 0.34 (0.1–0.69) | 0.43 (0.1–0.93) | 0.48 (0.1–0.96) |
| Protein C (U/ml) | 0.28 (0.12–0.44) | 0.31 (0.11–0.51) | 0.35 (0.17–0.53) | 0.42 (0.2–0.64) |
| Protein S (U/ml) | 0.26 (0.14–0.38) | 0.37 (0.13–0.61) | 0.36 (0.12–0.6) | 0.5 (0.22–0.78) |

*Source:* Modified from Andrew, M., Paes, B., & Johnston, M. (1990). Development of the hemostatic system in the neonate and young infant. *American Journal of Pediatric Hematology/Oncology, 12*, 95–104. https://doi.org/10.1097/00043426-199021000-00019.

**TABLE 13.5**

## NORMAL BLOOD LEVELS OF FIBRINOLYTIC COMPONENTS IN PREMATURE AND TERM NEWBORNS

| Fibrinolytic Component | Premature Infants | | Full-Term Infants | |
|---|---|---|---|---|
| | Day 1 Mean (boundary) | Day 5 Mean (boundary) | Day 1 Mean (boundary) | Day 5 Mean (boundary) |
| Plasminogen (U/ml) | 1.7 (1.12–2.48) | 1.91 (1.21–2.61) | 1.95 (1.25–2.65) | 2.17 (1.41–2.93) |
| Tissue plasminogen activator (ng/ml) | 8.48 (3–16.7) | 3.97 (2–6.93) | 9.6 (5–18.9) | 5.6 (4–10) |
| Alpha2-antiplasmin (U/ml) | 0.78 (0.4–1.16) | 0.81 (0.49–1.13) | 0.85 (0.55–1.15) | 1 (0.7–1.3) |
| Plasminogen activator inhibitor (U/ml) | 5.4 (0–12.2) | 2.5 (0–7.1) | 6.4 (2–15.1) | 2.3 (0–8.1) |

*Source:* Modified from Andrew, M., Paes, B., & Johnston, M. (1990). Development of the hemostatic system in the neonate and young infant. *American Journal of Pediatric Hematology/Oncology, 12*, 95–104. https://doi.org/10.1097/00043426-199021000-00019.

## INITIAL STEPS IN HEMOSTASIS

### Vascular Spasm

Initial hemostasis in a ruptured blood vessel consists of a vascular spasm resulting from multiple mediator interactions, nervous reflexes, and localized muscle spasm. Although nervous reflexes respond to pain, most vascular spasms are due to muscle contractions in the vessel wall secondary to direct injury. Vascular response to injury is present in an 8-week fetus and at term. It is equivalent to adult capillary fragility and bleeding time norms. This fact depends on gestational age, as evidenced by increased capillary fragility in preterm infants (Bagwell & Steward, 2020).

### Platelet Plug Formation

The second mechanism of hemostasis after vascular injury is platelet plug formation. Platelets meeting an injured vascular wall adhere to the wall and form a platelet plug. This hemostatic plug is the primary means of closing small vascular openings caused by the injury at the capillary and small-vessel levels. The platelets' ability to adhere on contact to a vascular wall requires a glycoprotein, von Willebrand factor (vWF), which is synthesized by vascular endothelial cells and megakaryocytes (Hall & Hall, 2020).

Platelets can also aggregate together to form large clumps. Aggregation is made possible by the platelet's small size, ability to modify its shape, and secrete many biochemical substances (platelet release reaction) that promote cohesion. When platelets and associated glycoproteins are activated by the excess release of these biochemical substances during stress, fibrinogen receptors appear on the platelet's surface, as seen in Figure 13.7. These receptors enhance the platelets' ability to bind fibrinogen, which cross-links the platelets, allowing them to aggregate. This provides a tight mesh or clot around an injured vessel, reducing the bleeding. After 32 weeks' gestation, average platelet counts are comparable to those of term infants and adults, but the ability of platelets to aggregate is relatively diminished. Understanding how fragile and premature some of the NICU patients are emphasizes the importance of care related to any invasive procedures that are necessary for these neonates.

### Coagulation

When bleeding cannot be controlled with a platelet plug, circulating plasma coagulation factors are triggered to form a network of fibrin that turns the existing plug into a hemostatic

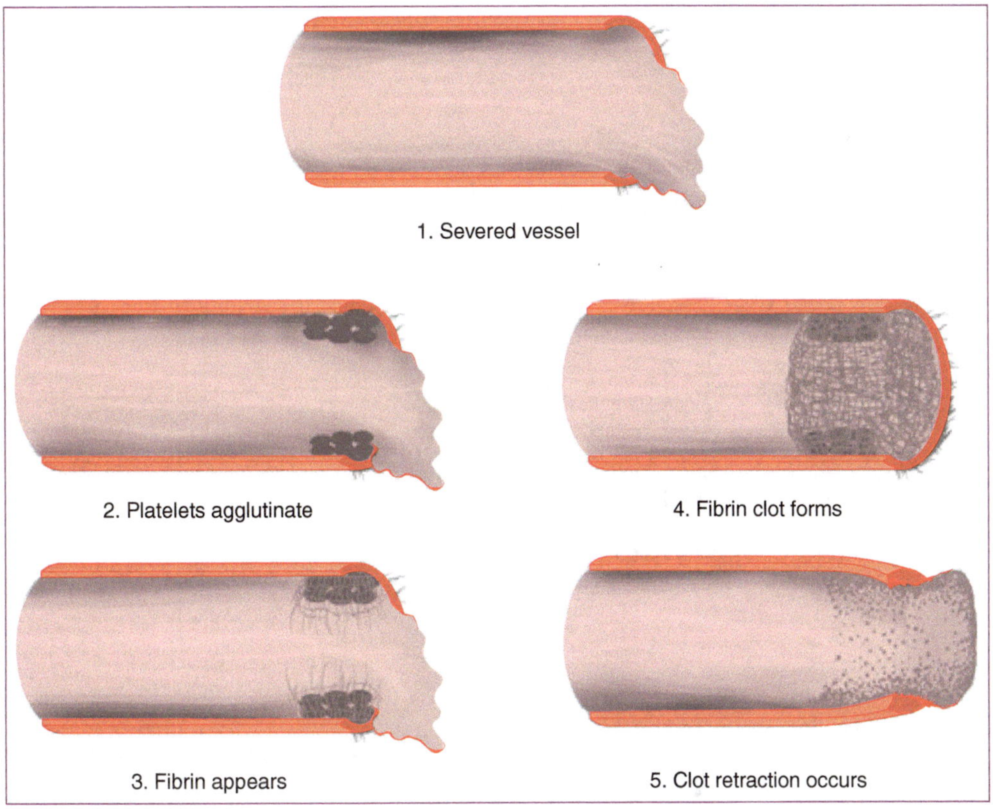


**FIGURE 13.7 When vessel wall injury occurs, the initial clotting process begins with forming a platelet plug.** Platelet activation stimulates fibrinogen receptors found on the surface of the platelets, which enhance their aggregation with other platelets and fibrinogen. The fibrin clot that forms retracts and occludes the damaged vascular wall.

*Sources:* Adapted from Hall, J. E. (2020). *Guyton and Hall textbook of medical physiology* (14th ed.). Elsevier; Witt, S. (1948). *Hemostatic agents.* Charles C. Thomas Publishers.

seal, which completes hemostasis. Fibrin threads, necessary for clot formation, can develop within 15 to 20 seconds in the presence of normal coagulation factors. Within 3 to 6 minutes after vascular rupture, the entire opening is occluded by a clot; within 30 to 60 minutes, the clot begins to retract, pulling the injured vascular portions together and further sealing the vascular end. This coagulation reaction involves several plasma proteins and three distinct phases: (1) formation of prothrombin activator, (2) activation of prothrombin to thrombin (formation of thrombin), and (3) conversion of soluble fibrinogen to fibrin (Hall & Hall, 2020).

**Phase I: Formation of Prothrombin Activator.** Prothrombin activator can be generated by two separate pathways: the intrinsic and extrinsic pathways. The intrinsic pathway is triggered by trauma or damage occurring inside the vessel or to the blood itself. The extrinsic pathway is triggered by the production of tissue thromboplastin generated by vessel wall damage. This bimodal pathway can be interrupted by a deficiency in platelets or any plasma coagulation factors or by the presence of inhibitors (anticoagulants) in the plasma. One of these pathways' complex and selective activation depends on the site, type, and injury severity.

Activation of the intrinsic pathway is slower because it lacks the major stimulus that the extrinsic pathway receives by the tissue thromboplastin release generated by vessel wall damage. The intrinsic pathway relies on blood trauma or injury within the vessel to alter platelets and plasma proteins and to convert dormant factors that are naturally found in circulating blood into active proteolytic enzymes (Figure 13.8). Each activated enzyme subsequently reacts with the succeeding factor, changing it into its activated form. The steps of *intrinsic* activation of coagulation are as follows:

1. An activator (blood trauma, injury within the vessel) activates Factor XII, converting it to Factor XIIa, while simultaneously damaging platelets, which causes a release of platelet phospholipids.
2. Factor XIIa, in conjunction with prekallikrein and high-molecular-weight kininogen, activates Factor XI, converting it to Factor XIa.
3. Factor XIa activates Factor IX, converting it to Factor IXa.
4. Factor IXa, platelet phospholipid, and Factor VIII combine to activate Factor X, converting it to Factor Xa.
5. Factor Xa combines with Factor V and platelet phospholipids to form prothrombin activator (prothrombinase), which releases thrombin from prothrombin. Calcium is required for this and the preceding two steps.

The extrinsic pathway can generate thrombin in seconds when an injury occurs outside the vascular space (Figure 13.9). Tissue thromboplastin (tissue factor), composed

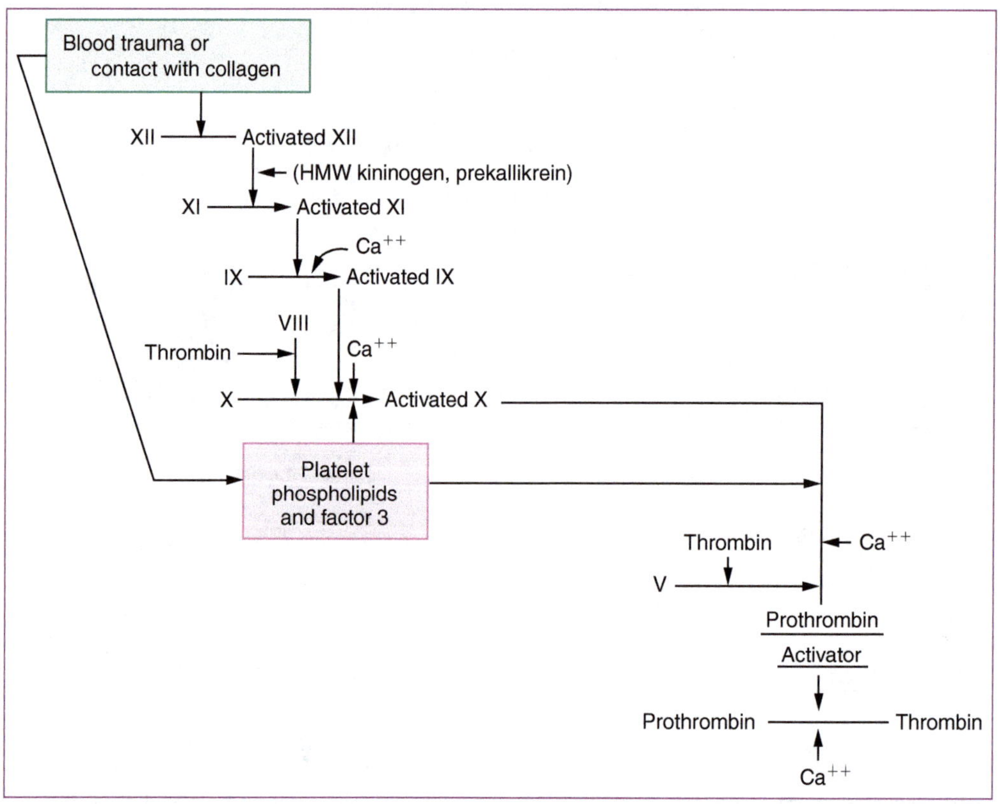


**FIGURE 13.8 The intrinsic pathway for initiating the clotting cascade is activated by trauma to the blood, injury within the vessel, or contact with collagen.**

HMW, high molecular weight.

*Source:* From Hall, J. E., & Hall, M. E. (2020). *Guyton and Hall textbook of medical physiology* (14th ed.). Elsevier.

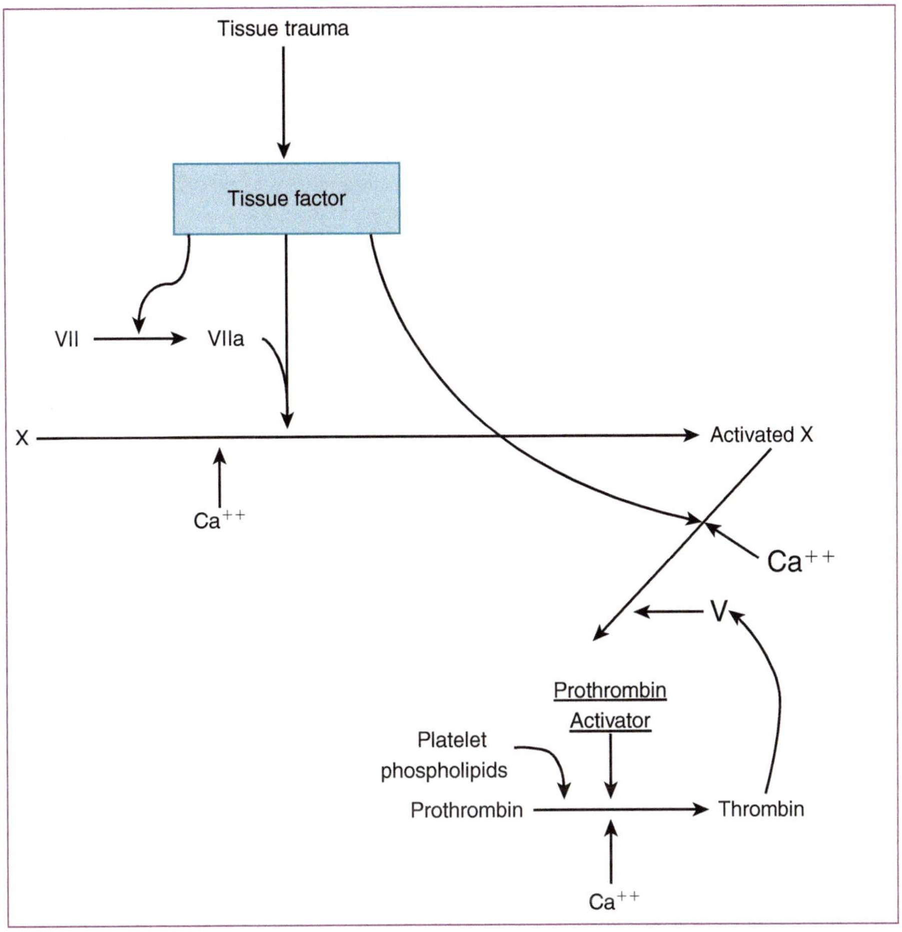


**FIGURE 13.9 The extrinsic pathway for initiating the clotting cascade can generate thrombin rapidly as a result of thromboplastin release from injured tissue.**

*Source:* From Hall, J. E., & Hall, M. E. (2020). *Guyton and Hall textbook of medical physiology* (14th ed.). Elsevier.

of glycoproteins and phospholipids, is produced when tissue is injured. When plasma encounters tissue thromboplastin, the initial intrinsic phases are bypassed, and an extrinsic pathway ensues as follows:

1. Tissue thromboplastin or tissue factor (Factor III) activates Factor VII to Factor VIIa. These two factors form a complex with glycoprotein in the presence of ionized calcium (tissue factor–Factor VIIa complex) that activates Factor X, converting it to Factor Xa.
2. In the presence of calcium, Factor Xa forms complexes with phospholipids and Factor V to form prothrombin activator.

From this point on, the intrinsic and extrinsic pathways are identical, with both proceeding to phase II.

**Phase II: Formation of Thrombin.** Prothrombin activator from either of the two pathways continues the clotting cascade by further influencing the breakdown of the unstable plasma protein prothrombin. Prothrombin (Factor II) is synthesized by the liver under the influence of vitamin K (VK), along with the other factors that form the prothrombin complex (Factors VII, IX, and X). When acted on by a prothrombin activator, prothrombin forms the potent coagulant thrombin. The newly formed thrombin stimulates the completion of the third and final coagulation phase. (Any factors missing or deficient during this process could alter the final clotting ability, such as Factor IX for hemophilia B type or refusal of VK. Please refer to the discussion later in this chapter.)

### Phase III: Fibrin Clot Formation

**Procoagulants.** Thrombin promotes the conversion of fibrinogen (Factor I), a protein produced by the liver, into fibrin by splitting off two peptides from the soluble fibrinogen molecule. This exposes two sites where other split fibrin molecules can cross-link, forming an insoluble fibrin chain. Fibrin stabilizing factor (Factor XIII, Hemophilia type A, the more severe types lack this or are deficient in this factor; please refer to discussions later in this chapter) further strengthens the tight bond of this developing fibrin mesh. Fibrin stabilizing factor is naturally found in the plasma and secreted by entrapped platelets. The forming fibrin clot begins to contract and retract with the help of platelets with actin-myosin action, the same action by which a muscle works. Extension of the clot into the surrounding circulating blood promotes further thrombosis. Thrombin from the clot can cleave prothrombin into more thrombin and enhance the production of prothrombin activator, thus acting as a potent biofeedback system for perpetuating the complex clotting cascade.

**Anticoagulants.** Throughout the entire coagulation pathway, the action of the activated enzymes is modulated at each stage by multiple and specific inhibitors (anticoagulants) so as not to lead to a hypocoagulable state. Consequently, coagulation balances coagulation factors and naturally occurring inhibitors/anticoagulants. Some of these anticoagulants are endothelial surface features that prevent coagulation until the vessel's endothelial wall is damaged. One such feature is the smoothness of the wall, preventing any adherence and subsequent activation, as well as the monomolecular layer of protein covering the wall, which repels plasma clotting factors and platelets.

Two inhibitors, alpha-1-antitrypsin, and C1 esterase inhibitor, interfere with the coagulation factors involved in the initial activation of the intrinsic pathway, as does Factor Xa despite its role in cleaving prothrombin into thrombin. Factor Xa rapidly binds with a tissue factor pathway inhibitor (TFPI) in the plasma. This complex, TFPI–Factor Xa, joins with the tissue factor–Factor VIIa complex to form a quaternary complex that inhibits further activation of Factor X by tissue factor (Bagwell & Steward, 2020).

Thrombin also acts as its inhibitor by stimulating the activation of protein C, which inactivates Factors V and VIII in the presence of another vitamin K--dependent inhibitor, protein S. A deficiency of these two proteins can cause neonatal thrombosis.

Other inhibitors of thrombin formation are: (a) fibrin threads created during clot formation, which absorb thrombin, thus removing it from circulation and eliminating its potential for further unnecessary or excess coagulation; (b) thrombomodulin, found on the endothelial surfaces of the body and in the plasma complexes with thrombin, which eliminates thrombin's ability to cleave fibrinogen; (c) alpha-2-macroglobulin (found in elevated levels in newborns), which inhibits proteases, including thrombin; (d) antithrombin III, which combines with thrombin, blocking the conversion of fibrinogen into fibrin; and (e) heparin cofactor II, which removes several activated procoagulants. Both antithrombin III and heparin are produced in the precapillary connective tissue of the lungs and liver (Albisetti & Monagle, 2021).

**Fibrinolysis.** Once a clot develops, it can be invaded by fibroblasts that lay down connective tissue throughout the clot, or it can dissolve. The dissolution process occurs by activating naturally occurring factors that lyse or break down the clot. Fibrinolysis is activated simultaneously with stimulation of the coagulation system, with powerful but inactivated anticoagulants built right into the clot. One of these anticoagulants, plasminogen, is manufactured by the liver, kidneys, and eosinophils. Under the influence of thrombin, activated Factor XII, tissue plasminogen activator (t-PA; located on the vascular endothelium), and urokinase plasminogen activator (u-PA; found in the urine), plasminogen is converted into plasmin, a proteolytic enzyme that breaks down fibrin into fibrin split products. Plasmin not only digests the fibrin chains but also deactivates fibrinogen; Factors V, VII, and XII; and prothrombin. Plasmin can be inactivated by its inhibitor, alpha-2-antiplasmin; its inhibitor can inactivate t-PA, plasminogen activator inhibitor-1.

In summary, both term and preterm newborns can create a balance between transitory deficiencies in the amount and function of various clotting factors, platelets, and anticoagulant factors. The homeostasis between clotting factors and anticoagulants places the newborn in a mildly hypercoagulable state at birth compared with older children and adults. Therefore, the newborn has no greater tendency to bleed but does have several differences regarding coagulation components and reserves, including gestational age–dependent variations in the concentrations of coagulation factors, anticoagulants, and fibrinolytics; shorter lifespan of components; and difficulty in quickly synthesizing any components (Albisetti & Monagle, 2021).

## ASSESSMENT OF HEMATOLOGIC FUNCTION

Because infants respond to a variety of problems similarly, many clinical findings (e.g., hypoglycemia, hypocalcemia, hypothermia, apnea, bradycardia, cyanosis, lethargy, poor feeding) warrant at least a complete blood count (CBC) to determine if a hematologic reason exists for these symptoms. With active bleeding, platelet counts, clotting studies (thrombin time, prothrombin time), fibrinogen levels, and measurements of products of fibrinolysis (e.g., D-dimer, fibrin split products, or fibrin degradation products) can shed light on the type of blood disorder potentially present and can direct the caregiver to the appropriate therapeutic response. These studies also provide a way to monitor and evaluate treatments. However, laboratory data are most helpful when used with clinical observation and physical assessment skills. Nurses play a vital role in recognizing early symptoms that may have hematologic etiologies.

Several physical findings can help determine the well-being and homeostasis of the hematologic system (Box 13.1). Abnormalities such as hematomas, abrasions, petechiae, and bleeding from the umbilical stump or gums should alert the nurse to the possibility of a hematologic abnormality. Hepatosplenomegaly can also indicate the abnormal breakdown of RBCs.

**BOX 13.1**

**PHYSICAL FINDINGS HELPFUL IN EVALUATING THE INTEGRITY OF THE HEMATOLOGIC SYSTEM**

Ecchymosis

Hematomas

Hepatosplenomegaly

Jaundice

Obvious blood loss—hemorrhage

Pallor

Petechiae

Plethora

Hepatosplenomegaly concurrent with hyperbilirubinemia and hemolysis can signal alloimmune problems (e.g., Rh and ABO incompatibilities) or acquired, congenital, or postnatal infection (e.g., cytomegalovirus [CMV], toxoplasmosis, herpes simplex virus [HSV] infection, or hepatitis). A bleeding disorder is discussed more in-depth later in the chapter.

## COMMON HEMATOLOGIC DISORDERS

### Blood Group Incompatibilities

Blood group incompatibilities were first recognized in the 1940s with the discovery of the Rh grouping and the first test for detecting antibody-coated RBCs, devised by Coombs in 1946. Please see the earlier discussion on Rh blood type and inheritance patterns. Before the introduction of Rh immune globulin (i.e., RhIgG, RhIG, RhoGAM, Rhophylac) in 1964 and its release for general use in 1968, Rh incompatibility accounted for one-third of all blood group incompatibilities. With the use of RhIgG, the frequency of Rh incompatibility has dropped significantly, and ABO has become the main blood group incompatibility, with sensitization occurring in 3% of all infants. Both incompatibilities involve maternal antibody response to fetal antigen, leading to fetal RBC destruction by hemolysis. Rh antibody response is elicited on exposure to antigen and does not exist spontaneously, whereas anti-A and anti-B antibodies occur naturally. These entities also differ in the severity of the effect on the fetus and newborn and in the treatment method.

Other minor blood groupings (e.g., Kell, C, E, Duffy, and Kidd) may also involve incompatibilities resulting in hyperbilirubinemia. Still, Rh and ABO incompatibilities are the most common, accounting for 98% of all cases. There are 400 known RBC antigens that can induce antibody production. Some of these antibodies are induced in response to the transfer of incompatible fetal blood cells into the maternal circulation during pregnancy. The Rh system alone has 40 discrete antigens, but only six (C, D, E, c, d, and e) are recognized as important. Maternal blood type is tested at an early prenatal visit; thus, if a mother receives proper prenatal care, common incompatibilities can be avoided in many cases (Bagwell & Steward, 2020).

### ABO Incompatibility

As discussed earlier in this chapter, the four major blood types are A, B, O, and AB, with the antibodies to the antigens of different blood types occurring naturally in the plasma (Table 13.2). Antigens or agglutinogens present on the fetal RBC surface of each blood type react with antibodies or agglutinins found in the maternal plasma of opposing blood types. Of the 30 common antigens involved in antigen–antibody reactions, the ABO antigens are one of two groups most likely to be a problem, the other being the Rh group (Hall & Hall, 2020).

With antigen and antibody in harmony, no RBC destruction occurs, but RBC destruction occurs when a conflicting antibody is introduced into the circulation. RBCs have multiple binding sites to which opposing antibodies can attach. An antibody can simultaneously attach to several RBCs, thus creating a clump of cells. This clumping of cells, known as *agglutination*, can cause occlusion of small vessels and impair circulation and tissue oxygenation. Fetal RBCs coated with antibodies attract phagocytes and macrophages that eventually destroy these agglutinated RBCs, usually through hemolysis by the reticuloendothelial cells in the spleen.

In a transfusion reaction, when conflicting blood types are mixed, the donor's RBCs are agglutinated, and the recipient's blood cells tend to be protected. The plasma portion of donor blood that contains antibodies becomes diluted by the recipient's blood volume, thus reducing donor antibody titers in the recipient's circulation. However, recipient antibody titers are adequate to destroy the donor RBCs by agglutination and hemolysis or by hemolysis alone. This describes the ABO incompatibility. In such cases, the maternal blood type is usually O, containing anti-A and anti-B antibodies in the serum, whereas the fetus or newborn is type A, B, or AB. Although incompatibility can occur between A and B types, it is not seen as frequently as O-A, O-B, or O-AB because of the globulin types of the antibodies. In the O-type mother, the antibodies are typically IgG, which cross the placenta, whereas type A or B mothers' antibodies are frequently IgM, which are too large to cross the placenta.

When transplacental hemorrhage (TPH) occurs between an ABO-incompatible mother and fetus, fetal blood entering the maternal circulation undergoes agglutination and hemolysis by maternal antibodies. This rapid response prevents the development of antibodies to other antigens present on fetal RBCs because a time lapse is required for activation of the immune system. Consequently, fetal RBCs that are Rh positive, in addition to being type A or type B, are destroyed by naturally occurring anti-A or anti-B antibodies before any maternal antibodies to Rh factor (anti-D) can be produced. This naturally occurring phenomenon is the basis for using RhIgG, in which extrinsic anti-D destroys fetal cells before the maternal immune system can produce antibodies (Fung-Kee-Fung et al., 2024).

Despite this destruction of fetal RBCs, maternal anti-A or anti-B antibodies of the IgG form can freely cross the placenta and adhere to the fetal RBCs. For this reason, ABO incompatibility can occur in the first pregnancy (40%–50% of total occurrences involve primigravidas) because TPH and inoculation of the mother with fetal blood are not necessary for the development of these naturally occurring antibodies. Because the A and B antigens on the fetal and neonatal RBCs are not well developed, only a small amount of maternal antibody attaches to the antigen. The resulting small amounts of IgG in the plasma do not stimulate activation of the complement system; hemolysis is minimal (Bagwell & Steward, 2020).

**Clinical Manifestations.** The chief symptom of ABO incompatibility is jaundice within the first 24 hours of life. Routinely, not every baby's blood type and Coombs tests (direct or indirect) are performed; however, when maternal blood type is O or Rh negative, the standard is to test the newborn to anticipate the potential early hyperbilirubinemia. The direct Coombs test measures the presence of antibodies on the RBC surface; the indirect Coombs test measures antibodies in the serum. Hemolysis and anemia are usually minimal, although signs of a mildly compensated hemolytic state are reflected in specific CBC values. There may be an elevated reticulocyte count (immature nucleated RBCs), and the peripheral blood smear may show evidence of spherocytes or RBCs lacking the normal biconcave, disclike shape of the normal RBC. The spherocytes appear thicker. These physical characteristics result in abnormal fragility under osmotic stress. Spherocytes are not distensible or compressible because they lack the normal amount of loose cell membrane, making them more susceptible to destruction in the splenic sinusoids.

On physical examination, hepatosplenomegaly can be observed, a reflection of extramedullary erythropoiesis generated by the fetus in response to significant hemolysis, which occurred chronically. To compensate for increased cell destruction, the liver and spleen manufacture RBCs for a more extended period than is usually seen in the fetus and newborn (please refer back to the earlier discussion in this chapter on erythropoiesis cite transition from the yolk sac to the bone marrow). Splenomegaly results from engorgement of the splenic sinusoids by hemolyzed RBCs.

**Treatment.** Because the antibodies involved in ABO incompatibility occur naturally, elimination of this type of incompatibility is virtually impossible. However, its effects on the fetus and newborn are much less dramatic and less life threatening than those of Rh incompatibility; therefore, amniocentesis and monitoring of amniotic fluid bilirubin levels, intrauterine transfusions, and early delivery are usually unnecessary. Nevertheless, problems associated with postnatal bilirubin clearance do arise, and phototherapy and possible exchange transfusion become part of the repertoire of care; therefore, a routine protocol to follow up for the hyperbilirubinemia is critical.

## Rh Incompatibility

Incompatibilities involving the Rh system are the second most common alloimmune problem, but the severity of complications far surpasses that of ABO incompatibility. Antibodies never occur naturally in the Rh system; exposure to the antigen is necessary to trigger the production of Rh antibodies. Such exposure occurs through maternal inoculation with fetal RBCs by TPH or through undetectable hemorrhage during labor, abortion, ectopic pregnancy, amniocentesis, chorionic villus sampling, or percutaneous fetal procedures. It cannot be overemphasized the critical need for a thorough prenatal history, which may identify risk factors for the development of ABO or Rh incompatibility that have gone undetected.

Spontaneous TPH allows fetal RBCs to pass into the maternal circulation, where antibodies develop in response to any conflicting RBC antigen the mother does not possess. The risk of immunization depends on the ABO status of both the mother and fetus and the size of the trophoblastic cells (TPC). Based on blood type, the risk for maternal Rh immunization in an ABO-compatible Rh-negative mother and Rh-positive fetus is 16%. In contrast, an ABO-incompatible pregnancy with a Rh-negative mother and Rh-positive fetus runs a 1.5% to 2% risk with each pregnancy. If the volume of TPH is less than 0.1 ml RBCs, the overall risk for immunization is 3%; if the hemorrhage is greater than 5 ml, the risk increases from 50% to 65%.

The maternal Rh antibody is slow to develop and initially may consist exclusively of IgM, which cannot cross the placenta due to the larger size. This is followed by the production of IgG, which can cross the placenta into the fetal circulation. The maximum concentration of the IgG form of antibody occurs within 2 to 4 months after termination of the first sensitizing pregnancy (Hall & Hall, 2020). Suppose initial immunization occurs shortly before or at the time of delivery; in that case, the first Rh-positive infant born to such a mother may trigger the initial antibody response in the mother, but this infant will not be affected. However, subsequent exposure to RBCs of Rh-positive fetuses produces a rapid antibody response in the mother (mostly IgG, which crosses the placenta). This response results in maternal antibody attachment to the fetal RBCs for the subsequent pregnancy. The affected RBCs undergo agglutination, phagocytosis, and eventually extravascular hemolysis in the spleen. The by-products of hemolysis, especially bilirubin, pass through the placenta into the maternal circulation to be metabolized and conjugated by the maternal liver. The rate of destruction of fetal RBCs depends on the amount of anti-D antibodies on the cells, the effectiveness of anti-D antibodies in promoting phagocytosis, and the capability of the spleen's reticuloendothelial system to remove antibody-coated cells. This explains why not all Coombs-positive infants display significant hemolysis and jaundice as dramatically as others.

## Erythroblastosis Fetalis

Fetal RBC hemolysis caused by Rh incompatibility results in the disease known as *erythroblastosis fetalis (EBF)*; significant consequences are anemia, hyperbilirubinemia, and perinatal death (Levine et al., 1941). The name is derived from the presence of immature circulating RBCs (erythroblasts) forced into the circulation of affected fetuses to compensate for rapidly destroyed fetal blood cells. (The Rh D–negative mother has become sensitized and thus, developed antibodies against the Rh D–positive antigens of fetal RBCs, which enter the fetal circulation to destroy fetal RBCs.) The severity of the disease depends on the degree of hemolysis and the ability of the fetus's developing erythropoietic system to counteract the ensuing anemia. To compensate for rapid destruction, the fetus continues to use extramedullary organs, such as the liver and spleen, which normally would have ceased RBC production after the seventh month of gestation. Because the RhIgG became available, with the improved early identification of maternal Rh D–negative status and proper administration of RhIgG to avoid maternal sensitization to fetal Rh D–positive status (Rh positive) over the years, the risk of D-immunization has decreased from 16% to less than 0.1%, reducing perinatal morbidity and mortality (Tobian & BenAvram, 2024). In regions where prenatal care is thorough, and the availability of RhIgG is sufficient, this condition is infrequently encountered today. However, it is not eradicated and requires awareness.

Formerly, RhIgG came from D-negative individuals who were sensitized after exposure to D-positive fetuses. Due to the enhanced use of RhIgG in D-negative mothers, decreasing the number of overall D-negative individuals who become sensitized, the number of individuals who can offer plasma to manufacture RhIgG decreased significantly, leading to RhIgG shortages. Various approaches have been made to secure RhIgG manufacturing, and the availability has met challenges.

In December of 2023, the Food and Drug Administration (FDA) reported shortages and associated concerns. The Association for the Advancement of Blood & Biotherapies recommends that institutions develop site-specific policies to prioritize their use, which are aligned with the recommendations by ACOG (Tobian & BenAvram, 2024).

**Clinical Manifestations.** The clinical manifestations of EBF are like those of ABO incompatibility but often are more intense. Jaundice results from an exaggerated rise in bilirubin due to the RBC destruction, with the premature infant exhibiting an earlier rise and a more prolonged period of elevation. Hepatosplenomegaly and varying degrees of hydrops may be found on physical examination (for overworking to compensate). Hydrops fetalis, a late sign, is a severe, total-body edema often accompanied by ascites and pleural effusions, which complicates the general condition, further affecting the cardiopulmonary status and other systems, leading to multisystem organ failure. Although the pathogenesis is not fully understood, it is thought to be the result of congestive heart failure and intrauterine hypoxia from severe anemia, portal and umbilical venous hypertension caused by hepatic hematopoiesis, and low plasma colloid osmotic pressure induced by hypoalbuminemia.

Altered hepatic synthesis can impair the production of vitamin K and vitamin K–dependent clotting factors, which predisposes infants to the likelihood of hemorrhage. Petechiae and prolonged bleeding from cord and blood sampling sites may be initial signs of clotting abnormalities. Transient hypoglycemia secondary to hyperplasia of the pancreatic islet cells is also associated with moderate to severe EBF. Products of RBC hemolysis are thought to inactivate circulating insulin, promoting increased insulin release and pancreatic beta-cell hyperplasia.

**Antenatal Therapy.** Adequate antenatal care is important in safeguarding the fetus that may be affected by EBF. The most recent recommendations include:

- All pregnant mothers should have blood group type and antibody screening completed at early prenatal visit after 8 weeks of gestation.
- Nonsensitized Rh D–negative mothers should receive 300 micrograms of Rho (D) immune globulin (RhIgG) at 28 weeks' gestation.
- Nonsensitized Rh D–negative mothers whose newborns are Rh D positive, an additional 120 to 300 mcg of RhIgG should be administered within 72 hours of delivery of the infant.
- When feto-maternal hemorrhage is confirmed, an increased dose of RhIgG may be recommended. (< 6 ml of fetal RBCs, 120 mcg versus if > 6–15 ml of fetal RBCs, 300 mcg). With hemorrhage over this amount, an additional 10 mcg should be added per additional 1 ml of fetal blood (Fung-Kee-Fung et al., 2024).

Potential obstetrical conditions occurring during the first or second trimester that may require RhIgG prophylaxis because they can increase the risk of sensitization by increasing the chances of TPH, are as follows:

- Therapeutic or spontaneous abortion of any type; the incidence of TPH is higher with therapeutic abortion (3 in 30 women may be sensitized)
- Any procedure that could cause TPH, such as an amniocentesis, chorionic villus sampling, or percutaneous umbilical sampling (risk is low when performed by an experienced professional)
- Ectopic pregnancies or hydatidiform moles
- Abdominal trauma
- Antepartum bleeding, as with placental abruption or placenta previa

Failure to administer RhIgG after such occurrences may leave these women at risk for sensitization.

**Treatment.** On delivery of an infant with EBF, assessment of the newborn's cardiorespiratory status is of utmost importance. Because of ascites, pleural effusions, and circulatory collapse, these infants often require airway stabilization by intubation and mechanical ventilation. If the circulating blood volume is low, anemia and volume depletion must be corrected. Nursing care requires heightened attention to the cardiorespiratory status and related ongoing and changing signs and symptoms. Laboratory findings are essential to be reviewed. Some laboratory data that are important to be obtained for any infants exhibiting the symptoms include the following:

- The mothers' and infants' blood and Rh types
- Coombs reactivity: The infant's RBCs are coated with anti-D antibodies, resulting in a positive direct Coombs test result; on occasion, the heavy coating of neonatal RBCs with antibody can lead to a false Rh typing (Rh negative); if the direct Coombs test result is positive, the infant should be considered Rh positive.
- The infant's hematocrit, reticulocyte count, and RBC morphologic characteristics: The presence of immature cells or spherocytes helps distinguish Rh incompatibility from ABO incompatibility.
- Plasma bilirubin levels: The initial cord-blood bilirubin level and the rate of rise determine the appropriate timing of any exchange transfusion needed to control bilirubin levels. Cord bilirubin levels are closely associated with the severity of the disease and the mortality rate.

## HYPERBILIRUBINEMIA

Bilirubin production begins as early as 12 weeks' gestation. Bilirubin is the final degradation product of hemoglobin, produced after completion of the natural life span of the RBC, coupled with immature erythropoiesis or premature destruction of blood cells, which can increase its production. The increased level of bilirubin causes visible jaundice. Hyperbilirubinemia or jaundice occurs in 80% of newborns at varying degrees. The American Academy of Pediatrics (AAP) published an updated Clinical Guideline for Management of Hyperbilirubinemia in 2022, replacing the previous recommendations published in 2004. The focus is placed on prevention, risk assessment, monitoring, and treatment of hyperbilirubinemia to avoid acute bilirubin encephalopathy and kernicterus, which is a permanent neurologic condition due to the unconjugated/free form of bilirubin crossing into the brain (Kemper et al., 2022).

## BRIEF BILIRUBIN PHYSIOLOGY

In RBC destruction, the aging or hemolyzed RBC membrane ruptures, releasing hemoglobin from the inside, which macrophages phagocytize. The hemoglobin molecule then splits into a heme and a globin portion. Bilirubin is derived from the degradation of the heme ring in the heme portion that heme oxygenase catalyzes. This unbound bilirubin (unconjugated or indirect) will bind to the albumin, which carries and transports the bilirubin to the liver, where the bilirubin becomes conjugated. Free bilirubin or unconjugated unbound bilirubin not attached to albumin can easily cross the blood–brain barrier, causing the damage seen in kernicterus.

The major route of fetal excretion of bilirubin is through the placenta (it is in the unconjugated form to pass through the placenta, and bilirubin production is noted as early as 12 weeks' gestation). In the newborn, the major routes of bilirubin excretion are through the intestine and the kidneys. The newborn liver plays a role in conjugating the albumin-bound transported bilirubin to excrete it through the intestine. When available albumin binding sites are saturated, or the albumin level is low, the binding sites are limited; bilirubin circulates freely in the plasma, thus increasing the free-flowing unconjugated bilirubin that can migrate into brain cells. The newborn liver's ability to conjugate is reduced during the first few days of life; however, a newborn can metabolize and process more than two-thirds of the bilirubin circulating in the body. As the production of bilirubin exceeds the newborn liver's capacity to conjugate and eliminate it, plasma levels of free bilirubin begin to rise, and jaundice becomes visibly noticeable (Bagwell & Steward, 2020).

When albumin-bound bilirubin reaches the liver, it is transferred across the cell membrane and into the liver cell. Two proteins, Y and Z, called *ligands*, affect bilirubin transfer from plasma to the liver. The bilirubin is either stored in the cell cytoplasm or removed from the ligands and conjugated in the hepatic endoplasmic reticulum. Conjugation is essential for the excretion of bilirubin into bile. Eighty percent of bilirubin is conjugated with glucuronic acid, becoming bilirubin glucuronide. Glucuronosyltransferase is the hepatic enzyme necessary to produce bilirubin glucuronide. Ninety-five percent of bilirubin glucuronide is excreted into bile and subsequently into the intestine (Bagwell & Steward, 2020).

Effective excretion of bilirubin from the intestine depends on the time needed to pass stool and the presence of substances that break down conjugated bilirubin. The newborn may have diminished bowel motility and delayed meconium passage, allowing more prolonged stool exposure to bilirubin glucuronidase. The action of this enzyme, in conjunction with the newborn's lack of the intestinal flora required to reduce bilirubin to urobilinogen, converts the conjugated form back to the unconjugated form, which is then reabsorbed by the intestine and enters the enterohepatic circulation where it returns to the liver for conjugation.

### Kernicterus

Kernicterus is a chronic and preventable form of acute bilirubin encephalopathy. The exact incidence of kernicterus is unknown, and it is known to vary among various global regions. One study in a large health system reviewed cases of severe hyperbilirubinemia among births ≥ 35 weeks' gestation from 1995 to 2011 ($n$ = 525409) and identified 47 infants who experienced ≥ 30 mg/dl total serum bilirubin (8.6 per 100,000 births) (Kuzniewicz et al., 2014). The recommendations when risk factors and follow-up assessment were implemented at a health systemwide scale (116 hospitals, $n$ = 1028817), cases/incidence of dangerous total serum bilirubin level > 30 mg/dl decreased significantly from 9 to 3 per 100,000 births (Mah et al., 2010). Another large health system also reported a decrease of serum total bilirubin ≥ 25 mg/dl among births ≥ 35 weeks from 65 to 24 per 100,000 births by adopting the screening and follow-up guidelines (18 hospitals, $n$ = 101272) (Eggert et al., 2006). These reports suggest the importance of systematic bilirubin screening and adherence to recommended guidelines to prevent kernicterus globally (Kemper et al., 2022).

The early signs of acute encephalopathy include lethargy or irritability and poor eating or alterations in muscle tone, in addition to increasingly severe jaundice. Kernicterus is permanent damage characterized by some or all of the following: cerebral palsy, upward gaze paresis, enamel dysplasia of deciduous teeth, sensorineural hearing loss, auditory neuropathy, dyssynchrony spectrum disorder, and specific known findings on brain magnetic resonance imaging (MRI). The risk for kernicterus increases as serum total bilirubin rises above 20 mg/dl, with the highest risk associated with serum levels above 30 mg/dl (Kemper et al., 2022).

Certain risk factors can influence bilirubin binding to albumin and increase the risk of kernicterus at lower bilirubin levels, including the following:

- Premature infants commonly experience relative hypoproteinemia and have fewer albumin-binding sites available for free bilirubin.
- Premature infants have shorter RBC lifespans, which increases the destruction of RBCs, leading to an increase in circulating bilirubin.
- The presence of other substances competing for available binding sites: Certain drugs (e.g., sulfonamides, cephalosporins, penicillins, salicylates, sodium benzoate) compete with bilirubin for binding sites or displace bilirubin loosely attached to binding sites. Of note, ibuprofen was found to displace bilirubin, raising unbound levels during in-vitro studies.
- Acidosis and hypoxia: Increased production of hydrogen ions and implementation of anaerobic metabolism can impede bilirubin binding. Albumin's ability to bind bilirubin drops to half its potential at a serum pH of 7.1 (Bagwell & Steward, 2020).

### Increased Red Blood Cell Breakdown

Excessive RBC destruction also occurs in neonatal bacterial and viral infections and intrauterine viral infections, especially those of the TORCH complex (toxoplasmosis, other agents, rubella, CMV, and HSV), have been implicated in the hemolytic destruction of RBCs. Other conditions prevalent in premature and term newborns can result in the extravasation of large amounts of blood (e.g., significant bruising, cephalohematoma, and pulmonary or intracerebral hemorrhages). These extravascular collections of blood cells increase the bilirubin load on a metabolically immature neonatal liver. This increased load often results in hyperbilirubinemia in the newborn and requires further assessment and risk-based vigilant screening.

## Interference With Bilirubin Conjugation

**Abnormal Bilirubin Excretion.** Any disease state resulting in abnormal bilirubin excretion can raise serum bilirubin levels significantly. This is seen in hepatic dysfunction secondary to such entities as hypoxia or asphyxia, bowel obstruction, ileus, and congestive heart failure. These conditions tend to elevate both the conjugated and unconjugated bilirubin levels. The diminished bowel motility associated with these conditions lengthens the time during which beta-glucuronidase, naturally present in the gut, can act on conjugated bilirubin in the stool. This enzymatic reaction converts conjugated bilirubin into the unconjugated form, which is reabsorbed into the intravascular compartment through the enterohepatic circulation. Any hepato-cellular damage associated with cholestasis and bacterial and viral infections can further impair the liver's ability to conjugate bilirubin (Bagwell & Steward, 2020).

**Breastmilk.** Feeding support will be further discussed under the prevention strategies aligned with the new hyperbilirubinemia management guideline, which will be presented in more depth later.

Breastmilk composition itself plays a role. Two substances found in breastmilk, pregnanediol, and nonesterified fatty acids, interfere with bilirubin conjugation or increase enterohepatic circulation, resulting in resorption of bilirubin from the intestine and elevating the overall bilirubin level as described previously. Typically described as "breastfeeding jaundice," it occurs in place of adequate volume intake, and this type of jaundice and hyperbilirubinemia may persist for as long as 3 months. This nonpathologic jaundice does not cause severely high levels of bilirubin. When reaching nearly 1 month of age, one study found these infants to have safe levels of hyperbilirubinemia with 34% $\geq$ 5 mg/dl, 9% $\geq$ 10 mg/dl, and 1% $\geq$ 12.9 mg/dl (Kemper et al., 2022).

## Revised AAP Clinical Guideline for Hyperbilirubinemia Management

The updated AAP clinical guideline for the management of hyperbilirubinemia in the newborn infant 35 or more weeks of gestation is the primary foundation for the evidence-based clinical guidance presented in this chapter (Kemper et al., 2022). The important pillars of this guideline include prevention, risk assessment, monitoring, and treatment.

### Prevention of Hyperbilirubinemia

It is important to prioritize prevention. Because hemolytic disease causes significant hyperbilirubinemia, often in a severe form, prevention must ideally begin during the pregnancy to identify mothers who are at risk for developing antibodies against their unborn child's RBC antigens. ABO typing and Rh status are critical information to avoid erythroblastosis fetalis or any ABO incompatibility.

Please follow the guidance in Figure 13.10.

Prevention also includes feeding support to prevent infants from developing exaggerated hyperbilirubinemia due to suboptimal intake. Breastfed infants' hyperbilirubinemia, which peaks at 3 to 5 days of age, is often inaccurately described as breastmilk jaundice, simply due to the intake being exclusively breastmilk. These situations are often accompanied by moderate to significant weight loss, indicating inadequate or suboptimal volume intake. Decreased intake also leads to dehydration and reduced stooling, which causes increased intestinal reabsorption of bilirubin back into the intrahepatic

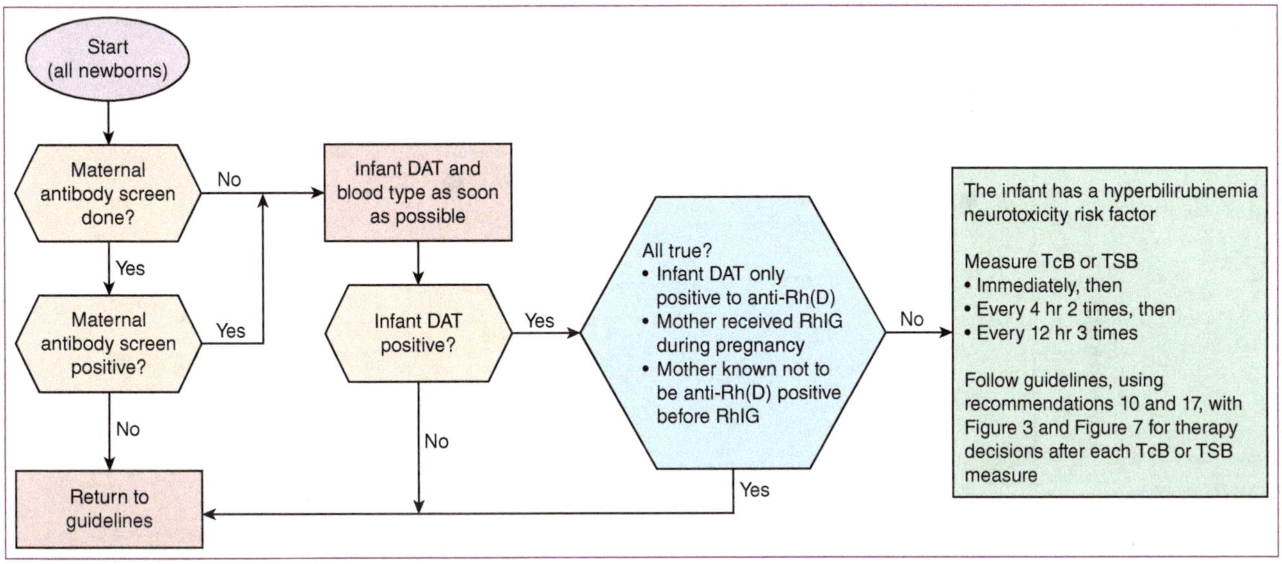


**FIGURE 13.10 Approach to identify newborns with maternal anti-erythrocyte antibodies and to guide early management.**

*Source:* From Kemper, A. R., Newman, T. B., Slaughter, J. L., Maisels, M. J., Watchko, J. F., Downs, S. M., Grout, R. W., Bundy, D. G., Stark, A. R., Bogen, D. L., Holmes, A. V., Feldman-Winter, L. B., Bhutani, V. K., Brown, S. R., Maradiaga Panayotti, G. M., Okechukwu, K., Rappo, P. D., & Russell, T. L. (2022). Clinical practice guideline revision: Management of hyperbilirubinemia in the newborn infant 35 or more weeks of gestation. *Pediatrics, 150*(3), e2022058859. https://doi.org/10.1542/peds.2022-058859.

circulation. Some recommendations include encouraging early feeding within an hour of birth and feeding at least eight times a day. Adequate hydration prevents significant hyperbilirubinemia. Oral provision of supplemental water or dextrose to decrease bilirubin concentration is not recommended either as a prevention or treatment strategy (Kemper et al., 2022).

### Risk Assessment

The identification of any risk factors is highly important, and the nurse's role is paramount. This section discusses some of the risk factors for hyperbilirubinemia; however, this is not an exhaustive list. Lower gestational age, including those who are termed late preterm infants (risk increases with each week that the infant does not advance toward full term; Stewart et al., 2019), those who become visibly jaundiced within 24 hours of birth, those with any skin injury, birth injury (e.g., hematoma, bruising) that would increase hemolysis, family history of exchange transfusion or phototherapy, any hereditary component that may suggest any RBC disorder (e.g., glucose-6-phosphate dehydrogenase [G6PD] deficiency), exclusive but suboptimal intake of breastfeeding, large for gestational age (LGA) infants, infants of diabetic mothers (IDMs), and infants with Down syndrome are risk factors. Risk factors are identified through observation, examination, laboratory results review, and thorough history taking. G6PD deficiency has been recognized as one of the most important causes of hazardous levels of hyperbilirubinemia with risk of kernicterus not only in the United States but globally. Even in an earlier U.S. study that explored the etiologies of infants with dangerous levels of total bilirubin ≥ 30 mg/dl, G6PD deficiency was a significant factor (Al-Bedaywi et al., 2024; Kuzniewicz et al., 2014).

### G6PD deficiency and Its Significance

G6PD deficiency is an X-linked recessive enzymatic disorder, one of the most common enzyme disorders known to humans. The G6PD enzyme protects the RBCs from oxidative stress and prevents intravascular hemolysis. When individuals are deficient in the G6PD enzyme, they are prone to hemolysis, and infants may have an acute rise, early or late onset, in the bilirubin. The prevalence of G6PD is more common in Sub-Saharan Africa (SSA), the Middle Eastern region, the Mediterranean, the Arabian Peninsula, and Southeast Asia. The prevalence of individuals with G6PD deficiency varies, yet it has been reported to be as high as 25% in some regions. Eleven to thirteen percent of Black males are affected by this condition, and 24% are carriers. In comparison, 4% of Black females are thought to be affected by G6PD deficiency (Al-Bedaywi et al., 2024; Kemper et al., 2022). With the increased migration of the worldwide population from one region to another, an ethnicity/race/genetic ancestry–conscious approach to practice has become more critical than ever. Because G6PD level can be falsely normal when the blood sample is obtained during or soon after a hemolytic event or if the infant already had an exchange transfusion, the recommendation is G6PD follow-up at least 3 months later when G6PD deficiency is suspected, but the initial results are normal (Kemper et al., 2022).

### Monitoring

Serum total bilirubin (STB) should be the definitive test rather than visual estimation alone, although visual assessment is a critical screening mode. Every newborn infant must be visually assessed for presence or jaundice every 12 hours after birth throughout the infant's stay. If visual assessment recognizes jaundice within 24 hours of birth, total serum bilirubin (TSB) or transcutaneous bilirubin (TcB) measurement should be completed immediately. The results should be plotted against the graph (Figures 13.11–13.15) to determine if the level is appropriate for the gestational age and hours since birth and is if the TSB or TcB is approaching the phototherapy threshold or exceeds its. Most facilities have implemented safeguards, and many well-baby care settings have a "24-hour lab order" that is incorporated into the

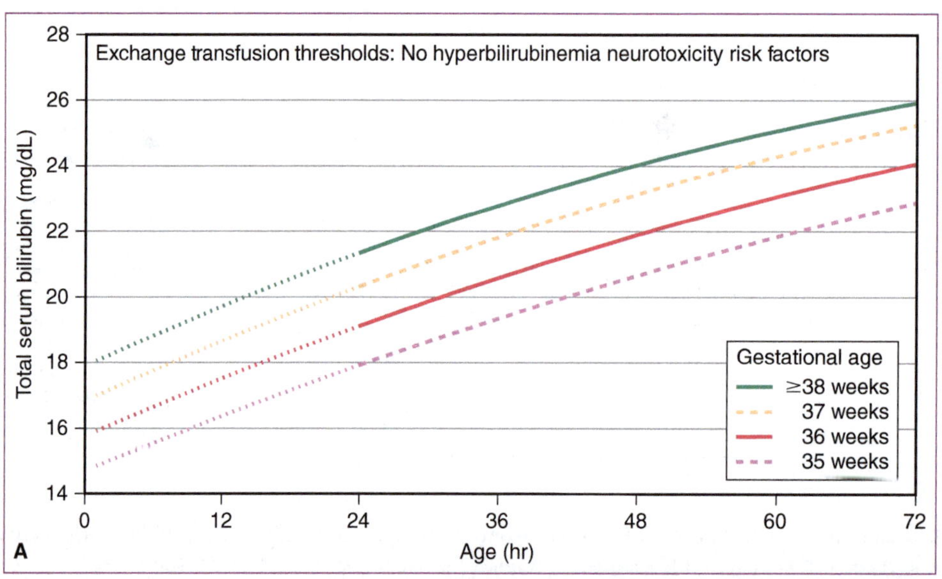


**FIGURE 13.11** (A). Phototherapy thresholds by gestational age and age in hours for infants with no recognized hyperbilirubinemia neurotoxicity risk factors other than gestational age up to 72 hours of age. (B). Phototherapy thresholds by gestational age and age in hours for infants with no recognized hyperbilirubinemia neurotoxicity risk factors other than gestational age from 3 to 14 days.

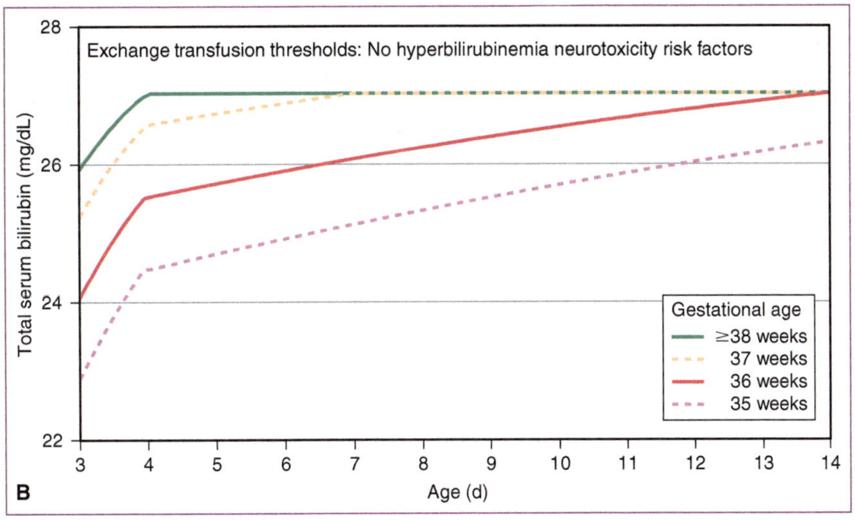


**FIGURE 13.11** *(continued)*

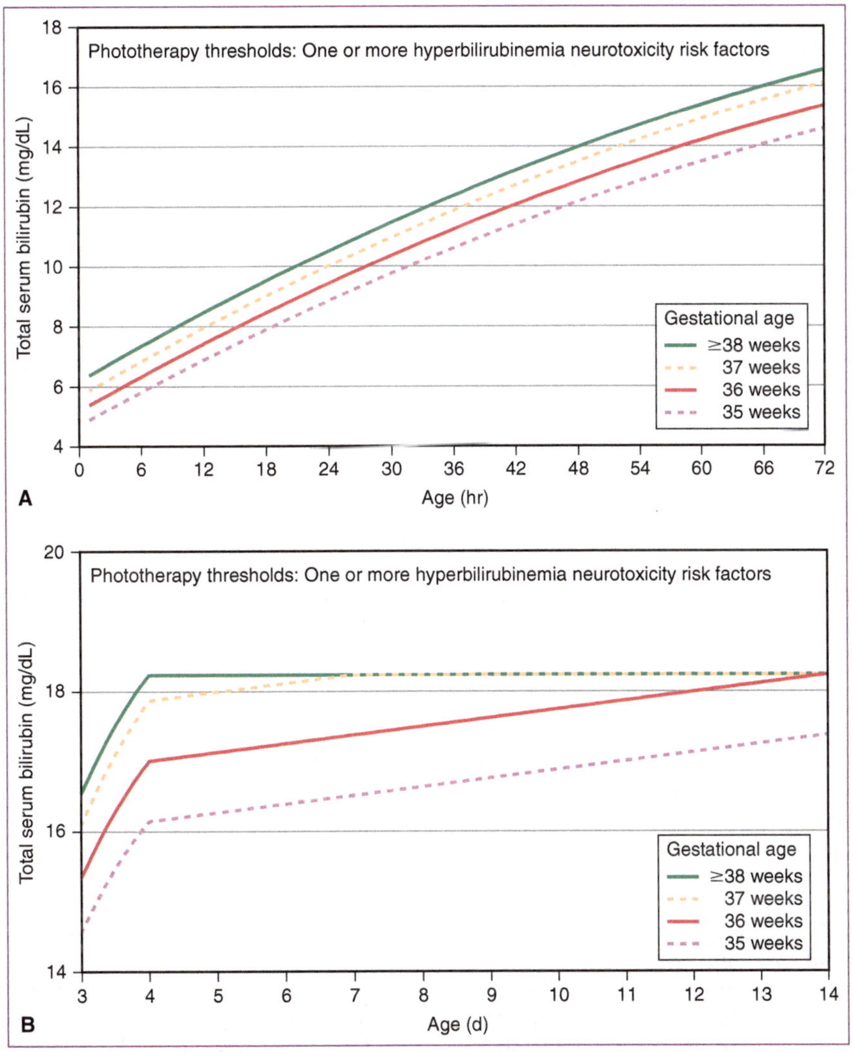


**FIGURE 13.12** (A). Phototherapy thresholds by gestational age and age in hours for infants with any recognized hyperbilirubinemia neurotoxicity risk factors other than gestational age up to 72 hours of age. (B). Phototherapy thresholds by gestational age and age in hours for infants with any recognized hyperbilirubinemia neurotoxicity risk factors other than gestational age 3 to 14 days.

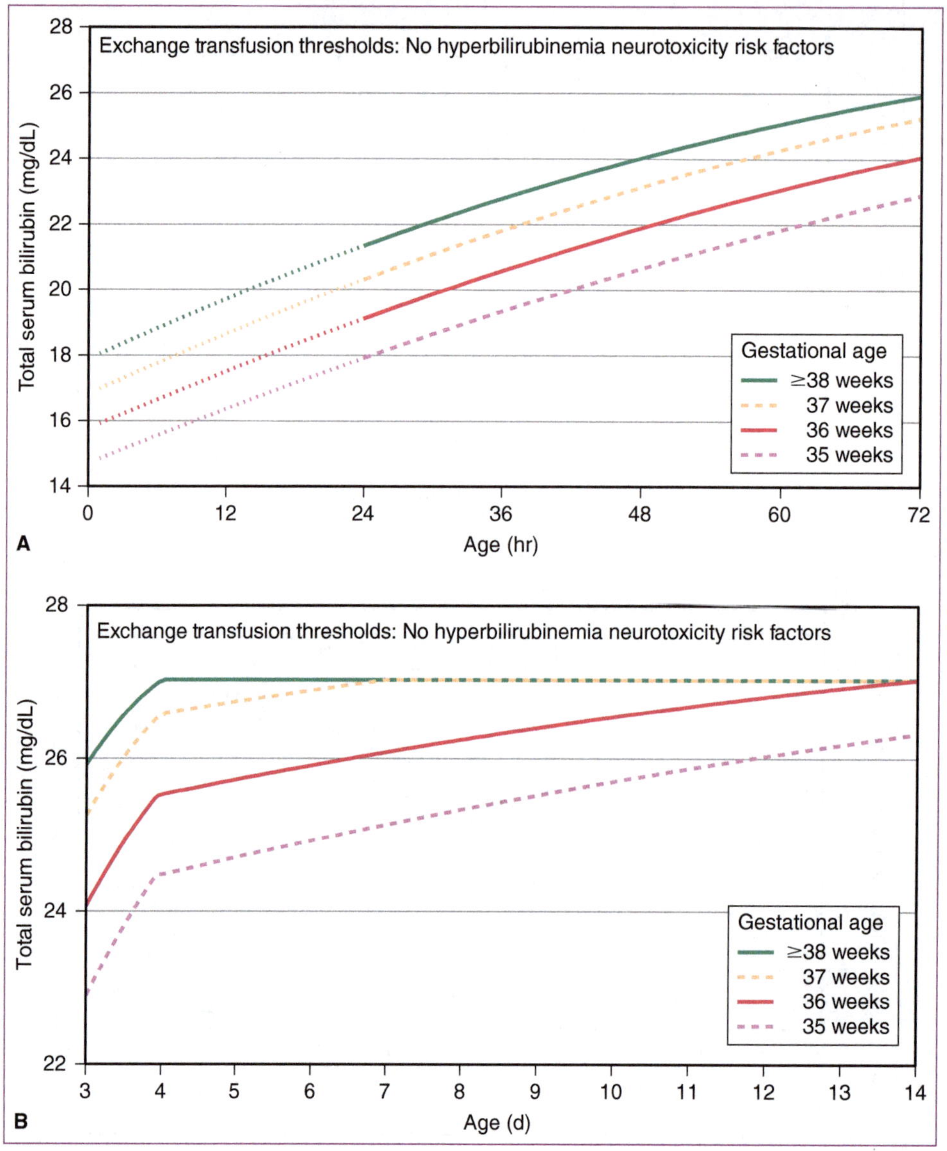


**FIGURE 13.13 (A). Exchange transfusion thresholds by gestational age for infants with no recognized hyperbilirubinemia neurotoxicity risk factors other than gestational age from birth to 72 hours. (B). Exchange transfusion thresholds by gestational age for infants with no recognized hyperbilirubinemia neurotoxicity risk factors other than gestational age from 3 to 14 days.**

admission order, where the STB and newborn screening test can be completed at the same time. It is important to review the institutional practice to ensure that a monitoring system is in place and risk assessment components are routinely included in infant information that nurses collect and document.

TcB is reported to have a sufficient correlation with TSB. However, it is known that some instruments may over- or underestimate the TSB when infants have greater skin melanin concentration. TSB is the definitive test. TSB is necessary if the TcB indicates a level exceeding the phototherapy level, or it is very close (< 3 mg/dl below) to the threshold. If TcB shows a level of ≥ 15 mg/dl, TSB is immediately warranted. The rate of increase in the bilirubin is also an important indicator to identify high-risk infants. A rapid rate is ≥ 0.3 mg/dl/hr during the first 24 hours and ≥ 0.2 mg/dl/hr post-24 hours.

In summary, the decision of when to initiate treatment is based on the gestational age, hours of age since birth, and any neurotoxicity risk factors that are identified. The AAP guideline specifically provides the risk factors for hyperbilirubinemia neurotoxicity as the following: (a) gestational age < 38 weeks; (b) albumin level < 3.0 g/dl; (c) isoimmune hemolytic disease (DAT positive), G6PD deficiency, or any other hemolytic condition; (d) sepsis; and (e) significant clinical instability during the previous 24 hours (Kemper et al., 2022). In assessing the infant's TSB or TcB, if the infant has any of these neurotoxicity risk factors, use the graph set that offers lower

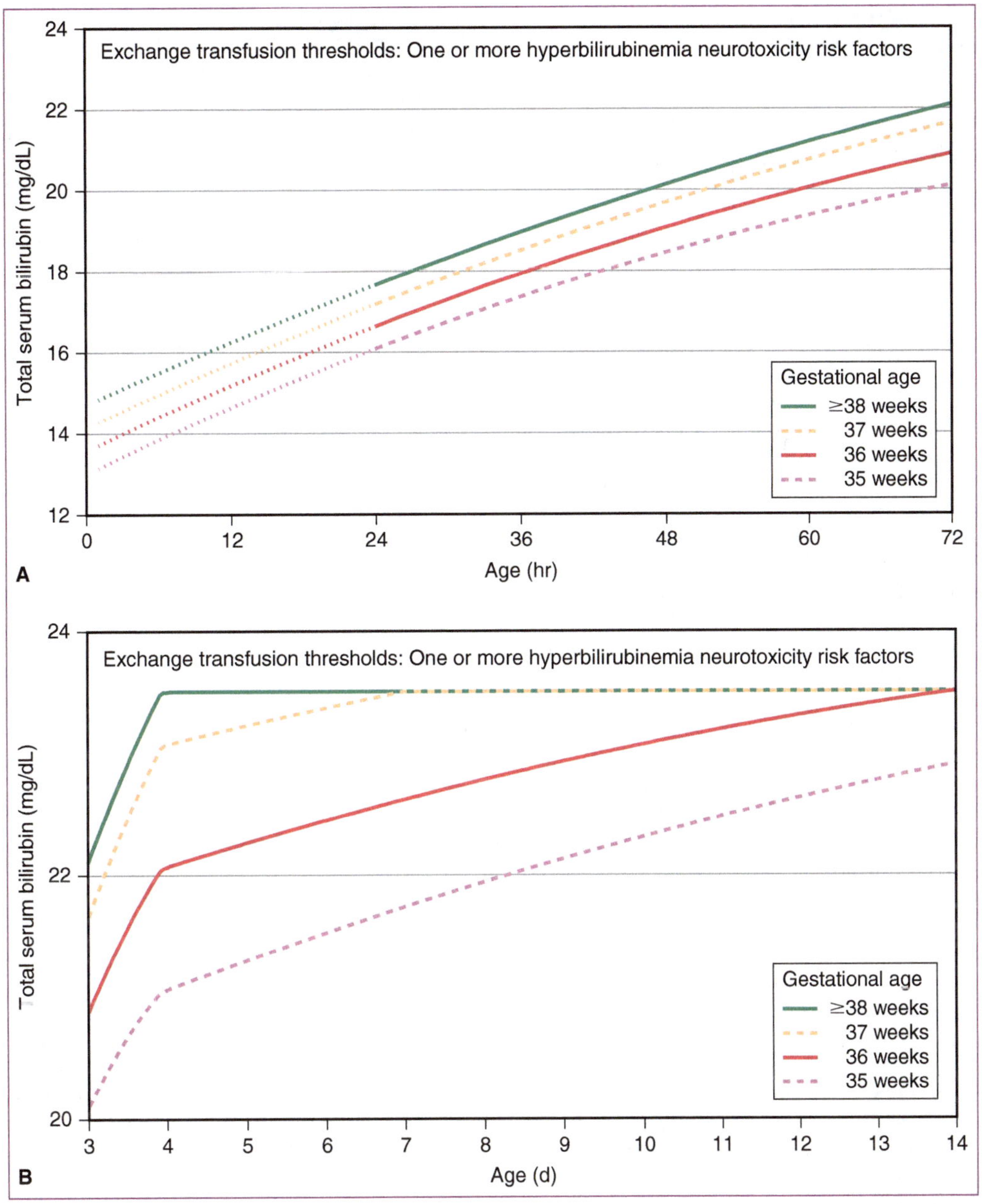


**FIGURE 13.14 (A). Exchange transfusion thresholds by gestational age for infants with any recognized hyperbilirubinemia neurotoxicity risk factors other than gestational age from birth to 72 hours. (B). Exchange transfusion thresholds by gestational age for infants with any recognized hyperbilirubinemia neurotoxicity risk factors other than gestational age from 3 to 14 days.**

phototherapy or exchange transfusion thresholds considering the risk factors (Figures 13.12 and 13.14). If no neurotoxicity is recognized, then refer to Figures 13.11 and 13.13.

## Follow-Up Monitoring

Newborns may be discharged early when the TSB is still below the phototherapy threshold, but it is still likely rising, suggesting that it would peak after the infant is home. How soon to plan the follow-up monitoring depends on how close the TSB is to the phototherapy threshold (Kemper et al., 2022). Individual facilities or care settings must have a coordinated monitoring system in collaboration with the healthcare providers/workers in the community when infants are discharged early because follow-up monitoring is still required. Infants' feeding status (optimal or suboptimal), stooling pattern, and weight are all important data at the time of discharge to determine the speed of follow-up bilirubin monitoring and parent education topics. Parents today can easily photograph their infant to note the skin color (visible jaundice level) or to recognize that the sclera of the eyes is not yellow at the time of discharge. Therefore, parents can realize visible changes to alert them. Parents are also informed of the critical need for optimal feeding during this period.

## Treatment of Hyperbilirubinemia: Phototherapy, Medication, and Exchange Transfusion

### Treatment: Phototherapy

When to begin phototherapy, according to the guideline, is based on the gestational age of the infant, the hours of life since birth, and any presence of hyperbilirubinemia neurotoxicity risk factors as previously mentioned. Once the TSB is recognized as reaching the phototherapy threshold or closely approaching the threshold, phototherapy is initiated. Phototherapy reduces the bilirubin level by converting the unconjugated bilirubin into a water-soluble form by several photochemical reactions such as photooxidation and photoisomerization to allow a direct excretion of bilirubin without hepatic metabolism. Photooxidation is the oxidation of bilirubin pigment, which is deposited in the skin, and converts the pigments into a colorless form that can be excreted in the urine. Photoisomerization is another function and it converts the bilirubin polymers in the skin into excretable isomers (Thomas & Abiramalatha, 2021)

The effectiveness of phototherapy depends on the intensity and quality of the light and how well the surface area of the infant's skin is exposed to the phototherapy light. Equipment differs from type to type, but it is important to expose the infant's surface area as much as possible. Intense phototherapy that reduces TSB more quickly while shortening the treatment time requires LED blue light (narrow-spectrum type with irradiance minimum of 30 μW/cm$^2$/nm at a wavelength of 475 nm). Light with a wavelength below 460 nm and above 490 nm may pose potential harm because unnecessary heat is generated. The primary objective of phototherapy is to reduce the likelihood of escalation of care to an exchange transfusion and protect the infants from developing harmful effects of hazardous TSB levels (Kemper et al., 2022).

**Home Phototherapy.** The guideline offers guidance on hyperbilirubinemia management for infants whose TSB level rises to the phototherapy threshold after going home. The decision must be made based on the region; however, following are specific criteria for home phototherapy with an LED-based phototherapy device: (a) gestational age ≥ 38 weeks; (b) ≥ 48 hours old; (c) clinically well with adequate volume intake; (d) no neurotoxicity risk factors; (e) no history of previous phototherapy; (f) TSB is no more than 1 mg/dl above the phototherapy threshold (if significantly higher, inpatient monitoring is necessary); (g) home use device that is appropriate is available; and (h) ongoing TSB monitoring is possible every day (Kemper et al., 2022).

In any transition to home situation, caregivers must carefully evaluate each infant's case, including the home situation, parental confidence/compliance, and overall psychosocial factors, to determine the infant's safety. If the infant is not feeding well, intravenous (IV) fluids must be established, and immediate hospitalization frequently ensues.

**Nursing Care of Infants Under Phototherapy.** For optimum therapy, phototherapy units should be checked for adequacy of light levels. Eye shields must be used to protect the infants' eyes from exposure to phototherapy lights, which may cause retinal damage. Phototherapy units and eye protection should be removed for short periods throughout the day to provide the infant with visual stimulation and developmentally appropriate interactions with the parents and caregivers. Infants undergoing phototherapy require all the standard care, such as monitoring the vital signs and assessment of general condition, including robustness for feeding or intake and output (voiding and stooling). Infants exhibit the following with acute bilirubin encephalopathy: hypertonia, arching, retrocollis (a form of cervical dystonia that leads to muscle contractions that make the neck extend backward), opisthotonos (head and heel bend backward and back is rigid and arches), and a high-pitched cry or apnea. Therefore, physical and overall assessment is highly important.

Premature, low birth weight (LBW), or SGA infants require more vigilance for temperature control and benefit from warmer or closed incubators to avoid hypothermia. Adequate fluid intake and compensatory fluid adjustments for increased insensible water and stool loss may be required to prevent dehydration in very small infants. Because phototherapy lights can alter blood bilirubin results, the lights should be turned off when drawing blood for a serum bilirubin check. When reporting the bilirubin levels to providers, the next STB must be discussed. If the TSB is high enough for phototherapy but not high enough for exchange transfusion, multiple phototherapy lights are used, and follow-up TSB is ordered within 4 to 6 hours or even 2 hours to assess the need for escalation of care.

When care escalation is anticipated, requiring exchange transfusion (TSB is 2 mg/dl below the exchange transfusion threshold), a decision must be made promptly to ensure that infants can be transferred to a setting where a higher level of neonatology care is available. The role of nurses in recognizing and communicating with the providers is essential.

### Treatment: Medication

IV immune globulin (IVIG) administration has been used, especially for Rh hemolytic disease, which causes significant hyperbilirubinemia; however, its efficacy has not been fully established (Wolf et al., 2020). Association of IVIG with harmful conditions has also been described (e.g., NEC); however, the 2022 AAP guideline does recognize the role of IVIG for infants who have positive DAT and for whom isoimmune hemolytic disease is causing significant hyperbilirubinemia (IVIG: 0.5–1 g/kg over 2 hours) (Kemper et al., 2022). Decisions are made for each situation by the clinicians/providers by weighing various factors. If the infant is far from any NICU where an exchange transfusion can be performed and transfer cannot be easily coordinated in a timely fashion, or excessive hemolysis is evident, priority must be carefully weighed to protect the infant from acute encephalopathy or kernicterus.

### Treatment: Exchange Transfusion

In today's NICU, thanks primarily to the dissemination of hyperbilirubinemia management guidelines, exchange transfusions are not performed frequently compared to the past from decades ago; exchange transfusion may be necessary if bilirubin levels start to approach levels threatening kernicterus despite phototherapy. The 2022 AAP guideline defines the escalation-of-care threshold as when TSB is 2 mg/dl below the exchange transfusion and states that the escalation-of-care is a medical emergency that requires immediate

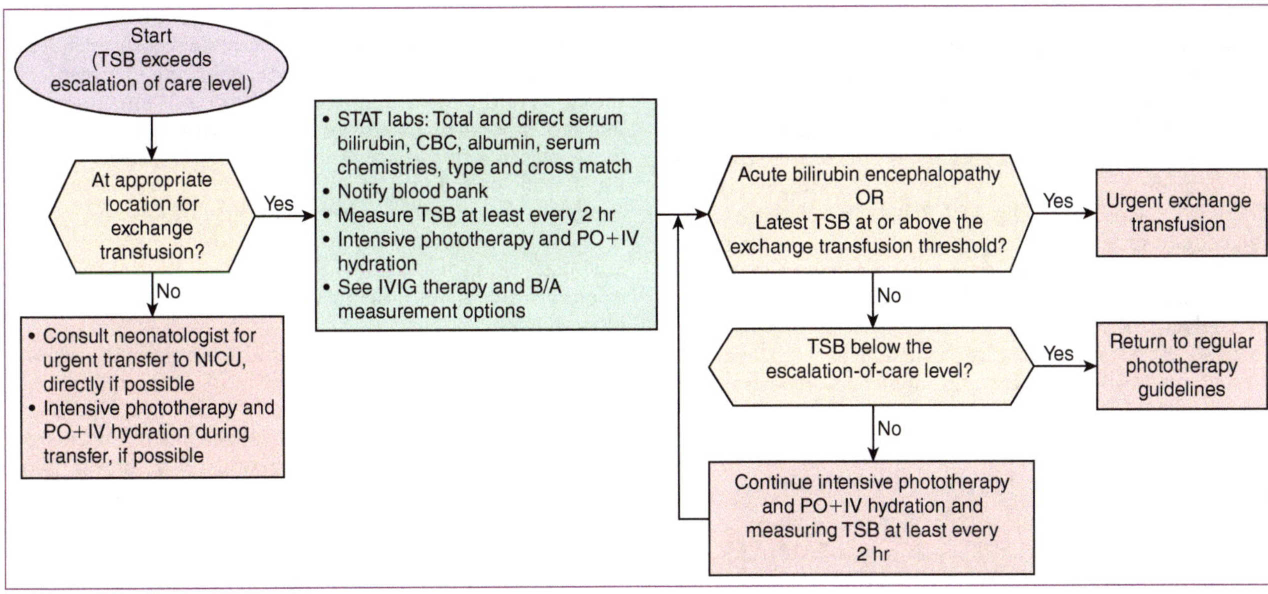


**FIGURE 13.15 Approach to escalation of care.**

The escalation-of-care threshold is 2 mg/dl below the exchange transfusion threshold.

B/A, bilirubin-to-albumin ratio.

*Source:* From Kemper, A. R., Newman, T. B., Slaughter, J. L., Maisels, M. J., Watchko, J. F., Downs, S. M., Grout, R. W., Bundy, D. G., Stark, A. R., Bogen, D. L., Holmes, A. V., Feldman-Winter, L. B., Bhutani, V. K., Brown, S. R., Maradiaga Panayotti, G. M., Okechukwu, K., Rappo, P. D., & Russell, T. L. (2022). Clinical practice guideline revision: Management of hyperbilirubinemia in the newborn infant 35 or more weeks of gestation. *Pediatrics, 150*(3), e2022058859. https://doi.org/10.1542/peds.2022-058859.

action. Every 2-hour monitoring of TSB is necessary during the escalation-of-care period. Please refer to Figure 13.15 for the recommendation on the escalation of care. Immediate labs that must be sent include TSB, CBC, albumin, chemistries, type, and cross-match. Blood banks must be informed of the emergency. IV access must be established, and D10W maintenance fluid should be initiated. If, at this point, the infant has not been recognized as needing phototherapy, multiple lights should be provided for intense phototherapy while waiting for the next step.

The 2022 AAP guideline includes the use of the bilirubin/albumin (B/A) ratio as an additional tool to guide in decision making. The B/A ratio is obtained by TSB (mg/dl) divided by serum albumin (g/dl). The threshold differs based on gestational age and risk factors. The B/A ratio has been reported to strongly correlate with the unbound free bilirubin level for infants ≥ 35 weeks' gestation and younger infants when serum is obtained prior to receiving phototherapy (Abe et al., 2021; Sato et al., 2012). The higher the B/A ratio, the higher the level of unbound free bilirubin circulating, threatening to cross into the blood–brain barrier, thereby increasing the risk of bilirubin neurotoxicity. In addition to all discussed previously, additional guidance in considering the need for exchange transfusion using the B/A ratio is:

- ≥ 8.0 and ≥ 38 weeks' gestation and no hyperbilirubinemia neurotoxicity risk factors, or
- ≥ 7.2 and ≥ 38 weeks' gestation and there is at least one hyperbilirubinemia neurotoxicity risk factor, or
- ≥ 7.2 and ≥ 35 to 37 weeks' gestation and no hyperbilirubinemia neurotoxicity risk factors, or
- ≥ 6.8 and ≥ 35 to 37 weeks' gestation and there is at least one hyperbilirubinemia neurotoxicity risk factor (Kemper et al., 2022).

Exchange transfusion removes bilirubin and the antibody-coated RBCs from the newborn's circulation. In addition, some of the circulating maternal antibodies and Rh-positive fetal RBC are removed while potentially normalizing the hematocrit. The recommendation is to use cross-matched washed PRBCs mixed with adult fresh-frozen plasma (thawed) at the hematocrit level of 40%. The plasma contains albumin, and this also aids in bilirubin removal.

Exchange transfusion is not without complications, such as vascular accidents, electrolyte or hematologic abnormalities, or cardiovascular compromise. Although the exchange process is performed slowly with caution, its effect on pressure changes, volume fluctuations, the cardiovascular system, and biochemical changes throughout the system is not to be taken lightly. Wolf et al. reported based on infants ≥ 23 weeks' gestation born from 1997 to 2016 ($n$ = 1247425) within one large health system in the United States and identified 1,252 infants (0.1%) to have received exchange transfusion. Over the course, the transfusion rate decreased from 0.3% to 0.05%. The most common postexchange transfusion adverse effects reported was thrombocytopenia (64%). Other effects noted include hyperkalemia (5%), hypocalcemia (2%), NECs (< 1%), seizure (2%), severe IVH (1%), and mortality (6%). Mortality was assessed for 1,161 out of 1,252 infants who received exchange transfusion. Infants ≤ 29 weeks' gestation had the highest mortality. Five of the infants who died developed IVH after the exchange transfusion (Wolf et al., 2020).

**Nursing Care of Infants During and After Exchange Transfusion.** The effect of not only the volume/pressure changes but also numerous biochemical alterations can result in morbidities and mortality (Wolf et al., 2020). An ongoing vigilance in performing physical assessments and monitoring vital signs is required. Highly important nurses' roles include frequent vital sign checks during the transfusion; timely follow-up of labs, especially TSB, CBC, and electrolytes as ordered; and prompt notifications of abnormal results to the providers. These infants should remain on the cardiorespiratory monitor during and after the procedure until stability is observed and a determination is made for safety. Increased apnea episodes, respiratory status changes, neurologic changes, and any vital sign changes require immediate reporting and interventions.

## Final Thoughts on Hyperbilirubinemia

This concludes the section for the hyperbilirubinemia and important management guidelines from the 2022 AAP recommendations. Hyperbilirubinemia, whether severe or mild, is a frequent finding seen in an estimated 80% to 85% of all newborns around the world. Readers are encouraged to become familiar with the risk factors as well as processes and tools for monitoring. An online tool called "PediTools" for the 2022 AAP guideline exists. It can be accessed at this link: https://peditools.org/bili2022/

The smart phone version is highly accessible for busy clinicians. The PediTool home page at https://peditools.org also provides numerous other online tools for other pediatric needs, such as growth calculation, which provides highly useful tools (Chou et al., 2020).

# ANEMIA

## Pathophysiology

Etiologies of neonatal anemia has three broad classifications: (1) blood loss (chronic and acute), (2) hemolysis, and (3) suboptimal or reduced production of RBCs. Hemorrhage may occur during any of the prenatal, perinatal, or postnatal period. Lastly, iatrogenic blood loss for sick infants is discussed (Driscoll, 2016; Ree & Lopriore, 2019; Stark et al., 2019). Most recent reviews advocate defining anemia when the hematocrit or hemoglobin is below the fifth percentile based on the reference population specific to the gestational age. Extremely preterm infants, such as 24 weeks' gestation, will have anemia at a much lower level of hematocrit or hemoglobin than term infants (Christensen et al., 2023).

### Anemia Due to Chronic Blood Loss

Chronic anemia can be caused by a chronic fetal to maternal hemorrhage (FMH). A full-term infant can be significantly anemic if 50 ml of blood was lost to the mother; however, for preterm infants, less blood loss to the mother would cause significant anemia. The Kleihauer–Betke test can be ordered on the mother to determine the presence of fetal RBCs in maternal circulation. If ABO incompatibility exists, sometimes this test proves negative because the mother's system removes incompatible fetal cells from her system.

Another chronic blood loss that leads to anemia is twin-to-twin transfusion, which can occur in monozygous (identical) twins who share the placenta (monochorionic). Sometimes, the cords of the twins or any multiples do not implant in the placenta in ways that share an equal network of blood vessels in the placenta they share. An unequal blood transfer occurs, leaving one as a donor twin and another the recipient. This condition causes one twin to become anemic (also hypovolemic) and the recipient to be polycythemic (and hypervolemic), adding stress on the cardiovascular system. Mortality is high if intervention is not done to stop the uneven transfer of the blood flow.

When born, newborn infants with chronic anemia, such as the case with fetal–maternal transfusion, may appear very pale; however, they may not present with the typical signs and symptoms of more apparent hypovolemia or shock seen in acute blood loss (shock, poor peripheral perfusion, poor respiratory effort or respiratory distress, tachycardia, pallor, lethargy, hypotension tachycardia, tachypnea). Severely anemic infants are visibly pale and no resuscitation effort at birth would bring the infant to pink up without RBC transfusion. In cases of chronic hemorrhage, infants have had significant time to become accustomed to the low level of hemoglobin and hematocrit. These infants may benefit from slower volume replacement to prevent fluid overload from burdening the cardiovascular system. Chronic anemia can also occur with congenital infection (Driscoll, 2016; Ree & Lopriore, 2019; Stark et al., 2019).

### Anemia Due to Acute Blood Loss

For acute blood loss, which could occur anytime during the prenatal, perinatal, or postnatal period, there are several common causes: any bleeding from procedures performed on the fetus that leads to bleeding, tight nuchal cord, abruptio placentae, cord prolapse, velamentous cord insertion (which can tear easily), subgaleal hemorrhage, or any other hemorrhage that leads to disseminated intravascular coagulation (DIC). Any condition that leads to the acute loss of the blood supply to the infants requires emergent volume replacement with PRBCs. Traumatic delivery or vacuum extraction or extensive scalp bleeding can result in hemorrhage in the subgaleal space because of the emissary vein rupturing. Significant blood loss can occur because the subgaleal space can hold up to 240 ml of blood. This represents the entire blood volume if the infant's weight is near 3 kg (80 ml/kg blood volume), leading to significant shock that requires immediate interventions. Hemorrhage into the liver, kidneys, spleen, or retroperitoneal space can also occur in association with traumatic and breech deliveries (Bagwell & Steward, 2020; Driscoll, 2016; Ree & Lopriore, 2019).

### Anemia Due to Hemolysis

Isoimmunization, as in ABO and Rh incompatibility, accounts for most cases of neonatal hemolysis and earlier discussions can be referenced. A reduced RBC lifespan caused by hemolysis is usually associated with a rise in the bilirubin level, with 1 g of hemoglobin yielding 35 mg of bilirubin. Infants who have received intrauterine transfusions or exchange transfusions for blood group incompatibilities are predisposed to anemia that develops within the first few months of life. The pathophysiology is bone marrow suppression, possibly due to the increased amount of hemoglobin received during the blood transfusions.

Bacterial sepsis and viral infections, especially congenital infections such as syphilis, rubella, toxoplasmosis, CMV, or herpes, once referred to as TORCH; and human immunodeficiency virus (HIV) and hepatitis, also cause hemolysis. Drug-induced RBC destruction, caused by either maternal ingestion or direct administration of the drug to the newborn, is another common cause of hemolysis. An example of this would be the hemolysis that could occur with the administration of iron supplements to an infant with vitamin E deficiency. G6PD deficiency and other hereditary causes, such as thalassemia, can also cause early destruction of RBCs, leading to anemia (Kemper et al., 2022).

### Suboptimal RBC Production

Premature infants have diminished function or effectiveness of hematopoiesis and reaction to the anemic state to respond by accelerating the hematopoiesis. In addition to the short lifespan of premature RBCs, these infants eventually become anemic.

### Iatrogenic Blood Loss From Blood Sampling

For sick infants, phlebotomy losses can account for significant blood loss. The sicker the infant, or the more premature the infant, the more frequent blood sampling is often required. Care providers must be prudent in deciding what laboratory tests are truly necessary, and the negative effect of the ordered laboratory tests on the infant's overall blood volume. Accurate recording of blood lost to sampling can be beneficial in assessing a sick infant's circulatory status and volume needs (Bagwell & Steward, 2020; Ree & Lopriore, 2019).

## Monitoring

It is recommended that preterm or sick infants have periodic monitoring to assess the trend to capture their state of anemia. It is essential to follow hematocrit and hemoglobin levels. After the acute hemorrhage, initial hematocrit and hemoglobin levels may be normal or near normal until hours later. Therefore, these must be followed up hours later (8–12 hours based on the initial results).

- Reticulocyte counts, when high, indicate chronic anemia. Increased numbers of immature RBCs reflect the degree of hematopoietic activity in response to anemia, and this response does not occur immediately in hours in response to the hemorrhage.
- Blood typing, Rh determination, and Coombs testing must be completed when chronic hemolysis is suspected (if this information is unavailable at the time of discovery of an anemic state).

## Management

Emergency transfusion is not always required. However, based on the history of how the infant lost the blood (e.g., acute loss versus chronic loss) or how severe the chronic loss resulted, and how symptomatic the infant is, all play a role in the clinical decision making regarding the treatment. In acute blood loss, volume replacement with PRBCs is indicated urgently. Even if it is not an acute loss, many cases, such as tight nuchal cord, benefit from vigilant monitoring and potentially urgent intervention. Rapid line placement for fluid replacement, volume expansion (with normal saline or blood transfusion), and blood sampling may require the use of the umbilical vein or artery. Central venous pressure measurements can help assess the degree of volume loss and the amount of replacement needed.

- If acute volume expansion is required, normal saline is the volume expander of choice at 10 to 20 ml/kg. If time allows, fresh frozen plasma or O-negative blood can be used at the dosing of normal saline until a type and cross-match replacement is available.
- After the infant's condition has been stabilized, laboratory tests and a physical examination should be performed to determine the cause of the anemia and to rectify the problem.
- Examining the placenta and maternal blood sample testing for fetal hemoglobin may be helpful in determining the cause of the blood loss.

With all newborns, the principles of care (provision of warmth, monitoring of vital signs, ongoing assessment, and accurate determination of intake and output) are essential to the well-being of the infant who has experienced any blood loss.

### Dietary Supplementation

The three major nutritional factors that affect RBC production are iron, folate, and vitamin E. Because all three increase in amount with increasing gestational age, premature birth predisposes the immature infant to anemia due to insufficient stores.

Without iron supplementation, the hematopoiesis necessary to maintain a normal hemoglobin level depletes the infant's iron reserves when birth weight is doubled. Various factors can contribute to iron deficiency anemia, such as LBW, low initial hemoglobin levels, and blood loss through trauma, hemorrhage, or sampling. In the term infant, exhaustion of iron reserves occurs typically by 20 to 24 weeks postnatal age, but this happens much earlier in the preterm infant. Iron stores needed for hemoglobin production are present in insufficient quantities at birth in premature infants, making supplementation necessary during the first 2 to 4 months to prevent iron deficiency anemia.

Folate is the generic description for folic acid and its related compounds. Folate is a component of the B-complex vitamins involved in the maturation of RBCs, particularly the synthesis of DNA, which controls nuclear maturation and division. Because bone marrow is one of the body's faster-growing and more proliferative tissues, folic acid deficiency diminishes bone marrow's ability to produce RBCs, resulting in megaloblastic anemia.

Vitamin E, an antioxidant, protects the RBC membrane from destruction due to lipid peroxidation. Deficiency of this nutrient shortens the cell's lifespan by exposing the unprotected, unsaturated membrane lipids to peroxidation and hemolysis. Infants are born in a state of relative vitamin E deficiency that is more intense in the smaller and more premature infants. Vitamin E is required in increasing amounts as the intake of polyunsaturated fatty acids increases. Deficiency becomes apparent in infants of birth weights less than 1,500 g at approximately 4 to 6 weeks, resulting in decreased hemoglobin levels ranging from 7 to 10 g/dl. The administration of iron supplementation in the presence of vitamin E deficiency will intensify the hemolytic response (Bagwell & Steward, 2020).

### Transfusion Therapy

In the past, of all preterm infants admitted to a NICU, approximately 90% received one transfusion in the first 6 weeks of life. Today, transfusions have declined due to the improved treatment and prevention of neonatal lung disease, the reduction of blood loss from blood gas and chemistry analysis (thanks to available cutaneous measuring devices), early protein and adequate iron supplementation, and the use of transfusion guidelines (Ree & Lopriore, 2019).

Although a critically ill infant is generally maintained with a hematocrit level above 40%, the benefits of transfusion therapy in the convalescent infant remain controversial. When the effects of transfusion therapy in the convalescent infant were studied, the elimination of symptoms attributed to anemia was not a consistent finding. Some studies show that, in premature infants with a hematocrit level below 30%, apnea, bradycardia, dyspnea, feeding difficulties, poor weight gain despite good calorie intake, lethargy, tachypnea, tachycardia, and increased cardiac output and oxygen consumption appear to be relieved by transfusion therapy. The threshold for when transfusion is needed is primarily based on the symptoms rather than a certain hematocrit level; however, monitoring the lactic acid levels may be used in some institutions or regions (to capture the body's response to the lowering hematocrit, which convert from own metabolism from aerobic to anaerobic). The establishment of transfusion criteria can effectively minimize donor exposure. These guidelines help determine which infants would benefit from transfusion based on symptoms, hematocrit value, and severity of illness (Bagwell & Steward, 2020; Ree & Lopriore, 2019).

## PHYSIOLOGIC ANEMIA OF THE NEWBORN AND ANEMIA OF THE PREMATURE INFANT

The physiologic regulator of RBC production, erythropoietin, falls to very low levels after birth because the relative intrauterine hypoxia that stimulated its release is no longer present. Erythropoietin levels remain low until another hypoxic stimulus occurs, one created by the normal drop in the hemoglobin level that marks the physiologic anemia of the newborn. This drop in the hemoglobin level is due to decreased marrow production of RBCs secondary to diminished circulating erythropoietin levels, a shorter lifespan of the neonatal RBC with destruction of fetal hemoglobin, and hemodilution caused by growth.

The drop in hemoglobin that prompts the postnatal rise in erythropoietin directly correlates with the infant's gestational age and birth weight (Figure 13.16). The smaller and more immature the infant, the lower the infant's nadir at an earlier postnatal age. The hemoglobin level in the term newborn reaches a nadir of 11.4 g/dl ± 0.9 in the first 2 to 3 months of

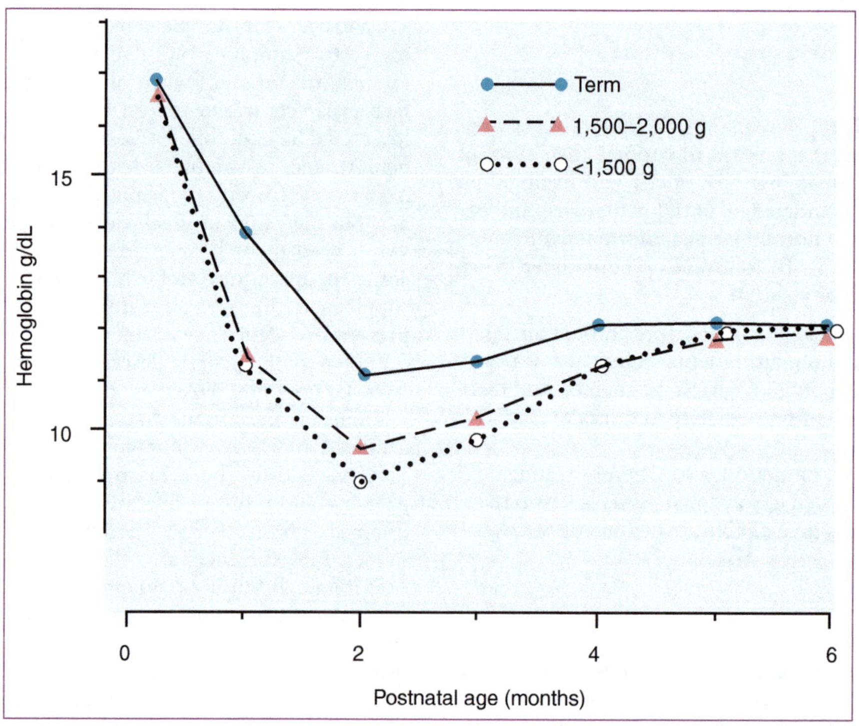


**FIGURE 13.16 Gestational age and birth weight are directly correlated with the timing of the postnatal drop in hemoglobin and with the nadir of the drop.** Shown here are the differences between term infants and two groups of preterm infants, one weighing 1,500 to 2,000 g and the other less than 1,500 g.

*Source:* From Brown, M. (1988). Physiologic anemia of infancy: Normal red cell values and physiology of neonatal erythropoiesis. In J. Stockman & C. Pochedly (Eds.), *Developmental and neonatal hematology* (pp. 249–274). Raven Press.

life. It plateaus at this level for approximately 2 more months before gradually increasing. Although there is no significant difference in cord-blood hemoglobin levels between term infants and preterm infants born after 32 weeks' gestation, the drop in hemoglobin occurs earlier in the preterm infant, is more precipitous, and reaches a lower nadir. Starting at 2 weeks of age, the preterm infant has a drop in hemoglobin of 1 g/dl/wk for the first several weeks; the nadir at 6 to 8 weeks of age is 2 to 3 g/dl lower than that of the term infant. An infant weighing 1,000 to 1,500 g at birth will have a mean hemoglobin nadir of 8 g/dl at 4 to 6 weeks of age.

Infants who have undergone exchange transfusion or multiple transfusions also have a more significant fall in their hemoglobin level in the first 3 months of life. This phenomenon may be due to improved oxygen delivery to tissue associated with replacing fetal hemoglobin with adult hemoglobin. Adult hemoglobin has less affinity for oxygen because of the structural difference of the globin portion of the hemoglobin molecule. This, coupled with the increased amount of 2,3-disphosphoglycerate in the blood, allows adult hemoglobin to release oxygen to the tissue more easily. Improved tissue oxygenation effectively lowers serum erythropoietin levels, decreasing RBC production. Consequently, an infant undergoing intrauterine transfusion, exchange transfusion, or frequent postnatal transfusions has improved tissue oxygenation and a decreased erythropoietin level.

The switch in the predominant site of erythropoietin production during fetal life from the liver to the kidneys occurs concurrently with the change in hemoglobin to a more mature form. Hepatic erythropoietin production in response to hypoxia is not as quick and effective as the kidneys' response, an adjustment that protects the fetus from overproducing RBC and polycythemia in utero. However, the persistence of this hepatic pathway after premature birth may be the reason the premature infant's hematocrit values reach a lower nadir, which persists longer compared to the term infant. Although erythropoietin levels are reduced in the early newborn period, the erythroid progenitor cells in the bone marrow are exceedingly sensitive to erythropoietin and respond rapidly as blood levels increase.

Numerous researchers worked tirelessly to bring human recombinant erythropoietin to the market, and equally, numerous trials have explored the use of pharmaceutical-grade erythropoiesis-stimulating agent (ESA) to prevent anemia in premature infants (Migliaccio, 2024; Ohlsson & Aher, 2020). The first human study of the ESA was on chronic renal failure patients on dialysis who were transfusion dependent primarily because the kidneys lost the ability to produce erythropoietin (Eschbach et al., 1987). The early use of ESA in preterm infants (within 8 days of birth) does reduce the number of RBC transfusions, the total volume transfused, and the donor exposures. Conflicting results were reported from two large trials. In summary, routine ESA use for premature infants is not currently recommended because the benefits identified are somewhat limited (Ohlsson & Aher, 2020).

## Treatment

Physiologic anemia does not usually require any form of treatment. With good nutrition, the hemoglobin level in the term infant should start to rise by 3 months of age. With adequate nutrition and iron supplementation, the hemoglobin level in the preterm infant should begin to increase by 5 months of age, eventually attaining hemoglobin values comparable to those of the term infant. This emphasizes the value and the need for the primary care that continues for newborn patients, not only for monitoring of growth and development or disease prevention but also for monitoring of the anemia status.

## Polycythemia

**Pathophysiology.** Polycythemia is defined as a peripheral venous hematocrit level over 65%. Recent changes in practice related to DCC have been named as the contributing factors of some cases of polycythemia and hyperbilirubinemia. However, not all the studies report the same results (Chaudhary et al., 2023; Eschbach et al., 1987; Prachukthum et al., 2023).

Although the fetus lives in a low-PO2 environment that should induce a polycythemic response, it protects itself by keeping hematocrit levels below 60%. This may be a function of the slower fetal hepatic response to hypoxia compared with the rapid renal response after birth. The average hematocrit on the first day of life is approximately 50% in the term infant and the preterm infant of more than 32 weeks' gestation and 45% in the preterm infant of less than 32 weeks' gestation.

The choice of sampling site can affect **hematocrit** values considerably, particularly during the early newborn period when peripheral circulation may be somewhat sluggish. Infants younger than 1 day of age either lack or have diminished cutaneous vasoregulatory mechanisms that reduce peripheral perfusion. Capillary blood sampling sites will have the highest **hematocrit**, followed by blood from a peripheral site, with central blood having the lowest **hematocrit** (Bagwell & Steward, 2020).

The main concern with polycythemia is that it can impair peripheral circulation by increasing blood viscosity and reducing the flow rate. As blood viscosity increases, vascular resistance increases in the peripheral circulation and the microcirculation of the capillaries throughout the body, including the lungs, leading to potential respiratory problems. With **hematocrit** levels below 60% to 65%, blood viscosity increases linearly, but viscosity exponentially increases at higher **hematocrit** levels (Bagwell & Steward, 2020).

The ability of RBCs to modify their shape to traverse the peripheral vascular bed successfully and microcirculation also affects the blood flow rate. The degree of deformability of the cell determines its ability to pass through small vascular spaces, the greater the deformability of the cell, the quicker its passage. Less deformable cells can increase blood viscosity by occluding small vessels, causing microcirculation sludging, leading to thrombosis and tissue ischemia.

**Active Polycythemia.** Regardless of the cause, tissue hypoxia elicits an increase in erythropoietin that stimulates RBC production. In the fetus, erythropoietin is produced initially by the liver and then by the kidneys, the adult production site. The kidneys' potential to release erythropoietin is active by 34 weeks' gestation. A renal erythropoietic factor reacts with a substance in the plasma to produce erythropoietin, the RBC stimulating factor. Hypoxia of the tissues adjacent to the renal tubules, where erythropoietin is made, is the potent stimulator of this factor's release.

Many factors can lead to tissue hypoxia associated with the active form of polycythemia. These factors include the following:

1. Maternal factors that result in reduced placental blood flow: Pregnancy-induced hypertension (PIH), older maternal age, maternal renal or heart disease, severe maternal diabetes, oligohydramnios, and maternal smoking (the mechanism is thought to be the production of carbon monoxide that crosses the placenta and induces a state of tissue hypoxia in the fetus)
2. Placental factors: Placental infarction, placenta previa, viral infections (TORCH), postdate, and placental dysfunction that results in SGA infant
3. Fetal syndromes: Trisomies 13, 18, and 21, and Beckwith–Wiedemann Syndrome

**Passive Polycythemia.** Passive polycythemia is a result of increased fetal blood volume caused by maternal–fetal transfusion, or twin-to-twin transfusion, with one twin being polycythemic and the other anemic. In a recent study, a DCC of 120 seconds was associated with an increased incidence of polycythemia (4.6% with 30 seconds of DCC versus 13% with 120 seconds of DCC) (Chaudhary et al., 2023).

**Clinical Manifestations.** Symptoms of polycythemic hyperviscosity are usually evident within the first few days after birth, reflecting the compromise of various organ systems. The findings that were most seen by the systems are as follows:

1. Neurologic symptoms include lethargy or irritability, hypotonia, tremulousness, exaggerated startle, poor feeding, vomiting, seizures or apnea.
2. Cardiovascular symptoms include cardiomegaly or ECG changes that indicate atrial or ventricular hypertrophy.
3. Respiratory symptoms include respiratory distress, central cyanosis, pleural effusions, pulmonary congestion/edema or persistent pulmonary hypertension.
4. Hematologic symptoms include hyperbilirubinemia, thrombocytopenia, high reticulocyte levels, coagulopathies, hepatosplenomegaly, or renal/cerebral vein thrombosis.
5. Gastrointestinal symptoms include poor feeding, distended abdomen, vomiting, distended intestines on radiographic studies, and possibly as serious as NEC.
6. Genitourinary symptoms include oliguria, hematuria, or proteinuria.
7. Metabolic symptoms include hypocalcemia or hypoglycemia.

The complications of polycythemia center around the increased resistance to blood flow related to hyperviscosity; blood flow to all organ systems is impaired by sluggish circulation. Pulmonary blood flow can be dramatically compromised, resulting in pulmonary hypertension, retained lung fluid, and respiratory distress syndrome (RDS). Taxation of the heart by an increased vascular load can lead to congestive heart failure and left-to-right shunting across the foramen ovale or ductus arteriosus. Impairment of blood flow to the bowel can lead to NEC (Bagwell & Steward, 2020).

**Treatment.** Although most infants with polycythemia are asymptomatic or minimally symptomatic, the hematocrit level and the presence of symptoms, even if minimal, should form the basis of treatment. Most neonates will need to be observed for cardiac and respiratory status, have hematocrit drawn every 6 to 12 or 24 hours based on the level of the symptoms, and be observed for signs of the problems noted in the previous list. For those with a hematocrit level between 65% and 75%, supportive treatment of fluid boluses of normal saline to prevent the hematocrit from increasing any further is needed. Partial exchange transfusions were standard treatment for infants who were symptomatic with hematocrit levels between 60% to 65% or for infants that were asymptomatic with a hematocrit level greater than 65% due to increased incidence of neurologic abnormalities or changes but are now controversial if they do more harm than good. The current recommendation is not to perform exchange transfusion routinely for asymptomatic infants with a hematocrit < 75% because minimal data is available that support the benefit for the infants when asymptomatic (Consortium., 2023).

**Collaborative Management of the Infant With Polycythemia.** Any infants who exhibit respiratory conditions should have a CBC to examine the hematologic etiologies of the condition. Respiratory support, if required, additional assessment and monitoring is needed, including obtaining blood gases. The infant should be adequately hydrated and closely monitored for hypoglycemia and hypocalcemia. A hematocrit value over 65% should prompt careful observation of the infant for any symptoms associated with hyperviscosity.

## MOST COMMON COAGULATION DISORDERS IN THE NEWBORN

### Vitamin K Deficiency

The liver produces most of the clotting factors, including those of the prothrombin complex. Adequate function of this complex requires vitamin K (VK) as a cofactor for the carboxylation of VK-dependent factors, II, VII, IX, X, and inhibitor proteins C and S. VK is required for the conversion of these VK-dependent proteins into active clotting factors, which then possess coagulating capabilities. VK is necessary for the conversion of prothrombin binding sites into forms that can bind calcium, which is required for the completion of many steps in the clotting cascade (Ayombil & Camire, 2020).

Sources of VK typically are through VK-rich food and the synthesis of $VK_2$ by intestinal bacteria in the bowel. Newborns are at risk for VK deficiency due to insufficient VK intake by mouth, especially if breastfed, limited and inadequate placental transfer of VK during pregnancy, and poor bacterial colonization of newborn colon. Maternal VK store or function of VK can be negatively affected when mothers are on anticoagulants, anticonvulsants, antibiotics, antituberculosis medications, including rifampicin, or isoniazid and warfarin by inducing human cytochrome P450 (CYP450) enzymes in the fetal liver. CYP450 is known to aid in the elimination of the common clinically used medications, and it affects VK function (Albisetti & Monagle, 2021; Hand et al., 2022).

Vitamin K–dependent factors reach approximately 30% to 70% of adult levels in the cord blood of term infants but quickly drop to half that amount if the infant is not given vitamin K. Because these factors are dependent on gestational age, the more premature the infant, the lower the levels at birth for reasons stated earlier. Vitamin K–dependent factors will slowly rise but do not reach normal adult levels until approximately 9 months of age. Administration of approximately 1 to 2 mg of vitamin K can prevent this decline and normalize the prothrombin time (Albisetti & Monagle, 2021; Bagwell & Steward, 2020).

Hemorrhage during the early neonatal period that can be attributed to a deficiency of VK–dependent factors is classified as VK deficiency bleeding (VKDB). The types of VKDB are described as early, classic, or late onset based on the timing of the bleeding. The rarest form presents within 24 hours with a serious presentation such as intracranial hemorrhage (ICH) or abdominal bleeding, and often, this form is associated with maternal medications such as anticonvulsants and antituberculosis medications, as mentioned earlier. The classic form of VKDB usually occurs during the first 2 to 7 days of life, often in breastfed infants. The presentations include nose bleeding, intestinal bleeding, oozing from postcircumcision or puncture sites, or umbilical stump bleeding. However, more significant bleeding could also occur. This VKDB that occurs within a week was common in the United States until 1961, when the AAP recommended administering vitamin K to all newborns at birth (Hand et al., 2022). The late-onset VKDB (incidence per 100,000 births: 10.5–80) presents after the first week of life, often in breastfed infants from past 1 week old to 6 months of age. The incidence appeared to peak in 2 to 8 weeks and occurs often in those infants who did not receive VK at birth or those who have underlying diseases (cystic fibrosis [CF], hepatitis, coeliac disease, bile duct atresia, intestinal malabsorption, or other rare conditions). The late-onset VKDB is more catastrophic: the most common presentation of late-onset VKDB is ICH (30%–60%); however, intestinal bleeding has also been reported (Albisetti & Monagle, 2021; Hand et al., 2022).

The cause of VKDB is now primarily due to parental refusal of the intramuscular (IM) VK at birth. Parental refusal of VK for newborns is increasingly challenging in clinical settings. The incidence of hemorrhage without prophylaxis per 100,000 births is estimated to be 250 to 1,700 for early VKDB and from 10.5 to 80 for late VKDB. Parents' refusal of IM VK ranged from 0% to 3.2% in U.S. hospitals, up to 14.5% in home births, and up to 31.0% in birthing centers (Loyal & Shapiro, 2020). A study reports that among those who refuse, the most common source of information that the decision to refuse is based upon internet information (70%) (Hamrick et al., 2016). While breastmilk has VK, it is inadequate to make up for the deficiency of VK that infants are born with.

Treatment for an active bleeding caused by VKDB of the newborn require either IV or subcutaneous VK. Infants may also require blood replacement or the use of stored plasma or fresh frozen plasma for immediate clotting factor replacement (10–20 ml/kg) and the use of prothrombin complex concentrates for severe bleeding or ICH. Recombinant activated factor VIIa (rFVIIa) has been shown to effectively correct coagulopathy in several cases of ICH due to VK deficiency, allowing corrective neurosurgery. The infusion dosage used ranged from 90 to 200 mcg/kg (Albisetti & Monagle, 2021). rFVIIa was initially developed as the treatment for hemophilia that becomes refractory to the specific factors by developing alloantibodies or neutralizing inhibitors against the factors. However, it has also been reported to be highly effective in stopping spontaneous pulmonary hemorrhage among very preterm and very low birth weight (VLBW) infants (Albisetti & Monagle, 2021; Cosar et al., 2017; Ljung et al., 2019).

Preterm infants are particularly at high risk for VKDB due to inadequate intestinal microbial colonization and immaturity of hematologic function or hepatic function. Understanding from the earlier discussions of hematologic development during fetal life, it is understandable that more premature infants may face challenges of bleeding; therefore, it is important that nurses at the bedside are vigilant and aware that parental refusal of VK places these infants at much higher risk of complications.

Pregnant mothers who are on certain medications that interact negatively with the VK synthesis are recommended to take supplemental VK during the third trimester. Evidence is not fully established if supplemental VK for pregnant mothers reduces certain types of VKDB; however, prenatal VK supplementation has been shown to elevate cord VK plasma concentration (Albisetti & Monagle, 2021; Hand et al., 2022)

## Hemophilia

**Pathophysiology.** Hemophilia A (HA) and B (HB) are the most common inherited bleeding disorders that are clinically indistinguishable. HA is the most frequently inherited coagulation abnormality, accounting for 90% of all genetically linked coagulopathies and 80% to 85% of all hemophiliacs, whereas HB occurs in 10% to 15% of cases. Both diseases are X-linked recessive disorders and are passed from mother to son. HA is caused by Factor VIII (FVIII) deficiency, and HB is caused by Factor IX (FIX) deficiency. Both FVIII and FIX factors are essential in normal thrombin production. They are needed to activate the pathway of Factor X, which converts prothrombin to thrombin. The absence of either factor severely impairs the body's ability to generate both thrombin and fibrin. A hemophiliac's problem is not bleeding more rapidly but abnormal clot formation. This results in hemorrhage with a potential for significant blood loss. When the clot forms, it is often fragile, and rebleeding can occur without proper treatment (Albisetti & Monagle, 2021). The severity of the disease is dependent on the baseline level of FVIII or FIX. The factor activity level of < 1% is associated with severe diseases, and individuals with the severe form of hemophilia experience frequent bleeding, whether spontaneous or injury related. Bleeding often occurs in the joints and muscles but also in soft tissues, predisposing hemophiliac patients to poor quality of life due to joint pain and even dysfunction (Mahlangu et al., 2023). Severe HA patients experience bleeding more frequently than severe HB patients. Severity scores on the symptoms are also higher for HA patients than HB. FVIII deficiency for HA is now known to be caused by mutations of the F8 gene (located at the end of the long arm of the Z chromosome in X28). The mutated F8 gene does not encode the FVIII properly (Dardik et al., 2023).

Newborns with hemophilia are at high risk for ICH and other bleeding complications. The factor activity level of > 5% is a mild disease; however, ICH can still be possible for these patients, leading to further morbidity (Moorehead et al., 2018).

**Diagnosis.** The Centers for the Disease Control and Prevention (CDC), Universal Data Collection System surveillance project at U.S. Hemophilia Treatment Centers, reported that 82% of the 547 infants had HA. Seventy percent of the infants were diagnosed within 1 month of birth. Bleeding from various sites (postcircumcision site, soft tissue, oral bleeding) prompted the diagnosis in 35% of the infants. Overall, 50% of hemophiliacs are believed to be diagnosed in the neonatal period (Kulkarni et al., 2017).

Laboratory tests will be needed to determine if the infant has hemophilia. Tests needed will be a partial thromboplastin time (PTT), which will be prolonged, both FVIII and FIX with the affected factor being decreased, and a prothrombin time (PT), a thrombin time, and a platelet count, which will be relatively normal. HA is easier to diagnose in the neonatal period than HB because FIX levels in newborns are reduced at birth, and in preterm infants, it can be mistaken as an HB diagnosis. Newborns with mildly low FIX levels are recommended for retesting. The use of cord blood is also recommended for these multiple tests, including genetic testing, to avoid multiple invasive sticks and iatrogenic blood loss (Moorehead et al., 2018).

Recognizing the carrier mother prenatally is highly helpful as well as obtaining history regarding any existing family member with hemophilia. Pregnant mothers who are carriers or have family history, and are therefore a potential carrier, must receive genetic counseling to review the pattern of inheritance in the family or to discuss the testing options. Carrier status cannot be determined simply by examining the FVIII or FIX levels and the carrier mother may be completely asymptomatic, making the carrier identification challenging (Moorehead et al., 2018).

Prenatal diagnosis is possible through amniocentesis or chorionic villus biopsy. The option of prenatal diagnosis for HA now has advanced from sampling of fetal blood at 20 to 22 weeks' gestation for FVIII levels to a fine-tuned early genetic analysis by fetal chorionic villus sampling to identify F8 gene mutations (as early as week 11–14). Not every patient resides within a reasonable distance from established hemophilia centers where experts are available. Not all the tests are available in all the regions, making the history taking and traditional genetic counseling highly important. With advances in molecular technology and other innovations, it is hoped that more definitive noninvasive tools will be available to identify F8 gene mutations (Dardik et al., 2023; Moorehead et al., 2018).

**Treatment.** Evidence is not established on the recommended mode of delivery of infants with hemophilia; however, the goal of the delivery care team must be to minimize the risk of ICH or any other serious complications. The high incidence of ICH at delivery accompanies hemophiliac infants, and one study reported 14 delivery-related ICH cases among the 457 infants registered in the database, in addition to other spontaneous ICHs (Kulkarni et al., 2017). Prenatal planning far in advance for the delivery is recommended, and delivery should be planned at a location with high-risk obstetrics, hematology, neonatology, and 24-hour services for blood banks/laboratories. The most significant risk factor associated with intra- or extracranial hemorrhage is by far the vacuum- or forceps-assisted vaginal delivery (Moorehead et al., 2018). If diagnosed prenatally, vacuum extraction, forceps, fetal scalp electrodes, and other potentially high-risk interventions should be avoided.

Postnatally, the goal in treating hemophilia is to raise the defective or deficient factor to a level that will prevent significant bleeding. For any considerable bleeding prior to diagnosis, fresh frozen plasma at 10 to 20 ml/kg should be given, and a specific factor should be given after diagnosis. To have replacement products be as free as possible of transfusion-transmissible diseases, it was once recommended that recombinant products be used rather than plasma-derived products when available and feasible (Bagwell & Steward, 2020; Roberts et al., 2004). A recent randomized trial revealed that children who were previously untreated who were receiving plasma-derived FVIII demonstrated decreased incidences of developing inhibitors compared to those who were receiving recombinant FVIII. Plasma-driven FVIII is preferred as the first-line treatment for these patients. For FIX, both plasma-derived and recombinant FIX are available, and no information exists regarding the inhibitor development among patients based on the type of FIX (Albisetti & Monagle, 2021).

Hemophiliac infants should receive vitamin K without delay, and if IM, a 27-gauge needle should be used. Newborn screening and hepatitis vaccinations should be completed according to routine care. Hepatitis B vaccination is effective when given subcutaneously or IM (Moorehead et al., 2018).

New factor concentrates and other therapies are in the pipeline for hemophiliac treatment, and clinical trials must be viewed as a meaningful discussion with parents of newly diagnosed or prenatally diagnosed hemophiliac patients. If any appropriate clinical trials are available that address the diagnostics, treatment, or follow-up, parents must be informed of the importance of clinical trials, especially involving newborns. Overall, clinical trials for new therapies involving newborns are highly limited globally (Degl et al., 2021; Sundquist Beauman et al., 2023). New gene therapy, monoclonal antibody, targeted molecular therapy, and gene therapy are on the horizon, and parents must be counseled and provided with information even if their infant may not receive the direct benefit immediately by enrolling in the clinical trial.

## Von Willebrand Disease

Von Willebrand disease (vWD) is a disorder of the von Willebrand factor (vWF) proteins, and it is one of the most frequently inherited bleeding disorders in humans (James et al., 2021). A partial or complete deficiency in this factor leads to mucocutaneous and postsurgical bleeding. If it is absent or markedly reduced, it can lead to bleeding in joints and muscles like HA due to the reduction of FVIII. vWF levels are high at birth and in the neonatal period; thus, the newborn bleeding due to vWD is rarely reported. Because vWF serves as a carrier for FVIII, those who do present with bleeding will have signs and symptoms consistent with FVIII deficiency. Diagnosis can be complex, and necessary laboratory tests should include CBC, PT/PTT, fibrinogen, and platelet-dependent vWF activity levels. Other additional workups may be needed. It is beyond the scope of this chapter, and detailed guidelines for diagnosis and treatment should be referenced (Albisetti & Monagle, 2021; James et al., 2021). The goal for vWD treatment is to increase FVIII concentration while normalizing the platelet adhesion (Albisetti & Monagle, 2021).

## Thrombocytopenia

Platelet transfusion has increased exponentially as the survival of premature infants has increased. The thresholds for the platelet transfusions are primarily based on the expert Opinion, and platelet reference values are not strictly set; most commonly, 150 to 450 × $10^9$/L is used as the normal range for newborns. A full-term newborn is reported to have a mean platelet count of 250 × $10^9$/L, and preterm infants are also reported to have similar platelet counts as older children and adults; however, more frequently, preterm infants' platelet counts are found to be lower than 150 × $10^9$/L (Deschmann & Sola-Visner, 2021; Ferrer-Marín & Sola-Visner, 2022; Ree & Lopriore, 2019).

Thrombocytopenia and its etiologies are primarily categorized as the following: decreased production of platelets, increased consumption of platelets, increased extravascular loss of platelets, or a combination of any of these factors. Thrombocytopenia that occurs early (early onset is within 72 hours of life) is usually caused by prenatal factors, primarily maternal conditions, such as preeclampsia, IUGR for various reasons (such as PIH), asphyxia or maternal drug ingestion (e.g., chloramphenicol, hydralazine, tolbutamide, and thiazides), placental infarction, and immune-mediated maternal platelet antibodies. It is very common to see an infant's platelets being low due to chronic exposure to maternal hypertension; however, they are not low enough to require transfusion.

Late-onset thrombocytopenia occurs more than 3 days after birth and is associated with bacterial sepsis or line-related thrombosis. Reference values for platelets, or ranges for what is normal in newborns, are unclear. Thresholds for prophylactic platelet transfusions across the global neonatal communities also widely differ from 10 to 25 × $10^9$/L. In case of infants when they are exhibiting bleeding or preparing for an invasive procedure, the thresholds for transfusion are higher at < 50 ×$10^9$/L (Deschmann & Sola-Visner, 2021; Ree & Lopriore, 2019).

One international randomized controlled trial on platelet transfusion reported results offering caution for prophylactic platelet transfusion. A total of 660 preterm infants (median gestation age of 26.6 weeks) with low platelet count at birth were randomized into two groups based on two different platelet count thresholds for transfusion. One group was assigned to receive platelet transfusion at 50 × $10^9$/L and another at 25 × $10^9$/L. Major bleeding or mortality within 28 days after randomization was found to be statistically higher for the group who received platelet transfusion with a higher threshold of 50 × $10^9$/L (odds ratio 1.57, 95% CI, 1.06–2.32, $p$ = .02), suggesting the potential harm in prophylactic platelet transfusion (Curley et al., 2019). Platelet counts alone in the absence of bleeding risk should not determine the need for platelet transfusion, and current evidence suggests the restrictive transfusion threshold of platelet count less than 25 × $10^9$/L. Typically, 10 ml/kg of the infant's weight is given over 2 to 3 hours to avoid large blood volume change leading to increased cerebral blood flow/intracranial pressure (Ferrer-Marín & Sola-Visner, 2022).

## Fetal and Neonatal Alloimmune Thrombocytopenia

The most common severe form of thrombocytopenia in fetuses and newborns is fetal and neonatal alloimmune thrombocytopenia (FNAIT), and this is also the most common reason for ICH in term infants. Because FNAIT presents with severe morbidity and mortality, this condition requires prompt diagnosis and management. FNAIT occurs when the following three conditions are met: (1) the incompatibility of fetal–maternal platelet-specific antigens (inherited by the father to the fetus); (2) maternal alloimmunization, which is the immune response to a fetal platelet that is incompatible with the mother leading to the development of IgG antibodies; and (3) the crossing of the maternal IgG alloantibodies through the placenta to the fetus. The maternal antibodies may also negatively affect the megakaryocytes in the fetal system, which may impede normal platelet production (Mitchell & Bussel, 2021)

As many as 37 platelet antigens can cause antibody reaction; the most frequent cases of FNAIT involve the antibody reaction against the human platelet antigen, HPA-1a. It is estimated that HPA-1a FNAIT occurs once in every 1000 live births. However, routine screening is unavailable for this condition, and the true prevalence is difficult to ascertain. In the western world, 2% to 3% of the population is reportedly HPA-1a negative. It is estimated that 10% of pregnant mothers who are HPA-1a negative develop antibodies against an FPA-1a positive fetus. Currently, estimating the level or severity of thrombocytopenia based on the anti-HPA-1a levels is not established, and study results are divided (Stam et al., 2023). As early as 16 weeks of gestation, fetal platelet antigens are recognizable; therefore, maternal alloantibody development, antibodies crossing the placenta into the fetal circulation, and subsequent destruction of fetal platelets can occur early in fetal life. Immune-mediated thrombocytopenia reportedly accounts for 50% of the severe thrombocytopenia cases in newborns (Mitchell & Bussel, 2021; Stam et al., 2023). The goal of the treatment is to identify the problem and to prevent the ICH to prevent morbidity and mortality further. The majority of FNAIT-related deaths are due to ICH (Mitchell & Bussel, 2021).

The family history of a former child with FNAIT may be the only clue to early identification because routine platelet counts are not performed on healthy newborns unless they are admitted to the NICU for other reasons, such as a respiratory condition. FNAIT screening is not done in most regions of the globe. It is important to note that FNAIT worsens in the second affected fetus than the first sibling and the FNAIT progresses significantly through the pregnancy. Specific management strategies for the fetal identifications of FNAIT are not within the scope of this chapter; however, the goal of treating the mother with known AIT typically consists of IVIG administration to the mother to reduce the antiplatelet antibodies. Postnatal treatment is based on the infant's clinical condition and the severity of the thrombocytopenia. Earlier, primarily matched maternal platelet transfusion was considered to be the best option for the treatment. More value is placed today on matched platelets from a nonrelative. Today, for most AIT cases, IVIG (1 g/kg/dose) and a random donor platelet transfusion (10–20 ml/kg) serve as a sufficient treatment. Additional use of methylprednisolone (1 mg IV q 8 hours) in conjunction with IVIG administration is viewed as a potentially superior option (Mitchell & Bussel, 2021). Further research is ongoing.

The nurse's role in clinical settings is to recognize symptoms such as petechiae, ecchymoses, hematoma, melena, hemoptysis, hematuria, hematemesis, oozing from the umbilical stump or IV puncture site, or postcircumcision site bleeding should be brought to the attention of the providers immediately for further investigation. Timely laboratory tests, as well as thorough history taking, are highly important.

## Disseminated Intravascular Coagulopathy

DIC is a process triggered by an underlying condition rather than a disease, and DIC is characterized by a hypercoagulable state in both small and large blood vessels throughout, with micro- and macrovascular clotting impeding the normal circulation. The triggering condition activates the clotting factors, which may release cytokines and other inflammatory mediators leading to the procoagulant state and then to the hypercoagulable state to produce clots throughout. While the body is in a hypercoagulable state, platelets and clotting factors are consumed or devoured by the hypercoagulation, which causes the loss of the normal mechanism to clot; therefore, uncontrolled hemorrhage results (Albisetti & Monagle, 2021; Costello et al., 2024; Tsantes et al., 2023).

In a healthy state, even for a premature infant, the physiologic balance of the coagulation mechanism and anticoagulant/fibrinolysis mechanism to maintain some level of equilibrium to not hypercoagulate or bleed. This balance is lost with certain illnesses, such as infection or trauma, and numerous derangements occur in various systems, including the coagulation system. Tissue factors such as thromboplastin (which activates the extrinsic pathway of clotting cascade) may be released into the body from vascular endothelial damage from trauma. Bacterial endotoxins and inflammatory factors, such as cytokine presence, can all activate the coagulation factors leading to thrombin/fibrin formation toward prohypercoagulability. These series of events suppress the natural anticoagulants, such as antithrombin, protein C, and tissue-factor inhibitors (Albisetti & Monagle, 2021).

In premature infants, DIC can occur secondary to respiratory distress, bacterial or viral infection, meconium or amniotic fluid aspiration, NEC, or even hypothermia. Among the term infants, DIC often develops due to traumatic delivery events such as placental abruption, which results in asphyxia, hypoxia, severe metabolic acidosis, hypotension, and shock (Albisetti & Monagle, 2021). Neonates' hemostatic system is in somewhat of a developmental coagulopathy, and this places the neonates at a higher risk for DIC when body systems are under stress and compromised due to various conditions mentioned previously (VanVooren et al., 2018).

### Diagnosis

There is no single laboratory test for DIC, but a combination of tests are needed that help to confirm DIC, which can be difficult to diagnose in the early stages. DIC can advance quickly, and multiorgan failure and death can occur when early recognition is not made. Healthcare professionals must be attentive and be aware of the DIC potential in critically ill patients (Costello et al., 2024). The best diagnosis is made when a clinical picture of the current disease state, delivery and maternal history, clinical course, and laboratory results are known. In a large Asian nationwide retrospective study, which reviewed 7,902 patients with DIC treated during a 10-year period, over 1,200 hospitals reported risks based on the asphyxia history. DIC patients who experienced asphyxia had significantly higher in-hospital mortality compared to the nonasphyxia group (19% versus 11%; $p < .001$). Also, the asphyxia group had more severe bleeding and required more extensive treatments. Vigilance is warranted in all ill patients (Kitaoka et al., 2024).

Clinical presentation is bleeding or oozing of various forms like HA or HB described earlier. Laboratory findings suggestive of clinically significant DIC are prolonged PT, PTT, thrombocytopenia, decreased coagulation factors (fibrinogen, FV, and FVIII) and inhibitors (antithrombin, heparin cofactor, protein C), and increased fibrinogen degradation products or split products (Albisetti & Monagle, 2021).

### Treatment

Successful treatment of DIC depends on correcting the underlying cause that led to DIC and providing necessary supportive treatment for adequate oxygenation to ensure optimal cardiorespiratory function. Platelet or plasma transfusions should only be offered when active bleeding or high risk for bleeding or those patients who require invasive procedures. The threshold for platelet transfusions commonly used today for actively bleeding cases is $< 50 \times 10^9$/L and 10 to $20 \times 10^9$/L for those not in active bleeding; however, they have the potential for the risk for bleeding. Other treatment includes fresh frozen plasma (15–30 ml/kg) and cryoprecipitate transfusion (rich in factors VIII, XIII, and fibrinogen), which would replace the coagulation factors. Heparin may be necessary when infants have extensive clotting, especially in large vessels (Albisetti & Monagle, 2021; Costello et al., 2024). Providing antithrombin or protein C, the natural anticoagulants may be of value; however, information is limited, no large trials have been conducted, and definite recommendations are unavailable (Albisetti & Monagle, 2021).

## Collaborative Management of a Coagulopathy

Minimizing invasive procedures leading to more bleeding is the priority in care. The administration of blood products and clotting factors (recombinant or plasma derived) should be carefully identified by two nurses. To ensure effective therapy and prevent further problems, conscientious monitoring of vital signs is critical, as is the monitoring of laboratory results throughout the infant's course of therapy. The administration of blood or blood products potentially causes fluid overload and other negative responses; therefore, the infant's hemodynamic state must be monitored closely. Although blood reactions in newborns are rare, they tend to occur within the first 15 minutes of blood or blood product administration. Signs of such reactions include rashes, tachycardia, hypertension, hematuria, cyanosis, and hyperthermia. Regular and frequent assessment of perfusion, skin color, tone, vital signs, and other routine physical assessments is highly valuable (Bagwell & Steward, 2020).

## SUPPORT OF THE FAMILY DURING THE CRISIS

No family expects their baby to be born prematurely or ill or that their infants would require neonatal intensive care. Parents must be informed in their native language to understand the information as it becomes available. Collaboration between the nursing team and providers, such as neonatologists, pediatricians, and neonatal nurse practitioners (NNPs), can offer medically necessary information and emotional support. When there is a sick infant in the NICU, it is important to enlist the support available at the institution, including the social service experts. Peer support offered by former NICU parents is also a valuable resource during a crisis (Pascual et al., 2024). Parents have a role in deciding their baby's care goals, but they cannot make an informed decision unless they have been presented with complete and reliable information. Often, not all information is available when discussing the critical condition with the parents, adding to parental stress. Frequent updates may offer additional support.

## SUMMARY

This chapter outlines the common hematologic neonatal problems along with evidence-based interventions. The nurse's role is crucial to improve outcomes. Anticipation of problems, extensive history taking, a thorough and ongoing assessment, and evaluation of treatment responses are key to providing the best possible care. Communication with parents of ill infants is an important/critical aspect of healthcare professionals.

## CASE STUDY 1

**Identification of the Problem.** An NNP, NICU RN, and respiratory therapist (RT) were called to a stat C-section due to fetal distress during labor. The mother had very limited prenatal care, and very little history was available. This infant was not slated to be admitted to the care of the neonatology team. The rupture of membranes (ROM) occurred approximately 18 hours before the C-section. The infant was believed to be approximately 36 weeks' gestation. Upon extraction of the baby, the neonatal team (NNP, RN from NICU, RT) recognized immediately that the infant was extremely pale and had likely experienced a fetal–maternal hemorrhage. The NNP decided to move the infant rapidly to the NICU and a central line was placed for further care (umbilical artery line).

**Assessment: History and Physical Examination.** Gestational assessment was aligned with 36 to 37 weeks' gestation at the most. The pale, white infant was not in apparent respiratory distress; however, the color remained white with oxygen administration due to the suspected and evident severe anemia. The infant did not have much activity, and the general tone was weak; however, the infant was not totally flaccid of limp (or floppy). Due to the emergent nature of the C-section, the mother was placed under general anesthesia and was not available to provide information. The infant was quickly extracted, and although the mother received general anesthesia, the infant was minimally depressed.

**Differential Diagnosis.** Based on how pale and white the infant was, fetal–maternal hemorrhage was suspected immediately, which would be the cause of severe anemia. Anticipating the need for immediate blood transfusion, the blood bank was notified by the operating room (OR) of this situation. The respiratory therapist was asked to set up a high-flow nasal cannula for the infant to provide supplemental oxygen. The infant did not require intubation.

- **Admission interventions.** A double-lumen umbilical artery line (5 French) was placed immediately. A blood culture and CBC with differential were drawn from the umbilical arterial catheter (UAC) and sent to the lab emergently. An x-ray was done to confirm the line placement and view the lungs and abdomen for abnormal findings. Lungs were clear, and no other abnormalities were found. The UAC was at the appropriate position. Fluids of $D_{10}W$ with heparin ½ unit/ml were hung at 65 ml/kg/d, anticipating the volume of blood to be transfused as soon as the PRBCs became available. The NNP at this facility discussed with the off-site neonatologist transferring this infant to a larger facility; however, due to poor weather conditions and the fact that PRBCs would soon be available at the facility where the infant was born, the decision was made to perform the blood transfusion at this facility to avoid delay. The parents were informed of all the factors that entered into the decision making and agreed.
- **Other considerations.** The family was informed of the urgent situation and the plan of care. The labor and delivery team was notified as well so that when the mother was alert and awake, the team could provide information on how the infant was doing and what was being done to meet the infant's needs. A Kleihauer–Betke test was requested to be drawn from the mother.
- **Initial diagnosis.** The lab reported critical lab values to the NICU. The hematocrit was 16.5% and the hemoglobin was 4.5 mg/dl, confirming the severe anemia, which was likely due to fetal–maternal hemorrhage. A cord blood gas was obtained, and the pH was 7.0 with a base excess of –14, demonstrating metabolic acidosis.
- **Management.** After discussing the general assessment of the infant with the neonatologist, the decision was made to transfuse 15 ml/kg of PRBCs over 3 hours immediately and repeat 8 hours later so as not to fluid-overload the

infant. The maintenance fluid volume was then carefully managed. The initial blood glucose was normal, and they remained normal. Metabolic acidosis was not urgently treated because the perfusion improved with the RBC transfusion and would likely normalize the metabolic acidosis.

- **The course.** After the first transfusion, the infant's color pinked up mildly, and oxygen saturation improved. After the second transfusion, the infant did not require a high-flow device; the skin color was pink, and the infant appeared as a well-appearing newborn. Trophic feeding was offered in a small volume when the infant began to show feeding cues. However, the regular feeding volume was held until 8 hours after the second transfusion.
- Follow-up labs. Hematocrit and hemoglobin were redrawn 8 hours after the second transfusion was completed. The hematocrit was 34%, and the hemoglobin was 10 mg/d. The infant remained well throughout the course and began to feed well. Vital signs were all normal. However, careful observation continued, considering the severe anemia and risk for NEC. A Kleihauer–Betke test performed on the mother was POSITIVE. Capillary blood gas was obtained during the follow-up hematocrit and hemoglobin, and the normalization of the pH was 7.35, and the base excess was –2. Improved oxygenation resulted from the RBC transfusion and improved the overall clinical status, including respiratory status.
- Follow-up care: The infant went home with the mother on day of life 4. The blood culture remained negative. The feeding went well, and all physical examination findings were normal. Follow-up care will be given by the primary care pediatrician that the mother selected, and a discharge summary will be sent. Due to the severe chronic anemia, the infant would be monitored closely for neurologic and physical development. The infant was also registered for the neurodevelopmental follow-up service offered by the neonatology practice at 3 months of corrected age.

## CASE STUDY 2

**Identification of the Problem.** A NICU nurse received a call to report to the labor and delivery unit to assist with transitioning a newly born term infant who was slow to transition after an unexpected vacuum-assisted delivery due to shoulder dystocia. Also, meconium-stained fluid was noted. The NICU nurse called the NNP on call to come right away after seeing that the infant required further intervention. Both arrived within 1 minute of each other when the infant was approximately 7 to 8 minutes old. Labor and delivery nurses reported a very difficult last 5 to 10 minutes requiring a vacuum-assisted delivery and how depressed the infant was due to being initially stunned from the delivery. Vigorous stimulation was given, and the infant did come around to be responsive by 1 minute (therefore, they did not call the NICU team until later). The infant cried. The heart rate was consistently above 100 beats/min throughout the delivery and initial resuscitation and stabilization. No chest compressions were needed at the time of initial resuscitation and stabilization. Mother reportedly spiked a fever to 102°F (38.9°C) a few hours prior to delivery. The mother's membranes had ruptured nearly 18 hours ago at home, and the mother presented to the hospital in labor a few hours after ROM occurred.

**Assessment: History and Physical Examination.** The infant required continuous positive airway pressure (CPAP), and meconium staining was visible. Also, the infant had irregular spontaneous breathing. Cephalohematoma versus caput, in addition to the significant head molding, was noted. Oxygen saturation was > 90% when CPAP was being administered. The infant's tracing was reportedly normal, without any issues, until the end of the delivery.

**Differential Diagnosis.** The term male had respiratory distress due to meconium aspiration and stress from vacuum-assisted difficult delivery. A cephalohematoma was noted. A rule-out sepsis for prolonged rupture of membranes (PROM) and maternal fever occurred. The infant was transferred to the NICU for immediate respiratory support and observation.

- **Admission interventions:** High-flow nasal cannula (HFNC) was placed on the infant at 6 L/min, and CPAP was being considered; however, the infant's respiratory status was stabilized on the HFNC at 6 L/min with adequate saturations requiring $F_IO2$ of 0.25. The work of breathing was easy. A peripheral IV was placed to provide 70 mg/kg/d with $D_{10}W$. An orogastric (OG) tube was placed as routine care for infants who are on HFNC or CPAP (or CPAP was rendered longer during the resuscitation). The RN assigned to the infant was asked to monitor the cephalohematoma. A chest x-ray was ordered and revealed mild appearance of meconium aspiration. A double-lumen umbilical artery catheter was placed when the cephalohematoma appeared to increase in size. A blood culture, CBC with differential, and arterial blood gas (ABG) were all obtained quickly.
- **Development of additional issues:** When the infant was about 2 hours of age, the cephalohematoma increased in size, and a subgaleal hemorrhage was suspected due to the increasing head circumference and fluctuating pooled fluid/blood in the infant's head. Tachycardia ensued due to blood loss into the subgaleal space. The RN reported fresh blood being aspirated from the OG tube and the umbilical stump. Careful supportive measures were considered. Hourly head circumferences were obtained, and coagulation studies were ordered.
- **Other considerations:** Family members were at the bedside and very involved with care. The information regarding the likely subgaleal hemorrhage, as well as the pending labs, were provided. The blood bank was notified immediately to alert them about the potential for DIC in this patient.

**Differential Diagnosis.** Rule out sepsis (CBC with differential not showing significant signs and symptoms for infection). Subgaleal hemorrhage was initially diagnosed; however, the head circumference stopped increasing in size and tachycardia did not worsen. Respiratory distress due to meconium aspiration remained stable without the need to increase $PaO_2$ or flow on HFNC. Initial hematocrit was 42% with hemoglobin of 10.5 mg/dl.

**Development of Management Plan.** Continue to observe closely for all the vital signs, perfusion, the size of head circumference, and overall neurologic findings.

- **The course:** PT and PTT were prolonged, and the fibrinogen level was low. Spontaneous cessation of DIC tendency was achieved without blood transfusion. The infant continued to wean down on HFNC on flow and remained on $F_IO_2$ of 0.21 to 0.23. Low urinary output and elevated creatinine (initially > 1.2 and returned to > 0.8) were noted until approximately 36 hours of age. However, the urinary output returned to normal on day of life 3. The infant began showing cues for feeding readiness, demonstrating an overall improvement in clinical status. Due to the improved respiratory status, a repeat chest x-ray was not ordered.
- **Follow-up labs:** The infant's lowest hematocrit was 32%. Due to the spontaneous cessation of gastric bleeding within a few hours, additional PT, PTT, fibrinogen, and other studies were withheld to prevent iatrogenic blood loss. The infant was on full feedings by day of Life 4, without requiring IV fluids. However, due to the subgaleal hemorrhage and low hematocrit, the infant was monitored carefully and was discharged from NICU directly to home on the day of life 6. Although the maternal blood type was O positive, and the infant was A positive and Coombs negative, due to the subgaleal hemorrhage, a sharp rise in bilirubin level was anticipated. The infant did develop moderate hyperbilirubinemia, requiring phototherapy for 2 days, delaying the discharge. While under phototherapy, the infant came off HFNC, went to room air, and continued to feed well. The appearance of the bleeding in the infant's head continued to improve with decreasing head circumference over the course. Blood culture remained negative.
- **Follow-up care:** The primary pediatrician was fully informed of the infant's delivery history, the clinical course while in NICU, and the results of all labs. The recommendation was made for iron supplementation to start earlier than typically done for term newborns and follow-up HCT/HGB later. The team felt that the spontaneous resolution of bleeding tendency in this infant did not warrant immediate investigation for hemophilia diagnosis given the history of traumatic delivery, as well as the meconium aspiration leading to respiratory distress. The family did not have a history of family members with hemophilia or any other bleeding problems. The infant's primary care continued with routine care, being aware of the low hematocrit and providing monitoring.

## ONLINE RESOURCES

CourseConnect

Resources for this chapter are online and available at www.springerpub.com/courseconnect.

## REFERENCES

References for this chapter are online and available at www.springerpub.com/courseconnect.

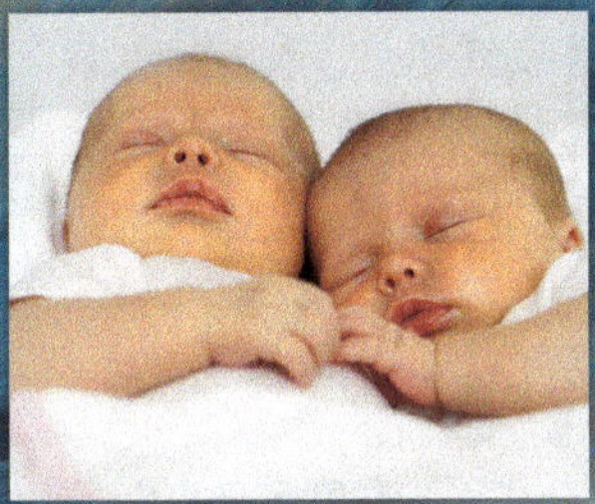

Stock.

CHAPTER 14

# Musculoskeletal System

Ashlea D. Cardin

## INTRODUCTION

The human body is astoundingly active, highly responsive, and constantly moving. The development of functional motor skills and integrated motor praxis is dependent upon the development and biomechanical maturity of the musculoskeletal system. The musculoskeletal system comprises bones, joints, ligaments, muscles, bursa, fascia, and tendons. From an anatomic structural standpoint, fetuses, infants, children, and adults differ in many ways: body size and mass proportions, growth rate and maturation, tissue thickness, body composition, bone density, muscle fiber type, joint structure development, muscle tone, posture, and bone, muscle, and ligamentous strength (Hunter et al., 2015; Kim, 2019; Williams et al., 2012). For fetuses, the buoyant uterine environment functions to support and reinforce musculoskeletal symmetry, strength, physical stature, range of motion (ROM), and muscle tone (Craighero, 2024; Franchak & Adloph, 2024; O'Brien, 2015). Flexible uterine walls assist in returning the infant from an extended posture to one that is flexed, midline, and supported circumferentially (Hunter et al., 2015). Additionally, the uterine environment supports hand-to-mouth activity, considered necessary for future participation in daily living activities such as feeding and playing.

This chapter provides a review of typical and atypical musculoskeletal development during the fetal and neonatal periods. Collaborative management is discussed, as well as the long-term implications of the functional and aesthetic concerns encountered with musculoskeletal anomalies.

Terminology used:

- Congenital anomalies: Major or minor, genetic or environmental, single or multiple, inherited or sporadic, lethal or nonlethal, isolated or patterned morphogenic defects of the organs or body parts that are identifiable pre-, peri-, or postnatally (Bacino, 2024; Cunningham et al., 2022; Sadlecki & Walentowicz-Sadlecka, 2023)
    - Malformation: Always congenital; refers to organ or body structures that are not formed, are partially formed, or abnormally formed. Major malformations have medical and/or social implications; minor have mostly cosmetic implications (Bacino, 2024).
    - Patterns: Grouped into syndromes, sequences, developmental field defects, or associations, this includes malformations that are grouped into recognizable diagnoses (Bacino, 2024). Syndromes are assumed to result from a single etiology, whereas sequences represent patterns of anomalies that can result from multiple etiologies (Bodamer, 2024).
    - Defect/birth defect: A physical or biochemical difference that is present at birth. Contemporary thought is that this term, while still common in medical literature and language (e.g., for specific conditions), should be used with caution because inclusive disability language guidelines state that some consider "defect," "birth defect," or "defective" offensive when describing a disability because they may imply that *the person* is deficient or inferior to others (National Center on Disability and Journalism [NCDJ], 2021).
    - Deformation/deformed: A typically developed structure that is changed, usually by restrictive extrauterine, intrauterine, or mechanical forces (Cunningham et al., 2022). A deformity is a condition in which the body part does not have the expected shape; this term should not be used as an adjective to describe a person (NCDJ, 2021).
    - Disruption: Structural defects that result from interruptions in typical development, often from vascular or mechanical forces such as compression, strangulation, or thrombosis (Bacino, 2024)
    - Dysplasia: Abnormal organization of cells into tissues (Bacino, 2024); two primary skeletal categories, including osteochondrodysplasia (abnormal development of cartilage and/or bones) and dysostoses (individual bone abnormalities)
    - Difference/limb difference/congenital difference: Contemporary phrases used to describe conditions in which fingers, hands, arms, legs, feet, or toes are missing or misshapen (NCDJ, 2021)

## EMBRYOLOGY

An extensive discussion of embryology is beyond the scope of this chapter; however, a brief review is provided. Prenatal development is divided into two stages: the embryonic period (first trimester) and the fetal period (second and third trimester) (Liu & Thompson, 2019). The embryonic period is characterized by maximal organogenesis and lasts from the end of the first week until the eighth week of gestation. Rapid cell division during organogenesis renders an organ vulnerable to disturbance, resulting in aberrant development. Functional and minor morphologic anomalies may occur at any time during gestation. The embryo originates from three cell layers: the ectoderm, the endoderm, and the mesoderm. The embryonic mesoderm gives rise to the articular, muscular, axial, and appendicular skeletal systems.

The articular system, or joints, can be classified into three types: fibrous, cartilaginous, and synovial. Fibrous joints are those in which two bones are separated only by dense fibrous connective tissue, as seen in cranial sutures. Cartilaginous joints (such as the symphysis pubis and between the intervertebral discs of the spine) have hyaline cartilage or fibrocartilage between the two bony surfaces. The elbow and knee are examples of synovial joints. The adjoining bone ends in these joints are covered with a thin cartilaginous layer and joined by a ligament lined with a synovial membrane. Ligaments hold bones together; the capsule encases the joint to provide support and protection. The synovial membrane secretes a lubricant referred to as *synovial fluid*, which is a source of nutrition for the articular cartilage. Synovial joints are the most mobile yet can withstand pressure and provide stability between the bones, especially during weight bearing. The articular system begins to develop during the sixth week of gestation, with functional joints present at the end of the eighth week. Joints allow motion to occur. Box 14.1 lists common terminology to describe types of motion and the planes in which motion occurs.

### BOX 14.1

### JOINT MOTIONS AND PLANES OF MOVEMENT

- Abduction: movement in the coronal plane that moves a limb laterally away from the body
- Adduction: movement in the coronal plane that moves a limb medially toward or across the midline of the body
- Dorsiflexion: movement at the ankle that brings the top of the foot toward the anterior leg
- Eversion: foot movement involving the intertarsal joints of the foot in which the bottom of the foot is turned laterally, away from the midline
- Extension: movement in the sagittal plane that increases the angle of a joint (straightens the joint); motion involving posterior bending of the vertebral column or returning to the upright position from a flexed position
- Flexion: movement in the sagittal plane that decreases the angle of a joint (bends the joint); motion involving anterior bending of the vertebral column

(continued)

### BOX 14.1

### JOINT MOTIONS AND PLANES OF MOVEMENT (*continued*)

- Horizontal abduction: holding the arm at shoulder height, moving the shoulder backward
- Horizontal adduction: holding the arm at shoulder height, moving the shoulder across body
- Hyperextension: continuation of extension beyond the normal range of motion
- Inversion: foot movement involving the intertarsal joints of the foot in which the bottom of the foot is turned toward the midline
- Palmar flexion: bending the wrist toward the palm
- Planes of movement:
  - Sagittal plane (lateral plane): a vertical plane running from front to back; divides the body or any of its parts into right and left sides; extension and flexion motions occur in this plane
  - Coronal plane (frontal plane): a vertical plane running from side to side; divides the body or any of its parts into anterior and posterior portions; abduction and adduction motions occur in this plane
  - Axial plane (transverse plane): a horizontal plane; divides the body or any of its parts into upper and lower parts; rotation occurs in this plane
- Plantar flexion: movement of the ankle toward the surface of the foot
- Pronation: movement that combines eversion, dorsiflexion, and abduction
- Scapular abduction: shoulder girdle protraction, or rounding the shoulders forward
- Scapular adduction: shoulder girdle retraction, or squeezing the shoulder blades together
- Supination: movement that combines inversion, plantar flexion, and adduction
- Trunk/neck lateral bending occurs to the right and left sides
- Ulnar and radial deviation: hand movement toward the little finger side and hand movement toward the thumb side
- Wrist extension/dorsiflexion: bending the wrist away from the palm toward the lower arm

*Sources:* Betts, J. G., Desaix, P., Johnson, E., Johnson, J. E., Korol, O., Kruse, D., Korol, O., Johnson, J. E., Womble, M., & Young, K. A. (2013). *Anatomy & physiology* (pp. 345–349). Rice University. https://opentextbc.ca/anatomyandphysiology/chapter/9-5-types-of-body-movements; Lippert, L. S. (2011). *Clinical kinesiology and anatomy* (5th ed.). F.A. Davis; National Cancer Institute. (n.d.). *Anatomical terminology*. https://training.seer.cancer.gov/anatomy/body/terminology.html.

Muscle origin and insertion, muscle fiber arrangement, types of muscle contraction, arthro- and osteokinematics, muscle tissue, and movement characteristics are important for clinicians to consider. Groups of myotubes, the primordia of skeletal or striated muscle, are apparent by the end of the eighth week of gestation. As the myotubes enlarge, the appearance of myofilaments is evident in interior regions. The growth of myofilaments leads to mature muscle fibers. Postnatal development of muscle fibers continues both in number and in size. Muscle development depends on proper innervation, evident at 8 to 10 weeks of gestation. Without this innervation, the muscles atrophy. The mother can detect intrauterine fetal movements at 16 weeks of gestation. Infants born prior to 31 weeks gestational age have immature muscle fibers, neuromuscular junctions, and diminished flexor tone. Muscle tone development occurs caudocephally, with lower extremity tone beginning at about 33 to 35 weeks postmenstrual age and upper extremity tone increasing around 35 to 37 weeks' gestation (Byrne & Garber, 2013).

The skeleton develops by intramembranous bone formation and endochondral ossification. It gives shape and support to the body, protects vital organs, and provides structure for muscular attachments. Bones are soft, develop cephalocaudally, and are made up of several types of tissue (fibrous, cartilaginous, osseous, nervous, and vascular). Upper limbs develop more quickly than the lower limbs, and several days elapse between the development of the upper limbs and that of the lower limbs. The vertebral column is initially of a cartilaginous form, with ossification beginning during the embryonic period and reaching completion in early adulthood. Ossification is evident in all long bones by 12 weeks' gestation, with arms, legs, fingers, and toes typically recognizable at this stage. The fetal period represents a time of further growth and development. At birth, an infant's skeleton is primarily cartilaginous and comprises more than 300 bones. The infant's bones will fuse and ossify throughout childhood and into adulthood, resulting in the 206 bones typically seen in an adult skeleton.

## POSITIONAL TERMINOLOGY

As an infant's body learns to move and reposition itself, it is imperative that clinicians and healthcare providers understand the infant's motoric developmental sequence and the terms that describe those changes from anatomic position:

- Anterior/ventral: front of the body or a position close to the front
- Posterior/dorsal: back of the body or a position close to the back
- Medial: toward the midline of the body
- Lateral: away from the midline of the body
- Supine: lying on back; face is upward
- Prone: lying on stomach; face is downward
- Side-lying: lying on side with neutral/midline orientation
- Distal: away from the trunk
- Proximal: toward the trunk
- Cephalic or cranial: close to the head
- Caudal: close to the feet
- Superior: refers to the position of a body structure above another
- Inferior: refers to the position of a body structure below another
- Superficial: position of relative depth; on top of
- Deep: position of relative depth; underneath
- Contralateral: refers to opposite side of body
- Ipsilateral: refers to same side of body
- Valgus: describes an abnormal position in which a distal body part is bent outward and away from the midline of the body
- Varus: describes an abnormal position in which a distal body part is positioned inward, toward the midline of the body
- Subluxation: incomplete dislocation or a displaced joint
- Dislocation: complete separation of one articulating joint surface from another
- Reduction: restoration of a body part to a normal position

## MUSCULOSKELETAL ASSESSMENT

The maternal history is reviewed for medical conditions (e.g., oligohydramnios, diabetes, thyroid disease), environmental or social health determinants (e.g., infections, nutrition), fetal movement during gestation or the birthing process, or uterine anomalies (e.g., septate or bicornate uterus) that may compromise fetal movement and growth. Also important is to consider a family history of musculoskeletal conditions.

Detailed observation is the key tool for assessing the neonatal musculoskeletal system. Visual inspection should begin in one body region—that is, cephalic or caudal—and progress along the body in an organized fashion from proximal to distal. For the initial examination (exam), place the infant in a quiet resting state to assess passive posture, resting tone, symmetry, positioning, and any obvious anomalies. Active movement by the infant allows the clinician to view muscle tone, movement quality, symmetry, and active ranges of motion (ROMs). Manipulation is used to assess ROM, including joint mobility. Caution should be taken when assessing infant ROM because it is often a stressful and potentially painful or harmful experience for the neonate. Radiologic studies as well as simple body measurements aid the healthcare provider in the identification of covert or hidden musculoskeletal deformities such as hip dysplasias and the absence of bony structures.

In developing a differential diagnosis, the clinician must be aware that a combination of anomalies present in the neonate may be a small part of a larger pattern or syndrome. Conversely, congenital anomalies that present in combination may be a coincidental finding (Box 14.2). Musculoskeletal conditions may be accompanied by acute and/or chronic pain, limitations in mobility, decreased functional ability, and reduced dexterity (World Health Organization, 2022).

## TYPES OF MUSCULOSKELETAL CONDITIONS

Abnormalities of the neonatal musculoskeletal system can range from a subtle brachydactyly (shortened fingers or toes) to congenital amputation, to a fatalistic form of osteogenesis imperfecta (OI) congenita. Causes range from uterine malpositioning of the fetus to autosomal dominant disorders.

**BOX 14.2**

**MUSCULOSKELETAL CONDITIONS**

- Arthrogryposis multiplex congenita, or multiple congenital joint contractures
- Congenital upper and lower limb differences that can be caused by maternal exposure to known risk factors, genetic abnormalities, growth restriction, or mechanical forces
  - Absence of limbs: *amelia*
  - Amniotic band sequence/syndrome: occurs when tears in the amnion get wrapped around digits, limbs, or other parts of the body
  - Congenital talipes equinovarus: "clubfoot"; characterized by hindfoot varus and equinus, midfoot cavus, forefoot adductus
  - Syndactyly: fingers and/or toes that failed to separate
  - Polydactyly/hyperdactyly: duplication of fingers and/or toes
  - Undergrowth (limb-reduction) or overgrowth of limbs
- Fractures and/or bowing
  - Birth trauma, including skull fractures
  - Greenstick fracture: occurs when one side of bone is broken and the other bent
  - Epiphysis/growth plate fracture
  - Bowing: angular deformity of bones, typically long bones
- Hip dysplasia or dislocation: instability of the femoral head in the acetabulum, allowing the hip joint to become partially or completely dislocated
- Positional deformities
  - Intrauterine
  - Acquired, i.e., from prolonged hospitalization due to medical complexity or acuity
  - Home based/postdischarge: from prolonged static positioning; examples include torticollis, plagiocephaly, hip contractures
- Orofacial clefts: incomplete closure of the palate and/or lip
- Craniosynostosis: premature closing/fusion of the fibrous cranial sutures
- Plagiocephaly: misshapen head; positional plagiocephaly results from a continuous external force that causes flattening (Blanco-Diaz et al., 2023)
  - Brachycephaly: wide, flattened back of head
  - Dolichocephaly or scaphocephaly: long, narrow head
- Structural disorders of the spine
  - Hemivertebrae: malformation of half of the vertebral body
  - Spinal conditions
    - Kyphosis: abnormally rounded upper back
    - Scoliosis: atypical curvature of spine
    - Lordosis: excessive in-curving at the base of the spine, or *swayback*

(*continued*)

**BOX 14.2**

**MUSCULOSKELETAL CONDITIONS (*continued*)**

  - Torticollis: congenital, positional, birth injury; tightness of the neck musculature causing the head to tilt to one side and rotate to the opposite
- Skeletal dysplasias: genetic bone and cartilage disorders affecting the fetal skeleton
  - Achondroplasia: *dwarfism* or short stature; most common dysplasia (Murton et al., 2023)
  - Hypochondroplasia; leads to limb-trunk disproportion
  - Thanatophoric dysplasia: lethal condition
  - Osteogenesis imperfecta congenita: "*brittle bone disease*", caused by hypomineralization
- Thrombocytopenia-absent radii syndrome: thumbs present, radius bones absent

Neurologic, infectious, and/or genetic conditions can affect musculoskeletal development, as can postprocedural disorders of the musculoskeletal system (e.g., birth trauma). Regardless of the clinical significance, an overt structural condition can become the focus of parental attention. Assessment of the musculoskeletal system—which can have multiple typical variants—and knowledge of pathogenesis, sequelae, treatment, and prognoses are imperative to the clinician. Delay in diagnosis and treatment may be implicated as a cause of a less than favorable outcome for the infant with a musculoskeletal anomaly. An atypical musculoskeletal system creates not only functional problems but, in some cases, outwardly visible differences as well. The type of dysfunction may significantly affect how the parent views the neonate and the infant's potential for positive growth and development. Family-centered caregiving, which includes appropriate family education by the healthcare professional, is paramount to a beneficial outcome because many musculoskeletal conditions require compliance with long-term therapy and possible surgical intervention.

## ARTHROGRYPOSIS MULTIPLEX CONGENITA

Historically, the term *arthrogryposis* (curved, hooked joint) has been used to describe a clinical appearance and diagnose various conditions (Figure 14.1). As a group of conditions, arthrogryposis multiplex congenita is considered rare, occurring in 1 out of every 3,000 to 12,000 births. The common denominator for more than 400 known conditions is the presence of multiple congenital joint contractures, which are typically characterized by decreased fetal movement (Lakhani et al., 2017).

### Pathogenesis

Classic arthrogryposis (also termed *amyoplasia*) describes limitation of movement in multiple joints that is present at birth. In distal arthrogryposis, the hands and feet are involved

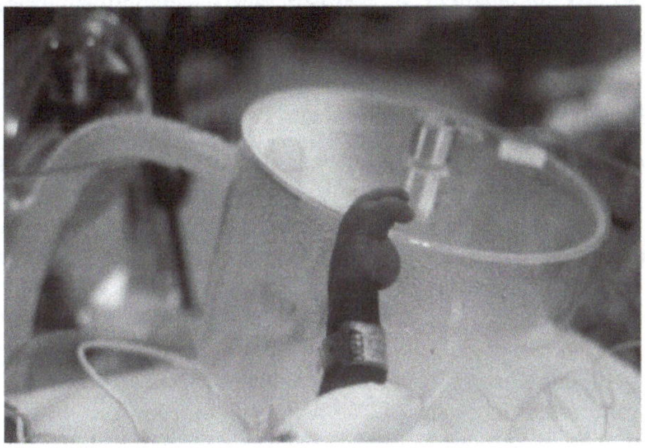

FIGURE 14.1 Distal fixed joints: arthrogryposis.

but larger joints are spared (Kimber, 2015). Due to the variety of comorbidities that may be associated with these conditions, the etiology is varied. With decreased movement, extra connective tissue forms around the joints of the fetus and fixes them in position. This may be related to abnormal development of the muscles, tendons, and/or joints, as listed in Table 14.1.

In some cases, the fetus may be prevented from normal movement due to restrictions within the uterus from multiple pregnancies or abnormalities of the uterine structure. Maternal diseases, such as myasthenia gravis or myotonic dystrophy, may be related to arthrogryposis, as well as the use of certain medications or infections in the mother. Intrauterine vascular compromise is another potential associated factor, with damage to developing muscles and nerves due to decreased blood flow (Chareyre et al., 2021). Finally, abnormalities of the fetus's central nervous system (CNS) may be a cause, such as spinal muscle atrophy or cerebro-oculo-facial-skeletal syndrome (Table 14.1).

**TABLE 14.1**

**ETIOLOGY OF DECREASED FETAL MOVEMENT**

| Category | Examples |
|---|---|
| ***Myopathic*** | |
| Abnormal muscle function secondary to failure of muscle formation or degeneration | Congenital muscular dystrophy<br>Absence of muscles |
| ***Neuropathic*** | |
| Abnormal nerve function or innervation that involves either CNS or the PNS | Drugs or toxins CNS malformations: decreased number of anterior horn cells |
| Abnormal connective tissue | Abnormal formation of bone, cartilage, tendons, or connective tissue |
| ***Mechanical Limitation*** | |
| Produces compression within the uterus | Twins; multiples<br>Amniotic rupture<br>Oligohydramnios<br>Benign uterine myomas |

CNS, central nervous system.
PNS, peripheral nervous system.

## Clinical Manifestations

Arthrogryposis is characterized by limited movement of the affected joints. The distal joints are more frequently affected than proximal joints. Talipes equinovarus (clubfoot) is almost universal, and the wrists are typically flexed. The elbows and knees can be in a flexed or extended position. Dimpling may be noted at the elbows and knees. Shoulders are internally rotated. Normal skin creases overlying the joints are often absent, suggesting an onset of arthrogryposis in the early intrauterine period. Changes in facial features may also be seen, including micrognathia (an undersized chin, which can interfere with breathing and eating).

## Diagnosis

A thorough evaluation is required to determine the cause of arthrogryposis. This process may begin prenatally. Decreased fetal movement and joint contractures are often seen on prenatal ultrasound. Polyhydramnios may be seen secondary to decreased fetal swallowing. Prenatal imaging may reveal other physical characteristics that lead to suspicion of certain syndromes. Amniocentesis may provide information leading to a genetic diagnosis. **Quality and Safety: A detailed family history is essential to detect evidence of an inherited disorder. Maternal pregnancy and labor/delivery history should be reviewed carefully.** Physical examination of the infant with a careful description of the affected joints is needed, as well as a detailed evaluation of the muscle mass, tone, and function of the nervous system. Radiographic and ultrasound evaluation is necessary to determine the presence of other congenital anomalies because this may help link the contractures to a specific syndrome. Detailed imaging of the brain and spinal cord is indicated. Muscle biopsy and nerve conduction tests may be recommended. Genetic testing is also required. If a specific genetic etiology or specific syndrome is detected, a more accurate assessment of long-term prognosis can be made.

## Management

Excluding infants with severe CNS dysfunction, infants with multiple congenital contractures have a good prognosis. The goal of management is to achieve and maintain an acceptable

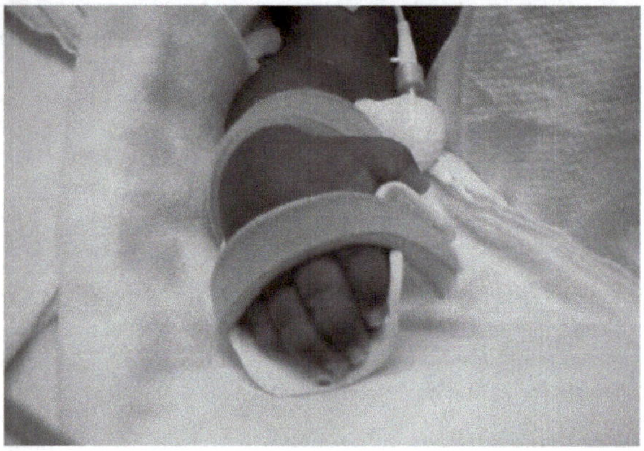

**FIGURE 14.2 Hand splint with arthrogryposis.**

ROM in the affected joints. During the newborn period, it is often a challenge to hold and care for these infants due to the extended or flexed position of the extremities and the reduced ability to manipulate the contracted limbs. Occupational and physical therapy should be initiated early in the neonatal period to begin strengthening muscles, improving ROM, and addressing challenges to daily living activities (occupations). Depending on the severity of contractures and positioning, splints and casts may be implemented, specifically molded and shaped for each limb (Figure 14.2). Occupational and physical therapy may be a lifelong process, and parents/familial caregivers can be taught techniques to use with the child. Family involvement is a key factor in therapy success for these infants. Creativity on the part of the healthcare professional, as well as on the part of the parents, complements efforts to manipulate the relatively rigid infant during feeding, sleeping, holding, and daily care activities. Parents may need referrals to agencies providing respite care or assistance from volunteers to maintain daily care needs.

## Prognosis

The long-term prognosis for multiple congenital contractures depends on the extent of involvement. Mortality rates are low for those without CNS involvement (1%–7%). For those with CNS involvement, perinatal mortality was 32% in a population of European infants (Hoff et al., 2011). Ventilator dependence at birth is associated with a poor prognosis (Chareyre et al., 2021).

## Amniotic Band Sequence

Amniotic band sequence (ABS, also referred to as amniotic rupture sequence or amniotic- or constriction band syndrome) is associated with asymmetric fetal deformities due to vascular disruption, pathogenic variants, or (primarily) entanglement of the infant in fibrous amniotic bands (Bodamer, 2024). Deformities that have been attributed to the ABS include congenital limb differences, syndactyly, constriction bands or rings, umbilical cord abnormalities, craniofacial anomalies such as cleft lip and palate, and rare visceral defects such as gastroschisis and omphalocele). Early fetal evaluation has linked ABS with CNS involvement, such as skull and brain malformations. **Emergency Alert: ABS can be fatal if organs are involved.**

## Pathophysiology

Etiologic factors in ABS are unclear. Part of the difficulty is that some of the same malformations with this sequence can also occur for other reasons. Thus, the exact cause is not always clear, but the primary theory is the association with early amnion rupture and fetal entanglement of the resulting fibrous bands.

Two theories—endogenous and exogenous—explain the primary cause of ABS (Nakashima et al., 2021). The endogenous theory postulates that the malformations are caused by an innate derangement of the primary embryonic cell layers from which the tissues and organs develop. According to the endogenous theory, the presence of amniotic bands is a late development with no clinical significance.

The exogenous theory contends that early amniotic rupture allows the fetus to move into close approximation to the chorion by entering the chorionic cavity. The ruptured amnion then forms fibrous strings or bands. These bands can adhere to the skin, thus altering normal morphogenesis (e.g., cleft lip or palate, omphalocele), or disrupt the vascular integrity, resulting in gastroschisis. Amniotic bands encircle normally developed structures, thus resulting in congenital amputations, constriction rings with lymphedema distal to the ring, and facial clefts in nonanatomic distribution. Postural malformations such as clubfoot are believed to be caused by the fetus's close approximation to the chorion.

Figure 14.3 is an example of an amniotic band constriction ring noted on an infant's arm with unilateral cleft lip and palate. Evidence of this constriction ring indicates that development of the lip and palate were at one time typical, but development was altered with the presence of amniotic bands.

## Diagnosis

Many clinicians believe that amniotic bands must be present for ABS to be diagnosed. Others, however, believe that the presence of fetal deformities in a nonanatomic pattern, without obvious bands, is sufficient to establish the sequence

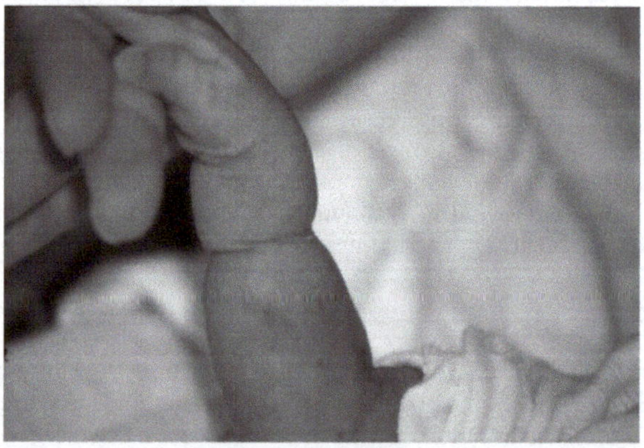

**FIGURE 14.3 Amniotic band constriction ring on the arm of a neonate.**

diagnosis. Congenital malformations, such as the visceral and craniofacial types, in the absence of amniotic bands may go undiagnosed as ABS because they could represent a faulty midline developmental pattern during the first trimester of pregnancy instead of the production of amniotic bands that constricted or restricted growth. The true incidence of this sequence, therefore, may be much higher than it generally appears—not only because of the difficulty in establishing a diagnosis but also because of the high mortality rate that exists during gestation.

## Collaborative Management

Notwithstanding the inherent problems associated with omphaloceles, gastroschisis, encephaloceles, clubfoot, syndactyly, and facial clefts, the clinician must be attuned to the unique complications of constricting bands. Constricting bands are usually associated with edema distal to the band. The resulting edema and vascular compromise contribute to complications such as skin breakdown, necrosis, thromboembolic formation that results from venostasis, and infection. **Quality and Safety: Care should include frequent vascular checks to assess perfusion. Trauma and tissue breakdown are discouraged through positioning and skin care. Observation for localized areas of necrosis is stressed.**

As with other musculoskeletal conditions and limb differences, the family may require emotional and psychological support. Families may be fearful that the infant's limb may require amputation or reduction because of necrotic tissue formation or infection. These fears may be justified, and the parents should be prepared for such a possibility. Complete surgical repair may not be possible during the infant's initial hospitalization, thus necessitating frequent hospitalizations during the early developing years. The delay in repair may necessitate families be taught to observe for vascular perfusion of an extremity, to recognize signs of infection, and to change dressings over open or healing areas. Preparation for discharge requires a multidisciplinary approach. The family may need surgical supplies, orthopedic or surgical consultations, occupational and/or physical therapy services, pediatrician and nursing follow-up for general well-child care, and social or financial services support to meet the long-term responsibilities of caring for their infant.

Multidisciplinary caregivers must provide opportunities for parent–infant bonding in preparation for discharge. While the infant is still in the hospital, the parents must be encouraged to touch and talk to the infant and to participate in the infant's care. They must also be encouraged to verbalize their feelings about their infant's condition. Every attempt should be made to address their fears, concerns, or misconceptions.

# CLUBFOOT

The classic clubfoot, talipes equinovarus, refers to an excessively plantar-flexed foot with hindfoot equinus (heel is pulled upward as if walking on the toes), forefoot adduction (toes are pointed inward), and midfoot supination. The term *clubfoot* may also be used to describe milder talipes conditions, including talipes calcaneus and talipes varus.

Highly common, clubfoot has an incidence of 1 in 1,000 live births. Males are affected nearly twice as often as females, and in infants with unilateral presentation, the majority appear on the right.

## Pathology

The precise mechanism of development of clubfoot has not been irrefutably established. Some researchers allude to the theory of intrauterine malposition (positional clubfoot), whereas others note a higher incidence of clubfoot in families with a positive history of the disorder (congenital clubfoot) or ascribe it to a genetic cause (syndromic clubfoot). One theory is that clubfoot is a multifactorial disorder involving a genetic predisposition coupled with environmental forces such as oligohydramnios, primiparity, macrosomia, and multiple fetuses.

## Clinical Manifestations

Clubfoot deformities are apparent at birth. The skin overlying the lateral aspect of the foot may be taut, whereas the medial aspect may have increased skin folds. The affected foot may be smaller in size than a normal foot. In older children, the calf muscle may be noticeably decreased in size. Milder talipes conditions may be returned to the neutral position by manipulation. The potential for pain also must be addressed.

## Collaborative Management

Early diagnosis by orthopedic specialists and treatment referrals to physical and occupational therapists is essential. In the neonatal period, joints, muscles, and ligaments may be more compliant to corrective manipulation without surgical intervention. This may involve serial casting or initiation methods of correction and maintenance, such as the Ponseti method (Smythe et al., 2017). **Emergency Alert: Difficulty with skin closure has been reported as a complication following correction of severe clubfoot.** This is especially true if the affected foot has received prior surgery. Special shoe splints or braces may be used toward the end of any successful treatment.

Parental education includes implementing routine newborn care for an infant wearing either splints or bilateral casts. Problems and solutions associated with clothing, sleeping, feeding, and bathing should be addressed. Parents' compliance with using splints may vary. Because consistent treatment is necessary for a favorable outcome, healthcare professionals must explore parental feelings and actions while providing anticipatory guidance.

# SYNDACTYLY

Fusion, or webbing, between two digits is referred to as *syndactyly*. This condition is the most common hand anomaly, with an incidence of 1 in 2,000 to 3,000 live births, and may be classified as simple or complex and complete or incomplete (Chouairi et al., 2020). Males are affected slightly more than females. Half of the time, both hands are involved in a symmetric presentation. Syndactyly of the fingers may be accompanied by syndactyly of the toes.

### Pathology

Although most occurrences of syndactyly appear to be through spontaneous mutation, familial predisposition has been reported, thus indicating an autosomal dominant pattern. Syndactyly may also be associated with specific syndromes such as Apert syndrome, a condition involving premature fusion of the cranial sutures (craniosynostosis).

There are four classifications of syndactyly. *Complete syndactyly* occurs when the fusion is from the base to the tip of the digit. Fusion that does not extend to the tip of the digit is termed *incomplete*. *Simple syndactyly* refers to digits connected by skin and soft tissue. Fused digits involving an osseous connection are considered *complex*. Abnormal nerve and vessel configurations may accompany complex syndactyly.

### Treatment

The type and timing of syndactyly treatment depend on its classification. Surgery is directed toward promoting normal function and appearance. Fingers should be separated before 18 months of age to prevent curvature of the fingers. If more than two adjacent digits are involved, surgery may include skin grafts and may be performed in stages to prevent vascular compromise (Chouairi et al., 2020).

### Prognosis

Prognosis is favorable for typical function and appearance, except in cases of complex syndactyly involving both bone and vascular and nervous tissue. These cases may be associated with some postoperative loss of function.

### Collaborative Management

Parents of infants with syndactyly are instructed in occupational and physical therapy, specifically in massage of the interconnecting skin. Massaging the webbed area prior to surgery allows some skin stretching, which permits easier repair. Referrals to certified hand therapists or plastic surgeons may also be indicated.

## POLYDACTYLY

Polydactyly, which may occur in isolation or within a syndrome, is any duplication of digits beyond the typical five. Also referred to as *hyperdactyly*, it is the second most common hand anomaly, with an incidence between 0.37 and 1.2 per 1,000 live births, depending on race (Bubshait, 2022). Polydactyly is believed to be caused by duplication of a single embryonic limb bud.

The two most common types of nonsyndromic polydactyly are preaxial (PPD) and postaxial (PAP) (Bubshait, 2022). Preaxial polydactyly is less prevalent and includes a wide array of finger duplications. Postaxial polydactyly is characterized by extra digits on the ulnar side of the hand. Postaxial polydactyly may be further classified into three types: Type I is merely a rudimentary soft tissue mass connected by a piece of tissue or pedicle. Treatment of this type involves simple excision, which can typically be done prior to discharge from the nursery per the parents' request. To avoid any residual skin tag after excision, infants are often referred to plastic surgery for a more complete removal. Type II is a partial duplication with the involvement of the phalanges. Type III, a rare occurrence, involves complete duplication of the metacarpal and phalanges. In addition to PPD and PAP, central axial polydactyly is rare but includes the ring, long, or index finger duplication. Central axial polydactyly is often associated with complex syndactyly.

### Collaborative Management

Treatment of polydactyly types II and III centers around functional capacity first and appearance second. The infant is observed for which duplication is dominant and most functional, and efforts are made to remove the least functional counterpart. If both duplicated digits appear equally functional, surgery should be used to promote aesthetic appearance. Reparative surgery often begins before 18 months and should be completed by 3 years of age.

## BIRTH TRAUMA

Birth trauma encompasses both mechanical and asphyxial events occurring during delivery. This trauma may be due to pressure and distortion. Mild, transient, or disabling trauma can occur despite exemplary obstetrical care; encouragingly, birth trauma rates are declining but still occur in approximately 2.6% of live births (Chaturvedi et al., 2018). A positive association exists between birth trauma and macrosomia, prematurity, breech presentation, shoulder dystocia, cephalopelvic disproportion, and vacuum extraction.

### Clinical Manifestations

Birth trauma includes subdural and intracerebral hemorrhage, abrasions, ecchymoses, erythema, cephalohematomas, caput succedaneum, fractures (especially of the clavicle), skeletal and spinal cord injuries, shoulder dystocia resulting in brachial plexus damage, and nerve palsies (Cunningham et al., 2022). Clavicular fractures are the most common fractures diagnosed as birth trauma. Clavicles are at an increased risk for fractures during shoulder dystocia in a vertex presentation or with arms extended during a breech delivery (Högberg et al., 2020; Liu & Thompson, 2019). **Quality and Safety: Physical examination findings related to birth trauma may appear only as bruising, abrasions, and petechiae that overlie the affected part.** Further diagnostic methods should be used when the infant exhibits pain on movement, limited motion, and abnormal passive positioning of an extremity or head movement.

Skull fractures may present as cephalohematomas. Skull fractures are most often linear and typically involve the parietal bones. Symptomatic evidence of a non-depressed skull fracture may resemble signs of increased intracranial pressure (ICP) secondary to epidural hemorrhage. Clinical presentation may include changes in muscle tone, hypertonicity or hypotonicity, arching of the back with the head in hyperextension, and respiratory compromise. Usually, no treatment is indicated for asymptomatic skull fractures. Depressed skull fractures, however, may require elevation of the depressed area.

**Emergency Alert:** **A rare but possible fatal delivery complication is subgaleal hemorrhage.** This may present as a cephalohematoma with a small area of swelling on the scalp as early as 4 hours of age. This often progresses and, unlike the cephalohematoma, crosses suture lines and involves the nape of the neck. The volume of blood loss may be high, causing hypovolemic shock. Vertebral fractures may be incurred in difficult breech deliveries in which there is longitudinal traction in combination with a twisting motion.

The most common nerve injury attributed to birth trauma is brachial plexus damage and resulting nerve palsy. This injury involves damage to the network of nerve fibers in the neck and shoulders, referred to as the *brachial plexus*. The prognosis is variable: Up to 35% of children with brachial plexus palsy may demonstrate lasting functional impairment of the involved limb (O'Berry et al., 2017). Involvement may occur in the upper portion (Erb–Duchenne palsy), the lower portion (Klumpke paralysis), or both portions (complete brachial plexus palsy).

Erb–Duchenne paralysis is the most common form. The affected arm is limp and in a position of elbow extension and internal rotation. The Moro reflex is diminished, and the grasp reflex is intact. Klumpke paralysis involves paralysis of the hand and wrist and is uncommon in infants. Complete brachial plexus paralysis results in paralysis of the entire arm. With full nerve-root avulsion injuries, some sensory recovery may occur, but no motor recovery can be expected (Liu & Thompson, 2019).

### Diagnosis

Diagnosis of birth trauma is based on physical assessment findings. These are usually visible at birth or in the immediate postnatal period. When necessary, physical findings should be confirmed by radiologic evaluation to establish whether a fracture is present. For significant scalp swelling, radiographic assessment of the skull is indicated.

### Collaborative Management

Treatment of birth trauma depends on the type and severity of the trauma. Often, supportive measures may be the only intervention required. For instance, brachial plexus injuries may require supportive positioning or immobilization in a neutral position using braces or splints. Specialized treatment protocols may, however, be initiated by occupational and physical therapists under the direction of pediatric orthopedic and/or neurology specialists. Surgery may also be indicated in severe cases.

Clavicular fractures also respond to supportive management. Typically, the arm is flexed, and the elbow is held against the chest. This position limits movement, thereby decreasing pain and preventing additional trauma at the site. Callus formation stabilizes the fracture by 10 days of age. A hard, palpable knot can often be felt with this callus formation. Again, referral to orthopedists and occupational and/or physical therapists may be indicated, though most fractures heal spontaneously with no long-term effects.

### Parental Education and Support

Diagnosing a disorder resulting from birth trauma can evoke anxiety in a parent. How such information is taken from and conveyed to the family is important. Nonjudgmental, supportive care by health professionals and consistent primary care by one individual may diminish some anxiety and allow the parents to establish trust. Calm reassurance about the nature of the trauma is important. It also helps to allay fears that something was done incorrectly during the delivery process if parents understand that many of these injuries cannot be avoided or anticipated. Parental education is a prerequisite if the parents are to understand the need for continued long-term treatment, which may be required. Birth trauma injuries may require long-term follow-up care by orthopedists, neurologists, or occupational or physical therapists.

## DEVELOPMENTAL DYSPLASIA OF THE HIP

Unilateral (asymmetric) or bilateral developmental dysplasia of the hip (DDH) refers to any manifestation of hip instability, ranging from subluxation to complete dislocation. DDH remains a common problem despite almost universal neonatal screening. Although controversy surrounds the usefulness of clinical neonatal screening programs for the diagnosis of DDH, these programs have led to earlier diagnosis and treatment for many infants. Additional studies have noted improved diagnosis of hip dysplasia with the use of ultrasound. It is recognized that up to 88% of unstable hips will normalize without treatment. Early clinical exams and targeted ultrasounds for infants with high-risk factors are currently used primary screening tools. Infants with high-risk factors include those with a family member with congenital/developmental hip dysplasia, those with breech presentation, and those with feet deformities (Shorter et al., 2011).

### Incidence and Risk Factors

Reports of the incidence of DDH vary. The incidence of DDH in the United States is approximately 1 to 4 in 1,000 live births (Rosenfeld, 2024). Differences in DDH incidence rates across ethnic groups can be attributed to genetic, ethnic, and environmental influences. Other influential factors include the infant's age at the time of examination, the expertise of the examiner, and the definition used by the examiner for the diagnosis of DDH.

The incidence of DDH is increased in first-born children. This increase may be due to the unstretched uterine and abdominal muscles, oligohydramnios, and the high association of fetal breech positioning in primigravidas. A definite preponderance of DDH occurs in female children. The ratio of occurrence of DDH in girls to boys is 6 to 1. Females account for 80% of all cases of DDH. Factors contributing to this finding include the fact that twice as many females as males are present in the breech position, and females appear to have heightened laxity in response to maternal relaxing hormones.

Breech position remains a major contributory factor to the development of DDH. Specific incidences of DDH related to positioning are 0.7% for cephalic, 2% for footling, and 20% for single breech. Delivery methods do not alter the incidence of DDH for infants in the breech presentation. Breech-positioned infants delivered by cesarean section have the same predisposition to hip dislocation as those delivered vaginally. The left hip is involved three times more often than the right hip. Approximately 60% of DDH is on the left, 20% on the right, and 20% bilateral. This finding is attributed to the tendency of the fetus to lie with its left thigh against the maternal sacrum. This position forces the left hip into a posture of flexion and adduction. Thus, the joint capsule covers the femoral head more than the acetabulum (Figure 14.4).

For infants born with other musculoskeletal and congenital renal abnormalities, such as torticollis and Potter sequence, the incidence of DDH is increased. Congenital renal abnormalities can result in fetal oliguria (abnormally small amounts of urine), thus subsequently producing oligohydramnios. Oligohydramnios can cause postural deformities because of the mechanical pressure on the fetus. Torticollis, arthrogryposis, and metatarsus adductus are thought to result from intrauterine compression, as does DDH.

After 40 weeks' gestation, the femoral head in the typically developing infant is firmly seated in the acetabulum and remains positioned there by the surface tension of the synovial fluid. The hips of the infant are difficult to dislocate. Conversely, the infant with a dysplastic hip has a loosely fitting femoral head and acetabulum. Because of this pathophysiologic phenomenon, the femoral head can assume several abnormal positions in an infant with DDH. One such position is termed *subluxation*. Subluxation occurs when the femoral head can be moved to the edge of the acetabulum but not completely out of it. Another position is termed a *dislocatable hip*. A dislocatable hip exists when the femoral head can be displaced from the acetabulum by manipulation but returns to the acetabulum afterward. The femoral head can also be found completely dislocated at birth (Figure 14.5). Dislocated hips may or may not be reduced by manipulation.

DDH is a dynamic disorder that may improve or deteriorate with or without treatment. Thus, the joint may spontaneously dislocate and reduce (return to normal position) with normal neonatal movement. With time, this simple mechanism progresses in complexity secondary to adaptive changes. DDH can eventually progress either to permanent reduction, complete dislocation, or dysplasia (abnormal development). More than 60% of infants with hip instability stabilize within the first week of life, and 88% stabilize postnatally within the second month. Only 12% of infants with initial hip instability are considered to have DDH with the potential for progression.

When a complete dislocation occurs, pathologic changes occur to the femoral head, acetabulum, and ileum. This complete dislocation is due to the adaptive changes that occur in the adjacent tissue and bone. **Quality and Safety: When adequate treatment has not occurred, the long-term complication of dislocation is degenerative changes of both the femoral head and the acetabulum. Once adaptive changes occur, the risk for progressive degeneration despite treatment increases.** The subluxated hip, when not diagnosed in the neonatal period, is generally diagnosed in adolescence when the strain of puberty and rapid growth spurts occur.

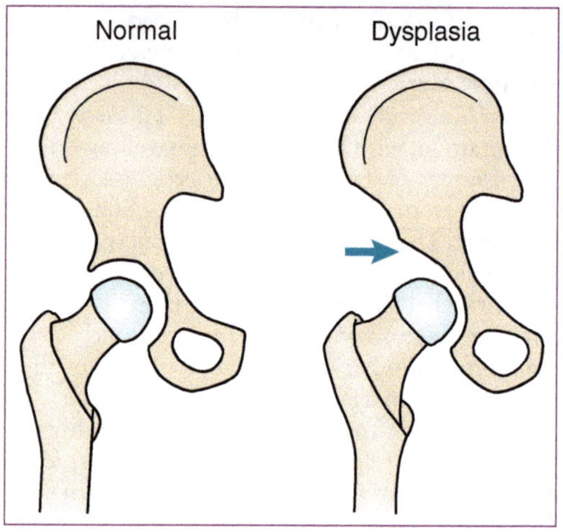


**FIGURE 14.4 Acetabular dysplasia of the hip.**

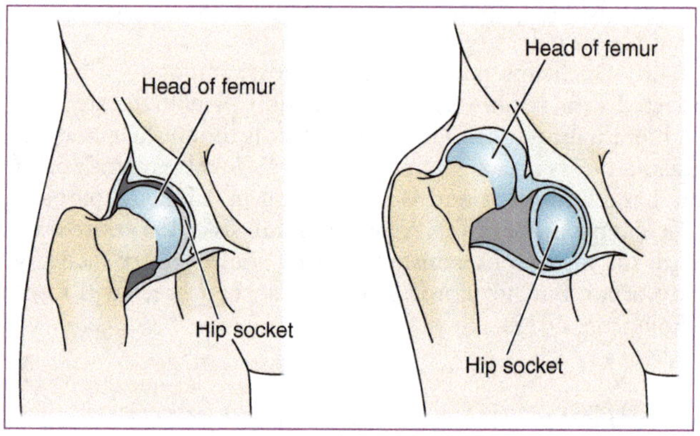


**FIGURE 14.5 Normal position of the femoral head and hip socket (left), and hip dislocation (right).**

With subluxation, the femoral head is laterally displaced and pushed upward into the joint; it is not entirely out of the acetabulum. As the child grows and increased weight bearing occurs, the femoral head slides around and moves to the joint's edge. Degenerative changes result from this continual sliding. Early arthritis is a common complication in those with DDH, often requiring surgical intervention for improved mobility (Stelzeneder et al., 2012).

## Diagnosis and Clinical Manifestations

In the neonatal period, the Ortolani and Barlow maneuvers help diagnose DDH (Williams et al., 2016). The Ortolani test is used to determine dislocation in the hip of a newborn, and the Barlow test is used to determine whether the hip is dislocatable (Barlow, 1962; Ortolani, 1976). In practice, both procedures are done in sequence. For examination, the infant is placed on a firm surface in the supine position.

The infant should be relaxed and quiet. Only one hip should be examined at a time. To perform the Ortolani test, the clinician stabilizes the infant's pelvis with one hand and, with the other hand, grasps the infant's thigh on the side to be tested. The examiner's middle finger is located over the greater trochanter (lateral aspect of the upper thigh), and the thumb is across the knee. The infant's hip is flexed to 90 while bending the knee. The infant's leg is then gently abducted with an anterior lift. In a positive Ortolani test, a *clunk* is heard with abduction. This clunk occurs as the dislocated femoral head slides over the posterior rim of the acetabulum and into the hip socket. Next, the hip is adducted, and, for the infant with DDH, a second clunk can be heard as the femoral head is displaced out of the acetabulum.

False-positive diagnoses of DDH have occurred when the examiner misinterprets a normal *click* (high-pitched sound) for a clunk. A click is not a sign of DDH. Clicks may be heard as a result of snapping of ligaments or tendons, and the majority are normal.

Barlow's test determines hip instability and identifies those hips that can be dislocated upon manipulation. Both hips and knees are flexed, with the hip to be tested in slight adduction. The examiner's middle finger remains positioned as for the Ortolani test over the greater trochanter. The thumb is, however, located over the medial aspect of the infant's lower thigh. The thumb exerts gentle pressure posteriorly and laterally (down and out). For the infant with DDH, the femoral head can be felt to move out of the acetabulum with the typical clunk. The hip can then be reduced by the Ortolani maneuver or simply by releasing thumb pressure and abducting and flexing the hips.

When the femoral head is subluxated, the examiner may observe a sliding motion in the hip joint during physical examination. This sliding motion can be characteristic of an unstable hip joint. Most cases of unstable hips spontaneously resolve without treatment.

The American Academy of Pediatrics (AAP) Committee on Quality Improvement has issued guidelines to assist in diagnosing and managing infants with DDH. All newborns should receive a screening exam. The Barlow and Ortolani maneuvers are not useful after 8 to 12 weeks of age. Ultrasonography is not recommended as a universal screening tool but is helpful as a targeted screening tool. If the physical exam of the neonate is equivocal, a repeat exam should be performed at 2 weeks of age. Certain physical signs that would result in an equivocal hip exam for DDH would include a persistent soft click. A referral to an orthopedic specialist is required if the Ortolani/Barlow exam is positive with a hip clunk at 2 weeks of age. This is not an emergency but should be completed in a timely matter over the next few weeks. The infant presenting at 2 weeks with a persistent soft click should receive ultrasonography of the hip within the next 3 to 4 weeks or referral to an orthopedic specialist at this time. For the infant who exhibits a normal hip exam with the resolution of the soft hip click, routine screening with well-baby checks during the first year of life is the recommendation. It is important to note that, according to the AAP recommendations, a newborn discharged before 48 hours of age should receive a repeat hip exam 2 to 4 days after discharge.

If the family has a history of DDH, the incidence increases to 9.4/1,000 in males and 44/1,000 in females. Because of this increased risk, even with a negative hip exam, an ultrasound at 6 weeks should be considered, or an x-ray of the hips at 4 months can be an alternative (Morey, 2001).

## Collaborative Management

Collaborative management aims to achieve and maintain the reduction of the unstable hip. The sooner treatment is implemented, the greater the chance for a successful outcome. Various splinting devices are used to treat DDH in infants. Examples of splints include the Pavlik harness, von Rosen splint, Denis Browne hip adduction splint, and Frejka pillow splint. The most commonly used splint for neonates is the Pavlik harness.

The Pavlik harness allows for spontaneous hip and lower extremity movement while maintaining the reduction of the hip joint. It can be worn comfortably during all aspects of newborn care, including diaper changes. The Pavlik harness can be adjusted for growth. It is indicated for use in newborns and infants up to 6 months of age. The use of the Pavlik harness is contraindicated for infants who are able to stand and for infants whose hip joints are not reducible by manipulation. A major factor influencing the success of the Pavlik harness is parental compliance with the treatment. With this condition, extensive parental education is imperative.

## Parent and Family Education and Support

In addition to providing information regarding the pathology and treatment goals of DDH, the nurse should allow the parents to remove and reapply the harness while under supervision. Referrals to physical therapy and/or occupational therapy may also be indicated. Parental support groups can help parents adjust to the infant's temporary condition. Parents should also be educated in the procedure used to reduce the dislocated hip because complete reduction must be achieved before the harness is applied.

## Long-Term Consequences and Complications

As with most therapeutic treatments, the potential for iatrogenic complications exists. Complications observed following DDH treatment include avascular necrosis, redislocation, and acetabular dysplasia. Complications can result from either inadequate or overly aggressive treatment. **Quality and Safety: Delaying surgery is associated with poorer clinical outcomes, including a limited range of motion, gait disturbances, and possible radiologic abnormalities (Alnamshan et al., 2018).**

**Emergency Alert: An additional complication that has been reported with the use of the Pavlik harness is the development of brachial plexus palsy (Mostert et al., 2000).** The tension of the shoulder harness appears related to this complication. The harness may be applied too tightly or may not be modified with the infant's growth, thus causing downward pressure on the brachial plexus nerves and subsequent neuropathy.

Alternatives to harnessing include surgical and nonsurgical reduction of the hip followed by casting. A hip spica cast is most often used with these infants. **Quality and Safety: Care then includes observance for poor pedal pulses, decreased peripheral circulation, pain, skin excoriation or abrasions, and possible development of respiratory infections resulting from decreased mobility.** An adjustment in car seats is required with the harness, and any casting and parental education should be documented prior to discharge of the infant, or a specialized car seat may be needed for safe transport of the infant.

## HOSPITAL-ACQUIRED POSITIONAL DEFORMITIES: SUPPORTING THE MUSCULOSKELETAL SYSTEM OF THE PREMATURE INFANT IN THE NEONATAL INTENSIVE CARE UNIT

Infants born early are often at a motoric disadvantage. According to Celik et al. (2018), "Disorders in the processing of the signals coming from the proximal sensory systems (vestibular, proprioceptive, tactile) lead to problems in the production of an adaptive response, the development of postural control and movement coordination, and the motor development and the arrangement of the awake-orientation status—all of which affect the development of play, social participation, education, and self-care occupations" (p. 2). Regarding musculoskeletal implications, Sweeney and Gutierrez (2002) state that "alignment and shaping of the musculoskeletal system occur during each body position that infants experience while in neonatal intensive care. Neonatal nurses and physical therapists can play a major role in designing, modeling, and teaching positioning strategies that promote skeletal integrity, postural control, and sensorimotor organization" (p. 58). They continue, describing positioning procedures used by neonatal intensive care unit (NICU)–based healthcare professionals to prevent extremity malalignment, skull deformities, and motor delays.

Infants admitted to the NICU are typically premature and/or medically fragile; therefore, they often demonstrate signs of motoric instability during their hospital stay. Motoric *stability* is indicated by consistent muscle tone appropriate for postconceptual age; controlled activity, including the smooth movement of extremities and head; smooth postural changes; demonstration of bright-eyed alertness and visual attention; and attempts to self-regulate through foot clasp (bringing feet together), grasping, bracing, holding on, hand to head or mouth activity, trunk tucking, or sucking. *Instability* is demonstrated through tremors, twitches, startles, coughs, sneezes, yawns, sighs, seizures, flaccidity, hyper/hypotonicity, hyperflexion, frantic activity, fluctuating tone, or eye floating (disorganized eye movements).

Both medical and familial caregivers can support infant musculoskeletal development through recognition of the signs and symptoms of instability and through the use of the following interactions to promote motoric stability: (a) containing the infant's extremities using hands, blankets, positioning aids, and so forth, to promote gentle flexion of the trunk and all extremities; (b) positioning the infant with extremities flexed toward midline and hands on the face or head; (c) moving the infant slowly to encourage organized position changes; (d) keeping the infant in contact with the bed during movement, if possible; (e) allowing opportunities for the infant to use their hands and feet to push against surfaces, grasp objects, clasp hands together, and suck; (f) varying infant positions; (g) lifting the infant in prone or side-lying (as opposed to supine) position to promote fetal tuck and calm; (h) providing daily opportunities for prone tummy time as medically appropriate (Danner-Bowman & Cardin, 2015); (i) performing swaddled bathing; and (j) referring to occupational and physical therapy for specialized evaluation and treatment recommendations.

## CRANIOSYNOSTOSIS

The bones that constitute the skull are joined with fibrous joints. These joints are lined with a thin layer of fibrous tissue. Separation of these joints allows for remodeling of the skull at the time of delivery and for rapid head growth during the early developmental years. The skull has five main sutures: coronal, lambdoidal, squamosal, sagittal, and metopic. The signal for closure of these sutures remains unclear but is believed to be secondary to multiple factors. The various sutures of the skull begin to close clinically in the first year of life, and the process continues into childhood. Complete ossification of these sutures is anticipated in the second or third decade of life. Figures 14.6 and 14.7 illustrate the newborn's cranial sutures.

Premature closure of any suture in the skull results in a clinical condition called *craniosynostosis*. The early closure of a cranial suture typically starts at one point and progresses along the suture line. Premature closure may occur prenatally or postnatally. Only one suture may be prematurely fused, or multiple sutures may be involved. Simple craniosynostosis, which involves one suture, generally occurs as an isolated defect. Complex craniosynostosis describes the premature closure of two or more sutures. This is usually associated with genetic syndromes such as Apert syndrome or Crouzon syndrome.

### Pathology and Clinical Characteristics

Clinical characteristics depend on which suture is affected. The closure of one suture does not allow growth in that area but generally increases growth in the other areas of the skull. The sagittal suture is the most commonly affected suture. When this suture is involved, the head presents as dolichocephalic, with a long and narrow appearance of the skull and increased length from front to back. Bossing of the frontal and occipital regions is also seen. The coronal suture is the second most common suture involved in premature closure. Bilateral closure of the coronal suture leads to the clinical appearance of a skull that is wide from side to side but short from front to back (also termed *brachycephaly*). Unilateral closure of a coronal suture results in plagiocephaly, with prominence of the forehead on the unaffected side, because the skull grows in this direction. The forehead is flattened, and the eyebrow is raised on the affected side. Bilateral lambdoidal craniosynostosis could be identified with a flattened occipital region. In contrast, unilateral lambdoidal craniosynostosis has a flattened area on one side of the occiput and appears asymmetrical compared to the other. Long-term supine positioning of the infant can also produce this appearance.

Positional asymmetric skull appearance, unrelated to abnormal suture closure, may be seen in infants with a neuromuscular defect that will not allow the child to move their

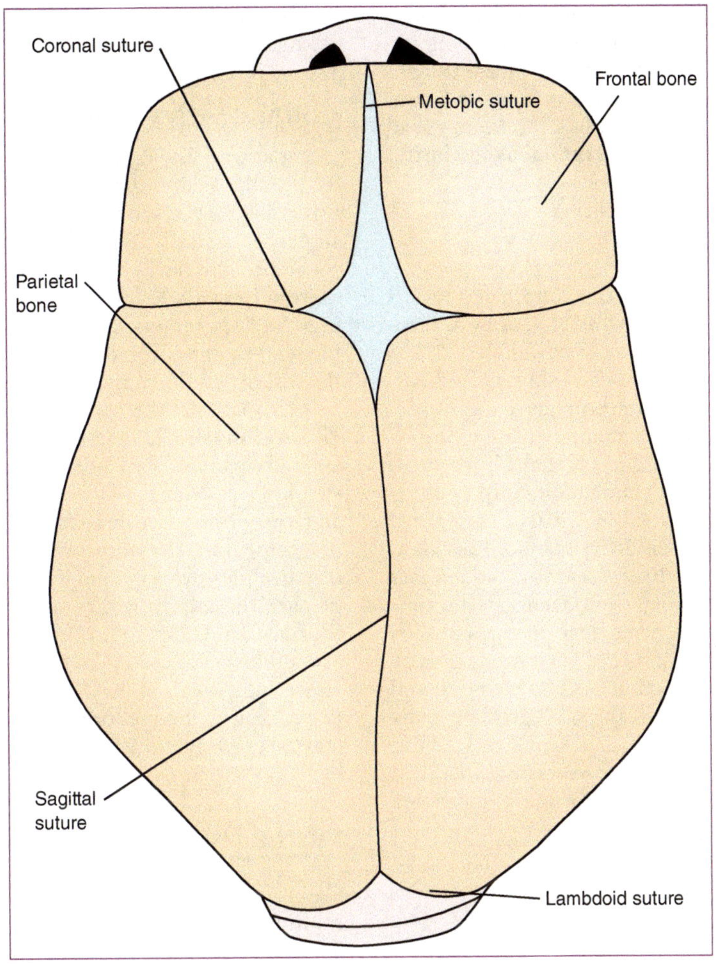


**FIGURE 14.6 Superior view of neonatal cranial sutures.**

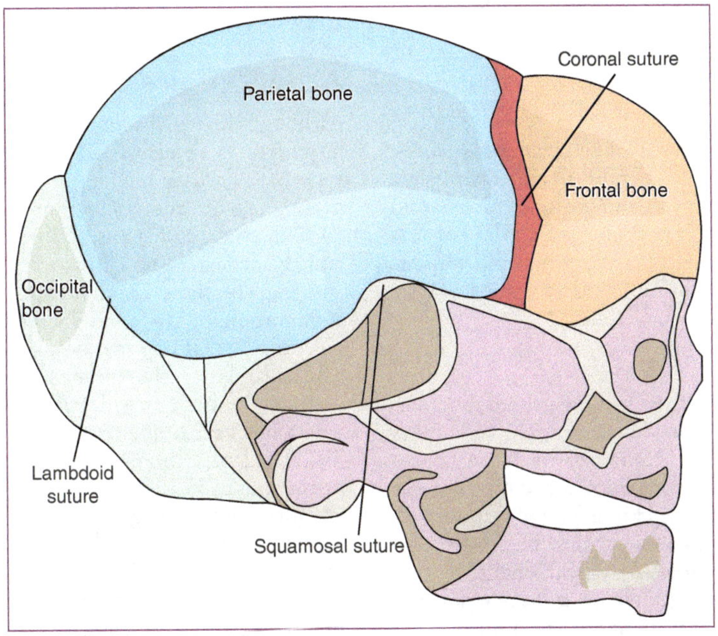


**FIGURE 14.7 Lateral view of neonatal cranial sutures.**

head from side to side spontaneously. Congenital torticollis (Danner-Bowman & Cardin, 2015) can result in an asymmetrically flat occipital region as the infant tilts the head toward the affected side. Isolated metopic craniosynostosis will produce a deformity with a narrow, protruding forehead. Facial development of the skull is affected, and orbital hypotelorism is also noted with this defect.

## Diagnosis and Management

Diagnosis is preceded by suspicion of the abnormal physical appearance of the skull, by plagiocephalometry, or by anthropometric measurements with a caliper (Siegenthaler, 2015). There is persistent or progressive abnormal skull growth, often with the head circumference intact for age. Craniosynostosis is usually confirmed with a computed tomography (CT) scan of the skull, with three-dimensional CT required for a more detailed preoperative examination. Surgery is required to correct this defect. This will occur in a specialized pediatric hospital with a multidisciplinary team of providers. The complexity of the procedure increases with the number of sutures involved and the cranial remodeling at the time of surgery. The type of repair is dependent on the suture(s) involved. Surgery occurs in early infancy (3–9 months of age). The goal is to achieve early correction of the synostosis and avoid extreme cranial deformities as the skull grows rapidly in the first year of life. In recent years, endoscopic procedures have shown good results in reducing the excessive blood loss and extended hospital stays that were previously associated with the repair of craniosynostosis.

# CONGENITAL MUSCULAR TORTICOLLIS

Congenital muscular torticollis, with an incidence of 0.4% in all live births, is a rare musculoskeletal condition with unknown pathogenesis. It is known to be primarily a disorder of the sternocleidomastoid muscle.

## Pathophysiology

Several theories exist as to the cause of congenital torticollis, including genetics, atypical uterine positioning, neurogenic disorders, and ischemic injury to the sternocleidomastoid muscle. Whatever the cause, this pathologic disorder consists of a fibrous contraction of the sternocleidomastoid muscle. Typically, the ipsilateral trapezius muscle is atrophied.

## Diagnosis

Congenital torticollis can present within the neonatal period. Presentation may include a 1- to 3-cm hard, palpable mass in the neck on the affected side accompanied by an abnormal head position. Infants with congenital torticollis tilt their heads to the affected side, and the chin is pointed upward in the opposite direction. Facial asymmetry may be a later sign. The face and skull on the affected side appear smaller.

In children with untreated congenital torticollis or cases with torticollis unresponsive to therapy, the shoulder on the affected side is raised to compensate for the atypical head positioning. This form of compensation may lead to cervical and lumbar scoliosis as well as chronic back pain.

## Collaborative Management

Occupational and/or physical therapy for congenital torticollis is traditionally instituted immediately. Because congenital torticollis may resolve naturally within the first year of life, surgery is typically delayed, pending therapy results.

Severe fibrosis of the sternocleidomastoid muscle may require surgery (Nilesh & Mukherji, 2013). In one study, however, 98% of infants diagnosed with torticollis responded to physical therapy. The duration of therapy was dependent on the severity of the muscular fibrosis (Lee et al., 2011).

Occupational therapists, physical therapists, and orthopedic surgeons should be consulted to assist in the management and subsequent follow-up of these infants. Family members should be provided with a functional home exercise program and counseled regarding the possibility of a neck brace to be postoperatively worn by the infant. It may be the nurse's responsibility to coordinate outpatient consultations and to prepare the family with discharge instructions. In addition, the nurse must determine whether the family lives in an area accessible to follow-up care. If not, a referral to social services, Individuals with Disabilities Education Act (IDEA) Part-C Early Intervention services, or financial counseling may be needed so the family can participate in follow-up.

# SKELETAL DYSPLASIA

*Skeletal dysplasia* is a term used to identify a group of clinical conditions that involve abnormal endochondral ossification. It includes achondroplasia, hypochondroplasia, and thanatophoric dysplasia, all of which present with short-limbed skeletal dysplasia at varying ages of development. The estimated incidence is 15.7 in 100,000 births (Bacino, 2024).

## Achondroplasia

Although the word *achondroplasia* was once used to describe any form of dwarfism, it is now recognized as one distinct type of dwarfism having characteristic features. Achondroplasia has an autosomal dominant pattern of inheritance (Wilkin et al., 1998) and is the most common nonlethal skeletal dysplasia. Most cases occur by spontaneous mutation, so many of these children have parents of typical stature. A mutation of the gene encoding fibroblast growth factor receptor-3 (FGFR3) has been implicated in this disorder. In achondroplasia, the infant's body has trouble converting cartilage to bone (ossification). The incidence of achondroplasia has varied due to multiple forms of skeletal dysplasia diagnosed as achondroplasia. One risk factor for spontaneous mutation that involves achondroplasia appears to be advanced paternal age.

Infants with achondroplasia can be identified at birth with a rhizomelic shortening of the extremities. In other words, when the arms are viewed, the upper arm (humerus bone) will appear more severely shortened compared to the lower arm (radius and ulnar bones). The same holds for the lower extremities, where the thigh (femur) will appear more severely shortened than the lower leg (tibia and fibular bones). The infant with achondroplasia also presents with a disproportionately large head with frontal bossing and a depressed nasal bridge. The hands are small, with a trident configuration that describes the appearance of the fingers and an increased spacing between the long and ring fingers (Horton & Hecht, 2011). Identification of mild hypotonia and limitation of elbow extension with laxity in most other joints are also noted. These neuromuscular and skeletal anomalies, including mild hypotonia, rhizomelia, joint laxity, and reduced elbow extension, can delay gross motor milestones but generally progress toward age-appropriate skill over the first few years of life. Commonly associated health problems include apnea, recurrent ear infections, and obesity. Central intelligence is normal in most cases.

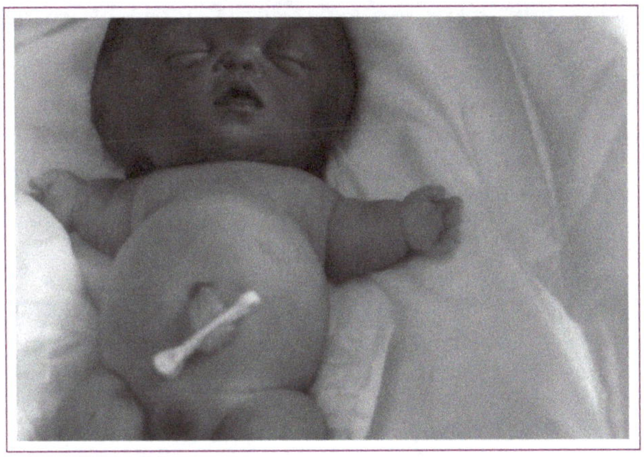

**FIGURE 14.8 Thanatophoric dysplasia: narrow thorax and protuberant abdomen.**

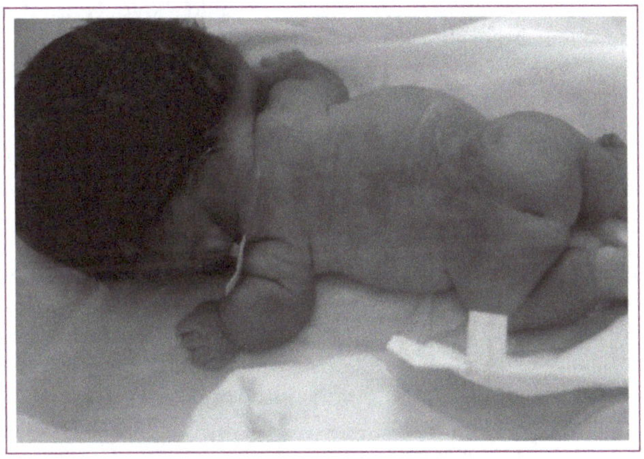

**FIGURE 14.9 Thanatophoric dysplasia: shortened lower extremities.**

## Hypochondroplasia

Hypochondroplasia is similar to achondroplasia but considered milder. It may be rarely noted at birth, because the infant's length is often age appropriate. The short stature becomes clinically apparent around 24 months of age. This condition is rarely diagnosed in the neonatal period but may present with macrocephaly. Children and adults experience similar orthopedic complications as individuals with achondroplasia. Some of these include joint and lower back pain, limited range of motion at the elbows, and bowing of the lower extremities.

## Thanatophoric Dysplasia

Thanatophoric dysplasia is the third in this series of common skeletal dysplasias. The name of this disorder is derived from the Greek word *thanatos*, meaning *death bearing*. It is a lethal defect and is often compared to OI, type II, in terms of its clinical scenario after birth (Stembalska et al., 2021). Death usually occurs within a few hours or days, secondary to respiratory failure from severe pulmonary hypoplasia. The clinical presentation of thanatophoric dysplasia describes a fetal environment of reduced fetal movements and polyhydramnios. Hypotonia in the neonate with macrocephaly, often presenting as a cloverleaf-shaped skull, is believed to be secondary to early fusion of the coronal and lambdoidal sutures. The limbs are short and bowed with severe brachydactyly or short digits. The thorax is very narrow and short, reminding the clinician of the abnormal pulmonary development and severe pulmonary hypoplasia. The abdomen has a protuberant appearance (Figures 14.8 and 14.9). Almost all cases of thanatophoric dysplasia result from a new genetic mutation, with a low risk of recurrence in subsequent pregnancies. As with other skeletal dysplasias, there is a defect in the *FGFR3* gene.

## Differential Diagnosis

The differential diagnosis of a neonate with shortened stature includes achondroplasia, OI type II, thanatophoric dwarfism, asphyxiating thoracic dysplasia, lethal short limb–polydactyly syndromes, and achondrogenesis. In achondroplasia, the child has markedly shortened limbs and often bowing of the lower limbs. Still, radiographic studies do not show evidence of multiple fractures and long bone crumbling, as seen in OI type II. Thanatophoric dwarfism and achondrogenesis, both typically fatal in the neonatal period, are characterized by an extremely narrow chest and marked defective ossification, respectively (Shirley & Ain, 2009). These disorders may be detected prenatally through ultrasound identification of the abnormal skeletal features.

## Management

Management of infants with skeletal dysplasias depends on the long-term outcome for the specific type of dysplasia. With nonlethal varieties, complications are primarily neurologic and involve the spinal nerves. The anatomic configuration of the intraspinal canal results in pressure on the spinal cord and nerves. This pressure produces chronic backache and, in the most severe scenario, paraplegia. Referrals to occupational and physical therapists, along with long-term orthopedic follow-up, can reduce some of the complications.

**Quality and Safety: If changes in the spinal column do occur, the child is at greatest risk for the development of increased respiratory difficulties, mobility problems, daily activity (occupational) challenges, self-concept and self-esteem concerns, physical pain, and central or peripheral nervous system (PNS) neuropathies.** Other common long-term complications include recurrent otitis media, hearing loss, dental overcrowding, and sleep apnea, which may present in childhood (Sisk et al., 1999).

Limb-lengthening techniques are sometimes used in the management of skeletal dysplasias. This has been done to reduce the functional and psychosocial difficulties associated with very short stature. Limb lengthening is arduous and surgically complex (Sheridan et al., 2020), with lengthy rehabilitation periods. Often, the physical outcome does not match the desired result, so the benefit of these procedures remains to be determined (Wright & Irving, 2012).

Because children with achondroplasia have a different appearance than their peers, any exaggeration of the condition can add to a faulty self-concept. As the child grows, continual assessment by healthcare professionals and the parents concerning the personal image that the child is developing is a prelude to positive self-esteem. Positive support from parents during the neonatal period is vital.

## OSTEOGENESIS IMPERFECTA

OI, sometimes called *brittle bone disease*, is a connective tissue disorder causing bone fragility and deformities (Forlino & Marini, 2016). It is caused by a genetic mutation affecting collagen, the major extracellular protein, wherein children experience fractures, osteoporosis, and mineral bone loss. The incidence of this disorder is about 1 per 20,000 births. Collagen is found in bone, sclera, ligaments, skin, and teeth. In this disorder, all of these tissues may be affected (Sillence & Danks, 1978).

The clinical presentation of OI varies greatly, depending on the particular type. There is also a wide range of severity and symptoms within each type. The original classification system described by Sillence and Danks (1978) outlines four basic types of OI; today, this classification has expanded to over 20 identified types, each categorized by defects in collagen, bone mineralization, protein abnormalities, collagen processing and cross linking, osteoblast lineage abnormality, or newer forms of OI (Balasubramanian, 2024).

### Types of Osteogenesis Imperfecta and Clinical Presentation

OI type I has an autosomal dominant inheritance pattern. In general, type I is the mildest type of OI, but the clinical appearance of individuals may range from mild to severe, even within the same family. A small number of individuals with this type may present with fractures in the neonatal period. An increased rate of fractures may be seen as the child begins to walk. People with this type are generally of typical height and stature. Sclerae are blue, and the teeth are also affected. Hearing loss may occur in adults with type I OI (Bishop, 2010). Premature or accelerated bone loss following menopause is also seen.

OI type II is also referred to as the *lethal perinatal type*. This is an autosomal recessive disorder that generally results in death either in utero or in the perinatal/neonatal period. The likelihood of prenatal diagnosis is increased with type II, due to the multiple fractures and bowing of extremities seen in utero. **Emergency Alert: Death can occur secondary to damage to vital organs (brain, liver, and lungs) that are not protected by the fragile bony structures.** Severe respiratory distress is seen secondary to the narrow and shortened ribcage. Infants with type II OI are small for gestational age with shortened bodies and legs, with the head appearing large for body size. The extremities tend to be shortened and deformed with multiple fractures. Radiographs may demonstrate multiple fractures, both old and new. Ribs and smaller bones may also appear thin and difficult to discern radiographically. Birth trauma may include the maceration of the head and limbs.

OI type III is a severe form with an autosomal recessive inheritance pattern. This is the most severe type for those surviving the neonatal period. Multiple fractures of the long bones may occur both before and after birth. There is a significant deformity of the bones over time, with scoliosis and hearing loss. Sclerae may be blue. Infants with type III may have typical height and weight at birth. This deteriorates over time, with very short stature seen in childhood/adulthood. The severe deformities of the spine and thorax seen in type III can restrict breathing, leading to significant respiratory complications in adulthood. These problems may shorten life expectancy (Marini, 2011).

OI type IV is similar to type I in that it is an autosomal dominant disorder with variable penetrance. OI type IV resembles type I in terms of presentation. Newborns rarely have identified fractures, but many fractures occur as the child begins to ambulate, with increased weight bearing. These infants also present with growth that is average for gestational age. The growth pattern can change as the child matures, secondary to increased bowing of extremities and kyphoscoliosis, with a short stature comparable to typical height at maturity with the milder forms of type I. OI type IV can also progress to a more severe form, depending on the degree of kyphoscoliosis and vertebral compression fractures, often resembling type III. Unlike type III, the lifespan in type IV is not affected.

As stated earlier, additional types of OI have been identified since the original classification system was developed. These are described as types V (moderate in severity), VI (extremely rare), and VII, VIII (white sclerae), which do not have defects in the collagen genes. However, the clinical features and management are similar to the other types of OI.

### Diagnosis

OI may be suspected prenatally if there is a positive family history. Fractures and other skeleton deformities may be seen on ultrasound before birth at around 20 weeks (Van Dijk & Sillence, 2014). After birth, the diagnostic process is based mainly on physical exam findings of fractures and deformities of the extremities. While the preferred method of diagnosis involves molecular genetic testing, a skin biopsy may also be used to provide a definitive diagnosis through examination of collagen (Steiner et al., 2013).

## Collaborative Management

**Quality and Safety:** **Neonates with OI should be handled very gently to avoid causing new fractures and to reduce the pain of existing injuries.** They should be lifted during care while gently supporting the buttocks and head. Infants should never be lifted by pulling the extremities or with hands under the armpits. With diaper changes, it is essential never to lift the infant by the ankles but to move the diaper by lifting the buttocks. When dressing these infants, the caregiver should gently bring the garments over the arms and legs while avoiding pulling the extremities through the sleeves and legs of the garments. Simple garments with wide openings for extremities are best. At discharge, a special car bed that allows prone or supine positioning may be required (Osteogenesis Imperfecta Foundation, n.d.).

Feeding ability may be compromised in these infants due to respiratory compromise and difficulty with positioning and handling. Gentle rubbing should be used for burping to avoid rib fractures. If these infants require prolonged immobilization during the healing of fractures, measures to protect the skin and facilitate frequent repositioning may be used, such as gel pads or foam wedges. **Quality and Safety:** **Pain management is also an important part of the care plan when fractures are present.** IV medications or oral sucrose may be used, as well as other nursing measures, to improve comfort and positioning (McLean, 2004). Referrals to occupational therapy, physical therapy, and palliative care may be indicated.

The long-term medical management of patients with OI is focused on avoiding fractures and correcting deformities of bones while maintaining maximal mobility and physical function. Intravenous bisphosphonates have shown some benefit by improving bone volume, though this does not change the essential collagen defect (Monti et al., 2010). Growth hormone has also been used with the milder types of OI.

# THROMBOCYTOPENIA-ABSENT RADIUS SYNDROME

Thrombocytopenia-absent radius (TAR) syndrome is characterized by the bilateral absence of radii and severe thrombocytopenia in the neonatal period. Hypoplasia or absence of the ulna may also be seen. The thumbs are always present in this syndrome (Scott & Montgomery, 2011). Congenital heart disorders and renal anomalies occur in a significant percentage of these patients. Skeletal differences of the lower limbs may also be present, although this is highly variable.

## Pathology

This disorder's inheritance pattern is uncertain, although a microdeletion on chromosome 1 is part of the genetic signature. The most remarkable pathology occurs in the neonatal period and correlates to the severity of thrombocytopenia, which can lead to intracranial and gastrointestinal hemorrhages (Sola et al., 2000). Thrombocytopenia is significant in many patients, with counts as low as 10,000. Hematologic complications improve with age, hence the reduced mortality and morbidity associated with this syndrome after the first year of life. Platelet counts are generally normal by childhood. If no significant intracranial hemorrhage occurs in the neonatal period, intelligence is expected to be typical for age.

Complications occurring from atypical hand and arm development may be encountered as the child matures. These include fine and gross motor developmental delays. Many children affected with this syndrome require some adaptive device, or they may learn to compensate with their existing limbs. Referrals to occupational and physical therapy are indicated for specialized assessment and treatment.

## Management

The primary management in the newborn period centers on the platelet levels. Because of the increased risk of bleeding, platelet transfusions may be required. In addition, handling and phlebotomy via heel sticks should be kept to a minimum to reduce bruising. Cow's milk allergy is seen in many patients with TAR syndrome. The introduction of cow's milk may lead to the worsening of thrombocytopenia, and this factor should be considered in management (Toriello, 2011).

# SUMMARY

The human body is active, responsive, and constantly moving. The development of its functional motor skills depends on the development of the musculoskeletal system. Although most musculoskeletal differences or conditions in the newborn are nonlethal, they may become the focus of the parent's or family's attention. Understanding the development of the musculoskeletal system and pathologic differences can assist the clinician in teaching and supporting the family and the infant. In addition, recognizing subtle asymmetries can prompt the clinician to evaluate for additional associated anomalies that could have serious genetic implications. This chapter helps identify the epidemiologic and clinical aspects of infant musculoskeletal conditions to improve clinician understanding of the defect and provide guidelines for management based on pathology, complications, and prognosis. However, the awareness that musculoskeletal development is best supported in a family-centered environment and in collaboration with parents eager to maximize their child's potential is of equal importance.

## CASE STUDY

■ **Identification of the Problem.** Female infant born at term gestation is noted on initial physical exam to have abnormalities of the upper extremities.

■ **Assessment: History and Physical Examination.** The infant was born by vaginal delivery at 37 weeks' gestation to a 16-year-old Caucasian female, G1 P0. The mother received late and limited prenatal care, with the pregnancy remaining unacknowledged until the third trimester secondary to young maternal age. Delivery was uncomplicated. The 1-minute Apgar score was 9, and the infant did not require resuscitation or other special care at delivery. The birth weight was 2,850 g. Infant was noted on general inspection to have abnormalities of the upper extremities.

Physical exam on admission to the transition nursery:

- GENERAL: pink, well-developed female infant, vital signs in the normal range, oxygen saturation was 98% on room air
- Head, ears, eyes, nose, and throat (HEENT): normocephalic, anterior fontanelle open and flat, eyes normal, ears normally formed, nares patent, palate intact
- LUNGS: bilateral breath sounds clear and equal, good respiratory effort
- Cardiovascular (CV): Regular respiratory rate (RRR), soft murmur, good peripheral perfusion, femoral and pedal pulses palpable
- Abdomen (ABD): soft, active bowel sounds, no organomegaly or masses, three-vessel cord
- Genitourinary (GU): normal-term female features, patent anus
- Neurologic (NEURO): appropriate tone for gestational age, active and responsive
- NECK: full ROM, no masses
- SPINE: intact
- EXTREMITIES: bilateral malformed upper extremities with thumbs present, lower extremities appropriate for age
- SKIN: pink, scattered petechiae over the trunk and face

**Differential Diagnosis.** In this patient, the physical exam findings led to a strong suspicion of TAR syndrome. Immediate evaluation would be indicated to assess platelet count, which can be very low with a risk of hemorrhage. Cranial ultrasound should be done to rule out intracranial bleeding. Evaluation of the skeletal structure of the upper extremities would also be needed. An echocardiogram should be performed to rule out cardiac conditions, which are present in a large percentage of patients with this disorder.

### Diagnostic Tests

1. Complete blood count (CBC) with differential: White blood cells (WBCs) 12.7, hematocrit 39%, platelet count $28{,}000/mm^3$
2. X-rays of upper extremities: bilateral absence of radii, with hypoplasia of the ulnae bilaterally; the humeri were present and normal bilaterally; x-rays of lower extremities revealed no abnormalities
3. Echocardiogram: patent ductus arteriosus (PDA), no significant structural abnormalities
4. Cranial ultrasound: no evidence of intracranial hemorrhage

### Development of Management Plan

- Platelet transfusion
- Gentle handling of the infant to avoid bruising and bleeding
- Close monitoring of the platelet count

**Implementation.** The infant was transferred to NICU to obtain a peripheral IV and to have the necessary studies completed. The platelet count was repeated 12 hours after the transfusion with a value of $49{,}000/mm^3$. The infant received an additional transfusion of platelets with an improvement to $72{,}000/mm^3$. The infant remained hospitalized for an additional week while receiving ad lib breastfeeding. She remained stable. Repeat cranial ultrasound at 7 days of age was again normal.

**Evaluation of Effectiveness.** The infant was discharged home at 10 days of age with a platelet count of $80{,}000/mm^3$. She returned to the newborn outpatient clinic 3 days later with a platelet count of $43{,}000/mm^3$. An additional platelet transfusion was given in the outpatient clinic with no complications. The platelet count on a follow-up visit the next day was $85{,}000/mm^3$. The infant continued to receive periodic follow-up visits for CBC monitoring over the next 3 months. She required no further platelet transfusion.

**Outcome.** The infant was seen at 6 months of age in the newborn follow-up clinic and showed typical growth and development. The platelet count was normal.

## EVIDENCE-BASED PRACTICE

Osteogenesis imperfecta, often called *brittle bone disease*, is a condition caused by a genetic mutation affecting collagen. The complications of OI stem primarily from bone fractures. Treatment focuses chiefly on preventing fractures, thereby minimizing pain and improving long-term mobility and function. A number of research studies have investigated the use of bisphosphonates to reduce fracture rates in patients with OI. Bisphosphonates act by decreasing the activity of osteoclasts, thereby reducing the rate of bone resorption. These drugs are used successfully in adults with osteoporosis to improve bone strength and density.

A review by Bishop (2010) examined the early use of IV pamidronate in neonates in the first year of life. The drug was given on a cyclical basis at varying intervals. A reduced rate of fractures was seen in these infants, as well as improved growth. No severe side effects were documented. There are concerns regarding the difficulty of maintaining reliable central venous access in a small infant. Also, the long-term effects of this therapy remain unknown. It should be noted that the drug does not change the process of abnormal collagen formation.

Growth hormone, which is known to stimulate bone growth and collagen synthesis, has also been examined as a potential treatment for OI. A review by Monti et al. (2010) examined the available information. Data from limited studies suggested that growth hormone could improve growth and exert a beneficial effect on muscle mass and strength, thereby improving capacity for exercise; no increased rate of fractures was noted. This increase in physical activity in OI patients may improve skeletal health and overall physical well-being. Growth hormone is considered

(continued)

## EVIDENCE-BASED PRACTICE (*continued*)

a promising therapy in patients with moderate forms of OI. Patients with the more severe types of the disorder did not see a benefit.

Research in the arena of genetics is very promising. Investigators hope to identify more specific causative factors at the molecular level, as well as to explore the possibility of manipulating the disorder's genetic expression. Bone marrow transplant is also being examined as a potential treatment. Limited data suggest that bone marrow transplant can be used to introduce stem cells into the body that can produce normal bone. These modalities remain in early stages of development.

### References

Bishop, N. (2010). Characterising and treating osteogenesis imperfecta. *Early Human Development*, *86*, 743–746. https://doi.org/10.1016/j.earlhumdev.2010.08.002

Monti, E., Mottes, M., Fraschini, P., Brunelli, P., Forlino, A., Venturi, G., Doro, F., Perlini, S., Cavarzere, P., & Antoniazzi, F. (2010). Current and emerging treatments for the management of osteogenesis imperfecta. *Therapeutics and Clinical Risk Management*, 6, 367–381. https://doi.org/10.2147/tcrm.s5932

OI, osteogenesis imperfecta.

## ONLINE RESOURCES

CourseConnect

Resources for this chapter are online and available at www.springerpub.com/courseconnect.

## REFERENCES

References for this chapter are online and available at www.springerpub.com/courseconnect.

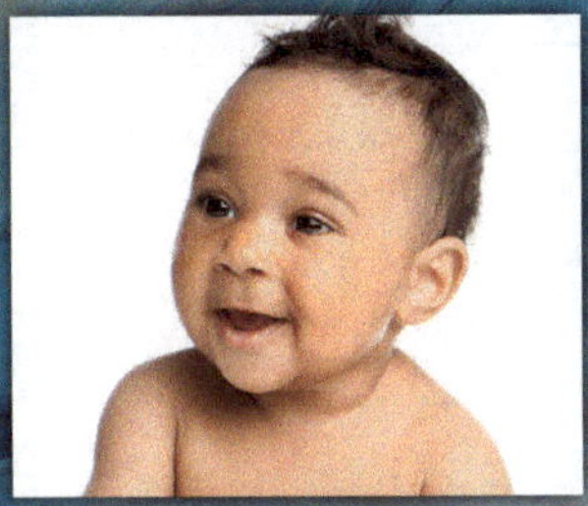

Source: New Africa/Adobe Stock.

CHAPTER 15

# Neurologic System

**Pamela A. Harris-Haman**

## INTRODUCTION

The central nervous system (CNS) is an extraordinarily complex system. CNS normal function is critical to the activity of every organ and the integration of systems that coordinate physiologic and neurobehavioral processes. Neonatal neurologic dysfunction can arise from insults that occur before, during, or after birth. Such insults can affect the infant's survival in the perinatal and neonatal periods and have implications for later developmental and cognitive outcomes. Alterations in neurologic function have significant immediate and long-term consequences for the infant and family. Early recognition of infants at risk for neurologic dysfunction and prompt implementation of appropriate interventions are crucial for both survival and reduction in long-term morbidity. This chapter examines the structural and functional development of the CNS in the embryo, fetus, and neonate and the basis for common congenital and developmental anomalies. Neurologic assessment of the neonate, related diagnostic techniques, and selected pathophysiologic problems that affect the central and peripheral nervous systems are also presented. The neurologic problems examined include neonatal seizures, intracranial hemorrhage, brain injury in preterm infants, hypoxic-ischemic encephalopathy (HIE), structural alterations, and birth injuries. Figure 15.1 shows the general structure of the newborn brain.

## CNS DEVELOPMENT AND STRUCTURAL ABNORMALITIES

Many neurologic disorders are related to defects in the development of the CNS. CNS development can be divided into six stages: (a) neurulation, (b) prosencephalic development, (c) neuronal proliferation, (d) neuronal migration, (e) organization, and (f) myelination. These stages overlap, and development progresses at different rates in various sections of the CNS. Embryologic CNS development begins shortly after fertilization, and maturation continues after birth until adulthood. The CNS is one of the earliest systems to begin development and one of the last to reach maturity. The stages of CNS development are summarized in Table 15.1. CNS development is controlled by developmental genes in a complex cascade of signaling molecules, neurotropic growth factors, and vitamins (such as vitamin A and folic acid) that mediate gene expression along the anterior–posterior axis of the embryo (Gressens & Hüppi, 2025; Yuskaitis & Pomeroy, 2022).

### Neurulation

Neurulation is the process by which the formation of the central neuroaxis, that is, the brain and spinal cord, occurs as a result of inductive events within the dorsal aspect of the embryo (Table 15.1). The inductive events are separated into two stages: primary neurulation, the events related to the formation of the brain and spinal cord excluding the caudal segments of the lumbar region; and secondary neurulation, the events related to caudal neural tube formation (Blackburn, 2018; du Plessis & Volpe, 2025).

Primary neurulation occurs during the first 3 to 4 weeks of gestation and involves the formation of the neural plate, neural folds, and neural tube. This process leads to the formation of the primitive brain and spinal cord except the lower sacral and coccygeal segments. The CNS arises as a thickening of the ectoderm on the dorsal portion of the embryo at about 18 days' gestation. The brain and spinal cord develop from this thickening, which is called the *neural plate*. The neural plate invaginates, forming the midline neural groove along the dorsal surface of the embryo. The parallel folds of tissue on either side of this groove are called the *neural folds*. The neural folds eventually form the forebrain, midbrain, hindbrain, and spinal cord. By the end of the third postconceptional week, the neural folds fuse to form the neural tube. The cranial portion of the lumen of the neural tube forms the ventricles; the caudal portion forms the central canal of the spinal cord. The tissues of the neural tube interact with surrounding mesoderm tissues (somites) to stimulate development of the bony structures of the CNS—the skull and vertebrae (Blackburn, 2018; du Plessis & Volpe, 2025; Torchia & Persaud, 2024). In the

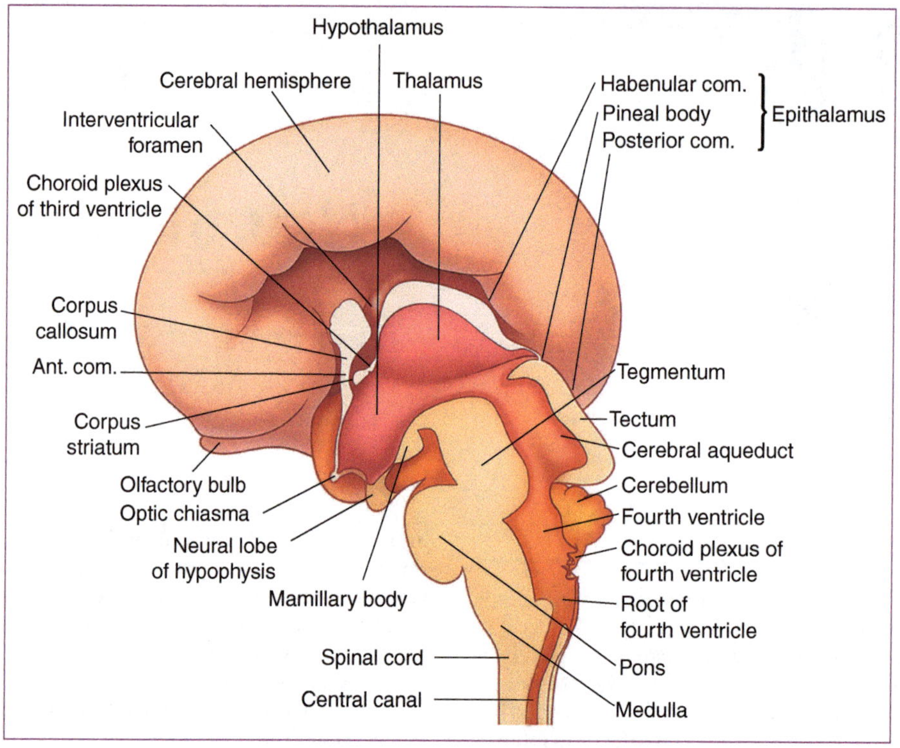


**FIGURE 15.1 Cerebral anatomy.**

fusion of the neural folds, some of the neuroectodermal cells on the upper margins are not incorporated into the neural tube. These cells form the neural crest, which lies between the neural tube and the surface ectodermal layer. The neural crest tissue forms the peripheral nervous system (PNS), which includes the cranial, spinal, and autonomic system ganglia and nerves, Schwann cells, melanocyte (pigment) cells, meninges, and skeletal and muscular components of the head (du Plessis & Volpe, 2025; Torchia & Persaud, 2024).

Closure of the neural tube begins in the occipitocervical region (at the level of the future hindbrain and cervical junction) at about 22 days' gestation (du Plessis & Volpe, 2025). The neural folds do not fuse simultaneously; fusion proceeds in cephalic and caudal directions. For several days, the neural tube is fused toward the central area but is open at both ends. The end areas are known as the *rostral* (anterior) and the *caudal* (posterior) neuropores. The cranial end of the neural tube closes at approximately 24 days' gestation. Fusion of the cranial portion contributes to the formation of the forebrain. The caudal neuropore, which is in the future lumbosacral area, closes in a rostrocaudal direction at approximately 26 days' gestation (du Plessis & Volpe, 2025). Once both neuropores are closed, the neural tube is a closed, fluid-filled system that has no further connection to the amniotic cavity unless a defect is present. Alterations in neural tube development and closure give rise to neural tube defects (NTDs). Because differentiation of the surrounding mesodermal tissue (somites) into vertebrae, cranium, and dura depends on interaction with the neural tube, NTDs involve not only the neural elements but also the bony structures and meninges (Blackburn, 2018; du Plessis & Volpe, 2025; Torchia & Persaud, 2024).

Secondary neurulation consists of two sequential phases: canalization and regressive differentiation. These phases form the spinal cord of the sacral and coccygeal segments. Canalization begins at 28 to 32 days' gestation and continues through the seventh week of gestation and involves the development of the lower lumbar, sacral, and coccygeal areas from an undifferentiated cell mass at the caudal end of the neural tube. Vacuoles develop that gradually coalesce, enlarge, and contact the caudal end of the neural tube. The second phase, regressive differentiation, begins about the seventh week and continues until sometime after birth. Regressive differentiation is characterized by regression of much of the caudal cell mass, leaving behind the ventriculus terminalis, which is located in the conus medullaris, and the filum terminale (Blackburn, 2018; du Plessis & Volpe, 2025).

**Disorders of Neurulation.** Congenital anomalies that arise during the period of neurulation result from alterations in neural tube closure, of which 80% occur at either the cranial or caudal end, or alterations in surrounding tissues under development during this period (du Plessis & Volpe, 2025; Torchia & Persaud, 2024). Alterations in neurulation are often accompanied by alterations in vertebral, meningeal, vascular, and dermal structures and include craniorachischisis totalis, anencephaly, encephalocele, spina bifida occulta, and cystica (meningocele, myelomeningocele [MMC], and myeloschisis), and Chiari type II malformations (Blackburn, 2018; du Plessis & Volpe, 2025). NTDs are one of the most common CNS malformations. The incidence of NTDs varies with ethnicity, diet, geographic area, and socioeconomic status; prevalence has decreased with increased folic acid intake by childbearing women (du Plessis & Volpe, 2025).

**TABLE 15.1**

**STAGES IN THE DEVELOPMENT OF THE CNS AND RELATED DEVELOPMENTAL DEFECTS**

| Stage | Peak Period of Occurrence | Examples of Developmental Defects |
|---|---|---|
| Primary neurulation | 3–4 weeks' gestation | NTDs, anencephaly, encephalocele, spina bifida cystica (MMC, and myeloschisis), dermal sinus, Arnold Chiari malformation |
| Prosencephalic development | 2–3 months' gestation | Holoprosencephaly, holotelencephaly, agenesis of the corpus callosum |
| Neuronal proliferation | Cerebrum: 3–4 months' gestation (may continue to term for interneurons)<br>Cerebellum: 2–10 months postnatally | Micrencephaly vera, macrencephaly, neurofibromatosis, other neurocutaneous disorders, tuberous sclerosis |
| Neuronal migration | Cerebrum: 3–5 months' gestation (may continue to term for interneurons)<br>Cerebellum: 4–10 months | Schizencephaly, lissencephaly, pachygyria, polymicrogyria<br>Joubert Syndrome |
| Organization | 5–6 months' gestation—first years postnatal (continues for many years postbirth) | Alterations in brain development secondary to the effects of Down syndrome and trisomy 13, 14, and 15; behavioral alterations; intellectual disabilities |
| Myelination | Birth to 8 months' gestation—first years postnatal (continues for many years postbirth) | Brain hypoplasia, neurologic deficits, leukodysplasias, cerebral white matter dysplasis, cerebral white matter disease of prematurity |

MMC, meningocele, myelomeningocele; NTDs, neural tube defects.

*Sources:* Compiled from Blackburn, S. T. (2018). *Maternal, fetal and neonatal physiology: A clinical perspective* (5th ed.). Elsevier; du Plessis, A. J., & Volpe, J. J. (2024). Neural tube development. In J. J. Volpe, T. E. Inder, B. T. Darras, L. S. de Vries, A. J. du Plessis, J. J. Neil, & J. M. Perlman (Eds.), *Volpe's neurology of the newborn* (7th ed., pp. 3–37). Elsevier; Gressens, P., & Hüppi, P. S. (2025). Normal and abnormal brain development. In R. J. Martin, A. A. Fanaroff, & M. C. Walsh (Eds.), *Fanaroff and Martin's neonatal-perinatal medicine: Diseases of the fetus and infant* (12th ed., pp. 980–1010). Elsevier Saunders; Yuskaitis, C. J., & Pomeroy, S. L. (2022). Development of the nervous system. In R. A. Polin, S. H. Abman, D. H. Rowitch, W. E. Benitz, & W. W. Fox (Eds.), *Fetal and neonatal physiology* (6th ed., pp. 1297–1318). Elsevier Saunders.

Disorders of neurulation arise from genetic, nutritional, and/or environmental influences (Blackburn, 2018; du Plessis & Volpe, 2025; Gressens & Hüppi, 2025; Yuskaitis & Pomeroy, 2022). A familial incidence and an increased genetic susceptibility within immediate families are seen. The risk for an NTD increases from a 2% to 5% recurrence risk for siblings compared to 0.1% risk in the general population. The risk increases to 10-fold with two or more affected family members (Copp & Greene, 2022). In addition, the risk of NTD is greater if the previously affected family member had a lesion at T11 or higher. In the general population, increased risk of NTD is associated with maternal diabetes, maternal obesity, prior miscarriages, maternal folate deficiency, and maternal exposure to drugs such as valproic acid and folic acid antagonists such as trimethoprim and carbamazepine (du Plessis & Volpe, 2025).

Folic acid supplementation at conception reduces the rate of NTDs (Breitkopf & Hill, 2019; Viswanathan et al., 2023). Up to 50% to 72% of NTDs may be preventable with adequate folate supplementation (du Plessis & Volpe, 2025). Folate is a cofactor for enzymes needed in DNA and RNA synthesis. It is essential to a cell's ability to methylate proteins, lipids, and myelin for cell proliferation and growth and the actions of other B vitamins (Breitkopf & Hill, 2019; Viswanathan et al., 2023). Women of childbearing age are recommended to consume 0.4 mg of folate daily; for women who previously have had an infant with NTD, the recommendation is 4 to 5 mg daily (American Academy of Pediatrics Committee on Genetics, 1999; Viswanathan et al., 2023).

Antenatal screening for NTDs involves maternal serum alpha-fetoprotein screening (MSAFP) and ultrasound examination, or, more commonly, just second-trimester ultrasound (American College of Obstetricians and Gynecologists [ACOG], Committee on Practice Bulletins-Obstetrics, 2017; Kim et al., 2022). Analysis of MSAFP is performed between 15 and 20 weeks' gestation, with the optimal time between 16 and 18 weeks' gestation. Alpha-fetoprotein screening (AFP) is a major fetal glycoprotein, like the albumin produced in the fetal liver from 6 weeks' gestation; concentrations of AFP peak at 13 to 15 weeks' gestation. Usually, the AFP concentration of the cerebrospinal fluid (CSF) is significantly higher than that of the amniotic fluid; therefore, when CSF leaks into the amniotic fluid, as occurs with an open NTD, the AFP level of the amniotic fluid and maternal serum is elevated. MSAFP is done much less frequently due to improvements in ultrasonography and increased use of second-trimester fetal anatomic assessment; the detection rate is 96% (ACOG, 2017). Fetal ultrasound can be used for detection by the end of the first trimester, although the detection rate is lower (ACOG, 2017; Kim et al., 2022). If MSAFP screening is used, elevated AFP levels are followed up with examination by fetal ultrasound to determine if the elevated AFP levels are the result of open NTD or other causes, such as open abdominal wall defects (gastroschisis and omphalocele), congenital nephrosis, or fetal demise (ACOG, 2017).

## Prosencephalic Development

Prosencephalic development, or ventral induction, involves early brain and ventricular system development, which occurs during the second to third month of gestation (peaking at 5–6 weeks). The brain develops from the cranial end of the neural tube, beginning at the end of the fourth week. During this period, the three primary brain bulges (or vesicles) and cavities are formed after the fusion of the neural folds in the cranial area.

Primary brain bulges are the forebrain (prosencephalon), the midbrain (mesencephalon), and the hindbrain (rhombencephalon). During the fifth week, the forebrain divides into two secondary vesicles, the telencephalon, and the diencephalon, and the hindbrain divides into the metencephalon and the myelencephalon. Derivatives of each of these structures form the structures of the definitive brain. The third and fourth ventricles are formed from cavities within the rhombencephalon and diencephalon; the aqueduct of Sylvius links these two ventricles. The lateral ventricles arise from cavities in the cerebral hemispheres and are connected to the third ventricle by the foramen of Monro (see Figure 15.1). Early growth of the neural tube is the most rapid in the forebrain region. To give these structures space to grow, the neural tube bends at several points, forming the mesencephalic (midbrain area), cervical (junction of the hindbrain and spinal cord), and pontine flexures (Dean & Doherty, 2024; Torchia & Persaud, 2024). The cerebellum arises from the rhombencephalon.

**Disorders of Prosencephalic Development.** Malformations during this period generally arise around the fifth to sixth week of gestation. Infants with these anomalies have a poor prognosis, and many are lost in early pregnancy or are stillborn. Malformations of the forebrain include holoprosencephaly and holotelencephaly. Holoprosencephaly is an abnormality in cleavage of the hemispheres that arises from genetic or possibly environmental alterations. Failure of horizontal, transverse, and sagittal cleavage of the prosencephalon disrupts the formation of the telencephalon and the diencephalon and their derivatives. The resultant brain has a single monoventricular cerebral mass enclosed by a membrane; aplasia of the optic tract with the absence of the olfactory tracts and bulbs and agenesis of the corpus callosum are also characteristic. Microcephaly, hydrocephaly, and facial anomalies also may be seen (Dean & Doherty, 2024; Torchia & Persaud, 2024). With holotelencephaly, the parts of the brain that develop from the telencephalon form a single spheroid structure; the diencephalon and its derivatives are less affected. Congenital hydrocephalus and agenesis of the corpus callosum can also arise during this period. Face development is associated with prosencephalic development of the CNS; consequently, alterations in brain development often result in facial malformations (Dean & Doherty, 2027).

## Neuronal Proliferation

Development of neurons and glial cells involves proliferation in the germinal matrix (GM); migration (to their final destination) in the next stage of CNS development; differentiation of glial cells (during the period of organization) into specific cell types; alignment of neurons; and the development of interneuron and glial–neuron relationships. Cerebellar neurons arise within the cerebellar GM. The peak period of neuronal proliferation in the cerebral area lasts from 2 to 4 months' gestation, followed by glial proliferation beginning at 15 weeks' gestation, and in the cerebellum from 2 months' gestation to 10 months postnatal age (Yuskaitis & Pomeroy, 2022). During this stage, further development occurs in the cerebral subventricular and ventricular zones, where neurons and glial cells are derived from stem cells in the cerebral GM. Initial proliferation involves primarily neurons and radial glia, which are needed for neuron migration. The proliferation of other glia and their derivatives (astrocytes and oligodendrocytes) occurs intensively during the stage of organization, which occurs between 5 and 8 months' gestation. During the most intense period of proliferation, before 32 to 34 weeks' gestation, the periventricular area receives a large proportion of the cerebral blood flow. This area is vulnerable to hemorrhage (see the section on Germinal Matrix Hemorrhage–Intraventricular Hemorrhage) in preterm infants (Blackburn, 2018; Fleiss et al., 2018; D'Gama et al., 2025).

**Disorders of Neuronal Proliferation.** Disorders of proliferation arise from inadequate or excessive proliferation of neuronal derivatives, glial derivatives, or glial cell derivatives. Insults may alter the neuronal-glial stem cells, which reduces the number of neurons or glial cells, or may alter cell growth, which results in smaller cells. The resulting disorders include micrencephaly, macrencephaly, and neurofibromatosis. Micrencephaly may be due to a reduction in either the size or number of stem cells (Dean & Doherty, 2024; D'Gama et al., 2025). Micrencephaly vera is associated with a small brain caused by a decrease in the size of the proliferating units due to genetic or environmental factors and occurs between 2 to 4 months' gestation. These infants often do not have marked neurologic deficits or seizures during the neonatal period, and in general, the brain is well formed; however, the infants later manifest mental delays. Genetic factors associated with micrencephaly vera include autosomal recessive or dominant trait, X-linked recessive trait, or translocation. Micrencephaly vera is related to environmental factors such as irradiation, metabolic alteration, maternal rubella, fetal alcohol syndrome (FAS), maternal cocaine use, and maternal phenylketonuria with elevated phenylalanine levels during pregnancy.

Macrencephaly results in a large brain size because of excessive proliferation of neuronal or nonneuronal elements, or a combination of both. Macrencephaly is associated with genetic disorders, including Beckwith–Wiedemann syndrome, Sturge–Weber syndrome, Weaver syndrome, and achondroplasia; chromosomal disorders such as Klinefelter and fragile X syndromes and partial trisomy of chromosome 7; and neurocutaneous disorders, such as neurofibromatosis. Neurofibromatosis is an autosomal dominant genetic disorder involving excessive proliferation of nonneuronal elements in the CNS and mesodermal structures of the body, with cutaneous stigmata (Blackburn, 2018; Dean & Doherty, 2024; D'Gama et al., 2025). Neurofibromatosis often presents with alterations to skin pigmentation (café-au-lait macules), Lisch nodules of the iris, buphthalmos (enlarged eyeball), skin nodules, and multiple benign neurofibromas. Infants with more than five café-au-lait macules larger than 5 mm in diameter at birth should be further evaluated for neurofibromatosis. Neurofibromatosis is associated with learning disabilities and, later in life, possible development of skeletal abnormalities, vascular disease, CNS tumors, or malignant peripheral nerve sheath tumors (Blackburn, 2018; D'Gama et al., 2025).

## Neuronal Migration

The peak period for the neuronal migration stage is 3 to 5 months' gestation in the cerebrum and 4 to 10 months' gestational postnatally in the cerebellum (Yuskaitis & Pomeroy, 2022). This stage is characterized by the movement of millions of cells from their point of origin in the subependymal GM of the periventricular region to their eventual loci in the cerebral cortex (see Figure 15.1) and similar movements of neurons within the cerebellum from their point of origin to their final location. The process of neuronal migration is critical to the formation of the neocortex, gyri, and deep nuclear structures. The gyri and sulci development follows a predictable pattern linked to gestational age. At 21 to 25 weeks' gestation, the central ventricles are large, and the brain is agaric; gyral development begins by the end of this period (Blackburn, 2018; D'Gama et al., 2025).

The mechanisms that guide neuronal migration are not entirely understood, but they are mediated by signaling proteins, surface molecules, and receptors on the neurons and the radial glia. The radial glia assists in the migration of the neurons to both the cortex and the cerebellum. Radial glia guides migrating cells and later transforms into astrocytes (D'Gama et al., 2025). The cerebral cortex has essentially achieved its full complement of neurons by 24 weeks' gestation; however, gamma-aminobutyric acid (GABAergic) neuron migration continues until the near term (D'Gama et al., 2025; Fleiss et al., 2024). Later migration predominantly involves glial cells.

**Disorders of Neuronal Migration.** Errors or exogenous insults before or after birth can alter the migration of neurons and glial cells. Alterations in migration can result in hypoplasia or agenesis of the corpus callosum, agenesis of a part of the cerebral wall (schizencephaly), or gyral anomalies (pachygyria, lissencephaly, and polymicrogyria). The preterm infant may be especially vulnerable to gyral alterations. The rapid development of the gyri begins at 26 to 28 weeks' gestation and continues through the third trimester into the postbirth period. The development of gyri results in a marked increase in cerebral surface area (D'Gama et al., 2025; Fleiss et al., 2024).

## Organization

The peak period for organization is about the fifth month of gestation to a few years after birth. However, organizational processes continue throughout childhood, particularly in the cerebellum. Some processes, such as synaptogenesis, continue until death. Organizational processes allow the nervous system to act as an integrated whole. These processes include (a) establishment of subplate neurons; (b) attainment of the proper alignment, orientation, and layering of cortical neurons; (c) arborization or differentiation and branching of axons and dendrites; (d) differentiation of glial cells; (e) development of synaptic connections ("wiring" of the brain) with balancing of excitatory and inhibitory synapses; (f) gyral development; and (g) cell death and selective elimination of neuronal processes (Blackburn, 2018; Fleiss et al., 2024; Haynes et al., 2025b).

Subplate neurons are critical structures in the neocortex development, with maximal size and vulnerability reached within 24 to 32 weeks' gestation (Fleiss et al., 2024; Haynes et al., 2025b). Thus, subplate neurons are vulnerable to perinatal injury. Subplate neurons serve as transient "way stations" by providing a place of synaptic contact for axons that ascend from the thalamus. Other areas in which connecting cortical neurons are not yet in place are a site of initial synaptogenesis between regions where cortical connections are not yet fully formed become initial sites of synaptogenesis between cortical areas, generate axons that form the corpus callosum, and are crucial for guiding axons to their final targets and establishing functional interconnections across the brain (Fleiss et al., 2024; Haynes et al., 2025b). Subplate neurons may be damaged in preterm infants with periventricular leukomalacia (PVL) (Fleiss et al., 2024).

Glial cells serve as supportive structures with the CNS. The three forms of glia are (a) myelin-producing glia (oligodendrocytes in the CNS; Schwann cells in the PNS); (b) guiding glia (radial glia for neuron migration during CNS development; Schwann cells for guiding peripheral nerves); and (c) "cleanup" glia (astroglia and microglia), which remove waste and dead tissue. Astroglia also provide support for neurons, assist in integrating information within the CNS, and are important in the structure and function of the blood–brain barrier. Astrocyte proliferation peaks at 26 to 28 weeks (Fleiss et al., 2024). Microglia are capable of phagocytosis function as brain macrophages and may be involved in developmental apoptosis (Blackburn, 2018; Haynes et al., 2025b). When activated by inflammation or ischemia, as occurs with white matter injury (WMI), microglia can lead to further cellular injury. During the premyelinating period, oligodendrocytes are especially vulnerable to hypoxic-ischemic injury (see the section on White Matter Injury in Preterm Infants in this chapter) (Back & Volpe, 2025; Fleiss et al., 2024).

Cell death and selective elimination of neuronal processes are important in adjusting the size of individual neurons to their anticipated need. It is also an important component of brain plasticity in infants. In the developing brain, neuronal processes targeted for elimination can be saved if they are needed because of damage to other processes; by this means, functional ability is preserved. Excitatory neurotransmitters, such as glutamate, mediate neural development and organization by acting on N-methyl-D-aspartate (NMDA) receptors and, also likely, on GluR2- deficient alpha-amino-3-hydroxyl-5-methyl-4-isoxazolenpropionic acid (AMPA) receptors and by opening voltage-dependent calcium channels (Haynes et al., 2025b).

A striking increase in the cerebral cortical volume and gyral changes occurs during this period of development and with organization of cortical neurons, especially from around 28 to 40 weeks' gestation. During this time, there is a fourfold increase in cortical gray matter volume (Haynes et al., 2025b).

**Disorders of Organization.** Organization of the brain is susceptible to insults from errors of metabolism, abnormal chromosomes, and perinatal insults. Organizational processes are particularly vulnerable in the preterm infant being cared for in an intensive care unit (ICU) during this period. Alterations in arborization and wiring of the brain can lead to hypersensitivity, poorly modulated behavior, and all-or-nothing responses. Alterations in organization are seen in infants with Down syndrome/trisomy 21, who have abnormal development of the axons and dendrites and altered synaptic formation, fragile X syndrome, Angelman syndrome (microdeletion on the long arm of maternal chromosome 15), Duchenne muscular dystrophy, intellectual disabilities (with or without seizures), and Rett syndrome.

## Myelination

The myelination stage involves developing myelin sheaths around nerve fibers in the nervous system. Oligodendrocytes myelinate the nerve fibers of the CNS, and Schwann cells myelinate the nerve fibers of the peripheral nerves. The lipoprotein plasma membranes of these cells wrap themselves around the nerve fibers for several layers. Myelination of fiber tracts tends to occur before the maturation of functional ability (Haynes et al., 2025a, 2025b; Torchia & Persaud, 2024).

Myelination begins early in pregnancy and continues into adulthood. Myelination predominates between 8 months' gestation and 2 years of age, with the peak period thought to be occurring within the first 8 postnatal months of life. However, myelination continues into adolescence and early adulthood (Haynes et al., 2025a). This process begins before birth in the peripheral areas, first in the peripheral motor nerves and then in the peripheral sensory nerves. Myelination begins before birth in the CNS, moving upward from the brainstem and cerebellum. In the CNS, myelination occurs first in the sensory areas and then in the motor areas. Myelination of ascending pathways in the spinal cord, brainstem, and thalamus is completed by about 30 weeks' gestation, and myelination from the thalamus to the cortex is completed by 37 weeks (Haynes et al., 2025a). From birth to adulthood, myelination proceeds within the cerebral hemispheres with the development of higher associative and sensory functions. Myelination is important in most nerve tracts in the CNS because it insulates individual fibers to enhance the specificity of connections, increases the number of alternative pathways, and markedly increases the transmission speed (Blackburn, 2018; Haynes et al., 2025a). This has implications for neonatal pain management, particularly for preterm infants.

**Disorders of Myelination.** Myelination is susceptible to damage from diverse exogenous influences, particularly malnutrition, which can lead to neurologic deficits in which hypoplasia of the cerebral white matter occurs. Primary hypoplasia of the white matter with vacuolization of the myelin occurs in inadequate postnatal nutrition, congenital hypothyroidism, 18q-syndrome, and amino and organic acidopathies such as maple syrup urine disease (MSUD), homocystinuria, and phenylketonuria. This defect in myelination can lead to severe neurologic deficits (Haynes et al., 2025a).

# NEUROLOGIC ASSESSMENT

Assessing the infant's neurologic functioning is one of the initial steps in evaluating an infant. This initial assessment sheds light on the infant's response to the transition to extrauterine life and the effect of perinatal events. This provides an opportunity to assess the infant for pathophysiologic problems of the CNS and PNS. Assessment of neurologic function and identification of dysfunction encompasses several components, including history, physical examination, neurologic examination, laboratory tests, and other diagnostic techniques.

## History

Risk factors noted in the maternal, obstetrical, and neonatal histories can be helpful in identifying infants at risk for neurologic dysfunction and specific pathophysiologic factors. Specific risk factors for each problem discussed here are identified later in individual sections. General maternal or family historical factors that must be examined include a family history of NTDs; chromosomal or genetic abnormalities or other malformations; maternal substance abuse; chronic maternal health problems; maternal age, nutritional status, and exposure to teratogens; and the outcome of previous pregnancies (Fanning, 2025).

Obstetrical risk factors include prematurity, postmaturity, placental problems (e.g., abruptio placentae and placenta previa), use of analgesia or anesthesia, and maternal problems (e.g., infection, hypertension, and substance abuse). A large for gestational age (LGA) infant, prolonged or precipitate labor, forceps delivery, and abnormal presentation increase the risk of birth trauma and hemorrhage. Alterations in intrauterine growth and polyhydramnios may be present in an infant with CNS malformation. Fetal distress, hypoxia, ischemia, and low Apgar scores are associated with intracranial hemorrhage and HIE (Back & Volpe, 2025; Blackburn, 2018; Inder & Volpe, 2025; Mrelashvili et al., 2025).

Because neurologic dysfunction also can arise from postnatal problems, the infant's postnatal history is evaluated for status at birth, whether resuscitation was required, ischemic or hypoxic episodes, shock, hypoperfusion with or without hemorrhage, infection, and metabolic or electrolyte aberrations. The infant's record is also reviewed for clinical signs, such as seizures or alterations in activity, tone, and state, associated with neurologic dysfunction (Fanning, 2025; Demauro & Hintz, 2025).

## Physical Examination

A comprehensive physical examination is a crucial component of assessing any infant at risk for, or showing evidence of, neurologic dysfunction. Infants are examined especially for evidence of infection and birth trauma, such as ecchymosis, edema, lacerations, and fractures. Temperature, blood pressure, color, and respiratory patterns are also assessed. The infant is examined for signs of vascular alterations, such as a port-wine stain along trigeminal nerve branches, which may indicate Sturge–Weber syndrome. The characteristics of the infant's cry (e.g., robustness, presence in response to aversive stimuli, and pitch) may also be useful. Funduscopic examination may be performed to assess for chorioretinitis (associated with intrauterine viral infection), papilledema (seen with cerebral edema, although less reliably in neonates), and congenital anomalies (Demauro & Hintz, 2025; Volpe & El-Dib, 2025a).

Specific parameters that are particularly important for the nurse to assess in infants with neurologic problems are (a) the head size, shape, and rate of growth; (b) the sutures and fontanelles; (c) whether major and minor anomalies are present; and (d) the vertebral column. Because CNS anomalies often are associated with other anomalies and syndromes, the infant is also examined for significant body anomalies and isolated or clustered minor malformations, such as low-set or abnormally shaped ears, micrognathia, and hypertelorism of the eyes. The vertebral column is inspected and palpated for evidence of NTDs. Signs indicating an underlying defect include hair tufts, dimples, and fistulae (Demauro & Hintz, 2025; Volpe & El-Dib, 2025a).

**Head Size, Shape, and Rate of Growth.** The monitoring and plotting of head circumference are basic components of healthcare for all infants, regardless of gestation or health status. The largest circumference is usually measured, the occipitofrontal circumference, about 1 cm above the eyes. The measurement is plotted on the appropriate growth grid for the infant's gender and gestation. The most accurate measurements are made with a metal or plastic tape marked in centimeters. Paper tapes tend to stretch and are less precise but can be used for initial screening and for infants whose head size raises no concern. The occipitofrontal circumference generally ranges from 32.6 to 37.2 cm in term infants. Infants with caput succedaneum or overriding sutures may need to be reassessed more frequently to assess for baseline changes. The head usually grows 0.1 to 0.6 cm/week in infants 24 to 40 weeks' gestation (Parker, 2021).

Serial measurements must be made to identify changes in the rate of growth as well as in size. Changes in the growth rate are important because an infant may significantly increase or decrease in head growth but remain within the 10th to 90th percentiles on standard head growth grids. The occipitofrontal circumference should be measured several times over the first days after birth to obtain an accurate baseline after molding and edema from birth have resolved. Head circumference is measured weekly on preterm or ill infants. More frequent measurements may be made if the infant is at risk of developing progressive ventricular dilatation. Head shape can also reflect perinatal events and specific anomalies. The forces of labor and delivery may deform the head, but these changes are transient and disappear within a few days. Infants with craniosynostosis (premature closure of one or more sutures) and hydrocephalus have abnormal head configurations (Fulton et al., 2024; Johnson, 2025).

**Sutures and Fontanelles.** The entire head is inspected and palpated, and each suture and fontanelle is assessed. The anterior fontanelle is evaluated while the infant is in a quiet state and a semi-upright or sitting position. The fontanelle should be open, soft, and flat. Pulsation may be felt normally in a newborn but can be associated with elevated blood pressure. **Emergency Alert: A sunken or depressed fontanelle is seen with dehydration, and a bulging fontanelle is noted with increased intracranial pressure (ICP).** The anterior fontanelle is usually diamond shaped and may be small at birth if molding and overriding of the sutures are present; the size increases within a few days to the usual dimensions seen in term infants (i.e., 3–4 cm long by 1–3 cm wide). The anterior fontanelle closes at 8 to 16 months of age. The anterior fontanelle may bulge slightly with increased tension when the infant cries and may be somewhat depressed when the infant is upright. The posterior fontanelle closes any time from 8 months' gestation to 2 months (closes 6–8 weeks after birth). If the posterior fontanelle is open at birth, it is 1 to 3 cm wide and has a triangular shape. The mastoid fontanelle, also known as the posterolateral fontanelle, can be found on either side at the intersection of the temporal, parietal, and occipital bones. These fontanelles usually close between 6 and 18 months of age. The sphenoid fontanelle or anterolateral fontanelle is located on either side of the skull at the intersection of the sphenoid, parietal, temporal, and frontal bones. Closure of these fontanelles usually takes place at around 6 months of age. In rare cases, A "third fontanelle" may be palpated along the sagittal suture between the anterior and posterior fontanelles; this is not a true fontanelle but a defect in the parietal bone. It can be palpated in normal infants but also seen in infants with congenital infections such as Rubella, Down syndrome, or hypothyroidism (Fanning, 2025; Lipsett et al., 2024; Volpe & El-Dib, 2025a). A 4- to 5-mm separation (up to 1 cm) of all the sutures except the squamosal (temporoparietal) suture is normal in the newborn. The squamosal suture should not be separated more than 2 to 3 mm, especially in the term or near-term (late preterm) infant. Overriding of the bones and molding from delivery may modify this finding in the first few days after birth. Abnormal findings include persistence of suture separation over time, increased separation of the sutures, and separation of the squamosal suture by more than 2 to 3 mm. With increased ICP, separation of the sutures occurs in a specific order: sagittal, coronal, metopic, lambdoidal, and squamosal; therefore, separation of the squamosal suture is the most clinically significant (Lipsett et al., 2024; Volpe & El-Dib, 2025a). Cranial bones are inspected and palpated to evaluate for fractures, extradural hemorrhage, edema, and uneven ossification of the cranial bones or craniotabes.

## Neurologic Examination

The neurologic examination is useful for evaluating the presence and determining the extent of neurologic dysfunction in neonates, monitoring recovery, and as a prognostic indicator. Factors such as gestational age, health status, the infant's state, medications, and timing of feedings must be considered in interpreting neurologic findings. Parameters examined in the assessment of neurologic status include level of consciousness, activity, tone, posture, reflexes, and evaluation of selected cranial nerves. The optimum state of the infant during a neurologic examination is quiet and alert after awakening naturally from a sleep state. It may be challenging to find such a perfect moment, and often, the infant must be aroused from a sleep state or quieted from a state of heightened arousal. It is essential to determine the state of the infant prior to a neurologic examination because the infant's level of alertness affects the interpretation of the infant's neurologic status (Fanning, 2025; Volpe & El-Dib, 2025a).

**Observation of State: Level of Consciousness.** Neurologic insults frequently alter the infant's level of consciousness. The level of consciousness may range from normal states of consciousness for gestation to hyperexcitability, irritability, lethargy, hyperalertness, and stupor or coma. The three clinical levels of consciousness that best correlate with outcome are hyperalertness, lethargy, and stupor or coma. In the hyperalert state, the infant has an increased sensitivity to sensory stimulation, with wide-open eyes but a diminished blink response and ability to fixate and follow. A lethargic infant responds to tactile and noxious stimuli, but the responses are delayed. A stuporous or obtunded infant's response is limited to noxious stimuli, and a comatose infant shows no response to tactile or noxious stimuli (Volpe & El-Dib, 2025a). Hyperexcitability and irritability are assessed by noting an infant's response to caregiving actions and medical procedures, as well as the baby's state between caregiving intervals, to assess the infant's ability to use self-consoling measures.

**Posture, Tone, and Activity.** Because normal tone requires integrated functioning of the entire nervous system, so CNS or PNS disturbances may manifest in alterations in neonatal position, tone, and activity. The infant is first assessed while lying in a resting position. A frog-leg position while supine is seen in immature infants, after breech delivery, and in infants who have experienced severe asphyxia or who have significant health problems or neuromuscular disorders (Volpe & El-Dib, 2025a). The quality and symmetry of activity with spontaneous and elicited movement are assessed. Alterations in symmetry of the trunk, face, and extremities at rest or with spontaneous movement suggest congenital anomalies, birth injury, or neurologic insult. Tight fisting is an abnormal sign. A cortical thumb (inside thumb on the closure of the hand) may be expected, but it is abnormal if persistent. Opisthotonos and decerebrate or decorticate posturing may also occur (Fanning, 2025; Johnson, 2025).

Abnormal movements include seizure activity, jitteriness, and tremors, although the last two findings often are normal. Tremors and jitteriness must be differentiated from seizures. The characteristic movements seen with tremors in neonates vary with the underlying disorder. Tremors associated with metabolic abnormalities are usually low-amplitude, high-frequency movements, whereas tremors associated with CNS complications are usually high-amplitude, low-frequency movements. Jitteriness is a common finding in infants because of the lack of myelination of the pyramidal tracts. A significant function of these tracts is to inhibit spinal reflexes. In neonates, these unmyelinated tracts respond to central arousal with generalized peripheral hyperexcitability. Jitteriness is stimulus sensitive and is not marked by gaze or eye deviations. The predominant movement in jitteriness is tremulousness, rather than the clonic movement seen in seizures, which ceases with passive flexion. Spontaneous or elicited movement can set off tremors. Tremors can also be associated with metabolic abnormalities, asphyxia, or drug withdrawal (Fanning, 2025; Keene et al., 2025).

Resting, passive, and active tone are assessed. Resting tone is evaluated by observing the infant at rest in a supine position. The passive tone is assessed by examining extensibility, which involves maneuvers used in the neuromuscular component of the assessment of gestational age. Evaluation of active tone consists of altering the infant's posture to obtain directed motor responses (Volpe & El-Dib, 2025b).

Common maneuvers are righting reactions of the legs and trunk and examination of neck flexors and extensors. Righting reactions are elicited by holding the infant upright with the feet on a firm surface. The infant's ability to straighten the legs and trunk is assessed. Neck flexors and extensors are assessed using the pull-to-sit maneuver (Fanning, 2025; Volpe & El-Dib, 2025a, 2025b). Infants with peripheral nerve injuries, neuromuscular disorders, alterations at the neuromuscular junction, and spinal cord injuries tend to be hypotonic and have muscle weakness. Infants with CNS disturbances secondary to asphyxia, intracranial hemorrhage, chromosomal disorders or other genetic defects, or metabolic disturbances tend to be hypotonic without muscle weakness (Yeo et al., 2024; Volpe & El-Dib, 2025a, 2025b). Hypertonia is seen less often than hypotonia in neonates with neurologic problems. Marked extensor hypertonia with arching of the back (opisthotonos) may be seen in association with severe hypoxic-ischemic injury, bacterial meningitis, or massive intraventricular hemorrhage (IVH) (Fanning, 2025; Johnson, 2025; Volpe & EL-Dib, 2025a, 2025b).

**Reflexes.** Primary and tendon reflexes may be diminished, absent, or accentuated in infants with neurologic dysfunction. Primary reflexes are affected by gestational age, but all are present to some degree by 28 to 32 weeks' gestation and include sucking, grasping, crossed extension, automatic walking (stepping), and the Moro reflex. These reflexes should be present, symmetric, and reproducible in the neonatal period and should gradually disappear during infancy. The tendon reflexes assessed in the neonate are the biceps, knee, and ankle jerk. All should be present after about 33 weeks' gestation but are not very helpful beyond confirming symmetry in the neonatal period (Hoppe & Bosse, 2024; Volpe & El-Dib, 2025a, 2025b).

**Examination of Selected Cranial Nerves.** A full cranial nerve assessment is generally not performed on the neonate. The function of these nerves can be evaluated using several relatively simple maneuvers: fixation and following, pupillary responses, doll's eye response, hearing, vestibular response, and suck and swallow (Table 15.2) (Fulton et al., 2024; Fanning, 2025; Johnson, 2025; Volpe & El-Dib, 2025a, 2025b).

**Clinical Signs Associated With Neurologic Dysfunction.** Clinical manifestations of neurologic dysfunction can be specific or nonspecific. Five types of clinical signs are seen in infants with neurologic problems: (a) CNS depression, (b) hyperirritability, (c) increased ICP, (d) seizures, and (e) movement alterations. Seizures are discussed later. Signs and symptoms of CNS depression, hyperirritability, increased ICP, and movement alterations are listed in Table 15.3.

## TABLE 15.2

### NURSING ASSESSMENT OF SELECTED CRANIAL NERVES IN THE NEWBORN

| Nerve | Assessment | Implications |
|---|---|---|
| Optic (II) | Blink in response to light (consistent by 28 weeks' gestation)<br>Fixation on object placed approximately 19 cm in front of infant's face (consistent by 32 weeks' gestation)<br>Follows object with eyes and by turning head (consistent by 37 weeks' gestation)<br>Examination of external eye | Visual system intact to the level of the superior colliculi (does not indicate visual cortex function)<br>Presence of vision |
| Oculomotor (III), trochlear (IV), and abducens (VI) | Funduscopic examination (ophthalmoscope set at 2–4 diopters)<br>Pupillary reactivity (equal and responsive to light; appears by 28 weeks') | Evaluation of abnormalities (e.g., cataracts, irregularities of size or shape, microphthalmos, or scleral hemangiomas) |

ICP, intracranial pressure.

*Sources:* Volpe, J. J., & El-Dib, M. (2025b). Injuries of the extracranial, cranial, intracranial, spinal cord, and peripheral nervous system structures. In J. J. Volpe, T. E. Inder, B. T. Darras, L. S. de Vries, A. J. du Plessis, & J. M. Perlman (Eds.), *Volpe's neurology of the newborn* (7th ed., pp. 1253–1282). Elsevier; and Volpe, J. J., & El-Dib, M. (2025a). Neurological examination: Normal and abnormal features. In J. J. Volpe, T. E. Inder, B. T. Darras, L. S. de Vries, A. J. du Plessis, J. J. Neil, & J. M. Perlman (Eds.), *Volpe's neurology of the newborn* (7th ed., pp. 293–323). Elsevier Inc.

## TABLE 15.3

### CLINICAL MANIFESTATIONS OF CNS DYSFUNCTION

| Alteration | Clinical Manifestations |
|---|---|
| CNS depression | Altered level of consciousness |
| | Weak, absent cry |
| | Weak, absent primary reflexes |
| | Poor feeding |
| | Decreased activity |
| | Decreased passive tone |
| | Decreased active tone |
| | Altered respirations |
| Hyperirritability | Sharp, excessive crying |
| | Difficult to console |
| | Low sensory threshold |
| Increased ICP | Irritability |
| | Lethargy |
| | Increased head circumference |

(*continued*)

## TABLE 15.3

### CLINICAL MANIFESTATIONS OF CNS DYSFUNCTION (*continued*)

| Alteration | Clinical Manifestations |
|---|---|
| | Palpable sutures, especially squamous |
| | Bulging, tense fontanelle |
| | Increased extensor tone of neck |
| | Downward deviation of eyes |
| | Vomiting (late) |
| | Dilated head veins (late) |
| | Decorticate posturing |
| | Opisthotonos |

CNS, central nervous system; ICP, intracranial pressure.

*Sources:* Data from: Fanning, B. A. (2025). Neurologic assessment. In C. L. Witt & C. M. Wallman (Eds.), *Tappero & Honeyfield's physical assessment of the newborn: A comprehensive approach to the art of physical examination* (7th ed.). NICU Ink; Volpe, J. J., & El-Dib, M. (2025a). Neurological examination: Normal and abnormal features. In J. J. Volpe, T. E. Inder, B. T. Darras, L. S. de Vries, A. J. du Plessis, J. J. Neil, & J. M. Perlman (Eds.), *Volpe's neurology of the newborn* (7th ed., pp. 293–323). Elsevier; and Volpe, J. J., & El-Dib, M. (2025b). Injuries of the extracranial, cranial, intracranial, spinal cord, and peripheral nervous system structures. In J. J. Volpe, T. E. Inder, B. T. Darras, L. S. de Vries, A. J. du Plessis, J. J. Neil, & J. M. Perlman (Eds.), *Volpe's neurology of the newborn* (7th ed., pp. 1253–1282). Elsevier.

## Diagnostic Techniques

Diagnostic techniques for infants suspected of neurologic problems include neurophysiologic studies, structural brain imaging and assessment of cerebral blood flow, and laboratory tests. Neurophysiologic studies used in the neurologic evaluation of the newborn include brainstem auditory evoked responses, visual evoked responses, somatosensory evoked responses, and electroencephalogram (EEG) and amplitude-integrated EEG (aEEG) (de Vries & Volpe, 2025). The brainstem auditory evoked response test reflects the electrical events generated in the auditory pathways detected via small external sensors and indicates the infant's response to an auditory stimulus. This test is easily performed and is currently the most often used technique for routine hearing screening in newborn nurseries. Visual evoked and somatosensory evoked responses are part of a more extensive neurologic examination to aid in determining the extent of the disturbance in the vision and peripheral sensation (de Vries & Volpe, 2025; Volpe & El-Dib, 2025a). EEG and aEEG will be discussed in the section on neonatal seizures.

Three types of brain structural imaging most often used are ultrasonography, computed tomography (CT), and magnetic resonance imaging (MRI). Head, or cranial, ultrasound examination is often used to evaluate intracranial structures. It is most frequently the imaging modality of choice to assess germinal and IVH in premature infants, with an estimated 90% accuracy level (de Vries & Volpe, 2025). Ultrasonography is portable, safe, convenient, and readily available at the bedside, utilizing nonionizing radiation with minimal/no need for sedation. Cranial and sagittal images can be evaluated using the anterior fontanelle and PVL through the posterior fontanelle. Doppler sonography, as part of a complete head ultrasound, can assess cerebral blood flow. Head ultrasonography is not generally helpful in evaluating the posterior fossa and intraparenchymal and meningeal areas (de Vries & Volpe, 2025; Kaufman et al., 2024; Pierson & Volpe, 2025). CT uses ionizing radiation and computerized image reconstruction to provide high-resolution images within a few minutes of scanning. A CT of the newborn brain provides information regarding calcifications and cranial bony abnormalities, most parenchymal disorders, hemorrhage or fluid in the subdural and subarachnoid spaces, and most posterior fossa lesions. The MRI, which uses nonionizing radiation, is useful for diagnosing many abnormalities, some of which may be missed by sonography or CT, such as partial agenesis of the corpus callosum, arteriovenous malformations, acute or chronic focal cerebral ischemic lesions (infarcts), venous thrombosis, PVL, hemorrhagic lesions, and virtually all lesions in the posterior fossa and spinal cord (de Vries & Volpe, 2025; Kaufman et al., 2024; Pierson & Volpe, 2025). Both CT and MRI require transportation and sedation, which may be detrimental to the critically ill infant. Using these modalities often necessitates waiting until the infant has recovered from the initial critical condition to be performed (de Vries & Volpe, 2025; Pierson & Volpe, 2025).

Laboratory tests are performed to assist in the diagnosis of specific neurologic disorders and to identify underlying causes. The CSF is examined for signs of hemorrhage (increased red blood cells, increased protein, decreased glucose, and xanthochromia) and to rule out infection (culture, turbidity of the fluid, and increased or decreased white blood cells, protein, and/or glucose) (Gomella et al., 2020). Xanthochromia often is a late sign and may reflect an elevated protein level rather than the presence of blood. Other laboratory evaluations include complete blood count (CBC) with differential (e.g., white and red blood cell counts, hemoglobin, hematocrit [Hct], neutrophils, bands, and platelet count), serum glucose and calcium levels, electrolyte levels, blood gases, and acid–base status. A sepsis workup or screening for toxoplasmosis, rubella, cytomegalovirus, herpes simplex, and syphilis is performed if intrauterine infection or neonatal sepsis and meningitis are suspected. A genetic workup and other metabolic studies are performed if errors of metabolism or other inherited disorders are thought to be present (Merritt & Gallagher, 2024; Pierson & Volpe, 2025).

# SPECIFIC NEONATAL NEUROLOGIC ISSUES

## General Management Principles

Management specific to each type of neurologic dysfunction is described in later sections. However, in the nursing care of infants with neurologic dysfunction, common nursing diagnoses and management techniques that must be considered with all infants and their families are included in the following list. Those marked with an asterisk (*) are discussed in other chapters.

1. Alteration in level of consciousness:
   - Monitor the infant's state, activity level, responsiveness, eye movements, head circumference, and vital signs; also monitor for seizure activity and signs of increased ICP.
   - Position the infant to promote skin integrity, prevent contractures, and reduce ICP (i.e., head in midline and slightly elevated).
   - Monitor fluid and electrolyte status.
   - Maintain adequate ventilation and perfusion.
   - Implement comfort measures.
   - Maintain an appropriate thermal environment.
   - Reduce environmental stressors.
   - Promote neurobehavioral stability.
2. Potential for injury related to trauma or infection:
   - Use sterile technique.
   - Position the infant to prevent contamination of defects or operative sites.
   - Monitor for signs of localized infection or neonatal sepsis.
   - Handle the infant gently.
   - Position the infant to reduce potential of trauma or contamination.
3. Impairment of skin integrity:
   - Position the infant in alignment and change position regularly.
   - Use foam, sheepskin, lambskin, or waterbeds.
   - Massage the skin gently to stimulate circulation.
   - Use appropriate skin care measures.
4. Alteration in comfort.*

5. Impaired mobility:
   - Position the infant in alignment and change position regularly.
   - Promote skin integrity.
   - Use gentle range-of-motion (ROM) exercises.
6. Alteration in thermoregulation.*
7. Alteration in nutrition.*
8. Promote neurobehavioral organization and development.*
9. Altered family processes.*
10. Grieving (family).*

## Anencephaly

Anencephaly is associated with failure of the anterior neural tube to fuse in the cranial area. The primary defect may involve failure of normal mesenchyme and cutaneous (i.e., skin, bone, and dorsal coverings) development (du Plessis & Volpe, 2025). Since the advent of antenatal diagnosis and folic acid therapy, the incidence of infants born with anencephaly has markedly declined. Because fusion of the anterior neural tube contributes to the forebrain, anencephalic infants have minimal development of the brain. The brain tissue that does develop is poorly differentiated and becomes necrotic with exposure to amniotic fluid; this results in a mass of vascular tissue with neuronal and glial elements and a choroid plexus marked by partial absence of the skull bones. Anencephaly is thought to occur before about 24 days' gestation, around the period of closure of the rostral neuropore (du Plessis & Volpe, 2025).

Anencephalic infants often have other anomalies. Three-fourths of these infants are stillborn; live-born infants usually die within the first postnatal month, generally by the end of the first week (du Plessis & Volpe, 2025; Dean & Doherty, 2024). Management of infants with anencephaly is supportive, involving the provision of warmth and comfort until the infant dies. Families require emotional support and assistance coping with their grief over the birth of an infant with a defect and their death.

## Encephalocele

Encephaloceles are "developmental disorders of cranial mesoderm ... associated with a cystic extracranial extension of meninges, neural tissues, and cerebrospinal fluid" (du Plessis & Volpe, 2025, p. 9). Encephalocele is thought to be a post-neurulation disorder involving a skull defect through which neural tissue protrudes (Dean & Doherty, 2024). Although this defect can occur in any region, approximately 70% to 80% occur in the occipital region (du Plessis & Volpe, 2025; Dean & Doherty, 2024). The sac protrudes from the back of the head or the base of the neck. The next most common area is the frontal region, involving the orbit, nose, and/or nasopharynx. Although uncommonly, encephaloceles can occur in the temporal or parietal areas (Gressens & Hüppi, 2025).

The protruding sac varies considerably in size; however, the size of the external sac does not necessarily correlate with the presence of neural elements. For example, a large occipital sac may contain minimal neural tissue, whereas a small sac may contain parts of the cerebellum or accessory lobes; some occipital lesions have no neural elements in the sac. Neural tissue generally displays normal gyration and white matter and is connected to the brain by a slender necklike structure (du Plessis & Volpe, 2025; Gressens & Hüppi, 2025). If the sac is leaking CSF at birth, immediate repair is necessary. If the defect is covered by skin, surgery may be delayed until a complete workup, including skull radiography, CT or cranial ultrasonography, MRI, and EEG, can be performed. Surgical closure helps prevent infection and facilitates feeding and other care.

Hydrocephalus, which may be present at birth or develop after surgical repair, occurs in 50% of occipital encephaloceles because of alterations in the posterior fossa (Gressens & Hüppi, 2025). Encephalocele may be associated with chromosomal abnormalities, such as trisomy 13, 18, and 21, Meckel–Gruber syndrome, or Walker–Warburg syndrome (du Plessis & Volpe, 2025). A ventriculoperitoneal shunt is inserted if hydrocephalus is present. Other management includes preventing infection and trauma and positioning to avoid pressure on the defect. Maintaining normal body temperature is essential, especially in infants with CSF leakage, because these infants are at risk for thermoregulatory problems caused by evaporative losses. Postoperative management includes assessment of ventilation and perfusion, comfort measures, monitoring of neurologic and motor function, promotion of normothermia, prevention of infection, positioning to prevent pressure on the operative site, and monitoring the site for CSF leakage. The mortality rate and later outcome are significantly better for infants with anterior defects than those with posterior defects. The prognosis is poor if significant brain tissue is contained within the sac (Dean & Doherty, 2024).

Families of infants with an encephalocele need initial and continuing support and counseling. Initial parental care involves assisting parents with the shock of the defect and its appearance and with their grief over having an infant with an anomaly and helping the parents deal with the outcome implications of this defect. Nursing care involves enhancing parent–infant interaction and involving parents in the infant's care when they are ready. Teaching before discharge includes skin care, positioning, exercises, handling and feeding techniques, and activities to promote growth and development.

## Spina Bifida

Spina bifida is a general term used to describe defects in the caudal neural tube closure that are associated with spinal cord and vertebrae malformations. Spina bifida arises from defects in the closure of the caudal neuropore during primary neurulation (open defects) or secondary neurulation (closed defects). Defects range from minor malformations of minimal clinical significance to major disorders that result in paraplegia or quadriplegia and loss of bladder and bowel control. The two primary forms of spina bifida are spina bifida occulta and spina bifida cystica.

Spina bifida occulta is a vertebral defect at L5 or S1 that arises from failure of the vertebral arch to grow and fuse between 5 weeks' gestation and the early fetal period. Frequently, only one vertebra is involved in the defect, and the spinal cord and nerves are not involved, so there are usually no neurologic symptoms. The dermal layer is intact over the vertebral defect; occasionally, the defect is indicated by a dimple or tuft of hair.

Incidence is difficult to determine because many are unrecognized due to minimal/no physical problems arising from this defect. Spina bifida occulta is often discovered in radiographs of the lumbar and sacral regions. A few individuals have underlying abnormalities of the spinal cord, the nerve roots, or both, such as diastematomyelia or dermal sinus (Torchia & Persaud, 2024). Diastematomyelia results from a bony spicule or cartilaginous band's division of the spinal cord or nerve roots in an anteroposterior direction. A dermal sinus is a tract of squamous epithelium that connects to the dura mater and is found in the midline, usually in the lumbosacral area, corresponding to the location of the caudal neuropore. A dermal sinus is occasionally recognized at birth, but more often, it is diagnosed later, after repeated episodes of meningitis (Copp & Greene, 2022; du Plessis & Volpe, 2025).

Spina bifida cystica is a generic term for NTDs characterized by a cystic sac containing meninges, spinal cord elements, or both, along with vertebral defects. Epithelium, or a thin membrane, covers the sac. As with anencephaly, the incidence has declined in recent years (ACOG, 2017; Torchia & Persaud, 2024). Spina bifida cystica can occur anywhere along the spinal column but is often seen in the lumbar or lumbosacral area. The three main forms of spina bifida cystica are MMC, and myeloschisis.

A meningocele involves a sac containing meninges and CSF, but the spinal cord and nerve roots are normal. Neurologic deficits are not typically associated with a meningocele. Meningoceles account for about 5% of spina bifida cystica (Torchia & Persaud, 2024).

MMC refers to a sac containing spinal cord or nerve roots, or both, in addition to meninges and CSF and accounts for 80% of spina bifida cystica. The incidence of MMC is 0.3 to 0.72 per 1,000 births (Cavalheiro et al., 2017). This defect occurs at around 26 days' gestation, around the time of closure of the caudal neuropore (du Plessis & Volpe, 2025). During development, the nerve tissues become incorporated into the sac wall, impairing the differentiation of nerve fibers. The spinal cord and/or nerve roots are displaced dorsally, and muscle and bony structure defects are present. These lesions are covered with skin meninges or both and are usually located in the lumbosacral area. The level of the impairment of the spinal cord dictates the severity of the neurologic deficit because the nerve tissues below the sac are impaired. The sensory level generally tends to approximate the motor level but may be several segments lower because of differences in the innervation pattern between sensory and motor fibers (Blackburn, 2018). Approximately 80% of these malformations occur in the lumbar area, the final area of neural tube fusion (du Plessis & Volpe, 2025). If the sac is covered with meninges, there is a risk of rupture during delivery, along with leakage of CSF and the risk of infection and dehydration. Individuals with MMC may have motor and sensory impairments of the lower extremities, bowel and bladder dysfunction, hydrocephalus, and spinal/leg alterations such as scoliosis and hip, ankle, and foot issues (Cavalheiro et al., 2017). Those infants with MMC have altered tone and activity of the lower extremities and may assume a froglike posture. In those infants with bowel and bladder involvement, dribbling of urine and feces may be noted. Many infants have associated Chiari type II malformations with a noncommunicating form of hydrocephalus (Gressens & Hüppi, 2025; Torchia & Persaud, 2025). Hydrocephalus is seen in up to 82% of infants repaired after birth (Cavalheiro et al., 2017).

Chiari type II malformations are defects in neural tube closure involving several anomalies, including displacement of the medulla, fourth ventricle, and lower cerebellum into the cervical canal; bony defects of the occiput, foramen magnum, and cervical vertebrae; and obstruction of the foramen magnum, leading to hydrocephalus (du Plessis & Volpe, 2025; Gressens & Hüppi, 2025). The resulting hydrocephalus is caused primarily by one or both of two defects—either a hindbrain malformation blocking the normal flow of the spinal fluid from the fourth ventricular outflow and/or through the posterior fossa, or there may be aqueductal stenosis disrupting normal spinal fluid flow. Chiari type II malformation occurs with most MMCs at the thoracolumbar, lumbar, and lumbosacral levels.

## Management

In utero, repair of MMC is performed before 26 weeks in some centers to reduce postnatal complications such as hindbrain herniation, hydrocephalus, and urologic dysfunction. In utero intervention is based on the hypothesis that long-term outcomes are related to both the primary defect (MMC) and secondary complications, such as damage to exposed neural tissue along with the development of Chiari II and hydrocephalus, and that in utero surgery may reduce this secondary damage (du Plessis & Volpe, 2025). Compared to postnatal surgical outcomes, prenatal surgery has demonstrated improvements in the need for hydrocephalus treatment (shunting) within the first year of life, improvement in hindbrain herniation, and improved motor outcomes with an increased likelihood of independent ambulation. Significant improvement in sensorimotor function has not been reported, and an increase in obstetrical complications, such as preterm labor, oligohydramnios, premature rupture of the membranes (PROM), and surgical risks involved, were reported in several small studies (Adzick et al., 2011; Danzer et al., 2016; Rimbos, 2024). To determine whether prenatal repair of MMC improved outcomes over postnatal surgical repair, a large, prospective randomized clinical trial, the Management of Myelomeningocele Study, was done at three maternal–fetal surgery centers (Adzick et al., 2011; Copp & Greene, 2022; Rimbos, 2024). This study showed that in utero repair of MMC reduced the need for postnatal shunting and improved motor outcomes at 30 months but was associated with maternal and fetal risks. Maternal risks included oligohydramnios, chorioamniotic separation, placental abruption, and spontaneous membrane rupture. Fetal complications included premature delivery, with an average gestational age of 34.1 versus 37.1 weeks in the postnatal surgical group, and nearly 13% delivered before 30 weeks' gestation (versus none in the postnatal surgical group), and respiratory distress syndrome (RDS), which was likely primarily attributable to prematurity. No other significant fetal/neonatal complications were reported for the in utero surgical group.

In utero surgery was associated with a decreased need for a ventriculoperitoneal shunt, less risk of moderate-to-severe brain herniation, improved motor function and ambulatory status, and improved mental development (Adzick et al., 2011; Copp & Greene, 2022). The prenatal surgical group required more procedures for delayed spinal cord tethering than did the postnatal surgical group. Parent-reported self-care and mobility were also significantly better in the prenatal surgical group than in the postnatal group. There were no differences in later cognitive scores between groups (Adzick et al., 2011; Copp & Greene, 2022). Long-term follow-up of infants with fetal surgery at 10 years of age found that 79% were community ambulators, 14% were wheelchair dependent, and 26% had normal bladder function (Danzer et al., 2016). Because fetal surgery requires a specialized, multidisciplinary team, it is only available in a limited number of centers and, as previously noted, is associated with increased maternal and fetal complications (Cavalheiro et al., 2017). Work is ongoing on improving surgery techniques, such as examining less invasive endoscopic techniques and using a cellulose patch to reduce maternal and perinatal complications (Cavalheiro et al., 2017; du Plessis & Volpe, 2025).

Immediate management for all NTDs includes stabilization and prevention of trauma and or infection of the sac, if present, and its contents. The infant is monitored for signs of sepsis, including systemic sepsis, localized infection, and meningitis. Warmth and hydration are provided, and fluid and electrolyte status are monitored. **Emergency Alert: These infants are at greater risk of hypothermia and dehydration because of the open lesion, which lacks the normal protective skin covering.** Infants with NTDs may have evidence of hydrocephalus at birth. Ultrasonography, CT, or MRI can be used to determine the ventricular system's size, rule out Chiari type II malformation, and monitor ventricular status and the development of hydrocephalus. Renal dysfunction may develop as a result of recurring urinary tract infections (UTIs). Infants with NTDs may also have cardiac, intestinal, orthopedic, and other neurologic anomalies (Blackburn, 2018; du Plessis & Volpe, 2025; Gressens & Hüppi, 2025).

The infant with NTD is positioned prone or on the side to reduce tension in the sac. A roll between the legs at hip level assists in maintaining abduction of the legs; a foot roll is used to maintain the feet in a neutral position. Change of position from prone to side lying or side to side, as well as ROM exercises, helps prevent skin breakdown and contractures. If the infant must be temporarily placed supine for a procedure, a donut roll can avoid pressure on the sac. Postoperative positioning also involves using the prone or side-lying position, maintaining body alignment, preventing hip abduction, and preventing pressure on the operative site withholding. Lumbar/sacral defects must be kept free of fecal or urine contamination. Meticulous skin care, with attention to keeping the skin clean and dry and removing urine and stool, helps prevent skin breakdown and infection. The timing and characteristics of urination and stool excretion are observed to help determine the degree of deficit.

For most infants with MMC, immediate closure and aggressive care constitute appropriate management (Cavalheiro et al., 2017; Dean & Doherty, 2024). Decreased rates of infection and better outcomes are reported, with MMC repairs occurring within 48 hours of birth (Cavalheiro et al., 2017). Unless the defect is severe or is associated with multiple life-threatening anomalies, more than 90% of infants with MMC survive the neonatal period. Immediate closure reduces the risk of infection and improves the prognosis by reducing further spinal cord and nerve tract deterioration. Early closure also facilitates caregiving. A large defect may require several surgical procedures for complete closure. If the defect is completely covered by epithelium, surgery may be delayed for a short period to further evaluate function. All infants with NTDs are evaluated and monitored for hydrocephalus. Urologic function and renal function are also assessed continually. All infants with spinal cord or nerve roots involvement, or both, require multidisciplinary follow-up and continuing care to deal with neurologic, urologic, orthopedic, and psychologic problems (Dean & Doherty, 2024).

Families of infants with NTDs need initial and continuing support and counseling. Initial parental care involves assisting parents with the shock of having an infant with a defect and its appearance and with their grief over having an infant with an anomaly. Nursing care also involves enhancing parent–infant interaction and involving the parents in the infant's care when they are ready. Teaching before discharge includes skin care, positioning, exercises, handling and feeding techniques, and provision of activities to promote development. Parental referral to peer parent-to-parent support groups and spina bifida associations should be considered.

The prognosis associated with NTDs varies with the level and severity of the defect. However, these limitations are changing due to improved perinatal management and new technologies, and more children are ambulatory now than they were previously. The prognosis has also improved with the current early and aggressive treatment of infants, especially in those without major cerebral lesions, hemorrhage, infection, high spinal cord lesions, or advanced hydrocephalus (Dean & Doherty, 2024; du Plessis & Volpe, 2025).

## NEONATAL SEIZURES

Neonatal seizures are the most common neurologic sign during the neonatal period and are more common in the newborn stage than at any other time in childhood. Neonatal seizures have unique pathophysiology and electrographic findings, resulting in clinical manifestations that can be different compared to older age groups (Farmania et al., 2020; Krawiec & Muzio, 2025). The reported incidence of neonatal seizures is approximately 1 to 5.5 per 1,000 live term births (Krawiec & Muzio, 2025), 5 per 1,000 incidence for neonates of 31 to 36 weeks gestational age, 54.9 per 1,000 for neonates of 28 to 30 weeks gestational age and 85.6 per 1,000 for neonates < 28 weeks gestational age (Pisani et al., 2020). Neonatal seizures usually are acute, with a third occurring on the first day and another third on the second day of life, then disappearing within the first few weeks after birth. Perinatal hypoxia-ischemia is generally reported to account for 50% to 60% of all neonatal seizures and is the most common cause of seizures for term newborns; IVH is the most common cause of seizures for preterm newborns (Keene et al., 2025; Pisani et al., 2020).

Seizures are abnormal synchronous neuronal discharges within the verbal cortex. This can be due to excessive excitatory or deficiency inhibitory neuronal discharges. Due to its immature state, the neonatal brain is prone to seizures due to an imbalance of neuronal excitation over inhibition. Several factors result in this imbalance. The primary factor is the developmental state of the neonatal neuron. In the neonatal brain, the chloride concentration is intracellularly high with a reversal of the chloride ion gradient. Thus, when the gamma-aminobutyric acid (GABA) receptor is stimulated, chloride ion channels open, and there is an efflux of chloride ions, and depolarization of the neuron occurs through an influx of sodium and calcium ions. Other factors involved in this imbalance include the development of excitatory synapses before inhibitory synapses and the early maturation of voltage-gated ion channels specific to depolarization (Farmania et al., 2020; Krawiec & Muzio, 2025).

Seizures are not a disease in themselves but a sign of underlying disease processes that have resulted in an acute disturbance within the brain. There is increasing evidence suggesting that these seizures exacerbate brain injury, which increases the necessity for prompt recognition, efficient observation and monitoring methods, and effective therapeutic interventions (Abend et al., 2025; Keene & Glass, 2024). If left untreated, these disorders can lead to permanent damage of the CNS or other tissues. Disease processes associated with seizures in the neonate include primary CNS disorders, hypoxic-ischemic events, systemic diseases, and metabolic insults. Seizure activity may be an acute, recurrent, or chronic phenomenon. Recurrent or continuous seizures increase the risk of neurologic damage from the seizure activity itself (Keene & Glass, 2024).

## Pathophysiology

Seizures result from excessive, synchronous electrical discharges or depolarization in the brain that produces stereotypic, repetitive behaviors. Depolarization and repolarization of the nerves are caused by the movement of sodium and potassium across the cell membrane. The inward migration of sodium ions ($Na^+$) results in depolarization; repolarization is produced by the outward migration of potassium ions ($K^+$). These processes require an energy-dependent pump and energy in the form of adenosine triphosphate (ATP). The specific mechanism that causes neonatal seizures is unknown but might be the result of one or more of the following mechanisms: (a) disturbances in energy production and the $Na^+$-$K^+$ pump, (b) altered neuronal membrane permeability to sodium, and (c) imbalances in excitatory and inhibitory neurotransmitters (Abend et al., 2025; Farmania et al., 2020; Keene & Glass, 2024). A disturbance in energy production, with changes in the movement of $Na^+$ and $K^+$ across the neuronal membrane, may lead to an imbalance between depolarization and repolarization. The movement of $K^+$ (repolarization) unbalances the movement of $Na^+$ (depolarization).

Changes in energy production may result from hypoxemia, ischemia, and/or hypoglycemia. Alterations in the permeability of the neuronal membrane to sodium can occur with hypocalcemia. Calcium typically binds with proteins in the cell membrane to inhibit $Na^+$ movement. A decrease in calcium availability would increase the inward movement of $Na^+$ and lead to depolarization. Hypomagnesemia also increases membrane permeability to $Na^+$; alkalosis or hyponatremia also leads to seizures through this mechanism. Imbalances in neurotransmitters lead to a relative excess of excitatory neurotransmitters (glutamate or acetylcholine) over inhibitory neurotransmitters (GABA) and increase the rate of depolarization. This can occur as a result of an excess of excitatory substance (associated with hypoxemia, ischemia, and hypoglycemia) or a deficiency of inhibitory substances. Pyridoxine deficiency leads to an inhibitory neurotransmitter deficiency by depressing the activity of the enzyme responsible for the synthesis of GABA. Elevated levels of excitatory inhibitors derived from ammonia are seen in infants who have liver dysfunction after severe hypoxic-ischemic events (Abend et al., 2025; Farmania et al., 2020; Keener & Glass, 2024).

## Biochemical Effects of Seizures

Seizures result in increased energy expenditure, which leads to the following sequence of biochemical events: (a) breakdown of ATP to adenosine diphosphate with the release of energy; (b) increased glycolysis, stimulated by adenosine diphosphate, with the conversion of glycogen to glucose; (c) increased production of pyruvate, which is used by the mitochondria in ATP production; (d) increased oxygen and glucose consumption; (e) increased production of lactate from pyruvate, stimulated by increased adenosine diphosphate; and (f) lactate/$H^+$-stimulated local vasodilation, which increases local blood flow and substrate availability (Abend et al., 2025; Keene & Glass, 2024). Increased blood pressure associated with seizures also increases cerebral blood flow and substrate availability. Seizures result in a marked decrease in brain glucose concentrations because the cells replenish ATP supplies by using the available glucose. Repetitive seizures in the neonate eventually alter brain lipid and protein metabolism and energy metabolism, reducing total brain DNA, RNA, protein, and cholesterol. In animal models, these deficiencies impair cellular proliferation, differentiation, and myelination. Effects in the human neonate are unclear but of concern. Brain damage caused by seizure activity could be the result of alterations in protein metabolism or the energy supply, or it could be the result of damage from asphyxia or edema. The extent to which these changes occur in the human newborn with recurrent seizures is controversial; mounting evidence suggests that seizures are associated with less favorable neurobehavioral outcomes (Abend et al., 2025; Keene & Glass, 2024).

## Seizures in Neonates Compared With Those in Older Children and Adults

Seizures are expressed differently in neonates than in older individuals because of structural and functional differences in the neonatal brain (Abend et al., 2025; Blackburn, 2018). The peak time for organizational processes in the brain is from the sixth month of gestation to 1 year after birth; therefore, term and especially preterm infants have relatively immature brain organization. This lack of organization results in an inability to propagate and sustain generalized seizures. For example, the neonate's brain lacks the arborization and synaptic connections (wiring) necessary for a firing neuron to recruit adjacent neurons to fire synchronously. The lower rate of nerve conduction, limited myelination, and fewer connections between neurons alter the threshold for neuron firing and the ability to propagate seizures (Abend et al., 2025; Blackburn, 2018; Keene & Glass, 2024).

The neonate has increased inhibitory synapses compared with excitatory synapses, which may be a protective mechanism because it reduces the chance that a generalized seizure will be propagated in the cerebral cortex. As a result, cortical seizures are rare in neonates (Abend et al., 2025; Blackburn, 2018). The newborn has more excitatory (glutamate) than inhibitory neurotransmitters. In addition, GABA, the main inhibitory neurotransmitter in adults, is excitatory in the newborn. The glutamate level is increased (the brain needs it for neuronal development and organization), maturation of the inhibitory system is delayed, and the number of NMDA receptors that respond to glutamate is increased (Blackburn, 2018; Farmania et al., 2020). Seizure activity in these infants is more likely to be generated in areas of the brain that are more mature, such as the temporal lobe and subcortical structures, especially in the limbic region. The limbic area above the corpus callosum is one of the oldest parts of the brain in embryologic development. This area is involved with behaviors such as sucking, drooling, chewing, swallowing, oculomotor deviations, and apneic episodes, behaviors typical of those seen with subtle seizures in the neonate (Abend et al., 2025; Blackburn, 2018).

## Assessment

Seizures are a clinical manifestation associated with various underlying pathologic processes (Table 15.4), including hypoxia, ischemia, hypoglycemia, hypocalcemia, intracranial hemorrhage, infection (meningitis, congenital viral infections, viral encephalopathy), congenital anomalies of the CNS, and

**TABLE 15.4**

**MAJOR CAUSES OF NEONATAL SEIZURES**

| Cause and Frequency (% of Total) | Usual Age at Onset (Days) | Predominant Type of Seizure |
|---|---|---|
| Hypoxic-ischemic injury (38% [Abend et al., 2025]; others 50%–60%) | After 1 or more (often 6–18 hours following birth); 90% in the first 72 hours | Subtle (all), generalized tonic, multifocal clonic |
| Perinatal stroke (18%); AIS most frequent; CSVT | | |
| Hypocalcemia (15%) | Early: 1–3 days; late 4–7 days | Usually focal or multifocal |
| Neonatal-onset epilepsy (13%) | | |
| Neonatal genetic epilepsy syndrome (6%) | | |
| Intracranial hemorrhage (11%) | | |
| IVH | Most within first 3 days; later with late-onset IVH | Subtle progressing to generalized tonic with severe IVH |
| SAH | 2–3 | Any type |
| SDH | 1–2 | May be focal |
| Hypoglycemia (10%) | 1–3 | Usually focal or multifocal |
| Infections (5%–10%) | | |
| Bacterial meningitis | 4–7 | Any type; may be tonic |
| Viral encephalopathy | 2–15 | Any type |
| Congenital viral infection | 3–7 | Tonic, myoclonic |

*(continued)*

**TABLE 15.4**

**MAJOR CAUSES OF NEONATAL SEIZURES (*continued*)**

| Cause and Frequency (% of Total) | Usual Age at Onset (Days) | Predominant Type of Seizure |
|---|---|---|
| CNS malformations (< 5%–10%) | 2–10 (often not until several months of age) | Tonic, myoclonic |
| Drug withdrawal (rare) | 3–34 | Tonic or myoclonic |
| Local anesthetic intoxication[a] (uncommon) | Before 1 (1–6 hours after birth) | Tonic |

[a] Caused by accidental injection of local anesthetic into the scalp during placement of paracervical block.

AIS, arterial ischemic strokes; CNS, central nervous system; CSVT, cerebral sinovenous thrombosis; IVH, intraventricular hemorrhage; SAH, subarachnoid hemorrhage; SDH, subdural hemorrhage, pudendal, or epidural blocks or during injection of local anesthetics at delivery.

*Sources:* Abend, N. S., Wusthoff, C. J., Jensen, F. E., Inder, T. E., & Volpe, J. J. (2025). Neonatal seizures. In J. J. Volpe, T. E. Inder, B. T. Darras, L. S. de Vries, A. J. du Plessis, J. J. Neil, & J. M. Perlman (Eds.), *Volpe's neurology of the newborn* (7th ed., pp. 381–448). Elsevier; Farmania, R., Garg, D., & Sharma, S. (2020). Status epilepticus in neonates and infants. *Annals of Indian Academy of Neurology, 232*(6), 747–754. https://doi.org/10.4103/aian.AIAN_189_20; Kenne, J. C., & Glass, H. C. (2024). Diagnosis and treatment of acute symptomatic seizures in the neonate. In J. M. Perlman (Ed.), *Neonatal questions and controversies: Neurology* (4th ed., pp. 145–164). Saunders/Elsevier; Pisani, F., Spagnoli, C., Falsaperia, R., Nagarajan, L., & Ramantani, G. (2020). Seizures in the neonate: A review of etiologies and outcomes. *Seizure: European Journal of Epilepsy, 85*, 48–56. https://doi.org/10.1016/j.seizure.2020.12.023.

other metabolic disturbances, such as alkalosis, hypomagnesemia, hypernatremia, and hyponatremia. Less common causes of seizures are drug withdrawal from opiates or barbiturates, genetic disorders of amino and organic acid metabolism, kernicterus, hyperviscosity, and local anesthetic intoxication (Abend et al., 2025; Farmania et al., 2020; Keene & Glass, 2024; Keene et al., 2025).

Seizures can be difficult to recognize in neonates because the clinical manifestations often are subtle and can be associated with other disorders or can involve individual behaviors such as grimacing, startling, sucking, and twitching. Seizures can also occur with minimal or no outward signs, leading to an increasing reliance on EEG or aEEG. Recognition of seizures in the neonatal period requires careful, continuous assessment by the nurse of all at-risk infants. Clinical manifestations may include abnormal movements or alterations in tone of the trunk or extremities; abnormal and repetitive facial, oral, tongue, or ocular movements such as blinking, lip smacking, or chewing motions; and increases in blood pressure and apneic events (Abend et al., 2025; Keene et al., 2025; Krawiec & Muzio, 2025). Specific examples of each of these are listed in Table 15.5.

## Types of Seizures

Various classifications of neonatal seizures are used, some focusing primarily on clinical and behavioral manifestations and others on the presence or absence of echocardiogram correlates (Keene & Glass, 2024; Krawiec & Muzio, 2025). Increasing evidence supports a combination of clinical categories with electrographic confirmation, especially with the recent advances in digital technology that make it possible to archive and review vast amounts of data generated by bedside video-EEG monitoring (Abend et al., 2025; Keene & Glass, 2024). The addition of simultaneous, continuous video-EEG and aEEG (method of displaying one or two channels of compressed and filtered EEG readings) monitoring may refine the diagnosis and management of newborns, with seizure activity categorized within traditional classifications. The aEEG monitoring technique is a relatively easy method of detection of seizure activity and is in use with increasing regularity and reliability for monitoring the neurologic status of infants with HIE (Abend et al., 2025; Farmania et al., 2020; Weeke et al., 2024).

Determining the etiology of the seizure is essential because it will provide the opportunity to administer specific treatment and for prognostic information. Many etiologies may cause neonatal seizures, but relatively few etiologies account for the majority of neonatal diagnoses. Seven tertiary care pediatric centers in the United States comprising the Neonatal Seizure Registry consortium collected prospective data related to etiology for 426 newborns with seizures who underwent continuous EEG (cEEG). This study found that 38% of the newborns experiencing seizures related to HIE, 18% with ischemic stroke, 13% with neonatal-onset epilepsy, 11% with intracranial hemorrhage, 6% with neonatal genetic epilepsy syndrome, 4% with congenital cerebral malformation, and 3% with benign familial neonatal epilepsy (BFNE). In addition, 59% of the newborn subjects experienced greater than seven electrographic seizures, and 16% developed status epilepticus. There was no significant difference in the number of seizures between preterm and full-term newborns or among the three most common causes of seizure (HIE, ischemic stroke, and intracerebral hemorrhage) (Abend et al., 2025).

**TABLE 15.5**

**TYPES OF NEONATAL SEIZURES**

| Type | Specific | Generalized |
|---|---|---|
| Focal clonic | Repetitive rhythmic contractions. Can involve the face, upper or lower extremities, neck or trunk.<br>Cannot be extinguished by the physical suppression of movement or limb repositioning.<br>May migrate to other areas of body within the same seizure. Most commonly contralaterally but can occur ipsilaterally. | Seizure activity is diffuse, bilateral, and synchronous. |
| Focal tonic | Continuous but transient extremity posturing or asymmetric posturing of the trunk or neck. May include horizontal eye deviations. | May mimic decerebrate posturing, (upper and lower extremity tonic extension) or decorticate posturing, (upper extremity flexion and lower extremity extension). |
| Myoclonic | Nonrepetitive contractions. Involves flexor muscle groups of the extremity, most commonly the upper extremity, trunk, diaphragm, or face. | Seizures may appear as bilateral, jerking at the flexor muscles of the upper and lower extremities. |

*Source:* From Krawiec, C., & Muzio, M. R. (2025). Neonatal Seizure(Archived). In *StatPearls*. StatPearls Publishing.

Traditional clinical seizure classification identifies the following seizure types: subtle, tonic, clonic (multifocal or migratory and focal), and myoclonic (Abend et al., 2025; Keene et al., 2025). Subtle seizures are the most common type of seizure seen in neonates, particularly among preterm infants. This type of seizure is often missed because the clinical manifestations may be difficult to recognize and distinguish from other events. The behaviors most commonly seen with subtle seizures are (a) tonic, horizontal deviations of the eyes with or without nystagmoid jerking; (b) repetitive blinking or fluttering of the eyelids; (c) drooling, sucking, or tongue thrusting; and (d) swimming or rowing movements of the arms with occasional bicycling movements of the legs. Apnea may occur but usually is the result of the underlying cause of the seizure in the preterm rather than of the seizure and rarely occurs as an isolated seizure event (Abend et al., 2025; Keene et al., 2025; Keene & Glass, 2024; Krawiec & Muzio, 2025).

The most common form of tonic seizure is generalized, which usually involves tonic extension of all the extremities but is sometimes limited to a single extremity or manifested by tonic flexion of all limbs. Generalized tonic seizures can be confused with decorticate or decerebrate posturing. Other signs may include eye deviations, apnea, and occasional clonic movements. This type of seizure is the one seen most frequently in preterm infants, especially those with IVH and hypoxic-ischemic insults. Apnea, decerebrate-type postures, or both often accompany generalized tonic seizures. Occasionally, focal tonic seizures may occur, characterized by sustained asymmetric posturing of the limbs, trunk, or neck. Focal tonic seizure activity may be challenging to differentiate from voluntary movement (Abend et al., 2025; Fanning, 2025; Keene & Glass, 2024; Krawiec & Muzio, 2025).

Clonic seizures may be multifocal or focal. Because multifocal or migratory clonic seizures involve the cortex, they are more characteristic of term infants but occasionally may be seen in older preterm infants. This type of seizure involves rhythmic, jerky, clonic movements of one or more limbs that migrate to other parts of the body randomly. Multifocal clonic seizures can be confused with jitteriness. These seizures are associated with diffuse hyperexcitability of the cortex, such as occurs with metabolic derangements (Abend et al., 2025; Keene et al., 2025).

Focal clonic seizures are also seen more frequently in term than in preterm infants. This form of seizure is characterized by localized clonic jerking that is usually present in one limb or the face. Focal clonic seizures may be associated with focal traumatic CNS injuries, such as cerebral contusions and infarcts, or may be a response to a severe metabolic disturbance or asphyxia and occur in combination with other seizure types (Abend et al., 2025; Fanning, 2025; Keene & Glass, 2024; Krawiec & Muzio, 2025).

Myoclonic seizures are uncommon in term infants and are rarely seen in preterm infants. These seizures are characterized by single or multiple sudden jerks with flexion of the upper (most common) or lower extremities and occasionally the trunk and neck. Myoclonic seizures are most often seen with inborn errors of metabolism or other metabolic problems (Fanning, 2025; Keene et al., 2025; Krawiec & Muzio, 2025).

## Management

Management of neonatal seizures has two goals: (a) to determine and treat the underlying cause and (b) to protect the infant from injury during and after the seizure. Determining the cause involves an assessment of the perinatal and neonatal history, a physical examination, laboratory evaluation, and other diagnostic studies. Previous events that may indicate the underlying cause include the delivery history, bleeding, birth trauma, hypoxic-ischemic events, exposure to infectious agents and other teratogens, maternal substance abuse, and postbirth illnesses.

The physical examination includes evaluating the infant's general health and neurologic status. Routine laboratory studies include electrolyte levels, glucose, calcium, magnesium, and blood urea nitrogen (BUN) levels, Hct value, blood gases, and pH. A blood culture and lumbar puncture are also often performed. A lumbar puncture helps to rule out both infection and CNS bleeding. Other laboratory and diagnostic studies may include screening for congenital viral infections, amino acid screening (for inborn errors of metabolism), CT, ultrasonography, MRI, skull radiography, or EEG. The results of a continuous video-EEG can provide information for the prognosis, more so in a term than a preterm infant (Abend et al., 2025; Fanning, 2025; Keene & Glass, 2024).

**Quality and Safety: Seizures must be recognized, seizure activity must be documented, and the infant must be protected and supported during and after the seizure.** Observing and documenting seizure activity involves noting and recording (a) the time the seizure begins and ends; (b) the body parts involved (e.g., extremities, eyes, head); (c) a description of motor movement, eye deviations, and pupillary reactions; and (d) the infant's respiratory status, color, state, level of consciousness, and postictal status. **Emergency Alert: During the seizure, the infant's airway must be maintained, vital signs monitored, and the infant assessed for adequacy of respiration and heart rate to maintain ventilation and perfusion.** To protect the infant from injury during the seizure, the nurse should not force anything into the infant's mouth or try to restrain the infant's extremities. If possible, the nurse should try to turn the infant's head to the side. After the seizure, the infant's condition should be monitored, and supportive care should be provided to maintain ventilation, oxygenation, adequate fluids, glucose, and warmth. The nurse should also assess the infant for signs related to the events that can cause seizure activity in the neonate to help determine the cause of the seizure and prevent additional seizures (Fanning, 2025; Keene & Glass, 2024).

The overall goal of treatment of neonatal seizures is to prevent long-term brain damage through management of the underlying cause of the seizures and cessation of the clinical and electrical seizure activity (Abend et al., 2025; Keene & Glass, 2024). Treatment of the underlying cause of the seizure is a priority for preventing more seizures and neurologic damage. Continually monitoring blood gases, acid–base status, serum glucose, and fluid and electrolyte status is important for any seizure infant. Regardless of the cause, infants who have seizures require intravenous (IV) glucose administration because seizure activity depletes brain glucose and energy supplies (Abend et al., 2025; Blackburn, 2018; Keene & Glass, 2024). Alterations in oxygenation and acid–base status can occur as a complication of the apnea associated with a seizure or the physiologic consequences of seizure activity. Fluid and electrolyte management should be appropriate to the underlying cause of the seizures. For example, fluids are restricted initially in infants with cerebral edema and perinatal hypoxic-ischemic injury (Abend et al., 2025; Keene & Glass, 2024).

The issues of when to treat with anticonvulsant drugs, which drug or combination of drugs to use, and duration of treatment are controversial (Keene & Glass, 2024). Recurrent or prolonged seizures require treatment with anticonvulsants to reduce the risk of brain injury. The current consensus remains that the first-line anticonvulsant used for seizure control in the newborn continues to be phenobarbital; phenytoin (Dilantin) is the second line if seizures persist. Drugs used include fosphenytoin (recommended for IV use over phenytoin) and benzodiazepines such as lorazepam and midazolam. Phenobarbital, phenytoin, and fosphenytoin doses may be given incrementally to reach therapeutic blood levels, which must be monitored carefully to maintain the therapeutic effect and prevent toxicity. Refractory seizure may require alternative agents such as clonazepam, lidocaine, carbamazepine, diazepam, valproate, or primidone (Abend et al., 2025; Farmania et al., 2020; Keene & Glass, 2024). Other antiseizure drugs, such as lidocaine and bumetanide, are still under investigation due to cardiotoxicity and ototoxicity concerns (Pisani et al., 2020).

The length of treatment after seizure activity has been controlled and after the infant has recovered is undefined at this point. Often, the duration of treatment is clinically determined by the etiology of the seizures, the time taken, the dosage, and the number of medications required to control the seizure activity. It may range from hospitalization to 2 years postdischarge, provided no further seizure activity or perceived neurologic indication for extending treatment (Abend et al., 2025; Keene et al., 2025; Keene & Glass, 2024).

Anticonvulsants can be respiratory, myocardial, and/or CNS depressants and can compete with bilirubin for albumin binding; the infant's cardiorespiratory status, color, and neurologic status are monitored in addition to drug effectiveness. Parent teaching includes helping the family understand the cause and significance of the seizure or seizures and any planned diagnostic tests. Discharge teaching of parents includes recognition of seizure manifestations, care of the infant during and after a seizure, and administration of anticonvulsants (dosage and side effects) if administration of these drugs is to be continued after discharge.

## Outcomes

The overall prognosis for newborns with seizures has improved over the past several decades. A review of more than 2,000 cases of neonatal seizures in mostly full-term newborns from published reports before and after 1969 demonstrates that mortality has decreased from approximately 40% to 15% (Abend et al., 2025). The incidence of neurologic sequelae (intellectual disability, motor deficits [including cerebral palsy], and epilepsy) in survivors remains high at 20% to 35%, with no substantial improvement over the past several decades. The mortality rate for infants with seizures is potentially devastating, with a high risk of mortality (9%–15%) and poor long-term outcomes in terms of the development of epilepsy and neuro-cognitive sequelae. A review of children with a history of neonatal seizures demonstrated that 18% developed epilepsy, with nearly 70% having onset within the first year. Associated neurologic impairments were present in 81% of the children with epilepsy and included 18% with intellectual impairment, 6% with cerebral palsy, and 45% with both cerebral palsy and intellectual impairment. Another factor influencing the outcome after seizures in the newborn is the gestational age of the infant. Clinical seizures in preterm infants are commonly associated with more severe brain injury and, thus, a poor prognosis. Adverse outcomes occurred at twice the frequency in preterm than in term newborn infants. These outcomes included mortality (42% in preterm newborn infants compared with 16% in term newborn infants); postnatal epilepsy (48% in preterm newborn infants compared with 29% in term newborn infants); cerebral palsy (63% in preterm newborn infants compared with 25% in term newborn infants); and intellectual disability (52% of preterm newborn infants compared with 25% in term newborn infants) (Abend et al., 2025; Farmania et al., 2020).

The prognosis for infants who have seizures during the neonatal period is influenced by (a) the time of onset, (b) the cause of the seizure, (c) continuous video-EEG results, (d) responsivity to treatment, and (e) the frequency and duration of the seizures (Abend et al., 2025; Keene et al., 2025; Keene & Glass, 2024). Seizure onset less than 48 hours after birth is associated with a poor prognosis, whereas onset after 4 days generally has a good prognosis. Clonic seizures have a better prognosis than the other types. EEG results appear to be a better prognostic sign in term than in preterm infants (Abend et al., 2025; Keene et al., 2025; Keene & Glass, 2024). The best prognosis is seen in infants with seizures secondary to late hypocalcemia, hyponatremia, and uncomplicated subarachnoid hemorrhage (SAH). Other causes have a mixed prognosis. The poorest prognosis is seen with seizures associated with severe hypoxic-ischemic injury, grade III or grade IV IVH, herpes infection, some bacterial meningitis, and CNS malformations. Repeated or prolonged seizures can lead to brain injury by altering cerebral blood flow and delivery of oxygen and nutrients, depleting brain glucose and energy stores, and interfering with ventilation (Abend et al., 2025; Inder et al., 2025; Keene et al., 2025).

## HYPOXIC-ISCHEMIC ENCEPHALOPATHY

HIE is an injury to the brain caused by oxygen deficit resulting from systemic hypoxemia (decreased oxygen in blood supply), ischemia (diminished cerebral blood perfusion), or a combination of the two conditions. Hypoxemia and ischemia may occur simultaneously or sequentially, and it appears from recent evidence that ischemia is the more important of the two oxygen deprivation states in causing brain injury. In addition, the subsequent reperfusion of the affected brain area is when most of the injury to the brain occurs. Glucose deprivation also plays a part in the severity of brain injury (Mietzsch & Juul, 2024; Mrelashvili et al., 2025). HIE may occur secondary to prenatal, intrapartum, or postnatal insults in both preterm and term infants. The injury site varies with maturational changes in the brain's vascular anatomy and metabolic activity. In preterm infants younger than 32 to 34 weeks' gestation, hypoxic-ischemic damage is usually associated with germinal matrix hemorrhage–intraventricular hemorrhage (GMH/IVH). The incidence of severe forms of HIE has declined markedly due to advances in perinatal care. Most perinatal hypoxic-ischemic events are mild with minimal effects. The insult is significant enough to cause transient organ dysfunction in 2 to 5 per 1,000 live births and result in death or significant neurologic sequelae in 1 per 1,000 live births (Gillam-Krakauer et al., 2023; Mietzsch & Juul, 2024; Mrelashvili et al., 2025).

### Pathophysiology

After 33 to 34 weeks' gestation, blood flow and brain metabolic activity become less prominent in the GM and periventricular area and shift to the cortical area. Hypoxia and ischemia in older preterm and term infants, therefore, are more likely to damage areas of the peripheral and dorsal cerebral cortex. Five types of lesions have been identified in infants with HIE: (a) selective neuronal necrosis; (b) status marmoratus of the neurons of the basal ganglia and thalamus, with loss of neurons in these areas; (c) parasagittal cerebral injury; (d) PVL (primarily in preterm infants); and (e) focal or multifocal ischemic brain necrosis (Mietzsch & Juul, 2024; Mrelashvili et al., 2025).

The primary lesion for the hypoxic injury is neuronal necrosis in the cortices of the cerebrum and cerebellum, with damage to the gray matter at the depths of the sulci. Neurons of the brainstem may also be injured. Areas of necrosis may extend into the white matter and the gray matter of the basal ganglia. The primary ischemic injury occurs in the posterior portion of the parasagittal region secondary to watershed or border zone infarcts. The border zone is at the junctions of the anterior, middle, and posterior cerebral arteries and the superior and inferior cerebellar arteries. This area is farthest from the major cerebral vessels, which are the source of the blood supply for the brain. Thus, with localized ischemia, such as when the infant has systemic hypotension or hypoperfusion, this area receives the least amount of blood. With hypoxia and systemic hypotension, cerebral perfusion is maintained at first by cerebral vasodilation and redistribution of blood flow to the brain from other organs. If the hypoxia continues, cerebral blood flow is altered, energy is depleted, ischemia and edema develop, and neurophysiologic activity is disrupted. At the cellular level, neurologic injury is caused by energy depletion, accumulation of extracellular glutamate, and activation of glutamate NMDA receptors. This process occurs in two phases. The initial insult and effects of hypoxia lead to hyperpolarization with an influx of sodium, potassium, and water into the cell. This interferes with the cell's ability to produce an action potential, leading to failure of the sodium-potassium pump and cell edema. Calcium moves into the cell via voltage-dependent ion channels opened by the changes in the sodium-potassium pump. This reduces calcium currents and the release of neurotransmitters. These events may be protective mechanisms to reduce neuronal excitability and conserve oxygen. However, reperfusion and reoxygenation may lead to a buildup of free oxygen radicals and primary neuronal death. If the hypoxia and ischemia persist, NMDA receptors are activated, increasing intracellular calcium (entering the cell via glutamate-controlled ion channels). More glutamate is released and accumulates to toxic levels. Nitric oxide (NO) is also released and accumulates. NO, which at normal levels promotes vasodilation and increased blood flow, reaches toxic levels, producing excess free oxygen radicals and further activating NMDA receptors. NO combines with superoxide free radicals to make the toxic peroxynitrates, causing further cell damage. This late reperfusion phase (usually beginning 6–12 or more hours after the initial insult) is characterized by hyperexcitability and cytotoxic edema and damage caused by the release of free oxygen radicals and NO, inflammatory changes, and imbalances in inhibitory and excitatory neurotransmitters with secondary neuronal death due to necrosis or apoptosis (Gillam-Krakauer et al., 2023; Mrelashvili et al., 2025; Russ & Ostrem, 2023). After a hypoxic-ischemic insult, the entire cortex may initially be edematous, and further ischemic damage may occur due to compression of the cortex against the skull.

## Assessment

Most term infants with HIE demonstrate a characteristic pattern of neurologic findings over the first 72 hours of life, including seizures, altered levels of consciousness, altered tone, altered activity, irregular respirations, apnea, poor or absent Moro reflex, abnormal cry, poor suck, and altered pupillary responses and eye movements. Clinical signs categorizing the severity of HIE have been classified in three stages, first by Sarnat and Sarnat (1976), and are summarized in Table 15.6. Stage 1, mild HIE, is characterized by mild depression or hyperalertness, irritability, and sympathetic nervous system excitation (tachycardia, dilated pupils). These infants have good Moro and deep tendon reflexes and are generally symptomatic for less than 24 hours or so. Infants in Stage 2, moderate HIE, demonstrate lethargy interspersed with brief arousal, decreased tone, altered primary reflexes, and increased parasympathetic tone (bradycardia, decreased pupil size, and blood pressure) and may develop seizures. Infants in Stage 3, severe HIE, have varying levels of consciousness initially but then become stuporous or comatose. These infants have depressed deep tendon and Moro reflexes, as well as hypotonia, and most develop seizures. Seizures occur in up to 60% of infants with HIE, with a usual onset at 12 to 14 hours of age. The types of seizures most often seen are multifocal clonic seizures in term infants, although myoclonic clonic and/or subtle seizures may also be seen (Mietzsch & Juul, 2024; Mrelashvili et al., 2025).

**TABLE 15.6**

**STAGES OF HYPOXIC-ISCHEMIC ENCEPHALOPATHY**

| | Stage 1: Mild | Stage 2: Moderate | Stage 3: Severe |
|---|---|---|---|
| Level of consciousness | Hyperalert | Lethargic; obtunded | Stuporous |
| Pupils | Dilated | Constricted | Variable; unequal |
| Heart rate | Tachycardic | Bradycardic | Variable |
| Muscle tone | Normal | Mildly hypotonic | Flaccid |
| Myoclonus | Present | Present | Absent |
| Sucking reflex | Weak | Weak; absent | Absent |
| Salivary secretions | Sparse | Profuse | Absent |
| Moro embrace reflex | Strong | Weak; incomplete | Absent |
| Seizures | None | Common; focal or multifocal | Uncommon |

HIE, hypoxic-ischemic encephalopathy.

*Sources:* Compiled from: Mietzsch, U., & Juul, S. E. (2024). Neonatal encephalopathy. In C. A. Gleason & S. E. Juul (Eds.), *Avery's diseases of the newborn* (11th ed., pp. 824–842). Elsevier; Mrelashvili, A., Ferriero, D., Inder, T. E., & Volpe, J. J. (2025). Hypoxic-ischemic injury in the term infant: Clinical-neurological features, diagnosis, imaging, prognosis, therapy. In J. J. Volpe, T. E. Inder, B. T. Darras, L. S. de Vries, A. J. du Plessis, J. J. Neil, & J. M. Perlman (Eds.), *Volpe's neurology of the newborn* (7th ed., pp. 643–696). Elsevier; and Sarnat, H., & Sarnat, M. (1976). Neonatal encephalopathy following fetal distress: A clinical and electroencephalographic study. *Archives of Neurology, 33*, 696–705. https://doi.org/10.1001/archneur.1976.00500100030012.

## Management

Infants with HIE have multiorgan and multisystem problems that arise from the original hypoxic-ischemic insult (Mietzsch & Juul, 2024; Mrelashvili et al., 2025). As a result, the management of these infants is complex and requires a coordinated team effort. Acute management of infants with HIE focuses on delivery room resuscitation and stabilization and management of the primary problem and related alterations in the cardiovascular, pulmonary, gastrointestinal, and renal systems. Prompt identification and treatment of seizures are needed to prevent further alterations in ICP and cerebral blood flow. Management of these infants in relation to neurologic problems focuses on eliminating the cause of the original hypoxia, alleviating tissue hypoxia, and promoting adequate cerebral perfusion and brain oxygenation with the maintenance of an adequate glucose supply. Inotropic support may be necessary for adequate perfusion (Cannavo et al., 2023; Gillam-Krakauer et al., 2023; Mrelashvili et al., 2025).

Interventions are directed toward establishing ventilation and adequate perfusion and preventing or minimizing hypotension, hypoxia, acidosis, rapid alterations in cerebral blood flow and systemic blood pressure, and severe apneic and bradycardic episodes. Hyperoxia is also avoided because this state can result in cerebral vasoconstriction and diminished perfusion. The infant's neurologic status is continually monitored and documented, as are oxygenation, temperature, and blood pressure (Cannavo et al., 2023; Gillam-Krakauer et al., 2023; Mrelashvili et al., 2025). HIE must be differentiated from other neurologic dysfunctions caused by trauma, infection, or CNS anomalies. An extensive workup to define the type, extent, and location of the injury may include cranial ultrasonography, brainstem auditory evoked potentials, MRI, EEG, and measurements of cerebral blood flow, ICP, and the creatinine kinase level (Cannavo et al., 2023; Chalak et al., 2021).

Other monitored parameters are the serum and urinary electrolyte levels and osmolality, BUN, serum creatinine and glucose levels, and fluid and electrolyte balance. These infants are at risk for hypocalcemia secondary to the release of excessive phosphorus from the breakdown of ATP that occurs to produce energy; the need for energy arises in response to the stress induced by perinatal hypoxic-ischemic injury. The excess phosphorus is also related to the use of bicarbonate to correct acidosis induced by these events. After hypoxic-ischemic events, an infant is at risk for hypoglycemia due to the depletion of stores from high energy; therefore, the provision of adequate glucose for energy and interventions to reduce energy expenditure is essential. Fluid status and intake and output are monitored to prevent fluid overload and to reduce localized increases in pressure; fluids are restricted, although the effectiveness of this intervention has not been evaluated with clinical trials. Fluid management is critical not only for treating cerebral edema but also for managing the alterations in renal function and problems such as acute tubular necrosis that frequently accompany moderate-to-severe stages of HIE (Gillam-Krakauer et al., 2023; Cannavo et al., 2023).

Induced mild hypothermia has been shown to provide neuroprotection and reduce the extent of tissue injury and is increasingly the treatment of choice for infants greater than or equal to 36 weeks' gestation with moderate-to-severe HIE (Cannavo et al., 2023; Gillam-Krakauer et al., 2023; Mrelashvili et al., 2025). Potential mechanisms for these effects with hypothermic therapy include inhibition of glutamate release, reduction in cerebral metabolism, and preservation of high-energy phosphates. Additional neuroprotective mechanisms include decreases in intracellular acidosis and lactic acid accumulation, preservation of endogenous antioxidants, reduction in NO production, decrease in protein kinase inhibition, improved protein synthesis, reduction in leukotriene production, minimization of blood–brain barrier disruption, reduced brain edema, and apoptosis inhibition. Techniques studied include either selective head cooling or whole-body cooling to attain mild systemic hypothermia of 89.6°F to 93.2°F (32°C–34°C) core body temperature (Kasdorf & Perlman, 2024; Mietzsch & Juul, 2024; Mrelashvili et al., 2025; Russ & Ostrem, 2023). Infants are assessed to determine whether hypothermia criteria are met before initiating the cooling regimen. Current criteria used to determine if a newborn is a candidate for hypothermia are (a) term infants ≥ 36 weeks' gestation without major congenital anomalies, intrauterine growth restriction (IUGR; ≤ 1,800 g), or known chromosomal anomaly; (b) admitted at less than or equal to 6 hours of age to the neonatal intensive care unit (NICU); (c) assessed to be in Stage 2 moderate HIE, or Stage 3, severe HIE by neonatologist and/or pediatric neurologist (Mietzsch & Juul, 2024; Mrelashvili et al., 2025). The cooling regimen continues for 72 hours and is begun as soon as possible after birth, by 5.5 to 6 hours postbirth, and optimally before seizure activity is noted. Within 6 hours of birth is a therapeutic window demonstrated in sheep between insult and further cell death for neuroprotective interventions; early hypothermia studies indicate that cooling may be less effective if started after the onset of seizures or in infants with most severe EEG changes before therapy (Kasdorf & Perlman, 2024; Mietzsch & Juul, 2024; Mrelashvili et al., 2025; Russ & Ostrem, 2023).

Hypothermia therapy has multisystem effects in addition to the effects resulting from HIE (Table 15.7). The infants undergoing a cooling regimen, either selective head cooling or whole-body cooling, require optimal care and attention at the bedside; this intervention is only done in tertiary NICU settings. Transport delays are critical and should be avoided. Induced hypothermia is not recommended either before or during transport. Care should be taken so that the infants do not become hyperthermic with core temperatures greater than 98.6°F (37°C) (Cannavo et al., 2023; Gillam-Krakauer et al., 2023; Molloy et al., 2022).

Fluctuations in systemic blood pressure with increased ICP and altered cerebral hemodynamics can occur due to caregiving or environmental stress; therefore, developmentally supportive care of these infants to reduce stress is essential. As the infant recovers, opportunities for sensory experiences are an important part of care. These experiences can be introduced slowly and as the infant can tolerate them without becoming stressed and overloaded. Physiologic and neurologic status is monitored and documented at regular intervals. The infant is observed for changes in consciousness, tone, and activity and evidence of seizures. Seizures are recognized and treated

**TABLE 15.7**

**POTENTIAL PHYSIOLOGIC EFFECTS OF HYPOTHERMIA BY SYSTEMS WITH MEDICAL AND NURSING INTERVENTIONS**

| System | Potential Physiologic Effects | Medical and Nursing Interventions |
|---|---|---|
| Neurologic | Decreased cerebral blood flow | Observe for seizure activity |
| | Decreased cerebral metabolic rate | Monitor infant's state of arousal |
| | Reduces ATP requirements Decreases glutamate levels Decreases cellular influx of calcium | Monitor blood glucose<br>Monitor renal functions |
| | Amplitude and frequency | EEG, cEEG with video; aEEG |
| Respiratory | Decreased respiratory drive | Monitor respiratory rate, effort; may need intubation, ventilation |
| | Increased pulmonary vascular resistance | Monitor systemic blood pressure |
| | Increased $CO_2$ and $O_2$ solubility | Monitor blood gases (preferably arterial) |
| | Decreased $CO_2$ production and $O_2$ consumption | Adjust assisted ventilation as needed to prevent hypercarbia, hypoxia. |
| | Decreased $CO_2$ production and $O_2$ consumption Increased risk for hypocapnia and alkalosis | Adjust assisted ventilation as needed to prevent hypercarbia, hypoxia. Follow blood gases. |
| | Increased pH by 0.0016 for every 33.8°F (1°C) decrease in temperature | Monitor saturations with pulse oximetry to prevent hypoxia. |
| | Decreased minute ventilation to preserve normal $PaCO_2$ | Monitor saturations with pulse oximetry. Monitor ABG. |
| Cardiovascular | Decreased heart rate by 14–60 beats/min Sinus bradycardia | Monitor continuous cardiorespiratory monitoring. |
| | Increased systemic vascular resistance | Monitor invasive arterial blood pressure. |
| | Decreased cardiac output | Observe changes in perfusion status, urine output. |
| | Decreased intravascular volume | Maintain blood pressure within parameters with vasopressors, boluses. |
| | Potential for ECG changes: prolonged PR, QRS, QT | Monitor cardiac strips; obtain ECG as needed. |
| Renal | Decreased renal perfusion and glomerular filtration rate | Monitor fluid intake, urine output. |
| | Impaired salt and water reabsorption | Obtain electrolytes every 4–8 hours as needed. |
| | Diuresis | Monitor intake and output. |

*(continued)*

## TABLE 15.7

### POTENTIAL PHYSIOLOGIC EFFECTS OF HYPOTHERMIA BY SYSTEMS WITH MEDICAL AND NURSING INTERVENTIONS (*continued*)

| System | Potential Physiologic Effects | Medical and Nursing Interventions |
|---|---|---|
| | Potential for hypokalemia with increased intracellular uptake | Maintain normal potassium level. |
| | Potential for hyperkalemia during rewarming | Monitor EKG.<br>Monitor potassium. |
| | Potential for decreased calcium, magnesium, phosphorus | Monitor calcium, magnesium, and phosphorus. |
| Gastrointestinal | Decreased intestinal blood flow | Provide parenteral nutrition. |
| | Reduces GI motility and perfusion | *Begin enteral nutrition cautiously after rewarming; monitor for intolerance. |
| Hematologic | Decreased platelet count; Increased severity of thrombocytopenia | Monitor platelet count every 6–12 hours as indicated.<br>Monitor PT, PTT, fibrinogen, CBC. |
| | Increased activation and aggregation (clumping)<br>Increases blood viscosity | Monitor platelet count every 6–12 hours as indicated. |
| | Increased PT, PTT<br>Inhibits clotting factors<br>Increases risk for DIC | Monitor PT, PTT every 12–24 hours as indicated. |
| Immunologic | Impaired neutrophil release and function | Monitor CBC with differential at least every 24 hours. |
| | Decreased leukocyte chemotaxis | Monitor CBC. |
| | Decreased phagocytosis | Monitor CBC. |
| Integumentary | Causes peripheral vasoconstriction | Obtain renal function panel. |
| | Increased risk for hypercalcemia | |
| | Increased risk for SCFN and HAPI | Frequently observe skin. |

aEEG, amplitude-integrated EEG; CBC, complete blood count; cEEG, continuous EEG; DIC, disseminated intravascular coagulation; GI, gastrointestinal; HAPI, hospital-acquired pressure injury; PT, prothrombin time; PTT, partial thromboplastin time, SCFN, subcutaneous fat necrosis.

*Sources:* Compiled from: DiSalvo, M. L., Hargett, S. L., Jnah, A., & Newberry, D. (2020). System specific effects of therapeutic hypothermia with neonatal encephalopathy: Pearl for clinicians. *Neonatal Network, 39*(4), 205–214. https://doi.org/10.1891/0730-0832.39.4.205; Gilliam-Krakaur, M., Shah, M., & Gowen, Jr., C. W. (2023). Birth asphyxia. In *StatPearls* [Internet]. StatPearls. https://www.ncbi.nlm.nih.gov/books/NBK430782/?report=printable; Kasdorf, E., & Perlman, J. (2024). General supportive management of the term infant with neonatal encephalopathy following intrapartum hypoxia-ischemia. In J. M. Perlman (Ed.), *Neonatal questions and controversies: Neurology* (4th ed., pp. 131–141). Elsevier; Mietzsch, U., & Juul, S. E. (2024). Neonatal encephalopathy. In C. A. Gleason & S. E. Juul (Eds.), *Avery's diseases of the newborn* (11th ed., pp. 824–842). Elsevier; Molloy, E. J., El-Dib, M., Juul, S. E., Benders, M., Gonzalez, F., Bearer, C., Wu, W. W., Robertson, N. J., Hurley, T., Branagan, A., Cotton, C. M., Tan, S., Laptook, A., Austin, T., Mohammad, K., Rogers, E., Luyt, K., Bonifacio, S., Soul, J. S., Gunn, A. J. (2022). Neuroprotective therapies in the NICU in term infants: Present and future. *Pediatric Research, 93*, 1819–1827. https://doi.org/10.1038/s41390-022-02295-2.

promptly to prevent further injury. Positioning and skin care are important, especially for hypoactive, obtunded, or comatose infants. Physiologic and clinical effects and supportive measures for infants treated with hypothermia are summarized in Table 15.7.

Parents need initial and continuing support in dealing with their infant's critical illness, the lack of infant responsiveness if the infant is hypoactive, stuporous, or comatose, the possibility of death, and the implications for later neurologic deficits. Parent teaching focuses on promoting an understanding of the infant's health status and care and providing anticipatory guidance regarding changes in the infant's state and the outcome. The parents need to be shown how to interact with and care for their infant in a developmentally appropriate manner to promote opportunities for interaction while minimizing stressful events. The nurse can model this type of care for the parents and provide anticipatory guidance on how the infant's needs and care will change as the baby matures. Parents can also be involved in devising and implementing a developmental plan of care for their infant. Neuroplasticity bundles target potential brain injury and growth. Elements in these bundles generally include (a) empowering families through Family Integrated care (FICare); (b) optimizing nutrition; (c) developmental care; (d) skin-to-skin contact (SSC) and massage therapy; (e) positive stimulating sounds such as music therapy, reading programs, parental voice, minimizing disturbing noises, and enhancing physiologic sleep–wake cycles; and (f) encouraging positive social interaction (Molloy et al., 2022).

## Outcomes

The prognosis, which varies with the extent and severity of the insult and the resulting brain injury, ranges from perinatal death to severe neurologic impairment to minimal or no sequelae. Specific sequelae may not be apparent for several months or longer. Some infants make a significant recovery, although the rate and degree of recovery vary. MRI or CT can be used to assess the injury's location, degree, and extent (Lodygensky et al., 2024; Mietzsch & Juul, 2024; Mrelashvili et al., 2025). Sequelae of HIE in term infants are related to the site of injury (e.g., the cortex) and include intellectual disabilities, microcephaly, cortical blindness, hearing deficits, and epilepsy. Generally, infants with mild HIE do well. Infants with moderate HIE or severe HIE have a higher mortality rate and later cognitive and motor problems (Mietzsch & Juul, 2024; Mrelashvili et al., 2025).

The advent of hypothermia therapy as a treatment modality has improved the general outcome, especially for infants with Stage 2 moderate HIE. Most human studies report beneficial effects of hypothermia therapy in terms of improved survival and outcome with no significant adverse effects for infants with Stage 2 moderate HIE (Mietzsch & Juul, 2024; Mrelashvili et al., 2025). Therapeutic hypothermia is now considered routine care for infants with moderate-to-severe neonatal cephalic apathy. Improvements and support of NICU care during treatment reduce brain injury detection by modern imaging and improve survival and neurologic outcomes into middle childhood. The risk of adverse outcomes, despite therapeutic hypothermia, has fallen from about 45% in the original trials to about 29% in the recent randomized controlled trial period. The recent trial of late cooling found an overall risk of adverse outcomes of just 26% (Molloy et al., 2022; Victor et al., 2021). Therapeutic hypothermia can be distinguished into selective head cooling and systemic hypothermia. Systemic hypothermia is preferred because it cools all brain structures by cooling the central body and deep brain areas to similar temperatures (Cannavo et al., 2023). In a recent meta-analysis, therapeutic hypothermia reduced the risk of death or major neurodevelopmental disability at 18 months of age (Victor et al., 2021).

# BRAIN INJURY IN PRETERM INFANTS

Preterm infants are particularly vulnerable to brain injury, with the greatest prevalence of neurologic alterations seen in very low birth weight (VLBW) infants. These infants are at increased risk for cognitive, behavioral, motoric, vision, hearing, attentional, and socialization problems (Demauro & Hintz, 2025; Law et al., 2021; Lien, 2020; Pierson & Volpe, 2025). There is an increased risk of moderate-to-severe neurodevelopmental impairment after IVH grade 1 to 2 and IVH grade 3 to 4. Children with IVH grade 1 to 2 have higher risks of cerebral palsy cognitive, hearing, and visual impairment. Children with IVH grades 3 to 4 had markedly higher risks of cerebral palsy and motor, cognitive, hearing, and visual impairment. Children with WMI had much higher risks of cerebral palsy, motor, and cognitive impairment. Cognitive dysfunction continues into school age and adulthood (Rees et al., 2020).

The major etiologic events leading to brain injury in preterm infants are a combination of pathophysiologic events leading to specific injuries and an increased susceptibility to injury due to their stage of brain development, leading to interruption or disruption of brain development. The relative contributions of altered or delayed maturation versus specific injury are unclear. Developmentally, preterm infants are vulnerable to alterations in brain maturation and injury because they are born during peak brain growth and CNS organization and differentiation (Farmania et al., 2020). Exposure to pain and stress, opioids and other pharmacologic agents, and the NICU environment may also influence brain development and maturation in preterm infants (Blackburn, 2018).

The main pathophysiologic events leading to brain injury in preterm infants are hypoxia-ischemia and inflammation/infection (Inder & Volpe, 2025; Lien, 2020). The primary lesions seen in these infants are GMH/IVH, which may include periventricular hemorrhagic infarction (PVHI) and posthemorrhagic hydrocephalus, WMI (including PVL, often accompanied by gray matter damage with neuronal and axonal damage), and cerebellar injury (Back & Volpe, 2025; Molloy et al., 2022). PVL, accompanied by neuronal and axonal abnormalities, has been referred to as the encephalopathy of prematurity and is the most common brain injury currently seen in preterm infants (Cheng & Ballabh, 2021; Molloy et al., 2022).

Prevention of brain injury in preterm infants is a complex process that begins in the perinatal period with the prevention of preterm birth, perinatal asphyxia, and birth trauma. Neurocritical care should be provided for all premature infants to emphasize the prevention of specific insults or to remedy insults that have already happened. Neuroprotective strategies for preterm infants include the use of antenatal glucocorticoids, antenatal magnesium sulfate to reduce the risk of cerebral palsy, delayed cord clamping, maintenance of stable cerebral blood flow and oxygen delivery based on hemodynamic monitoring, and neonatal SSC (kangaroo care) (Doyle et al., 2009; Lien, 2020; Mietzsch & Juul, 2024). Currently under investigation are the use of melatonin and erythropoietin (Lien, 2020; Mietzsch & Juul, 2024; Molloy et al., 2022; Rees et al., 2022). Nursing management after birth involves recognizing factors that increase the risk of brain injury, implementing strategies to reduce these risks, and supportive care.

## Germinal Matrix Hemorrhage–Intraventricular Hemorrhage

GMH/IVH, or, most commonly, IVH, is the most common type of intracranial hemorrhage seen in the neonatal period (Back & Volpe, 2025; Inder et al., 2025). IVH is seen almost exclusively in preterm infants, particularly those weighing less than 1,500 g. Decreasing gestational age increases the risk and severity of IVH. The incidence of IVH in premature infants less than 1,500 g has remained stable for the past decade at 15% to 25% (Back & Volpe, 2025; Inder et al., 2025; Zhou et al., 2024). However, the risk of IVH and severe IVH is higher in more immature infants, especially those with birth weights less than 750 g (Inder et al., 2025). The significant risk factors for IVH in the neonate are prematurity and hypoxic events interrelated with the anatomic and physiologic processes that make the periventricular site particularly vulnerable. IVH occurs but is uncommon after 35 to 36 weeks' gestation because of the involution of the subependymal GM and alterations in cerebral blood flow patterns that occur after this time. Any perinatal or neonatal event that results in hypoxia or alters cerebral blood flow or intravascular pressure increases the risk of IVH (Inder et al., 2025). The location and severity of the hemorrhage classifies IVH. Several classifications are available (Back & Volpe, 2025). Using Volpe's system, a grade I or slight hemorrhage is characterized by isolated GM hemorrhage; a grade II or small hemorrhage by IVH with normal ventricular size; and a grade III or moderate hemorrhage IVH with ventricular dilation and hemorrhage in greater than 50% of the ventricle (Inder et al., 2025). PVHI or severe hemorrhage (also referred to as grade IV) involves both intraventricular and brain parenchyma hemorrhage IVH (Back & Volpe, 2025; Inder et al., 2025).

**Pathophysiology.** The neuropathophysiology of IVH involves a complex interaction of intravascular, vascular, and extravascular factors. In infants of less than 28 to 32 weeks' gestation, the hemorrhage generally arises from the subependymal germinal matrix at the head of the caudate nucleus near the foramen of Monro. On those rare occasions when IVH occurs in term infants, bleeding usually arises from the choroid plexus rather than from the GM (Inder et al., 2025; Yap & Perlman, 2024). The GM includes the tissue underlying the ependymal wall of the lateral ventricles. In many preterm infants, the hemorrhage begins as a microvascular event in the GM and is confined to the subependymal area. In the rest, the original hemorrhage ruptures into the lateral ventricles and then into the third and fourth ventricles. The blood eventually collects in the subarachnoid space of the posterior fossa, often extending into the basal cistern (see Figure 15.1) (Back & Volpe, 2025; Sharma et al., 2022). Rupture of the hemorrhage from the GM into the ventricles may serve a protective function by decompressing the hemorrhagic area and reducing further tissue destruction. Progressive ventricular dilation may occur due to obstruction of CSF flow by obliterative arachnoiditis or as the result of blood clots at the level of the aqueduct of Sylvius or the foramen of Monro. With severe hemorrhages such as periventricular hemorhhagic infarction (PVHI), blood may also be found in the periventricular white matter, with parenchymal lesions seen in 10% to 15% of VLBW infants with an increased risk of adverse neurodevelopmental outcomes (Inder et al., 2025). These parenchymal lesions are differentiated from PVL in that the circulatory disturbance is venous (versus arterial in PVL), hemorrhagic (uncommon in PVL), and asymmetric with a single large cyst (versus more symmetric findings with multiple small cysts with PVL) (Inder et al., 2025).

The neuropathologic consequences of IVH include (a) destruction of the GM and its glial precursor cells, including oligodendrocytes and late migrating GABAergic neurons; (b) infarction and necrosis of periventricular white matter; and (c) posthemorrhagic hydrocephalus (Back & Volpe, 2025; Inder et al., 2025) that alters cerebral brain development, myelination, and axonal maturation (Inder et al., 2025). Infants with IVH may also have PVL. However, PVL is usually a consequence of hypoxic-ischemic injury and thus may not be a result of the IVH (Inder et al., 2025).

**Intravascular Factors.** Intravascular hemodynamic factors play a prominent role in the pathogenesis of IVH. These factors include the distribution of blood to the periventricular region, pressure-passive cerebral blood flow, and venous hemodynamics. The stages of CNS development characteristic of preterm infants born at less than 32 to 33 weeks' gestation increase the risk of hemorrhage in the periventricular area (Blackburn, 2018).

**Periventricular Blood Flow.** The subependymal GM is a transient structure that begins to thin after 14 weeks, then increases to become the site of neuron and glia proliferation, and then involutes during the third trimester (Inder et al., 2025). This site is where neuroectodermal cells that serve as precursors for neurons (primarily before about 24 weeks' gestation) and glial cells develop. These cells subsequently migrate to their eventual locus in the cerebral cortex. Processes involved in the proliferation, differentiation, and migration of these cells result in a highly vascularized and metabolically active area. Before 32 weeks' gestation, a significant portion of the total cerebral blood flow goes to the periventricular GM, primarily to support neuroblast and glioblast mitotic activity and migration. Any factor that increases cerebral blood flow can result in overperfusion of the periventricular region. Cell proliferation and migration decline after 32 to 34 weeks' gestation; the GM becomes less prominent and receives a smaller proportion of the cerebral blood supply. After this time, a greater proportion of blood flow is to the rapidly differentiating cerebral cortex (Back & Volpe, 2025; Ballabh & de Vries, 2021; Blackburn, 2016; Inder et al., 2025).

**Cerebral Autoregulation.** The brain's blood vessels are normally protected from marked alterations in flow by autoregulatory processes. If cerebral autoregulation is intact, the arterioles constrict or dilate to maintain a constant cerebral blood flow despite fluctuations in systemic blood pressure. Hypoxia and hypoxemia in the neonate alter cerebral autoregulation. This can lead to a pressure-passive system in which cerebral blood flow varies directly with arterial pressure. Subsequent alterations in systemic blood pressure or cerebral blood flow, or both, are transmitted directly to the brain, particularly to the area receiving the greatest proportion of cerebral blood flow, that is, the fragile, thin-walled vessels of the GM in preterm infants. Thus, rapid fluctuations in systemic blood pressure or cerebral blood flow (i.e., moving from increased to decreased flow and vice versa) may increase the risk of vessel rupture (Back & Volpe, 2025; Leon et al., 2022; Inder et al., 2025). Altered hemodynamics with fluctuations in blood flow can occur with positive pressure ventilation, rapid volume expansion, hypercapnia, and possibly reduced Hct and blood glucose values. Increased systemic blood pressure and, potentially, cerebral blood flow, can also occur with caregiving events, such as handling, suctioning, and chest physical therapy (Inder et al., 2025; Leon et al., 2022).

**Venous Hemodynamics.** Increased venous pressure, arising from events such as myocardial failure or positive pressure ventilation, can also be transmitted directly to the capillaries of the GM. These events can impede cerebral venous return, leading to stasis and congestion, as well as increased venous pressure and vessel rupture. The point of vulnerability in the venous drainage system of the brain is at the level of the foramen of Monro and the caudate nucleus (the usual site of IVH). At this location, a U-shaped turn occurs in the venous drainage system where the confluence of the thalamostriate, terminal, and choroidal veins forms the internal cerebral vein, which empties into the great vein of Galen. This results in a sharp change in the direction of blood flow and predisposes to turbulent venous flow with stasis and thrombus formation and an area vulnerable to increased intravascular pressure (Inder et al., 2025). The pliable skull of the preterm infant can easily be deformed, obstructing the major venous sinuses and increasing venous pressure.

**Vascular Factors.** The capillary bed of the GM is immature and has large, irregular, thin-walled vessels, a feature that increases its vulnerability to rupture. The capillary walls thicken with increasing gestational age. The fragility of these vessels is due partly to the lack of thickness and strength of the basement membrane, limitations in pericytes that provide basement membrane support, and the lack of collagen and smooth muscle (Ballabh & de Vries, 2021; Walsh & Inder, 2022). The GM undergoes involution with the migration of the neuronal and glial cells and their derivatives. The immature capillary bed is remodeled into the definitive, mature capillary. The epithelial cells of these capillaries are dependent on oxidative metabolism and, thus, are easily injured by hypoxic events. This characteristic increases the likelihood of leakage or rupture if transmural pressure increases. Because these vessels require an adequate supply of oxygen to maintain their functional integrity, decreased cerebral blood flow can lead to hypoxic-ischemic injury. These vessels are also susceptible to ischemia because they tend to lie in the vascular border zone, or "watershed" area. Therefore, both increased and decreased cerebral blood flow can be involved in the pathogenesis of IVH (Ballabh & de Vries, 2021; Blackburn, 2018; Inder et al., 2025).

**Extravascular Factors.** The capillary bed of the highly vascularized GM is embedded in gelatinous material and is deficient in supportive mesenchymal elements, thus providing poor support for fragile blood vessels. In addition, excessive fibrinolytic activity occurs in the periventricular area. As a result, a small initial bleed may not clot off and be localized but instead may continue to enlarge and rupture into the ventricles, the cerebral parenchyma, or both (Ballabh & de Vries, 2021; Inder et al., 2025; Walsh & Inder, 2022).

**Assessment.** Perinatal events associated with fetal and neonatal hypoxia include maternal bleeding, fetal distress, perinatal hypoxic-ischemic injury, prolonged labor, maternal infection, preterm labor, and abnormal presentation. Neonatal hypoxic events, such as respiratory distress, apnea, and hypotension, further increase the risk of IVH. Events associated with impairment of venous return, increased venous pressure, or both, include assisted ventilation, high positive inspiratory pressure, prolonged duration of inspiration, continuous positive airway pressure (CPAP), and air leak. Venous pressure can also be increased by compression of the infant's skull during vaginal delivery, application of forceps, and use of constricting headbands. Rapid administration of hypertonic solutions (e.g., sodium bicarbonate and glucose), rapid volume expansion, hypernatremia, hypercarbia, caregiving interventions, and environmental stress can increase cerebral blood flow. Hypercarbia causes cerebral vasodilation, thus increasing blood flow. Hypertonic solutions given rapidly or in a large bolus alter osmotic gradients between the brain and the blood. Repeated or prolonged seizures raise blood pressure and can lead to hypoxia (Blackburn, 2018; Inder et al., 2025; Walsh & Inder, 2022).

Clinical manifestations of this disorder often are nonspecific and are not well correlated with later sonographic evidence of bleeding. Therefore, a high suspicion index and careful monitoring are important for infants at risk. The diagnosis is generally made by cranial ultrasound to determine the presence and severity of IVH and the progression of the hemorrhage, as well as to monitor later complications such as PVL, progressive ventricular dilation, and posthemorrhagic hydrocephalus (Back & Volpe, 2025; Walsh & Inder, 2022). Although CT scans and MRI can be used, cranial ultrasound is preferred because it does not involve ionizing radiation and is done at the bedside (Inder et al., 2025).

More than 90% of infants with IVH bleed within the first 72 hours after birth; less than 5% develop after 4 to 5 days. Extension of the hemorrhage may be seen during the first few days (Back & Volpe, 2025; Ballabh & de Vries, 2021). Late hemorrhages after a few days or weeks are seen primarily in preterm infants with severe, prolonged respiratory problems. A new hemorrhage or an extension of a previous one may develop in these infants. IVH may also develop before birth in some infants (Inder et al., 2025).

IVH signs and symptoms are often nonspecific and subtle. Clinical signs may include a full anterior fontanelle, changes in activity level, and decreased tone. Other clinical signs associated with IVH are impaired visual tracking, increased tone of the lower limbs, hypotonia of the neck, and brisk tendon reflexes (Back & Volpe, 2025; Inder et al., 2025).

Other than a declining Hct or failure of the Hct to increase after transfusion, laboratory evidence suggestive of IVH involves CSF findings indicative of hemorrhage: increased red blood cell levels, increased protein levels, decreased glucose levels, and xanthochromia (often a later finding and caused by increased protein). Extremely low CSF glucose levels, or hypoglycorrhachia, can be found several days to a week (usually between 5 and 15 days) after the hemorrhage in some infants.

The patterns of clinical manifestations seen in individual infants vary widely and range from silent or subtle to catastrophic. At one end of the continuum are infants with IVH who have only silent, subependymal bleeding with no or minimal clinical signs. This is the most common manifestation, which is often discovered during routine ultrasound screening. Other infants may demonstrate clinical manifestations, including alterations in consciousness or stupor, hypotonia, abnormal eye movements or positions, and altered mobility. These infants generally survive. Later developmental outcome varies, depending on the severity of the hemorrhage (Back & Volpe, 2025; Inder et al., 2025).

Catastrophic deterioration usually involves major hemorrhages rapidly evolving over several minutes or hours. **Emergency Alert: Clinical findings include stupor progressing to coma, respiratory distress progressing to apnea, generalized tonic seizures, decerebrate posturing, fixation of pupils to light, and flaccid quadriparesis.** Clinical presentation is a declining Hct value, bulging fontanelle, hypotension, bradycardia, temperature alterations, hypoglycemia, and syndrome of inappropriate antidiuretic hormone (SIADH). Infants with catastrophic hemorrhages have a high mortality rate and, if they survive, a poor prognosis for later development (Back & Volpe, 2025; Inder et al., 2025).

**Management of GMH/IVH.** Management of IVH involves prevention of hemorrhage in infants at risk, acute care of infants with current bleeding, pharmacologic therapies, and management of posthemorrhagic ventricular dilation. Routine ultrasound screening of infants at risk for IVH can identify infants with silent bleeding or bleeding associated with nonspecific, subtle symptoms. Prevention or risk reduction begins in the perinatal period, with the prevention of preterm birth, perinatal hypoxic-ischemic injury, and birth trauma. Administration of antenatal glucocorticoids to enhance fetal lung maturation is associated with a decreased incidence of IVH, perhaps due to improved cardiovascular stability (Back & Volpe, 2025; Blackburn, 2018; Inder et al., 2025).

Postbirth prevention and risk reduction must begin immediately at birth. Activities include resuscitation by a trained NICU team and interventions to prevent or reduce hypoxic or ischemic events; to prevent rapid changes in cerebral blood flow, to avoid both hypocarbia and hypercarbia fluctuations in systemic blood pressure, and hyperosmolarity; and to prevent or minimize fluctuations in ICP. By identifying these vulnerable infants, interventions can be instituted to prevent new bleeding or extensions of existing hemorrhage. Continual assessment of fetal and neonatal oxygenation and perfusion is important to recognize subtle alterations, and clinicians can intervene early to prevent cerebral hyperperfusion and stabilize cerebral blood flow and pressures. Prompt resuscitation at birth minimizes hypoxemia and hypercarbia, which can alter cerebral autoregulation. Hypertonic solutions and volume expanders are administered slowly, carefully monitoring vital signs and color. Activities that can increase ICP or cause wide swings in arterial or venous pressure are avoided or minimized when possible, especially during the first 72 hours of life. Because seizures can alter cerebral blood flow and ICP, they must be recognized promptly and treated (Back & Volpe, 2025; Inder et al., 2025; Yates et al., 2021).

Acute treatment of infants with IVH involves providing physiologic support by maintaining oxygenation, perfusion, normothermia, and normoglycemia. Physical manipulation, handling, and environmental stressors are minimized to reduce the risk of hypoxia and fluctuations in arterial blood pressure and cerebral blood flow. The infant's position is also important. The head is positioned in a neutral position in the midline or to the side, without flexing the neck. The head of the bed can be elevated slightly. The Trendelenburg position is avoided. Vital signs, blood pressure, tone, activity, and level of consciousness are monitored frequently. The care of infants with progressive ventricular dilation is discussed in the section on hydrocephalus. Developmental interventions, such as containment or swaddling during aversive procedures that includes endotracheal suctioning, may promote greater physiologic stability during these procedures and a more rapid return to baseline (Fanning & Annibale, 2019; Owens, 2005). Specific interventions are listed in Table 15.8.

IVH generally occurs in the first few days after birth, IVH prevention bundles have been developed and implemented for the first 48 to 72 hours in many units to minimize activities that increase ICP or lead to alterations in venous and arterial pressure or to hypoxemia and promote neutral head positioning (Fanning & Annibal, 2019; Lien, 2020; Razak et al., 2023; Malusky & Donze, 2011).

Pharmacologic therapies have been tried prophylactically to reduce the incidence of hemorrhage, to prevent more severe bleeding and/or neurologic damage, or both. Research findings have been inconsistent for most of these therapies (Inder et al., 2025). For example, prophylactic indomethacin has been reported to reduce the risk of IVH in some, but not all, studies (Inder et al., 2025).

Parent care involves recognition and discussion of parental concerns about their infant's immediate and long-term prognosis and teaching regarding IVH, as well as its implications and management. Parents need to be shown how to interact with and care for the infant at risk for IVH in a developmentally appropriate manner to promote opportunities for interaction while minimizing stressful events. The nurse can model this type of care for parents and provide anticipatory guidance in ways the infant's needs and care will change as the baby matures. Parents can also be involved in devising and implementing a developmental plan of care for their infant to reduce pain and environmental stressors.

**Management of Progressive Ventricular Dilation.** Because progressive posthemorrhagic ventricular dilation can develop, infants with a history of IVH are followed with serial cranial ultrasonography. Approximately 25% develop a slow, progressive ventricular dilation; 25% develop

## TABLE 15.8

### NURSING CARE TO REDUCE THE RISK OF GERMINAL MATRIX–INTRAVENTRICULAR HEMORRHAGE AND OTHER BRAIN INJURY IN PRETERM INFANTS

| Intervention | Rationale |
|---|---|
| Position the infant with the head in the midline (neutral alignment) and the head of the bed slightly elevated. | ICP is lower with the head in the midline and the head of the bed elevated 30°. |
| | Turning the head sharply to the side causes obstruction of the ipsilateral jugular vein and can increase ICP. |
| Avoid tight, encircling phototherapy masks. | Pressure on the occiput can increase ICP by impeding venous drainage. |
| Avoid rapid fluid infusions for volume expansion and rapid infusion of hypertonic solutions such as glucose.<br>(a) Know the normal BP for the infant's weight and age.<br>(b) If the infant is not hypovolemic, suggest dopamine therapy to maintain BP. | Rapid increases in intravascular volume can rupture the capillaries in the germinal matrix, and this risk may be even greater with a history of hypoxia and hypotension. Even modest, abrupt increases in BP may cause IVH. |
| Monitor BP diligently. Inform physician with a fluctuating pattern in the arterial pressure tracing. | The blood flow velocity in the anterior cerebral artery is reflected by the pattern of the simultaneously recorded arterial BP. |
| Monitor BP diligently. Inform physician with a fluctuating pattern in the arterial pressure tracing. | The blood flow velocity in the anterior cerebral artery is reflected by the pattern of the simultaneously recorded arterial BP. |
| Monitor closely for signs of pneumothorax, including:<br>(a) Increase in mean BP, especially increases in diastolic BP (early)<br>(b) Tachycardia (early)<br>(c) Hypotension and bradycardia (late)<br>(d) Changes in breath sounds<br>(e) Diminished arterial oxygen pressure ($PaO_2$)<br>(f) Increased arterial carbon dioxide pressure ($PaCO_2$)<br>(g) Shift in cardiac point of maximum impulse | Pneumothorax may precede IVH. The sum of hemodynamic changes caused by pneumothorax is flow under increased pressure in the germinal matrix capillaries. Changes in vital signs can be early indicators of pneumothorax. |
| Maintain temperature in neutral thermal range. | Hypothermia has been associated with IVH. |
| Suction only as needed. | Even brief suctioning episodes (20 seconds) can increase cerebral blood flow velocity, BP, and ICP and reduce oxygenation. |
| Avoid interventions that cause crying.<br>(a) Consider long-term methods of achieving venous access to avoid frequent venipuncture.<br>(b) Critically evaluate all manipulations and handling.<br>(c) Use analgesics for stressful procedures. | Crying can impede venous return and increase cerebral blood volume. |
| Reduce pain and stress.<br>(a) Regularly assess and monitor of pain.<br>(b) Minimize numbers of painful procedures.<br>(c) Implement pharmacologic and nonpharmacologic pain reduction therapies.<br>(d) Monitor the NICU physical and caregiving environment and reduce stressors. | Pain and stress may alter neurodevelopment and impair cortical and white matter development. Exposure to repeated pain may alter pain circuitry and responsivity. |

(*continued*)

**TABLE 15.8**

**NURSING CARE TO REDUCE THE RISK OF GERMINAL MATRIX–INTRAVENTRICULAR HEMORRHAGE AND OTHER BRAIN INJURY IN PRETERM INFANTS (*continued*)**

| Intervention | Rationale |
|---|---|
| Maintain blood gas values within a normal range.<br>(a) Use continuous noninvasive monitoring of oxygenation.<br>(b) Adjust the fractional concentration of oxygen in inspired gas ($F_IO_2$) as needed to maintain the transcutaneous oxygen pressure ($TcPO_2$) or pulse oximeter values within desired range.<br>(c) Avoid interventions that cause hypoxia. | Hypoxia and excessive hypercapnia are associated with the development of IVH. These events increase cerebral blood flow and may impair the neonate's already limited ability to autoregulate the cerebral blood flow. Hypoxia can injure the germinal matrix capillary endothelium. |

BP, blood pressure; ICP, intracranial pressure; IVH, intraventricular hemorrhage; NICU, neonatal intensive care unit.

*Sources:* Adapted from Bissinger, R. L., Annibale, D. J., & Fanning, B. A. (2019). *Golden hours: Care of the very low birth weight infant.* The National Certification Company; Owens, R. (2005). Intraventricular hemorrhage in the premature neonate. *Neonatal Network, 24*(3), 55–71. https://doi.org/10.1891/0730-0832.24.3.55.

a nonprogressive dilation; 50% do not develop ventricular dilation (Inder et al., 2025). Posthemorrhagic hydrocephalus develops after birth at varying times after the initial insult, usually in the first 4 to 8 weeks, and affects about 50% of those with grade 3 or 4 IVH (Back & Volpe, 2025; Chari et al., 2021). Head size can increase without increases in ICP (normopressive hydrocephalus) because of the neonate's soft, malleable skull and open sutures and fontanelle. A tense fontanelle may be noted when the infant is upright, while the fontanelle is typically soft. Progressive ventricular dilation initially may cause compression and damage to the cortex without causing any change in head size, which may be apparent only on ultrasound. Signs of increased ICP (e.g., bulging anterior fontanelle, setting-sun sign, dilated scalp veins, and widely separated sutures) tend to be later findings. In most infants, ventricular dilation occurs slowly, without increased ICP. Ventricular growth spontaneously arrests in approximately 65% (Inder et al., 2025). The remaining infants continue to demonstrate ventricular dilation and increased ICP.

The initial treatment for normopressive hydrocephalus may be observation because, in many infants, ventricular growth arrests spontaneously without therapy. Progressive ventricular dilation with increasing ICP is managed with a ventriculoperitoneal shunt or, if the infant is too ill or too small for surgery, with temporary ventricular drainage (Back & Volpe, 2025). A ventriculoperitoneal shunt is the shunt of choice in infants and children because this type is easy to insert, revise, and uncoil as the infant grows. One end of a radiopaque catheter is placed in the lateral ventricle, usually on the right side, and the other end is placed in the peritoneal cavity. The catheter contains a one-way valve that is palpable on the side of the head near the ear. The shunt may need multiple revisions during childhood for growth and malfunctioning. Significant complications of ventriculoperitoneal shunts are infection and obstruction. Too-rapid drainage of CSF immediately after insertion of the shunt can lead to herniation of the brain or subdural hematoma.

**Quality and Safety: After surgery, the infant is positioned on the side opposite the shunt, with the head of the bed flat or slightly elevated (15°–30°) to prevent rapid loss of CSF and decompression.** The position can be rotated to supine every few hours to prevent skin breakdown. The skin should be kept clean and dry. Once the site has healed, infants may be placed on a donut on the affected side. Pressure to the shunt valve should be applied only if ordered by the surgeons. Infants with a shunt are observed for signs of localized or systemic infection, ileus, signs of peritonitis, and shunt obstruction. Obstruction of the shunt leads to accumulation of CSF, enlargement of the head, and signs of increased ICP. Infection of the shunt may appear as localized redness or drainage around the incision, temperature instability, altered activity, or poor feeding. Fluid status, intake, and output are monitored, and the infant is observed for signs of dehydration from too-rapid loss of CSF. Signs of too-rapid decompression include a sunken fontanelle, agitation or restlessness, increased urine output, and electrolyte abnormalities (Joseph et al., 2017).

Parent teaching before discharge includes the infant and shunt care, especially positioning and skin care. Parents must be comfortable in handling and caring for their infant before discharge. They should know the signs of shunt malfunction, increased ICP, infection, and dehydration. Continuing follow-up care of the infant and parental support are important. Parents may be referred to parent groups for peer support.

**Outcomes.** The severity and extent of the hemorrhage and the presence of associated problems (e.g., RDS, perinatal hypoxic-ischemic injury, and sepsis) influence mortality and morbidity. Infants with a history of IVH are also at risk for developing posthemorrhagic ventricular dilation, which may be normopressive or associated with increased ICP. Infants with small or mild hemorrhages survive and generally have a good outcome, with a low incidence of major neurologic sequelae and posthemorrhagic ventricular dilation. However, these infants may have a higher risk of neurodevelopmental issues than infants without IVH (Back & Volpe, 2025; Chari et al., 2021). Mortality and the risk of progressive ventricular dilation are increased in infants with moderate hemorrhages and still higher in infants with severe hemorrhages, especially infants with <750 g birth weight (Inder et al., 2025; Zhou et al., 2024). Although infants with severe hemorrhages tend to have significant motor and cognitive deficits, some seem to escape substantial long-term sequelae. The incidence of neurologic sequelae ranges from 15% to 25% in infants with moderate hemorrhage to 50% with grade III hemorrhage and 75% with PVHI (Inder et al., 2025; Zhou et al., 2024). Sequelae include cerebral palsy, developmental delay, sensory and attention problems, learning disorders, and hydrocephalus (Walsh et al., 2017; Zhou et al., 2024).

## White Matter Injury in Preterm Infants

WMI and its associated neuronal and axonal alterations is the most common severe neurologic insult seen in preterm infants (Inder & Volpe, 2025). White matter hypoxic-ischemic injury involves both cystic and noncystic focal necrotic lesions as well as diffuse WMI with damage to the premyelinating oligodendrocytes, astrogliosis, and microglial infiltration (Back & Volpe, 2025; Inder & Volpe, 2025). This injury is referred to as PVL. Leukomalacia relates to changes in the brain's white matter that are reflective of softening. Focal cystic necrotic lesions are seen in less than 5% of infants between 24 to 32 weeks' gestation; the more common diffuse noncystic lesions associated with disturbances in myelination are seen on MRI in about one-third of infants between 24 to 32 weeks' gestation, accounting for 25% of survivors (Miller & Back, 2025; Pierson & Volpe, 2025). WMI is often associated with IVH, but it is a separate lesion that may also occur without IVH. IVH may contribute to developing PVL via the increased formation of free radicals (Ballabh & de Vries, 2021; Inder et al., 2025). PVL is a symmetric, nonhemorrhagic, usually bilateral lesion caused by ischemia from alterations in the arterial circulation. The time of onset is variable; however, the time of peak vulnerability is prior to 32 weeks' gestation.

WMI is often accompanied by secondary alterations in the brain characterized by axonal and neuronal alteration that may include damage to the thalamus, basal ganglia, cerebral cortex, subplate neurons, and cerebellum, which together are referred to as the *encephalopathy of prematurity* ( Miller & Back, 2025; Inder & Volpe, 2025; Pierson & Volpe, 2025). Encephalopathy of prematurity is characterized as multifaceted gray and white matter lesions in the preterm brain that reflect acquired and developmental factors in combination (Inder & Volpe, 2025). This results in decreased volume of the cerebral cortex, cerebral white matter, alterations in the basal ganglia and thalamus, and altered thalamic and gyral development (Inder & Volpe, 2025). Risk factors include any event during the prenatal, intrapartum, or postbirth periods that result in cerebral ischemia; this includes asphyxia, IVH, hypoxia, hypercarbia, hypotension, cardiac arrest, and infection (in which the action of endotoxins diminishes blood flow) (Miller & Back, 2025).

**Pathophysiology.** PVL begins with ischemic necrosis of the white matter dorsal and lateral to the external angles of the lateral ventricles, especially in the border zone area, but may extend into the cortical white matter. The border zone is the area farthest from the original source of the cerebral blood supply and, thus, is most susceptible to ischemic damage from diminished cerebral blood flow (Back & Volpe, 2025). Pathologic changes begin with patchy areas of focal ischemic coagulation that may occur as early as 5 to 8 hours after the initial hypoxic-ischemic insult. This is followed within a few days by proliferation of macrophages and astrocytes, along with endothelial and glial infiltration. Later changes include thinning of the white matter and liquefaction in the central portion of the necrotic area, cavitation, cystic changes, and decreased myelination (Back & Volpe, 2025; Miller & Back, 2025).

Pathogenesis of WMI involves the interaction of three maturation-dependent factors: (a) immature vascular supply to the white matter that reduces oxygen delivery to vulnerable areas of the brain; (b) impairments in cerebral autoregulation, leading to pressure-passive cerebral circulation; and (c) vulnerabilities of the premyelinating oligodendrocytes to damage from reactive oxygen and nitrogen species (free radicals), glutamate, adenosine, and cytokines (Back & Volpe, 2025; Cheng & Ballah, 2021). Damage to the premyelin-producing oligodendrocytes leads to release of cytokines (indicating an inflammatory process), glutamate, and free radicals. Oligodendrocyte development and survival are impaired, leading to hypomyelination with subsequent motor, cognitive, and behavioral neurodevelopmental problems. Axonal damage and disruption also occur. Perinatal infection and an inflammatory response with the release of proinflammatory cytokines are also thought to play a prominent role in the pathogenesis of PVL, with potentially potentiating effects of hypoxia and inflammation (Back & Volpe, 2025; Cheng & Ballah, 2021).

**Assessment.** WMI is multifactorial and arises from a compilation of prenatal or postnatal insults or both. Risk factors include factors leading to hypoxia-ischemia (fetal metabolic acidosis, RDS, cardiac insufficiency from a large patent ductus arteriosus, sepsis, and congenital heart disease) and hypotension and inflammation (intrauterine infection, necrotizing enterocolitis, and neonatal sepsis (Miller & Back, 2025; Pierson & Volpe, 2025; Sevensky et al., 2021). Often, no clinical findings are specific to WMI or PVL during the first weeks of life unless the damage is severe. Cranial ultrasonography can identify infants at risk for, or who have, early signs of WMI. However, ultrasound is not as sensitive in diagnosing PVL as it is with IVH. MRI can identify changes early and is especially useful with noncystic and diffuse WMI and neurodevelopmental prognosis (Inder & Volpe, 2025; Lodygensky et al., 2024; Pierson & Volpe, 2025). Infants at risk for WMI should undergo serial cranial ultrasound examinations, again at discharge and with later follow-up. MRI may benefit ongoing follow-up, especially for infants with severe damage with the increased association of neuromotor abnormalities and developing ventricular enlargement (Ballabh & de Vries, 2021; Inder & Volpe, 2025; Lodygensky et al., 2024). As the infant matures, neurologic and motor deficits become apparent.

**Management.** Prevention strategies include prevention of preterm birth, use of antenatal glucocorticoids, and prompt stabilization and resuscitation at birth to maintain adequate ventilation, perfusion, and oxygenation (Lien, 2020; Pierson & Volpe, 2025). Initial management focuses on recognizing and treating the primary insult and its attendant complications and preventing further hypoxic-ischemic damage and inflammation (Blackburn, 2018; Ballah & de Vries, 2023). This involves preventing or minimizing hypotension, hypoxia, acidosis, and severe apneic and bradycardic episodes (Pierson & Volpe, 2025). Head ultrasound (HUS) and MRI are used serially to diagnose WMI/PVL and follow its progression in at-risk infants. Later management involves care related to residual problems, such as spastic diplegia and hydrocephalus. Nursing interventions focus on acute management of the primary problem and supportive care for the infant and parents. Nurses have a significant role in identifying signs of hypoxia and ischemia and instituting interventions to prevent further ischemic damage. These interventions are like those described earlier and in Table 15.8. Environmental stressors may increase the risk for the development of IVH and subsequent PVL or may cause associated developmental problems. Developmental and environmental interventions, therefore, are important aspects of nursing care.

Parents need initial and continuing support in dealing with their infant's illness and the risk of later neurologic problems. Parent teaching focuses on promoting an understanding of the infant's health status and care and providing anticipatory guidance and follow-up care. The parents should be shown how to interact with and care for their infant in a developmentally appropriate manner to foster parent–infant interaction and promote infant organization and development. The nurse can model this type of care for the parents, collaborate with parents in identifying stressors and soothing strategies, and provide anticipatory guidance as the infant's needs and care change.

**Outcomes.** Infants with WMI usually survive. Those who die in the neonatal period usually do so from the original hypoxic, hemorrhagic, or infectious insult rather than from WMI/PVL per se. Infants with WMI are at higher risk for later developmental problems, including cognitive deficits, language impairment, attentional dysfunction, cerebral visual impairment, and autism (Cheng & Ballah, 2021; Pierson & Volpe, 2025; Zhou et al., 2024). These infants are also at risk for spastic diplegia, especially those with multifocal cystic lesions around the lateral ventricles. In infants with spastic diplegia, descending fibers from the motor cortex cross the affected area around the ventricles. Because the leg motor fibers are closest to the ventricles, spastic diplegia of the leg is the most common sequela. With the extension of the damage, arm involvement with spastic quadriplegia may occur. Infants with diffuse WMI are more likely to develop visual, cognitive, and neurobehavioral impairments (Sevensky et al., 2021).

## Cerebellar Injury in Preterm Infants

The cerebellum is one of the later structures to mature, with critical developmental events occurring at the end of the second and beginning of the third trimester, accompanied by a rapid growth spurt from 24 weeks through the third trimester and birth (Limperopoulos et al., 2025). The cerebellum is important for the development of cognitive, learning, language, behavior, and motor function; it functions as a node in the distribution of neural networks with interconnections with the thalamus and parietal and prefrontal cortex; it integrates sensory information; and it is vital in socialization skills. Because the cerebellum undergoes rapid growth, complexity, and critical developmental processes during the time preterm infants are in the NICU, especially those who are VLBW, they are at risk for cerebellar injury. These injuries may alter motor and language development and cognitive, socioemotional, and behavioral function and increase the risk of attentional and autism spectrum disorders (Limperopoulos et al., 2025).

Mechanisms proposed for the alterations seen in the cerebellum in VLBW infants include: (a) direct injury (usually due to cerebral hemorrhage) leading to atrophy and reduced growth of the cerebellum; (b) indirect cerebellar injury or underdevelopment associated with cerebral injury; and (c) impaired cerebellar development, without evidence of direct or indirect injury, due to unknown causes (Blackburn, 2018). Cerebellar underdevelopment and hemorrhage are seen primarily in infants born at less than 28 weeks. These infants may have bilateral, usually symmetric, decrease in cerebellar volume. The exact etiology of cerebellar hemorrhage in preterm infants includes factors similar to that of GMH/IVH, including pressure-passive cerebral blood flow, increased venous pressure, fragility of the cerebellar germinal matrix blood vessels, and vasoocclusive injuries (Blackburn, 2018; Limperopoulos et al., 2025). Cerebellar injury may occur concurrently with PVL or IVH.

# BIRTH INJURIES

Traumatic injury to the CNS or PNS can occur during the perinatal or postnatal period. Most of these injuries happen during the intrapartum period and may occur with perinatal hypoxic-ischemic events. Perinatal events most frequently associated with birth injury include midforceps delivery; shoulder dystocia; low forceps delivery; birth weight exceeding 3,500 g; and a second stage of labor lasting longer than 60 minutes. The incidence of injury has declined markedly in recent years due to improvements in obstetrical care and increased use of cesarean sections for abnormal presentations. Birth injuries can also arise from trauma during a cesarean section or resuscitation. Compression or pressure injuries from an unusual fetal position usually cause injuries that occur before the intrapartum period. The risk of injury to the CNS or PNS is greater with malpresentation (especially breech), prolonged or precipitate labor, prematurity, multiple gestation, shoulder dystocia, macrosomia, and instrumental delivery. The most prevalent types of injury to the nervous system are extracranial hemorrhage, intracranial hemorrhage, skull fractures, spinal cord injury, and peripheral nerve injury (Hoppe & Bosse, 2024; Volpe & El-Dib, 2025b).

## Extracranial Hemorrhage

Caput succedaneum and cephalohematoma are the most common types of birth injury and the most benign. Caput succedaneum is characterized by soft, pitting, superficial edema several millimeters thick and overlies the presenting part in a vertex delivery. This edematous area lies above the periosteum and thus crosses suture lines. The edema consists of serum, blood, or both. Infants with caput succedaneum may also have ecchymosis, petechiae, or purpura over the presenting part. Caput succedaneum occurs in infants after a spontaneous vertex delivery or after the use of a vacuum extractor. This type of extracranial hemorrhage requires no care other than parent teaching regarding its cause and significance. It resolves within a few days after birth with no sequelae. Cephalohematoma occurs in 1.5% to 2.5% of newborns (Hoppe & Bosse, 2024; Volpe & El-Dib, 2025). It involves subperiosteal bleeding, usually over the parietal bone but possibly over other cranial bones. Cephalohematoma usually is unilateral but can be bilateral. This type of hemorrhage is seen most often in males, after the use of forceps; after a prolonged, difficult delivery; and in infants born to primiparas. The characteristic finding is a firm, fluctuant mass that does not cross the suture lines. The mass often enlarges slightly by 2 to 3 days of age. Approximately 5% of infants with unilateral and 18% with bilateral cephalohematomas have a linear skull fracture underlying the mass (Hoppe & Bosse, 2025; Volpe & El-Dib, 2025). In rare cases, an infant may have a subdural or SAH.

Caput succedaneum and cephalohematoma over the occipital bone must be differentiated from encephalocele. In contrast to extracranial hemorrhage, an encephalocele is characterized by pulsations, increased pressure (tenseness) with crying, and the appearance of a bony defect in radiographic studies (Fanning, 2025; Volpe & El-Dib, 2025). Infants with a cephalohematoma generally have no symptoms. Management includes parent teaching and monitoring for the development of hyperbilirubinemia. Occasionally, an infant with a large cephalohematoma becomes anemic. These infants should also be monitored for symptoms of intracranial hemorrhage or skull fracture. Generally, cephalohematomas resolve between 2 weeks and 6 months of age, and most resolve by 8 weeks. Calcium deposits occasionally develop, and the swelling may remain for the first year (Karlson, 2024).

**Subgaleal Hemorrhage.** Subgaleal, or subaponeurotic, hemorrhage is the most serious form of extracranial hemorrhage in newborns (Dumpa & Kamity, 2023; Hoppe & Bosse, 2025; Volpe & El-Dib, 2025). Subgaleal hemorrhage occurs in 4 per 10,000 spontaneous vaginal deliveries and 59 per 10,000 vacuum-assisted deliveries. The incidence is also increased with precipitous deliveries, macrosomia, and severe dystocia and with failed vacuum deliveries requiring forceps. Use of soft silastic cups (rather than the rigid hard cup) with vacuum extractors is associated with fewer scalp injuries, although the soft cups are more likely to fail (Volpe & El-Dib, 2025; Hoppe & Bosse, 2024). Mortality is 17% to 25%; however, if the infant survives the hemorrhage and does not develop HIE, the hemorrhage usually resolves in 2 to 3 weeks and outcomes are good (Hoppe & Bosse, 2024; Inder & Volpe, 2025; Volpe & El-Dib, 2025).

Traction or application of intense shearing forces to the scalp pulls the aponeurosis from the vault and ruptures large emissary veins. Blood collects in a large potential space between the galea aponeurotica and the periosteum of the skull through which the large emissary veins pass (Karlson, 2024; Volpe & El-Dib, 2025). The area is called a *potential space* because it is not present until blood separates the galea aponeurotica from the periosteum of the skull. This space can quickly expand to accommodate 260 to 280 ml of blood. Total newborn blood volume is 80 to 100 ml/kg, so this volume may be more than the entire blood volume of some newborns (Karlson, 2024; Volpe & El-Dib, 2025).

Subgaleal hemorrhage is a clinical emergency. These infants usually present at birth or within a few hours after birth (Dumpa & Kamity, 2023; Hoppe & Bosse, 2025; Volpe & El-Dib, 2025). Clinical findings include a firm, ballotable head mass that crosses sutures and fontanelles (often extending from the orbital ridge around the ears to the neck) and increases in size after birth. Each centimeter of enlargement is estimated to be equivalent to 40 ml of blood loss (Hoppe & Bosse, 2025; Volpe & El-Dib, 2025). The mass mimics edema and shifts with head repositioning. Infants usually show signs of pain on manipulation of the scalp or head. Infants may present with a rapidly falling Hct, anemia, hypovolemia, pallor, hypotension, tachycardia, tachypnea, hypotonia, and other signs of shock (Hoppe & Bosse, 2025; Karlson, 2024; Volpe & El-Dib, 2025). Management includes rapid recognition, cardiovascular and respiratory monitoring, administration of blood and volume expanders, and control of bleeding (Hoppe & Bosse, 2025; Volpe & El-Dib, 2025).

## Other Types of Intracranial Hemorrhage

In addition to IVH, several other clinically important types of intracranial bleeding can occur in the neonate, including primary SAH, subdural hemorrhage (SDH), and intracerebellar hemorrhage. These types of hemorrhage arise from trauma or hypoxia during the perinatal period.

**Primary SAH.** Primary SAH is the most prevalent form of intracranial hemorrhage in neonates and the least clinically significant for most infants. SAH occurs in both preterm and term infants but is more common in preterm infants. SAH may occur alone (primary SAH) or as a secondary event with other forms of intracranial hemorrhage. For example, with IVH, blood moves into the subarachnoid space via the fourth ventricle (Inder et al., 2025; Pierson & Volpe, 2025).

**Pathophysiology.** Primary SAH consists of bleeding into the subarachnoid space that is not secondary to subdural or intraventricular bleeding. In neonates, the source of the bleeding is venous blood; in older children and adults, SAH usually involves arterial blood. With primary SAH, blood leaks from the leptomeningeal plexus, bridging veins, or ruptured vessels in the subarachnoid space (Inder et al., 2025). This type of hemorrhage is associated with trauma or asphyxia. Trauma that causes increased intravascular pressure and capillary rupture is the underlying causal event in most term infants with SAH. In preterm infants, SAH usually is the result of asphyxial events. Factors that place an infant at risk for SAH include birth trauma, prolonged labor, difficult delivery, fetal distress, and perinatal hypoxic-ischemic events (Inder et al., 2025; Pierson & Volpe, 2025).

**Assessment.** Three clinical presentations have been described for infants with SAH (Inder et al., 2025). The most common is a preterm infant with a minor SAH. These infants are asymptomatic. The hemorrhage is discovered accidentally, for example, during a lumbar puncture, as part of a sepsis workup. With the second type of clinical presentation, term or preterm infants may show isolated seizure activity at 2 to 3 days of age, or preterm infants occasionally may present with apnea. Between seizures, the infant appears and acts healthy ("well baby with seizures"). Infants in both of these groups survive and usually do well developmentally. The third type of clinical presentation involves infants with a massive SAH that has a rapid and fatal course. This presentation is rare and is often associated with both a severe asphyxial event and birth trauma. Blood in the CSF on lumbar puncture indicates the possibility of SAH, but true hemorrhage must be distinguished from a bloody tap. MRI and CT also can help confirm the diagnosis; ultrasonography is unreliable with SAH (Inder et al., 2025).

**Management.** Management of these infants begins with efforts to prevent or reduce the risk of trauma and hypoxia during the perinatal period to reduce the risk of development of SAH. Infants with SAH are observed for seizures and other neurologic signs during the early neonatal period. Nursing care is primarily supportive and includes maintaining oxygenation and perfusion and providing warmth, fluids, and nutrients. Nursing management involves helping the parents to understand the basis for, and cause and prognosis of, SAH, as well as the care of their infant.

**Outcomes.** Generally, infants with SAH survive, and asymptomatic infants do well. Up to half of symptomatic infants with severe, sustained traumatic or hypoxic injury with further damage to the CNS have neurologic sequelae (Inder et al., 2025; Limperopoulos et al., 2025). Hydrocephalus occasionally develops in infants with a history of SAH due to obstruction of CSF flow by adhesions. These infants should undergo repeat ultrasonographic examinations to monitor ventricular dilation.

**Subdural Hemorrhage.** SDH is a common hemorrhage seen in newborns; however, recognition of this hemorrhage is important because an immediate intervention for large SDH can be lifesaving (Dumpa & Kamity, 2023; Inder et al., 2025). The incidence of SDH has declined markedly due to improvements in obstetrical care. This decrease has been particularly notable in term infants (Inder et al., 2025). Risk factors include precipitous, prolonged, or difficult delivery, use of midforceps or high forceps, prematurity, cephalopelvic disproportion, and macrosomia. SDH is seen more often in infants born to primiparas, possibly because of the more rigid birth canal. Infants with abnormal presentations (e.g., breech, foot, brow, or face) are also at higher risk for SDH (Dumpa & Kamity, 2023; Hoppe & Bosse, 2024; Inder et al., 2025; Pierson & Volpe, 2025).

**Pathophysiology.** SDH in newborns is almost always caused by trauma during the perinatal period. Unilateral or bilateral bleeding occurs between the dura and the arachnoid. The bleeding occurs over the cerebral hemispheres or posterior fossa with or without lacerations of the tentorium or falx cerebri (see Figure 15.1). The cerebral hemispheres are the most common site for SDH. Bleeding usually occurs over the temporal convexity, with rupture of superficial cerebral veins or of "bridging" veins between the superomedial aspect of the cerebrum and the superior sagittal sinus. Because the superficial veins over the cerebrum are poorly developed in the preterm infant, this type of hemorrhage is seen less often in these infants. Bleeding over the posterior fossa involves bleeding below the tentorium and compression of the brainstem. Dural tears at the junction of the falx and tentorium near the attachment of the great vein of Galen are also associated with compression of the brainstem and midbrain (Inder et al., 2025; Pierson & Volpe, 2025).

**Assessment.** SDH must be distinguished from other types of intracranial hemorrhage and neurologic problems. This differentiation often can be accomplished by evaluating the infant's history and presentation and, if the infant is having seizure activity, by ruling out other causes. SDH over the cerebral hemispheres is often associated with SAH. SDH also occurs with extracranial hemorrhages, such as cephalohematoma and subgaleal, subconjunctival, and retinal hemorrhages; skull fractures; and brachial plexus or facial palsies. MRI or CT can assist in confirming the diagnosis; CT appears to be the imaging modality of choice (Dumpa & Kamity, 2023; Inder et al., 2025; Pierson & Volpe, 2025).

Clinical signs of SDH relate to the bleeding site and the hemorrhage's severity. Three patterns are seen in infants with bleeding over the cerebral hemispheres (Inder et al., 2025). The first pattern is seen in most neonates with SDH; these infants have a minor hemorrhage and are asymptomatic or have signs such as irritability and hyperalertness. With the second pattern, primarily focal seizures develop during the first 2 to 3 days of life. Other neurologic signs that may be seen include unequal hemiparesis, unequal pupils that respond sluggishly to light, full or tense fontanelle, bradycardia, and irregular respirations. The third pattern is seen in a few infants with no or nonspecific signs in the neonatal period but in whom signs appear at 4 weeks to 6 months. These infants generally show poor feeding, failure to thrive, altered level of consciousness, increasing head size as a result of continued hematoma formation, and, occasionally, seizures caused by chronic subdural effusion. Infants with abnormal neurologic signs from birth often have bleeding over the posterior fossa with tentorial lacerations. Signs include stupor or coma, eye deviation, asymmetric pupil size, altered pupillary response to light, tachypnea, bradycardia, and opisthotonos. As the clot enlarges, these infants rapidly deteriorate, with signs of shock appearing over minutes to hours. The infant becomes comatose and has fixed, dilated pupils and altered respirations and heart rate, which culminate in respiratory arrest. Infants with small tears in the posterior fossa may have no clinical manifestations for the first 3 to 4 days of life. The clot gradually enlarges during this time until signs of increased ICP appear. As the brainstem becomes compressed, the infant's condition deteriorates, and oculomotor abnormalities, altered respiration, bradycardia, and seizures occur (Inder et al., 2025).

**Management.** Infants with a history of perinatal trauma or other risk factors are observed for seizures and other neurologic signs. Care is primarily supportive and includes maintaining oxygenation and perfusion and providing warmth, fluids, and nutrients. Nursing management also involves helping the parents to understand the basis for and the cause and prognosis of this type of hemorrhage, as well as the care of their infant.

Symptomatic infants with bleeding over the temporal convexity and increased ICP may require surgical evacuation if the infant's condition cannot be stabilized neurologically. Massive posterior fossa hemorrhage requires craniotomy and surgical aspiration of the clot (Inder et al., 2025). Infants at risk for SDH should be monitored carefully over the first 4 to 6 months after birth for late signs of bleeding and hematoma formation. Monitoring these infants includes observing their head size, growth, feeding, activity, and level of consciousness, as well as monitoring for seizure activity.

**Outcomes.** The prognosis varies with the location and severity of the hemorrhage. Infants with asymptomatic bleeding over the cerebral hemispheres do well, as do most infants with transient seizures in the neonatal period if no associated cerebral injury is present. Early diagnosis with CT or MRI has improved the outcome for infants with posterior fossa hemorrhage. Most infants with bleeding over the tentorium or falx cerebri die; severe hydrocephalus and neurologic sequelae usually develop in those who survive (Inder et al., 2025).

**Intracerebellar Hemorrhage.** Intracerebellar hemorrhage is rare and is thought to be multifactorial, with primary importance of birth trauma (breech or forceps delivery) and circulatory events. These hemorrhages occur in both term and preterm infants but are more common in preterm infants. Intracerebellar hemorrhage is seen during autopsy in infants with a history of perinatal hypoxic-ischemic events or severe RDS (or both) and IVH (Dumpa & Kamity, 2023; Inder et al., 2025).

Two presentations have been described. Many infants are critically ill from birth, with rapidly progressive apnea, a declining Hct value, and death within 24 to 36 hours. Other infants are less ill initially, and symptoms develop up to 2 to 3 weeks of age. Clinical manifestations include apnea, bradycardia, hoarse or high-pitched cry, eye deviations, opisthotonos, seizures, vomiting, hypotonia, and diminished or absent Moro reflex. Hydrocephalus often develops in these infants as early as the end of the first week after birth. The prognosis is poor in survivors, especially those born prematurely or with severe hemorrhage (Cain et al., 2020; Inder et al., 2025).

**Perinatal Stroke.** Ischemic strokes are more common in the perinatal period than at any other time of life. They are the leading cause of hemiplegic cerebral palsy, yet until recently, have been poorly understood and oftentimes not diagnosed in the neonatal period. Perinatal arterial ischemic stroke occurs in between 1 in 1,100 and 1 in 4,000 term births. Cerebral sinovenous thrombosis with or without infarction occurs in 2.6 to 12/100,000 term births. Hemorrhagic stroke occurs less frequently than ischemic strokes 1 in 63,000 births. Approximately 80% of neonatal strokes are ischemic, and 20% are cerebral sinovenous thrombosis (CSVT) or hemorrhage (Cain et al., 2020; Rivkin et al., 2025; Steggerda & de Vries, 2021). Evidence suggests that preterm infants are just as likely, if not more likely, than term infants to experience perinatal ischemic stroke. Stroke affects about 1 in 140 preterm births up to and including 34 weeks' gestation. Perinatal arterial ischemic strokes (AISs) account for 80% of diagnosed strokes in the neonatal period; the remaining 20% result from CSVT (Cain, 2020; Rivkin et al., 2025).

Perinatal stroke was defined in 2006 by the National Institute of Child Health and Human Development and the National Institute of Neurological Disorders as the result of a focal disruption of cerebral blood flow secondary to arterial or venous thrombosis or embolism occurring between 20 weeks' gestation and 28 postnatal days (Rivkin et al., 2025). Perinatal strokes are further classified as fetal or neonatal. Fetal stroke is defined as having occurred between 20 weeks' gestation and the onset of labor or cesarean section, and neonatal stroke as having occurred between the onset of labor and actual delivery. Presumed perinatal ischemic strokes are those identified by neuroimaging in infants greater than 28 days as having had a focal infarction at some point between 20 weeks' gestation and postnatal day 28 (Cain et al., 2020; Rivkin et al., 2025).

Risk factors for perinatal stroke seem to be multifactorial and are still being identified to determine which factors are associated with a predilection for or direct causation of stroke. Risk factors being studied can be grouped into maternal, pregnancy/labor-related, and fetal or neonatal conditions (Cain et al., 2020; Rivkin et al., 2025; Steggerda & de Fries, 2021). Maternal risk factors include thrombophilias (factor V Leiden, factor VIII, protein S deficiency, protein C deficiency, prothrombin mutation, and antiphospholipid antibodies), preexisting conditions such as thyroid disease, diabetes mellitus, or gestational diabetes or history of infertility. Pregnancy/labor-related risk factors implicated in perinatal stroke include significant maternal trauma, primiparity, placental abnormalities, oligohydramnios, decreased fetal movement, prolonged rupture of membranes, chorioamnionitis, prolonged second stage of labor, or assisted delivery (vacuum or forceps). Fetal or neonatal risk factors include fetal distress during labor, cord abnormalities (tight nuchal or body cord, true cord knot), thrombophilias (same as maternal), congenital cardiac defects, and corrective surgery (Cain et al., 2020; Rivkin et al., 2025; Steggerda & de Vries, 2021). In addition, there may be a gender effect on the incidence of stroke, with male gender being a risk factor over female gender (Rivkin et al., 2025).

The timing of the initial insult determines the clinical signs and symptoms of perinatal stroke. Seizures occur in 85% to 92% of affected newborns and are often the earliest manifestation of a perinatal stroke in an otherwise healthy-appearing newborn. Most seizures happen within the first 72 hours of life; approximately 50% are focal motor, 33% are generalized motor, and 17% are subtle (Rivkin et al., 2025). Physical examination may reveal a bulging and/or pulsatile fontanelle, dilated head and neck veins, papilledema, asymmetric movements or primitive reflexes, or seizurelike activity. Transient hemiparesis or generalized tone anomalies, such as hypotonia, are seen in the early newborn phase. Other symptoms of stroke are hypotonia and apnea, which are generic symptoms of any aberration in the newborn period, necessitating differential diagnosis from hypoxic, metabolic, and infectious disorders. Infants not diagnosed during the newborn stage are typically identified at a median of 6 months when the asymmetry of reach and grasp is noted. Seizures occurring after 28 days and language delays have also been reported (Rivkin et al., 2025; Steggerda & de Vries, 2021).

Diagnostic workup includes a thorough history, newborn assessment, laboratory tests, and cardiac and neurologic imaging. An echocardiogram and electrocardiogram may be used to assess for cardiac dysfunction or rhythm disorders.

EEG and neuroimaging are indicated to evaluate for perinatal stroke (Rivkin et al., 2025; Steggerda & de Vries, 2021). During the past decade, rapid advances in using good-quality early cranial ultrasonography and MRI with diffusion-weighted sequences have facilitated improved and rapid diagnosis in the neonatal period, allowing for earlier identification, treatment, and support of the affected newborn. Treatment of perinatal stroke is supportive and is directed at minimizing secondary brain injury and optimizing outcomes. Blood glucose, temperature, ventilation, oxygenation, blood volume, and pressure should be normalized. Hyperthermia and hyperthermic environment should be avoided. Seizures are documented and treated aggressively (Rivkin et al., 2025; Steggerda & de Vries, 2021).

The outcome for infants with perinatal stroke varies with the area of the original insult. It is estimated that 20% to 70% of hemiplegic cerebral palsy cases are associated with perinatal stroke, with the spasticity more marked in the upper extremities. Intelligence is within normal parameters for two-thirds of affected infants (Cain et al., 2020).

## Skull Fracture

Skull fractures are uncommon in the neonate; however, when they do occur, they consist of two types: linear and depressed (Choi et al., 2023; Hoppe & Bosse, 2025; Schroeder et al., 2024). Skull fractures occur in utero, during labor, with forceps delivery, or during prolonged, difficult labor with compression and battering of the fetal skull against the maternal ischial spines, sacral promontory, or symphysis pubis (Choi et al., 2023; Hoppe & Bosse, 2025; Schroeder et al., 2024). The fetal skull can often tolerate mechanical stressors relatively well because it is flexible, malleable, poorly ossified, and less mineralized than the adult skull. Depressed fractures occur after forceps delivery but occasionally are seen after vaginal or cesarean birth. Compression of the skull causes buckling of the inner table without a break in the continuity of the skull. Linear fractures usually occur over the frontal or parietal bones. These fractures are often associated with extracranial hemorrhage, may underlie a cephalohematoma, and are generally asymptomatic. Skull radiographs are required to diagnose (Choi et al., 2023; Hoppe & Bosse, 2025; Schroeder et al., 2024; Volpe & El-Dib, 2025). Intracranial hemorrhage rarely complicates linear fractures.

A depressed skull fracture is a visible, palpable depression or dent in the skull, usually over the parietal area. These fractures are often described as resembling a ping-pong ball because the depression does not involve any loss of bone continuity. Unless underlying cerebral contusion or hemorrhage is present, no other signs or symptoms are seen (Choi et al., 2023; Schroeder et al., 2024; Volpe & El-Dib, 2025).

In some infants with a depressed fracture, the fracture elevates spontaneously within the first week. Most clinicians recommend manually elevating an uncomplicated depressed fracture that does not elevate spontaneously within a few days. After this time, manual elevation is more difficult or impossible. Surgical intervention is usually necessary if manual elevation fails, if the fracture is more severe and bone fragments are in the cerebrum, if neurologic deficits exist, or if ICP is increased.

Linear fractures heal spontaneously with no sequelae unless underlying cerebral damage or a growing fracture is present. Basal fractures are associated with high mortality and poor developmental outcomes. Infants with depressed fractures that are small or treated early (or both) have a good prognosis. Infants with large fractures, especially if treatment is delayed, have a greater risk of sequelae. Unless a depressed fracture has lacerated the dura (a rare occurrence), neurologic deficits in these infants are usually caused by cerebral injury from the original trauma, a hypoxic event, or both, rather than by the fracture (Choi et al., 2023; Volpe & El-Dib, 2025). Infants with skull fractures should undergo regular evaluation of growth and development during infancy and early childhood.

Nursing assessment includes monitoring infants identified with skull fractures for signs of neurologic dysfunction, intracranial hemorrhage, meningitis, and seizures, although these findings are rare. Parents usually are concerned about their infant's appearance (with a depressed fracture) and the possibility of brain damage. They need support and teaching. Infants with uncomplicated linear fractures require no special management. Follow-up monitoring is usually recommended so that a growing fracture and development of a leptomeningeal cyst can be ruled out (Schroeder et al., 2024; Volpe & El-Dib, 2025). Infants with basal fractures are treated for shock and hemorrhage.

## Spinal Cord Injury

Spinal cord injuries are uncommon and usually occur in the midcervical to lower cervical and upper thoracic areas. Injury can occur at any point along the cord. Spinal cord injuries are caused by excessive traction, rotation, and torsion of the vertebral column and neck. Injury usually does not result from compression but rather from stretching of the spinal cord, which is less flexible than the bony vertebral column. Damage to the spinal cord ranges from complete transection to laceration, edema, hemorrhage, and hematoma formation. Hemorrhage into the lining of the arteries may result in thrombosis, infarction, and ischemic cord damage. Risk factors are breech delivery (major factor), dystocia, macrosomia, and cephalopelvic disproportion (Habek, 2021; Volpe & El-Dib, 2025, 2018b).

Infants with partial spinal cord injury have subtle neurologic signs and variable degrees of spasticity. Infants with high cervical or brainstem injuries are stillborn or die shortly after birth from respiratory depression, shock, and hypothermia. Infants with midcervical or upper cervical injury may be stillborn, born with marked respiratory depression, or have respiratory depression, with the neurologic injury going unrecognized until flaccidity, immobility of the legs, urine retention, or all three are noted. If born alive, these infants usually die within the first week, after the development of progressive central respiratory depression that is often complicated by pneumonia. Other findings in this group of infants include relaxation of the abdominal wall, absent sensation in the lower half of the body, absent deep tendon and spontaneous reflexes, brachial plexus injury, and constipation. This group also includes infants with injuries at the C8 to T1 level who usually survive and may have transient paraplegic paralysis at birth. Infants with mild injury may recover most or all their function. Infants with moderate-to-severe damage are paraplegic or quadriplegic and have permanent neurologic damage (Volpe & El-Dib, 2025).

Initially, clinical manifestations are those of spinal cord shock, with hypotonia, weakness, flaccid extremities, sensory deficits, relaxed abdominal muscles, diaphragmatic breathing, Horner syndrome (ipsilateral ptosis, anhidrosis, and miosis), and a distended bladder. Infants with low cervical lesions have shallow, paradoxical respirations; these infants do not sweat. The skin over the affected area is dry and warm. Pinprick and deep tendon reflexes are absent. Areflexia may be noted over the upper and lower extremities in some infants. The degree of neurologic insult often cannot be accurately evaluated until the infant has recovered from the initial period of spinal shock and any edema or hemorrhage has been reabsorbed (Volpe & El-Dib, 2025). After several weeks or months, paraplegic autonomic hyperreflexia develops and is characterized by periodic mass reflex response. This results in tonic spasms of extremities, spontaneous micturition, and profuse sweating over the paralyzed area (Volpe, 2018a).

Initial management focuses on stabilization, treatment of associated problems (e.g., asphyxia, hemorrhage, shock), and management of respiratory depression. Infants with midcervical to upper cervical or brainstem lesions require assisted ventilation. Parents are in shock initially and need time to grieve. They need continuing support and teaching regarding infant care. Ongoing management of these requires a multidisciplinary team that includes disciplines of nursing, medicine, neurology, neurosurgery, physical therapy, orthopedics, urology, social work, and psychology. Ultrasonography, CT, or MRI may be performed to determine the level and extent of injury (Volpe & El-Dib, 2025).

Skin integrity over the paralyzed area must be maintained to prevent pressure areas and skin breakdown. Thermoregulation may be a problem because evaporative loss through the skin is reduced over the affected body parts in the initial period of the recovery process. The infant is positioned and repositioned regularly to promote normal alignment of body parts and prevent the development of contractures and decubiti. The affected areas should be kept clean and dry and massaged with gentle, passive ROM exercises. These infants need meticulous bowel and bladder care to prevent UTIs and skin excoriation. Glycerin suppositories at regular intervals can help normalize bowel function. Infants are also monitored for signs of respiratory infection and pneumonia. Parental teaching before discharge focuses on normal baby care issues and concerns, as well as the special needs of a paralyzed infant.

The prognosis depends on the injury's level and severity, but it is generally poor. Higher lesions (cervical/upper thoracic) are associated with a high mortality rate, and lower lesions (lower thoracic and lumbosacral) may result in significant morbidity with bladder and bowel dysfunction (Dumpa & Kamity, 2023). Many infants with spinal cord injury are stillborn or die shortly after birth, particularly those with midcervical to high cervical or brainstem injuries. Those who survive have varying degrees of residual paralysis, respiratory problems, and bowel and bladder dysfunction, depending on the level of the injury. Most surviving infants have a spastic quadriplegia. Infants with intercostal muscles and diaphragm involvement are often ventilator dependent (Volpe & El-Dib, 2025).

## Peripheral Nerve Injuries

Peripheral nerve injuries result from stretching, compression, twisting, hyperextension, or separation of nerve tissue (Dunbar et al., 2021; Leblebicioglu & Pondaag, 2024; Volpe & El-Dib, 2025). Injury can occur before, during, or after birth. Damage can range from nerve swelling to complete peripheral degeneration (with later total recovery) to complete division of all structures. More common sites affected are the brachial plexus and the facial, phrenic, radial, median, and sciatic nerves. This injury is seen predominantly in term or LGA infants (Dunbar et al., 2021; Volpe & El-Dib, 2025).

Injury to the radial nerve usually results from compression of the nerve caused by a fracture of the humerus during a breech delivery or by intrauterine compression of the arm. The infant has a wrist drop with a normal grasp reflex. Recovery usually occurs over the first few weeks to months. Median and sciatic nerve injuries are typically postnatal iatrogenic events. Median nerve injury can be a complication of brachial or radial arterial punctures. These infants have diminished pincer grasp and thumb strength and a flexed fourth finger. Recovery is variable. Sciatic nerve injuries are often permanent. They arise from trauma from a misplaced intramuscular injection or ischemia from an injection of hypertonic solutions into the gluteal muscle. Infants with this injury have diminished abduction and distal joint movement. Hip adduction, rotation, and flexion are unaffected (Dunbar et al., 2021; Leblebicioglu & Pondaag, 2024; Volpe & El-Dib, 2025).

**Facial Nerve Palsy.** Facial nerve palsy has an incidence of 10 per 1,000 live births (Dumpa & Kamity, 2023). The facial nerve of the newborn is superficial after it emerges from the stylomastoid foramen. As a result, the nerve is vulnerable to compression injury at this site or as it traverses the ramus of the mandible. The temporofacial and cervicofacial nerve branches are most often involved. The injury is most common on the left. Injury to the peripheral nerve is caused by trauma from oblique application of forceps, prolonged pressure on the nerve during labor from the prominent maternal sacral promontory, or pressure from an abnormal fetal posture. Although some investigators have not found any differences in incidence between forceps and spontaneous vaginal deliveries, others have noted a correlation between the type of forceps and the incidence of injury. A favorable prognosis indicates that the injury involves hemorrhage or edema within the nerve sheath rather than actual disruption of the nerve fibers. (Volpe & El-Dib, 2025).

Facial nerve paralysis must be distinguished from asymmetric crying facies and nuclear agenesis. Asymmetric crying facies result from the absence of the depressor muscle at the angle of the mouth. These infants close their eyes normally when crying, but their mouths do not move down and out. They suck without dribbling. This disorder is generally benign. Nuclear agenesis (Möbius syndrome) is a more significant disorder characterized by congenital paralysis of the facial muscles (Volpe & El-Dib, 2025).

Clinical manifestations vary, depending on whether the injury is to the central nerve, the peripheral nerve, or the peripheral nerve branch. The complete peripheral nerve injury results in a unilateral inability to close the eye or open the mouth. The lower lip on the affected side does not depress during crying, nor does the forehead wrinkle. The affected side appears full and smooth, with obliteration of the nasolabial fold. These infants dribble milk while feeding. The infant may be unable to close the eye on the affected side. Central injury usually results in a spastic paralysis of the lower portion of the face contralateral to the side of CNS injury without involvement of the eyes or forehead. Peripheral nerve branch injury results in varying degrees of paralysis of the forehead, eye, or lower face, depending on the branch involved. The paralysis is apparent at birth or within 1 to 2 days after birth.

Nursing management involves parent counseling and teaching and prevention of complications. The eye on the affected side is patched, and 1% methylcellulose eye drops are instilled every 3 to 4 hours to prevent corneal damage. Dribbling with sucking can be a transient problem. A neurosurgical consultation is recommended if no improvement is noted by 7 to 10 days or if further loss of function occurs. With partial degeneration, physical therapy, massage, or electrical stimulation may be used, although efficacy of these therapies is controversial and not well documented. Electromyography, nerve excitability, or nerve conduction latency examinations may evaluate the extent of the damage (Leblebicioglu & Pondaag, 2024).

Almost all infants recover entirely. Improvement usually is apparent by 1 to 4 weeks, and complete recovery occurs after several months in most infants. Infants with severe nerve regeneration have a longer recovery period and may occasionally require later cosmetic surgery (Volpe & El-Dib, 2025).

**Brachial Plexus Injury.** Brachial plexus palsy involves injury of the C5 to T1 nerve roots and is seen almost exclusively in term infants. The incidence ranges from 0.5% to 2%, or approximately 2.5 per 1,000 live births. (Dumpa & Kamity, 2023; Volpe & El-Dib, 2025). Injury to the brachial plexus results from excessive lateral flexion, rotation, or traction on the neck. The degree of injury varies, ranging from edema and hemorrhage of the nerve sheath to avulsion of the nerve root from the spinal cord. With mild-to-moderate injury the axons are shattered, but the nerve sheaths remain intact. This degree of intactness of the nerve sheaths promotes regeneration of the nerve by 3 to 4 months, with full recovery by 3 to 15 months in most infants. Severe injuries result in radicular rupture or intraspinal tearing of the nerve and division of the nerve into radicles. If radicular rupture occurs, the root loses contact with the spinal cord. These injuries do not recover spontaneously (Dunbar et al., 2021; Leblebicioglu & Pondaag, 2024; Volpe & El-Dib, 2025).

Brachial plexus injuries usually are unilateral and on the left side. Fracture of the clavicle may occur in conjunction with this type of injury. Brachial plexus injury can be seen in uncomplicated deliveries and after cesarean birth; however, this injury is usually associated with vaginal delivery of LGA infants, shoulder dystocia, breech presentations, and prolonged labor or difficult delivery. Spontaneous injuries may occur from compression of the shoulder as the shoulder passes over the sacral prominence (Dunbar et al., 2021; Leblebicioglu & Pondaag, 2024; Volpe & El-Dib, 2025).

Clinical manifestations vary with the location and severity of the injury. Signs of injury usually are apparent from birth but may be delayed for several days to a few weeks in some infants. The major types of injury are Erb (Erb–Duchenne) palsy, an injury of the upper plexus involving C5 to C7, and Klumpke palsy or lower plexus injury at C5 to T1 C8-T1 (Dumpa & Kamity, 2023; Tappero, 2025; Volpe & El-Dib, 2025). With Erb palsy, the shoulder and upper arm are involved, and denervation of the deltoid, supraspinous, biceps, and brachioradialis muscles occurs. The arm lies passively at the infant's side, abducted and internally rotated, and the forearm is pronated. The wrist and fingers are flexed. This posture is referred to as the "waiter's tip" position. The Moro reflex is absent, and the biceps and radial reflexes are diminished or absent on the affected side; the grasp reflex is normal.

Klumpke palsy is seen primarily in breech infants whose arm has been hyperabducted and delivered with the head affecting the flexors of the wrist and hand. Cervical sympathetic fibers may also be affected; sweating and sensation are absent in the affected hand and arm. The infant holds the affected arm at the side of the thorax with the hand in a claw hand posture. The Moro and grasp reflexes are absent, and the triceps reflex is diminished or absent on the affected side; biceps and radial reflexes are present. If the T1 root is affected, the infant manifests Horner syndrome (Tappero, 2025; Volpe, 2025).

Erb–Klumpke (total) palsy is characterized by entire arm and hand involvement as a result of injury to the nerve roots of the brachial plexus from C5 to T1. Complete paralysis of the upper and lower arm and hand, flaccidity, and accompanying sensory, trophic, and circulatory changes are noted. Deep tendon and Moro reflexes are absent. If the C4 roots are also affected, an associated phrenic nerve (diaphragmatic) paralysis occurs. Involvement of the T1 root leads to Horner syndrome in about one-third of these infants (Dunbar et al., 2021; Leblebicioglu & Pondaag, 2024; Volpe, 2025).

Initial management focuses on protecting the arm until localized edema and pain subside. MRI or CT is used to visualize the degree of injury. The affected arm should not be splinted or immobilized because it has not proven beneficial to prevent contractures and further stretching of the plexus, as had previously been thought. After edema subsides, at about 7 to 10 days, physical therapy gradually is instituted as the infant can tolerate it. Gentle passive ROM exercises have been shown to minimize formation of contractures and to reduce permanent disability. These infants have continued physical therapy consisting of massage and exercise over the first months until total or partial recovery occurs (Volpe, 2018a). Infants with a brachial plexus injury should be evaluated for associated problems, including fractures and respiratory difficulty secondary to phrenic nerve paralysis. If improvement is not noted within the first few months, electromyography and nerve conduction studies are performed to determine the extent of the damage, to follow recovery, and to determine whether surgical intervention is needed (Volpe, 2025). Infants with brachial plexus injuries often experience considerable pain during movement of the affected arm in the first few weeks after birth. Nursing management is directed at reducing passive and active movement of the arm and providing comfort measures to reduce pain. The paralyzed arm is supported in a position of relaxation. Parent teaching regarding positioning, prevention of contractures, and exercise is essential.

Prognosis depends on the level and severity of the injury. Approximately 65% to 95% of infants have full recovery with supportive care. Many infants recover by 3 to 4 months of age and more than 90% of infants recover by 2 to 3 years of age. Erb palsy, the most common type of injury, has the best prognosis for full recovery. Infants with total paralysis are most likely to have residual paralysis. Residual functional deficits include alteration in abduction and external rotation of the shoulder; restricted movement of the elbow, forearm, and hand; and hand weakness. These functional impairments can lead to abnormal muscle development and arm growth (Dunbar et al., 2021; Leblebicioglu & Pondaag, 2024; Volpe & El-Dib, 2025).

**Phrenic Nerve Palsy.** Phrenic nerve palsy is caused by injury of the cervical nerve roots at C3 to C5. The injury results from tearing of the nerve sheath, which is accompanied by edema and hemorrhage. Phrenic nerve palsy may occur as an isolated event or in association with brachial nerve palsy. Risk factors, especially breech delivery, are like those for brachial plexus injury. Paralysis of the diaphragm is a result of damage to the phrenic nerve. The injury usually is unilateral and on the right side. Because the diaphragm is paralyzed, infants with phrenic nerve injury have dry tachypnea, asymmetric chest motion, and diminished breath sounds. This phenomenon must be differentiated from CNS, cardiac, and pulmonary problems (Dumpa & Kamity, 2023; Dunbar et al., 2021; Leblebicioglu & Pondaag, 2024; Volpe & El-Dib, 2025).

Infants with mild-to-moderate phrenic nerve injury may have early respiratory difficulty, suggestive of hypoventilation that stabilizes or improves. The infant may have recurrent episodes of cyanosis and dyspnea. Respiratory efforts result in primarily thoracic movement with minimal or no abdominal excursions, opposite of the normal newborn breathing pattern. Infants with complete avulsion or bilateral injury have severe respiratory distress from birth, with tachypnea, apnea, and a weak cry (Volpe & El-Dib, 2025).

Management focuses on promoting ventilation and oxygenation. Infants are not enterally fed initially until respiratory status improves. Infants with severe distress require positive pressure ventilation or continuous positive airway pressure for support until recovery occurs. Surgical plication of the diaphragm is performed if no improvement is noted or if the infant is still ventilator dependent at 4 to 6 weeks of age (Dunbar et al., 2021; Leblebicioglu & Pondaag, 2024; Volpe & El-Dib, 2025).

The infant is positioned on the affected side. If the infant cannot be fed, adequate fluid and calories must be provided. Feeding is instituted gradually, most likely by gavage tube initially. When oral feeding is started, feed slowly and give ample opportunity for rest and monitoring of respiratory status. Because recovery takes several months, parents must be taught feeding, positioning, and comfort techniques. The developmental needs of infants requiring prolonged hospitalization must be met; sensory input and play activities appropriate to their maturity and health status must be provided. Most infants recover by 6 to 12 months of age. Other infants recover clinically but have residual abnormalities of diaphragmatic movement on radiography (Dunbar et al., 2021; Leblebicioglu & Pondaag, 2024; Volpe & El-Dib, 2025).

## SUMMARY

Infants with neurologic dysfunction present a significant challenge to the neonatal nurse. The neurologic conditions may range from life-threatening conditions, such as perinatal hypoxic-ischemic injury and intracranial hemorrhage, to those with transient problems, such as an isolated seizure, and those with chronic issues, such as NTDs. To optimally care for these infants and their families, nurses must understand the basis for, and the implications of, specific types of neurologic dysfunction; they must recognize the clinical manifestations of these types of dysfunctions and respond appropriately in collaboration with other healthcare professionals.

Nursing care of infants who have or are at risk for neurologic dysfunction involves assessing and monitoring the infant's neurologic status and responses to the extrauterine environment, as well as subtle signs that may indicate a change in status. Nursing management of the infant involves activities to address alterations in the level of consciousness, the potential for injury related to trauma or infection, impairment of skin integrity, alterations in comfort, impaired mobility, alterations in thermoregulation, alterations in nutrition and fluid and electrolyte status, and promotion of neurobehavioral organization and development. Nurses must also deal with their responses and those of the families of infants who may die during the neonatal or early infancy periods or whose short-term and long-term outcomes may be altered by the extent of neurologic insult. The nurse must also assess family coping, interactive processes, knowledge, and grieving to assist the family in coping with the birth of an ill infant and, for many families, with the uncertainty or certainty of long-term neurologic deficits in their infant.

## CASE STUDY 1

■ **Identification of the Problem.** Term female infant vaginal delivery with vacuum assist; presented with apnea, no tone, requiring resuscitation intervention.

■ **Assessment: History and Physical Examination.** The term female infant was delivered vaginally to a 24-year-old G2 P1 woman following prolonged labor at term after an uncomplicated pregnancy. The vaginal delivery was assisted with a vacuum apparatus. Gestational age was term with a birth weight of 3.3 kg.

Upon delivery, the infant was limp, cyanotic/pale, and apneic. The infant was successfully resuscitated following the Neonatal Resuscitation Program (NRP) guidelines; the infant required 2 minutes of positive pressure ventilation by T-piece resuscitator to initiate effective ventilation when spontaneous respirations were noted; the infant received 10 minutes of CPAP via the T-piece resuscitator; heart rate was greater than 100 beats/min by 1 minute of age. Pulse oximetry was initiated at 1 minute of age, reading 44% oxygen saturation initially and gradually improved to 85% by 5 minutes of life; room air was used throughout resuscitation.

The infant remained pale with thready pulses and poor peripheral perfusion at 10 minutes of life; spontaneous respiratory rate 40 to 60 seconds with easy respiratory effort without CPAP; pulse oximetry saturations 88% to 94%; heart rate 160 seconds. The infant was brought to the NICU for ongoing care.

Apgar scores were $4^1$, $6^5$, $8^{10}$.

## Physical Examination on Admission to the NICU

GENERAL: pale with thready pulses, poor peripheral perfusion; heart rate 180 beats/min. Respiratory rate 46, shallow; saturations 88% to 92% in room air

HEAD, EARS, EYES, NOSE, AND THROAT (HEENT): increasingly boggy, enlarging scalp hematoma; eyes open, no blink; pupils reactive to light; positive red reflex and normal facies

RESPIRATORY (RESP): lung fields bilaterally clear and equal to bases; gasping respiratory effort

CARDIOVASCULAR (CV): rate regular with no murmur noted; poor peripheral perfusion, capillary blood refill time greater than 5 seconds and thready pulses were noted

ABDOMEN (ABD): abdomen soft and nontender with no hepatosplenomegaly or masses palpable; three-vessel cord; the anus appeared patent

GENITOURINARY (GU): normal female infant genitalia

NEUROLOGIC (NEURO): decreased responses, with eyes open and unblinking; extremities were well formed; muscle tone was markedly decreased

SKIN: pale with general cyanotic undertones, pronounced circumoral and acrocyanosis

EXTREMITIES: well-formed; 10 digits per extremity; generalized cool and mottled

## Differential Diagnosis

- Subgaleal hemorrhage
- Perinatal hypoxic-ischemic injury
- Shock
- Disseminated intravascular coagulation (DIC)
- Intracranial hemorrhage
- Sepsis screen
- Congenital cardiac defects screen

## Diagnostic Tests

*Laboratory Tests:*

- CBC/differential: WBC 10.3, segmented cells 44; bands 1; Hct 21%, platelet count 168,000/mm$^3$
- Coagulation (DIC) panel: prothrombin time (PT) greater than 100 seconds, partial thromboplastin time (PTT) greater than 100 seconds, fibrinogen 54 mg/dl, and D-dimers 2 to 4 mg/ml
- Blood, tracheal, and surface cultures for bacterial and/or viral infections: all negative

*Imaging Tests:*

- Head CT scan (performed within 4 hours of age): extensive blood within the extracranial soft tissues, mild IVH and SAH
- Transcranial Doppler and nuclear medicine flow scan (performed at 24 hours of age): no cerebral blood flow
- EEG (performed on day of life 3): absence of cortical activity

## Working Diagnosis

- Extensive subgaleal hemorrhage with hematoma
- Based on clinical, laboratory, and imaging findings, data from history and physical assessment

## Development of Management Plan

- Continuous monitoring of arterial blood pressure, vital signs, and neurologic status, every 2 to 4 hours Hct, platelet count, PT/PTT, and fibrinogen
- Maintenance fluid support; fluid boluses to support intravascular volume
- Ensure adequate blood volume, clotting factors: colloids (fresh frozen plasma with cryoprecipitate, whole blood, packed red blood cells, platelets) as needed to treat DIC, anemia
- Respiratory support with mechanical ventilation as needed
- Vasopressors to maintain adequate blood pressure and cerebral blood flow
- Antibiotics until cultures negative for 72 hours

## Implementation

- Implementation of management plan: (immediately after initial assessment in the NICU)
- Umbilical arterial and venous catheters were placed, and 10 ml/kg normal saline was given for volume expansion
- Dopamine 10 mcg/kg/minute initiated by 1 hour of life; was initiated because of low blood pressure and ongoing poor perfusion; weaned to 5 mcg/kg/minute by 36 hours
- Labs were drawn via the umbilical arterial catheter: arterial blood gas, CBC/differential, and DIC panel, transfusion panel (type and cross for transfusion)
- The scalp hematoma noted to be rapidly enlarging during this time
- The infant immediately intubated and given an emergency blood transfusion of 15 ml/kg
- Multiple blood transfusions, fresh frozen plasma with cryoprecipitate, whole blood and packed red blood cell transfusions, and normal saline boluses given to normalize the coagulation studies by 24 hours of age, with a total of 476 ml neonatal red blood cells, 8 U of cryoprecipitate, and 140 ml of fresh frozen plasma

## Evaluation of Effectiveness

- Respiratory status stable by 2 hours of life
- Blood pressures were normalized by 2 hours of life
- Metabolic acidosis and coagulation panel results were normalized within the first 24 hours of life
- Severe brain involvement was suspected on day of life 2, with dismal results of the Doppler and flow scan and flat EEG results

**Outcome.** Brain death was determined on day of life 3. Life support was terminated on day of life 4. The autopsy was remarkable for an extensive subgaleal hematoma and moderate SAH and SDH.

## CASE STUDY 2

**Identification of the Problem.** A 6-day-old former term infant turned blue at home on day of life 4 and was admitted to the local hospital.

**Assessment: History and Physical Examination.** A 6-day-old former-term neonate was delivered vaginally following an uncomplicated pregnancy with a birth weight of 2,990 g. Prenatal laboratory results were remarkable for positive group B streptococcus (GBS) vaginal culture, for which the mother received prophylactic perinatal antibiotics. The infant did well after delivery, breastfed vigorously, and was discharged home with the mother on day 2 of life. At the time of admission, the infant's weight was 2,950 g, occipitofrontal circumference was 33 cm, and length was 49.5 cm.

After initial admission to the local hospital, the infant was screened for sepsis (normal CBC and differential, negative cultures for viral and bacterial sepsis). On day 2, at the local hospital, the infant had a seizure consisting of lip-smacking, apnea, cyanosis, and bicycling of lower extremities; was given 10 mg/kg phenobarbital; and was taken to CT, which showed a right IVH. The infant was transferred to the NICU of the tertiary care hospital.

### Physical Examination

GENERAL: vital signs within normal limits; somewhat sleepy and irritable with handling

HEENT: anterior fontanelle large and soft, with sutures split to just above eyebrows, lateral sutures proximate; pupils equal and reactive to light; bilateral positive red reflex; sunset eyes when crying; nares patent bilaterally; palate and clavicles intact

LUNGS: clear and bilaterally equal; easy work of breathing with spontaneous respirations

CV: heart regular rhythm and rate, no murmur; peripheral pulses 2+ in all extremities, good peripheral perfusion; capillary blood refill time ~3 seconds

ABD: abdomen was soft and nontender; liver right costal margin; no hepatosplenomegaly or masses palpable; umbilical stump dry

GU: normal male genitalia; testes bilaterally descended; well-developed scrotum

NEURO: arched with handling, moved all extremities with increased tone; occasional tongue thrust; positive sunset eyes, positive gag reflex, positive blink response; no clonus

EXTREMITIES: well-formed with good muscle mass, 10 digits/extremity

SKIN: pale pink; good turgor and healing areas from previous lab draws and intravenous access attempts; no petechiae or rashes were noted

SOCIAL: maternal history is significant, for a cousin died of "fits" at 3 months of age; other relatives experienced frequent bone fractures or sundown eye signs; father is reportedly short-statured with short-statured children

### Differential Diagnosis

- Seizures of unknown etiology
- Rule out herpes simplex infection and other viral or bacterial meningitis
- Rule out brain structure abnormalities
- Rule out nonaccidental trauma (NAT)
- Rule out intracranial and IVH
- Hypoventilation of unknown etiology

### Diagnostic Tests

*Laboratory Tests:*

- CBC/differential: WBC 10.6, segmented cells 27, bands 0, Hct 60.2%, platelet count 254,000/mm$^3$
- Electrolytes: sodium 132, potassium 4.7, chloride 96, bicarbonate 29, calcium 11.9, ionized calcium 1.42, phosphorus 2.9, alkaline phosphorus less than 5, ammonia 45, lactate 2.2, BUN less than 1, and serum glutamic-oxaloacetic transaminase 33
- Blood and central spinal fluid bacterial and viral cultures: negative
- Urine drug screen: negative

*Imaging Tests:*

- Serial EEGs: excessive background discontinuity and prominent high-amplitude spikes and polyspikes, but no seizures; repeat EEG (hospital day 7) significantly improved but still mildly abnormal due to focal moderate amplitude, midline vertex, and negative spikes without seizure activity
- MRI of the brain: hemorrhage located either in subependymal location or cavum velum interpositum not consistent with shear injury
- Head CT: placement of the hemorrhage in the right thalamic area with extension into the lateral ventricles and stable ventricle size

*Consults (pediatric specialists):*

- NAT team: ophthalmic examination: normal without ocular hemorrhages; skeletal radiographic study no fractures; evidence of metaphyseal fraying in the lower extremities consistent with developing rickets
- Neurology, metabolic, and endocrine services

### Working Diagnosis

- Six-day-old infant with seizures due to probable congenital hypophosphatasia
- Possible endocrine disease
- Possible sepsis
- Possible metabolic disease

### Development of Management Plan

- Monitor the infant.
- Provide respiratory support as needed.
- Laboratory results effectively ruled out sepsis, meningitis, electrolyte imbalances, and metabolic disease as etiologies for seizure activity.
- The extremely low-alkaline phosphorus, low phosphorus, and high calcium and ionized calcium levels were indicators for endocrine disease.

- EEG was moderately abnormal due to excessive background discontinuity and prominent high-amplitude spikes and polyspikes, but no seizures and improved by hospital day 7.
- Imaging results ruled out NAT and other structural causes for the clinical presentation of seizurelike activity.
- Skeletal radiographic study gave further support for endocrine disease due to the early radiographic indication for rickets.
- NAT team concluded that the seizures were not caused by brain injury due to NAT.
- Neurology service concluded that the etiology of the seizures was not structural or related to brain injury but most likely due to pyridoxine deficiency or some endocrine or metabolic syndrome.
- Endocrinologists considered the seizures to be related to hypophosphatasia.
- Provide fluid, and nutritional support with a low-calcium formula.
- Initiate vitamin D supplements to delay bone decalcification and rickets.
- Provide teaching and support for the parents.
- Arrange follow-up with the primary care provider and the pediatric neurology, orthopedic, and endocrinology services.

### Implementation

- During the examination phase, pyridoxine was given for a seizurelike event on hospital day 2 that included bicycling, sneezing, and clonic–tonic movements with paroxysmal respiratory pattern.
- Maintenance pyridoxine was given until hospital day 10, when it was determined the seizures were caused by hypophosphatemia.
- The infant was nothing by mouth (NPO) with peripheral IV fluids until a special low-calcium formula could be delivered, and vitamin D supplements were started to delay bone decalcification and rickets.

### Evaluation of Effectiveness

- At the time of discharge, the infant was taking good amounts of the formula by nipple and gaining weight slowly.
- The mother was learning what little there is to know about this rare congenital disease and learning to prevent fractures as much as possible.
- Follow-up care was arranged with the primary pediatrician, neurology, orthopedics, and endocrinology.

### Outcome

- The prognosis for symptomatic congenital hypophosphatasia is poor, with death usually occurring within the first year of life. Parents initially denied being told about the infant's condition at first follow-up visit with the primary pediatrician; however, the parent was feeding the infant the correct formula and following all discharge instructions.

## CASE STUDY 3

**Identification of the Problem.** A term infant male was limp and not breathing after home-birth delivery.

**Assessment: History and Physical Examination.** The infant boy was born at 40 6/7 weeks by vaginal delivery to a 24-year-old, G1 P0 > 1 woman at home with a certified nurse midwife present. Prenatal laboratory results and history were unremarkable with negative GBS status. The pregnancy was uncomplicated. Membranes were spontaneously ruptured with clear fluid approximately 11 hours prior to delivery, and no maternal fever was documented; the mother received antibiotics about 4 hours prior to delivery. Active pushing in second stage was 4 hours, followed by shoulder dystocia after the infant's head was delivered. The infant was limp and apneic after delivery. The certified nurse midwife performed mask-delivered positive pressure ventilation with room air with improvement in respiratory effort. Apgar scores were $1^1$, $2^5$, $4^{10}$, $5^{15}$ per the nurse midwife report.

The infant was emergently brought to the NICU.

Admission weight: 3,765 g, head circumference: 37 cm, and length: 54 cm.

HEENT: anterior fontanelle was soft, flat, sutures opposed, proximate with a right cephalohematoma; eyes equal and reactive to light with a positive red reflex; nares bilaterally patent; palate and clavicles intact

RESP: breath sounds coarse bilaterally, slightly decreased over the lower right lung field.; increased work of breathing with increased subcostal and substernal retractions, slight tracheal tug, and flared nares

CV: mildly tachycardic, no murmur; peripheral pulses 1+ in all extremities; poor peripheral perfusion and capillary blood refill time of greater than 4 seconds; low-borderline cuff blood pressure

ABD: abdomen soft and nontender; no hepatosplenomegaly or masses palpable; three-vessel cord

NEURO: responsive and alert on admission

EXTREMITIES: well-formed; slightly decreased muscle tone

SKIN: pale pink and slightly mottled, with acrocyanosis and circumoral cyanosis

**Differential Diagnosis.** The differential diagnoses for an infant following a difficult delivery with positive pressure ventilation include:

- Respiratory distress versus transient tachypnea of the newborn
- Rule out pneumothorax
- Rule out HIE
- Rule out intracranial hemorrhage
- Sepsis screen
- Shock
- Rule out seizures
- Congenital cardiac defects
- Metabolic and/or endocrine defects

## Diagnostic Tests

*Laboratory Tests:*

- CBC with differential: WBC 11.7, segmented cells 33, bands 2; Hct: 56; platelets: 156,000/mm$^3$
- Blood cultures for bacterial and viral growth: negative
- Electrolytes, lactic acid, and ammonia levels, amino acid assays and urine organic acids, and liver function tests: normal

*Imaging Tests:*

- Chest radiography: small right pneumothorax
- Head CT (24 hours of life): no evidence of hydrocephalus, ischemia, or intracranial hemorrhage
- Serial EEGs (48 hours of life): moderately to severely abnormal EEG due to discontinuous low-amplitude background with asynchrony and frequent, subclinical, electrographic seizures from midline vertex and left central region. Second EEG: (72 hours) improvement from initial EEG with no electrographic seizures. There were positive, sharp transient waves that were of concern for underlying structural abnormalities and can be consistent with anoxic and hypoxic events as reflected with clinical presentation. Third EEG (5 days): abnormal due to predominantly right temporal sharp waves and possibly two brief electrographic seizures.
- MRI (11 days): abnormalities on T2 and diffusion-weighted imaging (DWI) consistent with perinatal HIE

*Consult:*

- Pediatric neurology: seizures due to HIE, and rhythmic extremity movement

## Working Diagnosis

- Seizures due to HIE
- Respiratory distress
- Pneumothorax

## Development of Management Plan

The management plan included:

- Monitoring
- Nasal CPAP to support respiratory effort
- Respiratory support with mechanical ventilation as needed
- Chest radiograph confirmed right pneumothorax
- Needle aspiration was performed for small amount of air
- Chest tube insertion if indicated
- Chest radiographs as needed
- Place umbilical arterial and venous catheters if needed for access
- Fluid support; initiate feeds
- Peripheral IV fluids at 80 ml/kg/day maintenance
- Fluid bolus 10 mg/kg normal saline as needed
- Monitoring for abnormal activity showed pneumothorax resolved; infant initially improved but on day 2 of life developed apnea, tonguing, lip smacking
- Lactic acid and ammonia levels, amino acid assays, and urine organic acids
- Expedite state newborn screen testing
- Sepsis screen
- Antibiotics

**Implementation.** Implementation of management plan (immediately after initial assessment in the NICU):

- Antibiotics were given for 48 hours for the sepsis screen.
- Right pneumothorax was reduced with needle aspiration and resolved without further intervention.
- Seizure activity was noted on day of life 2, confirmed with EEG, given phenobarbital 15 mg/kg, with resolution of the seizure.
- Subsequently was intubated at approximately 36 hours of life for a prolonged apnea event requiring positive pressure ventilation, then given another 15 mg/kg phenobarbital loading dose and initial lorazepam (Ativan) dose to control seizures.
- Metabolic etiology was ruled out with normal lactic acid and ammonia levels and normal amino acid assays and urine organic acids results.
- State metabolic screening results were normal.

## Evaluation of Effectiveness

- Neurologic examination deteriorated over the first 4 days, with the infant presenting with no gag, no corneal reflex, passive hypertonicity, active hypotonia, consistent and rhythmic hyperventilation, and periodic apnea, clonic–tonic movements of predominantly the left extremities by the end of day 3 of life, and persisting through day 5 of life.
- Maintenance phenobarbital was initiated on day 3 of life, and lorazepam was given periodically for seizure activity during days 4 to 5 of life. Seizures were no longer observed after day 5 of life; infant gradually improved clinically with improved passive and active tone, improved gag and positive corneal reflex.
- Extubated on day 6 of life to high-flow nasal cannula of 2 L/minute flow of room air; weaned quickly to room air without nasal cannula flow.
- Feeds of expressed mother's milk had been initiated per gavage tube on day 3 of life; infant was tolerating full volume by day 7 by gavage every 3 hours. Breastfeeding and nipple feeds were initiated on day 8, but the infant needed most of his feeds by gavage at discharge on day 18. Follow-up care was arranged for a neurology clinic and EEG 1 month after discharge.

**Outcome.** Infant was discharged with phenobarbital and gavage feeds; was breastfeeding well, gaining weight, and thriving at the neurology follow up appointment at 1 month of life.

## EVIDENCE-BASED PRACTICE

HIE is the major cause of encephalopathy in newborns. HIE is an injury to the brain caused by oxygen deficit resulting from either systemic hypoxemia or ischemia or a combination of the two conditions. The hypoxemia and ischemia may occur simultaneously or sequentially, and it appears from recent evidence that ischemia is the more important of the two oxygen deprivation states in causing the brain injury. Subsequent reperfusion of the affected brain area has been shown to be the time at which most the injury to the brain occurs. Glucose deprivation also plays a part in the severity of the brain injury. HIE causes transient organ dysfunction in 4 to 6 in 1,000 live births and results in death or significant neurologic deficits in 1 per 1,000 live births. Traditionally, the newborns affected by have been treated symptomatically of the resultant multiorgan and multisystem effects. A recent development in proactive treatment with the use of controlled hypothermia has proven to be effective for newborns with moderate-to-severe HIE (Back & Volpe, 2025).

Induced mild hypothermia is increasingly the treatment of choice for infants greater than or equal to 36 weeks' gestation with moderate-to-severe HIE in addition to establishing ventilation and adequate perfusion and preventing or minimizing hypotension, hypoxia, and acidosis; rapid alterations in cerebral blood flow and systemic blood pressure; and severe apneic and bradycardic episodes in providing supportive care. Mild hypothermia is induced using either selective head cooling or whole-body cooling. A systematic review and meta-analysis of seven randomized controlled trials including 1,214 newborns done by Tagin et al. (2012), provided evidence that hypothermia with either total-body cooling or selective head cooling improves survival and protects neurodevelopment in newborns with moderate-to-severe HIE. Simbruner et al. (2010) reported that in their randomized controlled trial involving 129 newborns, of which 111 participated in neurodevelopmental follow-up at 18 months, hypothermia treatment provided strong neuroprotective effect for infants with severe HIE. Improved survival and neurodevelopmental outcome at 18 months of age have been reported in multiple trials of therapeutic hypothermia, and currently, it is the only neuroprotective strategy for neonates suspected to have suffered an intrapartum hypoxic-ischemic event.

Selective hypothermia, if begun within 6 hours of life and carefully controlled within a tertiary level NICU environment for 72 hours while providing multisystemic and multiorgan support, appears to reduce mortality and improve morbidity for newborns with moderate-to-severe HIE (Abate et al., 2021).

### References

Abate, B. B., Bimerew, M., Gebremichael, B., Kassie, A. M., Kassaw, M. W., Gebremeskel, T., Bayih, W. A. (2021). Effects of therapeutic hypothermia on death among asphyxiated neonates with hypoxic-ischemic encephalopathy: A systematic review and meta-analysis of randomized control trials. *PLoS One*, *16*(2), e0247229. https://doi.org/10.1371/journal.pone.0247229

Back, S. A., & Volpe, J. J. (2025). Encephalopathy of prematurity: Pathophysiology. In J. J. Volpe, T. E. Inder, B. T. Darras, L. S. de Vries, A. J. du Plessis, J. J. Neil, & J. M. Perlman (Eds.), *Volpe's neurology of the newborn* (7th ed., pp. 547–591). Elsevier.

Simbruner, G., Mittal, R. A., Rohlmann, F., Muche, R., & neo.nEURO.network Trial Participants. (2010). Systemic hypothermia after neonatal encephalopathy: Outcomes of neo.nEURO.network RCT. *Pediatrics, 126*(4), e771–e778. https://doi.org/10.1542/peds.2009-2441

Tagin, M. A., Woolcott, C. G., Vincer, M. J., Whyte, R. K., & Stinson, D. A. (2012). Hypothermia for neonatal hypoxic ischemic encephalopathy: An updated systematic review and meta-analysis. *Archives of Pediatrics and Adolescent Medicine, 166*(6), 558–566. https://doi.org/10.1001/archpediatrics.2011.1772

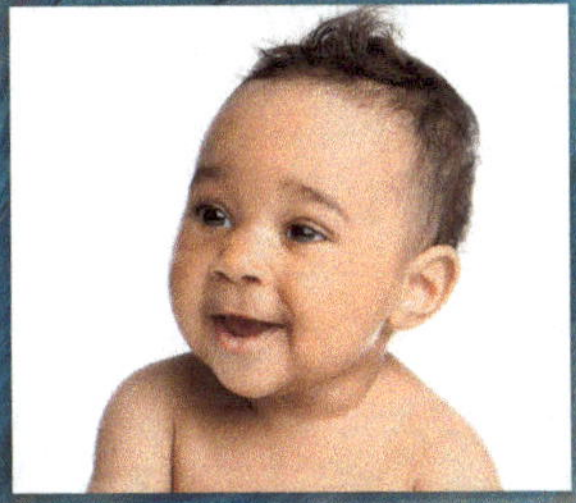

Source: New Africa/Adobe Stock.

## PARENT VOICES

### Heather McKinnis

**When Owen was born at 25 weeks, he was so tiny but so perfect in our eyes. Each ultrasound that first week of his life showed worsening degrees of brain bleeds. When the day 7 scan showed that the bleeding had spread beyond his ventricles and into his brain tissue, we were devastated. By that time, I had read so much about IVH and my one consolation was that his wasn't grade IV. I knew what that ultrasound may mean for my child. Bilateral grade IV IVH is the worst bleed he could have. Our doctors sat us down and went through every single limitation and challenge he may face. They explained the risks over the next weeks and then**

(*continued*)

## PARENT VOICES (*continued*)

**his delays as he grows. Not once, during those conversations, did one person give us hope. I understand the need for realistic and statistically based information, but as an overwhelmed and terrified first-time mom, I needed someone to give me a glimmer of hope for my baby. That one person was our nurse, Barb. After a couple of weeks of stable head ultrasounds and encouraging development from Owen, she encouraged me to just stop anxiously waiting for the bad and to enjoy the good. She told me to watch my baby. He responded to my voice, calmed at my touch, and moved both sides of his body. She reminded me how incredible the brain is and the amazing things she's seen in her time in the NICU. She did not tell me he was going to be OK. She did not give false hope or negative statistics. She held my hand, hugged me when I cried, and helped me find hope in a bleak situation. Owen is now 8 years old. He's healthy, happy, and thriving with his peers. I tell him about Barb often and how she was the first person to see his incredible potential.**

## ONLINE RESOURCES

CourseConnect

Resources for this chapter are online and available at www.springerpub.com/courseconnect.

## REFERENCES

References for this chapter are online and available at www.springerpub.com/courseconnect.

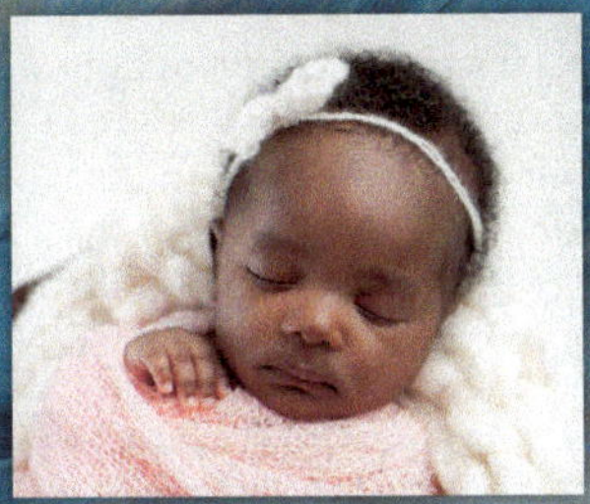


CHAPTER 16

# Auditory System

Denise McFadden

## INTRODUCTION

Hearing is a fundamental prerequisite to cognitive, social, and emotional development. Any temporary or permanent impairment from birth to 18 months of age can profoundly affect early language development (Shojaei et al., 2016). Auditory development, in particular, the development of speech, depends on exposure to a rich acoustic and linguistic environment. Hearing newborns recognize their mothers' voices because they are accustomed to hearing them in utero. Sensory deprivation affects the acquisition of communication skills, even though the hearing loss may be corrected. Screening newborns early for hearing impairments can reduce permanent deficits (Bower et al., 2023). A study of childhood language development and academic achievement reported that hearing impairment has a significant effect on the development of a child, as evidenced by limited speech. Hearing impairment can cause speech delays associated with lower academic achievement (Cree et al., 2024).

Approximately 16.5 per 10,000 live births demonstrated hearing loss (CDC, 2023).

## EARLY SCREENING FOR HEARING LOSS

Historically, screening for hearing loss in infants and very young children was limited to observations of behavioral responses to sounds, such as the ringing of a bell outside of a child's view. This method was fraught with difficulty and delay in early identification of hearing loss. Great strides have been made toward Universal Newborn Hearing Screening (UNHS) through early identification. State and federal levels promote a prescriptive plan to test newborns at regular intervals (Grosse et al., 2017). Since the initial Joint Committee Position Statement on Infant Hearing (Joint Committee on Infant Hearing, 1994) through subsequent revisions (Joint Committee on Infant Hearing, 2019) based recommendations on available evidence, supported the practice of UNHS. UNHS is widely accepted globally in developed countries and is considered a standard of care (Edmond et al., 2022).

## ANATOMY OF THE EAR

The ear is the anatomic unit involved in hearing and equilibrium. It consists of three parts: the external ear, the middle ear, and the inner ear. The external ear comprises the auricle (pinna) and the external ear canal (Figure 16.1). A complex cartilage framework gives structure to the auricle. Because of this anatomic position, the auricle is susceptible to trauma from external forces. The external ear canal is curved posterosuperiorly and anteromedially. The canal is oval, and the long axis is positioned superoinferiorly. Normally, the outer portion of the canal is cartilaginous, and the medial portion is bony. Before 34 weeks' gestation, the pinna is a slightly formed, cartilage-free double thickness of the skin. In the newborn, however, most of the canal is cartilaginous and collapsed (AlMakadma et al., 2023). As ear development ensues, the cartilage becomes firmer, making the outer two-thirds of the canal more patent (Figure 16.2). Cerumen glands and tiny hairs are present in the outer portion of the cartilaginous canal. The medial two-thirds of the canal lies immediately over

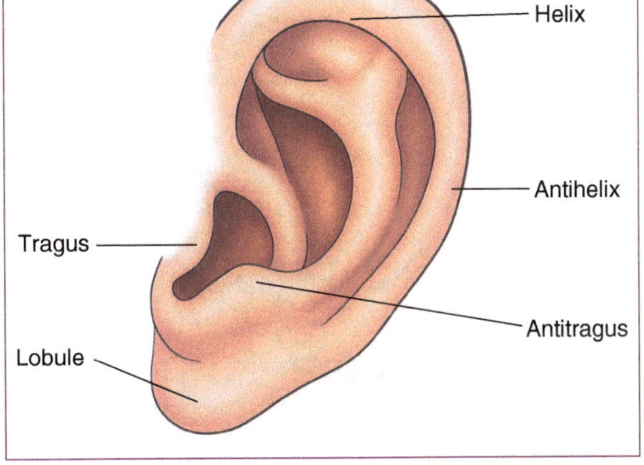


FIGURE 16.1 Anatomy of the external ear.

a bony area called the *osseous region*. The external auditory meatus assumes an irregular path from the concha to the tympanic membrane.

At the termination of the external canal is the eardrum, or tympanic membrane, which forms the boundary between the outer and the middle ear (Figure 16.3). The tympanic membrane has a complicated shape that loosely resembles a flat cone and moves with changes in air pressure. Because the tympanic membrane is oval and translucent, the middle ear structure can often be visualized through it. The short and long processes of the malleus are attached to the fibrous layer of the tympanic membrane and are visible on the lateral surface. In the middle ear, the malleus, incus, and stapes occupy the region between the tympanic membrane and the oval window of the middle ear. During the otoscopic examination, the long process of the incus can often be seen through the tympanic membrane. The middle ear cavity is an air-filled space connected by an air cell system posterior to the mastoid and by the eustachian tube anterior to the nasopharynx. Neither of these is in a dependent position for drainage of fluids. Ciliated columnar cells cover the walls of the tympanic cavity and mastoid air cells. Secretory cells are distributed throughout the middle ear, with the greatest number in the eustachian tube. The stapedius and the tensor muscles of the tympanic membrane attach in the middle ear to the malleus and the stapes by tendons. The chorda tympani nerve passes across the posterior surface. The medial wall of the middle ear cavity contains the oval and round windows. Between these two windows, the lower portion of the cochlea forms a prominence known as the *promontorium tympani* on the medial wall of the middle ear.

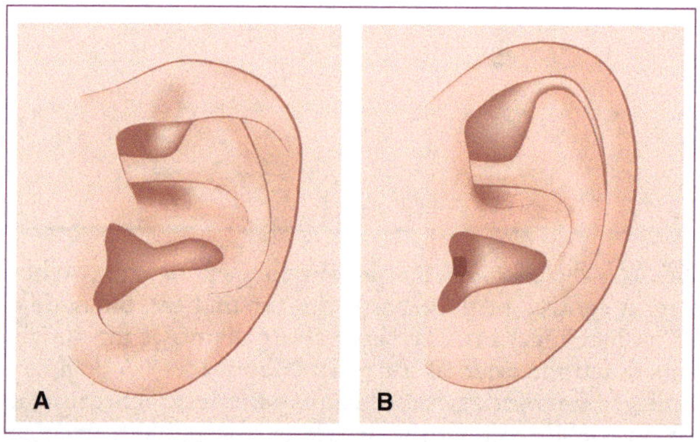


**FIGURE 16.2 Premature (A) and full-term (B) ear.**

*Source:* Adapted from Schreiner, R. L., & Bradburn, N. C. (1987). *Care of the newborn* (2nd ed.). Raven Press.

The inner ear consists of a bony labyrinth composed of three parts: the semicircular canals, the vestibule, and the cochlea. A dense, bony capsule in the petrous protein of the temporal bone surrounds these hollow spaces; this capsule contains perilymph and endolymph. Each semicircular canal has a dilated portion at the end, referred to as the *ampulla*, which includes the crista ampullaris, a vestibular sense organ. In the vestibule, the utricle and saccules are formed; these structures contain sensory endings essential for maintaining equilibrium.

The cochlea is a tubular structure with 2.5 turns; it closely resembles a snail shell, having a base and an apex. The cochlea

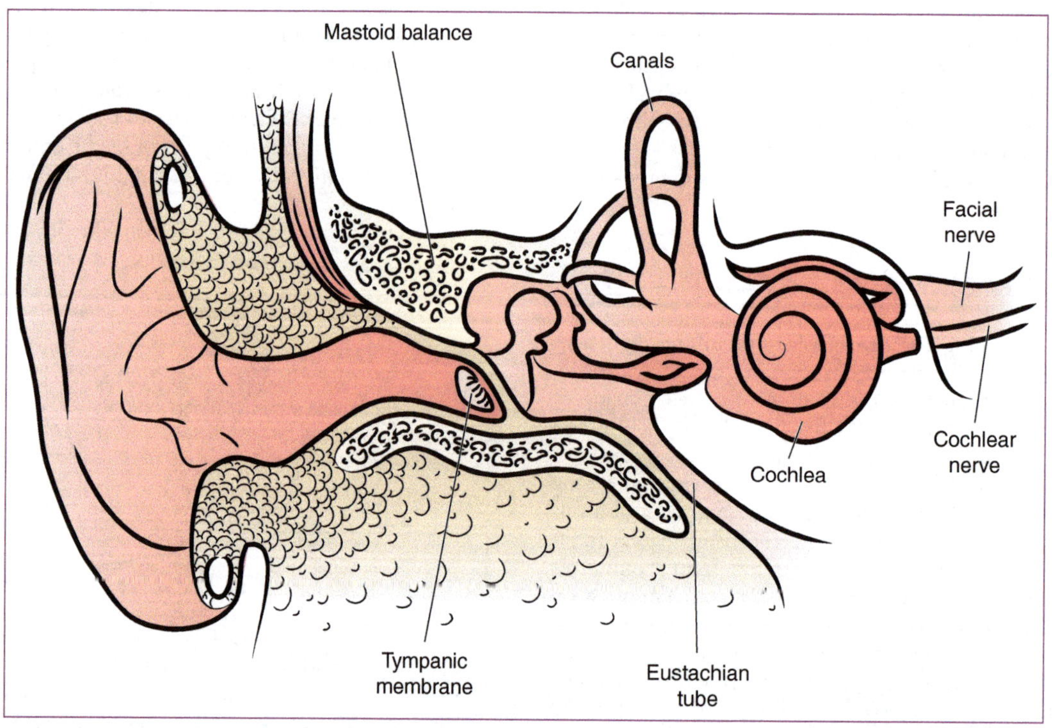


**FIGURE 16.3 General framework of the outer, middle, and inner ear.**

*Source:* Redrawn from Pappas, D. (1985). *Diagnosis and treatment of hearing impairment in children.* College-Hill Press.

is divided into the scala vestibuli, the scala media, and the scala tympani. The scala vestibuli begins at the oval window, and the scala tympani terminates at the round window. The basilar membrane side of the duct gives rise to the organ of Corti, the organ of hearing. The organ of Corti includes hair cells and supporting cells; attached to the hair cells is a gelatinous membrane called the *tectorial membrane*.

The membranous labyrinth of the inner ear is composed of connective tissue filled with endolymph that forms in the bony labyrinth. Afferent nerve fibers attach hair cells of the cochlea and the vestibular labyrinth to the neurons of the auditory system, the spiral ganglion, and the Scarpa ganglion in the temporal bone. Efferent nerve fibers from the ganglia form the auditory and vestibular division of the eighth cranial nerve and exit the temporal bone on its posterior surface to enter the brainstem.

## PHYSIOLOGY OF AUDIOLOGIC FUNCTION

### External Ear

The external ear consists of the auricle (pinna) and the external auditory meatus (external canal). The primary function of the external ear is to funnel sound to the tympanic membrane. Absence of the auricle contributes to difficulty in sound localization.

### Middle Ear

Advancing sound entering the auditory canal directly strikes the tympanic membrane. This membrane and the ossicles serve as transmitters from the outer ear to the inner ear. The malleus, which is continuous with the tympanic membrane and is connected with the incus and stapes, moves the ossicles. Ossicles transfer sound energy into the inner ear through the oval window, which holds the stapes through an angular ligament.

The middle ear is lined with respiratory mucosa composed of ciliated columnar epithelial cells, supporting cells, and secretory cells. Secretory cells secrete mucus that forms a complex mucous layer. The cilia of the middle ear interact with the mucus by transporting mastoid and middle ear secretions through the eustachian tube to the nasopharynx, where they are swallowed. This mechanism is known as the *mucociliary transport system*. Glycoproteins in the mucus determine the viscosity and elasticity of the middle ear mucus. A too-thick or too-thin mucus impedes the effective transport of bacteria and cellular debris from the mastoid and middle ear cleft; this transport protects against ear infections. In addition to serving as an exit for secretions into the nasopharynx, the eustachian tube equalizes the pressure between the middle ear and the ambient atmosphere.

### Inner Ear

Before this point in the hearing mechanism, all of the sound energy is contained in the air-filled spaces of the external and middle ear. From the stapes onward, the pathway for sound moves through fluid-filled spaces. When sound is transferred from the tympanic membrane to the inner ear, the stapes create a fluid wave that is transmitted to the round window. This transmission creates fluid waves that travel from the basal aspect of the cochlea to the apex. As the fluid wave moves, it displaces the basilar membrane. Maximum movement of the basilar membrane occurs at the point specific to the frequency of sound entering the ear; high-frequency sounds cause a minimal disturbance at the basal end of the cochlea, and low-frequency sounds cause a minimal disruption at the apex.

Vibrations in the basilar membrane cause movement of the organ of Corti. This organ contains receptor hair cells that are on the basilar membrane. Vibrations of the hair on the hair cells cause either polarization or depolarization, depending on the direction of the bend. When sufficient depolarization occurs, action potentials are produced and propagated along the auditory pathway to the auditory cortex. The cochlea provides input by coding information about loudness and frequency in the action potentials sent to the cortex, giving meaning to the sound. Hair cells of the spiral organ of Corti are stimulated as they touch the tectorial membrane. Hair cells act as transducers that convert mechanical energy into electrical impulses; this action occurs in the fibers of the spiral ganglion. Axons of these cells become the auditory nerve (vestibulocochlear nerve). Nerve fibers pass to the medulla, the pons, and the midbrain, and finally to the temporal lobes of the cortex, where the impulses are interpreted as sound.

The vestibular system is similar to the auditory system. Fluid moves within the vestibular labyrinth when the head moves. The semicircular canals respond to angular acceleration (rotation), and the utricle and saccule respond to linear acceleration (position). Movement of the endolymph exerts force on the hairs of the sensory cells of the cristae and the maculae. Depolarization of the sensory cells produces action potentials, which are transmitted to the vestibular cortex. The vestibular apparatus functions in conjunction with proprioception and visual orientation to maintain balance.

## HEARING LOSS

The American Speech-Language-Hearing Association (ASHA) (n.d.) defines hearing loss as “problems in the outer, middle, or inner ear.” Hearing loss represents a spectrum of hearing loss classified as mild, moderate, severe, or prolonged.

### Types of Hearing Loss

The types of hearing loss have been classified according to the location of the problem. Loss may be one of three types: *conductive, sensorineural,* or a *combination* of these. Conductive losses arise from conditions that affect the outer and middle ear; sensorineural loss results from inner ear disorders; and combination losses result from disruptions in both areas of the ear.

*Conductive hearing loss* exists when the outer or middle ear dysfunction disrupts the typical sequence of sound localization and vibration. The external auditory meatus frequently becomes occluded by cerumen (wax), which impedes the transmission of sound. Otitis media, an infection of the middle ear, is the most common cause of conductive hearing loss. Fluid accumulates (effusion) in the middle ear, preventing the tympanic membrane and ossicular chain from vibrating normally. Hearing loss may fluctuate or become permanent. Congenital deformities of the outer ear also can inhibit the neonate's ability to hear. Because the external ear functions to funnel sound, variations in the structure and protrusion of the pinna may contribute to conductive hearing loss. A missing or deformed pinna can result from a malformation of the auricular folds. Atresia of the auditory meatus or abnormal development of the ossicular chain may arise from defective development of the brachial chain (Liao & Chen, 2022). Infants with *conductive hearing loss* have difficulty hearing low-frequency sounds (i.e., those in the 125–500 Hz range). Management of neonates with conductive hearing loss is directed toward early observation, detection, and intervention to eliminate the source of infection, remove the blockage, and provide amplification, restoring normal hearing.

*Sensorineural hearing impairment* results from damage to the sensory nerve endings of the cochlea or dysfunction of the auditory nerve (eighth cranial nerve). A typical characteristic of inner ear dysfunction is the inability of the inner ear to interpret fluid changes in the cochlea. Sensorineural hearing loss may manifest as a congenital inner ear abnormality, resulting in congenital deafness. Other conditions that may cause sensorineural hearing loss are trauma to the inner ear, the effects of certain drugs, prolonged exposure to loud noise, infections, infectious conditions such as measles, and the effects of aging (Sowula et al., 2021).

## IDENTIFICATION OF THE HEARING-IMPAIRED INFANT

### Physical Examination

The physical examination of the infant should be performed in a quiet, warm, draft-free area appropriate for observation and inspection of auditory structures and function. Observing the infant's behavior before examining the ear yields baseline assessments. The alert, normal, full-term newborn reacts by turning toward the sound of human speech or the ring of a bell; this infant also startles to the stimulus of a loud noise. Observation of the preterm infant is deferred to a later time, before discharge, when the behavioral response has matured. Infant response alone provides only a crude estimate of neonatal hearing ability.

### Inspection of the Ear

Inspection of the ear begins with the medial and lateral surfaces of the pinna and the surface of the scalp, face, and neck. Development of the pinna correlates with the infant's gestational age. At term, the pinna of the newborn is well shaped and has sufficient cartilage to maintain normal shape and resistance (see Figure 16.2). Before 34 weeks' gestation, the pinna has a slightly formed double skin thickness. The relationship of the pinna to the other structures of the head and face is important in the initial assessment. With normal placement, the helix is located at the level of the outer canthus, and the tragus is roughly level with the intraorbital rim. Low-set auricles frequently are associated with abnormalities of the urinary system. Unilateral conductive hearing loss may be present in children with normal-size pinnae and unilateral absence of the superior crus or in patients with a fused antihelix-helix; thickened, hypertrophied earlobes; a "cup" ear; and a protruding pinna. The pinna may be abnormally small (microtia) or absent (anotia). Atresia (closure of the external auditory canal) may be observed. The condition is classified as mild, indicating a small ear canal; medium, suggesting that a bony atretic plate has replaced the canal with ossicular malformation; or severe, indicating a small or absent ear canal and middle ear space.

Several combinations of atresia and microtia may be seen; therefore, all children with these abnormalities should be suspected of having middle ear abnormalities. These infants may also have sensorineural hearing loss. Atresia often is observed with cranial, facial, mandibular, or acrofacial dysostoses. Abnormalities of the skeletal system or chromosomal aberration may also be accompanied by atresia. Aural atresia may be associated with facial, labial, or palatal clefts. Infants with atresia often have conductive hearing loss related to the inability of the ear canal to transmit sound. Preauricular abnormalities, including pits or tags (Figure 16.4) and branchial fistulas, are often accompanied by external or middle ear malformations. These appendages may be present with an otherwise normal-appearing pinna. Preauricular tags or pits usually require only cosmetic surgery or excision if draining.

The pinna should be inspected for its location and relationship to other facial structures. Normal attachment is to the side, level with the middle-third of the face, and fixed in position to the lateral aspect of the external auditory canal. The major convolutions of the pinna are the helix, antihelix, tragus, antitragus, and lobule. The lobule of the external ear has no cartilage. The pinna's placement angle is almost vertical; if the angle is more than 10 degrees off normal, it is considered abnormal. The superior helix is located at the outer canthus of the eye, and the tragus is roughly level with the infraorbital rim.

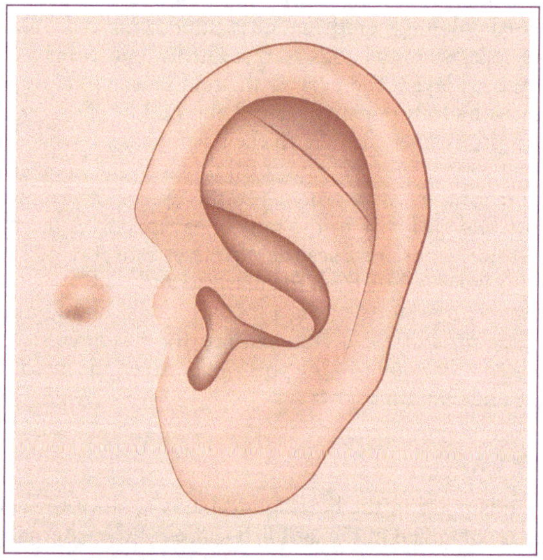

**FIGURE 16.4 Preauricular tag.**

*Source:* Adapted from Schreiner, R. L., & Bradburn, N. C. (1987). *Care of the newborn* (2nd ed.). Raven Press.

Low-set auricles are frequently associated with other abnormalities of the first and second branchial clefts and with abnormalities of the urinary system. Other abnormalities that may be noted are skin tags, sinuses, or pits, often associated with other auditory or renal malformations. The pinna frequently may be observed to have bruising from a forceps delivery. Depending on the degree of bruising, the discoloration should subside within the first week of life.

The external auditory meatus should then be observed for patency. Atresia or stenosis of the external meatus may be seen. This abnormality results in conductive hearing loss because sound transmissions are blocked; the condition should be noted as part of the physical findings.

## Inspection of the Middle Ear and Tympanic Membrane

The depths of the external meatus can be examined with a brightly illuminated pneumatic otoscope. Vernix caseosa is frequently encountered in the neonate's ear canal. The otoscope is introduced into the ear canal by exerting gentle traction posterosuperiorly on the auricle. In the neonate, the tympanic membrane lies in a nearly horizontal plane. The tympanic membrane is visualized through the collapsed neonatal ear by gently dilating the ear canal with the speculum as the cartilaginous canal is traversed. The tympanic membrane should be examined for thickness, vascularity, and contour. All areas, including the area above the short process of the malleus (pars flaccida), should be visualized for completeness. Normally, the tympanic membrane appears translucent. White shadows of the ossicles can usually be seen through the membrane. The mobility of the tympanic membrane can be assessed by applying intermittent pressure through a bulb or by blowing through a polyethylene tube connected to an otoscope.

Otitis media can occur in the first days of life and can be diagnosed by otoscopic examination. Otitis media often manifests as a poorly mobile, bulging, yellow, opacified tympanic membrane. Complications of otitis media are common. Otitis media with middle ear effusion may cause hearing loss, perforation of the tympanic membrane, and possibly intracranial complications, including meningitis, encephalitis, and brain abscess (Gendeh et al., 2019). Middle ear effusion occurs in both outpatient and inpatient groups of neonates.

## Inspection of the Head and Neck

The head and neck anatomy should be assessed for deficits as part of the screening process for all neonates. Ear anomalies associated with head and neck anomalies may occur due to a primary regional defect, secondary to a primary defect in an area contiguous to the temporal bone, as part of an inherited defect involving the skeletal system, or as part of a chromosomal disorder. Malformations of the head and neck may be relatively simple or complex. Any neonate with a defect, even a minor one, should be closely examined for hidden significant malformations.

**Nose.** Examination of the nose should be directed toward identifying suspicious defects, such as unusual broadness with a flat base and a short length (saddle nose), small nostrils, and notched alae. Deformities of the nose often appear, along with other craniofacial abnormalities.

**Mouth.** Defects in the oral cavity are the most common defect associated with hearing impairment. A child with cleft lip and/or palate has a deficiency in the palate musculature that is primarily related to the inability of the tensor muscle of the velum palatinum to dilate the eustachian tube actively during swallowing. Hearing problems may be observed in patients with cleft palate, depending on the patient's age on examination and the means of the exploration. A cleft lip or palate leaves the child vulnerable to fluid effusion and, consequently, to varying degrees of hearing loss. The consequences of effusion raise the rate of otitis media, of which 50% to 90% of incidences have been reported. The hearing loss associated with cleft lip or palate generally is conductive; however, sensorineural and combination losses have been reported. Infants younger than 12 months of age who had cleft palate that was surgically repaired often have a detectable degree of hearing loss. The degree of loss is directly related to the severity of the palatal defect.

**Eyes.** Deformities of the eyelids are the most common abnormality involving the eyes. A variation in eyelid configuration has been noted in which the upper eyelid forms an almost vertical curve at the level of the medial limit of the cornea and fuses with the lower eyelid. The distance of the two medial angles is increased. These findings typically are noted in Waardenburg syndrome, an autosomal dominant disorder that results in mild-to-severe sensorineural hearing loss in 50% of patients. The hearing loss may be unilateral or bilateral and progressive.

Epicanthal folds, which are true vertical folds extending from the nasal fold into the upper eyelid, are commonly noted in infants with Down syndrome or trisomy 21. Other physical features seen in Down syndrome are low-set ears, small pinnae, and a narrow external ear canal. Infants with this syndrome tend to have recurrent otitis media and anomalies of the middle ear ossicles. Hearing loss is high, and the condition may be sensorineural, conductive, or combination.

**Hair.** An unusual hair texture or hairline should raise suspicion in assessing abnormalities associated with hearing loss. Twisted hair (pili torti) has been associated with sensorineural hearing loss. The hair may be twisted, dry, brittle, or easily broken. Aberrant scalp hair patterns may also be significant.

**Neck.** Defects of the neck that may be associated with hearing impairment are branchial cleft fistulas and a mildly webbed or shortened neck. Not all infants with defects of the head or neck also have hearing impairments; many variations may be observed in the normal neonate population. The presence of such defects does increase the risk of hearing impairment, however, and should be followed up in the child's long-term interest.

## History

The importance of a comprehensive history for identifying the infant at risk cannot be overemphasized. The newborn carries a history extending back to the time of conception and is influenced by both perinatal events and parental genetic composition. Gathering data on the infant's history is the first step in identifying infants at risk for hearing impairment. A thorough history of familial hearing loss, present at birth or in childhood through adolescence, is significant.

## Family History

More than 50 types of hereditary hearing loss have been described. A significant number of hearing impairments may be classified as genetically based. Hereditary hearing loss must be identified based on a thorough medical and family history, which should include the following components:

1. Determination of the cause and circumstances under which the hearing impairment was first noticed: Many different circumstances surrounding the onset of the hearing loss may cause it to be labeled as congenital or hereditary, or both. An example of hearing loss that is hereditary and not congenital is Alport syndrome, an autosomal dominant trait resulting in deafness that begins in preadolescence.
2. A complete family history: This should include a history of previous and current pregnancies.
3. An extended family history of data relating to hearing impairments of both immediate and extended family members.
4. A thorough physical examination: The head and neck regions should be examined for abnormalities.
5. Selective testing procedures for assessing possible causes of sensorineural hearing loss.

A questionnaire can obtain information on familial hearing loss from the mother. Although the questions may easily be asked orally, the form provides a structure that ensures consistency and is the preferred data-gathering method in most settings. The questionnaire should be given to all new mothers and should be completed prior to discharge. The questionnaire provides an excellent opportunity for educating the mother on normal speech and language development.

# HEREDITARY HEARING LOSS

## Autosomal Dominant Inheritance

Autosomal dominant inheritance accounts for 10% to 25% of cases of hereditary hearing impairment. The hearing loss may be unilateral or bilateral, and males and females are affected equally. Autosomal dominant hearing disorders vary in severity ("variable expressivity") and in the progression of hearing loss. A typical example of an autosomal dominant hearing disorder occurs in Waardenburg syndrome, characterized by hypertelorism, a high nasal bridge, synophrys, and hypoplastic alae nasi. Pigmentation abnormalities include a white forelock, partial albinism, hypopigmentation of the fundi, blue irises, and premature graying. This syndrome has severe bilateral sensorineural hearing loss with integumentary system involvement. The histopathologic characteristics are the absence of the organ of Corti and atrophy of the spiral ganglion.

Another example of an autosomal dominant hearing loss with incomplete penetrance and variable expression occurs in Treacher-Collins syndrome. Major features of the syndrome include facial anomalies; small, displaced, or absent external ears; external auditory canal atresia; and poorly developed or malformed tympanic ossicles. Deafness generally is complete and conductive.

Klippel-Feil syndrome, if familial, is another example of autosomal dominance with variable expression. The characteristics of this syndrome are craniofacial disorders, fusion of some or all of the cervical vertebrae, cleft palate (occasionally), and severe sensorineural hearing loss. Crouzon disease is another disorder in which hearing loss is attributed to autosomal dominance with variable expression. An abnormally shaped head, a beaked nose, and marked bilateral exophthalmos caused by premature closure of the cranial sutures characterize this disease. Hearing loss may be conductive because of middle ear deformities or sensorineural abnormalities.

## Autosomal Recessive Inheritance

Autosomal recessive inheritance accounts for about 40% of childhood deafness. An estimated one in eight individuals is a carrier for a recessive hearing impairment. The incidence of recessive inheritance is higher in marriages of recent common ancestry, such as siblings or cousins. This type of union increases the possibility that each parent will be carriers of an identical defective gene that may express itself as an abnormal trait. Hearing loss in people with an autosomal recessive gene tends to be more severe than in those with autosomal dominant inheritance because most cases of recessive hearing loss are associated with the Scheibe deformity of the cochlea. With Scheibe dysplasia, the entire organ of Corti is rudimentary; hair cells are missing, and the supporting cells are distorted or collapsed. The vestibular membrane is usually collapsed. Pendred syndrome, a condition marked by hearing loss and goiter detected in the first 2 years of life, is an example of an autosomal recessive disorder.

**X-Linked Disorders.** Approximately 3% of hereditary deafness is due to the X-linked mode of transmission (Giannantonio et al., 2020). The mutant gene is on the X chromosome, and males transmit only Y chromosomes to their male offspring; therefore, only males are affected. The female is the carrier and has the chance to transmit the gene to 50% of her sons, who manifest the disease, and 50% of her daughters, who carry the abnormality. Hearing loss characteristically is not present at birth but develops in infancy to varying degrees. X-linked hearing losses, with exceptions, are sensorineural, and some retention of hearing in all frequencies often occurs. Recessive, or X-linked, Duchenne muscular dystrophy is an example of this type of disorder. Characterized by muscle wasting, the severe infantile form of muscular dystrophy is also associated with mild-to-moderate sensorineural hearing loss.

**Cytogenetic Disorders.** Cytogenetic disorders are caused by structural changes in one or more of the chromosomes or by errors in the distribution of the chromosomes. Down syndrome (Trisomy 21), which is caused by an extra chromosome 21, is the most common chromosomal aberration syndrome, with an incidence of 1 in 600 to 800 births. Approximately 5% of cases of Down syndrome are due to translocation and fusion of part of chromosome 21 to chromosome 14. Children with trisomy 21 have a high incidence of hearing loss.

Characteristic otologic findings that have an effect on the hearing performance of these children during the early years are a high incidence of (a) stenosis of the external auditory canal, (b) serous otitis media, and (c) a cholesteatoma-persistent growth of squamous epithelium from the ear canal into the middle ear or mastoid through a tear in the tympanic membrane. The narrowed segment is located at the junction of the cartilaginous and bony portions of the canal. With increasing age, the canal has been noted to assume a more typical appearance as the thickened tissue recedes.

The degree of hearing loss in these infants varies but is rarely profound. On examination of the aperture, some of these children are found to have congenital ossicular malformations and destruction caused by inflammations arising from chronic infection.

Intellectual disability is a clinical condition frequently seen with Down syndrome or trisomy 21. The effect of the otologic handicap on the developmental potential of these children is uncertain. **Emergency Alert: Early and frequent monitoring is imperative because of the high incidence of hearing loss in this group.** Collaborative research studies need to be done to identify factors affecting the otologic problems of infants with Down syndrome and to devise early strategies to optimize these infants' potential (Manickam et al., 2016).

## Differential Diagnosis

No differential diagnosis exists for deafness, although generally, a differential diagnosis to determine the etiology of the hearing impairment is listed.

## Diagnostic Tests

- Laboratory testing is not of benefit in the diagnosis of deafness; however, if a genetic syndrome is suspected, biochemical evidence may be of benefit in determining the etiology.
- Connexin-26 is a genetic marker for deafness (Xu et al., 2023).
- Laboratory testing for perinatal infections such as syphilis and other toxoplasmosis, other agents, rubella, cytomegalovirus (CMV), and herpes simplex (TORCH) infections may be indicated.
- For bilateral hearing loss, markers for general inflammatory disease, sedimentation rate, rheumatoid factor, or 68-kDa protein, a marker especially for autoimmune ear disease, may be evaluated.
- Computed tomography (CT) scanning and magnetic resonance imaging (MRI) may establish a malformation of the cochlea or cochlear nerve. MRI scanning may be used to identify an enlarged vestibular aqueduct in the case of a sensitive ear in a child with a minor head trauma who presents with deteriorating hearing.

# SCREENING METHODS FOR IDENTIFICATION OF HEARING LOSS

Neonatal Hearing Screening is the standard of care in hospitals throughout the United States and developed countries worldwide (ASHA, 2018). The primary focus of hearing screening for neonates (ages 0–6 months) is but one part of a comprehensive Early Hearing Detection and Intervention (EHDI) program of service. The primary focus includes newborn hearing screening as early identification of infants likely to have hearing loss and who will require further evaluation. The secondary purpose is to identify newborns with medical conditions who can present with late-onset hearing loss to establish a plan for continued care monitoring of their child's hearing status for this family unit (Joint Committee on Infant Hearing, 2019; NCHAM, 2019). The EHDI guidelines include hearing screening completion by 1 month of age, diagnosis of a hearing impairment, selection and fitting of a device within 1 month of confirmation of a hearing loss if parents choose that option, as well as entry into early intervention (EI) services by 6 months of age.

In the past 15 years, programs and procedures for screening newborns have been developed, modified, and improved. The goal of any screening program is to accomplish the task rapidly, accurately, and economically. EHDI refers to screening every newborn for hearing loss before hospital discharge. All 50 states and the District of Columbia have EHDI laws or voluntary compliance programs that screen hearings. The EHDI program creates, operates, and continuously improves a system. In addition, institutions are advised to use the risk factors associated with permanent congenital, delayed-onset, and/or progressive hearing loss in children. Box 16.1 is a guide to identifying infants whose history indicates that degenerative disease or intrauterine infection may cause progressive,

### BOX 16.1

### RISK FACTORS ASSOCIATED WITH PERMANENT CONGENITAL, DELAYED ONSET, AND/OR PROGRESSIVE HEARING LOSS IN CHILDREN

1. Family history of permanent childhood hearing loss
2. Neonatal intensive care for 2 days or more or any of the following: extracorporeal membrane oxygenation-assisted ventilation, exposure to ototoxic medications (gentamicin and tobramycin) or loop diuretics (furosemide/Lasix), and hyperbilirubinemia requiring exchange transfusion
3. In-utero exposure to infections such as CMV, herpes, rubella, syphilis, and toxoplasmosis
4. Craniofacial anomalies, including those that involve the pinna, ear canal, ear tags, ear pits, and temporal bone anomalies
5. Syndromes associated with hearing loss or progressive or late-onset hearing loss, such as Waardenburg, Alport, Pendred, Usher, and neurofibromatosis
6. Neurodegenerative disorders such as Hunter syndrome
7. Culture-positive postnatal infections associated with sensorineural hearing loss, including confirmed bacterial and viral meningitis
8. Head trauma
9. Chemotherapy
10. Recurrent or persistent otitis media
11. Concerned parent; child may have hearing loss

*Source:* Adapted from U.S. Preventive Services Task Force. (2008). Universal screening for hearing loss in newborns. U.S. Preventive Services Task Force recommendation statement. *American Family Physician, 122*(1), 143–148. https://doi.org/10.1542/peds.2007-2210.

fluctuating, or late-onset hearing loss. In these cases, it is recommended that the child have follow-up for 2 years in addition to initial screening.

The Joint Committee on Infant Hearing (2019) has endorsed universal screening of all newborns. In all cases, before discharge, the parents should be informed about speech and hearing milestones. They should be provided information about community agencies available for long-term follow-up if needed (Figure 16.5).

## Peripheral Measurements of Hearing Function

Assessment of hearing function in the neonate has focused on a two-tiered approach in which the evoked otoacoustic emissions (OAEs) test is used initially, and the automated auditory brainstem response (ABR) test is used as a follow-up for infants who show hearing impairment on the initial screening. OAEs are low-intensity sounds that can be measured

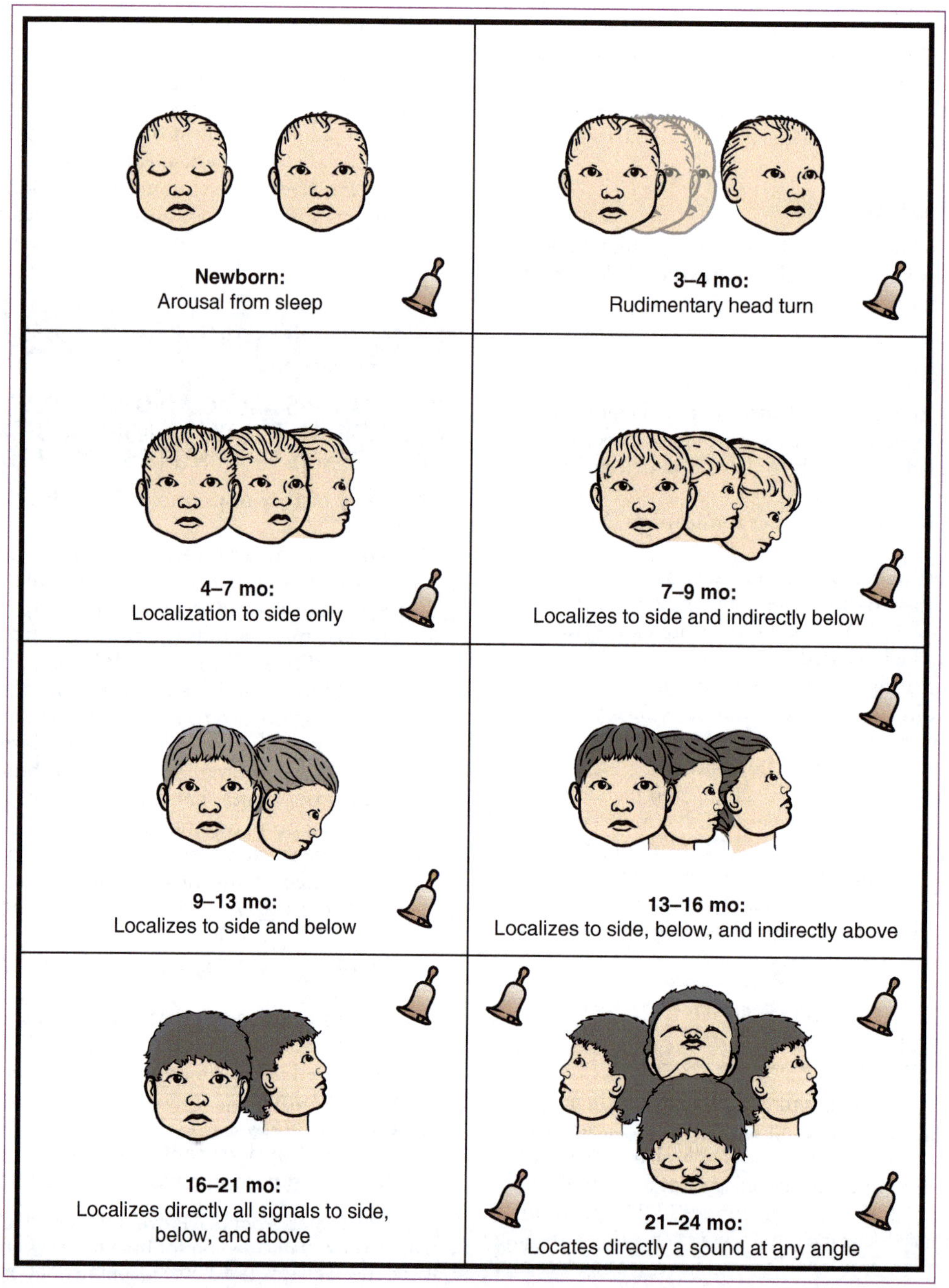


**FIGURE 16.5 Maturation of auditory response.**

*Source:* Redrawn from Northern, J. L., & Downs, M. P. (2002). *Hearing in children* (5th ed.). Lippincott Williams & Wilkins.

by placing a sensitive microphone in the ear canal. Hearing screening using OAEs is quick, inexpensive, and relatively accurate. Newborns delivered at home or a birthing center without hearing screening facilities must have some referral mechanism for newborn hearing screening and follow-up mechanisms.

If hearing impairment is detected on the OAE test, the ABR test can confirm the validity of that result. The ABR test records the electrical potentials that arise from the auditory nerve system. During this test, disk electrodes are attached to the vertex and mastoid areas, and repetitive sounds are presented to the ear in the form of clicks caused by a direct current pulse. The recorded response is a sequence of waves representing the auditory nerve's action potential. The wave latencies in at-risk infants tend to show smaller and more prolonged responses. The absolute latency of the ABR waves depends on the intensity of the click stimulus. Reducing the click stimuli from 60 dB to 30 to 40 dB identifies hearing thresholds. The absence of all waves indicates the presence of a peripheral lesion.

An abnormal ABR result may be defined as one that shows an absence of response at 40 dB or a wave V latency that exceeds the norm by two standard deviations. Wave V responses are used to determine abnormality because they are highly repeatable in infants and show little variability in normal-hearing subjects. The ABR test appears sensitive in that no false-negative results have been reported. Considering that any screening method should be quick, inexpensive, and easily administered and allow for easy interpretation of a large number of infants, the drawback to the ABR test is that it is more costly than the OAE test. Nevertheless, the ABR test can be justified as the initial neonatal hearing test, especially in preterm or high-risk infants. The Joint Committee on Infant Hearing (2019) specifies that an audiologist should supervise the infant hearing screening program.

In some infants whose initial ABR test results are passing but the infants meet risk criteria, continuing audiologic follow-up and management may be appropriate as designated by the U.S. Preventive Services Task Force (USPSTF) for the following 3 years. Those infants include one with risk factors associated with possible progressive or fluctuating loss, such as a family history of progressive hearing loss, CMV infection, and persistent fetal circulation.

Infants who do not demonstrate a repeatable ABR wave V to the signal presented at 40 dB in at least one ear should have a comprehensive hearing evaluation at no later than 6 months of age. This follow-up includes a general physical examination of the head and neck, otoscopy, identification of relevant physical abnormalities, and laboratory tests for perinatal infections. A comprehensive audiologic evaluation may include additional evoked potential evaluation and acoustic immittance measurements. Although precise data on hearing sensitivity cannot be obtained until the infant can respond to operant conditioning test procedures at approximately 6 months of age, habilitation should not be delayed.

Infants can be fitted with hearing aids before 3 months of age. Attention to early identification, amplification, and education does not necessarily ensure speech and language acquisition but certainly facilitates it, even in the most profoundly hearing-impaired child.

## Development of a Treatment Plan for the Hearing-Impaired Neonate

Hearing screening of all infants should be completed before discharge or no later than 1 month of age. Those not passing the newborn screening should undergo audiologic and medical evaluation before 3 months of age for confirmatory testing. If a diagnosis is confirmed, a treatment plan and habilitation can begin. **Quality and Safety: Infants whose history indicates they are at risk for late-onset hearing loss should be observed by periodic audiologic testing for 3 years.** For the infant with a confirmed hearing loss, efforts are directed at treatment. Per Public Law 99, EI services are (a) evaluation and assessment and (b) development of an individualized family service plan. The full evaluation plan is to be completed within 45 days of referral. This plan may include various methods to treat serous otitis media, a significant cause of temporary conductive hearing loss. For infants with permanent conductive hearing loss, amplification with a hearing aid may facilitate stimulation in the early critical period. Infants can be fitted with a hearing aid device as soon as the impairment is diagnosed. In addition to amplification, the family should be taught total communication skills to enhance interaction between the sender and the receiver. The basic premise is to use every means to communicate, such as gesturing, touching, and attending to stimuli.

An infant with severe-to-profound hearing impairment who is not at risk for recurrent otitis media and who does not get satisfactory results with a hearing aid is a candidate for cochlear implants (discussed in the "Cochlear Implants" in this chapter). For the hearing-impaired infant, multiple referral sources exist in which a multidisciplinary approach optimizes the infant's potential for growth and development.

## Cochlear Implants

Cochlear implants are not new, but they are increasingly used to treat infants with severe sensorineural hearing loss. Cochlear implants are electronic devices surgically implanted in the inner ear and bypassing the ear's damaged part to deliver electrical signals to the hearing nerve. A cochlear implant system comprises a microphone, an external sound processor, a transmitter, an internal cochlear receiver, and an electrode array. The external sound processor captures sound with a microphone and converts the sound to digital information. The digital signal is sent to the internal receiver and converted to electrical signals, stimulating tiny inner ear electrodes. The electrodes send the electrical signal to the hearing nerve. The brain then interprets these signals as sound. Implants work only if some spiral ganglion cells are present to transmit the auditory signal. The comfortable sound level is an issue for patients of any age with any cochlear implant. This sometimes is difficult to determine in infants, who cannot provide feedback as to what they are hearing.

Cochlear implants are Food and Drug Administration (FDA)-approved for adults and children as young as 12 months of age. Research has shown that earlier implantation is associated with better speech and language development (Culbertson et al., 2022). **Quality and Safety: It is critical that infants with hearing loss be diagnosed and EI be initiated without delay.** The later the child receives the implants, the more likely it is that speech and language development will be delayed.

Hearing screening is a task for a team of professionals that includes pediatricians, otolaryngologists, audiologists, neurologists, and nurse practitioners. Local public health agencies may provide services such as data collection and referral. Many large metropolitan medical centers have speech and hearing centers as part of a broad base of services ranging from diagnosis to rehabilitation.

## Implementation and Evaluation

The multidisciplinary, multiservices approach should be instituted only when all components are available to the infant and the family (ASHA, 2018). In addition to qualified professionals and services, other factors influence the management and habilitation of the hearing-impaired infant. These factors can facilitate or hamper entry into the system and compliance with the treatment regimen (Box 16.2).

### BOX 16.2

#### FACTORS INFLUENCING THE MANAGEMENT AND HABILITATION OF THE HEARING-IMPAIRED INFANT

**Factors That Facilitate Management and Habilitation**

Acknowledging the parents' sense of loss and feelings of inadequacy: a nonalarmist style of communication

Interpretation of test results and proposed plan of care

Information about expected developmental skills, suggestions for promoting skills, and a timeframe for follow-up

Encouragement to seek out and dialogue with other parents of hearing-impaired infants

Teaching the family total communication skills (gesturing, touching, and attending) to support interaction with the infant

Expeditious arrangements for referral

Parental involvement, offering a wide range of programs that are family centered and family focused

**Factors That Hamper Management and Habilitation**

Long waiting lists

Proximity to resources

Difficulty scheduling appointments

Parents being unaware of the plan of care

Focus on the child later, rather than the infant sooner

Parents wanted more involvement

Decision making that was therapist centered, not family centered

Poor communication between speech and hearing departments

## Parental Support

Support for the parents of a hearing-impaired child is based on the foundation of trust and acceptance between the practitioner and the family. Notifying parents that their child has a hearing impairment is a highly traumatic and deeply disturbing situation, one that often provokes denial. Problem identification is frequently delayed because the parents cannot admit something is wrong. Some practices in the diagnostic workup for hearing impairment favor separating the parents from the diagnostic process. OAE and ABR testing may foster denial because the findings are abstract, and parents need to have visible, tangible evidence of the impairment. The practitioner plays a major role in reiterating, interpreting, and reinforcing the information conveyed by the audiologist. Sensitivity to the parents' need to grieve the loss of the "perfect child" is important. Acceptance of the handicap can be aided by enlisting the parents as co-diagnosticians. Asking the parents what they think the problem is and making them part of the decision-making process objectifies the diagnoses and aids future compliance with the habilitative regimen. Balancing the ability to provide medical options with knowing the parent is the ultimate decision maker promotes better outcomes (DesGeorges, 2016). By listening to the parents' feelings of inadequacy and by indirect teaching, practitioners can help the parents acquire more fruitful coping strategies. An asynchrony may develop that can retard the infant's ability to acquire language even beyond the limits of the hearing loss itself. The family can be taught total communication skills (gesturing, touching, and attending) to support interaction with the infant.

# OUTCOME MEASURES

Outcome measures of the treatment program include early identification and implementation of a comprehensive habilitation plan to maximize communication potential and parental acceptance of the infant's condition. Teaching, role modeling, and clearly communicating with the family and integrating them as part of the healthcare team—including the follow-up—will improve the infant–family interactions.

# SUMMARY

Because of the countless efforts of many, 98% of the babies born in the United States and its territories receive hearing screening in the newborn period (CDC, 2023). Successful outcomes for children with hearing loss are within reach as a result of advanced knowledge, skills, and hearing technology available to these children and their families. Only 75% of newborns who did not pass the hearing screening test received diagnostic audiologic follow-up (Office of Disease Prevention and Health Promotion, n.d.). Clearly, positive outcomes can only be achieved if babies identified with hearing loss receive appropriate EI services in a timely manner. That is the challenge that lies in the future.

## PARENT VOICES

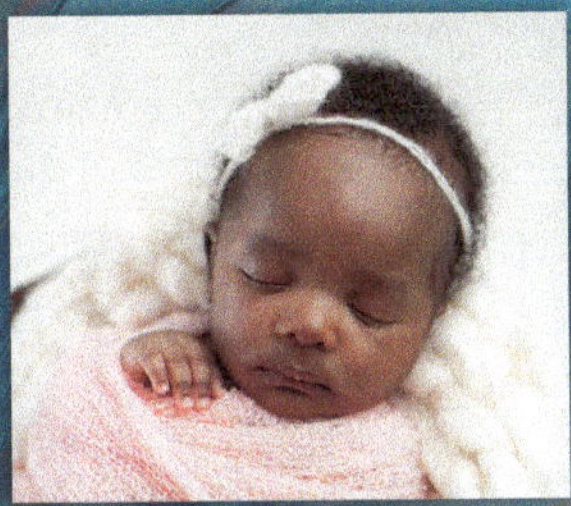

*Source:* Katrinaelena/Adobe Stock.

### Keira Sorrells

**Aside from having the most wonderfully supportive lactation nurses in our unit, the neonatal therapists were equally incredible. I will never forget when I walked in for a visit and our primary nurse said she had scheduled an appointment for the occupational therapist (OT) to teach me infant massage. This was a highlight of our time in the NICU, where the OT gently coached me and encouraged me to care for my daughter using the healing power of touch. She taught me important cues to look for, as well as potential areas for concern, as we worked together. Being able to provide this type of massage for my daughter allowed me an additional manner in which to bond, empowered me to feel more like a "real" mom, and was something I continued to do for my daughter on into her toddler years.**

## ONLINE RESOURCES

CourseConnect

Resources for this chapter are online and available at www.springerpub.com/courseconnect.

## REFERENCES

References for this chapter are online and available at www.springerpub.com/courseconnect.

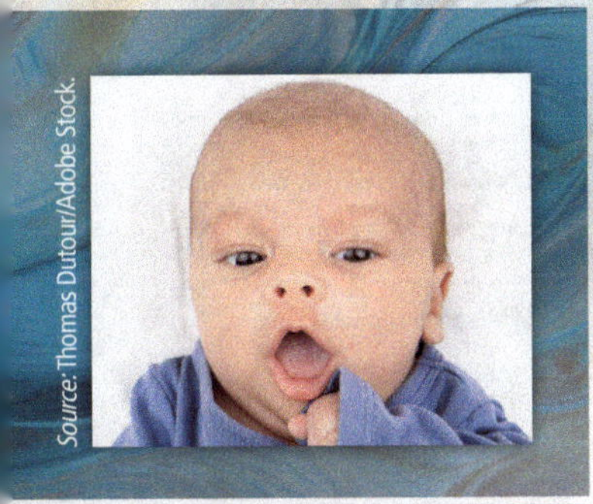



CHAPTER 17

# Ophthalmic System

Lori Baas Rubarth and Jocquelin V. Jones

## INTRODUCTION

Newborn eyes develop during intrauterine life, making them susceptible to malformation, deformation, and disruption injuries. Congenital anomalies, congenital infections, and prematurity can affect visual acuity, leading to blindness. Other maternal or neonatal diseases can affect the eyes. Early detection and treatment of eye disorders are essential for the best possible outcome for the newborn.

This chapter outlines the embryologic development of the eye, reviews the methods of assessment of a newborn's eyes, describes specific ophthalmic disorders of the eye, and describes diseases that can affect the eyes, including prematurity. Nursing care of the patient and family will be discussed.

## EMBRYOLOGY

Eye development begins during early embryogenesis with the formation of a single eye field or optic sulcus on the neural plate within the forebrain area (Schoenwolf et al., 2021). Many transcription factors early in development regulate and induce eye development. Without these transcription factors and other enzymes or proteins, anomalies can occur. The initial single-eye field is stimulated by the sonic hedgehog protein to split into two separate optic fields. Without this early splitting stimulation, holoprosencephaly (failure of the brain to split into two hemispheres) and cyclopia (a single, midline eye) would occur (Schoenwolf et al., 2021). Lack of transcription factors leads to anomalies such as anophthalmia (absence of the eye) or microphthalmia (small eye).

The eye develops from the following embryonic tissues: ectoderm, neuroectoderm, neural crest cells, and mesoderm. The lens develops from the ectoderm during the 5th to 7th week. The cornea develops from ectoderm and mesoderm. The pigmented epithelium and part of the retina develop from neuroectoderm. The ciliary and iris muscles, part of the choroid, and the sclera develop from neural crest cells. Part of the choroid also develops from mesoderm (see Figure 17.1).

At about 22 days after fertilization, lateral grooves form, which marks the early placement of the eyes in the embryo (Schoenwolf et al., 2021). Bilateral invaginations of the neural

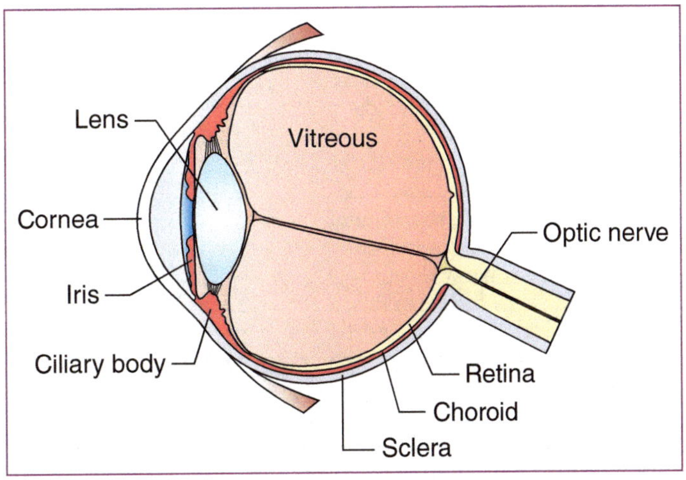



**FIGURE 17.1** Anatomy of the eye.

tube occur with the formation of the optic vesicles. These two optic vesicles remain in contact with the developing brain via the optic stalk (later becoming the optic nerve). By about 32 to 34 days, the optic vesicles change shape to appear as a "goblet" with an additional invagination of ectoderm inward becoming the lens of the eye (Schoenwolf et al., 2021, p. 480). The fibers within the lens become transparent with the assistance of crystallins, which are soluble proteins within the eye. With the invagination of the optic cup, there are two layers formed, which develop into the inner retina containing rods and cones and the outer melanin layer containing pigmented epithelium. These two layers of the retina do not fuse completely but can separate, causing a retinal detachment with many types of trauma to the head. Both layers expand over the lens from the edges of the optic cup, becoming the iris. The color of the iris is either light blue or gray at birth but becomes fully developed with increased pigment by about 6 months of age.

Cellular differentiation and development continue within the eye throughout fetal life. Macular differentiation occurs during the 6th month, and the fovea centralis, the area needed for sharp, high-acuity vision, does not mature until months into the postpartum period (Schoenwolf et al., 2021). Therefore, the term newborn's vision is present but limited during the first few days and weeks of life. Newborns are most interested in high-contrast shapes that are about 8 to 12 inches from the eyes.

The eyelids develop as surface ectoderm folds over the cornea by about the 6th week of fetal life. The eyelids fuse together by the 8th week but separate again sometime between the 5th and 7th months of fetal life. The lacrimal glands form from ectoderm but are still immature until about 6 weeks after birth (Schoenwolf et al., 2021). Tear production in newborns is limited until that time.

## ASSESSMENT AND EXAMINATION TECHNIQUES

### History

With an evaluation of the eye, it is important to understand the background of neonatal eye disorders (see "Other Disorders That Affect the Eyes" in this chapter). Understanding these disorders can assist the nurse in determining whether there are any risk factors for eye problems such as maternal diabetes, prematurity, alcohol consumption, or congenital diseases. The nurse can question the parents or view the maternal medical record to determine known family, maternal, or perinatal risk factors associated with vision problems. Look specifically for exposure to infectious diseases such as gonorrhea, chlamydia, rubella, or cytomegalovirus (CMV), which are known to cause significant eye problems in newborns. Look at the perinatal history for signs of hypoxia or anoxia (e.g., low Apgar scores) or other conditions associated with possible damage to the brain, including vision. Parents who have had a previous preterm birth may already have knowledge of or experience with retinopathy of prematurity (ROP). Nurses also need to understand the terminology involved in newborn eye assessment (Table 17.1).

**TABLE 17.1**

**NEWBORN EYE ASSESSMENT TERMINOLOGY**

| Definitions | |
|---|---|
| Amblyopia | Known as "lazy eye," where one eye wanders from a straight line of vision |
| Aniridia | Much or all the iris is missing |
| Anisometropia | A major difference in refractive error between the eyes |
| Anophthalmos | Complete absence of the ocular tissue within the orbit |
| Anti-mongoloid slant | An inner canthus that is higher than the outer canthus |
| Blennorrhea | Excessive mucus discharge from the eye |
| Brushfield spots | Speckled iris; frequently associated with Down syndrome |
| Coloboma | Defect or opening that results from failure of part of the eye to close during embryogenesis; can occur in the iris or eyelids |
| Ectropion | A condition in which the eyelid is turned outward |
| Endophthalmitis | Inflammation of the internal eye tissues and fluid |
| Epicanthal fold | Skin that appears to overlap and partially obscuring the inner canthus |
| Epiphora | Excessive tearing |
| Esotropia | Inward deviation of the eyes, presents as "cross-eyed" |
| Exophthalmos | An eye that appears to be bulging |
| Exotropia | Outward deviation of the eyes |
| Fovea | Center of macula where the eyesight is the sharpest |

*(continued)*

**TABLE 17.1**

**NEWBORN EYE ASSESSMENT TERMINOLOGY (*continued*)**

| Definitions | |
|---|---|
| Heterochromia | Pigmentation of the two irises is different |
| Hyperopia | Far-sighted |
| Hypertelorism | Increased interorbital distance or wide space between the eyes |
| Inner canthus | The angle of the eyelid nearest the nose |
| Interpupillary distance | The distance between the centers of each pupil |
| Leukocoria | "White" reflex, instead of red |
| Microphthalmia/ microphthalmos | Small eyes |
| Mongoloid slant | An outer canthus that is higher than the inner canthus |
| Myopia | Near-sightedness |
| Nystagmus | The involuntary rhythmic or oscillating movements of the eyes |
| Outer canthus | The outer angle of the eyelid |
| Palpebral fissure (width) | Width of the eyelid opening from inner canthus to outer canthus (fissure = opening) |
| Proptosis | Bulging of the eyes (exophthalmos) |
| Ptosis | Drooping of the upper eyelid |
| Strabismus | Cross-eyed; a condition where the eyes aim in different directions |
| Synophrys | An abnormal extension of the eyebrows so that they meet in the middle (midline) |
| Telecanthus | Widened space between the inner canthi of the eyelids |

## Examination

After birth, a screening examination of the eye is indicated. A full eye exam is not practical or indicated unless the newborn presents with some eye pathology. A knowledge of eye anatomy is important for examination of the eye (Figure 17.1). For a newborn screening exam, the external eye, eyelids, pupillary response, and red reflex are the major components. During the exam, the newborn should be quiet, awake, and alert. Dimming the lights or a darkened room will assist with the pupillary assessment exam. Holding the infant upright can facilitate the spontaneous opening of the eyes. It is important to protect the eye from injury and still evaluate as much of the eyes as possible. This requires a gentle opening of the eyes without stress on the infant and without scratching of the eyes. One hand is usually used to open the eyelids with two fingers, while the other hand holds the ophthalmoscope or light source. A second examiner is helpful during an examination of the eyes. Premature infant eye exams may be delayed until approximately 32 weeks of gestation or longer for evaluation of the pupils and retina.

### External Eye

Examination of the external features of the eye begins with inspection. Newborn eyes are examined for shape, symmetry, and size, as well as the presence of eyebrows and eyelashes. The eyes should appear clear, symmetric in size, and without discharge.

### Eyelids

The eyelids are examined for movement, redness, swelling, colobomas or other abnormalities. Infants with an inability to open their eyelids or who have ptosis (drooping) of one or both eyelids can develop amblyopia and poor visual development. Infants must be able to view images on the retina during the first months of life for normal vision to occur (Pineles & Isenberg, 2021). Deprivation amblyopia due to drooping eyelids can lead to poor vision. The presence of unusual folds (e.g. epicanthal folds near the inner canthus) and the slant of the eye (upwards or downwards) should be noted.

### Pupils

The pupils are examined for size, shape, symmetry, and reaction to light. An examination with an ophthalmoscope is indicated to check for the red reflex. The color, clarity, and intensity of the red reflex should be checked and compared bilaterally. In dark-skinned infants, the red reflex may be more of a dull red or gray rather than a bright red (Adams, 2021; Toli et al., 2021). Different races or ethnicities have different layers of retinal pigment, which can appear darker depending on the reflected light, but no studies have compared these differences (Subhi et al., 2021). It can be difficult to obtain a red reflex on premature infants under 28 weeks of gestation due to cloudy corneas, cloudy vitreous, and the vasculature of the lens. A "white" reflex (leukocoria) would indicate a blockage of light getting to the retina. The differential diagnosis of leukocoria includes cataract, retinoblastoma, persistent fetal vasculature, retinal detachment (from ROP or Norrie disease, Peter's anomaly, and Coats disease) (Pineles & Isenberg, 2021; Oatts et al., 2024). If dark spots are noted, this could be due to cataracts, retinal damage, or retinal hemorrhage.

**TABLE 17.2**

**EXTERNAL EYE DIMENSIONS (TERM NEWBORN)**

| | |
|---|---|
| Interpupillary distance | 33–46 mm (average 39 mm) |
| Inner canthal distance | 13–26 mm (average 20 mm) |
| Palpebral width (medial to lateral canthus) | 17–22 mm (average 18 mm) |
| Pupil size (in darkened room) | 2.5–4.4 mm |
| Premature (26–28 weeks) size | 3.0–5.0 mm |
| Cornea size (horizontal diameter) | 9–10 mm<br>< 9 mm = microcornea<br>> 11 mm = megalocornea |

*Sources:* Adapted from: Jones, K. L., Jones, M. C., & del Campo, M. (2022). Normal standards—Facial measurements. In *Smith's recognizable patterns of human malformation* (8th ed., pp. 973–998). Elsevier; Örge, F. H., & Salem, Z. M. (2024). Examination and common problems in the neonatal eye. In R. J. Martin & A. A. Fanaroff (Eds.), *Fanaroff & Martin's neonatal-perinatal medicine: Diseases of the fetus and infant* (12th ed.). Elsevier, Table 99.22; Pineles, S. L., & Isenberg, S. J. (2021). Eye disorders: Growth and development of the eye. In J. P. Boardman, A. M. Groves, & J. Ramasethu (Eds.), *Avery & MacDonald's neonatology: Pathophysiology and management of the newborn* (8th ed., pp. 891–904). Wolters Kluwer, Figure 58.3 and pp. 891–892; and Scanlon, J. W., Nelson, T., Grylack, L. J., & Smith, Y. F. (1979). A system of newborn physical examination (p. 57). University Park Press.

A significant variation between the two eyes would need further retinal assessment. The onset of pupillary constriction in response to light can be elicited by about 30 to 34 weeks' gestation. Interpupillary distance and pupil size can also be assessed (Table 17.2).

## Cornea

The cornea is the clear layer covering the pupil and the iris. The two corneas are examined for clarity and size (see Table 17.2). A cloudy cornea may be caused by congenital glaucoma, inborn errors of metabolism, or congenital stromal corneal dystrophy. Preterm or low birth weight (LBW) infants may also have a transient haziness of the cornea during the first week of life. A cloudy cornea is almost always indicative of a serious eye problem. Trauma at birth from forceps can also result in injury to the cornea, giving the cornea a hazy appearance.

## Iris and Lens

The iris is examined for coloboma and color. The iris or eye color of newborns is usually blue, gray, or light brown. Black infants have darker iris colors due to earlier melanin deposition. The full deposition of color in most infant eyes occurs by 6 months of age. Heterochromia is a color variation where the two eyes are different colors, or it can be that there are two colors within the same eye. Heterochromia can be a clue to the development of other disorders, including Sturge–Weber syndrome (with port-wine stain), Waardenburg syndrome, or Hirschsprung disease, and would indicate the need for further follow-up (Oatts et al., 2024). The iris is examined for coloboma resembling a keyhole within the pupil. The presence of coloboma may also indicate a need to look for abnormalities in other systems, such as fetal alcohol syndrome (FAS). Infants with FAS can have colobomas, cataracts, and microphthalmos. The presence of these findings should alert the nurse to look for other features of the syndrome. The maternal history should also be reevaluated for alcohol use during the pregnancy.

The lens is located behind the iris. A cataract results in a cloudy or white, opaque lens. A pediatric ophthalmologist needs to evaluate any cataract found in a newborn as soon as possible to determine if it is visually significant. Surgery would be performed to remove vision-threatening cataracts as soon possible.

## Sclera

The sclera is examined for color and hemorrhages. The sclera of term infants should be white in color. The infant sclera can take on a bluish-white appearance in the premature infant due to the thinness of the sclera. In term infants, a blue sclera is indicative of possible osteogenesis imperfecta. Subconjunctival hemorrhages are frequently visualized on the sclera of normal, healthy-term infants following a vaginal delivery due to the pressure changes throughout the birthing process resulting in small, capillary breakage. They present no significant long-term complications.

## Eye Movements

It is also important to note the infant's eye movements during the exam. In the neonate, the location or position of the eyes varies with immaturity and/or activity. Many infants display deviations in eye movements, exhibiting exotropia, esotropia, or nystagmus (see Table 17.1). These are types of eye wandering or twitching movements of the eye that occur in almost all infants and are considered normal during the newborn period. These eye movements should disappear within the first few months of life. Any persistent deviation needs to be evaluated.

## Vision

The infant's vision can also be assessed immediately after birth. Infants will look around at objects in the environment. Newborns can follow an object when placed in front of them. A term newborn's vision is immature. Determining a newborn's visual acuity cannot be done easily and will not be discussed as an examination method in this textbook. However, understanding the infant's vision progression is necessary for caring for these infants. All newborns are born with some degree of myopia or nearsightedness and appear to see best at about 8 to 10 inches from their faces. Infants appear to enjoy highly contrasted (black and white) objects, especially faces in the environment (Brown et al., 2015; Oatts et al., 2024). Infant vision improves during the first year of life.

Premature infants have a higher incidence of refractive errors, including myopia, hyperopia, and astigmatism (Kaya et al., 2017; Zhu et al., 2017). Many of these eye disorders are corrected with eyeglasses.

### Measurements

During an eye exam, it can be difficult to assess whether an eye is larger or smaller than normal. Therefore, certain measurements can be taken and compared to published data (see Table 17.2). These measurements can be obtained during an eye exam. The interpupillary distance and the width of the palpebral fissure can be determined, and abnormal values can indicate an underlying syndrome, such as the small eyes of FAS. The interpupillary distance determines whether the eyes are spaced correctly. Hypotelorism and hypertelorism are abnormalities where the eyes are either too close together or widely spaced. The palpebral fissure is the eye opening and can be determined if the opening appears smaller than normal.

### Retinal Examination

Although routine retinal examinations on all normal newborns are not indicated, a retinal exam or ophthalmology consult is indicated for the premature infant at risk for ROP or if physical exam findings suggest serious problems, such as cataracts or glaucoma. In addition, a retinal exam can be done with an ophthalmoscope and pupil dilation if needed to rule out abuse or trauma in older infants. Many newborns born by spontaneous vaginal deliveries will have retinal hemorrhages after birth, most often bilateral, between the optic discs and the macula (Oatts et al., 2024). The risk of retinal hemorrhage is greater with vacuum-assisted and instrument-assisted deliveries with a vacuum (about 50%) and decreased with an uncomplicated cesarean section (Cleveland Clinic, n.d.). Most retinal hemorrhages from birth resolve within one to 6 weeks; however, resolution of retinal hemorrhages may be delayed if labor is induced or forceps are used for the delivery (Oatts et al., 2024). Shaken baby syndrome would need to be part of a differential diagnosis of retinal hemorrhage seen after a month or longer of age.

**Eye Drops.** Specific eye drops are used routinely to dilate the eyes in newborns who require a retinal examination. These medications, which are adrenergic agonists (phenylephrine) and cholinergic antagonists (cyclopentolate), can be absorbed into the newborn's systemic circulation. Complications from dilatation medications need to be observed in the premature or term infant undergoing a retinal exam. These systemic effects are hypertension, tachycardia, arrhythmias, feeding intolerance, seizures, and skin rashes (Oatts et al., 2024). As a result, intracranial and intraventricular hemorrhage (IVH), necrotizing enterocolitis (NEC), and other major insults can occur, especially in a premature infant.

To decrease infant absorption, excess medications must be readily cleaned away from the skin to prevent systemic absorption. Applying pressure to the lacrimal sac for 1 to 2 minutes after instillation may minimize reabsorption.

After a retinal examination, the infant's eyes should be shielded from light or covered with eye shields until the pupils return to normal size. Dilated eyes exposed to bright lights may cause pain, distress, agitation, apnea, or bradycardia (Oatts et al., 2024).

# NEONATAL CONJUNCTIVITIS

Neonatal conjunctivitis or ophthalmia neonatorum ("pink eye") is an eye infection or inflammation of the conjunctiva or covering of the eyes, causing redness, swelling, and discharge within the first 4 weeks or 30 days of life. It can occur due to a bacteria, virus, or other pathogen, often in the vaginal canal at birth. Aseptic conjunctivitis can occur because of a chemical reaction to eye medication administered after birth, which rarely occurs with erythromycin ointment. The incidence of septic neonatal conjunctivitis with either gonorrhea or chlamydia in the United States is low (about 1%–2%) (Gomella, 2020). Chlamydial infection has replaced gonorrhea as the most common cause of eye infection in the United States and many other countries. Gonorrhea remains the most serious type of conjunctivitis in the United States. Septic neonatal conjunctivitis usually manifests with a discharge that develops shortly after birth. Because the origins of newborn conjunctivitis can vary, it is important to determine the exact cause of the infection. In some cases of conjunctivitis, rapid treatment is important to prevent vision loss.

The presentation of neonatal conjunctivitis varies with the cause of the inflammation or infection. Some findings, such as purulent eye discharge and erythema and edema of the eyelids, are present in almost all cases. Transient tearing or watery discharge may be noticed early in the infection process.

## Eye Prophylaxis for Ophthalmia Neonatorum

Most of the United States has required prophylaxis against newborn gonorrheal conjunctivitis for many years. Today, some states allow parents to refuse prophylactic eye treatment at birth for their newborns, such as in New York and Tennessee. Erythromycin ophthalmic ointment (0.5%) has been the only CDC-recommended therapy for prophylaxis of ophthalmia neonatorum available in the United States in recent years (American Academy of Pediatrics [AAP], 2024; Gomella, 2020).

Silver nitrate ($AgNO_3$) was used initially in 1881 as the prophylactic agent against ophthalmia neonatorum caused by *Neisseria gonorrhea* and other bacteria. One drop of 1% $AgNO_3$ into the eyes of newborns prevented gonococcal infection, corneal scarring, and possible blindness. During the early 1900s, many state legislatures passed laws requiring physicians to treat all newborns with a $AgNO_3$ solution to prevent blindness in newborns. Although penicillin was discovered in the late 1940s, $AgNO_3$ remained the main prophylactic agent until the mid-1990s. Silver nitrate was effective against *Neisseria gonorrhea* and most bacteria but not effective against chlamydia organisms. For this reason, erythromycin ointment is now used for routine prophylaxis in newborn eyes after birth. Erythromycin and tetracycline ointments are both effective against a variety of microorganisms, including chlamydia and gonorrhea. Still, they must be inserted into the eye and must be done soon after birth to prevent gonorrhea from invading the eye and possibly causing blindness (AAP, 2024; Oatts et al., 2024).

There has been discussion in the literature as to whether eye prophylaxis with any medication is still needed (AAP, 2024; Franco & Hammerschlag, 2023). Obstetric physician groups and their associations have promoted the screening of pregnant women for gonorrhea and chlamydia during each pregnancy. Therefore, prophylaxis of all newborns may no longer be necessary if the pregnant woman gets screened and then treated for either of the sexually transmitted infections (STIs). The treatment of all infants with antibiotics leads to resistant strains of organisms, making it more difficult to treat the patients. There is controversy, but at this point, the AAP has determined that continuing to prophylactically treat all patients to prevent blindness in those infants whose mothers did not have prenatal care or were without adequate screening or treatment (Curry et al., 2019; Franco & Hammerschlag, 2023).

Universal erythromycin prophylaxis mainly protects against *Neisseria gonorrhea* conjunctivitis. The AAP supported the continued use of universal neonatal eye prophylaxis in compliance with the CDC and U.S. Preventive Services Task Force (USPSTF) (AAP, 2024; Curry et al., 2019). The AAP Policy Statement on home birth deliveries reconfirmed that every newborn infant should receive eye prophylaxis against gonococcal ophthalmia neonatorum, as directed by local laws and regulations, whether born at home or in the hospital (Curry et al., 2019; Watterberg, 2021; Watterberg et al., 2020). Other countries are evaluating the need for eye prophylaxis. A few countries eliminated routine eye prophylaxis without an increase in ophthalmia neonatorum or blindness (Nolt, et al., 2022).

Recently, parents have questioned the necessity of many of the routine perinatal practices performed in the hospital. One of these practices is the eye ointment prophylaxis. Many parents will agree to the eye ointment if applied after the mother has had time to bond with her newborn, look into the eyes, and have the infant "see" her and the father. Usually, waiting about an hour is acceptable for the parents to administer the ointment. But it cannot be forgotten, which is why most facilities mandate giving it immediately after birth. If a mother declines to have the eye ointment applied to her infant's eyes after birth, a detailed history of negative screenings for *Neisseria gonorrhea* and *Chlamydia trachomatis* would need to be obtained and documented in the medical record (Nolt, 2022). There should also be a discussion with the parent(s) concerning the need to get immediate care if any eye discharge is noted after discharge. The main goal is to prevent newborn ocular complications.

There have been shortages of erythromycin (0.5%) ophthalmic ointment in the United States. Most other ocular medications have not been recommended for prophylaxis; therefore, if the erythromycin ointment is not available and a parent's test for gonorrheal infection is positive or not available at discharge, the newborn should be given one dose of ceftriaxone. A dose of 25 to 50 mg/kg IV or IM should be given prior to discharge, with a maximum dose of 125 mg (Gomella, 2020; Nolt et al., 2022).

## Chlamydial Conjunctivitis (Inclusion Conjunctivitis)

*Chlamydia trachomatis* is the most common cause of conjunctivitis in the newborn. The bacteria are transmitted from the infected mother to the infant at birth, and conjunctivitis may appear at about 5 to 14 days of life (Gomella, 2020; Oatts et al., 2024). The condition may be mild or moderate, and with proper treatment, it resolves within 6 weeks. Pneumonitis or chlamydial pneumonia can occur with conjunctivitis. Clinical symptoms of conjunctivitis include swelling of the eyelids and an initial watery discharge progressing to a mild, mucopurulent discharge. Chronic infection can lead to more serious consequences, such as conjunctival scarring, adhesions of the eyelid, and deposits of connective tissue under the cornea, which can result in blindness (Gomella, 2020).

Generally not a serious eye infection, a chlamydial pneumonia can develop, resulting in long-term respiratory consequences. Systemic therapy with oral erythromycin for 3 weeks is often necessary to eradicate the organism from the respiratory tract.

## Gonorrheal Conjunctivitis

Routine prophylaxis of newborns has greatly reduced the incidence of gonorrheal conjunctivitis. Because of the potential for blindness, early detection and prompt treatment are critical. Gonorrheal conjunctivitis typically manifests in the first 3 to 5 days after birth as an acute, purulent, bilateral conjunctivitis with eyelid edema (Lieberman et al., 2023). If not treated appropriately and quickly, the infection may progress to corneal ulceration, endophthalmitis, and perforation of the globe (Oatts et al., 2024). Gram stains and cultures should be performed routinely in all cases of neonatal conjunctivitis. The presence of *Neisseria gonorrhea* confirms the diagnosis. Treatment consists of the administration of IV or IM antibiotics and the application of topical antibiotics to the eye.

## Staphylococcal Conjunctivitis

Staphylococcal conjunctivitis is a bacterial infection usually acquired during vaginal delivery or by contact with an infected individual. Symptoms normally appear about 2 to 4 weeks after birth. In most cases, the conjunctivitis is mild and produces a purulent discharge. It may progress to corneal ulceration, endophthalmitis, or generalized skin infection. The diagnosis is made with cultures and Gram stain. Because staphylococci can be found in the conjunctiva of healthy neonates, laboratory results should be interpreted cautiously. Treatment includes application of topical antibiotic ointment and cleansing of exudate from the eyelids.

## Herpes Simplex Conjunctivitis

Herpes simplex infection at birth may be a feature of either localized or systemic disease. The newborn is usually infected during passage through the birth canal. Infants with herpes conjunctivitis exhibit eyelid swelling, inflammation, and corneal opacification. The onset of conjunctivitis usually occurs about 2 to 14 days after birth (Kabani & Kimberlin, 2018). The disseminated form of the disease may also lead to chorioretinitis, microphthalmia, cataracts, optic atrophy, apnea, respiratory distress, and death (James & Kimberlin, 2015). This disease should always be kept in mind when the mother or father has a history of genital herpes. Treatment should be instituted immediately upon diagnosis. Systemic treatment (IV) is necessary for infants whose conjunctivitis has spread to become a systemic infection.

### Infectious Conjunctivitis Caused by Other Microorganisms

Some case reports have described neonatal infectious conjunctivitis caused by other more unusual microorganisms. This is a rare occurrence but has been seen with a term infant readmitted at 10 days of age with conjunctivitis caused by *Neisseria meningitides*, a gram-negative meningococcal disease (Chacon-Cruz et al., 2017) and another term infant presenting on day of life 12 with conjunctivitis caused by *Neisseria cinerea* (Lieberman et al., 2023). These infants require local and systemic treatment. *Neisseria meningitidis* can cause a serious, systemic infection with significant morbidity and mortality and needs to be considered in an ill infant with purulent conjunctivitis.

Premature infants in the neonatal intensive care units (NICU) frequently are colonized with *Pseudomonas aeruginosa* or a variety of *Candida* species. These infants often will develop a purulent mucus discharge from the eyes. The infants may also develop simultaneous systemic infections. Eye involvement is usually limited to chorioretinitis that resolves with systemic antifungal therapy but requires both local and systemic treatment because there is poor penetration into the eye vitreous from the systemic circulation (AAP, 2024). The very low birth weight (VLBW) infants are at risk for more serious and deadly complications of any infection; therefore, they require adequate initial and rapid treatment. Conjunctivitis has also occurred in preterm infants with coagulase-negative *Staphylococcus*, *Klebsiella pneumonia*, *Escherichia coli*, methicillin-susceptible or -resistant *Staphylococcus aureus*, *Enterococcus* species, and various types of viruses. Ophthalmology consultation is also recommended for systemic or local conjunctival infections.

## LACRIMAL DYSFUNCTION

### Obstructed Nasolacrimal Duct

Blockage of the nasolacrimal duct occurs when the duct fails to canalize at the entrance to the nose, leaving a thin membrane. This blockage occurs in about 5% of all newborns and is a common cause of chronic conjunctivitis in infants (Oatts et al., 2024). After a month of age, the infant shows excessive tearing and mucus discharge in the inner canthal region. Pressure on the lacrimal sac area usually causes pus or mucus to exude from the opening. Because the problem resolves spontaneously in most affected infants by 6 months of age, conservative treatment involving lacrimal massage and application of topical antibiotics is recommended. Dacryocystitis can occur because of this temporary obstruction. Dacryocystitis is a secondary infection of the lacrimal sac. Obstruction that lasts beyond 6 to 12 months may require lacrimal probing. Nasolacrimal duct blockage should be differentiated from other causes of conjunctivitis, a foreign body on the eye, or corneal injury.

### Mucocele

Mucoceles occur because of the one-way valve effect at the end of the nasolacrimal duct. Mucus accumulates, or amniotic fluid is trapped in the nasolacrimal sac, and the infant develops a bluish mass in the inferomedial region of the eyelid. This swelling is most often confused with a hemangioma. If simple massage does not decompress the mucocele, probing the nasolacrimal duct may be necessary.

## CONGENITAL DEFECTS

### Aniridia

Aniridia is a severe ocular abnormality that manifests as a bilateral absence of the iris. Cataracts, corneal pannus (fine blood vessel growth on the cornea), macular dysfunction, and glaucoma usually accompany the defect. Most of these infants have significantly diminished visual acuity. About a third of infants with the noninherited form of aniridia eventually develop Wilms' tumor of the kidney (Pineles & Isenberg, 2021).

### Persistent Hyperplastic Primary Vitreous

Persistent hyperplastic primary vitreous is a unilateral disorder that affects both genders equally. It results from the persistence of the hyaloid vessels that connect the optic nerve and the posterior surface of the lens during fetal development. It should be considered in the differential diagnosis of leukocoria. The involved eye is usually small with an absent red reflex. Surgery may improve the eye's integrity, and useful vision is sometimes restored.

### Nevus Simplex and Hemangioma of the Eyelid

Nevus simplex vascular malformations are relatively common lesions in newborns and tend to occur on the eyelids and nape of the neck. They are sometimes referred to as "salmon patches" or "stork bites". They usually disappear over time and require no treatment (Gomez & Admani, 2023). The larger and deeper strawberry hemangiomas tend to enlarge, stabilize, and then regress by the time the child is between 5 to 10 years old. The hemangiomas are vascular malformations that usually are elevated and reddish purple at their peak size. The larger and deeper hemangiomas are called *cavernous hemangiomas*, which usually grow under the skin. No treatment is usually necessary, but it would depend on the location of the growth. Superficial tumors of the eyelid may cause cosmetic and visual problems. Parents often are concerned with hemangiomas on the face or near the eyes/eyelids and want them removed, but no treatment is the best option to prevent scarring. Pressure on the eye from a hemangioma tumor may result in significant astigmatism and, subsequently, amblyopia. Hemangiomas may be treated with surgical removal, radiation, or steroid injections. Tumors that are exclusively cosmetic should be allowed to regress without intervention.

Another type of hemangioma is called the port-wine stain because of its dark-purple pigmentation and location on the face. It is also called *nevus flammeus* and is associated with

Sturge–Weber syndrome. These birthmarks are extensive and usually removed with laser therapy.

## Ptosis

Ptosis is a drooping of one or both eyelids due to neurologic, muscular, or mechanical factors. If the ptosis is significant enough to cover all or part of the pupil, amblyopia may result. If bilateral ptosis is present, the infant may have slowed motor development and delayed ambulation later in life. Congenital ptosis is usually caused by an abnormality in the development of the levator palpebrae muscle, but other causes may be related to third nerve palsy or congenital Horner syndrome (Oatts et al., 2024). A thorough family history should be obtained, as well as ruling out birth trauma to the cervical ganglion. Direct trauma to the eyelid or a tumor in the eyelid may also cause ptosis. Surgical repair corrects this defect.

## Congenital Glaucoma

Primary congenital glaucoma occurs when there is a rise in the intraocular pressure causing enlargement of the eye with a cloudy cornea. This increased pressure results in damage to the optic nerve. Glaucoma is rare in newborns, but because of the potential for blindness, it must be detected early and treated. The newborn shows tearing, light sensitivity, eyelid spasms, and a large, cloudy cornea. The diagnosis can often be missed in the newborn period but diagnosed at about 2 to 3 months of age, at which time consultation with a pediatric ophthalmologist is essential. Conditions associated with glaucoma include trisomy 21, congenital rubella, Marfan syndrome, neurofibromatosis, oculodentodigital syndrome, Rieger syndrome, Sturge–Weber syndrome (about 50% of these infants will have glaucoma), Rubinstein–Taybi syndrome, and Weill–Marchesani syndrome (Örge & Salem, 2024; Sánchez-Espino et al., 2023).

Congenital glaucoma must be differentiated from other diseases that have similar symptoms. Nasolacrimal duct obstruction involves tearing but does not cause light sensitivity or a cloudy cornea. Difficult labor or forceps injury may damage the cornea and cause temporary clouding, but the intraocular pressure is not elevated, which is a hallmark feature of glaucoma. The large eyes of the infant with congenital glaucoma may appear beautiful to the parents, but health professionals should be alert to the possibility of this disease.

The abnormality in congenital glaucoma is a deformity of the filtering system that controls the level of intraocular pressure in the eye. Congenital glaucoma is treated surgically. The results usually are good, but parents must be educated about the need for continued monitoring of this condition throughout the child's life.

## Congenital Cataracts

The causes of significant lens opacity in the newborn are numerous. Cataracts are a significant cause of blindness because they may interfere with the process of visual development early in the infant's life. For this reason, visually significant cataracts must be detected and treated before they cause amblyopia, which may be unresponsive to the most persistent treatment.

Heredity is an important cause of congenital cataracts. A thorough family history is critical in determining the cause of the lens opacity. The inheritance pattern may be autosomal dominant, or recessive, or sex linked. Maternal history of diabetes, x-ray exposure, or malnutrition may be an important factor in cataract formation. In premature infants, transient cataracts or insignificant opacities are commonly seen because of remnants of developmental tissues. ROP can lead to cataracts in premature infants. Several inborn errors of metabolism cause cataracts, including galactosemia, Alport syndrome, Fabry disease, and Lowe syndrome (Ryzewski et al., 2021). Intrauterine rubella, CMV, toxoplasmosis, or herpes simplex infection are associated with neonatal cataracts.

Cataract surgery early in life is critical to the infant's visual rehabilitation. Useful vision is especially difficult to achieve in eyes with monocular cataracts. It is important for nurses to work closely with the infant's parents. The parents' persistence in handling contact lenses and amblyopia therapy often determines the outcome of their child's vision.

## Retinoblastoma

Retinoblastoma is a rare disorder and the most common eye neoplasm in childhood. Many tumors (about 60%) occur sporadically without a family history of the disease (somatic mutation), and the remainder are due to germline or inherited *RB1* gene transmission (Graeber, 2020). Retinoblastoma occurs in approximately 1 in 14,000 to 30,000 live births in the United States, with higher rates in other countries, such as India and Africa (Graeber, 2020; Oatts et al., 2024). Most retinoblastomas occur unilaterally, with only about 25% bilaterally, and most children are diagnosed before their second birthday (Oatts et al., 2024). With an earlier diagnosis or bilateral diagnosis, the more likely the gene is inherited from one of the parents (Dockery et al., 2023; Shields et al., 2021).

The most common presenting symptom is leukocoria. The tumor is highly malignant and may spread to the bone marrow, central nervous system (CNS), or other organs. Untreated patients rarely survive. The standard treatment for advanced cases of retinoblastoma is enucleation (removal of the eye). Less severe cases or cases diagnosed early can be treated with radiation, chemotherapy (intraarterial, intravitreal, or intracameral), transpupillary thermotherapy, or cryotherapy (Ancona-Lezama et al., 2020). Children with this tumor require close follow-up for possible recurrence after treatment. Parents must be educated about the disease so that they are aware of the need for constant monitoring of their child. Genetic testing of parents for the gene mutation is highly recommended for the best follow-up of the child.

# CONGENITAL INFECTIONS

## Cytomegalovirus Infection

Most infants with CMV will be asymptomatic. However, in infants with symptomatic disease, ocular lesions may include chorioretinitis, optic nerve atrophy, strabismus, cataracts, macular scarring, and visual impairment or blindness. Many infants with symptomatic CMV disease will have moderate-to-severe visual impairment (Khazaeni, 2017). Parents should be advised to seek routine eye screenings during childhood and later in life.

## Rubella

Congenital rubella, or German measles, has virtually been eliminated in the United States due to its vaccination program. However, the virus can still be found in other parts of the world; therefore, with international travel and parents withholding vaccinations, rubella has come back. The rubella virus is responsible for many eye complications, including cataracts, glaucoma, and microphthalmia, often together. The majority of newborns with congenital rubella have hearing, eye, and cardiac defects. Parents of a child with congenital rubella must understand that vision problems may occur at any time, and their child must be screened regularly.

## Herpes Simplex Virus

Herpes simplex virus (HSV) causes a wide variety of eye disorders in newborns. Though skin vesicles are the main sign of a HSV infection in the newborn, eye damage and CNS manifestations can also occur. An eye exam would be essential if skin lesions are present. Eye conditions that can be seen with a HSV infection are conjunctivitis, chorioretinitis, and cataracts (Kabani & Kimberlin, 2018; Oatts et al., 2024).

## Varicella

Although rare, congenital infection caused by varicella, commonly known as chickenpox, produces eye anomalies in more than half of affected infants. These defects include microphthalmia, chorioretinitis, cataract, nystagmus, anisocoria (unequal pupils), and Horner syndrome (Obi, 2024).

## Toxoplasmosis

*Toxoplasma gondii* is a parasitic organism with an affinity for brain and eye tissue. As with many other congenital infections, ocular anomalies vary depending on fetal age at the time of infection. The most common clinical presentation is chorioretinitis (often bilateral). Chorioretinitis is part of the classic triad of congenital toxoplasmosis with hydrocephalus and intracranial calcifications. Ocular manifestations occur in about 75% of newborns with toxoplasmosis and, in some infants, can be the only sign of infection (Oatts et al., 2024; Pineles & Isenberg, 2021). Other signs that can occur in the newborn are microphthalmia, strabismus, retinal scarring and detachment, and blindness (Pineles & Isenberg, 2021). A history of cleaning out cat litter boxes during pregnancy may be helpful in the diagnosis of toxoplasmosis because cats are the host for this parasite.

## Lymphocytic Choriomeningitis Virus

Another viral infection, lymphocytic choriomeningitis virus (LCV), can also cause ocular defects. LCV is a single-strand RNA virus found in rodents, including house mice and hamsters. Outbreaks of LCV infection associated with mice tend to occur in trailer parks, inner-city dwellings, and substandard housing. The virus is probably transmitted by airborne droplets and food contaminated by rodent urine or feces. It also may be transmitted by the bite of an infected animal (Kinori et al., 2018).

Congenital LCV results in many ocular findings, including generalized chorioretinitis leading to scarring, optic nerve atrophy, nystagmus, and strabismus. Eye abnormalities may be the first or only manifestation noted initially with this viral infection (Kinori et al., 2018). Newborns with congenital infections are at significant risk for neurologic damage and death.

## Endogenous Endophthalmitis

Endogenous endophthalmitis is a rare complication that can occur in neonates with systemic sepsis, usually premature or VLBW infants. Infants with sepsis have many microorganisms in their bloodstream. These organisms can cross into the eye and cause vision loss or blindness (Papudesu et al., 2020).

# RETINOPATHY OF PREMATURITY

ROP is a vasoproliferative disease of the retina affecting preterm infants. It affects the normal development of retinal vascularization and is the leading preventable cause of blindness and visual impairments in infants and young children. In 1942, Dr. Theodore Terry first reported the proliferation of abnormal blood vessels in the retina of a newborn. Terry described the disease as a grayish-white vascular membrane or a fibrous growth behind the lens that progressed to retinal detachment in premature infants. The condition was named *retrolental fibroplasia*, and the name was changed to ROP in 1984 by the International Classification of Retinopathy of Prematurity (ICROP), an international committee charged with providing a uniform classification system for the disease. This original classification system used a standard description of the location of retinopathy (using zones and clock hours), the severity of the disease (stage), the presence of special risk factors (plus disease), and the features of regression (International Committee on Retinopathy of Prematurity, 1984).

The ICROP published updates to the original classification in 2005, and in 2021, the committee presented a third edition (Chiang et al., 2021). This latest version improved the language used for diagnosing and classifying ROP due to the newer, current imaging technologies and therapies for treating ROP (e.g., anti–vascular endothelial growth factor [VEGF] injections). The new classifications also clarified the terms *regression* and *reactivation*, defined *persistent avascular retina*, as well as recommending that each eye be classified separately (Table 17.3). In describing the three zones, the committee added an area described as the "posterior zone II" (Figure 17.2).

Aggressive ROP (A-ROP) is a new term that replaced aggressive posterior retinopathy of prematurity, a term to describe a severely rapid, progressive form of ROP located in zone I or posterior zone II that quickly progressed to stage 5 ROP if left untreated. The clinical characteristics of A-ROP are the rapid development of neovascularization and severe plus disease without the typical progression of the stages of ROP. Eyes with A-ROP often develop a form of stage 3, which includes extraretinal neovascularization. The diagnostic features for A-ROP are the tempo of the disease and the presence of vascular abnormalities, not the location of the disease, which is why the term was changed. A-ROP was originally

**TABLE 17.3**

**STAGES AND CLASSIFICATIONS OF RETINOPATHY OF PREMATURITY**

| | |
|---|---|
| **Zones** | There are three zones on the retina with the addition of posterior zone 2 (added in 2021). **(See Figure 17.2)** |
| **Stage** | **Finding** |
| 1 | Demarcation line at avascular retina |
| 2 | Ridge with height and width at avascular retina |
| 3 | Ridge with fibrosis extending into vitreous (extraretinal neovascular proliferation) |
| 4 | 4A: Partial retinal detachment with fovea attached<br>4B: Partial retinal detachment with fovea detached |
| 5 | Complete retinal detachment |
| **Pre–plus disease** | Abnormal vascularization with some dilation and/or tortuosity of retinal vessels but less than that seen with plus disease |
| **Plus disease** | Dilation and tortuosity of retinal vessels |
| **Aggressive ROP** | A rapid development of neovascular proliferation and severe plus disease |
| **Extent** | Number of clock hours (12 sectors—12, 3, 6, and 9 per zone) of ROP in both eyes |
| **Late phases** (without treatment or after treatment) | Regression = Disease involution and resolution<br>Reactivation = Reoccurrence of a previous phase of the disease<br>Long-term sequelae = The occurrence of complications of disease or treatment, e.g., late detached retina, peripheral avascular retina, retinal holes, macular abnormalities, and other retinal or macula/fovea changes, and glaucoma |

*Sources:* Adapted from: Chiang, M. F., Quinn, G. E., Fielder, A. R., Ostmo, S. R., Chan, P., Berrocal, A., Binenbaum, G., Blair, M., Campbell, J. P., Capone, A., Chen, Y., Dai, S., Ells, A., Fleck, B. W., Good, W. V., Hartnett, E., Holmstrom, G., Kusaka, S., Kychenthal, A., ... Zin, A. (2021). International classification of retinopathy of prematurity. *Ophthalmology, 128*(10), e51–e68. https://doi.org/10.1016/j.ophtha.2021.05.031, Table 1, e51–e68. Oatts, J. T., de Alba Campomanes, A. G., & Binenbaum, G. (2024). Eye and vision disorders. In C. A. Gleason & T. Sawyer (Eds.), *Avery's diseases of the newborn* (11th ed., pp. 1391–1413). Elsevier, Table 96.5, p. 1408; & Pineles, S. L., & Isenberg, S. J. (2021). Eye disorders: Growth and development of the eye. In J. P. Boardman, A. M. Groves, & J. Ramasethu (Eds.), *Avery & MacDonald's neonatology: Pathophysiology and management of the newborn* (8th ed., pp. 891–904). Wolters Kluwer, Table 58.3, p. 900; Sabri, K., Ells, A. L., Lee, E. Y., Dutta, S., & Vinekar, A. (2022). Retinopathy of prematurity: A global perspective and recent developments. *Pediatrics, 150*(3), Table 1, p. 4.

described as affecting extremely premature infants, but it is increasingly occurring in larger preterm infants and areas beyond the posterior retina. The disease has a higher incidence in underdeveloped countries (Chiang et al., 2021).

ROP was responsible for an epidemic of blindness in young children in the 1940s and early 1950s until the link to supplemental oxygen therapy was made in 1952. Subsequently, the practice of limiting oxygen administration in the care of premature infants led to the near disappearance of the disorder; however, cerebral palsy and death increased. Improvements in neonatal health care in the past 35 years have increased the survival of tinier and sicker infants. As technology helped these smaller infants survive, the rate of ROP rose. The younger the gestational age and the lower the birth weight, the stronger the correlation with the incidence of ROP. Results from the Cryotherapy for Retinopathy of Prematurity (CRYO-ROP), LIGHT-ROP, and ET-ROP multicenter trials revealed that ROP occurs in 65% to 70% of premature infants with birth weights of 1,250 g or less (Early Treatment for Retinopathy of Prematurity Cooperative Group [ET-ROP], 2003, 2005; Reynolds, 2010; Reynolds et al., 2002).

Despite the improvements in healthcare, the incidence of ROP is increasing globally. A study in U.S. centers over

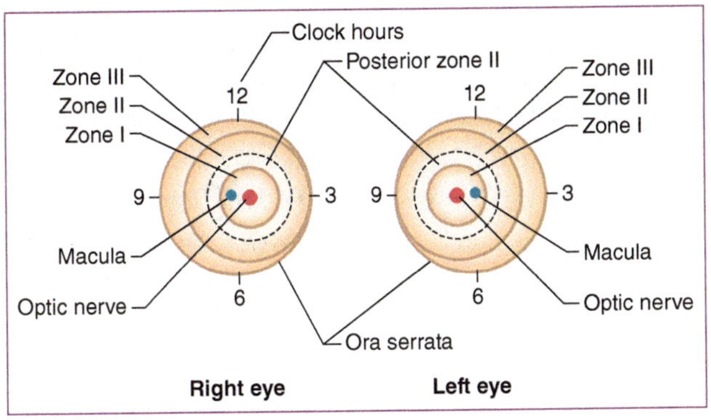


**FIGURE 17.2 Diagram of zones of the eyes.**

a 12-year period showed an increased incidence of ROP by about 5% during those years (2000–2012), and a Dutch study (2009–2017) conducted over 8 years showed an increased incidence of 6.5%. To date, approximately 30,000 to 50,000 children worldwide have lost their vision due to inadequate treatment for severe ROP (Modrzejewska & Bosy-Gasior, 2023).

## Pathophysiology

ROP is a disease caused by an abnormal adaptation of normal maturational processes in the face of physiologic stress. The disease develops gradually and is divided into five stages of increasing clinical severity (Table 17.3). Some ophthalmologists use the term stage 0 if the retina's vascularity is immature.

The key factor in the development of ROP in premature infants is the developing retinal blood vessels. The pathophysiology of ROP occurs in two phases. Phase I has delayed growth of the retinal vascularity following preterm birth. Phase II occurs when the hypoxia created during phase I causes retinal ischemia and stimulates the release of growth factors that contribute to the abnormal growth of blood cells in the eye. Retinal vascularization begins at the optic nerve at about 16 weeks of gestation and retinal vascular development continues slowly spreading out to the retinal periphery (ora serrata retinae), with complete development at 40 weeks of gestation (Fevereiro-Martins et al., 2023).

An incompletely vascularized retina has a peripheral avascular zone that varies with the degree of immaturity of the retina. In-utero growth of retinal blood vessels is stimulated by the release of vascular endothelial growth factor (VEGF) and insulin-like growth factor-1 (IGF-1). VEGF is found at the front line of the growing retinal blood vessels, whereas IGF-1 is maintained at a constant level in the retina microenvironment. VEGF is a cytokine regulated by oxygen (hypoxia). IGF-1 is a nonoxygen-regulated cytokine involved in regulating endothelial cell survival and proliferation. Preterm infants have low IGF-1 levels, which inhibit the normal growth of retinal vascularization (Oatts et al., 2024).

Following preterm birth, the normal growth of the retina vascularity stops, and some of the already-developed vessels are lost. The retina, however, remains metabolically active and becomes hypoxic because of the lack of blood vessels. This hypoxia becomes a potent inducer of new vessel growth (neovascularization) by stimulating the expression of VEGF at 30 to 33 weeks' postmenstrual age (Oatts et al., 2024). As the new blood vessels proliferate, they tend to grow into the vitreous, causing bleeding and the formation of fibrous tissue.

Many preterm infants in the NICU receive supplemental oxygen to treat their respiratory distress. The hyperoxia caused by oxygen use suppresses VEGF and IGF-1, resulting in retinal neovascularization.

As the preterm infant matures, the growing retina triggers a release of VEGF; IGF-1 levels will also rise. This creates an environment for new vessel growth (neovascular proliferation) that leads to the progression of retinopathy. Milder degrees of ROP are often transient and regress once the abnormal stimuli are removed or corrected. Moderate retinopathy can lead to excessive fibrous tissue formation or scarring in the peripheral retina, which may lead to reduced vision. In severe cases of ROP, fibrous tissue development may lead to retinal detachment and blindness. Severely affected neonates may also have leukocoria, glaucoma, or both.

## Risk Factors

Though the preterm birth rate in the United States has been stable over the past few years at about 10–11% (Martin et al., 2025), the incidence of ROP continues to rise, possibly due to the increased use of resuscitation of extremely premature infants at lower gestations (21–23 weeks). Although many risk factors for ROP have been identified, gestational age of less than 30 weeks, small for gestational age, and birth weight of less than 1,500 g remain the most important factors leading to the development of ROP secondary to the underdevelopment of the retinal vascular system (Bezman et al., 2023). ROP incidence strongly correlates with weight and gestational age at birth. Infant retinal vascularization is dependent on VEGF, which is triggered by IGF-1. In utero, IGF-1 levels are high and drop after birth; therefore, premature infants have low IGF-1 levels. Low levels inhibit the normal growth of retinal vascularization during the first phase of ROP. When IGF-1 levels increase with increasing postmenstrual age, it triggers VEGF to produce new blood vessels in the eye.

A multicenter study, which included more than 4,000 preterm infants who weighed less than 1,251 g, demonstrated that the risk for ROP decreased by 27% for each weight gain of 100 g and the ROP risk decreased by approximately 19% with each 7 days' increase in gestational age (Bezman et al., 2023). As mentioned previously, ROP is a multifactorial disease with prematurity, low birth weight, and hyperoxia being the biggest contributing risk factors. However, other possible risk factors include both maternal and postnatal factors: infertility, pregnancy-induced hypertension (PIH), thyroid diseases, chorioamnionitis, premature rupture of membranes (PROM), sepsis, respiratory distress syndrome (RDS), continuous positive pressure ventilation, and IVH (Reynolds, 2010).

Over the past decades, several studies have examined the correlation between oxygen saturation and the risk and progression of ROP. Raghuveer and Zackula (2020) performed a meta-analysis of oxygen saturation and ROP by reviewing four key ROP studies: Surfactant, Positive Pressure, and Pulse Oximetry Trial; Supplemental Therapeutic Oxygen for Pre-threshold Retinopathy of Prematurity Trial; Benefits of Oxygen Saturation Targeting Trial; and the Canadian Oxygen Trial. The results showed the lower oxygen group had a reduced risk for severe ROP, but a higher risk of mortality compared to the higher oxygen group. The AAP recommended a target oxygen saturation range of 90% to 95% in extremely low birth weight (ELBW) infants (Gantz et al., 2020; Nyugen et al., 2024; Raghuveer & Zackula, 2020).

Recent studies have suggested the important role of nutrition in ROP prevention. Meeting the nutritional needs of a preterm infant with enteral and parental nutrition is imperative to promote growth, a healthy immune system, and a healthy vascular retina. A maternal breastmilk diet may decrease the risk of ROP because it has a higher concentration of IGF-1 than formula (Darlow & Husain, 2019). Anderson-Berry et al. (2024) demonstrated that providing early enteral feeds during the first 6 weeks of life was associated with a lower risk of any stage of ROP or severe ROP. The participants were 7,483 infants at 29 facilities with a mean weight of 1,100 g and a mean gestation age of 28 and 6/7 weeks. Parental nutrition, in combination with enteral feeds, including trophic feeds, was considered a good option for best outcomes in high-risk infants.

Although most ROP occurs in premature infants, rare cases of the disease have been reported in full-term infants, stillborn infants, and infants who have not received supplemental oxygen. Many premature infants with variations in the Norrie disease gene, a gene responsible for an X-linked form of congenital retinal detachment or dysgenesis, were more likely to develop severe ROP with possible retinal detachment. Each individual carries genetic predispositions to certain disorders, but less is understood about the genetic proclivities toward outside effects such as trauma, hypoxia, and premature birth (Scruggs et al., 2023). Infants with Norrie disease often are blind at birth or within the first few months of life, and it usually occurs with term male infants.

## Screening for Retinopathy of Prematurity

Prematurity is the number one associated risk factor for ROP and timely screening is imperative for prevention, early detection, and appropriate follow-up of significant disease. Despite the international effort to standardize ROP and the efforts of several multicenter, randomized clinical trials, no universally accepted guidelines exist for the screening of premature infants. Screening protocols vary from institution to institution, among different countries, and even with the level of development of the countries. Recommended screening guidelines for the United States were recommended by the AAP, the American Academy of Ophthalmology, and the American Association of Pediatric Ophthalmology and Strabismus (Fierson et al., 2018) (Table 17.4).

ROP screening should include an indirect binocular ophthalmoscopy (IBO) of the retina and sclera indentation to assess the retinal periphery. A pediatric ophthalmologist or a retinal specialist should perform the procedure. This procedure remains the most common diagnostic approach for screening and diagnosing ROP. However, a wide-field digital camera (RetCam) is being used as an alternative to indirect ophthalmoscopy for screening infants for ROP and combined with IBO. More diagnostic tools and techniques are used for

**TABLE 17.4**

**RETINOPATHY OF PREMATURITY SCREENING GUIDELINES IN THE UNITED STATES**

| Recommending Group | Infant Criteria | First Examination Date | | |
|---|---|---|---|---|
| American Academy of Pediatrics, American Academy of Ophthalmology, and American Association of Pediatric Ophthalmology & Strabismus | • Birthweight < 1,500 g or gestational age < 30 weeks<br>• Selected infants between 1,500 to 2,000 g with an unstable clinical course | ***Gestational Age at Birth*** | | ***Age at Initial Exam*** |
| | | 22 weeks | 9 weeks | |
| | | 23 weeks | 8 weeks | |
| | | 25 weeks | 7 weeks | |
| | | 25 weeks | 6 weeks | |
| | | 26 weeks | 5 weeks | |
| | | 27–30 weeks | 4 weeks | |
| | | > 30 if high risk | 4 weeks | |

*Sources:* Fierson, W. M., & American Academy of Pediatrics Section on Ophthalmology, American Academy of Ophthalmology, American Association for Pediatric Ophthalmology and Strabismus, & American Association of Certified Orthoptists. (2018). Policy statement—Screening examination of premature infants for retinopathy of prematurity. *Pediatrics, 142*(6), 1–9. https://doi.org/10.1542/peds.2018-3061.

retinal examination to diagnose and monitor ROP. Ultrasonography, ultrasonography biomicroscopy, fundus photography, optical coherence tomography, optical coherence tomography angiography, and fundus fluorescein angiography are diagnostic tools for retinal examination that have offered new and innovative options for the diagnosis and monitoring of ROP (Agarwal et al., 2021). The use of smartphone technology for digital imaging and artificial intelligence both offer innovative tools for imaging, detecting, and monitoring ROP that may be helpful with telemedicine screening for ROP in underserved areas or underdeveloped countries. Retinal digital imaging is a reasonable alternative but not a substitution for a direct examination by an onsite ophthalmologist (Oatts et al., 2024).

Premature infants are extremely vulnerable, and retinal examinations can be physiologically stressful for the infants, caregivers, and families. ROP exams are time consuming for the ophthalmologist and costly for the medical system. In preparation for the procedure, the infants are administered a mydriatic agent (e.g., phenylephrine 2.5%, cyclopentolate 0.5%, or tropicamide 0.5%) that is instilled in the eye topically for pupil dilation approximately 30 to 45 minutes prior to the exam. A topical anesthetic, such as 0.5% proparacaine HCl ophthalmic solution, should be instilled in each eye to dull the corneal and conjunctival sensitivity and decrease the newborn's pain before the exam. A lid speculum and a sclera depressor, individually sterilized for each infant's examination, are used to visualize the peripheral retina and ora serrata, the anterior border of retinal vascularization or retinopathy (Figure 17.3). Examinations are performed with the binocular indirect ophthalmoscope and 30-diopter lens, first evaluating the posterior pole and then the periphery with sclera depression. The examiner should assess for the presence or absence of ROP disease, its location and extent, and the presence or absence of plus disease. Aggressive ROP and the location should be carefully documented at the time of examination according to ICROP-3 classifications (Chiang et al., 2021).

When utilizing the RetCam for ROP screening, the same eye drops must be utilized to dilate the pupils and anesthetize the area. The eyelid speculum is also used, but the scleral depressor is not needed. A water-soluble gel is applied as a barrier between the eye and the lens (Figure 17.4). Retinal images taken by the RetCam camera can be stored, transmitted to an

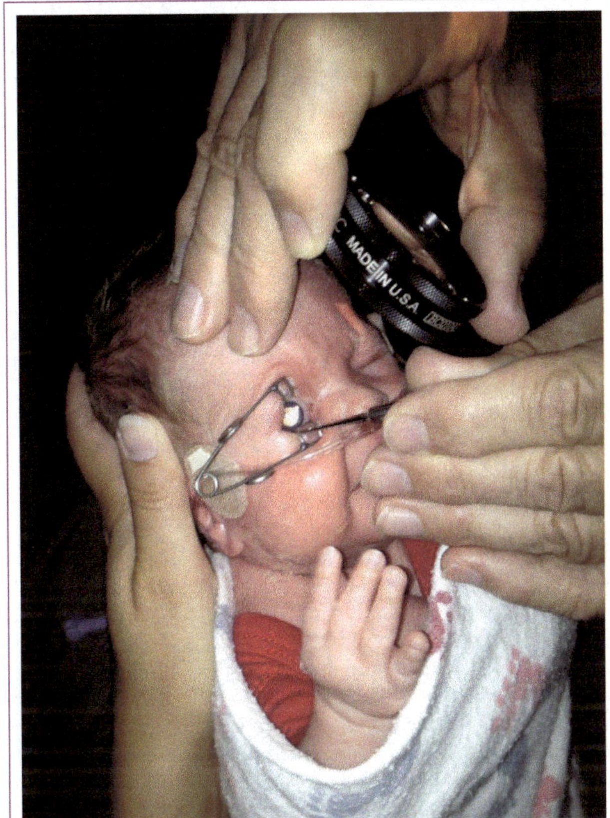

**FIGURE 17.3** **Premature infant during eye exam undergoing indirect ophthalmoscopy using eyelid speculum and sclera depressor.**

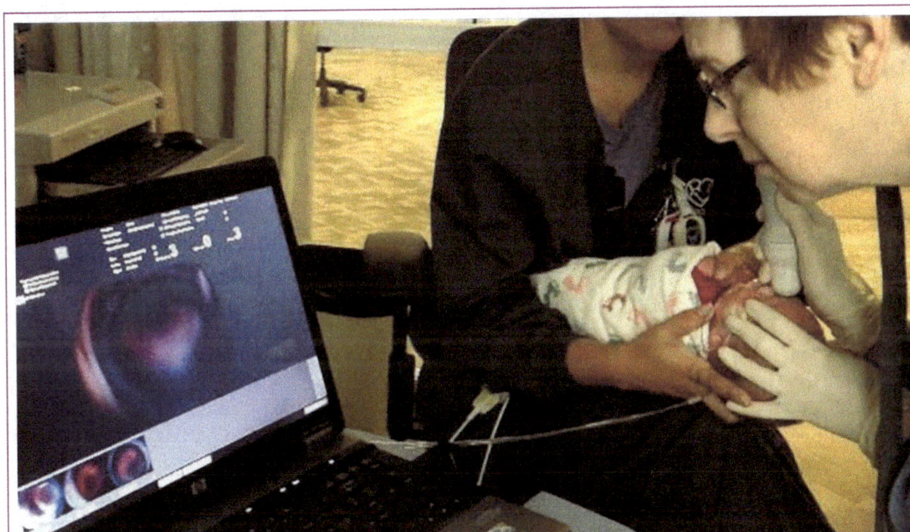

**FIGURE 17.4** **Premature infant during retinal evaluation using the RetCam.**

expert, reviewed, analyzed, and sequentially compared over time, and are helpful for telemedicine purposes.

The timing of eye exams can be frustrating for the NICU staff and the ophthalmologist. Often, the ophthalmologist may arrive to examine an infant when the infant is due to eat, the infant has just completed his feeding, or during the infant's scheduled "quiet time." Use of the RetCam allows examinations to be scheduled at the convenience of the NICU staff. The RetCam screenings are less traumatic for the infant and provide a digital image as a permanent form for documenting the disease process for the electronic health record.

## Treatment

Environmental lighting in NICUs has been implicated as a contributing factor in the development of ROP. Although there have been some clinical studies that claimed to show a relationship between lighting and ROP there were also studies that contradicted this claim (Reynolds et al., 1998). Also, the studies had many limitations. Despite no significant evidence, many NICUs continue to institute reduced environmental lighting and shielding of incubators as part of a developmental approach to care.

ICROP has never recommended treatment guidelines for premature infants. The treatment guidelines were developed by physicians after two landmark studies, the CRYO-ROP study and the ET-ROP study. The 1986 multicenter CRYO-ROP trial led to the definition of threshold and prethreshold ROP. Threshold disease was considered the minimum disease needed for treatment. The threshold defined by the CRYO ROP study was characterized by stage 2 in zone I or II involving greater than or equal to five contiguous or eight cumulative clock hours with plus disease. If untreated, there was a 50% risk of poor outcomes. High-risk prethreshold, type I ROP as defined by the ET-ROP study, was characterized by zone 1 any stage with plus disease or zone I stage 3 without plus disease or zone II stages 2 or 3 with plus disease (ET-ROP, 2003, 2005).

Treatment for ROP has evolved over the years. Laser photocoagulation has been the current gold standard of care for ROP. Laser ablation of the peripheral avascular retina can prevent progression to retinal detachment. Prior to laser photocoagulation, cryotherapy was the primary choice of treatment for ROP. Recently, laser photocoagulation with or without anti-VEGF- agents has become a first-line or second-line treatment for ROP (Bezman et al., 2023).

Today, the current treatment recommendations are still based on the results of the ET-ROP study published in 2003, which used earlier intervention. Intervention should be done with the development of Type 1 prethreshold ROP, which is defined as any stage with plus disease in zone I, OR stage 3 without plus disease in zone I, or stage 2 or 3 with plus disease in zone II (Oatts et al., 2024).

Cryotherapy was developed in Japan in the 1970s. It gained popularity in the United States in the 1980s after the release of data from the Cryotherapy for ROP Study. Cryotherapy is a surgical procedure involving the insertion of a probe cooled with liquid nitrogen on the medial aspect of the eye. Confluent spots on the avascular retina are ablated (destroyed by freezing), reducing the release of angiogenic factors that appear to induce retinal vasoproliferation.

Laser photocoagulation delivered through an indirect ophthalmoscope replaced cryotherapy as the treatment of choice for ROP. The advantages of laser photocoagulation therapy included the technical ease of performance and its usefulness in posterior ROP, which was difficult to treat with cryotherapy and required less eye manipulation. The procedure could be performed in either the operating room or within the NICU. Sedation and/or anesthesia could be utilized, depending on the preferences of the ophthalmologist and anesthesiologist and the medical condition of the infant. Laser photocoagulation has reduced the incidence of blindness but rarely improves visual acuity. Complications include myopia, scar tissue, inflammation, and peripheral visual field loss (Fevereiro-Martins et al., 2023).

The current use of intravitreal anti-VEGF drugs, which inhibit the VEGF, has been successful in the treatment of ROP. The drugs used are bevacizumab, ranibizumab, and aflibercept. Aflibercept is the only medication that is FDA approved for the treatment of ROP. However, over the past decade, anti-VEGF medications have become popular in the treatment of ROP. The Bevacizumab eliminates the angiogenic threat of retinopathy of prematurity (BEAT-ROP) study published in 2011 demonstrated that the incidence of retreatment for ROP occurred much later after intravitreal injection of bevacizumab when compared to laser photocoagulation (Mintz-Hittner et al., 2011). Although bevacizumab is the most commonly used anti-VEGF medication, there is a concern about delayed neurodevelopment. Other studies have shown ranibizumab and aflibercept may be safer alternatives. According to the Comparing Alternative Ranibizumab Dosages for Safety and Efficacy in Retinopathy of Prematurity Study (AAPOS and AAO Hoskins Center for Quality Eye Care; Stahl et al., 2022), ranibizumab was identified as an effective anti-VEGF alternative to bevacizumab. In comparison, ranibizumab has been shown to not suppress systemic VEGF levels, thus limiting unwanted effects on organs, such as the brain and lung, that are still undergoing development at the time of ROP treatment (Stahl et al., 2022).

Administration of the anti-VEGF medications decreases the high levels of VEGF in the vitreous gel, which are not reduced by conventional laser therapy. Development of peripheral retinal vessels continues after treatment with intravitreal anti-VEGF injections, whereas conventional laser therapy leads to the permanent destruction of the peripheral retina. Other benefits include less dependence on the surgeon's experience and expertise, injections can be performed under local anesthesia, treatment time is shorter, and there is a lower risk of myopia (Dammann et al., 2023).

Despite the wide usage of anti-VEGF injection and the success rates in the treatment of ROP, there is concern that these agents may enter the systemic circulation and alter the VEGF serum values. This may have an effect on the neurodevelopment of premature infants. Anti-VEGF therapy requires long and frequent follow-up for regression and reactivation of the disease. Harnett et al. (2022) discussed the ICROP-3 updates that included the terms *regression* and *reactivation*. Both of these conditions are associated with anti-VEGF therapy and should be closely monitored. Regression of ROP can occur rapidly after anti-VEGF therapy, and reactivation usually occurs following anti-VEGF therapy but may occur later than the natural course of ROP. Current recommendations require monitoring infants after anti-VEGF therapy until they reach at least 65 weeks' postmenstrual age or throughout the child's life.

Systemic propranolol, IGF-1 replacement, and omega-3 polyunsaturated fatty acid supplementation are the newer preventive strategies being evaluated. Newer, emerging therapeutic options have the potential to complement current therapies and improve treatment outcomes. Low plasma levels of IGF-1 are associated with the risk of ROP. Recent studies indicate that the combination administration of Recombinant Human Insulin-Like Growth Factor with its binding protein-3 could possibly increase the plasma levels of IGF-1 during the development of ROP (Bezman et al., 2023). Although anti-VEGF agents have had a positive effect on the treatment of infants with ROP, both regression and reactivation of the disease tend to occur after anti-VEGF therapy more often than with laser photocoagulation and should be closely assessed and documented with timely follow-up exams, as discussed previously (Chiang et al., 2021).

Retinopathy of prematurity may transition to retinal detachment in 15% to 30% of infants with ROP, but the incidence has decreased due to improved screening and proactive laser treatment (Nuzzi et al., 2017). The corrective treatment is surgery for the repair of the detached retina. Scleral buckling, vitrectomy, or both, with or without lensectomy, are the techniques most often used.

ROP is a preventable disease, and approximately 25% to 30% of those affected develop long-term eye complications, including abnormal retinal function, strabismus, and, in severe cases, blindness (Fevereiro-Martins et al., 2023). Infants with advanced stages of ROP are at the highest risk for blindness. Studies have shown that infants treated with both laser therapy and anti-VEGF had a higher incidence of myopia. Severe ROP is associated with delayed maturation of the eye and lower longitudinal IQ scores during the first 18 years of life. Neurodevelopmental delays vary with the type of treatment. The anti VEGF agent bevacizumab is a risk factor for neurodevelopmental delays (Raghuveer & Zackula, 2020). Severe ROP is a predictor of long-term sequelae that can affect several aspects of a child's growth and development.

The survival rates for premature infants have increased with infants born at gestational ages between 22 and 24 weeks. This population is at high risk for ROP and severe ROP. An examination of data from a 2008 to 2012 cohort of premature infants from the Neonatal Research Network Centers showed that infants born at 22 to 28 weeks of gestation had a 56% incidence of ROP. Infants born at 22 to 24 weeks of gestation had an incidence of ROP and severe ROP of 90% and 43%, respectively (Raghuveer & Zackula, 2020). As this population continues to grow, the incidence of ROP will continue to rise. It is imperative that evidence-based prevention strategies and adherence to ROP screening guidelines be implemented in the clinical management of preterm infants.

### Collaborative Care

ROP is a preventable disease that can contribute to poor outcomes in the neonatal population. Primary prevention begins in the delivery room and should be embedded in the daily management of care until discharge. When a preterm infant delivery is expected or occurs, it is very important for the providers in the NICU to introduce the risks and strategies in care to prevent ROP and what it may entail. As the literature explains, ROP is a developmental disease, and prevention and management require an interdisciplinary team approach that includes NICU providers, occupational therapists (OTs), physical therapists (PTs), nutritionists, pharmacy staff, and parents. Each team member contributes a unique set of skills and knowledge that creates a holistic approach to the prevention and management of ROP. Infants who acquire ROP and treatment require timely follow-up and long-term screening as both inpatients and outpatients. Prior to discharge, the ophthalmologist and family should have an established relationship to ensure proper outpatient follow-up eye appointments.

Over the years, many NICUs have developed and implemented programs using ROP protocols, as well as a staff coordinator. Understanding ROP, the purpose of the screening examinations, treatment, and the importance of follow-up is an important aspect for everyone involved in the care of premature infants. The ROP staff coordinators can provide ongoing education for the healthcare team and is instrumental in identifying the infants who meet ROP screening criteria and scheduling those screening exams. The role could also include preparing the clinical staff and the parents for the screening procedure, treatment, and follow-up care.

A major concern with the ongoing management of ROP is when an infant is transferred back to the referring hospital. The infant has the potential risk of a missed follow-up appointment. NICU providers have developed ROP tracking systems and required documentation of the timing of future eye examinations on an infant's daily progress notes. This may not occur at the lower level (primary or secondary) referring hospital. Another trend over the past decade has been to give the parents a letter with the outpatient ophthalmology appointment time and date listed, which then would require a parent's signature upon discharge. The eye examinations are essential for preventing worsening ROP and possible blindness in these post-NICU infants.

ROP is a disease that requires an interdisciplinary approach with primary, secondary, and tertiary care. Preventive measures after preterm births and adherence to evidence-based recommendations for ROP screening and treatment are imperative to limit the poor outcomes associated with this disease. Early parental involvement and communication with a pediatric ophthalmologist establish parental awareness of possible eye disorders and an understanding of the importance of regular eye examinations after discharge. The NICU providers are responsible for coordinating a comprehensive discharge plan that includes outpatient eye appointments for ROP follow-up, other specialty clinic follow-up as needed, and a developmental follow-up clinic for early detection of possible neurodevelopmental delays. Many families may benefit from referral to community resources, support groups, and special programs for children with visual problems.

## OTHER DISORDERS THAT AFFECT THE EYES

### Fetal Alcohol Spectrum Disorders

Maternal ingestion of alcohol during pregnancy results in fetal alcohol spectrum disorders, including the most severe type, FAS or prenatal alcohol exposure. Infants with FAS have mental deficiencies (CNS damage), dysmorphic facies, and severe intrauterine growth restriction (IUGR). The abnormalities of the eyes common in infants with FAS include microphthalmia, short palpebral fissures (in about 60%), hypertelorism (telecanthus), coloboma, strabismus, ptosis, epicanthal folds, optic nerve hypoplasia, small optic discs, retinal vessel tortuosity, diminished visual acuity, and some infants can develop blindness (Tsang et al., 2022).

## Zika Virus

Zika is a mosquito-borne virus discovered in Uganda in the 1940s, but it has now been found in South America, Central America, and even the United States. Adults bitten by a Zika-infected mosquito often develop only a mild version of the disease. Zika virus can also be transmitted to the fetus if the mother was infected with the virus during pregnancy. The fetus can develop brain damage and death, depending on the extent of the exposure and infection.

Infants who are exposed to the Zika virus in utero can develop several congenital malformations. The most common is microcephaly, but about a third of these infants can also develop some type of abnormal development of the eye, including microphthalmia, nonpurulent conjunctivitis, anterior uveitis, congenital glaucoma, cataracts, inflammation of the optic nerve, lens subluxation, iris colobomas, damage to the retina (chorioretinal atrophy) or optic nerve, macular atrophy, intraocular calcifications, or even blindness (Labib & Chigbu, 2022; Marquezan et al., 2018). These eye defects appear to be caused by changes in the neural crest cells during eye development in utero (Schoenwolf et al., 2021).

## Maternal Diabetes

Although maternal diabetes is recognized for its teratogenic effects, craniofacial anomalies are rarely reported. Infants of diabetic mothers (IDMs) should be carefully examined for the presence of oculoauriculovertebral spectrum (OAVS) disorders, including displaced inner canthi, lens opacity, microphthalmia, coloboma of eyelids or iris, optic nerve hypoplasia, tear duct obstruction, and ocular lipoma (Kokhanov, 2022; Singhal & Tripathy, 2023). It has been suggested that OAVS (or Goldenhar syndrome) occurs as a result of abnormal development of the first and second branchial arches with faulty neural crest cell migration or alteration of the *Pax3* gene path with hyperglycemia, which could occur in diabetic women with poor control during pregnancy (Kokhanov, 2022).

### Intraventricular Hemorrhage and/or Periventricular Leukomalacia

IVH with or without periventricular leukomalacia (PVL) is associated with eye abnormalities in premature infants. Visual impairments, including ROP, were common in infants with IVH, including strabismus, nystagmus, small visual field, and optic nerve damage (Khanna et al., 2022). Increased cranial pressure on the developing eye and optic nerve with hydrocephalus-associated IVH can cause even more visual acuity problems. There is an increased incidence of eye movement disorders (strabismus and/or nystagmus), worsened visual acuity impairment, and damage to the optic nerve with PVL (Khanna et al., 2022).

## Maternal Hypertension

A recent study in China (Zhu et al., 2024) found a higher incidence of strabismus among children born to mothers with hypertensive disorder of pregnancy or poorly controlled blood pressure. It may be advantageous to observe eye movement disorders in children born to mothers with hypertension and/or preeclampsia during pregnancy.

## SUMMARY

Visual disturbances, although sometimes difficult to detect in newborns, can have a dramatic effect on a newborn's behavioral and psychosocial development. PVL and severe IVH with hydrocephalus can cause serious eye disease in premature infants. Significant advances are being made every day in the diagnosis, treatment, and follow-up of ELBW infants. Neuroprotective bundles and caffeine may improve long-term vision outcomes by decreasing the incidence of IVH and PVL. Visual morbidity continues to be a concern as these small neonates survive the NICU.

Treatment of vision problems requires collaborative efforts among the neonatal healthcare team, the ophthalmologist, and the families. Clear, consistent communication between healthcare providers and parents, parental education, and good follow-up are essential to the quality of care.

## CASE STUDY

**Identification of the Problem.** Premature infants, especially those weighing less than 1,500 g, are at risk for complications from immature development of the eyes and the effects of supplemental oxygen on the developing eyes. As a result of the supportive therapies used in the NICU, ROP can develop. This case study presents a patient born at 25 weeks' gestation who is presently 11 weeks of age or 36 weeks' corrected gestational age. Due to his early birth, the infant has chronic lung disease (CLD), is on a mild diuretic, and continues to require a low amount of oxygen via nasal cannula. The plan is to discharge to home within 5 to 7 days.

**Assessment: History and Physical Examination.** The male infant was born on June 4, 2022, at 25 weeks' gestation, to a 23-year-old gravida 1, para 0 mother whose pregnancy was complicated by preterm labor. the mother received prenatal care and delivered spontaneously by vaginal route following 2 days of unsuccessful tocolysis treatment and rupture of membranes approximately 15 hours prior to birth. The infant was born with minimal respiratory effort, requiring intubation, bagging, and surfactant treatment in the delivery room, but was extubated to nasal continuous positive airway pressure (CPAP). By 4 hours of age, he required moderate ventilation, and his condition deteriorated, requiring high-frequency oscillatory ventilation by 24 hours of age. He received a second dose of surfactant and remained on ventilation for approximately 3 weeks. He was weaned to nasal CPAP, high-flow oxygen, and low-flow oxygen. He remains on 200 to 250 ml/min of oxygen via nasal cannula. He had umbilical lines placed after birth, peripherally inserted central catheter line for 12 days, started on nasogastric feedings that were well tolerated, and advanced to full feedings. He has been nippling feeds with occasional apnea and bradycardia.

## Physical Examination

- GENERAL: preterm, male infant
- HEAD, EARS, EYES, NOSE, AND THROAT (HEENT): slight dolichocephaly, anterior fontanel soft and flat with widened sagittal sutures; eyes clear, no drainage or redness; pupils reactive to light; positive red reflex both eyes (OU); eyes and ears normoset with palate intact
- RESPIRATORY: lung fields clear and equal bilaterally; minimal respiratory effort; respiratory rate = 48 with saturations 89% to 93% on 200 ml/L nasal cannula oxygen
- CARDIOVASCULAR: regular rate and rhythm with no murmur; pulses strong, regular and equal in all extremities; good peripheral perfusion 2+/4+ and capillary blood refill time less than 3 seconds
- ABDOMEN: soft and nontender with no masses palpable and positive bowel sounds throughout; liver edge down 2 cm below right costal margin; no splenomegaly; patent anus
- GENITOURINARY: normal male genitalia with testes descended into scrotum bilaterally
- NEUROLOGIC (NEURO): awake and active; cries when distressed or disturbed; sleep pattern appropriate for near-term infant; normal tone and responsiveness for gestational age
- EXTREMITIES: moves all four extremities with normal range of motion; hips—no click; clavicles—no crepitus; good muscle tone of all extremities; 10 digits per extremity
- SKIN: pink, warm, dry, and intact; no rashes or bruising noted; mucous membranes pink and moist

Premature infants are at risk for many complications due to their immaturity and treatments.

## Premature Diagnoses

- RDS—can develop into CLD
- Hypoglycemia
- At risk for patent ductus arteriosus (PDA)
- Possible sepsis/pneumonia
- At risk for IVH
- At risk for ROP
- Apnea of prematurity
- Anemia of prematurity

## ROP Examinations

| Dates | Age (Weeks) | Gestational Age (Weeks) | Results | Plan |
|---|---|---|---|---|
| July 16 | 6 | 31 | Immature vascularity in both eyes (stage 0, zones II–III bilaterally) | Follow-up in 2 weeks |
| July 30 | 8 | 33 | Stages 1–2, zone II with questionable plus disease | Follow-up in 1 week |
| August 6 | 9 | 34 | Stages 2–3+, zone II on right; stage 2+, zone II on left | Referral for laser treatment |
| August 8 | 9½ | 34½ | Stage 3+, zone II bilaterally | Laser photocoagulation was performed |

*Note:* According to the American Academy of Pediatrics, the first eye examination would be done at 6 weeks' gestation.

## Discharge Diagnoses

- Premature male infant
- CLD
- Apnea of prematurity
- ROP

### EVIDENCE-BASED PRACTICE

## Prevention of Blindness

The importance of clinical trials and research studies can be seen in the prevention of blindness in newborn infants. Numerous studies and clinical observations have allowed physicians and other providers to realize the effects that various treatments (and nontreatments) have had on the health and well-being of children. Newborns rarely participate in comparative clinical trials because we are trying to treat a disorder or disease and want the most effective treatment. Newborns are considered a vulnerable population for research. Many parents may not wish to consent

(*continued*)

## EVIDENCE-BASED PRACTICE (*continued*)

to a change in treatment modalities, and we cannot treat infants differently if it puts them at risk. However, always searching for the best and most recent studies is imperative to providing the best care.

Eye infections in the neonate can cause blindness if untreated. In the late 1800s, it was found that providing prophylactic treatment of newborn eyes with $AgNO_3$ drops can prevent the newborn from developing *Neisseria gonorrhea* from an infected mother. Providing eye drops after birth prevented blindness from this STI that can affect an infant's long-term development. Although penicillin was discovered in the late 1940s, $AgNO_3$ continued to be used as the main prophylactic agent due to the low cost and overall benefits for many children. In the 1980s to 1990s, erythromycin replaced $AgNO_3$ for newborn eye prophylaxis due to the effectiveness of this antibiotic in preventing *Chlamydia trachomatis* infections. There were also considerations for using povidone-iodine as a prophylactic because it had a lower cost and less toxicity than $AgNO_3$ (Isenberg et al., 2002). Povidone-iodine is used in some third-world countries due to its lower cost and effectiveness with both gonorrhea and chlamydia eye infections. There has also been discussion about the need for eye prophylaxis over the years, both in 1958 and again in 2023 (Franco & Hammerschlag, 2023; Mellin & Kent, 1958). The USPSTF also published a reaffirmation to continue erythromycin prophylaxis at this time, even with the knowledge that its effectiveness against chlamydia conjunctivitis is not as effective as was initially thought (Curry et al., 2019). A Cochrane meta-analysis was also completed in 2020 (Kapoor et al., 2020) on eye prophylaxis. Continuing to improve care is a goal for providers of neonatal healthcare, and we must make sure our management of eye disorders is based on evidence (Yoo et al., 2023).

It was also found that oxygen given to premature babies can result in ROP, leading to detached retina and blindness. The treatment of oxygen for newborn respiratory distress was found to possibly lead to blindness in those infants who develop severe ROP. Again, the use of many studies has allowed the medical community to develop effective treatments to either stop or control the development of this devastating effect of oxygen on the premature infant's retinas.

ROP is also one of the 12 core outcomes explored in the research on neonatal patients (Webbe et al., 2023). Without systematic clinical trials, the evidence needed to provide long-term care to newborns would be inadequate. As healthcare providers, we must continue to use our knowledge and resources to improve the healthcare of our youngest patients constantly.

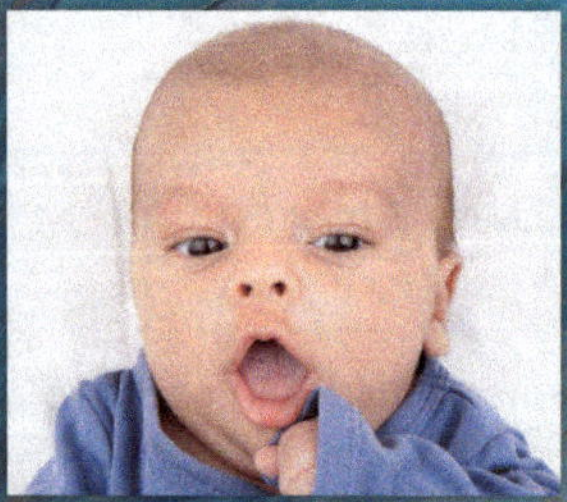
*Source:* Thomas Dutour/Adobe Stock.

## PARENT VOICES

### Jennifer Degl

**ROP had not been on my radar for the first 2 months that my baby was in the NICU. I had spent my time researching about what things could take her life and how to watch for signs and help prevent her from developing those complications. Once she was a few months old and relatively stable, and the doctors told me that she had passed the window of time where I had to be afraid every day, I was informed that she would likely develop an eye condition called ROP. All that was explained to me initially was that ROP is a disease of premature babies that causes abnormal blood vessels to grow in the retina. This growth can cause the retina to detach from the back of the eye, leading to blindness, and high levels of oxygen given to preemies exaggerate this condition. How is it that oxygen, needed for survival, can cause babies to go blind? It really does not make sense, but it is so. At first, my daughter had her eyes checked at the bedside every week, beginning at 8 weeks old. The eye specialist (pediatric ophthalmologist) told me that my daughter had between stage 3 and 4 ROP and that there was nothing to do but wait and try to lower her oxygen levels as much as possible, but that was not up to me. A few weeks later, she had developed stage 4 ROP. I was so afraid that my daughter would have tunnel vision or go completely blind, and there was nothing I could do about it. When my daughter was a little over 3 months old, the doctor told me that her ROP was improving. Each week, it continued to improve, and she was discharged from the NICU with only stage 1 ROP. We were instructed to follow up with a pediatric ophthalmologist. We saw the pediatric ophthalmologist every month for 1 year and then every 3 months and then every 6 months, and now we only go once a year. Today, at 6 years old, my daughter is cleared of ROP and only needs to wear glasses when she colors, reads, or does any close-up work.**

(*continued*)

## PARENT VOICES (*continued*)

### References

Curry, S. J., O'Leary, S. T., Aucott, S. W., Krist, A. H., Owens, D. K., Barry, M. J., & U.S. Preventive Services Task Force. (2019). Ocular prophylaxis for gonococcal ophthalmia neonatorum: U.S. Preventive Services Task Force reaffirmation recommendation statement. *JAMA*, *321*(4), 394–398. https://doi.org/10.1001/jama.2018.21367

Franco, S., & Hammerschlag, M. R. (2023). Neonatal ocular prophylaxis in the United States: Is it still necessary? *Expert Review of Anti-Infective Therapy*, *21*(5), 503–511. https://doi.org/10.1080/14787210.2023.2172401

Isenberg, S. J., Apt, L., Valenton, M., Del Signore, M., Culbillen, L., Labrador, M. A., Chan, P., & Berman, N. G. (2002). A controlled trial of povidone-iodine to treat infectious conjunctivitis in children. *American Journal of Ophthalmology*, *13*, 681–688. https://doi.org/10.1016/s0002-9394(02)01701-4

Kapoor, V. S., Evans, J. R., & Vedula, S. S. (2020). Interventions for preventing ophthalmia neonatorum. *Cochrane Database Systematic Reviews*, *9*(9), CD001862. https://doi.org/10.1002/14651858.CD001862.pub4

Mellin, G. W., & Kent, M. P. (1958). Ophthalmia neonatorum: Is prophylaxis necessary? *Pediatrics*, *22*(5), 1006–1015.

Webbe, J., Baba, A., Butcher, N. J., Rodrigues, C., Stallwood, E., Goren, K., Monsour, A., Chang, A. S. M., Trivedi, A., Manley, B. J., McCall, E., Bogossian, F., Namba, F., Schmolzer, G. M., Popat, H., Nguyen, K. A., Doyle, L. W., Jardine, L., Rysavy, M. A., … Offringa, M. on behalf of the Core Outcome Reporting in Neonatal Trials (Corint) Study Group. (2023). Strengthening reporting of neonatal trials. *Pediatrics*, *152*(3), 1–13. e2022060765 https://doi.org/10.1542/peds.2022-060765

Yoo, S. H., Rubin, S., Fredrick, D., & the AAP Section on Ophthalmology. (2023). *Century of changes: A commentary*. https://publications.aap.org/pediatrics/resources/24094/Commentary-From-the-AAP-Section-on-Ophthalmology?searchresult=1

## ONLINE RESOURCES

CourseConnect

Resources for this chapter are online and available at www.springerpub.com/courseconnect.

## REFERENCES

References for this chapter are online and available at www.springerpub.com/courseconnect.

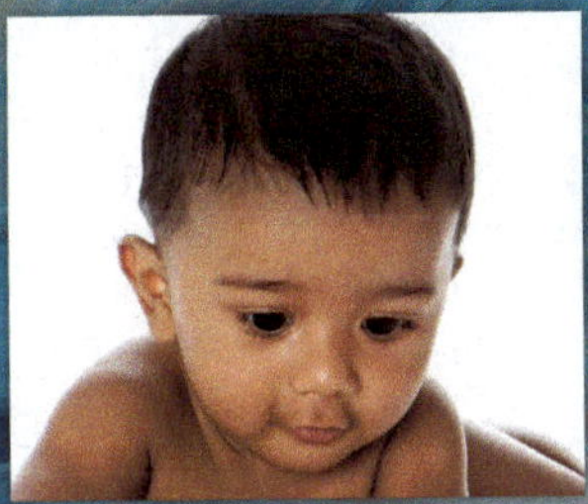

*Source:* lichtmeister/Adobe Stock.

CHAPTER 18

# Genitourinary System

Megan E. Glemza

## INTRODUCTION

Comprehensive nursing care of infants with renal or genital disorders requires a thorough understanding of normal anatomy and physiology. Development of renal and genital systems arises from shared structures; therefore, abnormalities in one system may indicate abnormal development in the other. Because nurses provide hands-on care to infants in both the newborn nursery and neonatal intensive care unit (NICU), they often first recognize abnormalities in the renal and genital systems. To readily identify such disorders and participate in collaborative management, nurses need a clear understanding of the normal anatomy and physiology of the genital and renal systems and the pathologic processes that may be present.

Kidneys function to maintain fluid, electrolyte, and acid–base balance and rid the body of nitrogenous and other waste products. Perinatal depression, prematurity, common neonatal medical management, and dehydration are only a few of the many factors placing the newborn at risk for renal compromise. Timely, accurate nursing assessment and intervention are necessary to ensure an optimal outcome.

This chapter outlines embryologic development and anatomy, physiology, and assessment of the genitourinary (GU) system. It also describes various abnormalities and disease processes commonly identified in the neonatal period, including pathophysiology, risk factors, clinical manifestations, diagnosis, collaborative management, and prognosis.

## EMBRYOLOGIC DEVELOPMENT OF THE UROGENITAL SYSTEM

During the first weeks of gestation, the mesoderm is divided into three segments: lateral, intermediate, and paraxial. The intermediate mesoderm separates from the paraxial mesoderm and migrates ventrally because the nephrogenic cords are located on either side of the primitive aorta. Cells on the dorsal end of the nephrogenic cords join to form the urogenital ridges from which components of both the urinary and genital structures are developed.

### The Urinary System

The urinary system consists of the kidneys, ureters, urinary bladder, and the urethra. Development of the primary excretory organ begins around the fourth week of gestation, with the production of fetal urine by week 10. At approximately 36 weeks, renal anatomic development is completed. Functional maturity increases after birth and continues until approximately 2 years of age.

Development of the kidneys occurs with the progressive formation of three unique nephric structures within the nephrogenic cord: the pronephros, the mesonephros, and the metanephros. The pronephros or primitive kidney develops during the first month of gestation and then gradually degenerates, thus contributing to the duct system for the next developmental stage. The pronephros has no excretory function.

The second excretory organ to develop is the mesonephros. Mesonephric development begins at the caudal end of the pronephros during the fourth to sixth weeks of gestation. The mesonephros contain thin-walled glomeruli and functional tubules. Ultra-urine is produced by these mesonephric nephrons at 8 to 10 weeks' gestation. Mesonephric nephrons located more cranially along the nephrogenic cord begin to degenerate because those located more caudally are still developing. During this time, approximately the fourth week, the gonadal blastema begins to form in the genital ridge located on the medial aspect of each mesonephros, thus creating a urogenital ridge between the developing kidney and the genitals. As the mesonephric structure begins to involute in a caudal direction, it leaves a duct system for the following stage. In addition, the mesonephric duct eventually matures into the epididymis, vas deferens, and ejaculatory duct in the male or the vestigial Garner in the female. Failure of the mesonephric duct to develop may result in anomalies in both the urinary and genital systems (Fong & Beritto, 2024).

The third and final stage of kidney development, beginning in the fifth week of gestation, is the formation of the metanephros, or definitive kidney. The metanephros develops from the induction of the metanephrogenic blastema (metanephric mesoderm) by the ureteric bud. The ureteric bud, also called the *metanephric diverticulum*, is an outgrowth of the mesonephric duct, and the metanephrogenic blastema originates from the lower segment of the nephrogenic cord. As this stage progresses, the stalk of the ureteric bud becomes the ureter. The development of the renal pelvis, major and minor calices, and, finally, the collecting tubes occurs through the continued elongating and branching of the cranial end of the ureteric bud. At the ends of the collecting tubules, the cells of the metanephric blastema clump and stimulate the formation of the glomerulus, proximal tubule, loop of Henle, and distal tubule, which eventually empties into the collecting duct, thereby forming a nephron (Torchia & Persaud, 2024).

To complete the formation of the urinary system, a bladder and urethra are formed. The epithelium of the bladder and most of the urethra derive from the embryologic hindgut. The expanded terminal end of the hindgut is the cloaca. The allantois, an outgrowth of the yolk sac, is attached to the ventral side of the cloaca. The urorectal septum creates a compartmentalized cloaca comprising the anorectal canal and the urogenital sinus. Except for the bladder trigone—the area between the urethra and the ureters—the bladder arises from this urogenital sinus. The primitive structures regress, fibrose, or become part of the newly formed structures. The point of origin of the ureteric bud marks the point of insertion for the ureters. The ureters, formerly the metanephric ducts, then open bilaterally into the urinary bladder as the developing bladder reabsorbs the distal portions of the mesonephric ducts into its dorsal wall (trigone).

The allantois narrows into a fibrous band called the *urachus* that runs from the apex of the bladder to the umbilicus. Abnormalities of the urachus occur when it either remains patent or forms an urachal sinus. A patent urachus may occur in association with other anomalous conditions and may allow the development of a functional kidney by alleviating the effects of urinary obstruction. An urachal sinus is usually an isolated anomaly and causes leakage of urine from the umbilical stump.

Urethral development in the male and female begins in the same manner. The urogenital sinus is visible at 6 weeks and consists of a narrow portion near the bladder, the pelvic urethra, and an expanded portion near the urogenital membrane (cloacal membrane), called the *phallic urethra*. Through several processes and stages, the phallic end of the urogenital sinus eventually becomes the bulbar and the penile urethra and the pelvic urethra develops into the permanent urethra and vagina. Differentiation of the urethra in the male and female fetus can be detected by 12 to 14 weeks' gestation.

Initially, the kidneys are located within the pelvic region. They make a gradual ascent into their final location in the flank position or lumbothoracic area. Normal renal ascent is achieved as the result of caudal growth of the fetal spine, lengthening of the ureter, molding of the renal parenchyma, and fixation of the kidney to the retroperitoneum (Torchia & Persaud, 2024). Failure of normal ascent of the kidneys results in abnormalities such as horseshoe kidneys or pelvic kidneys. Blood supply to the ascending kidneys changes from lower arteries that gradually regress to arteries that arise from the aorta.

In utero, the placenta functions as the excretory organ for the fetus. Functional kidneys are, therefore, not necessary for fetal homeostasis. Consequently, pathologic problems such as aplastic, hypoplastic, and otherwise nonfunctioning kidneys may only be detected after birth. Fetal urination, swallowing, and breathing all affect amniotic fluid volume. Excretion of fetal urine contributes significantly to amniotic fluid volume, especially during the third trimester. A reduction in fetal urine excretion results in oligohydramnios. Failure of the fetus to swallow amniotic fluid due to gastrointestinal obstruction or central nervous system (CNS) anomaly results in overaccumulation of amniotic fluid or polyhydramnios. Abnormalities in amniotic fluid volume can, therefore, signal pathology in various fetal organ systems.

A balance between genetic influences, cellular mediators, and the interaction of various molecular mechanisms is necessary for kidney development. Depending on the timing of development, insult or failure of the primitive structures to grow or to branch appropriately may result in a variety of uropathies, including dysplasia and renal agenesis.

## PHYSIOLOGY OF KIDNEY FUNCTION

Kidney structure includes the cortex, the major and minor calices, and the renal pelvis (Figure 18.1). The kidney is divided into two sections: the outer renal cortex and the inner medulla. The kidney functions to regulate fluid and electrolyte balance and arterial blood pressure, as well as to excrete toxic and waste substances. These regulatory mechanisms are intimately tied to the formation of urine that involves three basic processes: ultrafiltration of plasma by the glomerulus, reabsorption of water and solutes from the ultrafiltrate, and secretion of certain solutes into the tubular fluid (Koeppen & Stanton, 2018).

The nephron is the functional unit of the kidney and is the site of urine formation. It consists of a glomerulus (Bowman's capsule and glomerular capillaries) and a renal tubule that has three sections: a proximal convoluted tubule, the loop of Henle, and a distal convoluted tubule (Figure 18.2). After urine is produced by the nephron, it drains into the minor and

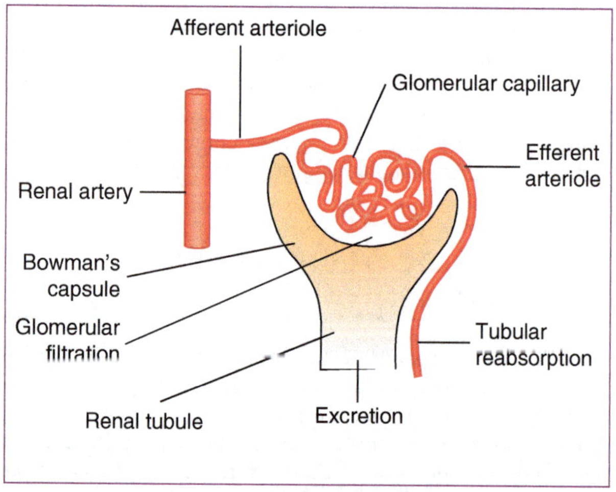


**FIGURE 18.1 Glomerular apparatus.**

*Source:* From Guyton, A. C., & Hall, J. E. (1997). *Human physiology and mechanisms of disease* (6th ed.). Saunders.

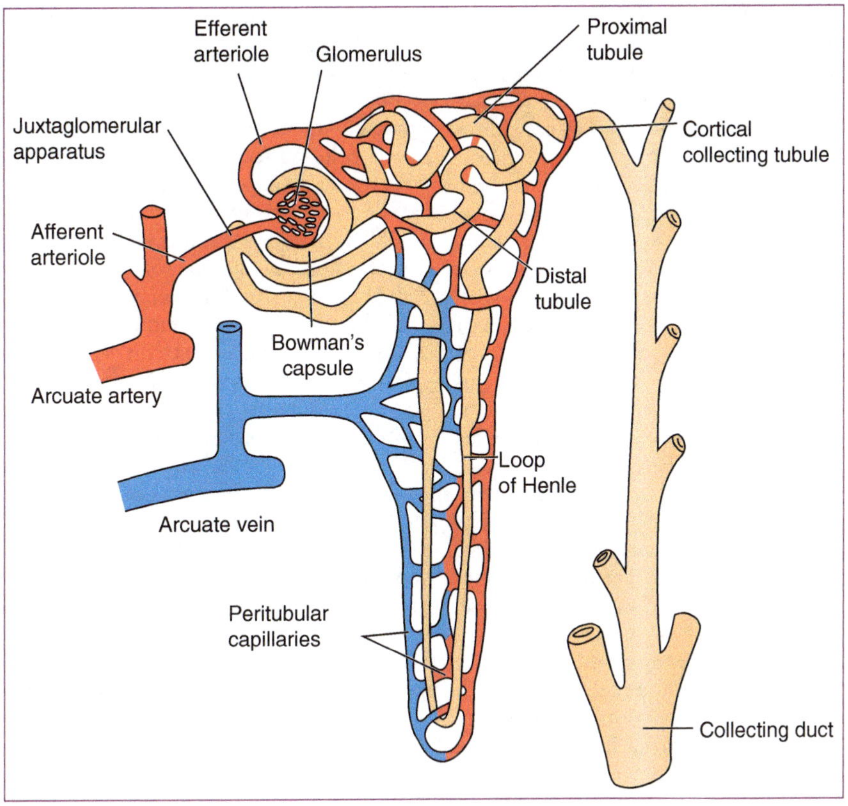


**FIGURE 18.2 Anatomy of the nephron.**

*Source:* From Guyton, A. C., & Hall, J. E. (1997). *Human physiology and mechanisms of disease* (6th ed.). Saunders.

major calyces. From there, it drains into a single large cavity called the *renal pelvis*, then out through the ureter, and finally into the bladder.

Nephron formation (nephrogenesis) begins during the second month of gestation and is anatomically completed by approximately 34 weeks' gestation. Although anatomic formation may be complete, functional immaturity of the nephrons continues throughout infancy. At the completion of nephrogenesis, each kidney contains approximately 800,000 to 1.2 million nephrons. Nephrogenesis begins deep within the renal cortex near the medulla in the juxtamedullary region and continues outwardly (Fong & Beritto, 2024). The juxtamedullary nephrons differ from the superficial cortical nephrons in that their glomeruli are larger, the loop of Henle is longer, and the efferent arteriole forms a more complex vascular system. The less mature superficial cortical nephrons make up most nephrons, whereas the more mature juxtamedullary nephrons account for a very small percentage of the total number. Altered renal function in the premature infant may, therefore, be caused by both anatomic and physiologic immaturity.

## RENAL BLOOD FLOW

Urine formation begins with blood flow. The pressure-driven process of ultrafiltration depends on optimal arterial pressure and is regulated by the dilation and constriction of afferent and efferent arterioles (Koeppen & Stanton, 2018). Adequate renal blood flow is, therefore, essential to renal function. During the first 12 hours of life, 4% to 6% of the cardiac output goes to the kidney, which increases to 8% to 10% over the next few days. This is compared to the 25% of cardiac output that reaches the adult kidney. Renal blood flow not only provides oxygen and nutrients to the kidneys but also affects the rate of solute and water reabsorption by the proximal tubule, participates in the concentration and dilution of the urine, and delivers substrates for excretion in the urine.

The left and right renal arteries arise from the aorta. After entering the kidneys, they divide and branch multiple times to eventually give rise to the afferent arterioles. Each nephron receives one afferent arteriole that divides and forms the glomerulus. The distal ends of the glomerular capillaries merge to form the efferent arterioles that carry blood away from the glomerulus. The efferent arterioles divide and form the peritubular capillaries, which surround the tubular parts of the nephron in the renal cortex. Other vessels called the *vasa recta* also arise from the efferent arterioles to surround the tubular parts of the nephron in the renal medulla. The peritubular capillaries empty into the venous system and eventually leave the kidneys as the renal vein. The fetus and infant have a decreased renal blood flow due to increased renal vascular resistance and decreased mean arterial pressure. Renal vascular resistance is elevated in the fetus because fetal renal function is required only for the production of amniotic fluid (Blackburn, 2017). Renal blood flow increases with both advancing gestational and chronologic age.

## GLOMERULAR FILTRATION RATE

As blood flows into the kidney via the renal artery, it is directed into the afferent arteriole and carried into the glomerulus. The glomerulus consists of the glomerular capillaries and Bowman's capsule. Plasma driven through the glomerular capillaries is filtered through the filtration barrier, and the protein-free plasma, or ultrafiltrate, is forced into the Bowman's capsule or leaves via the efferent arteriole and enters the renal vein. To produce ultrafiltrate, the glomerulus functions as a filtering site. Glomerular capillaries are lined with epithelial cells called *podocytes*, forming one of the layers of Bowman's capsule (see Figure 18.2). The endothelial cells of the glomerular capillaries are covered by a basement membrane and surrounded by podocytes. The basement membrane, podocytes, and the endothelial cells of the glomerular capillaries form the filtration barrier. The epithelial cells of this filtration barrier express negatively charged glycoproteins and contain many small openings called *fenestrations*. The size of the fenestrations inhibits the passage of large proteins, such as blood cells and platelets, but they are highly permeable to the passage of water, small solutes, urea, and glucose. In addition, positively charged large proteins are repelled by the cationic cell membrane (Koeppen & Stanton, 2018).

The glomerular filtration rate (GFR) is the rate at which fluid is filtered through the glomerulus. Because it is equal to the sum of all filtration rates of all nephrons in both kidneys, the GFR reflects kidney function, and a decrease in GFR signifies renal disease. Oncotic and hydrostatic pressures (Starling forces) drive the ultrafiltration process. Oncotic pressure is osmotic pressure generated by large proteins or colloids. Hydrostatic pressure is the pressure exerted by fluids in equilibrium and depends on arterial pressure and vascular resistance (Koeppen & Stanton, 2018). Oncotic pressure in Bowman's space is nearly zero because ultrafiltrate is nearly protein free (Dias et al., 2014). Filtration at this level is, therefore, driven by hydrostatic pressure across the glomerular capillaries. Hydrostatic pressure within Bowman's space and glomerular oncotic pressure oppose glomerular hydrostatic pressure in the capillaries. The GFR is proportional to the sum of hydrostatic and oncotic pressures existing along the renal capillaries multiplied by the ultrafiltration coefficient. The difference between the permeability of the glomerular capillary and the glomerular surface area available for filtration is the ultrafiltration coefficient (Koeppen & Stanton, 2018). GFR is, therefore, affected by changes in arterial blood pressure, vascular resistance, concentration of plasma proteins, and glomerular capillary permeability. Alteration in the permeability of the glomerular capillaries may result from inherent damage to the capillary, thus altering the pore size or changing the electrical charge within the membrane. GFR may also be negatively affected by urinary system obstruction.

Fetal GFR is relatively low due to increased renal vascular resistance and decreased renal blood flow, then rapidly increases during the first few hours following birth. GFR increases with both advancing gestational and chronologic age due to the increased number and growth of the nephrons and reaches full-term levels by 32 to 35 weeks' gestation (Blackburn, 2017). In the preterm infant, functional maturation is determined by conceptional age, not postnatal age. When corrected for body surface area, GFR is often less than 15 ml/min/1.73 $m^2$ at 28 weeks' gestation and rises to 30 ml/min/1.73 $m^2$ at term (Yanik et al., 2015). GFR does not rise due to an increase in the number of nephrons, but rather, it is believed to reflect a decrease in vascular resistance and an increase in glomerular surface area. Even in term infants, GFR is low compared to an older infant or child. This low GFR is adequate in normal circumstances, but in conditions such as sepsis, hypoxia, or the administration of nephrotoxic medications, the GFR may not meet the physiologic needs of the infant. Medications administered prenatally can also have detrimental effects on fetal GFR and subsequent neonatal renal function. Examples include prostaglandin inhibitors (indomethacin), nonsteroidal antiinflammatory drugs (NSAIDs), diuretics, and antibiotics, especially aminoglycosides and angiotensin-converting enzyme (ACE) inhibitors (Gubhaju et al., 2011).

Assessment of GFR is important in evaluating renal function. One method of assessing GFR is a measurement of the renal clearance of a substance. Renal clearance represents a volume of plasma completely cleared of a substance by the kidneys over a specified period (Koeppen & Stanton, 2018). Various substances are used as markers for measuring GFR. These substances must have the following characteristics: (a) freely filter across the glomerulus into Bowman's space; (b) not be reabsorbed or secreted by the nephron; (c) not be metabolized or produced by the kidney; and (d) not alter GFR (Koeppen & Stanton, 2018). Creatinine, a by-product of muscle metabolism, also meets the marker criteria and is the most used marker for estimating renal function in neonates; however, it may not be the best measure of GFR (Kastl, 2017). Because creatinine readily crosses the placenta, levels obtained during the first week reflect maternal levels (Filler et al., 2016; Kastl, 2017). After birth, the GFR in term infants increases as renal blood flow increases and vascular resistance decreases. This increase in function generally occurs over the first week of life and results in a drop in creatinine levels to nearly 0.4 mg/dl, depending on clinical status and gestational age. GFR does not increase as drastically until the completion of nephrogenesis. Therefore, premature infants do not demonstrate the same decline in serum creatinine levels as infants born after 36 weeks' gestation (Kastl, 2017). Small increases in serum creatinine levels may indicate a significant decrease in GFR. Monitoring trends in serial creatinine levels may render a more accurate evaluation of renal function.

Regulation of renal blood flow and, consequently, GFR is achieved by hormonal and sympathetic nervous system (SNS) influences. The renal vessels, including the afferent and efferent arterioles, are highly innervated by sympathetic nerve fibers. Mild stimulation of the SNS does not cause a change in renal vascular tone. Under severe physiologic stress caused by significant fluid loss, activation of the renal sympathetic nerve fibers causes vasoconstriction of the renal arteries, which decreases GFR.

Hormonal control is exerted mainly via activation of the renin–angiotensin–aldosterone system (RAS). The RAS plays a significant role in blood pressure regulation and sodium homeostasis and is found in the fetus, beginning at about

3 months' gestation. Renin is an enzyme found in high levels in the plasma and is produced and stored in specialized cells of the juxtaglomerular apparatus. Newborns have a significantly higher renin level than adults due to the neonate's altered GFR, increased vascular resistance, and decreased renal blood flow.

When renal blood flow is diminished due to decreased arterial pressure, the vessel walls of the afferent arterioles are less stretched, and the release of renin is stimulated. Release of renin causes the production of angiotensin I from angiotensin, which is then converted by ACE to angiotensin II. Angiotensin II stimulates the secretion of aldosterone by the adrenal cortex. Aldosterone triggers increased sodium and water reabsorption, thereby increasing extracellular fluid volume and renal perfusion (Figure 18.3). The goal of the renin–angiotensin cycle is to maintain an adequate systemic blood flow to supply the body's vital organs (Tortora & Derrickson, 2017).

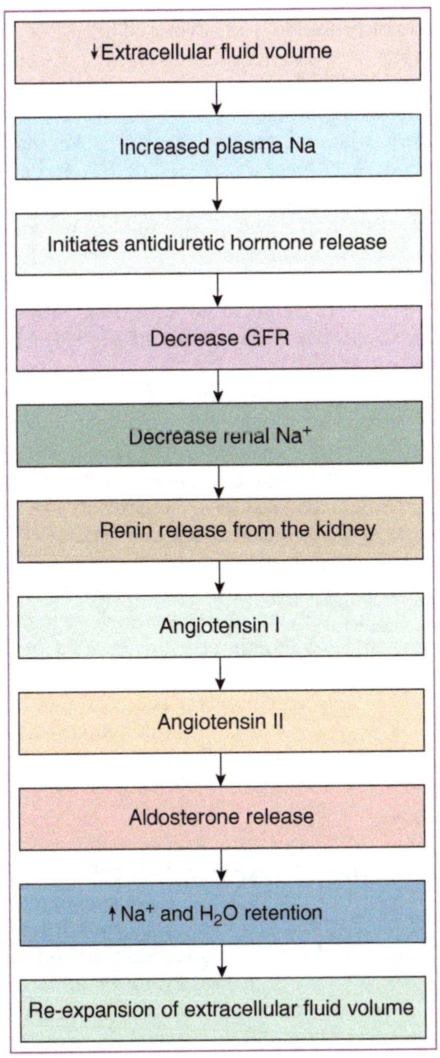


**FIGURE 18.3 The renin–angiotensin–aldosterone regulation of extracellular fluid.**

GFR, glomerular filtration rate.

## SECRETION AND REABSORPTION

The kidneys control fluid and electrolyte balance by reabsorption and secretion of sodium and water. The four segments of the nephron—the proximal tubule, loop of Henle, distal tubule, and the collecting duct—determine the composition and volume of urine.

Nephron formation begins in the medullary area, which is the thin ascending portion of the nephron that controls reabsorption. The medullary area is not fully formed in the neonate. By birth, nephron formation has extended from the medullary to the juxtamedullary area. The descending portion of the tubular system, which controls urine secretion, is, therefore, more fully developed than the ascending segment at birth. Thus, a newborn's ability to concentrate urine is decreased because although urine secretion occurs readily, reabsorption is limited. Infants are, therefore, more likely to lose sodium, glucose, and other solutes in their urine. This process is further altered in preterm infants, resulting in possibly significant fluid and electrolyte disturbances.

Tubular reabsorption, secretion, and excretion are closely tied together and function to maintain internal homeostasis and regulate fluids and electrolytes. Tubular reabsorption is the process whereby substances from the tubular lumen move into the capillary system through simple diffusion and active transport. Many of the body's nutrients, electrolytes, and 99% of the filtered water are reabsorbed, thus achieving a balance for continued growth and normal physiologic function. Simple diffusion involves movement of substances down a gradient, from an area of higher concentration to an area of lower concentration. Active transport requires energy derived directly from adenosine triphosphate because the net movement of substances is against a gradient. Molecular structures may link together to piggyback, or carry one another, across the membrane. Sodium first undergoes simple diffusion across the tubular membrane and then is transported via active transport by the sodium pump into the interstitial fluid. Because sodium filtration depends on GFR, a higher GFR increases sodium reabsorption into the vascular space. If the extracellular fluid volume increases, sodium reabsorption is decreased.

Water follows sodium ions across the membrane and into the capillary bed. This type of transport of a second substance is called *secondary active transport*. Simple facilitated diffusion is similar to active transport in that a carrier substance is used, but the net movement is not against a gradient. Glucose is a substance that secondary active transport carries along with sodium across the membrane. Glucose is reabsorbed by the proximal tubules, appearing in the urine only when the renal threshold or the maximal tubular transport capacity has been exceeded or when the permeability of the filtering capillaries has been altered. Amino acids, water-soluble vitamins, albumin, and lactate are also transported in this manner.

Tubular secretion moves substances such as potassium and hydrogen from the epithelial lining of the tubules' capillaries into the interstitial fluid and, finally, into the tubular lumen. Tubular excretion is the process whereby substances enter the filtrate that will eventually exit the body as urine. Ions such as potassium, which are secreted in the distal tubule (a portion is also reabsorbed in the proximal tubule), find their way into the urine when the body has no need for higher concentration levels. The movement of hydrogen ions influences the excretion of potassium; therefore, metabolic acidosis and alkalosis affect the potassium level. **Quality and Safety: Hormones and drugs, especially diuretics, can also affect the movement of potassium with aldactone causing potassium secretion and the thiazides resulting in potassium excretion.** Other filtrates present in the urine include urea, creatinine, and other ions not needed by the body.

# ASSESSMENT OF THE GENITOURINARY SYSTEM

## History

A thorough family history is imperative for all infants suspected of having a congenital anomaly of the kidneys and urinary tract (CAKUT). A spectrum of urogenital problems, including the kidneys, ureter, bladder, and urethra, has an inheritance pattern, suggesting a genetic predisposition. The history should focus on family members who have had a renal transplant or have undergone dialysis, those with a history of renal failure, and those with cystic kidney disease or anomalies of the GU system. A review of family history should also include fetal or neonatal deaths and the presence of individuals with external genitalia abnormalities, such as hypospadias, ambiguous genitalia, or undescended testicles. The prenatal history should be reviewed for antepartal factors associated with renal abnormalities, including oligohydramnios, an abnormal prenatal ultrasound, or perinatal depression. Once identified, the goal is to support and preserve the function of the kidneys and urinary tract, and prompt evaluation from pediatric nephrology, urology, and genetics services (Fong & Beritto, 2024).

The neonatal history should include the following questions:

1. Has the infant urinated, and if so, how long following delivery? Normal voiding occurs within the first 24 hours of life. Note whether the infant voided in the delivery room.
2. Has the infant undergone any significant hypoxic episodes that decreased renal blood flow?
3. Is the fluid intake sufficient relative to the infant's clinical status, gestational age, and immediate environment (radiant warmer or humidified incubator)? A radiant warmer can increase insensible water losses, thereby increasing fluid requirements.
4. Is the infant under treatment for jaundice? (Phototherapy can increase insensible water losses.)
5. Is the infant experiencing any bleeding or increased gastrointestinal losses from nasogastric suctioning, vomiting, diarrhea, or increased ostomy output?
6. What is the specific gravity of the infant's urine? (Normal range is 1.003–1.015.)
7. What is the infant's gestational and chronologic age?
8. Has the infant received any nephrotoxic medications?
9. What is the infant's blood pressure? (Hypotension can indicate volume depletion, whereas hypertension [HTN] may be associated with an underlying renal abnormality.)

# PHYSICAL ASSESSMENT

Physical examination should include inspection, palpation, and percussion. Auscultation is generally not useful in the assessment of the renal system.

## Inspection

Observation of the abdominal region is essential in infants suspected of having renal abnormalities. One should note the presence of abdominal distention, including whether the distention is localized to one side or is generalized. Any abdominal asymmetry is considered an abnormal finding. The presence of a renal abdominal mass is more likely to be GU in origin (Fong & Beritto, 2024). The presence of bladder distention should also be noted. Although mild abdominal protuberance in the neonate may be normal due to the relative weakness of the abdominal musculature compared to infants who are several months older, an absence of muscle tone is characteristic of prune-belly syndrome. The umbilicus should be assessed for hernias and/or drainage. If possible, the urinary stream should be assessed. A continuous, straight stream of urine is considered normal.

The external genital and perineal area should be carefully examined. Peritoneal tissue leading to the anal opening should be intact and smooth in appearance. Any abnormal openings, depressions, or swellings should be noted. The anus is normally located midline and can be tested for patency by gentle insertion of a gloved, well-lubricated small finger. Gentle stroking of the anal tissue and observation for anal sphincter constriction tests the anal wink, indicating adequate muscle tone.

Male infants require inspection of the skin covering the scrotum for color and the presence of rugae, edema, or ecchymosis. If the infant is full term, the scrotal sac should be full, and rugae should be present. The premature male infant exhibits a generally flaccid, smooth scrotal sac. The scrotum is generally darkly pigmented, without bluish discoloration that could denote disruption of circulation to the area, indicating the possible presence of testicular torsion. An enlarged or edematous scrotum may accompany a hydrocele (a trapping of fluid in the tunica vaginalis) or may result from pressure during the birth process, especially during a breech delivery. If a hydrocele is suspected, scrotal transillumination with a good light source, such as a transilluminator or a flashlight, helps determine the presence of fluid. When transilluminated, fluid will allow light to pass through what appears as a highly lightened area.

Penile size, resting position, and position of the urinary meatus should also be assessed. An abnormally large or small penis may indicate a genital abnormality. A micro penis is suspected when the penis measures less than 2 to 2.5 cm in length and can be associated with renal, genital, and chromosomal abnormalities. Priapism, or a constantly erect penis, is also an abnormal finding. The urinary meatus should be located midline on the ventral portion of the glans penis. Dorsal or ventral placement of the meatus can occur anywhere along the shaft of the penis and is considered abnormal. A urinary meatus located on the dorsum of the penis is known as an epispadias and a hypospadias if the opening is displaced along the ventral penile surface. A hypospadias can be associated with a downward curvation, bowing, or chordee of the penis. The foreskin of the uncircumcised male may be gently retracted for accurate observation of the meatal location and then returned to its unretracted state to avoid swelling and possible decreased penile circulation. Careful consideration should be taken to never forcefully retract the foreskin.

Female infants require inspection of the labia, clitoris, urinary meatus, and external vaginal orifice. The labia minora in the term infant should be well formed, and the labia majora should be present and extend beyond the labia minora. As gestational age decreases, the labia majora is smaller, and in premature infants, the labia minora may be larger than the labia majora. The labia may be darkly pigmented and is of no clinical significance. Because the labia may not be fully developed in premature infants, the clitoris in infants born preterm may appear prominent but, if normally sized, is considered normal. The urinary meatus should be patent and anterior to the vaginal orifice. The vagina should be inspected for patency, and any vaginal secretions should be noted. A white, milky vaginal secretion in the first few days of life, followed by pseudomenses or slight vaginal bleeding, is a normal finding. A hymenal tag may be present, usually disappearing within a few weeks, and is a normal finding.

In both males and females, bruising and swelling of the genitalia may occur following a breech delivery. Ecchymosis and sometimes hematomas may also occur after traumatic delivery. These birth-related findings are transient and can be expected to resolve within several days. The inguinal areas should be assessed for the presence of an inguinal hernia. The genital and peritoneal regions must be observed to ensure that there is a clear differentiation of the sexes. If not, ambiguous genitalia must be considered (see Chapter 10, "Endocrine System").

## Palpation

This portion of the physical examination may be stressful to the infant and thus is best left until the end of the examination. Place the infant in the supine position with the knees and hips flexed and provide a means of non-nutritive sucking for the infant. This position generally places the infant at ease and facilitates the relaxation of the abdominal muscles. The abdomen is then gently palpated with a gradual downward movement, anteriorly to posteriorly. To palpate the kidneys, place the fingers of one hand along the flank while the thumb palpates the abdomen. This allows the examiner to trap the kidney's pole between the fingers and the thumb (ballottement). Deep palpation is required to manually assess the kidneys and is, therefore, reserved only for infants suspected of having a GU or renal abnormality. The kidneys are only reliably palpated in the first 1 to 2 days of life (Witt & Wallman, 2024).

In males, palpate the scrotal sac for each testis and cord. If the testis is absent, palpate along the canal to assess its location. The scrotal sac may be palpated by gently pressing the tissue between two fingers, one on the anterior surface and the other on the posterior surface. The gentle movement of the fingers upward over the scrotum until the testes are detected bilaterally indicates whether one or both testes are descended and their location in relationship to the internal ring in the inguinal canal. Until 28 weeks' gestation, the testes are abdominal organs, and between 28 and 30 weeks, they begin to descend into the inguinal canal. The cremasteric reflex, recoil of the testes toward the inguinal canal, may be elicited by gentle stroking of the upper thigh or scrotal sac.

## Percussion

If bladder distention is palpated or observed, percussion should be performed. This technique is useful in determining whether the area is fluid filled or a solid mass. If the bladder is filled with fluid, percussion will invoke a somewhat tympanic sound, while a dull sound will be noted if the mass is solid. Percussion may also be used over the entire abdominal region. Examination of the abdomen and gastrointestinal system is discussed in depth in Chapter 8, "Gastrointestinal System".

## Related Findings

All infants should be examined for general characteristics suggesting renal abnormalities. Severe oligohydramnios sequence facies (flattened, beaklike nose; wide-set eyes; micrognathia; disproportionately large ears; and short neck) accompanied by abnormal positioning of the hands and feet, hip dislocation, arthrogryposis, and pulmonary hypoplasia are associated with oligohydramnios and may indicate a markedly reduced fetal kidney function. Because genetic syndromes commonly have associated renal abnormalities, one should assess for characteristics consistent with the presence of genetic abnormalities. A single umbilical artery is present in up to 1% of newborns (Fong & Beritto, 2024). **Quality and Safety:** **Historically, the presence of a single umbilical artery was thought to be strongly associated with renal abnormalities, and therefore, a renal ultrasound was recommended. Recent evidence has suggested that the association is not as strong as previously thought and that an ultrasound may only be indicated in infants with other symptoms of renal disease (de Boom et al., 2010).** Assess for atypical external ears because preauricular tags have been associated with urinary tract abnormalities. Meningomyelocele and other neural tube defects may cause decreased or absent bladder innervation, resulting in a neurogenic bladder and bladder distention. If untreated, the associated urinary stasis may result in a urinary tract infection (UTI). Syndromes associated with renal and genital problems are listed in Table 18.1.

## Urine Collection

Urine collection is a relatively simple procedure in the neonate, and several adhesive-backed collection bags are currently available. When placing urine collection bags, care should be taken not to include the rectum or the scrotum within the bag's opening. The penis should not be left in urine because infection and skin irritation may occur. To maintain skin integrity, care should be taken to avoid skin irritation when using adhesive-backed collection bags. Cotton balls can

**TABLE 18.1**

**SYNDROMES ASSOCIATED WITH THE DEVELOPMENT OF UROGENITAL DISORDERS**

| Syndromes | Renal Component | Genital Component |
|---|---|---|
| Severe oligohydramnios sequence | Renal agenesis | Absence of vas deferens, seminal vesicle, upper vagina, uterus |
| Meckel syndrome | Polycystic kidneys | Ambiguous genitalia<br>Hypoplastic phallus<br>Cryptorchidism |
| Trisomy 21 | Cystic kidneys and other renal anomalies | Hypoplastic penis and scrotum<br>Cryptorchidism |
| Trisomy 18 | Dysplastic renal system | Hypoplastic clitoris and labia minora<br>Cryptorchidism |
| Turner syndrome | Horseshoe kidney | Infantile genitalia<br>Duplications of the collecting system |
| Prune-belly syndrome<br>Urinary tract dysplasia | Bladder and ureter dilation | Patent urachus<br>Cryptorchidism |
| Errors of metabolism | Renal tubular dysfunction | Galactosemia<br>Tyrosinemia<br>Glycogen storage (von Gierke) disease |
| Adrenogenital syndrome | Masculinization of the female clitoral hypertrophy | Incomplete masculinization of the male<br>Hypospadias<br>Hypoplastic penis<br>Cryptorchidism |

be placed inside diapers to catch a small specimen for dipstick analysis or measurement of specific gravity. Many institutions now use super-absorbent disposable diapers, which can potentially alter the result of urine tests. Nursing research is needed to evaluate the accuracy of specific laboratory tests when using these newer products.

When sterile urine specimens are required for culture, a suprapubic bladder tap or urethral catheterization must be performed. The performance of a suprapubic tap requires minimal equipment and time. The lower abdomen is prepared with an antimicrobial solution and allowed to dry. If the infant has voided within the previous hour, the attempt should be delayed until the infant's bladder is full. If severe dehydration, abdominal congenital anomalies, inguinal hernias, or distention are present, a suprapubic tap may be contraindicated. Nonpharmacologic and/or pharmacologic pain relief should be provided. The procedure is usually performed with a 3-ml syringe and a 23- to 25-gauge straight needle. The needle is placed midline, 1 to 1.5 cm above the symphysis pubis, and is inserted perpendicularly or at a slight angle, pointing toward the head. Entry into the bladder is determined when resistance decreases as the needle is inserted. A slight traction on the plunger facilitates the aspiration of urine into the syringe. If no urine is obtained on the first attempt, a second attempt should be delayed until sufficient urine buildup has occurred. At the completion of the procedure, pressure should be applied over the puncture site until all evidence of bleeding has ceased.

**Emergency Alert:** **Suprapubic aspiration can result in complications, including uterine and bowel perforation, trauma to other portions of the renal system, and infection. The procedure is not recommended for neonates with clotting disorders or disseminated intravascular coagulation (DIC).** Urethral catheterization may also be performed to obtain sterile urine specimens. After prepping the area with an antimicrobial solution, a 3.5- or 5-French feeding tube or urinary catheter is coated with lubricant and inserted into the urethra until urine returns. Discarding the initial 1 to 2 ml of urine obtained may increase the accuracy of the culture results. Because bagged specimens have a significant risk of contamination, they are not recommended for Gram stain or culture.

## Urinalysis

One of the first steps in a urogenital workup is a urinalysis of freshly voided urine. Variables normally assessed in a urinalysis include color, pH, specific gravity, white blood cells (WBCs), blood, and protein. Urinalysis includes gross assessment as well as dipstick and microscopic evaluation. The urine is most often straw colored, but this may be altered by the type and amount of solutes. Dipstick testing of urine can provide a wide range of information. This test requires that one to two drops of urine be placed on the dipstick, or the stick may be dipped into a urine specimen. The results are generally obtained within 30 seconds to 1 minute; however, the exact timing required is based on the manufacturer's suggested procedure and can be found in either the instruction manual or on the dipstick bottle itself. In addition to pH, specific gravity, protein, and blood, the dipstick test may also assess the presence of leukocytes, nitrites, glucose, bilirubin, and ketones in the urine. The presence of leukocytes and nitrites can be indicative of a UTI.

Renal regulation of acid–base balance has previously been discussed. Urinary pH values range from 4.5 to 8, and reflect the kidney's attempt to maintain acid–base balance. The newborn initially excretes alkalotic urine with a pH of approximately 6. Urine pH values in the newborn should be evaluated in relation to the serum bicarbonate values. Production of alkaline urine with documented metabolic acidosis may indicate renal pathology.

Specific gravity indicates the kidney's ability to concentrate and dilute urine, and normal levels typically range from 1.001 to 1.015. Because infants have a decreased ability to concentrate urine, specific gravity measurements in the newborn can be misleading. High specific gravities can be an indication of either dehydration or high solute excretion. Excretion of glucose and protein in the urine may artificially increase the specific gravity in the newborn. Urine osmolality, the number of solute particles dissolved in a given volume of solution, is a more accurate measure.

## Urine Chemistries

Urine chemistries can be helpful in determining fluid and electrolyte balance when compared to serum electrolyte levels. Sodium excretion is very high in the fetus and premature infant but tends to decrease with increasing gestational age. While the term infant conserves renal sodium and renal sodium loss is small, sodium loss in the premature infant can be very high, necessitating correction in intravascular fluids or feedings. The increased sodium loss in premature infants is related to impaired reabsorption of sodium in the renal tubules, as well as unresponsiveness to aldosterone.

The glomerulus freely filters potassium, but urinary potassium levels are low because most of the filtered potassium is reabsorbed by the proximal tubule and, to a lesser extent, the loop of Henle. Urinary potassium levels reflect the amount secreted by the collecting tubule. As a result, an increased potassium load can significantly increase serum potassium levels. Hyperkalemia can be a life-threatening situation and is defined as a potassium level greater than 6 mEq/L. Infants who are extremely low birth weight (ELBW) (<1,000 g) are at a higher risk of hyperkalemia due to a reduced GFR, acidosis, and an immature tubular response to aldosterone.

## Blood Urea Nitrogen and Creatinine

Evaluating blood urea nitrogen (BUN) and creatinine levels is essential when assessing renal function. Creatinine is a breakdown product of creatinine phosphate in the muscles. The glomerulus freely filters it, and creatinine levels are the most common indicator of GFR. Creatinine levels at birth are relatively high and reflect maternal levels, gestational age, and the infant's GFR. The level may temporarily increase on day 1, but then begins to decrease over the first few weeks of life (Yanik et al., 2015). The more immature the infant, the higher the initial creatinine level and the longer it takes to reach normal levels. Serial levels are necessary to accurately evaluate renal function. Although these indices are not absolute indicators of long-term renal dysfunction, they can be used to identify and treat acute problems. During the first few days of life, BUN levels should not be greater than 20 mg/dl. Elevated BUN levels can result from significant dehydration, ingestion of high-protein loads, and renal dysfunction. Table 18.2 summarizes blood and urine chemistries in both term and preterm infants.

**TABLE 18.2**

**DIFFERENCES IN RENAL FUNCTION BETWEEN FULL-TERM AND PRETERM INFANTS**

| | Preterm | Full-Term |
|---|---|---|
| Creatinine clearance 1 week after birth (ml/min/1.73 $m^2$) | 11 ± 5 (GA 25–28 weeks)<br>15 ± 6 (GA 29–34 weeks) | 46 ± 15 |
| Plasma creatinine 1 week after birth (mg/dl) | 1.4 ± 0.8 (GA 25–28 weeks) | 0.5 ± 0.1 |
| Maximum urine osmolality (mOsm/kg $H_2O$) | 400–700 | 600–900 |
| Proteinuria (mg/$m^2$/d) | 86–377 | 68–309 |
| Plasma bicarbonate (mEq/L) | 19.5 ± 2.9 | 21.0 ± 1.8 |
| Mean fractional excretion of sodium (%) | 4 (GA ≤30 weeks) | ≤2 |

GA, gestational age.

*Source:* Modified from Springate, J. E., Fildes, R. D., & Feld, L. G. (1987). Assessment of renal function in newborn infants. *Pediatrics in Review, 9*(2), 51–56. https://doi.org/10.1542/pir.9-2-51.

## Urine Culture

Urine culture in the newborn is used to assess for UTI. UTIs are common in infants and can occur in association with urinary tract deformities due to sepsis or when organisms have been introduced via invasive procedures. To maintain the sterility of the specimen, either in-and-out catheterization or a suprapubic tap should be used to obtain urine cultures.

# RADIOLOGIC EVALUATION

Radiologic examination includes a variety of tests available for determining anatomic and physiologic function.

## Renal Ultrasonography

One of the safest and most common tests to evaluate for the presence of renal anomalies is ultrasonography. Ultrasound is readily available, is noninvasive and inexpensive, and can detect most structural renal abnormalities. The two-dimensional mode and Doppler imaging are the usual techniques. The two-dimensional mode may be used to determine kidney structure, and Doppler imaging provides information relative to blood flow in the renal arteries and veins. Ultrasonography is useful in identifying renal obstruction, hydronephrosis, the presence of renal calculi, and, in some cases, advanced parenchymal disease.

## Prenatal Ultrasound

Currently, the majority of pregnant women undergo prenatal ultrasounds between 16 and 20 weeks' gestation. Seventy percent of renal and urinary tract anomalies are diagnosed during prenatal ultrasound (Dias et al., 2014). Prenatal ultrasound is proficient in providing information regarding amniotic fluid volume, degree of urinary tract obstruction, as well as the presence of hydronephrosis. The presence of abnormally sized kidneys, renal cysts, hydronephrosis, abnormal bladder size, and oligohydramnios suggests significant renal or urinary tract abnormality. Amniotic fluid is predominantly produced by the kidneys, and anhydramnios or severe oligohydramnios may be indicative of severe kidney disease (Dias et al., 2014). Normal amniotic fluid levels are critical for normal lung development, and severe oligohydramnios can result in pulmonary hypoplasia.

Prenatal diagnosis of renal abnormalities provides an opportunity for family counseling and, if necessary, allows the family time to make treatment decisions, including elective termination if the anomaly is incompatible with life. It also allows maternal transfer prior to a tertiary care center so that the infant can be provided optimal care in the delivery room and immediately following delivery. Because of prenatal diagnosis, treatment of neonatal renal disease may be initiated prior to the onset of symptoms, potentially improving long-term prognosis. Prenatal diagnosis of renal abnormalities can cause significant family stress, and families require honest, accurate information. To become a source of this information, nurses must understand the disease process and treatment options for renal abnormalities.

Prenatal ultrasound also provides an opportunity for in-utero treatment of certain disorders. Placement of a vesicoamniotic shunt (a shunt placed in the bladder to drain urine into the amniotic fluid) can be used to increase amniotic fluid volume and reduce the complications of oligohydramnios (Figure 18.4) (Clayton & Brock, 2018). The goals of in-utero shunting include restoring adequate amniotic fluid volume for lung development and preserving renal function by relieving obstruction. This procedure is associated with varied success, and complications include dislodgement, premature labor, urinary ascites, and chorioamnionitis (Morris et al., 2015; Nassr et al., 2017).

## Voiding Cystourethrogram

During a voiding cystourethrogram (VCUG), a urinary catheter is placed into the bladder, contrast material is instilled, and fluoroscopy is then used to monitor bladder filling and voiding mechanisms and to assess for the presence of vesicoureteral reflux (VUR) (Choi et al., 2016). VCUGs are primarily used to evaluate for the presence of VUR but can also assess bladder and urethral function and anatomy. They are commonly performed in infants with recurrent UTIs, hydronephrosis, or hydroureter (Fong & Beritto, 2024).

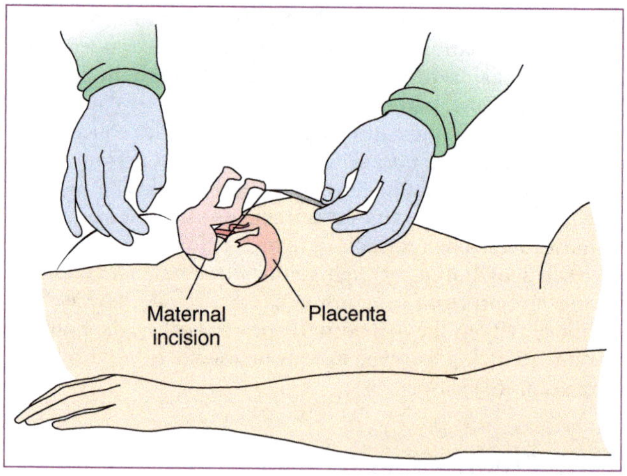


**FIGURE 18.4** **Fetal surgery to prevent hydronephrosis.**

## Renal Scintigraphy With Dimercaptosuccinic Acid Scan

This test (also known as DMSA) is considered the gold standard for assessing the renal parenchyma and is usually performed to evaluate renal function and assess for renal damage. It involves IV administration of a small amount of radioactive material (radioisotope). The most commonly used radioisotope is usually technetium-99m mercaptoacetyltriglycine ($^{99m}$Tc-MAG-3). The radioactive isotope is taken up by the renal parenchyma to identify regions of decreased uptake, representing inflammation or renal scarring. It is used to visualize kidney mass and the ureter and bladder outline. In premature infants, contrast material should only be used when necessary because the hyperosmolarity of the solution can lead to further renal compromise.

## Diuretic Renography

A diuretic renography is another radionuclide test that is used to differentiate between obstructive and nonobstructive uropathies and to assess renal function. A radioisotope injection is administered, followed 15 to 30 minutes later by a diuretic injection. The diuretic facilitates the movement of the radioisotope through the renal system, and a gamma computer tracks the isotope's movement. If urinary obstruction is present, the isotope's progress is slowed or impeded and is shown as retention of the radioactive substance. If dilation exists along the renal system, urine is retained at the ureteropelvic junction (UPJ) until overflow occurs with diuretic action. Stretching of the muscle fibers at this point causes strong contractions, release of urine, and rapid movement of the isotope with a sharp, immediate decline in isotope concentration. In a normal kidney, the isotope takes about 25 minutes to clear the system.

## Computed Tomography and Magnetic Resonance Imaging

Computed tomography (CT) and magnetic resonance imaging (MRI) provide high-resolution cross-sectional imaging and may be useful for providing additional information in the setting of complex urological abnormalities (Garcia-Roig et al., 2016). In addition, fetal MRI is becoming more accepted and adds significant value to characterize GU abnormalities prior to birth (Sefidbakht et al., 2020).

# MANAGEMENT

## Fluid, Electrolytes, and Nutrition

When renal failure is suspected, serum electrolytes, phosphorus, and calcium levels should be monitored as frequently as clinically indicated to prevent derangement. Fluids should be carefully managed relative to the clinical presentation and response to therapy.

Abnormalities in fluid status, including both dehydration and overhydration, are common and must be carefully monitored. Nursing management involves the ongoing assessment and reporting of signs and symptoms consistent with abnormalities in hydration. Daily or twice-daily weights may be required to determine excessive fluid retention or loss. Accurate intake and output must be measured, and urine specific gravities should be frequently monitored. The presence of edema due to fluid overload can be assessed by observing for the presence of periorbital edema and edema of the hands, feet, labia, and scrotum. Pitting should be determined by gentle fingertip depression into the suspected edematous site.

Hyponatremia is common and is usually related to fluid overload and increased antidiuretic hormone (ADH) production (Jetton & Sorenson, 2017). A sodium level less than 120 mEq/L can result in seizures and must be treated with sodium replacement therapy. **Quality and Safety:** **Careful monitoring of fluid status and restricting fluid intake to insensible water loss plus urinary output is imperative to prevent hyponatremia in infants with severe oliguria.**

Due to oliguria or anuria, hyperkalemia is also a potential complication of renal failure, and maintenance of appropriate potassium levels is imperative.

**Emergency Alert:** **If hyperkalemia is associated with ECG changes, it may result in a medical emergency; careful cardiac monitoring is essential to detect any abnormal rhythms or patterns resulting from alterations in potassium levels (Bonilla-Felix, 2017).** Potassium should not be added to parenteral fluids until an appropriate urine output has been established. The goals of hyperkalemia management are to decrease myocardial excitability, enhance cellular potassium uptake, and facilitate potassium excretion. Administration of IV calcium gluconate aids in decreasing myocardial excitability. Cellular uptake of potassium can often be achieved through combined administration of glucose and insulin, as well as administration of sodium bicarbonate alone (1 mEq/kg). These measures are the only temporary solutions to the problem because they do not remove the excess potassium from the body. Exchange transfusions and administration of a cation-exchange resin such as Kayexalate can facilitate potassium excretion. The administration of Kayexalate binds the serum potassium and actively removes it from the body (Bonilla-Felix, 2017). Each gram per kilogram administered will decrease the potassium level by 1 mEq/L. The mechanism of action is an exchange of a sodium ion for a potassium ion; hypernatremia, fluid overload, and congestive heart failure are potential side effects of Kayexalate. Kayexalate administration is not an immediate solution for hyperkalemia because its effect takes several hours. If the hyperkalemia is severe or if conventional therapies are unsuccessful, dialysis may be necessary.

Because of decreased excretion, hyperphosphatemia may also occur with renal disease, causing severe hypocalcemia and even tetany. Aluminum hydroxide is a treatment option by binding phosphorus in the intestines, but dialysis is often indicated for the treatment of severe hyperphosphatemia. A low-phosphorus formula such as Similac PM 60/40 (Abbott Nutrition, Chicago, IL) or Simulated milk adapted (SMA) formula (Wyeth Nutrition, Florham Park, NJ) may be indicated in infants receiving enteral nutrition.

Hypocalcemia is common and, if symptomatic, can be treated with calcium supplements. Close nursing observation is necessary during IV administration because rapid administration can precipitate cardiac arrest. Vitamin D supplementation is a useful adjunct for the correction of calcium levels through the facilitation of intestinal calcium absorption during enteral feedings. Metabolic acidosis often occurs in conjunction with renal disease due to decreased secretion and increased production of hydrogen ions. Sodium bicarbonate is indicated if the pH falls to less than 7.2.

Growth and nutrition may be compromised due to the necessary fluid and protein restriction, necessitating meticulous attention to nutrition and fluid status. A positive nutritional status positively affects both the short- and long-term outcomes of infants with renal disorders. If fluid restriction is necessary, attempts should be made to increase total caloric consumption without increasing the overall fluid volume. Kidney dysfunction in neonates has unique nutritional demands. The overall goal of nutritional therapy is to preserve a positive nitrogen balance while avoiding increases in nitrogenous waste products and increased BUN levels. Protein intake should be determined by overall caloric intake and BUN levels, and recommendations usually include 1.5 to 2.5 g/kg/d and increased up to 3.5 g/kg/d depending on gestational age and catabolic state of acute illness (Nesargi et al., 2024).

## Skin Management

Impaired skin integrity is common, especially in the presence of severe edema. The infant's position should be changed every 2 hours to decrease the effects of dependent edema and to improve circulation. The skin around any operative site should be inspected with every dressing change for signs of irritation or infection and should be kept clean and dry to prevent skin breakdown and infection.

## Respiratory Management

Due to oligohydramnios, respiratory compromise is common in infants with alterations in urinary elimination. During fetal life, insufficient amniotic fluid is linked to decreased development of the respiratory tree (see discussion on severe oligohydramnios sequence syndrome). Varying degrees of lung hypoplasia may exist, resulting in potentially significant respiratory distress.

Before extensive therapy is initiated for the treatment of renal anomalies, careful evaluation of respiratory status should be performed (see Chapter 6, "Respiratory System"). Measures to improve renal function may not be considered if respiratory capacity is insufficient to support life.

## General Preoperative Management

If surgical intervention is indicated, preoperative care is directed toward achieving and maintaining fluid and electrolyte balance and ensuring hemodynamic stability. An ongoing assessment for signs of a UTI, including poor feeding, temperature instability, cyanosis, and other subtle signs of infection, is necessary. Surgery should be delayed until the infant is free from any possible infection, including UTIs.

## General Postoperative Management

Postoperatively, nursing management is again focused on careful assessment and monitoring of fluid and electrolyte status as well as the hemodynamic system. Vital signs, including blood pressure, pulse, and respiration, should be monitored every 2 to 4 hours after the initial postoperative period. Accurate measurement of fluid intake and output is critical. Dressings should be inspected for bloody drainage or secretions. Initially, a small amount of bleeding at the site is common, but prolonged or heavy bleeding should be reported to the medical team. Depending on the infant's clinical status, feedings can usually be resumed.

If renal function is at risk due to a blockage at the level of the ureter, surgical placement of a nephrostomy tube may be indicated (Hwang et al., 2018). Generally, nephrostomy tubes are considered only for severe bilateral obstruction with renal failure or if there is evidence of renal insufficiency in a severely obstructed unilateral kidney (Lang et al., 2015). Because the renal system is highly vascularized, the chance of bleeding and infection is increased. After nephrostomy tube insertion, pink-tinged or even urine with visible bloody streaks is common. The tubes are located within the renal pelvis, and they should not be irrigated. Tubes should be connected to a closed drainage system to maintain sterility. A clean dressing surrounding the tube maintains the position and protects the underlying skin. Upon removal, urine leakage at the site for up to 48 hours is considered normal.

## Parental Support

Parental response to a critically ill infant will vary and must be addressed individually. Consenting to a major surgical procedure on their infant so early in life may be very difficult. Infants with congenital anomalies of the kidneys and urinary tract are also at increased risk for premature birth with associated comorbid conditions (Fong & Beritto, 2024). The parents must be given accurate information regarding their infant's prognosis and should be encouraged to express their concerns. The use of an interdisciplinary team is essential. Collaboration among the neonatologist, pediatric urologist, nurse, clergy, and social worker will help parents adjust to this frightening situation. If the infant's clinical status is terminal, early identification and involvement of their support network, including family, friends, and clergy, can assist the parents in coping with the reality that their child may not survive. For the family's needs to be met, the bedside nurse must anticipate their needs and respond appropriately (Purdy et al., 2015).

The general principles of collaborative management have been outlined. The remainder of the chapter addresses the most common GU neonatal problems.

# URINARY TRACT INFECTIONS

## Pathophysiology

UTIs are common in infants and are defined as infection of the kidney and/or the bladder. Infection occurring in the kidney is called *pyelonephritis*, whereas infection of the bladder is *cystitis*. The presence of a UTI results in acute morbidity in the neonatal population and, if not properly treated, can result in long-term sequelae, including decreased renal function, renal scarring, and HTN. The presence of a UTI can also be a sign of an underlying renal abnormality (Arshad & Seed, 2015).

## Risk Factors

The incidence of UTIs is 7% to 15% in infants less than 30 days old, and the risk is even higher in infants born premature or who are critically ill (Bonadio & Maida, 2014). UTIs are more common in male infants, potentially due to an increased risk of UTI in uncircumcised males (Morris & Wiswell, 2013). Traditionally, it was thought that UTIs were strongly associated with the presence of VUR, but recent evidence has refuted this assumption. The risk of a UTI is increased in infants with a neurogenic bladder that is associated with neural tube defects, including meningomyelocele, and occurs when the bladder lacks innervation and, therefore, fails to completely empty.

## Clinical Manifestations

During the first 1 to 2 months of life, clinical manifestations of UTIs are often nonspecific and subtle and include temperature instability, poor feeding, cyanosis, abdominal distention, poor weight gain, hepatomegaly, jaundice, and fever. The presence of a UTI should be routinely considered in late-onset sepsis evaluations (Coggins & Glaser, 2022).

## Diagnosis

Initial examination of the infant suspected of having a UTI includes a thorough family and perinatal history. Any positive familial history of pyelonephritis or nephritis, as well as maternal infections, should be noted. Neonatal procedures, including suprapubic bladder taps and bladder catheterization, should be noted along with the dates these procedures were performed in order to estimate the incubation time for possible infection. Infants with signs of a UTI may have nonspecific inflammatory markers, including an elevated or decreased WBC count, a left shift on complete band count, and an elevated C-reactive protein (CRP). A urinalysis or dipstick positive for either leukocytes or nitrites should be considered evidence of a UTI until urine culture results are obtained. The presence of protein and blood in the urine suggests a UTI but is not conclusive.

A urine Gram stain and culture should be obtained using either suprapubic aspiration or sterile bladder catheterization. Bagged urine specimens should never be used for culture purposes due to the high likelihood of contamination (Coggins & Glaser, 2022). False-positive culture results obtained from bagged specimens can lead to misdiagnosis and inappropriate treatment. Any bacteria obtained from a suprapubic aspiration must be considered diagnostic, whereas urine obtained via catheterization can have up to $10^5$ colony-forming units (CFUs) before a UTI is diagnosed. Because of the strong possibility of systemic infection, a blood culture should also be obtained. All Gram stains and cultures should be obtained prior to the initiation of antibiotic therapy, allowing appropriate diagnosis and identification of pathogens (Coggins & Glaser, 2022).

## Prognosis

With prompt diagnosis and treatment, the prognosis is generally excellent for isolated UTIs. If left untreated, the potential for serious complications, including severe damage to the renal system, exists, including renal scarring, decreased renal function, and HTN (Stein et al., 2015). The prognosis of infants with underlying renal abnormalities is dependent on the severity and type of abnormality.

## Collaborative Management

Prompt treatment is imperative to prevent complications, including renal scarring, which can lead to HTN or permanent kidney failure. Empiric broad-spectrum IV antibiotic therapy should be initiated following completion of the diagnostic workup and continued for 7 to 14 days IV (Roberts et al., 2011). Following identification of the infective organism on culture and specification of sensitivities, antibiotic coverage may be adjusted. A repeat urine culture should be obtained 48 to 72 hours following initiation of treatment. The majority of UTIs are caused by *Escherichia coli*; however, *Klebsiella*, *Pseudomonas*, *Proteus*, *Enterococcus*, *Staphylococcus*, and *Candida* are becoming more common as causative agents in the NICU (Arshad & Seed, 2015). UTIs commonly occur in conjunction with systemic sepsis, and it may be difficult to determine whether the UTI is a result of sepsis or is the underlying cause.

Historically, infants diagnosed with a UTI underwent a VCUG to assess for VUR because of a presumed association between VUR and UTIs. Evidence now exists that the risk of recurrent UTI is not significantly affected by VUR, and the American Academy of Pediatrics (AAP) currently recommends that a VCUG not be performed following the first UTI unless the renal ultrasound indicates the presence of abnormalities, including hydronephrosis, renal scarring, severe VUR, or obstructive uropathy (Flannery et al., 2017; Roberts et al., 2011). A VCUG is also indicated if the infant is affected by subsequent UTIs. A renal ultrasound is recommended following all UTIs. It is a safe and easy procedure that may provide important information regarding an underlying renal abnormality (Fong & Beritto, 2024). Controversy exists concerning the necessity of prescribing prophylactic antibiotic therapy to all infants until the presence of reflux has been eliminated. Prophylactic antibiotics do not completely prevent future UTIs or the scarring associated with reflux, and the risk of subsequent UTIs is not increased without prophylactic antibiotics (Roberts et al., 2011).

## Nursing Management

Nurses play a key role in monitoring infants in the NICU for symptoms of UTIs. When an infant exhibits symptoms or has other signs, including the presence of leukocytes, nitrites, blood, or protein in the urine, these should be reported to the medical team for further evaluation. If a VCUG is performed, it is important for nurses to appreciate that this procedure may be uncomfortable for the infant and stressful for the family. Nonpharmacologic interventions, such as sucrose nipples, swaddling, and non-nutritive sucking, should be provided, and while pharmacologic pain interventions are rarely required, they should be administered if the infant's pain scores are elevated. Discharge instructions for infants who have been diagnosed with a UTI should include signs and symptoms of a UTI, and parents should be instructed to seek medical care immediately if symptoms occur (Roberts et al., 2011).

# CIRCUMCISION

Circumcision is the removal of the prepuce from the glans of the penis. Although the function of the prepuce is not entirely understood, it is probably involved in protecting the glans. Circumcision is one of the most performed procedures in the United States, and approximately 89% of neonates are circumcised (Introcaso et al., 2013). There are currently three commonly utilized methods of circumcision: the Gomco clamp, the Plastibell device, and the Mogen clamp. The method utilized is generally dependent on the provider's individual preference and familiarity.

Until 1989, the AAP recommended against routine circumcision based on lack of medical indication for the procedure. In 1989, a multidisciplinary Task Force on Circumcision established by the AAP summarized the pros and cons of circumcision but did not make a specific recommendation regarding the necessity of routine circumcision (Schoen et al., 1989). In 1999, this same task force again summarized the existing scientific evidence, stating that although potential benefits to circumcision existed, there were insufficient data to recommend routine circumcision. They suggested that parents be provided with accurate and unbiased information and be allowed to make the decision whether or not to circumcise their child (Lannon et al., 2012). The World Health Organization (WHO) takes a more proactive stance, stating that circumcision should be considered an effective intervention for HIV prevention in areas with heterosexual HIV epidemics and a low rate of male circumcision (WHO, n.d.).

Males who are not circumcised as neonates are at increased risk of infection of the prepuce (posthitis) or glans (balanitis) or both (balanoposthitis) and obstruction of the urethra (phimosis) (Morris et al., 2017). Uncircumcised infants have a 9.9 times higher risk of UTI, and the lifetime UTI incidence increases from 8.8% to 32.1% in uncircumcised males (Morris & Wiswell, 2013). This increased risk is thought to be due to the higher periurethral colonization of bacteria in uncircumcised males that can be introduced into the urethral opening.

Circumcision is also associated with long-term benefits, including a decreased risk of HIV, and in the United States, it is estimated that routine neonatal circumcision would decrease the rate by 2,500 per year (Lei et al., 2015; Nelson, 2015; Sharma et al., 2018). The risk of human papillomavirus (HPV) may also be decreased. Circumcision has also been associated with a reduced risk of penile cancer. However, the American Cancer Society states that due to the low risk of penile cancer among uncircumcised males in the United States, circumcision should not be recommended only to prevent penile cancer (American Cancer Society, 2017).

Complications of circumcision are rare, occurring in less than 5% of cases (El Bcheraoui et al., 2014). Most complications are minor and include bleeding, pain, inadequate skin removal, and mild infection. Bleeding is by far the most common complication, occurring in 1% of infants undergoing circumcision (Krill et al., 2011). A hematologic workup is warranted in patients who have persistent or significant bleeding associated with the procedure. More serious complications, including amputation of the glans, glandular necrosis, and meatal stenosis, are rare (Krill et al., 2011). Complications occur most often when the wrong-sized equipment is used or when the clinician performing the procedure is inexperienced or untrained. Although the complication rate of circumcision is higher in older individuals, some suggest that parents provide consent for what may be considered a nonessential procedure and should be delayed until the child reaches adolescence and can make an independent, informed decision.

It is well known that performing circumcision without analgesia produces significant pain and physiologic stress, underscoring the need for appropriate procedural analgesia, which is recommended by the AAP. The use of a dorsal penile nerve block, a ring block, and eutectic mixture of local anesthetics (EMLA) have all been shown to decrease the pain associated with circumcision, with the dorsal penile nerve block being found most effective in pain control (O'Conner-Von & Turner, 2013). Effective adjuncts to nerve blocks include non-nutritive sucking, sucrose nipples, and padded chairs; these therapies should be provided in addition to more invasive pain relief.

### Nursing Management

Nursing care following circumcision includes assessment for symptoms of bleeding every 30 minutes for at least 2 hours. Assessment and documentation of the first void following circumcision are also necessary to evaluate for urinary obstruction related to penile injury or edema. Petroleum gauze should be applied to the circumcision site and should be changed frequently to protect the site and prevent bleeding. Parent education prior to discharge is necessary and should include care of the site as well as potential complications requiring medical care. Parents should be told that normal bathing is safe and be provided instructions regarding the petroleum-based dressing. Parents should also be advised to seek medical care if the child presents with pain, fever, lethargy, separation of the edges of the skin, unusual swelling or bleeding, and difficulty with urination.

## ACUTE KIDNEY INJURY

### Pathophysiology

Acute kidney injury (AKI), formally referred to as *acute renal failure*, is associated with a significant increase in both the mortality and the morbidity of infants in the NICU. AKI occurs when the GFR abruptly decreases or completely ceases, leading to impairment in fluid and electrolyte regulation and acid–base homeostasis. AKI can be defined as the rise in creatinine and decrease in urine output, including a serum creatinine level that rises by 0.3 mg/dl per day from baseline or a serum creatinine level greater than 1.5 mg/dl (Mattoo, 2024a).

AKI can be classified as prerenal, intrinsic, or postrenal. Prerenal failure is by far the most common, accounting for 75% to 80% of cases, and is caused by inadequate perfusion to a normal kidney (Nada et al., 2017). Increased fluid losses from hemorrhage may cause decreased perfusion, increased insensible water loss, third spacing, or decreased renal blood flow due to congestive heart failure, hypotension, or hypoxia (Mattoo, 2024a). Persistent hypoxia may lead to shunting of blood away from the kidneys toward the more critical organs of the body, causing renal hypoperfusion. Failure to adequately recognize and treat prerenal failure can result in permanent kidney damage.

Intrinsic renal failure results from damage to renal parenchyma and can occur due to progression of either prerenal or postrenal failure, infection, renal vein thrombosis (RVT), or nephrotoxicity from medications such as aminoglycosides, indomethacin, and amphotericin B (Soares et al., 2021). Acute tubular necrosis (ATN) is the most common cause of intrinsic renal failure and is a renal tubular cellular injury due to severe hypoxia, dehydration, sepsis, or blood loss (Mattoo, 2024a). Other causes of intrinsic renal failure include structural abnormalities of the kidney, including renal dysplasia and polycystic or multicystic kidney disease (MKD) (Nada et al., 2017).

Postrenal failure is caused by obstruction of the urinary tract with resultant disruption in antegrade urine flow (Mattoo, 2024a). Posterior urethral valves (PUVs), UPJ and ureterovesical junction (UVJ) obstruction, prune-belly syndrome, and neurogenic bladder can cause obstruction. Back flow of urine into the kidney pelvis can result in hydronephrosis and subsequent damage to the renal parenchyma.

### Risk Factors

AKI is common in neonates and is estimated to occur in 20% to 40% of neonates admitted to the NICU with incidence higher in extremely preterm infants (Mattoo, 2024a). Any condition that interferes with normal renal function can cause acute injury (Table 18.3). Perinatal asphyxia is also a common cause of AKI, with 30% to 56% of affected infants

**TABLE 18.3**

**MAJOR CAUSES OF ACUTE KIDNEY INJURY IN THE NEWBORN**

| Prerenal Failure | Intrinsic Renal Failure | Postrenal Failure |
|---|---|---|
| Systemic hypovolemia | ATN | Congenital malformations |
| Fetal/neonatal hemorrhage | Congenital malformations | Imperforate anus |
| Septic shock | Bilateral agenesis | Urethral stricture |
| NEC | Renal dysplasia | |
| Polycystic kidney disease | PUVs | |
| Dehydration | | Urethral diverticulum |
| Renal hypoperfusion | Glomerular immaturity | Primary VUR |
| Perinatal asphyxia | Infection<br>Congenital syphilis | |
| Congestive heart failure | Toxoplasmosis | Ureterocele<br>Megacystis megaureter |
| Cardiac surgery | Pyelonephritis | |
| Respiratory distress syndrome | Renal vascular<br>Renal artery thrombosis | Eagle–Barrett syndrome (prune-belly syndrome) |
| Pharmacologic | Renal venous thrombosis | |
| Tolazoline | DIC | Ureteropelvic junction obstruction |
| Captopril | | |
| Indomethacin | | Extrinsic compression |
| | Nephrotoxins | |
| | Aminoglycosides | Sacrococcygeal teratoma |
| | Indomethacin | |
| | Amphotericin B | Hematocolpos |
| | Contrast media | Intrinsic obstruction |
| | Intrarenal obstruction | |
| | | Renal calculi |

(*continued*)

**TABLE 18.3**

**MAJOR CAUSES OF ACUTE KIDNEY INJURY IN THE NEWBORN (*continued*)**

| Prerenal Failure | Intrinsic Renal Failure | Postrenal Failure |
|---|---|---|
| | Uric acid nephropathy | Fungus balls |
| | | Neurogenic bladder |
| | Myoglobinuria | |
| | Hemoglobinuria | |

ATN, acute tubular necrosis; NEC, necrotizing enterocolitis; PUVs, posterior urethral valves; VUR, vesicoureteral reflux.

*Source:* Modified from Vogt, B. A., & Dell, K. M. (2015). The kidney and urinary tract. In R. J. Martin, A. A. Fanaroff, & M. C. Walsh (Eds.), *Neonatal-perinatal medicine: Diseases of the fetus and infant* (10th ed., Vol. 1). Elsevier Saunders.

having AKI (Chock et al., 2018). Severity of asphyxia correlates with both the incidence and the severity of AKI, and the risk increases during hypothermic therapy.

## Clinical Manifestations

Acute renal injury should be suspected in all critically ill infants in the NICU, especially those with underlying risk factors for AKI. Cardinal symptoms of AKI include urine output less than 1 ml/kg/hr and an elevated creatinine level. However, oliguria is not always present because infants with nonoliguric kidney injury may have a normal or high urine output. The infant may also appear edematous due to fluid overload resulting from a decreased urinary output and be hypertensive from fluid overload or an increased secretion of renin and aldosterone from the damaged kidney. Physical examination may reveal a flank mass, abnormal genitalia, or the presence of other associated congenital anomalies.

Serum electrolytes will show an elevated BUN and creatinine level and, possibly, hyperphosphatemia, hyponatremia, acidosis, and hypocalcemia. Hematuria and proteinuria on urinalysis are also common signs of intrinsic AKI (Mattoo, 2024a). A urine to plasma osmolality ratio of 1:1 or less is also indicative of renal failure. Renal compromise can be detected in utero through the evaluation of fetal urine samples. The maximum fetal urine electrolyte levels considered within normal limits are sodium, 100 mEq/L; chloride, 90 mEq/L; and osmolality, 210 mOsm/kg. When these levels are elevated, renal failure is suspected.

## Diagnosis

AKI is often a manifestation of other underlying disease processes, and diagnosis is aimed at both determining the presence of AKI and identifying the causative element. The suspected contributing process determines specific diagnostic testing.

A careful prenatal, perinatal, and postnatal history is necessary when evaluating an infant with symptoms of kidney injury. Family history and prenatal history, including prenatal ultrasound results and amniotic fluid measurements, should be evaluated. Information should be collected regarding a history of perinatal depression, conditions associated with decreased renal blood flow, and administration of nephrotoxic medications.

Diagnosis of neonatal AKI is commonly based on manifestations of low urine output and abnormally elevated creatinine levels. Alternatively, the biomarker, serum cystatin C level > 2.2 mg/L can be useful to determine AKI because neonatal concentrations are not affected by maternal kidney function (Mattoo, 2024a). To differentiate between prerenal and intrinsic renal failure, a fluid challenge of 10 to 20 mg/kg of an IV isotonic solution may be administered. A urine output of at least 1 ml/kg/hr within 2 hours of the fluid infusion strongly suggests a prerenal cause for the kidney injury. The use of a diuretic following the fluid challenge may be necessary if urine output does not immediately increase. A fractional excretion of sodium (FeNa) and a renal failure index may be calculated to further differentiate between prerenal and intrinsic renal failure. A FeNa greater than 3% and a renal failure index greater than 3 suggest a prerenal etiology. Unfortunately, both indices are only accurate after 48 hours following delivery, suggesting a need for alternative mechanisms for AKI within the first 48 hours of life. Urinary biomarkers are under investigation and may be more specific markers for renal tubular damage (Mattoo, 2024a).

Postrenal AKI originating in the lower urinary system can be diagnosed by a positive urinary output following the placement of a urinary catheter. A renal ultrasound is indicated to evaluate the etiology of both intrinsic and postrenal failure. Other diagnostic testing is indicated by individual clinical manifestations and suspected underlying etiology of the renal failure.

## Prognosis

The prognosis of AKI is related to both the severity of the underlying disease and the ability to treat the underlying problem. The presence of AKI is an independent risk factor for infant mortality and is associated with both short- and long-term complications (Harer et al., 2017; Maqsood et al., 2017). At least 40% of infants diagnosed with AKI experience residual renal dysfunction and/or HTN with an increased risk for chronic kidney disease (CKD), and a long-term follow-up is necessary (Yanik et al., 2015).

## Collaborative Management

Early recognition and treatment of AKI may prevent further renal failure and improve outcomes, and therefore, the overall treatment goal is to prevent long-term complications. AKI is treated symptomatically until a definitive cause is determined to guide more specific treatment. Increasing renal perfusion through administration of increased intravascular fluids. **Quality and Safety: Despite the lack of evidence, low-dose dopamine has been used for decades to prevent or treat AKI in critically ill infants. There are potential adverse effects from dopamine use, and given no straightforward evidence, low-dose dopamine should not be considered an acceptable approach to treating AKI (Prideaux & Guillet, 2024).**

In infants with intrinsic AKI, fluid administration is limited to the replacement of insensible water losses, other fluid losses, and urine output. Accurate calculation of fluid intake, electrolytes, and urine output is vital to prevent fluid overload and subsequent HTN, edema, and hyponatremia. Hyponatremia can occur because of fluid overload due to oliguria and increased renal sodium losses in infants with nonoliguric renal failure (Misurac, 2017; Nada et al., 2017). Although treatment with fluid restriction is usually sufficient, if the infant is symptomatic or the serum sodium level is less than 120 mEq/L, correction with 3% hypertonic 5 ml/kg over 4 to 5 hours may be necessary (Nada et al., 2017). Hyponatremia unresponsive to treatment may require dialysis.

Because the kidney excretes excess phosphorus, hyperphosphatemia can occur in infants with renal failure. Treatment includes phosphorus restriction, the use of a low-phosphate formula, and the administration of oral calcium carbonate, which binds phosphate and prevents absorption (Nada et al., 2017). Hypocalcemia is also common and may require additional calcium supplementation.

The kidney excretes potassium; therefore, infants with intrinsic renal failure are at significant risk of hyperkalemia. Due to the possibility of cardiac rhythm abnormalities, hyperkalemia can be life threatening, and thus, potassium intake should be significantly limited or eliminated and the serum level carefully monitored (Nada et al., 2017). Fresh blood should be used for transfusions because older blood is more likely to contain hemolyzed cells, with a resultant elevation in potassium. Treatment of hyperkalemia includes administration of sodium bicarbonate and a combination of insulin and dextrose to drive potassium from the intracellular space into the extracellular space, thereby reducing the serum level of potassium. Administration of IV calcium can be used to protect the heart against arrhythmias but does not reduce the serum potassium level. Kayexalate can be administered rectally to increase the elimination of potassium through the intestinal tract. Kayexalate may be ineffective in infants less than 29 weeks' gestation and may be contraindicated due to a possible increased risk of necrotizing enterocolitis (NEC). Uncontrolled hyperkalemia is the most common reason that dialysis is necessary.

Because the kidneys excrete excess hydrogen from the body, metabolic acidosis is common in infants with intrinsic renal failure. Treatment with either additional sodium acetate in IV fluids or administration of sodium bicarbonate orally or parenterally may be necessary (Mattoo, 2024b). Sodium bicarbonate should be administered with caution due to its hypertonic nature and the possibility of increasing the risk of intraventricular hemorrhage in premature infants.

HTN secondary to fluid overload or increased renin secretion from the damaged kidney is common and may require treatment with sodium and fluid restriction. Antihypertensive agents, such as hydralazine, nicardipine, and nitroprusside, may be required if the HTN is severe and/or uncontrollable (Mattoo, 2024b).

Because many medications are eliminated through the kidney, certain drugs, including aminoglycosides, penicillins, cephalosporins, theophylline, indomethacin, tolazoline, amphotericin, and magnesium, should be used with caution and levels carefully monitored (Mattoo, 2024b).

Adequate nutrition is critically important to prevent catabolism and malnutrition but is challenging due to the necessary protein and fluid restriction. Because of their decreased sodium potassium and phosphorous loads, infants receiving enteral nutrition may benefit from feedings of breastmilk, Similac PM 60/40™, or SMA™. Infants with intrinsic renal failure are unable to excrete the by-products of protein breakdown with subsequent elevation in BUN and ammonia levels. Protein administration is thereby generally limited to 1 to 2 g/kg/d.

**Emergency Alert: If the infant's condition continues to deteriorate and high BUN and creatinine levels coupled with increasing ammonia levels are present, dialysis may be necessary.** Dialysis is a process that removes solutes by diffusion from across a semipermeable membrane (Rees, 2017). Dialysis is generally indicated when maximal medical therapy has failed, and specific recommendations include hyperkalemia, severe hyponatremia, acidosis, hypocalcemia, hyperphosphatemia, volume overload, and malnutrition (Nada et al., 2017; Rees, 2017; Selewski et al., 2015). Although survival of infants requiring dialysis has increased over the past several decades, it remains challenging in neonates.

Currently, two types of kidney replacement therapy are used in neonatal patients: peritoneal dialysis and hemofiltration. Peritoneal dialysis is simple, less invasive, is associated with improved hemodynamic tolerance, and is currently the most common type of dialysis performed in neonates (Mattoo, 2024b). During peritoneal dialysis, hyperosmolar dialysate is infused into the peritoneal cavity through a surgically placed Silastic Tenckhoff catheter, and following dialysis, the fluid is drained from the cavity. Depending on the need for solute and fluid removal, cycle time, dwell time, volume, and the osmolar concentration of the fluid can be adjusted.

Continuous hemofiltration is used when peritoneal dialysis is contraindicated, such as in infants with NEC or those who have undergone abdominal surgery (Mattoo, 2024). Hemofiltration is a continuous filtration process and includes continuous arteriovenous and continuous venovenous hemofiltration. Continuous arteriovenous hemofiltration (CAVM) involves the cannulation of both an artery and a vein. Blood is removed via the artery driven across a filter and replaced via the vein. Continuous venovenous hemofiltration involves either the cannulation of two veins or the placement of a double-lumen venous line, and a pump is used to draw blood into the filtration circuit.

### Nursing Management

Accurate calculation of fluid intake and output is vital to prevent fluid overload and its associated HTN, hyponatremia, and edema. Frequent monitoring of electrolytes is essential to assess for abnormalities, including hyponatremia, which, if severe, can result in seizures, and hyperkalemia, which may produce life-threatening cardiac arrhythmias. Careful monitoring for cardiac arrhythmias using bedside ECG monitoring in infants with intrinsic renal failure at risk for hyperkalemia is necessary. Vital signs, activity level, and color should be frequently assessed to ensure that subtle changes indicating anemia are promptly detected. Infants with renal failure are prone to infection due to multiple invasive procedures and their extended hospitalization and, therefore, should be monitored for signs of infection and any abnormality reported to ensure timely diagnosis and treatment.

Nursing responsibilities for infants on dialysis include monitoring the equipment, monitoring the cycles if performed manually, performing clotting studies, and administering heparin and other drugs via the dialysis apparatus. Catheter care includes maintenance of aseptic technique, prevention of hemorrhage and clotting, and observation of the insertion site for signs of infection or dislodgment. The infant should be observed for signs and symptoms of chemical imbalances during the entire dialysis procedure. Accurate measurement of fluid intake and output and electrolyte levels is critical. Fluid shifts affecting blood pressure and electrolyte balance can occur rapidly, causing cardiac arrhythmias, muscle spasms, seizures, and shock.

## SEVERE OLIGOHYDRAMNIOS SEQUENCE (FORMALLY POTTERS)

### Pathophysiology

Severe oligohydramnios sequence occurs in approximately 1 in 10,000 births, with an increased incidence in males. Defects associated with this syndrome can be due to bilateral renal agenesis resulting when the ureteric bud fails to divide and develop, culminating in the complete absence of the kidney (Phua & Ho, 2016). The etiology can also include completely dysfunctional kidneys due to autosomal recessive polycystic kidney disease (ARPKD), dysplastic kidneys, renal hypoplasia, and obstructive uropathies. The developing fetus continuously swallows amniotic fluid, which is absorbed by the gastrointestinal system and is then secreted into the amniotic cavity by the kidney. When there is little to no urinary output, severe oligohydramnios occurs, resulting in the deformities seen in severe oligohydramnios sequence. An adequate amount of amniotic fluid is also necessary for normal pulmonary development. In the presence of severe oligohydramnios, normal pulmonary development fails to occur, resulting in the development of hypoplastic lungs.

### Diagnosis

Infants are often born premature, small for gestational age, and in the breech position. Many affected fetuses are stillborn. The effect of severe oligohydramnios on the facies includes low-set, malformed ears and micrognathia, "senile" appearance, wrinkled skin, parrot-beak nose, and wide-set eyes with epicanthal folds. Depending on the degree of oligohydramnios, variable degrees of respiratory distress due to pulmonary hypoplasia are present. Contractures of the limbs due to intrauterine compression are common.

Severe oligohydramnios sequence is readily identifiable on direct observation because of its characteristic features. Prenatal history includes severe oligohydramnios and bilateral renal agenesis or other renal disorders. Regardless of prenatal ultrasound results, an abdominal ultrasound following birth is indicated to confirm the diagnosis.

### Collaborative Management

Severe oligohydramnios sequence is almost universally fatal due to pulmonary hypoplasia and subsequent respiratory failure. Due to the irreversible pulmonary hypoplasia, treatment does not include renal transplantation or long-term dialysis.

Assisting the family to cope during and after the death of their infant is the primary aspect of nursing care of infants with severe oligohydramnios sequence. The nurse should encourage parents to visit and hold their infant. Support from pastoral services or social work is imperative during this difficult time.

## UNILATERAL RENAL AGENESIS

### Pathophysiology

When one of the ureteric buds fails to form in utero, unilateral renal agenesis, or the absence of one kidney, occurs. The incidence of unilateral renal aplasia may be as high as 1 in 500 births and is often associated with other structural defects, such as VACTERL association (vertebral, anorectal, cardiovascular, tracheoesophageal, renal, and limb anomalies), caudal regression syndrome, and chromosomal abnormalities. This condition may often go undetected in the newborn period and may be an incidental finding later in life.

### Clinical Manifestations

If the unaffected kidney is normal, infants with unilateral renal agenesis are often asymptomatic (Ozcan, 2024). Unfortunately, the contralateral kidney is often abnormal, and findings of VUR, UPJ obstruction, renal dysplasia, and ureterocele are common. When the contralateral kidney is abnormal, symptoms are directly related to the type of renal abnormality. If the function of the remaining kidney is significantly decreased, the infant may exhibit signs of renal failure.

Diagnosis centers on confirmation of the presence of a single kidney and investigation of the contralateral kidney for abnormalities. This is best accomplished by renal ultrasonography, with future testing being determined by the results of the ultrasound.

### Collaborative Management

If kidney function is not compromised, no nursing care beyond normal newborn care is usually necessary. Information regarding the nursing care and treatment of the specific disorders affecting the contralateral kidney is contained in the appropriate section. The prognosis for infants diagnosed with unilateral renal atresia is excellent if the contralateral kidney is normal. If the remaining kidney is abnormal, the prognosis depends on the specific disease process.

## CYSTIC KIDNEY DISEASE

Cystic disease of the kidney occurs when normal kidney tissue is replaced with nonfunctioning cysts. These cysts may occur unilaterally or bilaterally, and the amount of cystic formation within each kidney determines the severity of the disease. Severely affected kidneys often have an associated ureteral agenesis. Cystic kidney disease includes polycystic kidney disease and MKD.

## POLYCYSTIC KIDNEY DISEASE

### Pathophysiology

Polycystic kidney disease is a bilateral process involving micro- or macroscopic cysts distributed throughout the renal parenchyma (Niaudet, 2024). There are two types of polycystic kidney disease: autosomal dominant polycystic kidney disease (ADPKD) and ARPKD. ADPKD rarely presents in the neonatal period, with symptoms presenting in the fourth to fifth decades of life. In contrast, ARPKD presents in the neonatal period with enlarged kidneys and replacement of the kidney parenchyma with nonfunctional cysts (Figure 18.5). The pelvis, calyces, and ureter are all normal (Baum, 2015). Liver involvement, including hepatic fibrosis, is nearly universal, but symptoms rarely occur in the neonatal period (Heidenreich et al., 2022).

### Risk Factors

The incidence of ARPKD is between 1 in 400 to 1 in 1,000 live births (Niaudet, 2024). ARPKD is a dominant inherited disorder presenting in the neonatal or early childhood period involving the *PKHD1* and *PKHD2* genes (Heidenreich et al., 2022). Seven to ten percent of cases are de novo (Niaudet, 2024).

### Clinical Manifestations

Symptoms include bilateral abdominal masses and HTN. Respiratory distress may also be present due to pressure from the enlarged kidneys on the diaphragm or from pulmonary hypoplasia due to oligohydramnios (Niaudet, 2024).

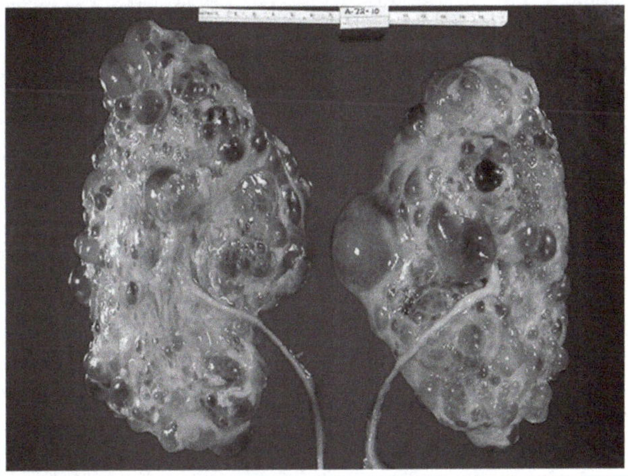

**FIGURE 18.5 Gross specimen showing polycystic kidney disease.**
*Source:* From Jnah, A. J., & Trembath, A. N. (Eds.). (2019). *Fetal and neonatal physiology for the advanced practice nurse.* Springer Publishing Company.

### Diagnosis

ARPKD may be diagnosed on prenatal ultrasound showing enlarged kidneys with increased echodensity. Postnatal diagnosis is through ultrasound findings of small cysts in the collecting ducts. After discussion with the family, a positive family history of ARPKD is often discovered.

### Prognosis

Many affected infants will die in the neonatal period, usually because of respiratory failure from pulmonary hypoplasia. Of those who survive the neonatal period, over 80% are alive at 10 years (Marlais et al., 2016). In those who survive the neonatal period, the disease rapidly progresses into end-stage renal disease, requiring dialysis and renal transplantation (Niaudet, 2024).

### Collaborative Management

Treatment of ARPKD is mainly supportive and includes treatment of renal failure, ventilatory support if significant respiratory distress is present, and treatment for HTN. HTN associated with ARPKD may be difficult to control, requiring treatment with fluid restriction and antihypertensive medications (Marlais et al., 2016). Nephrectomy may be indicated if severe respiratory distress occurs due to pressure on the diaphragm and/or lungs from the enlarged kidney (Misurac, 2017).

## MULTICYSTIC DYSPLASTIC KIDNEY DISEASE

### Pathophysiology

MKD is a severe form of kidney dysplasia characterized by a collection of different-sized noncommunicating cysts with a complete lack of renal function due to early obstruction of the ureter leading to kidney maldevelopment. MKD is generally a unilateral disease; if both the kidneys are affected, the prognosis is grim due to respiratory failure from pulmonary hypoplasia (Heidenreich et al., 2022).

### Risk Factors

MKD has an incidence of 4.3 in 10,000 (Winding et al., 2014).

### Clinical Manifestations and Diagnosis

Most cases are diagnosed via antenatal ultrasound (Heidenreich et al., 2022). If not diagnosed prenatally, most infants present with a palpable flank mass. Postnatal diagnosis is through renal ultrasound, indicating multiple noncommunicating renal cysts with no normal renal parenchyma or renal pelvis. A radionuclide renal scan will indicate a complete lack of renal function in the affected kidney. VUR and UPJ obstruction frequently occur in the contralateral kidney, requiring careful evaluation via ultrasound and VCUG (Tiryaki et al., 2013). The contralateral kidney is at risk for decreased function in the neonate and child.

### Collaborative Management

Historically, management included nephrectomy of the affected kidney to confirm the diagnosis and prevent HTN and renal malignancy. Spontaneous involution of the multicystic kidney occurs in 33% of cases, and therefore, conservative treatment is often recommended (Tiryaki et al., 2013). Follow-up care includes clinical and ultrasound assessment until complete involution of the kidney occurs (Heidenreich et al., 2022). Proponents of prophylactic nephrectomy argue that frequent follow-up is burdensome to both the family and child and that more cost is incurred than with early removal of the kidney (Tiryaki et al., 2013). Because long-term dysfunction in the remaining kidney is common, careful long-term evaluation for renal function is warranted.

## PRUNE-BELLY SYNDROME (EAGLE–BARRETT SYNDROME)

### Pathophysiology

Prune-belly syndrome consists of a triad of anomalies, including a lack of appropriate abdominal musculature, undescended testicles, and urinary tract malformations (Figure 18.6) (Wallner & Kramar, 2023). Associated urinary abnormalities include an enlarged, poorly functioning bladder; VUR; and urethral obstruction. The ureters may be tortuous and severely dilated, and the kidneys may be dysplastic due to urinary tract obstruction with reflux of urine into the kidneys. Other associated abnormalities include orthopedic, cardiovascular, and respiratory anomalies, as well as imperforate anus and patent urachus (Wallner & Kramar, 2023).

Two theories exist concerning the etiology of prune-belly syndrome. The first suggests that in utero, urethral obstruction results in a backflow of urine into the bladder, leading to severe bladder dilation. This extreme dilation places pressure on the abdominal muscles with subsequent abnormal

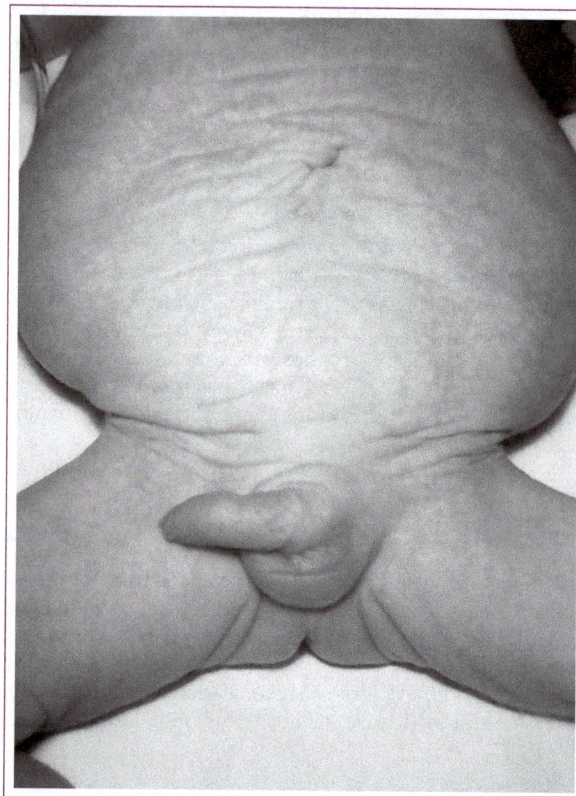

**FIGURE 18.6 A neonate with prune-belly syndrome.**
*Source:* From Clark, D. (2000). *Atlas of neonatology*. Saunders.

abdominal wall muscle development (Herman & Siegel, 2009). The second and most prevalent theory is that a generalized mesodermal abnormality occurs during the 4th to 10th weeks of fetal development. During this time, the bladder is taking shape and is being separated from the allantois, and the formation of the abdominal wall is occurring. The abnormal mesodermal development leads to the triad of defects seen with prune-belly syndrome (Misurac, 2017).

### Risk Factors

Prune-belly syndrome predominance is 20 times more common in males with an incidence of approximately 2 to 4 in 100,000 live births (Wallner & Kramar, 2023).

### Clinical Manifestations

If the abdominal muscles are severely weakened, the abdominal region may appear wrinkled, much like a prune's surface. Due to the lack of abdominal musculature, there may be visible bowel loops and observable spleen and liver. The abdomen will feel flaccid, and there will be a lack of muscle tone. A large, distended bladder and large kidneys will be present on palpation. Although the spleen is rarely palpable in neonates, one can often feel the spleen in infants with prune-belly syndrome is due to a lack of abdominal muscle tone. The liver may also be easily palpable, with more than 1 to 3 cm of liver appreciated even if no hepatomegaly is present. Bilateral cryptorchidism, undescended testes, are nearly universally present in males (Vricella & Coplen, 2017). There are likely multisystem effects, including pulmonary hypoplasia due to oligohydramnios may present with varying degrees of respiratory distress, and those with cardiac anomalies may have symptoms of congenital heart disease.

## Diagnosis

A diagnosis of prune-belly syndrome can be made as early as 11 to 13 weeks' gestation on prenatal ultrasound (Wallner & Kramar, 2023). Oligohydramnios may be present if fetal renal function is compromised. The presence of a distended bladder, dilated ureters, large kidneys, and an abnormal abdominal wall on prenatal ultrasound is highly suggestive of prune-belly syndrome. Following birth, the diagnosis of prune-belly syndrome is generally obvious upon initial examination. A postnatal ultrasound will indicate bladder and urethra distension, hydroureter, and hydronephrosis. Determination of renal function is necessary, and an electrolyte panel, including creatinine and BUN levels, should be obtained. Urinary output and fluid status must be meticulously monitored. Following stabilization, a VCUG is generally indicated to assess for VUR, and a radionuclide renal scan may be scheduled to determine the degree of renal function. MRI may be useful in further identifying anatomical and functional abnormalities (Garcia-Roig et al., 2016).

Woodard classified patients with prune-belly syndrome into three groups. The first group accounts for 20% of cases and presents with severe renal dysplasia and pulmonary hypoplasia and has a mortality rate of nearly 100%. The second group accounts for 40% of patients and presents with significant urinary tract abnormalities but adequate renal function. Future renal compromise may occur due to renal obstruction or infection. The third group, accounting for 40% of patients, presents with mild urinary tract abnormalities and normal kidney function (Woodard, 1978).

## Prognosis

The prognosis of prune-belly syndrome is directly related to the severity of any underlying renal dysfunction, whether there is pulmonary hypoplasia, and the presence of other associated anomalies. The mortality rate is 10% to 20%, and another 25% to 39% will develop chronic renal dysfunction, potentially requiring ultimate dialysis and transplantation (Seidel et al., 2015). Early diagnosis and intervention lead to improved survival rate (Wallner & Kramar, 2023).

## Collaborative Management

This triadic anomaly generally results in severe urinary tract complications. The bladder is usually extremely distended and has a large postvoid residual often requiring bladder decompression for prevention of stasis and resultant reflux of urine into the kidney. Bladder decompression generally requires bladder catheterization, and urethrotomy may be required if urethral obstruction is present. If urinary stasis results in UTIs, a vesicostomy may be indicated (Seidel et al., 2015). Other urinary tract correction is dependent on the type and severity of the underlying abnormalities. Postnatal management of severely affected infants requires early surgery. In some patients, the placement of a cystostomy button in the bladder is a safe and effective intervention to facilitate the drainage of urine (Wallner & Kramar, 2023).

The main goal of therapy is the preservation of existing kidney function. Urinary stasis, reflux, and infection can potentially lead to progressive deterioration in renal function. Careful monitoring and prompt diagnosis and treatment are necessary to preserve existing renal function. In infants with decreased renal function, careful attention to fluid and electrolyte balance, removal of wastes, and adequate nutrition for growth and development is required. Prophylactic antibiotics are usually recommended to decrease renal damage from UTIs.

The prenatal placement of a vesicoamniotic shunt may be considered in the presence of oligohydramnios, a large, distended bladder, and severe hydronephrosis when there is evidence of functioning kidneys. This procedure has been successful in decreasing the degree of oligohydramnios and its associated complications and improving subsequent renal function (Wallner & Kramar, 2023).

Muscle tone has been shown to improve with time, but abdominoplasty may be performed to improve the appearance of the abdomen and has been shown to increase self-esteem and improve abdominal strength (Seidel et al., 2015). The resultant improvement in abdominal strength may also decrease constipation associated with an inability to perform the necessary Valsalva maneuver required for intestinal evacuation. Strengthening the abdominal muscles may also decrease the number of respiratory infections occurring due to lack of abdominal support and an inability to produce an effective cough as well as to improve the child's posture.

Undescended testes are present in males affected with prune-belly syndrome, and orchiopexy is generally recommended prior to 6 months of age to avoid potential future testicular cancer; however, it is often delayed for 1 year to allow repair in conjunction with urinary tract reconstruction (American Urological Association guidelines; Kolon et al., 2014). Some recommend a nonoperative approach unless significant renal compromise is present, whereas others feel early urinary reconstruction to eliminate urinary stasis, correct reflux, and improve bladder drainage is necessary. Early urinary reconstruction, bilateral orchiopexy, and abdominoplasty may improve results (Wallner & Kramar, 2023).

## Nursing Management

If bladder distention and urinary retention continue when the infant is ready for discharge, parents should be taught to empty the infant's bladder by intermittent catheterization or use of the cystostomy button. Parents must also be educated regarding the signs and symptoms of a UTI, such as increased irritability with urination, temperature instability, increase or decrease in urine output, and cloudy or foul-smelling urine. Due to this risk, maintenance prophylactic antibiotics may be considered (Vricella & Coplen, 2017). They must understand the importance of early detection and intervention to prevent long-term renal compromise. If a vesicostomy or other urinary diversion procedure has been performed, parents will need specific discharge instructions regarding the care of the device.

Consideration of parental feelings concerning the physical appearance of their infant is mandatory. Because American culture places significant value on an individual's appearance, it may be difficult for parents to accept the loss of their "perfect" infant. Significant parental support from social and pastoral services may be necessary. To increase parent–infant interaction, nurses should attempt to include the family as much as possible in the daily care of their infant. Infants diagnosed with prune-belly syndrome often require frequent hospitalizations and several operative procedures, and it is necessary to prepare families for the long-term needs of their infant (Arlen et al., 2016).

## EXSTROPHY OF THE BLADDER

### Pathophysiology

Exstrophy of the bladder is a rare but severe congenital defect where the anterior abdominal wall fails to close at the point of the bladder (O'Kelly et al., 2018). It is theorized that the defect occurs due to an overgrowth of the cloacal membrane, which disrupts the closure of the abdominal wall. The timing of its rupture determines the severity of the defect. Exstrophy of the bladder is the most common condition in a spectrum of anomalies ranging from simple epispadias to classic bladder exstrophy (O'Kelly et al., 2018). The spectrum of anomalies involves the ventral body wall, genitalia, bony pelvis, and anus (Anand & Lotfollahzadeh, 2023).

### Risk Factors

The incidence of this defect is between 3 and 5 per 100,000 live births, with males being affected more often than females. There is a pattern for a genetic predisposition because the offspring of those affected by bladder exstrophy will have an increased incidence (Borer, 2023).

### Clinical Manifestations

In classic bladder exstrophy, all structures are displaced anteriorly, the bladder region appears open or uncovered, and the posterior wall of the bladder is exposed. Implantation of the ureters may be visible as urine continues to pass from the orifices. A concomitant defect exists in the genitalia, and males present with epispadias with a short, flat, and angulated penis. In the female, the labia do not meet in the midline, and there is a divided clitoris (Borer, 2023). Exstrophy of the bladder is generally isolated and not associated with other anomalies, and the kidneys are generally normal. Prolapse of the rectum may be evident prior to surgical correction. Failure of the pubic bones to meet anteriorly causes the hips to rotate outward. Cloacal exstrophy is the most severe expression in this spectrum of anomalies and presents with all the features of classic bladder exstrophy along with an omphalocele, imperforate anus, spinal defects, and UPJ obstruction (Borer, 2023). Neural tube defects and spinal dysraphisms are commonly present.

### Diagnosis

Prenatal ultrasound or MRI may suggest the presence of bladder exstrophy. However, a definitive prenatal diagnosis cannot always be made. Diagnosis often does not occur until after birth, when the defect is obvious on visual inspection (Borer, 2023) (Figure 18.7).

### Prognosis

Prognosis is generally favorable with most children leading nearly normal lives. Long-term complications include incontinence, upper urinary tract damage as well as sexual and fertility problems.

### Collaborative Management

Treatment goals for infants with exstrophy of the bladder include successful bladder and abdominal wall closure, urinary continence, preservation of the upper urinary tract, and normal-appearing genitalia. Prior to or immediately following delivery, the infant should be transported to a tertiary care facility experienced with care of the infant with this defect (Inouye et al., 2018). Because bladder exstrophy exposes the urinary tract to the environment, careful attention to the prevention of infection is essential both before and after surgical correction. Broad-spectrum antibiotic therapy is initiated prior to surgery and continued for at least 7 days. Because wound dehiscence is often caused by infection, strict observation of aseptic technique and aggressive management of infection is mandatory.

Repair may be accomplished in a single stage where the bladder is closed, the bladder neck is reconstructed, and the epispadias is repaired, usually around 6 weeks of life (O'Kelly et al., 2018). Repair may also be staged where there is a delay

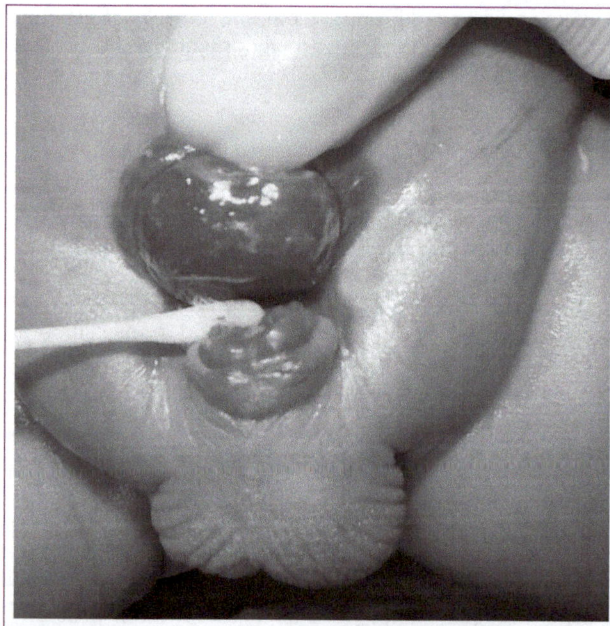

**FIGURE 18.7 An infant with exstrophy of the bladder.**
*Source:* From Clark, D. (2000). *Atlas of neonatology*. Saunders.

in epispadias repair and bladder neck reconstruction (O'Kelly et al., 2018). A suprapubic catheter and bilateral ureteral stents may be placed during surgery to allow drainage of urine while the bladder heals. In certain severe cases, a pediatric orthopedic surgeon may perform an osteotomy due to irregularities of the bony pelvis (Anand & Lotfollahzadeh, 2023). The infant may be immobilized for several weeks following surgery with traction to facilitate wound healing. VUR is common but can generally be managed conservatively (O'Kelly et al., 2018). Due to the increased risk of future pregnancies being affected, genetic counseling is indicated (Suzuki et al., 2017).

## NURSING MANAGEMENT

Immediately following birth, the exposed bladder should be covered with plastic wrap or a similar material to protect it from injury until closure is complete. The area should also be protected by avoiding gauze due to the possibility of becoming dry and adhering to the tissue, using a tie instead of a clamp for umbilical care, changing dressings as needed to prevent skin irritation, and using humidified incubators to prevent excess drying. Diapers should be kept folded well below the defect, to not only protect the area from irritation but to prevent wound infection. Evaluate the wound for bladder dehiscence.

## RENAL VEIN THROMBOSIS

### Pathophysiology

RVT is a rare occurrence in the neonate, potentially resulting in renal failure, renal atrophy, and HTN (Chan & Bhatt, 2023). The thrombus may be unilateral or bilateral and often extends into the inferior vena cava (IVC).

### Risk Factors

RVT occurs in approximately 2.2 per 10,000 live births (Guzman et al., 2023). RVT accounts for 10% of all thromboses in neonates. Although the presence of an umbilical catheter is a risk factor, the majority of RVTs are non–catheter related, and the exact etiology is often unknown (Guzman et al., 2023). Up to 80% of affected infants have one or more risk factors, including male gender, hyperviscosity and polycythemia, perinatal asphyxia, maternal diabetes, prematurity, dehydration, and infection (Bidadi et al., 2016). Most risk factors are thought to be related to an associated decreased kidney perfusion leading to vasoconstriction and a subsequent decreased venous blood flow and thrombosis. Neonates are at a higher risk for RVT than older children due to low renal perfusion pressure, decreased levels of natural anticoagulants, and lower levels of fibrinolytic components (Resontoc & Yap, 2016).

Up to 50% of affected infants have inherited prothrombotic risk factors, including hypercoagulation disorders such as protein C deficiency, homocystinuria, and Factor V Leiden (Resontoc & Yap, 2016).

### Clinical Manifestations

The mean age of onset is within the first 3 days following delivery. RVT often occurs in critically ill infants and may be incidentally discovered when the infant is imaged for other reasons. The classic triad of symptoms includes a palpable flank mass, hematuria, and thrombocytopenia, with a majority presenting with at least one of three of these symptoms (Chan & Bhatt, 2023). Other clinical manifestations include symptoms of decreased renal function, including decreased urinary output, elevated creatinine, and anemia (Brandao et al., 2011; Resontoc & Yap, 2016).

### Diagnosis

Diagnosis is through Doppler ultrasound showing an enlarged kidney. It also provides information regarding renal blood flow and may reveal the presence of a thrombosis located in the renal vein (Chan & Bhatt, 2023). A radionuclide renal scan may be performed to assess the function of the affected kidney. Because RVTs may not present with the typical triad of symptoms (flank mass, hematuria, and thrombocytopenia), a high degree of suspicion is necessary to increase the likelihood of prompt diagnosis and appropriate treatment.

### Prognosis

Prognosis depends on the extent of the thrombus and whether the lesion is unilateral or bilateral. RVT has the lowest risk for death in neonatal thromboembolic complications (Guzman et al., 2023). Although the mortality rate is relatively low (5%) and often related to the underlying critical nature of the infant rather than the RVT, the risk of both acute and chronic complications is significant (Brandao et al., 2011). Acute complications include adrenal hemorrhage, thromboembolism, and pulmonary embolism. HTN, renal atrophy, and chronic renal failure, including end-stage renal disease, are long-term complications (Guzman et al., 2023). HTN occurs in 19% to 22% of survivors and may require nephrectomy if severe (Lau et al., 2007). Chronic renal insufficiency occurs in up to 71% of affected infants, with 3% of infants ultimately experiencing end-stage renal failure (Lau et al., 2007).

### Collaborative Management

Treatment is dependent on the severity of the RVT, whether it is unilateral or bilateral, the location, impairment of renal function, and the extent of other comorbid conditions. Currently, no specific guidelines exist for RVT treatment, and therapy varies between institutions and individual clinicians. Therapy may include supportive care; degradation of the clot with urokinase, streptokinase, or tissue plasminogen activator; or anticoagulation with low-molecular-weight heparin (Chan & Bhatt, 2023). The decision making and collaboration with a pediatric hematologist will help guide individualized patient care. If signs of renal failure occur, careful monitoring of fluid and electrolyte status is necessary and treatment of any HTN. In severe renal failure, dialysis may be required. Due to the association of RVT with anticoagulant deficiencies, the infant requires a diagnostic workup for these disorders. All infants require long-term monitoring for HTN management, renal atrophy, and chronic renal insufficiency (Guzman et al., 2023).

### Nursing Management

Nurses are essential for the successful evaluation and treatment of RVT. They are often the first clinicians to recognize the presence of risk factors and clinical manifestations, and it is, therefore, necessary for nurses to have a strong knowledge base concerning RVTs. Careful monitoring for HTN is necessary as well as following dipstick urine analysis for hematuria and proteinuria. Strict monitoring of input and output, as well as electrolyte status, is also essential. The use of thrombolytic agents or heparin requires careful monitoring of coagulation status, and extreme caution is warranted when using these agents in very low birth weight (VLBW) infants due to the risk of intraventricular hemorrhage.

## HYDRONEPHROSIS

### Pathophysiology

Hydronephrosis, also known as *urinary tract dilation*, is the accumulation of urine within the renal pelvis and calices to the point of overdistention. If left untreated, this buildup of fluid can cause irreversible kidney damage. Hydronephrosis can be caused by obstruction of urine flow at the UPJ, the ureterovesical valve, or the urethrovesical valve. Nonobstructive abnormalities such as VUR and prune-belly syndrome can also cause hydronephrosis. Secondary etiologies include obstruction, such as kidney stones or tumors (Vincent et al., 2022). The severity of hydronephrosis is classified from grade I (mildest) to grade V (most severe), depending on the diameter of the renal pelvis (Fong & Beritto, 2024).

### Clinical Manifestations

Hydronephrosis is usually detected during a prenatal ultrasound. If the hydronephrosis is severe and bilateral, oligohydramnios may also be present. If diagnosis is delayed until after birth, hydronephrosis may present as a large, smooth, solid, palpable abdominal mass in the region of the kidney. Since the presence of an abdominal mass can signify many disease processes, including cystic kidney disease, urogenital tumors, and RVT, determination of the mass's etiology is essential.

Depending on the amount of functioning kidneys, infants with hydronephrosis may have a decreased or normal urine output. When only one kidney is involved, urine output may be normal because a single kidney is sufficient for adequate removal of water and waste. Severe bilateral hydronephrosis may present with signs and symptoms of kidney failure, including a low or nonexistent urine output as well as a high creatinine and BUN level. Infants born with bilateral severe hydronephrosis may also exhibit features consistent with severe oligohydramnios sequence syndrome, including pulmonary hypoplasia due to the presence of oligohydramnios. Because UTIs may be associated with hydronephrosis, infants may present with signs of an UTI, including fever, subtle signs of sepsis, hematuria, proteinuria, and the presence of WBCs on urinalysis (Baskin, 2023).

### Diagnosis

Hydronephrosis is most diagnosed on prenatal ultrasound and can be detected as early as 12 weeks' gestation by the presence of a dilated renal pelvis. Hydronephrosis is the most common renal abnormality detected prenatally and can be present in up to 4.5% of all pregnancies (Vincent et al., 2022).

The first diagnostic study indicated in infants suspected of having hydronephrosis or who have hydronephrosis on prenatal ultrasound is a postnatal renal ultrasound. In clinically stable infants, the ultrasound should be delayed until the infant is 3 to 4 days old because the newly born infant's relative dehydration may mask the presence of hydronephrosis (Choi et al., 2016). If bilateral hydronephrosis, unilateral severe hydronephrosis, or possible PUVs exist, an ultrasound should be performed within 1 to 2 days. A VCUG is recommended to assess for the presence of reflux if the hydronephrosis is moderate or severe (Baskin, 2023). Although the administration of prophylactic antibiotics for the prevention of UTI is somewhat controversial, many clinicians will prescribe them until the presence of reflux has been excluded.

### Prognosis

Prognosis depends on the underlying causative factor, the severity, and the presence of any permanent renal damage. Outcome ranges from complete resolution spontaneously to end-stage renal disease requiring dialysis and renal transplant. Most cases of hydronephrosis occur without significant obstruction and can be managed conservatively without surgery with most resolving spontaneously. Complications of hydronephrosis include HTN, UTI, and progressive renal damage (Oliveira et al., 2016). Antenatally diagnosed hydronephrosis can indicate obstruction or other serious abnormalities but can also represent a transient developmental change that may spontaneously resolve prior to birth. Even if resolved, postnatal imaging is required for at least 6 weeks (Choi et al., 2016).

### Collaborative Management

Preservation of renal function is the main goal of treatment, and treatment is dependent on the severity of the hydronephrosis. Mild-to-moderate hydronephrosis is usually managed conservatively with close ultrasound monitoring. A VCUG is generally indicated to evaluate for VUR (Choi et al., 2016). Although severe hydronephrosis is initially managed with conservative treatment, some cases will ultimately require pyeloplasty due to deteriorating renal function. When reflux is present, prophylactic antibiotics are often prescribed for UTI prophylaxis.

When severe hydronephrosis is prenatally diagnosed, vesicoamniotic shunting (placement of a catheter into the bladder to drain urine) may be performed to reduce oligohydramnios and its associated complications as well as to sustain kidney function. After birth, definitive surgery is necessary to correct the obstructive defect or to provide a diversion for urine flow (Vincent et al., 2022).

## Nursing Management

Careful assessment is imperative in infants diagnosed with hydronephrosis. Vital signs, including blood pressure, must be monitored at least every 4 hours and more frequently if unstable. Monitoring blood pressure is especially important because HTN is a common complication in infants with severe hydronephrosis. Fluid and electrolyte status, including serum creatinine and BUN, must also be carefully monitored. Fluid intake and output should be recorded at least every 2 to 4 hours.

# OBSTRUCTIVE UROPATHY

## Pathophysiology

When obstruction occurs in the urinary tract, changes referred to as *obstructive uropathy* can occur. Obstruction to urinary flow can cause reflux of urine into the kidney, with resultant hydronephrosis and irreversible kidney damage (Misurac, 2017). Urinary obstruction can be unilateral or bilateral and can occur at the UVJ, the UPJ, or due to PUVs (Figure 18.8). The most common cause of urinary obstruction is UPJ obstruction. UPJ obstruction occurs due to obstruction of urinary flow from the pelvis of the kidney into the ureter and is caused by stenosis of the ureter and/or its associated valves or by an insertion anomaly of the ureter (Choi et al., 2016). UVJ obstruction is caused by obstruction of flow from the ureter into the bladder.

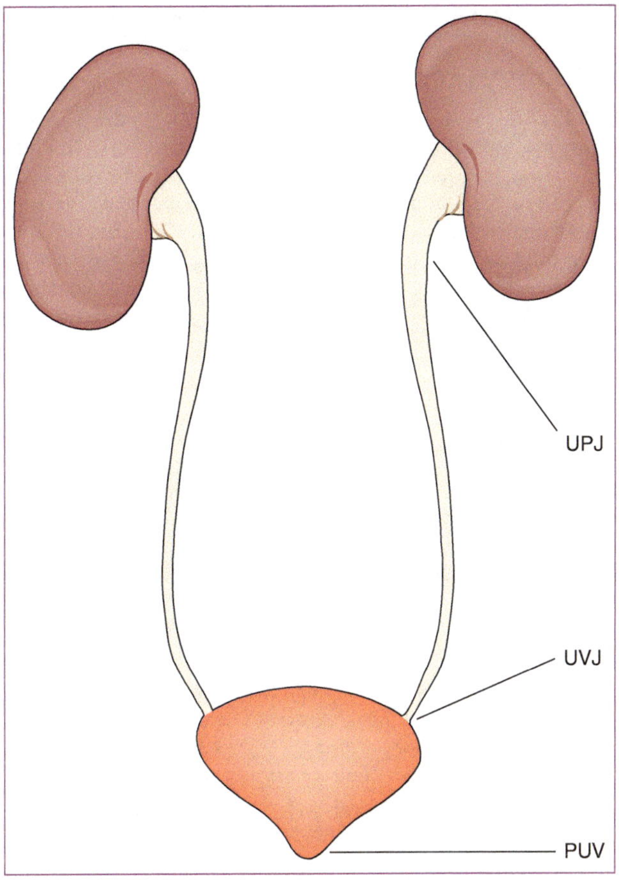


**FIGURE 18.8 Location of most common sites of congenital urinary tract obstruction.**

PUVs, posterior urethral valves; UPJ, ureteropelvic junction; UVJ, ureterovesical junction.

*Source:* From Chevalier, R. L. (2004). Perinatal obstructive nephropathy. *Seminars in Perinatology, 28,* 124–131. https://doi.org/10.1053/j.semperi.2003.11.009.

## Risk Factors

UPJ obstruction is the most common cause of obstructive uropathy, with an incidence of 1 in 2,000, and is increased in males (Epelman et al., 2012). Information concerning PUVs may be found in the later section of this chapter.

## Clinical Manifestations

Signs of urinary tract obstruction include symptoms of a UTI, or if significant hydronephrosis is present, an abdominal mass may be appreciated. Severe bilateral obstruction can also be associated with symptoms of renal failure.

## Diagnosis

Urinary tract obstruction can be diagnosed on prenatal ultrasound as early as 16 to 17 weeks' gestation with evidence of hydronephrosis (Oliveira et al., 2016). Ultrasound findings range from mild hydronephrosis to extreme obstruction with oligohydramnios.

Postnatal diagnosis is via renal ultrasound and may be followed by a VCUG to assess for reflux (Weitz & Schmidt, 2017). A radionuclide renal scan is recommended to assess renal function.

## Prognosis

Obstructive uropathy can result in chronic renal failure and is a common cause of pediatric kidney transplantations if bilateral (Misurac, 2017).

## Collaborative Management

Treatment depends on the severity of the obstruction and on whether the obstruction is unilateral or bilateral. If mild, conservative management is appropriate with frequent renal assessment. Prophylactic antibiotics may be indicated to prevent UTIs and the possibility of associated renal damage.

Surgical intervention may be indicated to relieve the obstruction. Insertion of a urinary diversion, such as a pyelostomy tube inserted into the renal pelvis, may be indicated (Hwang et al., 2018). Significant diuresis may follow urinary diversion, and thus, meticulous monitoring of fluid and electrolytes and replacement of losses are critical to avoid dehydration. Long-term follow-up is essential for the early detection of chronic renal problems.

Prenatal treatment, including insertion of a vesicoamniotic shunt, may be indicated if severe obstruction is present to increase the amniotic fluid volume and decrease the potential for renal failure. Complications of this procedure include shunt displacement and clogging of the shunt.

## POSTERIOR URETHRAL VALVES

### Pathophysiology

PUVs are the most common cause of urinary tract obstruction and cause severe obstruction uropathy, often resulting in end-stage renal failure. PUV occurs when urine is obstructed at the level of the bladder outlet due to the presence of enlarged membranous folds (Fishberg et al., 2018). Severity ranges from mild obstruction to severe disease, with obstructive uropathy and massive hydronephrosis. Urinary obstruction can increase pressure in the bladder and upper urinary tract, resulting in abnormal bladder function and renal injury (Holmes, 2023).

### Risk Factors

PUV is a rare disease occurring exclusively in males with an incidence of 1 in 4,000 to 1 in 8,000 live births (Holmes, 2023). The specific etiology is unknown. Other associated urinary tract anomalies, including VUR, are common.

### Clinical Manifestations

Neonatal symptoms of PUV include a palpable bladder, anuria or oliguria, a weak urinary stream, urosepsis, and urinary ascites. If severe oligohydramnios is present prenatally, respiratory symptoms due to pulmonary hypoplasia may be present (Holmes, 2023).

### Diagnosis

PUVs are often diagnosed on prenatal ultrasound with the presence of bilateral hydronephrosis, a distended bladder, a dilated posterior urethra, and a thickened bladder wall (Fishberg et al., 2018). Following delivery, an ultrasound is required to evaluate the presence and degree of hydronephrosis, the presence of bladder wall thickening, and the general health of the kidneys. However, the gold standard for diagnosis is through a VCUG, showing a dilated posterior urethra, a trabeculated bladder, VUR, and sometimes visualization of the enlarged valve leaflets. Renal scintigraphy for evaluation of renal function is usually deferred for approximately 4 weeks following birth to allow maturation of developing kidneys (Fishberg et al., 2018).

### Prognosis

The diagnosis of PUVs is associated with significant long-term morbidity, which is dependent on the amount of renal damage caused by the PUVs (Fishberg et al., 2018). In all, a percentage of infants diagnosed with PUV will progress to end-stage renal disease, often requiring dialysis and/or renal transplantation. Bladder dysfunction in childhood is common, including bladder overactivity, resulting in urgency, urge incontinence and nocturnal enuresis. The bladder can also become overdistended and overcompliant, causing ineffective bladder emptying and possibly requiring intermittent catheterization. Urethral strictures are also a possible complication occurring later in childhood (Silverii et al., 2024).

### Collaborative Management

The initial treatment of PUVs is immediate urinary diversion with either bladder catheterization or suprapubic diversion to relieve the obstruction and reduce the pressure on the urinary tract to maintain normal bladder and kidney function (Misurac, 2017). Due to the increased risk of long-term complications, suprapubic diversion is only performed if bladder catheterization is impossible or if early correction of the defect is impossible because of the infant's small size or if the urethra is too small, precluding insertion of the endoscope for valve ablation. The infant may also require stabilization, including administration of IV fluids, correction of electrolyte or acid–base abnormalities, and antibiotics to prevent infection. Mechanical ventilation may be required if pulmonary hypoplasia is present. The definitive treatment of PUVs is transurethral endoscopic ablation (rupture) of the enlarged valves (Caione & Nappo, 2011). Prophylactic antibiotics are often required to prevent UTIs and subsequent renal injury, and long-term follow-up is essential to monitor bladder and renal function.

Unfortunately, prenatal treatment is difficult to perform and has not been shown to improve the mortality or morbidity of infants with PUV. In cases of oligohydramnios-associated pulmonary hypoplasia, some clinicians favor prenatal treatment with urinary diversion to increase the amniotic fluid level (Morris et al., 2010). In the future, prenatal valve ablation may be possible, thereby avoiding the renal and urinary tract damage that often occurs early in gestation prior to diagnosis of the defect.

### Nursing Management

Immediately following delivery, the bladder should be catheterized under sterile conditions using a small 5- or 6-French feeding tube to allow passage through the constricted urethra. **Quality and Safety: The use of balloon catheters is contraindicated due to the possibility of bladder spasms.** Parents should be educated regarding the necessity of close postdischarge follow-up to ensure early detection of chronic renal disease and bladder dysfunction.

## HYDROCELE

### Pathophysiology

A hydrocele, the collection of fluid in the scrotal sac, is a common occurrence in neonates (Lao et al., 2012). The fluid originates from the peritoneal cavity, which communicates with the scrotum through a patent processus vaginalis. The only difference between the presence of a hydrocele and an inguinal hernia is the size of the processus vaginalis (Basta et al., 2015). If the processus vaginalis is small, only fluid can move into the scrotum, resulting in a hydrocele. Larger passageways may allow the escape of a bowel segment into the scrotum, resulting in an inguinal hernia.

### Risk Factors

The risk of a patent processus vaginalis is elevated with increased abdominal pressure secondary to a ventriculoperitoneal shunt or high ventilatory pressures and prematurity.

## Clinical Manifestations

Clinical manifestations include the presence of painless scrotal swelling that is readily transilluminated.

## Diagnosis

The most critical aspect of diagnosis is differentiating whether scrotal swelling is due to the presence of a hydrocele or the more serious diagnosis of either an inguinal hernia or testicular torsion. Upon palpation, inguinal hernias are generally reducible, whereas hydroceles are not. When transilluminated, the hydrocele will show a fluid-filled scrotum, whereas an inguinal hernia will appear as a solid mass. If the examiner encounters loops of the intestine near the vas deferens or the ductus deferens within the scrotal sac, an inguinal hernia is present. Ultrasound may also assist in differentiation (Basta et al., 2015).

## Collaborative Management

Treatment for hydroceles is rarely indicated; the majority will spontaneously resolve within 1 to 2 years due to the closure of the processus vaginalis (Basta et al., 2015). Indications for surgical correction generally include failure to resolve within the first year of life, although some surgeons will wait 2 years if there are no complications. Surgery entails drainage of fluid from the scrotal sac and closure of the processus vaginalis (Lao et al., 2012). Until the resolution of the hydrocele, the infant should be closely monitored for signs of intestinal herniation. If an inguinal hernia is suspected, surgical intervention is indicated.

## Nursing Management

Parents should be taught the signs of intestinal herniation and incarceration and the need for prompt medical attention if symptoms occur. These signs include the presence of a lump in the groin (this lump is especially noticeable when the infant is crying) and increased irritability. Careful attention must be paid to skin care of the edematous scrotum to avoid irritation and breakdown.

# INGUINAL HERNIA

## Pathophysiology

An inguinal hernia occurs when the intestines descend into either the inguinal canal or the scrotum through an open processus vaginalis (Lao et al., 2012) (Figure 18.9). During fetal life, as the testes descend into the scrotum, they bring a small part of the peritoneum, which is the processus vaginalis (Lao et al., 2012). When the processus vaginalis is open, fluid or intestines can pass through the opening, resulting in either a hydrocele or an inguinal hernia. The presence of a hydrocele

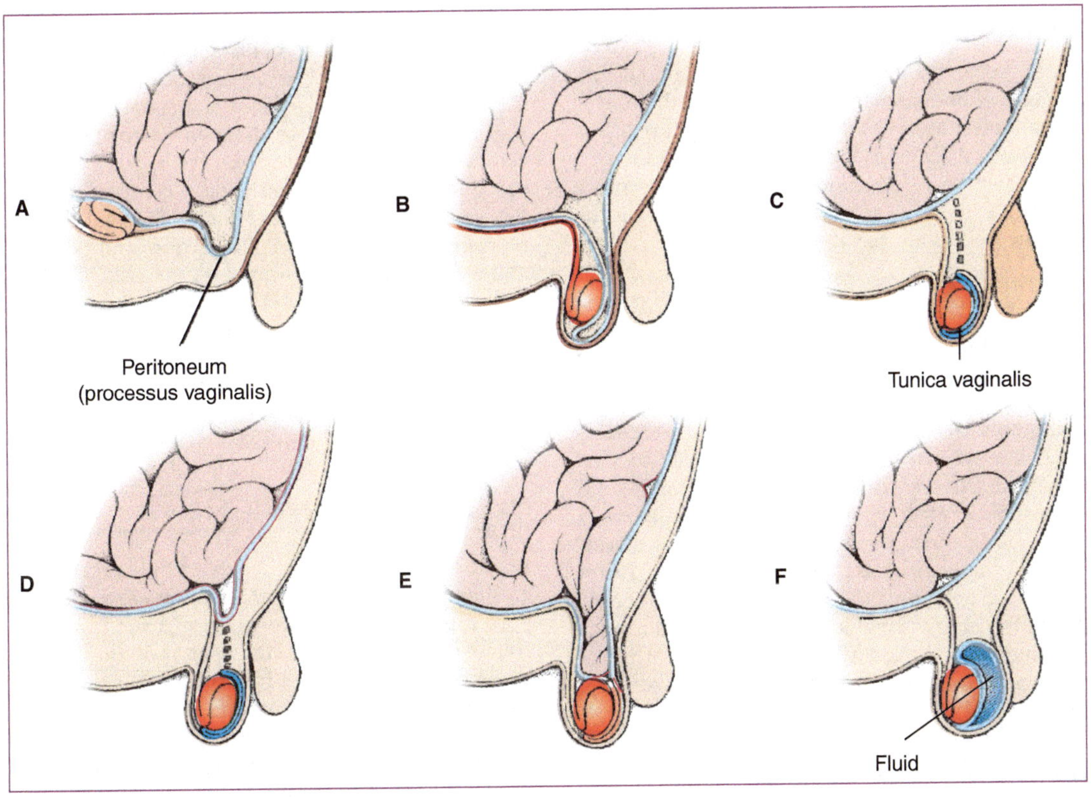


**FIGURE 18.9 Development of inguinal hernias.** (**A** and **B**) Prenatal migration of processus vaginalis. (**C**) Normal. (**D**) Partially obliterated processus vaginalis. (**E**) Hernia. (**F**) Hydrocele.

*Source:* From Hockenberry, M. J., Wilson, D., Winkelstein, M. L., & Wong, D. L. (2003). *Wong's nursing care of infants and children* (7th ed., p. 478). Mosby.

or inguinal hernia is dependent on the size of the opening. The processus vaginalis becomes obliterated between 38 and 48 weeks of gestational age.

## Risk Factors

Due to the presence of an open processus vaginalis during fetal life, the incidence of inguinal hernias is inversely related to gestational age and birth weight. In preterm infants, up to 10% to 30% are reported to have inguinal hernias (Kus et al., 2024), predominately affecting male infants (Youn et al., 2018). Sixty percent of inguinal hernias occur in the right inguinal canal and 15% are bilateral (Lao et al., 2012). Additional hernias can be observed during laparoscopic evaluation, leading to the need for bilateral repair in up to 73% of infants (Ramachandran et al., 2020). Additional risk factors include cystic fibrosis, congenital hip dysplasia, the presence of a ventriculoperitoneal shunt, and abdominal wall defects.

## Prognosis

The most severe complication of inguinal hernia is an incarcerated hernia with subsequent intestinal necrosis. The highest risk of incarceration occurs in early infancy, and the risk of incarceration in premature infants is up to 31% (Youn et al., 2018). When inguinal hernias are surgically repaired prior to incarceration, complications are rare. Reoccurrence after surgical repair can occur, especially in infants born premature (Ramachandran et al., 2020).

## Clinical Manifestations

The most common clinical manifestation of an inguinal hernia is the presence of an inguinal bulge or mass as the omentum of the small intestine slides through the open processus vaginalis (Cavaliere, 2024). Crying or increased abdominal pressure often causes the inguinal hernia to appear more prominent. When a hernia is reducible, the intestine can be gently manipulated back into the abdomen cavity.

## Diagnosis

The most important component of diagnosis is determining whether the mass is an inguinal hernia or other scrotal mass, including a hydrocele or testicular torsion. If the scrotum can be transilluminated, the mass may be either a hydrocele or an inguinal hernia (Cavaliere, 2024). Testicular torsion should be suspected if the scrotum contains a hard, solid mass. This is a surgical emergency and must be immediately reported to the surgical team. If it is not possible to distinguish between an inguinal hernia and a hydrocele, a rectal examination, while palpating the scrotum simultaneously, may reveal whether an intestinal loop is present in the scrotal sac rather than a fluid-filled hydrocele. The use of ultrasound may also prove helpful in differentiating between the two processes.

## Collaborative Management

Inguinal hernias should be reduced daily and as needed by applying gentle pressure to assess for incarceration of the hernia. An incarcerated hernia occurs when the intestines are caught within the processus vaginalis. Symptoms of incarcerated hernias include inability to reduce, vomiting, a firm and tense mass, inconsolable crying, and abdominal distention. When incarceration occurs, circulation is compromised, and intestinal necrosis is possible, necessitating an immediate surgical consult.

If the inguinal hernia is nonreducible, advanced attempts for reduction are often attempted. After the infant is well sedated and placed in the Trendelenburg position, ice packs are placed on the hernia to reduce intestinal edema. If gentle reduction is successful, surgery may be delayed for 24 to 48 hours. Surgery for incarcerated hernias includes reduction of hernia and, if necrotic bowel is present, resection of the affected intestine.

Because of the high risk of incarceration, it is generally recommended that surgical repair of inguinal hernias should be performed as soon as possible. Surgery may be delayed in premature infants due to the technical difficulty of operating and an increased risk of complications, including testicular atrophy and recurrent hernia. The exact timing of surgical intervention in the premature infant is controversial; however, many surgeons will correct the defect prior to discharge from the hospital (Peace et al., 2023). Although many surgeons advocate early repair, elective delayed repair after discharge from the NICU can also be considered by pediatric surgery secondary to increased perioperative risk in preterm infants (Peace et al., 2023). Timely access to elective outpatient inguinal hernia repairs is an important factor to consider when selecting this option (Kus et al., 2024).

Surgery may be performed either through an open procedure or through laparoscopic surgery (Ho et al., 2018). Surgical correction involves separation of the hernia sac from surrounding structures (Youn et al., 2018). The contralateral side may be explored to detect a patent process or a non–clinically evident hernia (Youn et al., 2018). Whether or not to explore the contralateral side is controversial. The goal of this exploration is to avoid future inguinal hernias, thereby reducing the risk of a second surgery and possible incarceration. However, it also increases the risk of infection, pain, and the cost of surgery. The risk of complications associated with surgical correction of inguinal hernias is generally low; however, premature infants are at high risk for postoperative apnea and should be monitored for at least 24 hours postsurgery. Apnea following surgery may decrease with use of spinal anesthesia.

# NURSING MANAGEMENT

Reduction of all inguinal hernias should take place daily, and an inability to reduce the hernia should immediately be reported to the medical and surgical team. The postoperative course is similar to following open procedures or laparotomy and includes observation for apnea and adherence to aseptic technique for suture line maintenance. The infant should be placed in a side-lying or supine position with the head turned to the side to prevent disruption of the suture line. Operative dressings should be observed for any drainage and bleeding and kept dry. The underlying skin should be regularly inspected for irritation and breakdown. Pain should be assessed every 4 hours, and appropriate pain management should be provided as indicated. Discharge is often 24 hours postsurgery, so parents must be instructed on proper surgical site and dressing care.

## TESTICULAR TORSION

### Pathophysiology

Torsion of the testicle occurs when the testis and coverings twist inside the scrotum, compromising blood flow and frequently resulting in a nonviable testicle (Hittelman, 2023).

### Risk Factors

The incidence of testicular torsion is 6.1 per 100,000 (Hittelman, 2023). Although it is most often unilateral, bilateral torsion can occur, resulting in a complete lack of testicular development (Nandi & Murphy, 2011). Risk factors include vaginal delivery, prolonged labor, gestational diabetes, macrosomia, and breech delivery, and it appears that fetal stress and mechanical factors may be the contributors.

### Prognosis

An 8.96% salvage rate for testicular torsion in the neonatal population has been reported. This may increase to 21.7% if surgery is emergent. Unfortunately, salvage of antenatally occurring torsion is extremely rare (Nandi & Murphy, 2011).

### Clinical Manifestations

Testicular torsion presents with unilateral acute pain and scrotal swelling. The scrotum is firm to the touch, tender, and often discolored. The abdomen may be significantly discolored and be either plethoric or cyanotic. The clinical presentation of testicular torsion is like other scrotal abnormalities, such as hydrocele, inguinal hernia, and trauma; however, it can often be distinguished due to the presence of scrotal discoloration and an inability to be transilluminated (Huang et al., 2024). Information related to testicular blood flow can be obtained via the use of color Doppler ultrasound. Because of the emergent need for surgical intervention, the diagnosis of testicular torsion must be considered in all infants presenting with scrotal swelling.

### Collaborative Management

The treatment of acute testicular torsion is immediate surgery to untwist the testicle and restore blood supply. Timing of the intervention is critical, and a delay in surgical intervention of 4 to 6 hours following initiation of symptoms offers little to no chance of testicular survival. If the torsion occurs antenatally, the chance for testicular survival is nearly nonexistent, and surgical intervention may be futile (Basta et al., 2015). The most important determinant in the decision to perform surgery is the appearance of the scrotum in the delivery room. If the scrotum appears normal initially and then becomes acutely painful, swollen, and discolored, immediate surgery is indicated to salvage the testicle. If the scrotum appears blue, hard, and painless immediately after birth, the torsion occurs prenatally, and the testicle has already become necrotic.

Controversy exists regarding the treatment of antenatally occurring testicular torsion. Some advocate conservative treatment with regular ultrasound examinations to monitor for testicular atrophy. Others suggest contralateral orchiopexy is necessary to prevent the possibility of torsion and subsequent necrosis of both testes (Nandi & Murphy, 2011).

### Nursing Management

The focus of nursing care is on keeping the infant as comfortable and quiet as possible. The abdominal girth should be measured every 4 hours to assess for distention. The infant should be supine with the head turned to the side or in a side-lying position to avoid excessive pressure on the abdominal and scrotal areas.

If surgery is required, nursing care is centered on the stability of the vital signs and prevention of infection. The suture line is generally small but still requires aseptic technique. The site should be assessed for edema, drainage, or discoloration.

## NEPHROBLASTOMA (WILMS' TUMOR)

### Pathophysiology

Wilms' tumor (nephroblastoma) is a well-encapsulated heterogeneous malignant tumor of the kidney. It is thought to be due to persistent nephrogenic embryologic cells that fail to develop appropriately. Wilms' tumor is associated with other anomalies, including aniridia (lack of development or absence of the iris), GU tract anomalies, and Beckwith–Wiedemann syndrome (Style et al., 2018).

### Risk Factors

The incidence of Wilms' tumor in neonates is rare, with the incidence increasing as the infant ages. It can be detected prenatally (Toussi et al., 2018). Wilms' tumor is generally a sporadic condition, but 1% of those affected have a family history of the disease (Powis, 2010; van den Heuvel-Eibrink et al., 2017).

### Clinical Manifestations

The typical presentation of Wilms' tumor is a unilateral smooth, solid abdominal or flank mass that does not cross the midline in an otherwise well-appearing infant (Powis, 2010). Microscopic hematuria may be present, and HTN may occur if associated renal artery stenosis or increased renin secretion is present (Smith & Chintagumpala, 2024).

### Diagnosis

Prenatal diagnosis is uncommon, and most are diagnosed after birth (Toussi et al., 2018). Prenatally, Wilms' tumor is associated with an increased risk of fetal distress, hydrops, and prematurity. Postnatally, the initial diagnostic procedure is an abdominal ultrasound to determine the origin of the abdominal mass. Either CT or MRI generally follows the ultrasound to make a definitive diagnosis and to determine the cancer stage (Powis, 2010). Biopsies are usually unnecessary in infants under 6 months of age.

## Prognosis

Prognosis is related to the stage of the disease and the size of the tumor. Children younger than 2 years generally have a very favorable prognosis, but the risk of complications is higher in neonates (Toussi et al., 2018).

## Collaborative Management

Because of the possibility that the encapsulated tumor may rupture and seed other areas of the body, repeated abdominal examinations should be avoided. Treatment of unilateral Wilms' tumor generally includes only nephroureterectomy in the neonate. If the tumor is bilateral, if shrinkage is necessary prior to removal, or if metastasis has occurred, chemotherapy may be required (van den Heuvel-Eibrink et al., 2017). **Quality and Safety: The diagnosis of cancer in a young infant can be devastating to the family. Clear, easy-to-understand information related to treatment and prognosis is required to assist parents to have realistic expectations related to their infant's diagnosis.**

## SUMMARY

An infant with a GU abnormality presents unique challenges to the neonatal care team. Although aberrations in the genital system are not life threatening, their appearance can be traumatic for parents. Urinary tract pathology, on the other hand, can result in emergent life-threatening events at any age. Renal abnormality and diseases manifesting in the neonatal period can have lifelong consequences. The neonatal nurse must be able to accurately assess and respond to alterations in renal function. Astute nursing care of the infant and parents is paramount to optimal management and outcome. Neonatal nurses are in the position to be the first members of the healthcare team to detect minor changes in neonatal physiologic functions that may signify the onset of significant compromise. To do this, the neonatal nurse must have knowledge of normal and abnormal renal and urinary tract physiology and pathophysiology. Parental support is another aspect of nursing care that is of major importance when caring for an infant with GU conditions. Timely assessment of parental coping mechanisms, alterations in parent–infant attachment, and evaluation of the parents' response to teaching provide vital information that will ultimately affect the infant's overall well-being.

## CASE STUDY

**Identification of the Problem.** Infant with an average urinary output of 0.4 ml/kg/hr for the past 24 hours.

**Assessment: History and Physical Examination.** The child is a 3-day-old, 900-g, 28-week gestational infant born to a 28-year-old gravida 1, para 0 mother. Blood type is A+, and all serologies, including Venereal Disease Research Laboratory (VDRL), HbsAg, GC (Gonorrhea, also known as the Clap), and HIV, are negative. The mother received good prenatal care during this pregnancy. No smoking, drug, or alcohol use was reported. Delivery was via cesarean birth due to placental abruption at 28 weeks' gestation. No antibiotics or prenatal steroids were administered prior to delivery. The infant required intubation at delivery because of apnea and low heart rate. Apgar scores were 4 at 1 minute and 8 at 5 minutes. The infant was transferred to the Level 3 NICU. The infant's problems included the following:

- Fluid, electrolytes, and nutrition: The infant is currently on minimal enteral feedings of 1 ml every 12 hours and tolerating these well; total fluid volume is 120 ml/kg/d of total parenteral nutrition.
- Respiratory: The infant received two doses of surfactant for a chest radiograph consistent with hyaline membrane disease. The infant remains intubated on moderate ventilatory settings.
- Cardiovascular: The infant has had several episodes of hypotension that have resolved spontaneously without treatment; heart rate is 175; current blood pressure has a mean arterial pressure of 28.
- Infectious disease: The infant is receiving ampicillin and gentamicin for suspected sepsis; no culture-proven sepsis.
- Hematologic: Hematocrit is 35%; under phototherapy for hyperbilirubinemia.
- Neurologic: A cranial ultrasound has been ordered for 1 week of life.
- Social: Parents are married; this is their first child; they are appropriately concerned and have been updated at the bedside daily.

**Physical Assessment**

- GENERAL: no obvious anomalies noted
- HEAD, EARS, EYES, NOSE, AND THROAT (HEENT): anterior fontanelle soft and flat; eyes clear without drainage, red reflex present; pupils equally reactive to light; nares patent bilaterally; no clefts or abnormalities of mouth noted; ear canals patent bilaterally
- CHEST AND LUNGS: heart rate regular without murmur; pulses equal in all four extremities; quiet precordium; capillary refill time is 2 seconds; lungs equal with fine crackles bilaterally
- ABDOMEN: soft and nondistended; positive bowel sounds auscultated in all four quadrants; no masses felt; umbilical cord normal; liver felt 2 cm below right intercostal margin
- GU: normal male infant; genitalia appropriate for gestational age
- SKELETAL: moves all extremities well; no obvious anomalies noted
- NEUROLOGIC: all reflexes present; tone appropriate for gestational age

**Differential Diagnosis.** The differential diagnosis of oliguria in this infant includes:

- Prerenal failure associated with decreased renal blood due to low systemic blood pressure or inadequate fluid intake
- Intrinsic renal failure due to the administration of nephrotoxic medications (gentamicin) or ATN due to perinatal depression related to the placental abruption as evidenced by the low Apgar scores

- Postrenal obstruction due to a neurogenic bladder related to fentanyl administration

**Diagnostic Tests.** Palpate the abdomen for the presence of a distended bladder and perform an in-and-out catheterization.

- Electrolytes: sodium 148; potassium 3.5; creatinine 0.4; BUN 10
- Weight is 780 g
- Gentamicin trough is 0.4 mg/L
- Urine specific gravity is 1,020, and no protein, blood, or WBCs are present in the urine

The next step should be administration of 10 to 20 ml/kg of normal saline via IV. Use of a diuretic after the fluid challenge may be necessary if urine output does not increase immediately after the fluid challenge.

**Working Diagnosis.** The bladder is not distended. No urine is obtained via in-and-out catheterization, thus ruling out postrenal failure.

Physical assessment is imperative for lack of abdominal masses that would possibly indicate an enlarged kidney and associated intrinsic renal failure. Tachycardia is present, possibly indicating mild dehydration. A borderline mean arterial pressure may indicate decreased intravascular volume or decreased systemic blood flow.

The infant has lost 120 g over the past 3 days.

Gentamicin level is normal and does not support the presence of intrinsic renal failure.

The sodium level and specific gravity are elevated, which are both consistent with prerenal failure.

The creatinine and BUN levels are normal. If elevated, they would support a diagnosis of intrinsic renal failure.

There is no blood or protein in the urine. The presence of these substances would also support a diagnosis of intrinsic renal failure.

The administration of a fluid challenge produced a urine output of over 1 ml/kg/hr, thus indicating a diagnosis of prerenal failure.

No other workup, such as a renal ultrasound, would be indicated at this time.

**Development of Management Plan.** Ensure administration of an adequate fluid volume by increasing fluid volume appropriately to ensure a urine output over 1 ml/kg/hr. Compensate for fluid losses due to insensible water losses, including losses from phototherapy.

Low-dose dopamine may increase renal blood flow.

Ensure appropriate renal blood flow by increasing mean arterial pressure. If increase in fluid volume does not increase blood pressure sufficiently, inotropes such as higher dose dopamine or dobutamine may be administered.

**Implementation and Evaluation of Effectiveness**

- Monitor skin turgor and fontanelles for signs of dehydration.
- Monitor serum electrolytes closely to ensure normalization of sodium levels
- Monitor vital signs every 3 to 4 hours to ensure normalization of blood pressure and heart rate.
- Carefully monitor intake and output to ensure that infant is receiving adequate volume to result in a urine output of over 1 ml/kg/hr.
- Perform daily or twice-daily weights.
- Monitor specific gravity to ensure resolution to a normal range.

## EVIDENCE-BASED PRACTICE

UTIs are common in infants and are defined as infection of the kidney and/or the bladder. They are estimated to occur in 0.1% to 2% of all newborns and in 20% of preterm and critically ill infants. UTIs can increase morbidity and, if not properly treated, can result in decreased renal function, renal scarring, and HTN (Arshad & Seed, 2015). Treatment of UTIs consists of antibiotic therapy, and traditionally due to concerns of VUR, a VCUG and prophylactic antibiotic therapy were recommended in all infants diagnosed with a UTI. Unfortunately, a VCUG is not a benign procedure and is associated with both infant pain and family stress.

Evidence now exists that the risk of recurrent UTI is not significantly affected by VUR, and the AAP currently recommends that a VCUG not be performed following the first UTI unless the renal ultrasound indicates abnormalities including hydronephrosis, renal scarring, severe VUR, or obstructive uropathy (Roberts et al., 2011). A meta-analysis of six studies including data on 1,091 infants indicated no benefit in providing prophylactic antibiotics to prevent future UTIs in infants with grades I to IV VUR, and there was insufficient data regarding use in infants with grade V VUR (Roberts et al., 2011). Furthermore, it is estimated that only 1% of infants diagnosed with a UTI has grade V VUR (Roberts et al., 2011). Therefore, the use of a VCUG or prophylactic antibiotic therapy is not recommended following an initial UTI (Roberts et al., 2011). If an infant is diagnosed with subsequent UTIs, a VCUG is required at that time (Roberts et al., 2011).

### References

Arshad, M., & Seed, P. C. (2015). Urinary tract infections in the infant. *Clinics in Perinatology, 42*(1), 17–28. https://doi.org/10.1016/j.clp.2014.10.003

Roberts, K. B., Downs, S. M., Finnell, S. M. E., Hellerstein, S., Shortliffe, L. D., Wald, E. R., & Zerin, J. M. (2011). Urinary tract infection: Clinical practice guideline for the diagnosis and management of the initial UTI in febrile infants and children 2 to 24 months. *Pediatrics, 128*(3), 595–610. https://doi.org/10.1542/peds.2011-1330

## ONLINE RESOURCES

CourseConnect

Resources for this chapter are online and available at www.springerpub.com/courseconnect.

## REFERENCES

References for this chapter are online and available at www.springerpub.com/courseconnect.

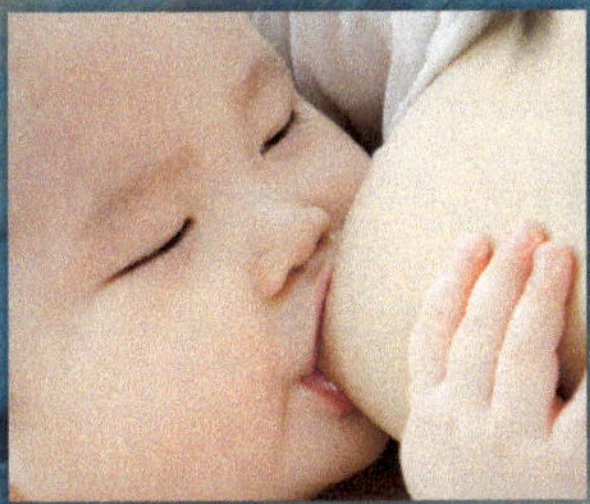

Source: Wong Sze Fei/Adobe Stock.



CHAPTER 19

# Fluids, Electrolytes, and Acid-Base Balance

Eric A. Raynal and Vivek Narendran

## INTRODUCTION

Maintenance of fluid, electrolytes, and acid–base balance are vital components of neonatal care. This is particularly true for very low birth weight (VLBW) infants because they require parenteral fluids for prolonged periods and have unique limitations related to their immature kidneys and skin. Rapid maturational changes in various organs and fluid shifts that occur after birth confound the issue further. Critically ill newborns are at additional risk for morbidity and mortality due to fluid and electrolyte imbalance.

## WATER

**Physiology.** Water is the main component of the human body. It is distributed both inside and outside the cells. Thus, the total body water (TBW) is a sum of intracellular water (ICW) and extracellular water (ECW). ICW is the total amount of water in all the body's cells. ECW is the total amount of water outside the cells, which includes the water in the interstitial space and the intravascular space (plasma).

The distribution of TBW between intracellular and extracellular spaces depends on the relative concentration of solutes (relative osmolality). The total number of solute particles in solution determines the osmolality of a solution. Osmolality values are expressed in osmoles or milliosmoles per kilogram of water (Osm/kg or mOsm/kg). Cell membranes are completely permeable to water but not to most solutes; therefore, water shifts from one compartment to the other until equilibrium is established between the osmolalities on both sides of the membrane. The osmolality of intracellular and extracellular spaces, therefore, is equal, although the composition of ICW is vastly different from that of ECW; for example, sodium ($Na^+$) is the major extracellular cation, whereas potassium ($K^+$) is the main intracellular cation. In each compartment, the main solute acts to keep water within the compartment:

- The volume of the intracellular compartment is maintained mainly by potassium salts and is regulated by the $Na^+/K^+$ cellular pump.
- The volume of the extracellular compartment is maintained mainly by sodium salts and is regulated by the kidneys.
- The volume of the intravascular compartment is maintained mainly by the colloidal osmotic pressure of plasma proteins and is regulated by the endocrine system and the kidneys.

**Changes in Water Distribution.** In the first trimester of gestation, TBW constitutes more than 90% of the body weight; however, its relative contribution to body weight declines as the fetus matures. TBW decreases to 75% at 36 weeks' gestation, 74% at 40 weeks' gestation, and approximately 60% to 65% at the end of the first year of life. The ratio of ECW to ICW also changes with growth. ECW declines from approximately 60% of body weight in the second trimester to about 45% at term. ICW increases from about 25% of body weight in the second trimester to approximately 33% at term. The decrease in TBW as the infant matures is attributed largely to the decrease in the ECW compartment (Figure 19.1).

Superimposed on the gradual contraction of ECW that occurs as the fetus approaches term is an acute expansion of ECW that occurs at birth. This is due to (a) placental transfusion, (b) reabsorption of fetal lung fluid, and (c) shifting of water and electrolytes from the intracellular to the extracellular space (Segar, 2020). The newborn at birth is, therefore, in a state of excess extracellular fluid, a condition that is particularly prominent in preterm infants (TBW and ECW are greater at lower gestational ages). After the first 24 to 48 hours of life, the infant undergoes a diuresis phase. This results in the loss of excess ECW, which is referred to as *physiologic weight loss* (5%–10% in term infants and up to 15% in very preterm infants). Any disruptions in this normal transition can lead to imbalances in fluid and electrolyte homeostasis, leading to morbidity. For example, in preterm infants, iatrogenic administration of large amounts of fluids can potentially increase the risk of a patent ductus arteriosus (PDA) requiring surgical intervention (Valentine et al., 2022), necrotizing enterocolitis (NEC) (Valentine et al., 2022), and bronchopulmonary dysplasia (BPD) (Starr et al., 2022).

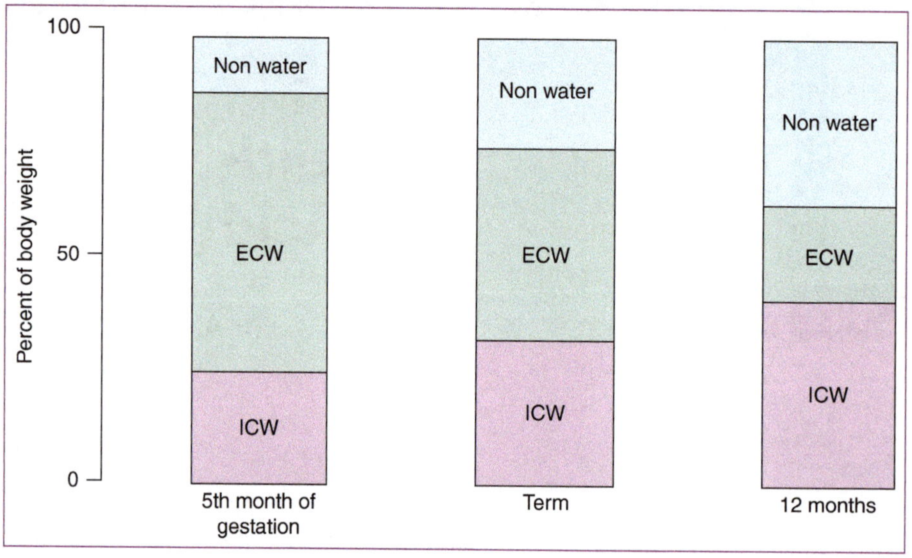


**FIGURE 19.1. Changes in body water distribution.** Note the relative decrease in the ECW compartment.
ECW, extracellular water; ICW, intracellular water.

**Water Balance and Requirements.** Water balance in neonates is under the direct control of antidiuretic hormone (ADH), which is also known as vasopressin. ADH is secreted by the hypothalamus when the serum osmolality is greater than 285 mOsm/kg or there is intravascular volume depletion. It regulates intravascular volume by changing water permeability of the collecting ducts in the kidneys. A mature adult kidney can concentrate urine up to a maximum of 1,500 mOsm/kg or dilute to a minimum of 50 mOsm/kg based on the body's fluid status. However, this concentrating ability is remarkably diminished in neonates. A term neonate can maximally concentrate urine up to 600 mOsm/kg and a preterm neonate to only 300 to 400 mOsm/kg (Lindower, 2017). This inability to sufficiently concentrate urine, proportionate to the demands of the body, predisposes neonates to a significant risk for water and electrolyte imbalances.

Maintaining optimal water and electrolyte composition depends on anticipating water losses and replacement with pertinent maintenance fluids. Table 19.1 highlights factors that affect water loss in neonates. Maintenance fluids are defined as

**TABLE 19.1**

**FACTORS AFFECTING WATER LOSS IN NEONATES**

| Increasing Water Loss | Decreasing Water Loss |
|---|---|
| ***Water Loss From the Skin*** | |
| Low gestational age | High humidity in incubator |
| Radiant warmer | Double-walled incubator |
| Hyperthermia | Plastic wrap while under radiant warmer at birth |
| Skin immaturity | Skin keratinization |
| Phototherapy | |
| Congenital defects (e.g., gastroschisis) | |
| ***Water Loss From the Respiratory Tract*** | |
| Tachypnea | Use of heated, humidified gas |
| Inadequate humidification | |
| ***Renal Water Loss*** | |
| Diuretic agents (e.g., furosemide) | Renal failure |
| Osmotic diuresis (hyperglycemia) | SIADH |
| CAH | Congestive heart failure |

(*continued*)

**TABLE 19.1**

**FACTORS AFFECTING WATER LOSS IN NEONATES (*continued*)**

CAH, congenital adrenal hyperplasia; SIADH, syndrome of inappropriate antidiuretic hormone secretion.

**TABLE 19.2**

**APPROXIMATE MAINTENANCE REQUIREMENTS FOR NEWBORNS MANAGED IN INCUBATORS IN THE FIRST WEEK OF LIFE**

| | Birth Weight | | | |
|---|---|---|---|---|
| **Time Period** | **< 750 g** | **750–1,000 g** | **1,001–1,500 g** | **> 1,500 g** |
| First 48 hours | 100–200 | 80–150 | 60–100 | 60–80 |
| Day 3–7 | 120–200 | 100–150 | 80–150 | 100–150 |

*Note:* Amounts are given as ml/kg/d.

the amount of water and electrolytes required to maintain a patient in a neutral water balance. These include replacement of urine, gastrointestinal losses, and insensible water loss (IWL). Preterm infants are particularly susceptible to water imbalances due to immature renal function, very high IWL through the skin and respiratory tract, higher body surface area to body mass ratio, and acuity of illness (Segar, 2020). Table 19.2 provides approximate requirements for the maintenance fluids (ml/kg/d) for infants up to a week of life. However, further titrations are made by assessing the clinical status of the patient and accounting for factors that might increase or decrease fluid loss. For example, phototherapy increases IWL, whereas the use of double-walled and humidified incubators reduces IWL. However, the use of newer devices for phototherapy combined with modern incubators has significantly decreased their effects on IWL (Maisels & McDonagh, 2008).

**Postnatal Adaptations.** Most preterm infants follow a progressive postnatal pattern of diuresis. For the first 24 to 48 hours of life, the glomerular filtration rate (GFR), urinary output (UOP), and sodium and potassium excretion are all very low. Water is lost mainly by IWL. The total fluid requirement is calculated to account mainly for the IWL (Tables 19.1 and 19.2) and supplementation with sodium, chloride, or potassium is rarely necessary. Because very preterm infants have significant skin (transepidermal) water losses, they are predisposed to hemoconcentration and hypernatremia even in this initial phase.

Beginning on day 2 to 5 of life, the UOP and sodium and potassium excretion increase abruptly. This transition seems to be triggered by atrial natriuretic peptide (ANP), which is released by myocardial cells in response to atrial stretching or filling. This occurs due to the physiologic decrease in pulmonary vascular resistance after birth that leads to increased venous return to the left atrium and the release of ANP. ANP, in turn, causes increased natriuresis (Modi, 2003). Water intake is adjusted to maintain a normal serum sodium concentration and to maintain total weight loss below 10% in term and below 15% in preterm infants. Sodium and potassium supplementation is also started.

Finally, UOP stabilizes after about day 5 of life. The goal of fluid and electrolyte intake is to maintain water and electrolyte balance and to provide nutrition for adequate growth. Preterm infants normally grow at a rate of 10 to 20 g/kg/d. Because three quarters of this new body mass is fluid, the total fluids given to an infant should provide a net positive balance of 10 to 15 ml/kg/d.

**Pathologic Fluid and Electrolyte Losses.** Certain clinical conditions predispose infants to pathologic fluid and electrolyte loss. Commonly encountered situations in the neonatal intensive care unit (NICU) include loss of gastric fluid due to Replogle tube placement or vomiting, loss of enteric fluids due to an ostomy, and fluid and electrolyte losses in stool. Table 19.3 highlights the electrolyte concentration of different body fluids and can be used to estimate specific electrolyte losses and for calculating replacements.

**TABLE 19.3**

**ELECTROLYTE CONTENT OF BODY FLUIDS**

| Fluid | Sodium (mmol/L) | Potassium (mmol/L) | Chloride (mmol/L) |
|---|---|---|---|
| Stomach | 20–80 | 5–20 | 100–150 |
| Small intestine | 100–140 | 5–15 | 90–120 |
| Bile | 120–140 | 5–15 | 90–120 |
| Ileostomy | 45–135 | 3–15 | 20–120 |
| Diarrheal stool | 10–90 | 10–80 | 10–110 |

*Source:* Adapted from Martin, R. J., Fanaroff, A. A., & Walsh, M. C. (Eds.). (2025). *Fanaroff and Martin's neonatal-perinatal medicine: Diseases of the fetus and infant* (12th ed.). Elsevier.

## ELECTROLYTES

**Sodium.** Sodium is the main extracellular cation, accounting for more than 90% of the solutes in the extracellular space. It is absorbed in both the small intestine and the colon; the largest amount is absorbed in the second portion of the small intestine, the jejunum. Sodium absorption involves several mechanisms:

- passive absorption along with glucose, secondary to the flow of water
- active absorption, uncoupled with glucose, involving the $Na^+/K^+$ pump
- active absorption in exchange for hydrogen ions ($H^+$)

The kidneys excrete sodium, which is first filtered by the glomeruli and later mostly reabsorbed throughout the tubules and the collecting ducts. Most sodium is absorbed with chloride ($Cl^-$), with lesser amounts absorbed in exchange with $K^+$ or $H^+$. Under normal circumstances, 96% to 99% of filtered sodium is reabsorbed. The main factors regulating sodium resorption are the oncotic and hydrostatic pressures in the peritubular capillaries of the kidneys. The mineralocorticoid aldosterone is also critical in maintaining sodium levels. When there is intravascular volume depletion, aldosterone is secreted by the renin–angiotensin–aldosterone system (RAS) in the juxtaglomerular cells of the kidney. Under the influence of the RAS system, sodium and water absorption is exchanged for $K^+$ and $H^+$. Although ADH does not directly affect sodium excretion, it can influence the serum sodium concentration indirectly because it regulates the excretion and resorption of free water.

**Emergency Alert: Fluctuations in sodium in preterm infants have been associated with increased risk of death and adverse neurologic outcomes at 18 months of age (Gervais et al., 2022).**

The sodium content of human and/or donor breast milk is insufficient to meet the daily requirement and support adequate growth. VLBW babies exclusively fed breastmilk often require enteral sodium supplementation to support growth (Isemann et al., 2016; Petersen et al., 2024). The sodium concentration in human milk ranges from 12 to 20 mEq/L. The recommendation for daily sodium intake in growing preterm infants is 3 to 5 mEq/kg/d (Koletzko et al., 2021). In the first few days of life, infants born at 22 to 23 weeks' gestation should receive extremely little sodium to reduce the risk of BPD (Costarino et al., 1992; Hartnoll et al., 2000). However, because of their high urinary loss of sodium, they may temporarily require 7 to 9 mEq/kg/d by the end of the first week of life (Segar et al., 2021). Thereafter, urinary losses in these infants decrease. The normal serum sodium concentration ranges from 130 to 150 mEq/L.

Disorders of sodium balance are listed in Box 19.1.

**BOX 19.1**

**DISORDERS OF SODIUM BALANCE**

**Hyponatremia**

VLBW infant-fed unfortified human milk or standard-term formula

Perinatal asphyxia

Renal failure, congestive heart failure

SIADH (associated with RDS, IVH, pneumothorax)

Diuretics

Sodium losses through the gut

Hypotonic fluid administered to mother during labor

Adrenal insufficiency (CAH)

**Hypernatremia**

Dehydration (vomiting, diarrhea, IWL through immature skin)

DI (central and nephrogenic)

Osmotic diuresis (hyperglycemia)

Iatrogenic (excessive administration of sodium-containing fluids)

Medication errors

CAH, congenital adrenal hyperplasia; DI, diabetes insipidus; IVH, intraventricular hemorrhage; IWL, insensible water loss; RDS, respiratory distress syndrome; SIADH, syndrome of inappropriate secretion of antidiuretic hormone; VLBW, very low birth weight.

**Hyponatremia.** Hyponatremia is defined as a serum sodium level below 130 mEq/L. There are three major mechanisms for this:

- increased sodium loss
- inadequate sodium intake
- inability to excrete excess water (dilution effect)

Therefore, it is important to first delineate the etiology of hyponatremia and assess volume status before instituting therapy. For example, an infant with hyponatremia due to the inability to excrete water because of acute kidney injury requires fluid restriction, while an infant with excessive urinary or stool water and sodium losses requires fluid replacement.

**Increased Sodium Loss and Inadequate Intake.** This is most seen after the first week of life in growing VLBW infants fed either unfortified human or donor breastmilk. These infants can have a negative sodium balance in the first weeks of life because of an inadequate sodium intake and transient unresponsiveness of the renal tubules to aldosterone (Baumgart & Costarino, 2000). Lower urine sodium concentrations (< 30–40 mEq/L) in these patients are suggestive of inadequate sodium intake (Gattineni & Baum, 2015). After the first week of life, VLBW infants may require up to 8 mEq/kg/d or higher to maintain a positive sodium balance. Usually, the lower the gestational age, the higher the sodium intake needed.

Abnormalities in either the production of aldosterone (congenital adrenal hyperplasia [CAH]) or the renal responsiveness to aldosterone (pseudohypoaldosteronism) can also lead to increased sodium losses and hyponatremia. Variable degrees of hyperkalemia and metabolic acidosis are associated with the previously noted disorders due to the influence of aldosterone on $K^+$ and $H^+$ excretion.

Extrarenal losses of sodium occur with vomiting and diarrhea. Loop diuretics such as furosemide are notorious for causing hyponatremia. Additionally, infants with ileostomies may have increased sodium losses.

**Inability to Excrete Excess Water.** In neonates, hyponatremia due to water retention (dilution) occurs after an acute kidney injury, leading to decreased GFR. This is seen after perinatal asphyxia or following nephrotoxic drug therapy. Another mechanism at play during perinatal asphyxia is the increased secretion of ADH (SIADH). Severe respiratory distress syndrome (RDS), intraventricular hemorrhage (IVH), and pneumothorax can also predispose newborns to hyponatremia due to SIADH.

Hyponatremia can also be iatrogenic secondary to excessive administration of hypotonic fluids to the mother during labor, feeding diluted formula, or following resuscitation with hypotonic fluids. Whenever the serum sodium concentration decreases, serum osmolality declines, causing water to move into cells (i.e., the intracellular space) to achieve an osmotic equilibrium between intracellular and extracellular fluid. This phenomenon also occurs in the brain cells, causing characteristic signs and symptoms of hyponatremia. Vomiting, lethargy, and apnea may occur with various degrees of hyponatremia. Seizures and coma are not seen unless the serum sodium concentration falls below 115 mEq/L.

Treatment is directed both at the underlying disorder and volume replacement with sodium chloride (NaCl)–containing solutions. The amount of sodium needed is calculated using this standard formula:

$$\text{Total sodium required (mEq)} = 0.6 \times \text{Weight (kg)} \times (\text{Desired serum } Na^+ - \text{Observed serum } Na^+)$$

**Quality and Safety: This correction is done slowly over several hours. The rate of correction should not exceed 10 to 12 mEq/L/d (or 0.5 mEq/L/hr).** The target is a serum sodium concentration of about 135 mEq/L. Rapid correction of hyponatremia puts the infant at risk for a condition known as central pontine myelinolysis.

This general rule has two exceptions:

- In the presence of overt or impending shock, normal saline should be given intravenously and rapidly at 10 to 20 ml/kg over 20 to 30 minutes; treatment is repeated until arterial blood pressure is normal for gestational age.
- If hyponatremic seizures are diagnosed, hypertonic saline (3%) should be infused. These seizures usually abate with correction in serum sodium concentration of 3 to 5 mEq/L. Care must be taken to avoid overcorrection.

**Hypernatremia.** Hypernatremia is defined as a serum sodium level over 150 mEq/L. It is caused by three major mechanisms:

- increased loss of free water (renal or extrarenal)
- decreased water replacement
- excess sodium intake

Whenever hypernatremia occurs, the serum osmolality increases, leading to water moving out of the cells into the extracellular space to achieve an osmotic equilibrium between intracellular and extracellular fluid. This shifting water balance results in volume depletion of the intracellular space. To counteract this phenomenon, brain cells (neurons) have the unique ability to generate new solutes called *idiogenic osmoles*. These substances (amino acids, polyols, trimethylamines) are synthesized by the brain cells as a protective response to serum hyperosmolality. Idiogenic osmoles are produced and catabolized slowly and, therefore, are effective only if hyperosmolality does not develop too rapidly. For this reason, correction of hypernatremia with hypotonic solutions should not be performed rapidly, because cerebral edema can occur due to the movement of water back into brain cells.

**Increased Loss of Free Water and Decreased Replacement.** This is referred to as *hypernatremia with dehydration*. Water loss in a neonate can occur through the immature skin, kidneys, or gastrointestinal tract. Hypernatremia due to excess IWL through the immature skin is particularly pronounced in VLBW infants. The magnitude of these losses is inversely related to gestational age. In VLBW infants, weight, UOP, serum sodium level, and glucose concentrations should be monitored closely. Adequate fluid replacement and sodium restriction during the first 3 to 5 days of life may prevent hypernatremia. IWL is minimized by using double-walled incubators with a high relative humidity.

Excessive renal water loss occurs when an increased amount of solute, such as glucose, needs to be excreted (osmotic diuresis) or secondary to diabetes insipidus (DI). DI is caused by either decreased production of ADH by the hypothalamus (central DI) or renal unresponsiveness to ADH (nephrogenic DI). In both conditions, the infant presents with hypernatremia, polyuria, decreased feeding, and poor growth. These infants frequently require periodic fluid replacements to compensate for ongoing renal losses. Water loss similarly may occur from the gastrointestinal tract following vomiting, diarrhea, or increased ostomy output.

**Quality and Safety: Hypernatremia with dehydration must be corrected slowly to avoid cerebral edema.** Intravascular volume should be restored relatively quickly with isotonic fluids, but water deficits should be corrected slowly with hypotonic fluids. Generally, serum sodium should not decrease by more than 0.5 mEq/kg/hr (or 10–12 mEq/kg/d).

**Excessive Sodium Administration.** This is referred to as *hypernatremia with overhydration*. Excessive sodium administration can be caused inadvertently by the administration of certain medications such as ampicillin, gentamicin, heparin, sodium bicarbonate, and fluids to keep central lines patent (Eibensteiner et al., 2020). VLBW infants are particularly at risk from these "large" sodium loads. Treatment of this iatrogenic form of hypernatremia involves sodium restriction by careful selection of maintenance and medication carrier fluids.

**Potassium.** Potassium is the main intracellular cation. Its concentration in cells is maintained by the membrane $Na^+/K^+$ pump, and it is involved in the regulation of cell membrane potential. Small variations in serum potassium concentration have significant effects, particularly on the myocardial cells.

Dietary potassium is mainly absorbed in the small intestine by passive absorption and is actively secreted in the colon. The kidneys excrete potassium, and most filtered potassium is reabsorbed in the proximal tubule. Potassium is then secreted by the distal tubules in exchange for sodium in a process regulated by aldosterone. Preterm infants with BPD who require chronic diuretic therapy (most diuretics are natriuretic) often need replacement with enteral potassium chloride (KCl) to correct their electrolyte imbalance because of chronic kidney losses of both sodium and potassium. The potassium requirement for preterm infants is 2.3 to 4.6 mEq/kg/d (Embleton et al., 2023). The normal serum concentration of potassium for all infants is 3.5 to 5 mEq/L.

Disorders of potassium balance are listed in Box 19.2.

**Hypokalemia.** Hypokalemia is defined as a serum potassium level below 3.5 mEq/L. It can be caused by increased renal losses (diuretics, renal tubular acidosis [RTA], and Bartter syndrome), increased gastrointestinal losses (diarrhea, vomiting, continuous nasogastric aspiration, and ostomy output), or inadequate intake. The use of potassium-sparing diuretics may decrease the incidence of hypokalemia in the NICU.

Hypokalemia manifests through its effects on muscle cells. Although abdominal distention, diminished bowel motility, weakness, and lethargy are described, the cardiac effects are of much greater concern. An electrocardiogram (ECG) is a better measure of severe toxicity than the serum potassium concentration. **Emergency Alert: ECG changes associated with hypokalemia include a depressed ST segment, a flattened T wave, and a prominent U wave. A prolonged P-R interval, widening QRS complex, and various arrhythmias may follow, if untreated.**

Treatment involves potassium replacement. KCl should be given very slowly (< 0.3 mEq/kg/hr) with frequent serum and ECG monitoring. Rapid intravenous (IV) administration of potassium may itself cause fatal arrhythmias.

**Hyperkalemia.** Hyperkalemia is defined as a serum potassium level over 6.5 mEq/L. It can be caused by an excessive intake of potassium, impaired excretion (renal failure, CAH, and pseudohypoaldosteronism), or severe metabolic acidosis (increased movement of potassium from the intracellular to the extracellular space). Factitious hyperkalemia may be associated with hemolysis (breakdown of red blood cells) when a non–free-flowing sample is collected via a heel stick and must be ruled out. Hyperkalemia occurs in approximately 50% of infants whose birth weight is less than 1,000 g and is thought to occur due to decreased activity of the $Na^+/K^+$ pump. Thus, potassium should only be added to IV fluids in the first few days of life once adequate UOP is established. Cardiac toxicity is a serious complication of hyperkalemia and is better reflected by ECG changes than by the serum concentration. The typical ECG sequence is peaked or "tented" T waves, the disappearance of P waves, and a widening QRS complex, which can fuse with the T wave to form a sine wave. Ventricular fibrillation and cardiac arrest may follow if the serum potassium level remains untreated. Treatment of hyperkalemia is generally recommended when > 6.5 to 7 mEq/L (Segar & Jetton, 2024) and emergently when electrographic changes are noted on ECG.

Treatment is directed at the underlying disorder. All potassium-containing fluids and supplements should be stopped immediately. Management of hyperkalemia with ECG changes includes the following:

- 10% calcium gluconate (100–200 mg/kg/dose, IV) is given to counteract the effects of hyperkalemia on myocardial cells (stabilizing the myocardial membrane against arrhythmias). It does not decrease the serum potassium concentration.
- Sodium bicarbonate (1–2 mEq/kg, IV) is given to raise the blood pH, and consequently increase potassium influx into cells.
- Nebulized beta-agonist (albuterol) is administered to increase the intracellular uptake of potassium.
- Infusion of glucose and insulin at a ratio of 4 g of glucose to 1 unit of insulin to increase intracellular uptake of potassium.
- Loop diuretics (furosemide; 1 mg/kg, IV) are given to increase renal excretion of potassium.

Binding resins (Kayexalate) are no longer used, especially in preterm infants, due to their associated risk of bowel injury (Segar & Jetton, 2024). Most other measures are transient, because they do not decrease total body potassium but shift it intracellularly. Therefore, if the serum potassium continues to rise and exceeds 8 mEq/L, dialysis (hemo- or peritoneal) or exchange blood transfusions (using a mixture of washed red blood cells and fresh frozen plasma) may be necessary.

**Chloride.** Chloride is the main inorganic anion in the extracellular fluid and, together with sodium, is responsible for maintaining plasma volume. Chloride is typically administered with $Na^+$ or $K^+$, either NaCl or KCl, in diet or IV fluids. Intestinal absorption is passive in the jejunum and occurs secondary to sodium absorption. In the ileum and colon, chloride is actively absorbed in exchange for bicarbonate ($HCO_3^-$). Normally, only minimal amounts of chloride are lost in the feces. Like sodium, it is filtered by the glomeruli and reabsorbed throughout the tubules and collecting ducts. Normally, 99% of the filtered chloride is reabsorbed.

**BOX 19.2**

**DISORDERS OF POTASSIUM BALANCE**

**Hypokalemia**

Renal losses: chronic diuretics, RTA, Bartter syndrome

Inadequate potassium intake

Gastrointestinal losses: vomiting, diarrhea, nasogastric aspiration, ostomy output

**Hyperkalemia**

Hemolyzed blood sample

Excessive intake

Impaired excretion: renal failure, CAH, pseudohypoaldosteronism

Potassium-sparing diuretics

Metabolic acidosis

CAH, congenital adrenal hyperplasia; RTA, renal tubular acidosis.

Chloride resorption is inversely related to bicarbonate resorption. Therefore, their serum concentrations are also inversely correlated, which keeps the total anion concentration ($Cl^-$ and $HCO_3^-$) constant and maintains electrical neutrality. For this reason, although chloride has no buffer effect, it plays an essential part in acid–base regulation. When chloride is retained in the body, the serum bicarbonate level declines, and metabolic acidosis follows. When chloride is lost from the body, the serum bicarbonate level rises, and metabolic alkalosis ensues.

The recommended enteral chloride intake for preterm infants is 3 to 8 mEq/kg/d (Embleton et al., 2023). Normal serum chloride concentrations are 90 to 112 mEq/L in full-term infants and 100 to 115 mEq/L in preterm infants.

Disorders of chloride balance are listed in Box 19.3.

**Hypochloremia.** Hypochloremia is defined as a serum chloride level below 90 mEq/L and is caused by either a diminished intake or increased loss of chloride (gastrointestinal or renal). Clinical manifestations include metabolic alkalosis, hypokalemia, and, when chronic, failure to thrive.

Insufficient intake has been reported due to the low chloride content of the inappropriately diluted formula. The diagnosis of insufficient intake is based on the dietary history and the absence of urinary chloride, which indicates a normal ability to retain chloride to compensate for the low intake. Chloride losses independent of sodium and potassium may occur from prolonged vomiting in the form of hydrochloric acid (HCl), for example, as seen in pyloric stenosis or continuous aspiration of gastric contents via nasogastric tubes (e.g., in NEC).

Congenital chloride diarrhea is a rare disorder of severe diarrhea, beginning at birth, caused by impairment of the active $Cl^-/HCO_3^-$ transport system in the ileum and colon. It is caused by a mutation in the *SLC26A3* gene responsible for encoding the exchange transporter in the intestine. However, these infants usually have normal electrolyte absorption in the jejunum. Analysis of stools shows an acidic pH and a significantly increased chloride concentration (> 90 mmol/L) (Di Meglio et al., 2021). Diarrhea is caused by the osmotic effect of excess chloride, which then leads to metabolic alkalosis and hypokalemia. Urine chloride is also decreased. Treatment involves lifelong supplementation and replacement of appropriate electrolytes. Other therapies include proton pump inhibitors and oral butyrate.

The most common cause of increased renal loss of chloride is diuretic therapy. **Quality and Safety: Chronic administration of furosemide, used often in the management of BPD, may cause chloride deficiency with secondary metabolic alkalosis.** Alkalosis, in turn, causes compensatory hypoventilation and an increase in the partial pressure of carbon dioxide ($PCO_2$) in the blood. This clinical picture can simulate pulmonary edema; however, the treatment should not be additional diuretic therapy but correction of the underlying hypochloremia.

Metabolic alkalosis with hypochloremia, hypokalemia, and hypercalciuria due to increased renal loss of chloride is the characteristic feature of Bartter syndrome. These infants also have failure to thrive and episodes of dehydration. It is caused by mutations directly or indirectly involving the $Na^+$-$K^+$-$Cl^-$ cotransporter. Timing of onset and symptoms help to categorize Bartter syndrome into neonatal (antenatal) and classic subtypes. Elevated prostaglandin E concentrations are observed in the urine. Electrolyte replacement with NaCl and KCl, maintenance of intravascular volume, and nonsteroidal antiinflammatory medications (NSAIDs; prostaglandin E2 antagonists) are the mainstays of treatment (Mrad et al., 2021).

**Hyperchloremia.** Hyperchloremia is defined as a serum chloride level over 115 mEq/L. It is caused by either bicarbonate depletion or by excessive chloride intake and is commonly associated with metabolic acidosis. Diarrhea is the most common cause of hyperchloremic metabolic acidosis, as chloride is absorbed with sodium, and bicarbonate is excreted with potassium in the intestine.

**Emergency Alert: Increased loss of bicarbonate occurs with RTA (type II or proximal type). In this condition, the renal threshold for bicarbonate drops and absorption of bicarbonate does not occur until the serum levels drop below approximately 15 mEq/L. The result is a hyperchloremic metabolic acidosis.** The condition is often self-limited because the proximal tubular length increases and function matures. The diagnosis is based on demonstrating a renal bicarbonate reabsorption threshold that is lower than normal.

Hyperchloremia may follow excessive administration of NaCl. Overtreatment with NaCl may be absolute, as in accidental errors in administration, or relative, as in renal failure, where the excretion is impaired. Finally, apparent hyperchloremia and increased serum concentrations of other electrolytes can occur with dehydration when there is a water deficit in relation to the solute.

**BOX 19.3**

**DISORDERS OF CHLORIDE BALANCE**

**Hypochloremia**

Decreased intake: inappropriately diluted formula

Increased gastrointestinal losses: vomiting (e.g., pyloric stenosis), continuous gastric aspiration

Congenital chloride diarrhea

Increased renal losses: diuretics, Bartter syndrome

**Hyperchloremia**

Increased bicarbonate losses: RTA

Excessive administration (with NaCl: absolute or relative)

Hypertonic dehydration (apparent hyperchloremia)

RTA, renal tubular acidosis.

**Calcium and Phosphorus.** Calcium (Ca) is the most abundant mineral in the human body and is an essential component of the skeleton. It plays a vital role in muscle contraction, neural transmission, and blood coagulation. Phosphorus (P) is equally necessary for bone mineralization. About 80% of phosphorus is present in the bones, and the remaining 20% is incorporated into energy storage molecules as adenosine triphosphate (ATP), which is essential for cell metabolism.

In the third trimester, the placental accretion of calcium is about 100 to 136 mg/kg/d, and that of phosphorus is 60 to 81 mg/kg/d. Unfortified human milk fails to provide comparable levels of minerals, predisposing premature infants to relative osteopenia, known as metabolic bone disease (MBD) of prematurity (Koletzko et al., 2021).

Recommendations for enteral intake in preterm infants are 120 to 200 mg/kg/d of calcium and 70 to 115 mg/kg/d of phosphorus (Embleton et al., 2023). With parenteral nutrition, a calcium intake of 32 to 80 mg/kg/d and a phosphorus intake of 31 to 62 mg/kg/d is recommended in the first few days of life and, once growing, increased to 64 to 140 mg/kg/d of calcium and 50 to 108 mg/kg/d of phosphorus (Mihatsch et al., 2018). **Quality and Safety: To avoid precipitation in the parenteral solution, the calcium concentration should be maintained between 500 and 600 mg/L (12.5–15 mmol/L), and the phosphorus concentration should be maintained between 390 and 470 mg/L (12.5–15 mmol/L).**

**Calcium.** Calcium transport in the intestine occurs by both passive and active processes. Active intestinal transport involves carriers called calcium-binding proteins. Vitamin D in its active form, 1,25-dihydroxyvitamin D, or calcitriol, is essential for the active process. Parathyroid hormone (PTH) is involved in the production of 1,25-dihydroxyvitamin D. Vitamin D deficiency and intestinal malabsorption due to any cause can impair calcium transport. **Quality and Safety: Corticosteroids diminish calcium absorption by inhibiting its transfer in the intestinal mucosa. Similarly, anticonvulsants can inhibit intestinal transfer of calcium (phenytoin) and interfere with vitamin D metabolism (phenobarbital, phenytoin).**

Calcium is present in the serum in three forms: ionized (50%), bound to proteins (mainly albumin, 40%), and complexed with organic and inorganic compounds (10%). The ionized calcium is the only biologically active form. The calcium bound to albumin serves as a reserve. Therefore, measuring the ionized calcium level is more clinically relevant than the total serum calcium concentration. The affinity of calcium to albumin is increased by metabolic alkalosis and decreased by acidosis. In addition, with every 1 g/dl decrease in serum albumin, the total serum calcium decreases by 0.8 mg/dl, but the ionized calcium remains unchanged. The serum calcium concentration is maintained within narrow limits by the action of PTH, 1,25-dihydroxyvitamin D, and calcitonin. PTH and 1,25-dihydroxyvitamin D increase the serum calcium level, while calcitonin reduces it. PTH secretion is driven by the serum ionized calcium concentration via the calcium-sensing receptors in the parathyroid cells.

The kidneys excrete calcium, and filtered calcium is reabsorbed in most segments of the renal tubules. PTH increases tubular resorption of calcium, whereas calcitonin increases calcium excretion.

Disorders of calcium balance are listed in Box 19.4.

**BOX 19.4**

**DISORDERS OF CALCIUM BALANCE**

**Hypocalcemia**

- *Early*
  - Preterm infant
  - Infant of diabetic mother
  - Perinatal asphyxia
  - Maternal anticonvulsant therapy
- *Late*
  - Hyperphosphatemia (increased dietary intake, renal failure)
  - Cow's milk–based feeding
  - Hypomagnesemia
  - Hypoparathyroidism
  - Vitamin D deficiency

**Hypercalcemia**

Excessive administration of calcium or vitamin D (or both)

Hypophosphatasia

Subcutaneous fat necrosis

Williams syndrome

Idiopathic hypercalcemia

Hyperparathyroidism

Bartter syndrome

Familial hypocalciuric hypercalcemia

**Hypocalcemia.** Neonatal hypocalcemia is defined as a serum ionized calcium concentration below 4.4 mg/dl (1.1 mmol/L) in full-term infants. For preterm infants, insufficient normative data at different gestational ages exists; therefore, a total serum calcium concentration below 7 mg/dl (1.75 mmol/L) remains a practical definition. Hypocalcemia is conventionally divided into early hypocalcemia, which occurs in the first 2 to 4 days of life, and late hypocalcemia, which occurs after the first 4 days, usually at about 1 week of age.

There is a physiologic fall in the calcium concentration during the first 48 hours of life. This is due to the abrupt interruption of maternal calcium supply and low dietary intake. In preterm infants, this fall in calcium is more rapid and inversely proportional to gestational age. Factors contributing to early hypocalcemia in preterm neonates include inadequate PTH release, decreased responsiveness of renal tubules to PTH, and relative resistance to 1,25-dihydroxyvitamin D.

Infants of diabetic mothers are at increased risk of hypocalcemia due to hypomagnesemia. Mothers with diabetes have increased losses of magnesium in the urine, which in turn causes fetal hypomagnesemia and secondary hypoparathyroidism (Hay, 2012).

Hypocalcemia in the first few days of life is also seen following birth asphyxia. These infants have increased serum calcitonin and a relative increase in phosphorus load due to reduced glomerular filtration. Treatment of associated acidosis with bicarbonate may further aggravate hypocalcemia in these infants due to increased calcium binding to albumin, as mentioned earlier.

Late hypocalcemia typically occurs by the end of the first week of life. It is seen more often in term than in preterm infants and is caused by the relative resistance of renal tubules to PTH. This leads to increased phosphate retention and hypocalcemia. Low serum magnesium levels lead to hypocalcemia due to their inhibitory effect on PTH secretion (see the section titled "Magnesium" later in the chapter). Infants fed cow's milk are also more prone to late hypocalcemia due to its high phosphorus content. Maternal vitamin D deficiency may be a predisposing factor; therefore, vitamin D supplementation (400 IU daily) for all exclusively breastfed infants is currently recommended. **Quality and Safety: Furosemide therapy can cause hypocalcemia and nephrolithiasis secondary to calciuresis.** Phototherapy is a risk factor for neonatal hypocalcemia, particularly in preterm infants, shown to be secondary to PTH suppression (Beser et al., 2023).

Neonatal hypoparathyroidism is characterized by low PTH, hypocalcemia, and hyperphosphatemia. It can be caused by structural abnormalities of the parathyroid glands, defects in the PTH molecule, or dysregulation of PTH secretion. In rare cases, late hypocalcemia can occur because of subclinical maternal hyperparathyroidism: maternal hypercalcemia leads to fetal hypercalcemia, which suppresses the fetal parathyroid glands. After birth, when the maternal source of calcium is no longer available, the suppressed parathyroid glands are unable to maintain a normal serum calcium concentration. Because maternal hyperparathyroidism is often asymptomatic, neonatal hypocalcemia may provide the initial clue to maternal disease.

Neonatal hypocalcemia may be asymptomatic or can cause symptoms such as irritability, tremors, poor feeding, muscle twitching, and seizures. Diagnosis of hypocalcemia is based on definitions outlined earlier. The serum magnesium level should also be measured due to its effects on calcium homeostasis.

Several factors complicate the choice of treatment for neonatal hypocalcemia:

- In most cases, the condition is asymptomatic and self-limited.
- It may be associated with seizures without being the cause of seizures.
- It may coexist with other perinatal complications, such as asphyxia and hypoglycemia, which can cause similar clinical signs.

If the hypocalcemia is asymptomatic, 10% calcium gluconate (9.4 mg of elemental calcium per ml) may be given enterally at a dose of 75 mg/kg/d divided into six equal doses. If hypocalcemia is symptomatic (e.g., seizures), 10% calcium gluconate must be given intravenously at a rate of 2 ml/kg over 10 minutes while the heart rate is continuously monitored, and the infusion stopped at any sign of bradycardia. For late hypocalcemia caused by increased phosphorus load, human milk or formulas low in phosphorus and supplementation with calcium are recommended. If associated with hypomagnesemia, serum magnesium should be corrected prior to treating hypocalcemia.

**Hypercalcemia.** Hypercalcemia is defined as a serum calcium level over 11 mg/dl (2.75 mmol/L) or an ionized calcium level greater than 1.45 mmol/L. Hypercalcemic disorders, such as subcutaneous fat necrosis, Williams syndrome, congenital hyperparathyroidism, neonatal Bartter syndrome, osteopetrosis, and familial hypocalciuric hypercalcemia, are all exceedingly rare among newborns. Hypercalcemia is usually iatrogenic and results from excessive administration of calcium or vitamin D or insufficient phosphorus intake (human milk diet). Therefore, before embarking on an elaborate differential diagnosis and expensive tests, one should carefully review the actual calcium, phosphorus, and vitamin D intakes.

Secondary hyperparathyroidism may be caused by maternal hypoparathyroidism or hypocalcemia, which leads to high PTH levels in the fetus. This condition is usually transient and resolves completely by 6 months of age. Primary hyperparathyroidism is caused by mutations in the *CASR* gene (Riccardi & Valenti, 2016). The type presenting in neonates is familial hypocalciuric hypercalcemia, characterized by abnormally low urine calcium and high PTH levels in the presence of elevated serum calcium.

Clinical signs of hypercalcemia are nonspecific and include constipation, polyuria, and bradycardia. Infants with long-standing hypercalcemia may present with failure to thrive. Nephrocalcinosis (calcium deposition in the renal parenchyma) and nephrolithiasis (renal stones) accompanied by hematuria are often the earliest presentation of hypercalcemia. Nephrocalcinosis is a common finding in VLBW infants due to the calciuric effects of commonly used drugs such as furosemide. Long-term outcomes for infants with nephrocalcinosis are unknown.

Treatment of hypercalcemia is as follows:

- Calcium and vitamin D supplementation is suspended, and dietary intake of calcium and vitamin D is restricted (human milk or vitamin D–free formula is given).
- Urinary excretion of calcium is promoted by fluid administration (about twice the maintenance requirement).
- In the case of vitamin D excess, glucocorticoids are given to reduce intestinal absorption and bone resorption of calcium.
- As a last resort, pamidronate can be trialed, although experience with bisphosphonates in newborns is limited. Pamidronate is generally given at a dose of 1 mg/kg as a single 4-hour IV infusion. Additional doses are given weekly, only, if necessary, as the serum calcium nadirs after administration by day 6 to 7.
- Dialysis may be needed in case of severe and refractory hypercalcemia.

**Phosphorus.** Phosphorus is absorbed mainly in the duodenum and jejunum by both active and passive diffusion. Absorption depends on the amount of phosphorus in the diet, the relative concentrations of phosphorus and calcium (excessive calcium can diminish phosphorus absorption and vice versa), and the presence of phosphorus-binding substances (e.g., phytates in soy-based formulas).

The kidneys excrete phosphorus under the control of PTH and fibroblast growth factor (FGF-23) activity. High levels of PTH and FGF-23 lead to hypophosphatemia due to their phosphaturic effects. Normally, about 95% to 99% of the filtered phosphorus is reabsorbed in term infants. Preterm infants have a greater fractional excretion of phosphorus in urine.

Disorders of phosphorus balance are listed in Box 19.5.

**BOX 19.5**

**DISORDERS OF PHOSPHORUS BALANCE**

**Hypophosphatemia**

MBD

Inadequate parenteral phosphorus administration

Malabsorption

Hyperparathyroidism

Familial hypophosphatemia: vitamin D–resistant rickets, X-linked hypophosphatemia

**Hyperphosphatemia**

Impaired excretion of phosphorus: renal failure

Hypoparathyroidism

Excessive parenteral or enteral administration of phosphorus

MBD, metabolic bone disease

**Hypophosphatemia.** Hypophosphatemia is defined as a serum phosphorus level below 4 mg/dl (1.29 mmol/L). It is a common feature in preterm infants with MBD, which is caused by insufficient intake of calcium and phosphorus. Adequate phosphorus levels are needed to cause apoptosis (programmed cell death) of hypertrophic cells in the bony growth plate. **Quality and Safety: Hypophosphatemia leads to the formation of abnormal bone tissue and MBD (Baroncelli et al., 2024).** Phosphorus deficiency can also result in muscle weakness and impaired white blood cell function.

In very rare cases, hypophosphatemia may be caused by neonatal hyperparathyroidism. In infancy, hypophosphatemia can occur due to disorders of vitamin D metabolism (vitamin D–dependent rickets) or defects in renal phosphorus transport (hypophosphatemic rickets).

Severe hypophosphatemia, a serum phosphorus level below 1 mg/dl (0.32 mmol/L), is uncommon and usually occurs only in newborns receiving parenteral alimentation with inadequate amounts of phosphorus. Respiratory failure and decreased myocardial performance have been described as possible consequences of severe hypophosphatemia.

**Hyperphosphatemia.** Hyperphosphatemia is defined as a serum phosphorus level over 7 mg/dl (2.26 mmol/L) and can be caused by ingestion of milk formulas containing high amounts of phosphorus, excessive parenteral administration of phosphorus, impaired phosphorus excretion (renal failure), or by defects in hormonal regulation (hypoparathyroidism). Severe hyperphosphatemia may cause metastatic calcifications and hypocalcemia. Management includes alimentation with human milk or with a low-phosphorus formula and calcium supplementation to increase the binding of phosphorus to promote its fecal excretion. Reducing the parenteral phosphorus intake usually resolves the hyperphosphatemia. In renal failure, 1,25-dihydroxyvitamin D, which exerts its effects independent of functioning renal tissue, can be given to counteract hypocalcemia secondary to hyperphosphatemia.

Supplementation with 1,25-dihydroxyvitamin D and calcium may be used to treat hypoparathyroidism in newborns arising from maternal hyperparathyroidism (transient secondary hypoparathyroidism) or permanent primary hypoparathyroidism (sporadic or hereditary).

**Metabolic Bone Disease.** This condition occurs primarily in VLBW infants and is associated with several prenatal and postnatal risk factors (Box 19.6). Early initiation of enteral nutrition, use of specialized preterm formulas, and parenteral supplementation of calcium and phosphorus have decreased the incidence of MBD. The relative calcium, phosphorus, and vitamin D content of commonly used enteral feeds for VLBW infants are given in Table 19.4. Management of MBD

**BOX 19.6**

**RISK FACTORS FOR METABOLIC BONE DISEASE**

**Prenatal**

Premature birth: abrupt cessation of placental calcium and phosphorus accretion

Intrauterine growth restriction

Preeclampsia

Maternal vitamin D deficiency

**Postnatal**

Inadequate intake of calcium and phosphorus

Medications: diuretics, methylxanthines, steroids

Vitamin D deficiency

Sedation or paralysis

**TABLE 19.4**

**CALCIUM, PHOSPHORUS, AND VITAMIN D CONTENT OF ENTERAL FEEDS**

| | Unfortified Human Milk (20 kcal/oz) | Fortified Human Milk (24 kcal/oz) | Preterm Formula (24 kcal/oz) |
|---|---|---|---|
| Calcium (mg/kg) | 37 | 184–218 | 210–234 |
| Phosphorus (mg/kg) | 21 | 102–125 | 107–130 |
| Vitamin D (IU) | 2.4 | 283–379 | 290–468 |

*Note:* For 160 ml/kg/d of feeds for an infant weighing 1,500 g.

*Source:* Adapted from Martin, R. J., Fanaroff, A. A., & Walsh, M. C. (Eds.). (2025). *Fanaroff and Martin's neonatal-perinatal medicine: Diseases of the fetus and infant* (12th ed.). Elsevier.

is centered on maximizing calcium and phosphorus intake. There are limited data to guide the dosing of calcium or phosphorus supplementation in addition to appropriately fortified human milk or preterm formula because it may pose a risk for molar ratio imbalance and promote forming a calcium soap with dietary fat or for precipitation with other nutrients (Koletzko et al., 2021). Serum 25-hydroxyvitamin D levels should be maintained above 20 ng/ml, and medications such as furosemide, dexamethasone, and caffeine should be judiciously used. Serum alkaline phosphatase may be used as an additional marker of MBD, with levels greater than 600 to 800 IU/L at 4 to 6 postnatal weeks being suggestive of MBD.

**Magnesium.** Magnesium is distributed primarily in the skeleton and the intracellular space. It is involved in energy production, cell membrane function, mitochondrial function, nerve conduction, and protein synthesis. In the serum, about a third of the magnesium is bound to albumin.

Magnesium is absorbed in the small intestine by both a passive and an active saturable mechanism. Absorption is related to intake, and approximately half of the dietary magnesium is absorbed. Under the influence of many hormones, the kidneys regulate the serum magnesium concentration, and normally, less than 5% of the filtered magnesium is excreted. PTH, calcitonin, ADH, and insulin increase magnesium reabsorption. Most magnesium reabsorption occurs in the ascending limb of the loop of Henle. PTH also mobilizes magnesium from the bone to increase the serum magnesium concentration. An acute decline in the serum magnesium concentration increases the secretion of PTH, but chronic magnesium deficiency reduces PTH secretion and may cause hypocalcemia.

The recommended intake for preterm infants is based on placental accretion rates of 3 to 5 mg/kg/d (Embleton et al., 2023). Preterm infant enteral absorption of magnesium is about 40%, so intake of 9.7 to 12.1 mg/kg/d of fortified human milk or formula is likely sufficient. The magnesium content of mature human milk is about 31 mg/L. In parenteral solutions, the concentration of magnesium should be maintained between 36 and 48 mg/L to avoid precipitation.

Disorders of magnesium balance are listed in Box 19.7.

**BOX 19.7**

**DISORDERS OF MAGNESIUM BALANCE**

**Hypomagnesemia**

- Infant of diabetic mother
- Intrauterine growth restriction
- Malabsorption syndromes
- Loop diuretics and aminoglycosides
- Isolated renal magnesium wasting

**Hypermagnesemia**

- Maternal treatment with magnesium sulfate (e.g., for tocolysis, preeclampsia)
- Excessive magnesium administration with parenteral nutrition
- Magnesium-containing antacids
- Magnesium therapy for neonatal pulmonary hypertension

**Hypomagnesemia.** Hypomagnesemia is defined as a serum magnesium level below 1.6 mg/dl (0.66 mmol/L). Hypomagnesemia may be the cause or effect of neonatal hypoparathyroidism. Magnesium transfer from the mother to the fetus is impaired in maternal disorders with placental insufficiency and predisposes neonates to hypomagnesemia. Infants of diabetic mothers (IDMs) have an increased incidence of hypomagnesemia because of maternal magnesium depletion (Hay, 2012). **Emergency Alert: Loop diuretics and aminoglycosides have been associated with renal magnesium wasting.** Isolated defects of intestinal malabsorption and renal wasting of magnesium have also been described.

Symptoms of hypomagnesemia are usually not apparent until the levels fall below 1.2 mg/dl (.49 mmol/L). The symptoms of hypomagnesemia are like those of hypocalcemia and frequently coexist in clinical practice. Neonatal hypomagnesemia is usually benign and transient (except in cases of malabsorption and renal wasting). It can cause hyperexcitability, tremors, and, occasionally, severe hypocalcemic seizures that are unresponsive to anticonvulsant medications and calcium replacement. They respond to a slow infusion of 50% magnesium sulfate 0.1 ml/kg. **Emergency Alert: Complications of magnesium administration include systemic hypotension and arrhythmias.** Treatment can be repeated with close monitoring of the serum magnesium concentration every 12 hours until normal magnesium levels are achieved. In cases of malabsorption syndromes, daily enteral supplementation of 50% magnesium sulfate 1 ml/kg may be required.

**Hypermagnesemia.** Hypermagnesemia is defined as a serum magnesium level over 2.8 mg/dl (1.15 mmol/L). Hypermagnesemia is usually secondary to excessive administration through parenteral nutrition or following maternal treatment with magnesium sulfate for tocolysis, neuroprotection, or seizure prevention in preeclampsia. Serum levels following maternal treatment seldom reach dangerous levels and gradually return to normal after several days. Rarely, magnesium-containing antacids can cause hypermagnesemia.

The most common presentation of hypermagnesemia is perinatal depression of the infant following maternal magnesium therapy. Clinical signs include hyporeflexia, lethargy, and respiratory depression. Hypermagnesemia can lead to decreased PTH and 1,25-dihydroxyvitamin D production, resulting in a fall in serum calcium concentration. Treatment of hypermagnesemia is usually supportive. It is essential to maintain adequate hydration to promote urinary excretion. Loop diuretics may also be used to aid renal elimination. Rarely, mechanical ventilation may be required to overcome respiratory depression.

## ACID–BASE BALANCE

Several complex physiologic processes are at work in a normal infant to maintain the pH within a tight range of 7.35 to 7.45. This pH range is essential for normal metabolic functioning, growth, and development. These processes are disrupted in critically ill neonates and preterm infants, leading to either acidosis or alkalosis. Preterm infants are especially at risk for acidosis due to their impaired renal ability to acidify urine and lower renal threshold for bicarbonate absorption when compared to term infants.

The following section discusses the two main processes that help maintain acid–base balance.

## Acute Compensation

Whenever acute changes in the acid–base status occur, two major buffering mechanisms come into play to restore pH to normal levels. First, the $H^+/K^+$ exchanger can alter the relative concentrations of $H^+$ and $K^+$ in the intracellular and extracellular spaces. For example, when there is acidosis (decrease in serum pH), this exchanger causes the $H^+$ ions to move intracellularly and $K^+$ to move extracellularly. Therefore, acute acidosis is often complicated and accompanied by hyperkalemia. The second buffering mechanism is via carbonic anhydrase, an enzyme that catalyzes the conversion of water ($H_2O$) and carbon dioxide ($CO_2$) to carbonic acid ($H_2CO_3$) and vice versa. The $H_2CO_3$ can dissociate to form $H^+$ and $HCO_3^-$ ions.

$CO_2$ crosses the blood–brain barrier and decreases the pH, activating central chemoreceptors that increase the respiratory drive (i.e., increased exhalation of $CO_2$). Similarly, alkalosis results in hypoventilation, leading to the retention of $CO_2$ to normalize the pH. It is important to note that respiratory compensatory mechanisms can only partially normalize serum pH. Therefore, if the serum pH is normal, a mixed acid–base disorder should be suspected rather than a compensated condition.

## Long-Term Compensation

The lungs and kidneys are responsible for the maintenance of long-term acid–base homeostasis. The lungs primarily release $CO_2$, a by-product of energy metabolism. The kidneys excrete a daily acid load of about 1 to 2 mEq/kg and more in pathologic processes such as sepsis or lactic acidosis. The kidneys also maintain acid–base balance by reabsorption and excretion of bicarbonate, which may be disrupted in conditions such as RTA.

## Metabolic Acidosis

Metabolic acidosis is defined as a serum pH of less than 7.30 with a normal $PCO_2$ level and decreased $HCO_3^-$ level. It is a common finding in preterm and critically ill neonates. It is divided into two categories based on anion gap: (a) *increased* anion gap metabolic acidosis and (b) *normal* anion gap metabolic acidosis (Box 19.8). Anion gap is defined as the difference between the measured cations (positively charged ions) and anions (negatively charged ions) in the serum. It can be calculated by the formula:

$$\text{Anion gap} = (Na^+ + K^+) - (Cl^- + HCO_{3^-})$$

**The normal anion gap is 8 to 16 mEq/L.**

### BOX 19.8

**CAUSES OF METABOLIC ACIDOSIS**

**Increased Anion Gap**

Sepsis, NEC

Hypoxia

Hypovolemic shock

Inborn errors of metabolism (organic acidemia, glycogen storage disease, galactosemia, mitochondrial defects)

Maternal salicylate use (e.g., aspirin, bismuth salicylate)

**Normal Anion Gap**

Renal tubular acidosis

Secretory diarrhea

Carbonic anhydrase inhibitors (e.g., acetazolamide, dorzolamide)

NEC, necrotizing enterocolitis.

The most common cause of increased anion gap metabolic acidosis is lactic acidosis. Endogenous lactic acid, a by-product of anaerobic metabolism, is produced in conditions with poor tissue perfusion as seen in sepsis, hypoxia, or NEC. Acidosis with increased anion gap can also be seen in the case of inborn errors of metabolism such as organic acidemias, glycogen storage disease, galactosemia, or mitochondrial defects. A condition unique to neonates is the *late metabolic acidosis* of prematurity. It is usually seen in the third week of life and is caused by the excess acid load following high-protein (casein/whey) formulas. This is primarily a self-limited condition and resolves as the kidneys mature.

Normal anion gap metabolic acidosis is commonly seen in RTA, diarrhea, and certain medications. In proximal RTA (type II), there is a defect in the bicarbonate reabsorption, while in distal RTA (type I), there is an inability to excrete $H^+$ ions. In diarrhea, there is an excessive loss of $HCO_3^-$ ions in the stool. Medications such as carbonic anhydrase inhibitors cause decreased uptake of $HCO_3^-$ in the kidneys. To maintain electrical neutrality, the serum chloride level is usually elevated in normal anion gap metabolic acidosis.

Treatment is aimed at correcting the underlying cause. Bicarbonate should be used with extreme caution because it can inadvertently increase $PCO_2$, with a consequential shift in the oxyhemoglobin dissociation curve to the left, leading to decreased oxygen delivery to the tissues and intracellular acidosis.

## Metabolic Alkalosis

Metabolic alkalosis is defined as a serum pH greater than 7.45 with a normal $PCO_2$ level and elevated $HCO_3^-$ level. The most common cause of metabolic alkalosis in preterm infants is chronic diuretic therapy for BPD. Depletion of the extracellular fluid volume leads to metabolic alkalosis by activation of the RAS leading to $Na^+$ absorption and $H^+$ and $K^+$ excretion

**BOX 19.9**

**CAUSES OF METABOLIC ALKALOSIS**

**Chloride Responsive**

Chronic diuretic therapy

Loss of gastric acid (gastric suctioning or excessive vomiting)

Congenital chloride diarrhea

**Chloride Resistant**

Early diuretic therapy

Excessive administration of base (bicarbonate, acetate, or citrate)

Bartter syndrome

in the renal tubules. Volume depletion also reduces the GFR and, thus, the amount of bicarbonate filtered. This is termed *contraction alkalosis*. Metabolic alkalosis is divided into two categories (Box 19.9): (a) chloride responsive and (b) chloride resistant. A urinary chloride level can help delineate the type.

Chloride-responsive metabolic alkalosis is associated with a low urinary chloride level and is seen after chronic diuretic therapy (furosemide acts by inhibiting the $Na^+$-$K^+$-$Cl^-$ cotransporter), excessive loss of gastric hydrochloric acid due to vomiting or prolonged gastric aspiration, and congenital chloride-wasting diarrhea (rare).

Chloride-resistant metabolic alkalosis is associated with a high urinary chloride level and is seen in early diuretic therapy, excessive administration of bicarbonate, acetate, or citrate, and Bartter syndrome (rare).

Mild-to-moderate metabolic alkalosis does not warrant therapy. Treatment is aimed at correcting the underlying cause. Metabolic alkalosis secondary to chronic diuretic therapy is treated by supplementing chloride, most commonly in the form of KCl, either enterally or parenterally. Discontinuation or reduction of the diuretic dose may also be required. Alkalosis due to loss of gastric acid is corrected by appropriate fluid replacement (normal saline or Ringer's lactate). Acetazolamide has been occasionally used for treatment in critically ill neonates, but the evidence is limited (Kalikkot Thekkeveedu et al., 2021).

## Respiratory Acidosis

Respiratory acidosis is an increase in $PCO_2$ associated with a decrease in serum pH. It is caused by conditions that decrease the respiratory drive (ventilation), leading to $CO_2$ retention. The most common causes are RDS, transient tachypnea of the newborn (TTN), pneumonia, meconium aspiration, and chronic lung disease. It can also be seen acutely in an obstructed or improperly positioned endotracheal tube. A strategy of permissive hypercapnia (respiratory acidosis) is often used in infants with chronic lung disease to minimize ventilator-associated lung injury and facilitate weaning of respiratory support.

## Respiratory Alkalosis

Respiratory alkalosis is a decrease in $PCO_2$ associated with an increase in serum pH. The most common cause of respiratory alkalosis in neonates is mechanical overventilation. A factitious decrease in $PCO_2$ is also observed whenever an air bubble is trapped in the blood gas specimen. True central hyperventilation (increased respiratory rate) requires further diagnostic workup because it is associated with intracranial pathologies and hyperammonemia.

## Identifying Acid–Base Disturbances

When one of the four conditions mentioned earlier is present in isolation, it is called a simple acid–base disorder. In these conditions, an appropriate respiratory or renal compensation occurs to counteract the primary abnormality to mitigate large changes in the serum pH. For example, a primary metabolic acidosis is associated with a respiratory compensation wherein $PCO_2$ levels decrease, and respiratory alkalosis ensues. Similarly, a primary respiratory acidosis is associated with compensatory renal changes (increase in secretion of $H^+$ ion) that lead to metabolic alkalosis. The respiratory compensation of primary metabolic abnormalities occurs rapidly, while metabolic compensation for a primary respiratory acid–base disorder occurs more slowly. There is an initial acute but modest renal response followed by a chronic renal response that usually takes 3 to 5 days. If the compensation in pH from a respiratory or renal process is greater or lesser than expected, a mixed acid–base disorder is suspected. For example, in a septic patient with metabolic acidosis due to poor perfusion, there may be associated respiratory failure leading to respiratory acidosis and a higher-than-expected $PCO_2$ level. Appropriate diagnosis of acid–base disturbances requires (a) identification of the primary abnormality (history, clinical examination, and laboratory data) and (b) assessment of the degree of secondary compensation. The expected values for appropriate secondary compensation for the various disorders are given in Table 19.5 (McPherson & Pincus, 2022).

## Nursing Management

Nurses have a vital role to play in the fluid and electrolyte management of infants admitted to the NICU. In addition to obtaining vital signs and monitoring intake–output and daily weights, they are responsible for securing peripheral and central vascular access to ensure the safe delivery of IV fluids and medications. **Quality and Safety:** **It is crucial for a bedside nurse to promptly recognize and report the signs and symptoms of fluid and electrolyte imbalance to avoid complications associated with inappropriate fluid administration.**

**Assessment and Evaluation in Fluid and Electrolyte Therapy.** The estimation of an infant's fluid and electrolyte needs depends on the gestational age, day of life (DOL), weight, and the underlying disease process. The needs of a 4-kg infant with perinatal asphyxia and seizures are vastly different from those of a 32-week, 1,750-g infant with RDS or a 24-week, 500-g infant with multiple complex problems. Each represents a different disease process along with varying

**TABLE 19.5**

**COMPENSATORY RESPONSE TO PRIMARY ACID–BASE DISTURBANCES**

| Acid–Base Disturbance | Primary Finding | Secondary Compensation |
|---|---|---|
| Metabolic acidosis | Every 1 mEq/L decrease in $HCO_3^-$ | Decrease in $Pco_2$ by 1.2 mm Hg |
| Metabolic alkalosis | Every 1 mEq/L increase in $HCO_3^-$ | Increase in $Pco_2$ by 0.7 mm Hg |
| Respiratory acidosis | Every 10 mm Hg increase in $Pco_2$ | Acute: increase in $HCO_3^-$ by 0.7 mEq/L<br>Chronic: increase in $HCO_3^-$ by 4 mEq/L |
| Respiratory alkalosis | Every 10 mm Hg decrease in $Pco_2$ | Acute: decrease in $HCO_3^-$ by 2 mEq/L<br>Chronic: decrease in $HCO_3^-$ by 5 mEq/L |

degrees of organ maturation, necessitating careful management of fluid and electrolytes to maintain homeostasis.

**Fluid Requirement.** Fluid needs of an infant can be calculated using body weight, body surface area, or caloric expenditure (Kliegman, 2024). In clinical practice, the total daily fluid requirement is approximated based on the gestational age, weight, and the infant's DOL. It is then further adjusted by accounting for past and projected losses. Factors that affect water loss in neonates are given in Table 19.1. An example of this is the term newborn infant with a large gastroschisis. This midline abdominal wall defect predisposes the infant to large IWLs because of the exposed abdominal organs. Similarly, a 24-week, 500-g infant with the typical "translucent" skin that has not yet formed a competent epidermal barrier is predisposed to dehydration due to large IWL through the skin. The fluid requirements for such an infant may be as high as 150 to 200 ml/kg/d. In contrast, a birth-asphyxiated full-term infant may need fluids restricted to no more than 40 to 50 ml/kg/d for the first 48 to 72 hours of life.

Environmental factors such as temperature and humidity also affect IWL. The use of radiant warmers increases IWL, while the use of a double-walled, well-humidified incubator significantly reduces IWL. Finally, it is critical for a nurse to double-check fluid orders to ensure that the correct fluids and rate are delivered. The approximate maintenance requirements of newborns in the first week of life (based on birth-weight) are given in Table 19.2.

**Fluid Output.** The underlying disease process dictates the frequency of fluid (intake–output) calculations, which are usually performed once a day. In neonates recovering from acute renal failure (polyuric phase), calculations may need to be done every 4 hours, whereas in conditions with decreased urine output (renal failure, nephrotoxic drugs) it may suffice to calculate every 12 to 24 hours. Urine output is measured and expressed in ml/kg/hr, and if output is less than 1 ml/kg/hr, the infant is diagnosed with oliguria.

For example, if a 32-week gestation 2-kg infant has 240 ml of urine in a 24-hour period,

$$UOP = 240 \text{ ml}/24 \text{ hr} = 10 \text{ ml/hr}$$

$$10 \text{ ml/hr}/2 \text{ kg} = 5 \text{ ml/kg/hr}$$

This is an adequate UOP for an infant of this weight and gestational age.

Neonates can also have significant fluid losses through vomiting, diarrhea, an ostomy, a gastric tube, a chest tube, and/or surgical wound drainage. In general, if the fluid loss from these sources exceeds 20 ml/kg in 24 hours, replacement fluids should be initiated to prevent fluid and electrolyte imbalances. Table 19.3 gives the electrolyte concentrations of different body fluids and can be used to guide the choice of replacement fluids.

**Infant Weight.** Weight is a sensitive indicator of overall fluid status. Infants are usually weighed daily; however, extremely low birth weight (ELBW) infants may be weighed more often (e.g., every 12 hours) because fluid requirements are recalculated based on weight changes. It is important to weigh infants accurately because inaccuracies can lead to misguided calculations and detrimental outcomes. Neonates should be weighed naked, with minimal extraneous equipment (e.g., ECG leads, probes), at the same time each day, and on the same scale. In-bed scales that give constant weight readouts simplify the weighing process and reduce infant stress. Birth weight is used to calculate daily fluid requirements during the first week of life because physiologic fluid shifts occur and affect daily weights. Once the infant regains birth weight, the daily weights are used to calculate fluid needs.

**Physical Examination.** The physical examination can reveal changes in the infant's fluid status and should be used in conjunction with laboratory data to plan interventions in fluid and electrolyte therapy. A general assessment of hydration status includes the infant's color, skin turgor, activity, mucous membranes, fontanelles, and capillary refill:

- *Color:* Pink and well perfused, rather than pale and mottled (indicates dehydration)
- *Skin turgor:* Good turgor, rather than "tenting" (indicates dehydration) or edematous and shiny (indicates fluid overload)
- *Activity:* Active with good tone, rather than lethargic and hypotonic (indicates dehydration or overhydration)
- *Mucous membranes:* Pink and moist, rather than dry and gray (indicates dehydration)
- *Fontanelles:* Soft and flat, rather than depressed (indicates dehydration) or tense and full (may indicate overhydration)
- *Capillary refill:* It is an important indicator of peripheral perfusion and hydration status. Normal capillary refill

time in neonates is less than or equal to 2 seconds. Capillary refill greater than 3 seconds is concerning for dehydration.

### Vital Signs

- **Heart rate: Tachycardia is a relatively early sign of dehydration.** Because a variety of other factors can also cause tachycardia in neonates (pain, anemia, or caffeine therapy), the heart rate trend is more useful in diagnosing fluid imbalance rather than absolute values at a moment in time.
- **Blood pressure: Hypotension and shock occur late in dehydration.** Acute changes in the mean arterial blood pressure are a significant risk factor for IVH in extremely preterm neonates.

**Laboratory Data.** The frequency of laboratory assessment depends on the clinical status of the infant. In most preterm and critically ill infants who require IV fluids, a daily basic metabolic panel (BMP) is obtained for the first 3 days of life. These assessments are made more frequently in infants with high fluid losses or with significant derangements in electrolytes. On the other hand, infants with relatively stable electrolytes, despite being on chronic diuretic therapy, may only require weekly checks.

Point-of-care assessment of urine specific gravity (normal 1.005–1.012) and acute changes in central hematocrit are also helpful in assessing hydration status at the bedside.

## CONSIDERATIONS FOR THE PERIVIABLE INFANT

Although a universally accepted gestational age range for the "periviable" infant does not exist, these infants represent the smallest and most fragile patients in the NICU. The typical gestational age range included are those infants born at 22 to 24 weeks; however, any ELBW infant born very prematurely may also warrant special attention. Fluid and electrolyte shifts, nutrition, and medications are critically important to monitor at least twice daily. With ongoing attention to detailed care and greater understanding of the physiology and pathophysiology unique to this population of NICU patients, survival has increased significantly over time. One review found that when compared to the 2008 to 2012 period, those infants born between 22 and 28 weeks at the same hospitals between 2013 and 2018 had increased survival to discharge by around 78% (Bell et al., 2022).

Renal and skin immaturity contribute to the significant water and electrolyte shifts during the first few days of life. Evidence to guide best practices is limited, but there is a trend toward an initial restriction of fluids and sodium to reduce rates of BPD, PDA, and NEC and improve survival. An accurate estimation of maintenance fluids needs is complicated by the competing interests of the infant's thermoregulatory environment (incubator versus radiant warmer), changing cardiopulmonary physiology, and any overlaying pathology.

The ideal thermoregulatory environment for ELBW infants is not known. Because initial water losses through the gastrointestinal and respiratory systems (using heated, humidified gas) are minimal, IWL can be attributed primarily to transepidermal water loss (TEWL). Infants born at 22 to 24 weeks' gestation may have an IWL of approximately 60 to 200 ml/kg/d, depending on their care environment. Higher humidities (80%–90%) achieved inside an incubator significantly reduce TEWL; however, delays skin maturation, impedes visualization and adherence of monitoring devices and may increase the risk for infections. Infants cared for under a radiant warmer with a plastic wrap covering (30%–40% humidity) have very large TEWL, leading to large fluid and electrolyte shifts associated with rapid skin maturation due to the xeric stress.

Urinary sodium losses are initially much higher in periviable infants. As discussed previously, sodium supplementation should initially be avoided for the first few days, but subsequently, higher amounts are needed to attain a positive sodium balance required for growth. Careful attention should be paid to the required iatrogenic sodium administration from flushes and transfusions. Potassium administration should be considered only after adequate UOP is established. Potassium supplementation is required to maintain a positive potassium balance when serum potassium is below 4 mEq/L.

Careful monitoring of intake and output, along with selective laboratory evaluation and serial weights, is critical to maintaining the careful balance of electrolytes and fluids in the periviable infant. Weights should be obtained at least daily using an incubator scale with careful attention to the minimum weight measurable by that scale. Serum electrolytes should be monitored approximately twice daily using a combination of point-of-care and laboratory methods, depending on the access and reliability of each technique. Urine output should be recorded every 6 hours. To make fluid adjustments more efficiently, a two-bag fluid system should be considered—the first with a starter nutritional solution (total parenteral nutrition) and the second with dextrose only. Colostrum should be introduced as soon as it is available and considered a medication rather than a source of fluid intake.

## SUMMARY

The care of infants with fluid and electrolyte balance alterations presents a management challenge for both physicians and nurses. A thorough understanding of the underlying pathophysiology and the rationale for therapy enables the healthcare team to provide more informed care for these infants and to anticipate and prevent problems.

## CASE STUDY

**Identification of the Problem.** A 24-week female infant with a birth weight of 500 g was born to a 30-year-old gravida 1 para 1 mother following preterm labor. Pregnancy was complicated by limited prenatal care, and maternal group B streptococcus status is unknown. The delivery occurred via a cesarean section under general anesthesia. Upon delivery, the infant was limp, blue, and apneic and required intubation and mechanical ventilation. Apgar scores were 2, 6, and 8 at 1, 5, and 10 minutes, respectively. Upon arrival to the NICU, the infant is placed in an isolette whose temperature and humidity are set to maintain a thermoneutral environment. The nurse obtains peripheral IV access and draws a screening septic workup. Umbilical venous and arterial lines are placed and the infant is given a dose of ampicillin and gentamicin. The infant is started on a $D_{7.5}W$ with amino acids at 80 ml/kg/d. Vital signs remain stable, and a BMP obtained at 24 hours of life is normal. Venous blood gas is pH 7.26, $PCO_2$ 49 mm Hg, and base deficit of –5. Bilirubin level is noted to be 8 mg/dl and the infant is started on phototherapy. On DOL 2, the infant's fluid goal is increased to 100 ml/kg/d, and 1/4 sodium acetate is added to fluids, but peripheral access is lost. The nurse also reports concerns with the umbilical venous line fluids repeatedly backing up and notices that the bed is soaked with clear fluid. Following this, the nurse places a peripherally inserted central catheter (PICC) and restarts IV fluids at the previous rate. A BMP obtained on DOL 3 shows $Na^+$ 161 mEq/L, $K^+$ 6.5 mEq/L, $Cl^-$ 129 mEq/L, $HCO_3^-$ 16 mEq/L, BUN 53 mg/dl, creatinine 1.26 mg/dl, glucose 73 mg/dl, and serum osmolality 345 mOsm/L.

## Assessment: History and Physical Examination

**Weight:** Birth weight 500 g, weight on DOL 2, 450 g. 10% weight loss.

**Vital signs:** Heart rate 180 beats/min; respiratory rate 60 breaths/min; blood pressures: systolic 40 mm Hg, diastolic 18 mm Hg; mean arterial pressure 25 mm Hg.

## Physical Examination

- GENERAL: decreased spontaneous activity
- HEAD, EARS, EYES, NOSE, AND THROAT (HEENT): normocephalic, anterior fontanelle slightly sunken
- RESPIRATORY: bilateral breath sounds equal and clear
- CARDIOVASCULAR: tachycardia with continuous murmur; pulses = +1; capillary refill ~3 seconds
- ABDOMEN: soft, round, and not tender to palpation, no hepatosplenomegaly noted
- GENITOURINARY: immature female genitalia
- SKIN: immature skin with developing areas of breakdown

## Differential Diagnosis

- Dehydration due to peripheral/central line malfunction (umbilical venous line repeatedly backing up with clear fluid soaking the bed, lack of IV fluids while PICC was being attempted)
- Excessive IWL due to immature skin and phototherapy (24-week infant with high bilirubin)
- Excessive administration of sodium (addition of 1/4 sodium acetate to fluids on DOL 2)

## Diagnostic Tests

- BMP
- Serum osmolality
- Urine specific gravity
- Blood gas
- Complete blood count

**Development of Management Plan.** The management plan involves evaluating the fluid status based on clinical examination and laboratory data. This extremely premature infant has lost 10% of birth weight on DOL 2, and on physical examination has signs concerning for dehydration. BMP on DOL 3 shows increased serum osmolality, hypernatremia, hyperkalemia, hyperchloremia, and metabolic acidosis. The most likely cause of hypernatremia is dehydration due to cessation of IV fluid delivery secondary to loss of peripheral and central venous access. Furthermore, a fluid goal of 80 to 100 ml/kg/d in the first 48 hours of life is inadequate for this ELBW infant weighing only 500 g due to high IWL through the immature skin. Phototherapy is an additional risk factor that augments the IWLs. Early sodium supplementation in the absence of adequate diuresis can increase the risk for hypernatremia.

The total fluid goal for this infant should be increased by about 40 to 60 ml/kg/d to correct dehydration. **Quality and Safety: Normal saline boluses should be avoided because ELBW infants at this age have poor cerebral blood flow autoregulation and are at significant risk for IVH.**

**Evaluation of Effectiveness.** Periodic assessment of the infant's weight, vital signs, and physical examination are critical. A BMP is repeated to evaluate the electrolytes 12 to 24 hours later. The correction of sodium levels should not be greater than 10 to 12 mEq/L/d (or 0.5 mEq/L/hr), due to the risk for cerebral edema. The infant is also monitored for signs of hyperkalemia and metabolic acidosis.

**Outcome.** After the fluid goal was readjusted and measures were taken to reduce IWL, the electrolyte abnormalities slowly corrected over a 48-hour period.

## EVIDENCE-BASED PRACTICE

Virtually all preterm infants need IV fluid infusions for a variable length of time, depending on the degree of prematurity and severity of complications. The optimal daily fluid requirements are tailored to the infant's needs. In 2014, Bell and Acarregui published a Cochrane review to determine the effect of varying levels of fluid intake on postnatal weight loss, morbidity, and mortality in preterm infants. Five randomized controlled trials evaluating different IV fluid intakes were included in the analysis.

The water intake in the "Restricted Fluids" group ranged from 50 to 122 ml/kg/d, while in the "Liberal Fluids" group it ranged from 80 to 169 ml/kg/d. The postnatal weight loss was significantly higher, along with a trend toward increased risk of dehydration in the fluid-restricted group. The risk of PDA (relative risk [RR], 0.52 and number needed to treat [NNT] was 7) and NEC (RR 0.43 and NNT was 20) was significantly lower in the fluid-restricted group. In addition, there was a trend toward reduced risk of chronic lung disease and IVH in the fluid-restricted group, but it did not reach statistical significance. There was no difference in mortality between the two groups.

The authors concluded that appropriately restricted fluid intake (without causing dehydration) in preterm neonates could potentially reduce the risk of PDA and NEC.

### Reference

Bell, E. F., & Acarregui, M. J. (2014). Restricted versus liberal water intake for preventing morbidity and mortality in preterm infants. *Cochrane Database of Systematic Reviews*, *2014*(12). https://doi.org/10.1002/14651858.CD000503.pub3

## ONLINE RESOURCES

**CourseConnect**

Resources for this chapter are online and available at www.springerpub.com/courseconnect.

## REFERENCES

References for this chapter are online and available at www.springerpub.com/courseconnect.

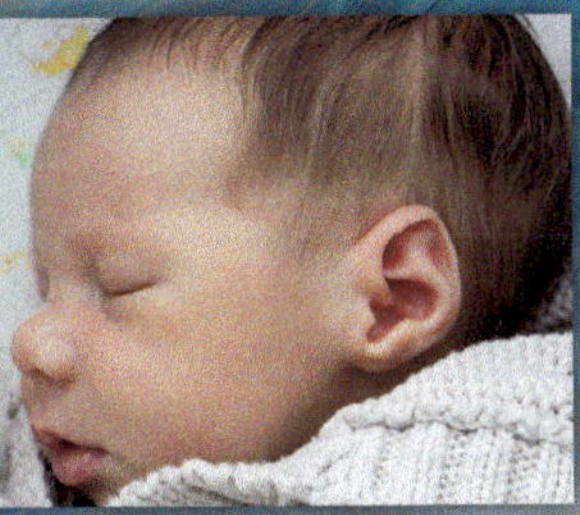

Source: giomatmicro /Adobe Stock.

CHAPTER 20

# Nutrition Management of Premature Infants

Kathryn Hanson and Georgia Haas

## INTRODUCTION

Meeting the nutritional needs of premature and sick infants is essential to their survival (Heird et al., 1972). Under conditions of total starvation, these infants have **reserves** for only 4.5 days, and daily provision of intravenous (IV) glucose will prolong survival for only about 7 days. Therefore, the mandate is to meet the basic nutrient requirements of these infants and to understand their metabolic limitations to avoid physiologic stress and morbidity related to the delivery of enteral and parenteral nutrition (PN). Nutrition management of the premature infant continues shortly after birth with IV fluids, PN, and/or enteral feedings, depending on the infant's gestational age and clinical condition. The third trimester of pregnancy, which premature infants miss, is a period of rapid growth and nutrient accretion (Cordova & Belfort, 2020). While the position statement of the American Academy of Pediatrics (AAP) states the goal for premature infant growth is to mimic the rate and composition of a fetus at the same gestational age, newer research is emerging that this may not be appropriate given the premature infant's environment and altered metabolic needs compared to the fetus (AAP Committee on Nutrition, 2014; Cordova & Belfort, 2020). The ideal pattern of preterm infant growth remains undefined, but various growth curves can be utilized clinically to monitor and assess the preterm infant's growth, each with their own advantages and limitations. The goal for the premature infant differs from that of the healthy term infant due to increased nutrient demands requiring fortification of human milk to meet nutrient needs. Due to illness and immaturity, PN and gavage feedings will commonly be needed. Premature infants are at nutrition risk for many reasons, including early birth, which limits nutrient stores such as calcium, iron, and fat; rapid growth, which increases nutrient demand; illness, which may alter nutrient needs, nutrient tolerance, and feeding modality; an immature gastrointestinal (GI) tract, which presents as decreased gut motility, decreased digestive abilities, and decreased tolerance of feedings; and cold stress, which increases energy demand.

After birth, all infants will initially lose weight due to fluid losses and low nutrient intakes, the preterm infant even more so than the term infant (Fenton et al., 2024). Once the birth weight is regained, the premature infant will gain weight that parallels the birth weight curve. Although the actual growth pattern will be more nuanced for each infant, the curve may not be linear and reflects their genetic potential, prenatal intrauterine environment, and postnatal course. Clinical assessment by knowledgeable providers is necessary to determine the appropriateness of growth for each infant. Nutrition and a neonate's nutritional status affect the growth patterns—both immediate and long term. There is mounting evidence suggesting that aberrant body composition in the neonatal period, both growth restriction and excessive postnatal weight gain, have adverse long-term health outcomes, including cognitive impairment and metabolic syndrome (Cerasani et al., 2020; Cordova and Belfort, 2020). This supports the need for good nutrition for the premature or sick neonate if short- and long-term complications are to be minimized.

This chapter starts with a brief review of the metabolism of nutrients, minerals, and vitamins in the neonate. It then discusses the developmental and physiologic issues unique to premature and sick infants. A discussion of neonatal nutrition with special emphasis on premature infants describes the challenges of providing appropriate nutrients. The various nutrition routes are included.

## MACRONUTRIENTS

### Protein

Protein must be broken down into amino acids to be absorbed. Protein digestion and absorption take place in the stomach, small intestinal lumen, and the intestinal cell, the enterocyte (Cruz & Neu, 2022). Protein digestion begins in the stomach by gastric acid, hydrochloric acid, and the enzyme pepsin. Protein digestion continues in the intestinal lumen by the presence of pancreatic enzymes in the form of peptides (a group of amino acids). In the enterocyte, the peptides are further broken down into amino acids. The amino acids and some small peptides are then absorbed into the blood. The intestines of the infant is immature, and intact proteins can cross into the bloodstream and perhaps induce an allergic reaction to milk protein. The openness of the intestinal wall to intact protein is greater in infants born at less than 33 weeks' gestation, but closure does occur a few days after birth (Cruz & Neu, 2022). In the fetus, gastric acid production has been found at 13 weeks' gestation, and gastric levels are lower in premature infants than levels seen in term infants. Gastric enzymes appear at 16 weeks' gestation, and pancreatic enzymes by 24 weeks' gestation. Protein digestion and absorption do not appear impaired with premature infants (Cruz & Neu, 2022).

## Fat

Food fat is mainly present as triglycerides, which are three fatty acids attached to the carbohydrate glycerol. Fat is digested in a two-step process in the intestine. The first step is to make the triglyceride water soluble with the mixing of bile salts from the liver. The second step breaks the triglyceride into two fatty acids and a monoglyceride by the pancreatic lipases, lingual lipase, gastric lipase, intestinal lipase, or milk bile acid–stimulated lipase present in human milk. The monoglyceride and free fatty acids can be directly absorbed into the enterocyte or entered by transporter protein for fatty acids (Cruz & Neu, 2022). Once in the enterocyte, triglycerides are made and are grouped with cholesterol, lipoproteins, and other lipids to form chylomicrons. The chylomicrons circulate by the lymphatic system into the blood system and then into cells throughout the body. Fat digestion and absorption are limited in infants due to decreased levels of bile salts and lipase levels. Bile acid levels are low due to decreased synthesis and decreased intestinal reabsorption. Fetal lipase levels are detected at 21 weeks' gestation but do not reach adult concentrations until 6 months of age in the term infant. Premature infants have lower lipase levels at birth than term infants. Fat is 40% to 50% of the dietary calories from human milk or infant formula, so it is a major component of intake by infants for their growth.

Medium-chain triglyceride (MCT) oil has been added to premature infant formulas. MCT oils do not require bile salts or pancreatic lipases to be digested and are absorbed directly into the bloodstream by the infant. The addition of MCT does not help the premature infant absorb more fat but may be helpful for infants with major absorption problems such as short gut syndrome.

## Carbohydrate

Carbohydrates must be in their simple form or as monosaccharides to be absorbed. Lactose is the major carbohydrate in human milk and is composed of the monosaccharides glucose and galactose. Starch consists of glucose polymers, and sucrose contains glucose and fructose. Digestion of carbohydrates begins in the mouth with salivary amylase to break it down into smaller-size carbohydrates or oligosaccharides. The digestion continues with human milk alpha-amylase when consumed and pancreatic amylase enzymes in the intestine. The final digestion occurs on the brush border of the enterocyte with the enzymes lactase, maltase, and sucrase used to break down lactose, starch, and sucrose. The monosaccharides are carried into the enterocyte by a transport protein and into the blood by a different transport protein. Premature infants have decreased levels of the enzymes lactase, maltase, and sucrase, but after birth with lactose-containing human milk, the lactase enzymes are increased by 2 weeks of age (Cruz & Neu, 2022). Formulas for premature infants contain a blend of lactose and glucose polymers that are well tolerated, whereas term formulas are typically 100% lactose. Infants who have intestinal damage following necrotizing enterocolitis (NEC) or have developed short gut syndrome may not tolerate lactose and will need a formula containing glucose polymers (corn syrup solids).

## Summary

The absorption of the three major nutrients is relatively inefficient in the preterm and the term infant. Diets such as human milk or premature infant formulas are well tolerated. For nurses, a basic understanding of these absorption mechanisms is essential to understand the rationale for various dietary adjustments.

# MICRONUTRIENTS

## Vitamins, Macrominerals, and Trace Minerals

Infants received most of their fat-soluble vitamin stores during the last trimester of pregnancy. Premature infants will have lower vitamin A, D, E, and K stores than the term infant. Premature infants do not absorb fat-soluble vitamins well because of their poor ability to digest and absorb fat (Leaf & Lansdowne, 2014). Premature infants have decreased bile salts and pancreatic lipase concentrations, both of which are needed for the absorption of fat and fat-soluble vitamins. Premature infants have increased vitamin needs due to limited vitamin stores, increased demand for growth, and limited absorptive capabilities.

Water-soluble vitamins—B complex and vitamin C—are less likely to create deficiency states owing to their relative availability and method of absorption in infants. Information on water-soluble vitamin needs is limited for the premature infant, and there is much to be learned (Leaf & Lansdowne, 2014).

The absorption of sodium, potassium, chloride, and bicarbonate across the intestinal mucosa in the infant appears to differ from that in the adult. Under normal circumstances, this difference appears to be of no consequence. In unusual circumstances, such as diarrhea, the increased intestinal permeability may lead to large intestinal losses of these electrolytes as well as water. This causes the infant to develop dehydration and electrolyte imbalance more rapidly than later in life. Basic requirements also vary in the infant because renal absorption and excretion of these minerals are not well regulated owing to organ immaturity, which is accentuated in premature infants.

Calcium absorption occurs by active transport and passive diffusion (Fogleman et al., 2012; Namgung & Tsang, 2019). Active transport depends on vitamin D. Passive diffusion of calcium may be enhanced by the presence of bile salts and lactose because they increase intestinal cell permeability. Calcium and vitamin D are important micronutrients for improving bone mineralization and reducing osteopenia of prematurity.

Zinc that is ingested, as well as that which is re-secreted from pancreatic and biliary secretions, is absorbed in the small bowel (AAP Committee on Nutrition, 2014). Absorption varies based on the bioavailability of the source and the presence of other minerals in the diet, such as iron and copper, which are known to interfere with absorption (Domellof, 2014). Zinc is an important element for growth and development in the preterm infant (Terrin et al., 2015).

## GASTROINTESTINAL FUNCTION OF THE PREMATURE INFANT

Research on the developing fetus has determined that much of the GI tract begins to function early in fetal life. Anatomically, the foregut and hindgut are present as early as 4 weeks' gestation, with the intestinal villi appearing at 8 weeks (Mahe et al., 2022; Munshi & Clark, 2022). It is clear, however, that even in the full-term infant, the GI tract is inefficient in its ability to propel, absorb, and utilize nutrients and maintain homeostasis during stress.

Developmentally, the issues of the premature infant begin with the inability to suck, swallow, and breathe in a coordinated fashion. This problem places a heavy burden on the caregiver to provide adequate nutrient intake via all artificial methods. Suck, swallow, and breath coordination matures around 32 to 34 weeks' gestation. There are many additional reasons this coordination can be delayed. For example, it is common to observe late coordination in infants who have cardiorespiratory disease and who are physiologically unstable. Another large group of infants who cannot regulate their own intake is those who remain on assisted ventilation. The sequence of the infant suck, swallow, and breathe pattern has been described as mature when the suck/swallow/respiration has a 1:1:1 to 2:2:2 pattern (Amaizu et al., 2008). This sequence not only presumes infant maturity but also depends on physiologic stability. Nonnutritive sucking has obvious differences from nutritive sucking, which make it only one of several indicators of feeding readiness.

The second physiologic issue of the premature infant is the absence or weakness of the gag and cough reflexes. This challenge increases the risks to premature infants when gastric enteral feedings are used. The risk of aspiration must be considered when the stomach is used for feeding. The assessment for the presence of the gag reflex is easy to do by direct observation while passing a feeding tube. It is nearly impossible to assess the adequacy of the gag reflex in preventing aspiration if vomiting or reflux occurs. **Quality and Safety: The risk of aspiration should be considered in all premature infants when started on enteral feeding.** Additionally, if the infant has vomiting issues, chronic loss of nutrients can become problematic. Reflux has frequently been linked as a cause of apnea. New research suggests that they often occur together, but it is apnea that leads to gastric reflux (Mitchell et al., 2022). During an apnea episode, the respiratory neural output is decreased, accompanied by relaxation of the lower esophageal tone, resulting in gastroesophageal reflux. On rare occasions, reflux can result in apnea.

The third challenge is the relative relaxation of the lower esophageal sphincter. The purpose of this sphincter is to allow food to pass into the stomach. Inappropriate relaxation may lead to reflux of food back into the esophagus (Khlevner et al., 2022). Inadequate sphincter function is an additional risk factor for all premature infants when orally fed.

Delayed gastric emptying is the fourth physiologic challenge in premature infants. Gastric emptying is relatively delayed in infants. This process is delayed in disease states, and nurses find that milk feedings are not predictably empty in preterm or sick term infants. This challenge may be the single limiting factor when the preterm infant is placed on enteral feeds in that little can be done toward feeding progression until stomach emptying occurs. If stomach emptying remains a limiting factor, it can be bypassed with transpyloric feedings.

Intestinal dysmotility is the fifth major challenge in the premature infant. Clinicians can observe improvement around 30 to 33 weeks' gestation and maturity of motility by 36 weeks' gestation (Khlevner et al., 2022). If there are central nervous system abnormalities, motility can be adversely affected. If intestinal motility is the limiting factor in the progression of enteral feedings, it should be identified as such before multiple formula changes are made. It is always essential to identify the specific challenge as the causative factor when addressing a plan to deliver enteral nutrients.

The incompetence of the ileocecal valve, the sixth challenge, must be assessed by the clinician. This valve acts as a barrier between small and large bowel contents, thus separating bacterial flora and regulating the time for the small bowel to absorb nutrients before its contents are delivered to the colon for water absorption. When reflux through this valve occurs, the small bowel is colonized with bacteria. With the presence of undigested nutrients in the small bowel and bacteria proliferation, hydrogen gas is produced. This mechanism is part of one sequence of events hypothesized to lead to NEC (Wilson-Costello et al., 2013).

The seventh and last challenge is the passage of the first meconium stool. Term infants should pass a stool within 48 hours of life (Clark, 1977). Many premature infants will pass their first stool within 48 hours of life, but some premature infants can take up to more than 1 week of age without problems (Verma & Dhanireddy, 1993). Term infants who have not stooled by 48 hours will need to be monitored and may need to be assessed for GI obstruction.

### Summary

The premature infant has many developmental and mechanical challenges that make using the GI tract difficult or impossible. The tract matures with postnatal age and physiologic stability and needs to be reassessed regularly. Feeding assessment needs to be monitored to make changes in feedings as indicated.

## PARENTERAL NUTRITION

### Indications

PN describes a form of providing nutrients—amino acids, dextrose, and intravenous lipid emulsion (ILE)—by an IV route rather than orally. PN is indicated for preterm neonates and infants who cannot receive estimated energy and nutrient requirements enterally (Robinson et al., 2023). Reasons an infant may not receive adequate nutrients enterally include immature bowel, congenital GI or cardiac anomalies, or other acquired GI illnesses, such as NEC or short bowel syndrome.

Infants are started on PN on the first day of life when slow feeding advancement is anticipated. Prompt initiation once intravascular access is obtained is indicated because infants rapidly develop protein and total energy deficits after birth. Early initiation of PN has been associated with less initial weight loss, glucose homeostasis, better nitrogen balance, and improved growth trajectory (Robinson et al., 2023). Starter or Stock PN, which contains a standard concentration of glucose, protein, and sometimes calcium, is used initially because it is rapidly available. Intravenous lipid emulsion may be provided on day 1 to provide essential fatty acids and promote nitrogen balance (Vlaardingerbroek et al., 2013). **Quality and Safety: Electrolytes are not indicated on day 1 of age.** Vitamins are not added to the standard starter PN solutions because they decrease the shelf life; but they are added to custom PN on subsequent days. PN nutrients can then be advanced as described in the following sections. Table 20.1 provides the guidelines for PN. Table 20.2 provides parenteral calculations.

**TABLE 20.1**

**GROWING PREMATURE INFANTS—PARENTERAL GUIDELINES: ENERGY, PROTEIN, MINERALS**

| Nutrient | Unit (kg/d, Except as Noted) |
|---|---|
| Energy, kcal | 90–115 (preterm)<br>90–100 (term) |
| Glucose, mg/kg/min | 8–12 (preterm)<br>8–10 (term) |
| Carbohydrate, g | 11.5–17.3 (preterm)<br>11.5–14.4 (term) |
| Protein, g | 3–3.5 (preterm)<br>2.5–3 (term) |
| Fat, g | 3 (preterm and term) |
| Calcium, mEq/kg/d | 2.5–4 (preterm)<br>1.6–3 (term) |
| Phosphorus, mmol/kg/d | 1–3 (preterm)<br>0.5–2 (term) |
| Magnesium, mEq/kg/d | 0.4–0.6 (preterm)<br>0.2–0.4 (term) |
| Sodium, mEq | 3–5 (preterm)<br>2–3 (term) |
| Potassium, mEq | 2-5 (preterm)<br>1.5-3 (term) |
| Chloride, mEq | 3–5 (preterm)<br>2–3 (term) |
| Zinc, mcg | 450 (preterm)<br>250 (term) |
| Copper, mcg | 20 |
| Selenium, mcg | 1.5–2 (preterm)<br>2 (term) |
| Chromium, mcg | 0.0006 |
| Manganese, mcg | 1 |

(continued)

**TABLE 20.1**

**GROWING PREMATURE INFANTS—PARENTERAL GUIDELINES: ENERGY, PROTEIN, MINERALS (*continued*)**

*Sources:* Data from American Academy of Pediatrics Committee on Nutrition. (2014). Nutritional needs of preterm infants. In R. E. Kleinman & F. R. Greer (Eds.), *Pediatric nutrition handbook* (7th ed., pp. 83–121). Vanek, V. W. (2015). Review of trace mineral requirements for preterm infants: What are the current recommendations for clinical practice? *Nutrition in Clinical Practice, 30*(1), 720–721. https://doi.org/10.1177/0884533614563353; Vanek, V. W., Borum, P., Buchman, A., Fessler, T. A., Howard, L., Jeejeebhoy, K., Kochevar, M., Shenkin, A., Valentine, C. J., Novel Nutrient Task Force, Parenteral Multi-Vitamin and Multi–Trace Element Working Group, & American Society for Parenteral and Enteral Nutrition (A.S.P.E.N.) Board of Directors. (2012). A.S.P.E.N. position paper: recommendations for changes in commercially available parenteral multivitamin and multi-trace element products. *Nutrition in Clinical Practice, 27*(4), 440–491. https://doi.org/10.1177/0884533612446706. A.S.P.E.N. position; Carlson, S., Hovasi Cox, J., Dumm, M., Gates, A., Groh-Wargo, S., Hodges, B., Johnson, M., Jones, A., Kavars, A. M., Lewis, A. E., Merlino Barr, S., O'Toole, G., Paul, E., Pepin, H. L., Phillips, S., Rohrer, A., Smith, C., Thompson, M., & Trumpower, E. (2023). *Pocket guide to neonatal nutrition* (3rd ed.) [review of pocket guide to neonatal nutrition]. Academy of Nutrition and Dietetics.

**TABLE 20.2**

**CALCULATIONS FOR PARENTERAL NUTRITION**

| Nutrient | Calculations |
|---|---|
| Dextrose | 3.4 kcal/g |
| Protein | 4 kcal/g |
| 20% Lipid | 10 kcal/g (which is 9 fat kcal and 1 glycerol kcal)<br>or<br>2 kcal/mL (1 fat g/5 mL) |
| GIR mg/kg/min | ([mL/kg/d] × [grams glucose/100 mL] × [1,000 mg/g])/1,440 min/d For example, infant receiving 130 mL/kg/d of 12.5% dextrose ([130 mL/kg/d] × [12.5 g dextrose/100 mL] × [1,000 mg/g])/1,440 GIR = 11.3 mg/kg/min |

GIR, glucose infusion rate.

## Energy

Energy intake of 40 to 60 kcal/kg/d is recommended for nitrogen balance during the first days of life (Meiliana et al., 2024). Energy intake should then increase to 60 to 120 kcal/kg, the goal for growth with PN. For enteral feedings, 105 to 130 kcal/kg/d will meet the needs of most premature infants (AAP Committee on Nutrition, 2014; Meiliana et al., 2024).

## Glucose

Glucose homeostasis is an issue for premature infants because they are at risk for both hypoglycemia and hyperglycemia. Premature infants are at risk for hypoglycemia due to poor glycogen stores, impaired gluconeogenesis, increased glucose need with acute illness (sepsis, respiratory distress), maternal therapy with beta-blockers, and hyperinsulinemia commonly seen with infants of diabetic mothers, perinatal stress, and growth-restricted infants (Burris, 2017). Conversely, premature infants are also at risk for hyperglycemia due to immature glucose tolerance in the setting of ongoing gluconeogenesis, reduced insulin production, increased insulin resistance, and acute stress/illness. Blood glucose levels should be monitored closely as parenteral glucose loads are advanced or weaned to ensure tolerance.

Neonates usually produce endogenous glucose at the rate of 3 to 5 mg/kg/min for the term infant and up to 8 to 9 mg/kg/min in the extremely low birth weight (ELBW) infant (Poindexter & Ehrenkranz, 2015). Due to impaired glucose tolerance in infants with very low birth weight (VLBW), PN starting glucose infusion rate (GIR) is recommended at around 4 to 6 mg/kg/min (AAP Committee on Nutrition, 2014). The GIR is then advanced slowly to a goal of 11 to 12 mg/kg/min to meet energy needs for growth (AAP Committee on Nutrition, 2014). Glucose can be advanced by 1 to 2 mg/kg/min (Carlson & Kavars, 2016). The addition of parenteral protein enhances insulin release and the tolerance of the glucose load (Thureen et al., 2003). By monitoring blood glucose loads, slowly advancing glucose loads, and providing parenteral protein, VLBW infants typically tolerate advancement to nutritional target goals. Occasionally, infants may require exogenous insulin to treat hyperglycemia, but this is avoided due to increased incidence of hypoglycemia and adverse outcomes with its use (Alsweiler et al., 2012; Beardsall et al., 2008; Robinson et al., 2023).

**Emergency Alert: Hypoglycemia can occur when inadequate glucose is provided, glucose is not delivered due to IV line infiltration, PN has been rapidly discontinued, or insulin has been administered.**

## Protein

The latest research recommends a protein target of 3 to 3.5 g/kg/d, resulting in normal plasma amino acid levels, increased nitrogen balance, and increased protein anabolism (AAP Committee on Nutrition, 2014; Denne & Poindexter, 2007; Robinson et al., 2023; Thureen et al., 2003). Early protein intake of 3 g/kg/d is associated with better gain in weight, length, and head circumference at 36 weeks postmenstrual age, and decreased incidence of head circumference less than the 10th percentile at 22 months corrected age (Poindexter et al., 2006).

Blood urea nitrogen (BUN) does not consistently correlate to parenteral protein intake during the first week of life. It should not be used to limit protein intake unless renal dysfunction is demonstrated by decreased urine output and elevated serum creatinine (Blanco et al., 2008; Radmacher et al., 2009; Ridout et al., 2005). BUN level can reflect hydration status, excessive protein intake, inadequate protein or energy intake, illness, renal function, and hepatic synthesis (Radmacher et al., 2009).

Parenteral protein is provided as amino acids, and pediatric solutions are recommended. These solutions provide a blend of amino acids to produce blood amino acid levels similar to those found in breastfed term infants or cord blood levels found in premature infants (Poindexter & Ehrenkranz, 2015). The premature infant's ability to synthesize cysteine, tyrosine, and arginine is limited, so these should be provided in the early diet. Cysteine is unstable in solutions, so it is added as cysteine hydrochloride. The addition of cysteine improves nitrogen balance and increases the acidity of the solution, which allows greater amounts of calcium and phosphorous to be added (Soghier & Brion, 2010).

## Lipids

IV lipids are given to provide essential fatty acids and kilocalories (Poindexter & Ehrenkranz, 2015; Robinson et al., 2023). Not providing lipids in the first week of life can result in biochemical fatty acid deficiency for premature infants with limited fat stores. IV lipids may be started at 1 to 2 g/kg on day 1 of life and advanced by 1 g/kg/d to a goal of 3 g/kg/d (AAP Committee on Nutrition, 2014). (Of note, certain short-term use lipids have a maximum dosage recommendation of 1 g/kg/d.) Infants who have decreased serum levels of lipoprotein lipase or experience metabolic stress may not clear lipids well. Infants most at risk include those who are small for gestational age, experience intrauterine growth restriction (IUGR), are early gestational age, are ELBW, have sepsis, or have received steroids (AAP Committee on Nutrition, 2014; Choi et al., 2015). Serum triglycerides may be monitored, but acceptable levels have not been determined (Neu, 2009). A level under 200 mg/dl has been suggested (AAP Committee on Nutrition, 2014).

In the United States, ILE is available as soybean oil emulsions (Intralipid), multicomponent soy oil, MCTs, olive oil, fish oil blend (SMOFlipid), and fish oil (Omegaven). Soy oil provides the essential fatty acids linoleic acid (omega-6 fatty acid) and linolenic acid (omega-3 fatty acid). Fish oil contains omega-3 fatty acids, docosahexaenoic acid, eicosapentaenoic acid, and vitamin E, which have antiinflammatory and antioxidant properties (Hojsak et al., 2016). The best ILE for neonates has yet to be established (Frazer & Martin, 2021). Historically, Intralipid was the only ILE available and has continued to be used widely. A known complication of ILE is the development of parenteral nutrition–associated liver disease (PNALD), which has been linked to the phytosterols contained in soy oil (Hojsak et al., 2016). Newer multicomponent ILEs contain less soy oil and theoretically could mitigate some of the risks of developing PNALD, though the data currently does not support that theory (Robinson et al., 2023). Once PNALD is established, dose reduction or alternate ILE is recommended (Hojsak et al., 2016). It is important to ensure that the appropriate dose of ILE is provided to prevent essential fatty acid deficiency (Robinson et al., 2023).

## Carnitine

Carnitine facilitates the transport of long-chain fatty acids into the mitochondria for oxidation. Premature infants have limited carnitine stores and a decreased ability to synthesize carnitine (Clark et al., 2017). Human milk and infant formula provide sources of carnitine, while parenteral solutions do not contain carnitine unless added. A 10 mg/kg/d dosage may be provided for infants receiving only PN for more than 2 to 3 weeks (AAP Committee on Nutrition, 2014; Hay et al., 2014).

## Fluid and Electrolytes

Premature infants have high and variable fluid needs based on birth weight, gestational age, clinical condition, and their environment (Curtis, 2025). **Quality and Safety: Constant monitoring and assessment are indicated to promote normal hydration status.** Monitoring includes body weight, fluid intake, urine output, stool output, other fluid losses, and serum electrolytes (Curtis, 2025). A weight loss of up to 15% is common in the first week of life (Curtis, 2025).

**Quality and Safety: Sodium is not added in the first few days of life to allow for the diuresis of the extracellular fluid, but IV saline infusions or flushes may be indicated.** These sources of sodium must be accounted for when prescribing PN sodium. The usual sodium requirement is 2 to 4 mEq/kg/d. Potassium is not needed on the first day of life but is added as renal function is established and serum potassium levels become normal. A potassium intake of 2 to 3 mEq/kg/d will usually meet the needs of the infants (Poindexter & Ehrenkranz, 2015). Chloride may be provided with sodium and potassium. Acetate is indicated when acidosis occurs (Poindexter & Ehrenkranz, 2015). All serum electrolytes require monitoring to ensure normal serum levels.

## Calcium, Phosphorus, and Magnesium

Calcium, phosphorus, and magnesium are needed for metabolic management and bone mineralization. Calcium and phosphorus should be provided at a 1 to 1.3/1 molar ratio of calcium to phosphorus to promote normal blood levels and bone mineralization (Carlson & Kavars, 2016). Calcium and phosphorus must be provided together instead of in alternate-day administrations to avoid urinary mineral wasting or abnormal blood calcium and phosphorus levels (Carlson & Kavars, 2016). Phosphorus is often not included in starter PN solutions. Phosphorus needs to be added to the following order of PN to avoid hypercalcemia and hypophosphatemia (Hair et al., 2016a).

## Vitamins

Pediatric multivitamin injections are available but are not designed for premature infants (AAP Committee on Nutrition, 2014). The dosage schedule is based on the infant's weight. Different manufacturers have slightly different components, and appropriate doses should be confirmed with unit dietitians and clinical pharmacists (AAP Committee on Nutrition, 2014). Parenteral vitamins are not available as single vitamins.

## Trace Minerals

Trace mineral guidelines are shown in Table 20.1. Trace minerals are available as multimineral packets or as separate minerals. Extra zinc is indicated for infants with intestinal losses and monitoring blood zinc levels may be helpful (Terrin et al., 2015). When cholestasis is present, copper and manganese intakes are decreased due to elimination of these trace minerals in the bile. With restricted copper intake, blood copper levels may need to be monitored to detect copper deficiency (Marquardt et al., 2012). Selenium and chromium intakes are limited with impaired renal function (AAP Committee on Nutrition, 2014).

# ENTERAL NUTRITION

Premature infants have increased nutrient needs to support fetal growth. Table 20.3 provides enteral nutrient guidelines. Enteral feedings are always the goal for the nourishment of premature infants. The infant should be evaluated daily for feeding advancement, milk fortification, and vitamin and mineral supplements.

## Oral Care With Colostrum

Providing oral care with the mother's colostrum or donor milk is recommended within the first 48 hours of life for infants who are nothing by mouth (NPO) or on enteral feeds

**TABLE 20.3**

**ENTERAL NUTRIENT GUIDELINES FOR VERY LOW BIRTH WEIGHT PREMATURE INFANTS (UNIT/KG/D)**

| Nutrient | Amount | Nutrient | Amount |
|---|---|---|---|
| Energy, kcal | 110–130 | Selenium, mcg | 7–10 |
| Protein, g | 3.5–4.5 | Iodine, mcg | 10–55 |
| Carbohydrate, g | 11–13 | Vitamin A, mcg | 400–1,000 |
| Fat, g | 4.55–8.1 | Vitamin D, IU | 400–1,000 |
| Calcium, mg | 120–200 | Vitamin E, IU | 2.2–11 |
| Phosphorus, mg | 70–120 | Vitamin K, mcg | 4.4–28 |
| Magnesium, mg | 8–15 | Vitamin C, mg | 16.5–41 |
| Sodium, mEq | 3–5 | Thiamin, mcg | 132–275 |
| Potassium, mEq | 2–5 | Riboflavin, mcg | 200–430 |
| Chloride, mEq | 3–5 | Niacin, mg | 1.1–5.5 |
| Iron, mg | 1–3 | Vitamin B6, mcg | 66–275 |
| Zinc, mg | 2–3 | Folate, mcg | 22–100 |
| Copper, mcg | 120–230 | Vitamin B12, mcg | 0.12–0.6 |
| | | Biotin, mcg | 3.3–15 |
| | | Pantothenic acid, mg | 0.6–2.1 |

IU, International Units.

[a] Vitamin D intake is per day.

*Source:* Data from Carlson, S., Hovasi Cox, J., Dumm, M., Gates, A., Groh-Wargo, S., Hodges, B., Johnson, M., Jones, A., Kavars, A. M., Lewis, A. E., Merlino Barr, S., O'Toole, G., Paul, E., Pepin, H. L., Phillips, S., Rohrer, A., Smith, C., Thompson, M., & Trumpower, E. (2023). *Pocket guide to neonatal nutrition* (3rd ed.) [Review of pocket guide to neonatal nutrition]. Academy of Nutrition and Dietetics.

(Shakeel, 2023). Colostrum can be provided by syringe or swab into the buccal pouch of the oral cavity. It is recommended to provide hands-on care at least every 6 hours (Shakeel, 2023). Benefits include immune and antioxidant provision, infection prevention, positive oral stimulation, and motivation to start and maintain supply (Garofalo & Caplan, 2019).

## Human Milk

The milk of choice for all infants is human milk. Pasteurized donor milk is preferred when the mother's milk is not available or sufficient (Parker et al., 2021). The human milk diet for premature infants results in a decreased incidence of mortality, sepsis, NEC, retinopathy of prematurity, and bronchopulmonary dysplasia, improved neurodevelopment, and a quicker time to full enteral feedings with fewer days of PN needed (Abrams et al., 2014; Carlson et al., 2023; Hair et al., 2016b; Meinzen-Derr et al., 2009; Schanler et al., 1999; Sisk et al., 2007; Sullivan et al., 2010; Vohr et al., 2007).

Pasteurized donor milk should be obtained from one of the donor human milk banks or commercial banks to ensure product safety. Donors are screened for infections, medications, drugs, or high-risk activities by history and blood tests. Informal milk sharing, which is the noncommercial sharing of breastmilk between mothers for feeding their infants, is becoming more common in the United States. Because these donors have yet to be formally screened, milk is unpasteurized and may have suboptimal collection and storage techniques. Thus, informal milk sharing is generally not recommended for the premature infant. Despite counseling, some families may still choose to provide informally shared milk to their infants. Some NICUs will have policies in place to ensure adequate education is provided and consent is obtained prior to feeding the preterm infant. Mothers who want to donate milk should be referred to one of the banks for proper screening. The Human Milk Banking Association of North America (http://www.hmbana.org) is a volunteer association that nonprofit Human Milk Banks may be a member of and whose members are required to meet the standards for human milk banking guidelines, set by the association guidelines (AAP Committee on Nutrition, 2014; Parker et al., 2021).

Human milk fortifier (HMF) is indicated for VLBW infants to meet their increased nutrient needs becauses human milk alone will not suffice. Additional calories, protein, calcium, phosphorus, and vitamin D are provided. There are both bovine-based and donor human milk–based HMF. They can be added as early as 40 to 60 ml/kg of human milk intake or feeding day 2. Earlier fortification has been associated with less weight loss, faster linear growth, and less head circumference decline (Salas et al., 2023). Bovine-based HMF is typically added to 22 or 24 kcal/oz. Donor milk fortifier is available at 24, 26, 28, or 30 kcal/oz. Table 20.4 compares human milk with the fortifiers fed at a standard volume of 160 ml/kg and at the usual milk kilocalorie concentrations.

## Infant Formulas

Premature infant formulas are more nutrient dense than standard infant formulas and contain nutrients in a more easily digested form. Table 20.5 shows a selected nutrient comparison. Premature infant formulas come as 20, 24, and 30 kcal/oz milk. The 20- and 24-kcal/oz milk will meet the needs of most premature infants. The 30 kcal/oz milk is indicated for infants who are fluid restricted. The 24 kcal/oz premature formulas are available as regular and high protein. See Table 20.5 for a comparison of formulas fed at a standard 160 ml/kg volume. Recent litigation has questioned the safety of preterm infant formulas, raising the question that starting these formulas too early could cause NEC.

## TABLE 20.4

### SELECTIVE NUTRIENT COMPARISON OF HUMAN MILK WITH FORTIFICATION—160 ML/KG*

| Nutrient | Koletzko 2021 (per kg) | Human Milk (20 kcal/oz) | Human Milk + Liquid Bovine Milk Fortifier (24 kcal/oz) | Human Milk + Donor Milk Fortifier (24 kcal/oz) |
|---|---|---|---|---|
| Energy, kcal | 110–130 | 107 | 128 | 128 |
| Protein, g | 3.5–4.5 | 1.4 | 3–4.2 | 3 |
| Calcium, mg | 120–220 | 37 | 186–190 | 194 |
| Iron, mg | 2–3 | 0.1 | 0.6–2.4 | 0.3 |
| Vitamin D, IU | 400/d | 2 | 189–253 | 5 |
| Phosphorus (mg) | 60–140 | 21 | 102–109 | 102 |

IU, International Units.

*Representing usual volume intakes and milk concentrations without vitamin and mineral supplementation.

*Sources:* Data from Carlson, S., Hovasi Cox, J., Dumm, M., Gates, A., Groh-Wargo, S., Hodges, B., Johnson, M., Jones, A., Kavars, A. M., Lewis, A. E., Merlino Barr, S., O'Toole, G., Paul, E., Pepin, H. L., Phillips, S., Rohrer, A., Smith, C., Thompson, M., & Trumpower, E. (2023). *Pocket guide to neonatal nutrition* (3rd ed.) [Review of pocket guide to neonatal nutrition]. Academy of Nutrition and Dietetics; Koletzko, B., Cheah, F. C., Domellöf, M., van Goudoever, J. B., Poindexter, B. B., & Vain, N. (2021). Scientific basis and practical application of nutritional care for preterm infants. *World Review of Nutrition and Dietetics, 122,* XIII–XIV. https://doi.org/10.1159/000514773; Abbott Nutrition: https://www.abbottnutrition.com/; Mead Johnson Nutrition: https://www.meadjohnson.com/; Prolacta Sciences: https://www.prolacta.com/en/.

## TABLE 20.5

### SELECTIVE NUTRIENT COMPARISON OF INFANT FORMULAS—160 ML/KG*

| Nutrient | Koletzko 2021 (per kg) | Standard (Term) (20 kcal/oz) | Premature High Protein (24 kcal/oz) | Premature Discharge (22 kcal/oz) |
|---|---|---|---|---|
| Energy, kcal | 110–130 | 108 | 130 | 119 |
| Protein, g | 3.5–4.5 | 2.2 | 4.3–4.7 | 3.3 |
| Calcium, mg | 120–220 | 84 | 215–234 | 125–143 |
| Iron, mg | 2–3 | 1.9 | 2.3 | 2.1 |
| Vitamin D, IU | 400/d | 65 | 195–390 | 83 |
| Phosphorus (mg) | 60–140 | 45–46 | 117–130 | 74–79 |

IU, International Units.

*Representing usual volume intakes and milk concentrations without vitamin and mineral supplementation.

*Sources:* Data from Carlson, S., Hovasi Cox, J., Dumm, M., Gates, A., Groh-Wargo, S., Hodges, B., Johnson, M., Jones, A., Kavars, A. M., Lewis, A. E., Merlino Barr, S., O'Toole, G., Paul, E., Pepin, H. L., Phillips, S., Rohrer, A., Smith, C., Thompson, M., & Trumpower, E. (2023). *Pocket guide to neonatal nutrition* (3rd ed.) [review of pocket guide to neonatal nutrition]. Academy of Nutrition and Dietetics; Koletzko, B., Cheah, F. C., Domellöf, M., van Goudoever, J. B., Poindexter, B. B., & Vain, N. (2021). Scientific basis and practical application of nutritional care for preterm infants. *World Review of Nutrition and Dietetics, 122,* XIII–XIV. https://doi.org/10.1159/000514773; Abbott Nutrition: https://www.abbottnutrition.com/; Mead Johnson Nutrition: https://www.meadjohnson.com/; Prolacta Sciences: https://www.prolacta.com/en/.

However, the Food and Drug Administration (FDA), Centers for Disease Control (CDC), and National Institutes of Helath (NIH) all agree that preterm infant formulas do not cause NEC and that these formulas are the most appropriate option for infants who do not have a sufficient supply of breastmilk (ASPA Press Office, 2024).

Premature discharge formulas are designed for the premature infant at discharge. The nutrient composition is between standard and premature infant formula composition. Studies on these formulas have been on infants less than 1,800 g birth weight (Carver et al., 2001; Koo & Hockman, 2006; Lucas et al., 2001). Studies have shown improved growth and poorer growth for premature infants fed premature discharge formula compared to the term formulas. There have been reports of better growth for infants fed these formulas for 6 to 9 months (Carver et al., 2001; Lucas et al., 2001). Premature infants who are formula fed should be evaluated on an individualized basis for these formulas at discharge (AAP Committee on Nutrition, 2014). A multivitamin should be continued upon discharge until the infant gets 1 L of formula daily; at this point, formula will meet micronutrient Dietary Reference Intakes (DRIs; www.nationalacademies.org). Iron supplementation should continue for premature infants until they are getting an adequate amount via iron-fortified solid foods.

Soy infant formulas are not recommended for premature infants because they have low mineral and vitamin content (Abrams & Committee on Nutrition, 2013).

Specialized infant formulas, including protein hydrolysates and free amino acid formulas, are used for infants with malabsorption problems, such as the short gut, who may not tolerate human milk. Vitamin or mineral supplementation may be needed with these formulas because they are not designed to meet the needs of premature infants.

### Feeding Management

Enteral feedings should be considered for all infants. Trophic feedings (which are small feedings for the purpose of feeding the gut and do not serve as a major nutrition source) are frequently used for infants who are VLBW or clinically stressed. Studies have ranged from 1 to 25 ml/kg/d, and human milk is the milk of choice for these feedings (AAP Committee on Nutrition, 2014). Reported benefits of early, small feedings include decreased incidence of indirect hyperbilirubinemia, cholestatic jaundice, and metabolic bone disease; increased concentrations of gastric hormones; quicker achievement of full feedings; faster maturation of intestinal motility patterns; increased lactase activity; and reduced intestinal permeability (Berseth, 1992; Dunn et al., 1988; Meetze et al., 1992; Shulman et al., 1998a, 1998b). By meta-analysis, the incidence of NEC was not increased with trophic feedings (Morgan et al., 2013). There is no standard time for the length of trophic feedings because the studies have used different lengths of time for trophic feeding, different days of life to initiate feedings, and different kinds of milk. However, having a standardized feeding guideline in place can reduce risks (Meiliana et al., 2024), though these guidelines often differ from center to center. Trophic feedings can be initiated with the umbilical catheters in place (Davey et al., 1994). Feedings are often advanced by 10 to 40 ml/kg/d for VLBW infants.

### Feeding Method

The feeding method for the infant will depend on the infant's gestational age, weight, clinical condition, and the experience of the nursery nursing staff (AAP Committee on Nutrition, 2014). The premature infant does not coordinate sucking, swallowing, and breathing until 32 to 34 weeks' gestation. Nasogastric and orogastric feedings are used for infants too young or ill to breast or bottle feed (AAP Committee on Nutrition, 2014). Transpyloric feedings are used for infants with emesis or other signs of intolerance without intestinal pathology present, but research is lacking to support this method for routine feeding of premature infants (AAP Committee on Nutrition, 2014; Watson & McGuire, 2013). Continuous milk infusion is needed for infants fed via transpyloric feedings because the intestine has limited compliance (Schanler & Anderson, 2008). Gastrostomy feedings may be indicated for infants with congenital anomalies or neurologic impairment (Sapsford & Smith, 2016).

Continuous and bolus feedings are used with gastric feedings, and numerous studies have suggested that each method is best (Premji & Chessell, 2011). One concern with continuous infusion is the reported loss of fat and calcium (Rogers et al., 2010). Therefore, bolus feedings are usually the preferred option if tolerated.

### Feeding Assessment

Feeding assessment is indicated for premature infants, who often do not tolerate feedings well and are at risk for illness. Consensus is lacking on the criteria to evaluate feeding tolerance (Schanler & Anderson, 2008). To assess feeding tolerance, the following need to be monitored: stools, emesis, apneic episodes, bradycardic episodes, temperature instability, and abominable change (Carlson et al., 2023). Gastric residuals are no longer used to assess feeding tolerance (Carlson et al., 2023).

## GROWTH AND GROWTH CHARTS

Daily weights, weekly lengths, and weekly head circumferences should be obtained and plotted on intrauterine growth curves. The intrauterine charts are developed from the birth weight, birth length, and birth head circumferences of a large group of infants (Fenton & Kim, 2013; Olsen et al., 2010). Premature infants can be plotted against these charts to assess how their growth compares to the goal of fetal growth (AAP Committee on Nutrition, 2014; Cordova & Belfort, 2020).

The Fenton chart is a fetal–infant chart that goes from 22 weeks' gestation to 50 weeks postmenstrual age (Fenton & Kim, 2013). The fetal portion is based on infants from Germany, the United States, Italy, Australia, Scotland, and Canada, and the 40 to 50 weeks is taken from the World Health Organization (WHO) growth charts. The Fenton chart is electronically available from the website (http://ucalgary.ca/fenton) (Figures 20.1a and 20.1b). Though Fenton has some

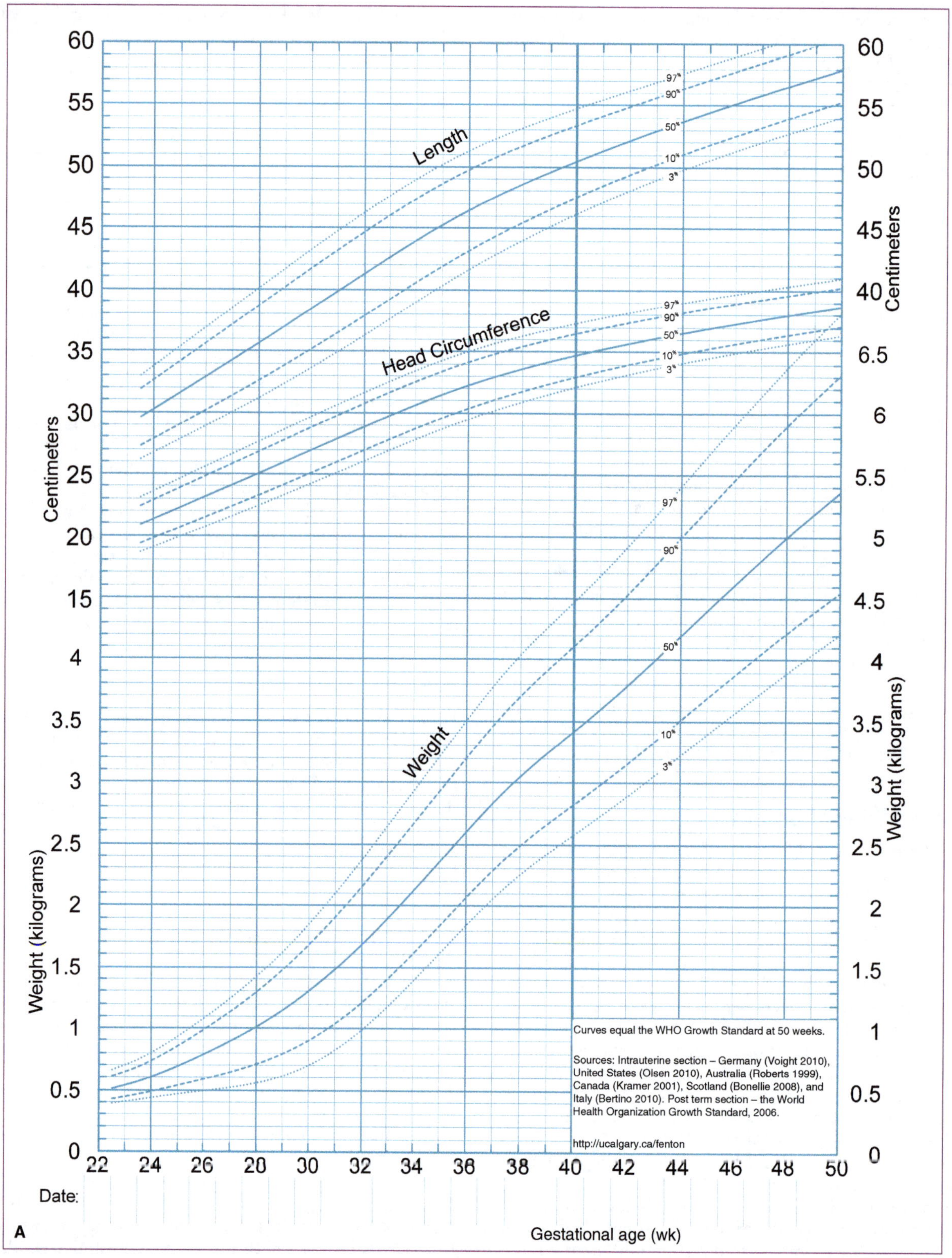


**FIGURE 20.1 (A) Fenton preterm growth chart for girls. (B) Fenton preterm growth chart for boys.**

WHO, World Health Organization.

*Source:* Reproduced with permission from Tanis R. Fenton, PhD. http://ucalgary.ca/fenton.

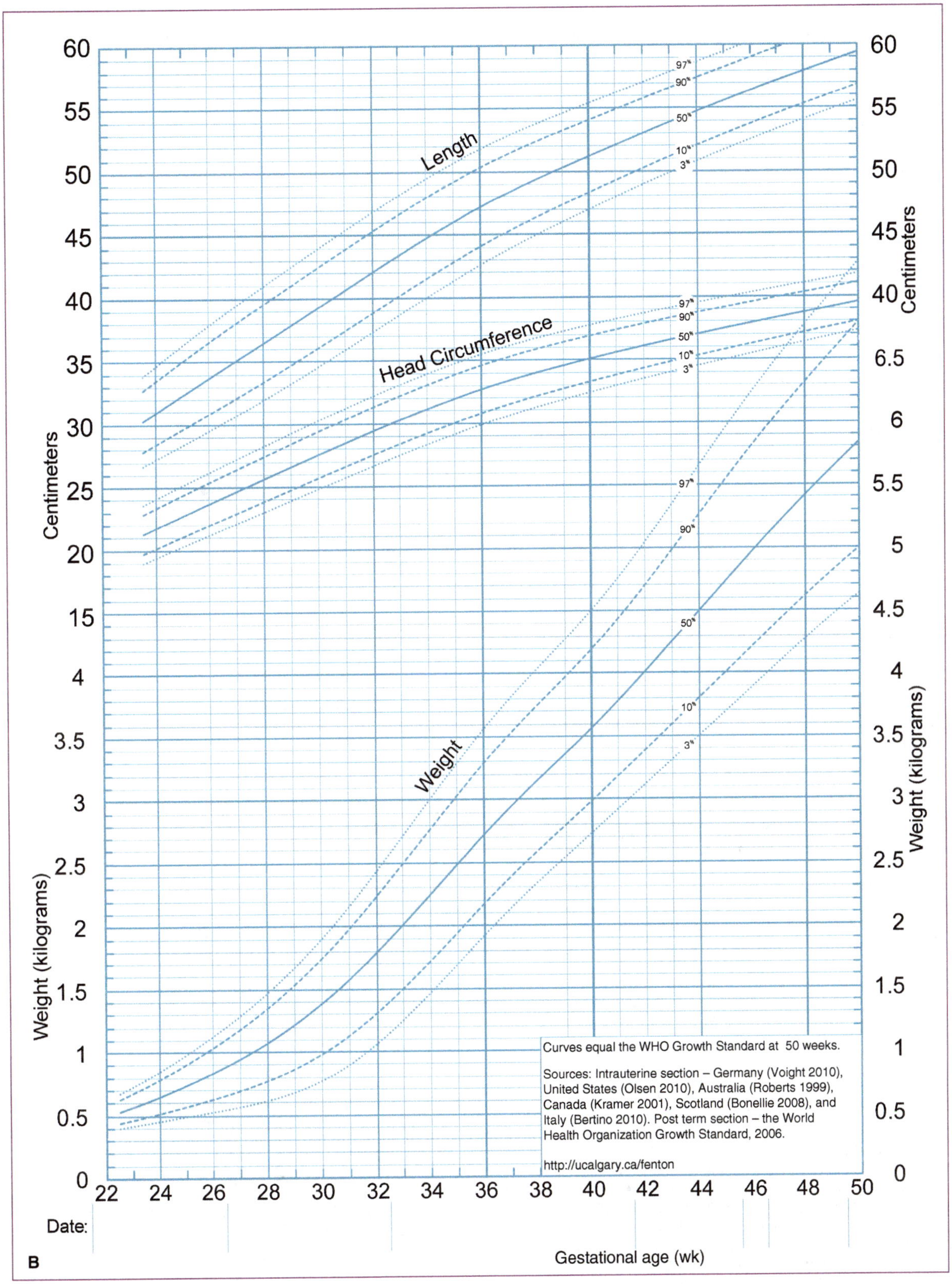


**FIGURE 20.1** (*continued*)

limitations, as do all of the growth charts, the AAP recommends that it be used for preterm infants in an attempt to match intrauterine growth patterns as closely as possible.

The Olsen chart is based on a large, racially diverse sample from the United States, from 23 to 41 weeks' gestation (Olsen et al., 2010). The gender-based charts include weight, length, and head circumference. These charts may be downloaded for individual patient use at the following: https://downloads.aap.org/DOSP/2022OlsenGAGrowthCurves.pdf

Once the premature infant reaches 40 weeks postmenstrual age, the WHO growth charts can assess catch-up growth (Grummer-Strawn et al., 2010). These charts are based on the growth of predominantly breastfed infants for the first year of life and represent ideal growth. The WHO growth charts can be downloaded from www.cdc.gov/growthcharts/who_charts.htm.

The INTERGROWTH-21st Project produced birth classification charts for the very preterm infants of 24 to 33 weeks' gestation and another chart from 24 to 42 weeks' gestation (Villar et al., 2016). Postnatal growth charts for premature infants were developed based on the growth of 201 infants born between 26 and before 37 weeks' gestation who were followed to 64 weeks' gestation (Villar et al., 2015). Infants were born in eight countries (Brazil, China, India, Italy, Kenya, Omen, United Kingdom, and the United States). Growth charts can be downloaded from https://intergrowth21.tghn.org/.

During the first week of life, premature infants can lose up to 14% of their birth weight, primarily due to expected fluid losses (Carlson et al., 2023). Goals for weekly rate of gain are given in Table 20.6. Though weights are obtained daily, it is important to look at the average weight gain per day over the week. Closely monitoring growth is essential to ensure the best growth for these high-risk infants and their future development because appropriate growth in the neonatal stage is associated with improved neurodevelopmental outcomes (Fenton et al., 2024). When poor growth occurs, an assessment of the etiology should be explored. Poor growth may be related to medical conditions or nutrition management. Medical issues that may contribute to poor growth include acidosis, hyponatremia, increased work of breathing, cold stress, anemia, infections, and the use of steroids (Anderson, 2012). These conditions require treatment before nutrition can be fully utilized. Issues related to nutrition are given in Box 20.1.

Of note, the term "extrauterine growth restriction," which was previously commonly used when describing preterm infants, is now considered outdated. Rather, it is recommended to consider an infant's genetic potential, provide optimal nourishment, and avoid overfeeding for these very small infants (Carlson et al., 2023).

## Biochemical Indices

Labs such as glucose, electrolytes, calcium, magnesium, phosphorus, triglycerides, BUN, liver enzymes, and alkaline phosphatase are routinely checked while an infant is on PN.

**TABLE 20.6**

**GROWTH GOALS**

| | |
|---|---|
| Weight gain | 15–20 g/kg/d for infants < 2 kg<br>20–30 g/d for infants > 2 kg<br>15–20 g/kg/d for infants 23–36 weeks gestation |
| Length gain | 0.9–1.1 cm/wk |
| Head circumference | 0.9–1 cm/wk |

*Sources:* Data from Fenton, T. R., Anderson, D., Groh-Wargo, S., Hoyos, A., Ehrenkranz, R. A., & Senterre, T. (2018). An attempt to standardize the calculation of growth velocity of preterm infants-evaluation of practical bedside methods. *Journal of Pediatrics, 196*, 77–83. https://doi.org/10.1016/j.jpeds.2017.10.005; Pereira-da-Silva, L., Virella, D., & Fusch, C. (2019). Nutritional assessment in preterm infants: A practical approach in the NICU. *Nutrients, 11*(9), 1999. https://doi.org/10.3390/nu11091999; Meiliana, M., Alexander, T., Bloomfield, F. H., Cormack, B. E., Harding, J. E., Walsh, O., & Lin, L. (2024). Nutrition guidelines for preterm infants: A systematic review. *JPEN—Journal of Parenteral and Enteral Nutrition, 48*(1), 11–26. https://doi.org/10.1002/jpen.2568.

**BOX 20.1**

**CONSIDERATIONS FOR POOR GROWTH—NUTRITION FACTORS**

Feeding intolerance—abnormal stools, excessive residuals, or emesis

Full nutrition just achieved that meets nutrient guidelines

**Nutrition Not Optimized**

Parenteral nutrient concentrations not adequate

Incorrect amount of fortifier not added to human milk

Incorrect calculations

**Human Milk**

Continuous infusions will lead to fat losses

Use of foremilk that is low in fat and kilocalories

**Ordered Diet Not Received**

Infant not able to consume adequate milk and is not supplemented with gavage feedings

Feedings held for tests

Volume of feedings ordered per kg has not kept up with weight gain

**Nutrition Solution Not Prepared Correctly, or Incorrect Milk Feeding Provided**

Intravenous fluid administration has been held to provide medication or blood

Ostomy output is excessive so parenteral fluids will need to be increased and enteral feedings decreased to meet infant's nutrition needs

*Source:* Data from Anderson, D. M. (2012). Nutrition for premature infants. In P. Q. Samour & K. King (Eds.), *Pediatric nutrition* (4th ed., pp. 53–69). Jones & Bartlett Learning.

Depending on disease state, age, and other factors, these labs may be drawn as much as daily or as little as monthly (Carlson et al., 2023). Typically, most labs are taken weekly to assess for nutritional deficiencies and adjust the PN order.

Being on PN for an extended period of time puts infants at risk for PN-associated liver disease, which can be monitored with labs. While on PN, serum conjugated bilirubin and serum alanine aminotransferase (ALT, serum glutamic-pyruvic transaminase) will be drawn weekly at baseline and then every 2 to 3 weeks during PN therapy to detect PN-associated liver disease. Serum calcium, phosphorus, and alkaline phosphatase activity levels are drawn on infants at risk for osteopenia, which includes VLBW infants and infants with a prolonged course of PN or milk intake of formula not designed for premature infants. If these levels are abnormal, the infant will require increased vitamin supplementation careful handling due to increased risk for fractures, and further laboratory and radiographic investigation is indicated (Lee & De Beritto, 2022). Hematocrit and hemoglobin levels should be monitored because VLBW infants are at risk for prematurity anemia (Holzapfel et al., 2023; Schanler & Anderson, 2008).

## POSTDISCHARGE NUTRITION

Prior to discharge, the infant's nutritional status should be assessed for present growth status, and feeding volume should allow for infant's actual volume intake, presence of any abnormal serum levels that require treatment, and the mother's desire to breastfeed. Depending on the infant's history regarding osteopenia, ability to nurse, and fluid allowance, the infant's feeding recommendation will be individualized. The infant should be placed on the discharge diet prior to discharge to assess growth and feeding tolerance to the plan. Parents must demonstrate their ability to feed their infant, administer supplements, and prepare special milk if indicated.

There are various options for feeding the preterm infant at discharge. Most NICU experts agree that if maternal milk is available, it should be utilized. The benefits of providing human milk outweigh the benefits of displacing it with preterm formula. Therefore, providing breastmilk, fortified breastmilk, or enriched breastmilk at discharge is the gold standard for growth, nutrient absorption, and many other factors.

Essential nutrients such as calcium and phosphorus are more bioavailable in human milk than in formula despite containing lower amounts of these nutrients. Studies have shown that infants who received the highest amount of human milk in their diet had the highest bone mineral content (Cohen & McCallie, 2012) and had improved whole-body bone size and bone mass (Fewtrell et al., 2009). Another study showed that infants fed a higher percentage of human milk had higher mental and psychomotor developmental index scores at 18 and 30 months of age (Vohr et al., 2007). Other benefits of providing more human milk over formula include preventing excessive weight gain (Cohen et al., 2015), simplifying breastfeeding at home, and allowing for more opportunities to feed at the breast.

However, there are instances in which discharging on some or all formula is most appropriate, such as if there is not enough supply of maternal milk, if an infant has a specific allergy or intolerance and requires a specialized formula, or if the infant consistently demonstrates poor growth on breastmilk. In general, discharge nutrition plans should be decided on a case-by-case basis.

Preterm infants on either breastmilk and/or premature discharge formula still need to be on multivitamins and iron supplements at discharge. For those on formula, supplementation can be stopped once the infant is getting 1 L formula, as mentioned earlier. For those on breastmilk, multivitamins can be discontinued at about 1 year of corrected age, and iron supplementation can be stopped once they get adequate iron via iron-fortified solid foods.

## SUMMARY

This chapter has reviewed the basic physiology of digestion and the importance of adequate neonatal nutrition for positive growth and development. Different routes of feeding, as well as different formulas and breastmilk feeding, have been discussed. Neonatal nutrition is a challenge but sets the course for a lifetime of health.

## ONLINE RESOURCES

CourseConnect

Resources for this chapter are online and available at www.springerpub.com/courseconnect.

## REFERENCES

References for this chapter are online and available at www.springerpub.com/courseconnect.

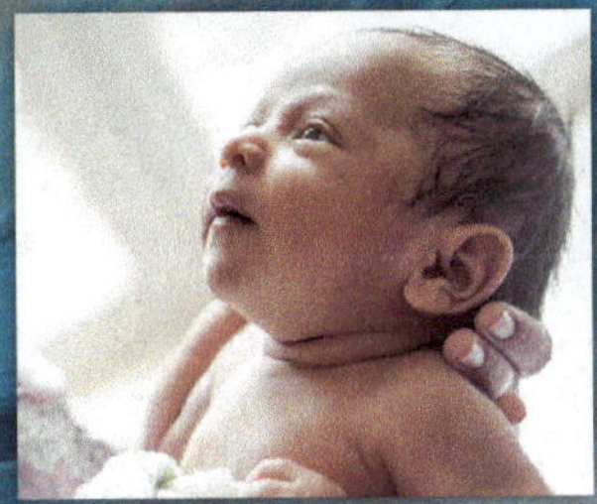

Source: Rohan Katwe/Adobe Stock.

CHAPTER 21

# Neonatal and Infant Pharmacology

Genevra Galura

## INTRODUCTION

Neonates and infants are not simply smaller versions of adult patients—especially when it comes to medication. Immature organ systems affect their response to medications and they can have rapid physiologic changes that contribute to unpredictable drug responses. Understanding infant pharmacology is essential to providing optimal care to these patients, particularly given the limitations in drug research and the risk of medication errors in this vulnerable population. This chapter reviews basic neonatal and infant medication therapy principles and discusses nursing implications.

## PEDIATRIC MEDICATION USE AND LABELING: HISTORICAL PERSPECTIVE

Compared to evidence for adult patients, there is a relative lack of quality evidence regarding drug safety and efficacy in pediatric and neonatal patients. Historically, most medications have not yet to be studied in this population before receiving Food and Drug Administration (FDA) approval. Medications are often prescribed off-label to pediatric and neonatal patients, meaning that they are prescribed outside of FDA labeling. Before 1997, more than 80% of medications approved in the United States did not have a pediatric indication (American Academy of Pediatrics [AAP] News, 2022). The Best Pharmaceuticals for Children Act (BCPA) of 2002 and the Pediatric Research Equity Act (PREA) of 2003 were laws passed by Congress that incentivized and required pediatric-specific medication labeling. Over 1,000 medications have since had labeling changes to include pediatric dosing information and indications.

Despite these advances, adequate safety, efficacy, or dosing information still needs to be improved for approximately half of drug products for children (Sachs et al., 2012). Data on neonatal patients remains particularly sparse. One study reviewed FDA databases and identified only 28 drugs studied in neonates and 24 related labeling changes since the implementation of BCPA and PREA (Laughon et al., 2014). These drugs are rarely used in the neonatal intensive care unit (NICU). Limitations in drug research and labeling for neonatal patients continue to make appropriate medication use in this population challenging.

## PEDIATRIC DOSING METHODS

Drug doses given to neonates and infants are not simply a fraction of those given to adults. Pharmacokinetic and pharmacodynamic changes in this population affect appropriate drug dosing. Because of this, drug dosing is dependent on patient-specific factors and highly individualized. The most common strategy for determining medication dosage is using the patient's body weight (usually presented as mg/kg/dose or mg/kg/day). Many NICUs utilize a standard practice for determining the patient's "dosing weight", which is used to calculate medication doses and may differ from the actual daily weight. The appropriate dose for neonatal patients is also dependent on age, which may be expressed in terms of gestational age (GA), postnatal age (PNA), and postmenstrual age (PMA) (Table 21.1). Neonatal organ function and

**TABLE 21.1**

**PEDIATRIC AND NEONATAL AGE TERMINOLOGY**

| Term | Definition |
|---|---|
| Gestational age | In weeks—elapsed time from first day of mother's last menstruation until birth |
| Postnatal age | In days—chronologic age after birth |

(continued)

**TABLE 21.1**

**PEDIATRIC AND NEONATAL AGE TERMINOLOGY (*continued*)**

| Term | Definition |
|---|---|
| Postmenstrual age | PNA plus GA at birth |
| Preterm infant | < 37 completed weeks GA at birth |
| Full-term infant | > 37 weeks GA at birth |
| Neonate | 0–28 days PNA or < 44 weeks PMA |
| Infant | 1 month–1 year of age |
| Child | 1–12 years of age |

GA, gestational age; PMA, postmenstrual age; PNA, postnatal age.

*Source:* Adapted from Engle, W. A., & American Academy of Pediatrics Committee on Fetus and Newborn. (2004, reaffirmed July 2021). Age terminology during the perinatal period. *Pediatrics, 114*(5), 1362–1364. https://doi.org/10.1542/peds.2004-1915.

body composition vary with each of these ages, making understanding of these terms essential in determining appropriate medication dose and frequency.

## ADVERSE DRUG EFFECTS AND MEDICATION SAFETY

Neonates and infants are a vulnerable population prone to medication errors and adverse drug events (ADEs). NICU medication error rates vary greatly, with estimates of 5.5 to 77.9 errors per 100 medication orders (Alghamdi et al., 2019). Errors may lead to patient harm, but many may be considered preventable. Patients admitted to the NICU may be at risk for medication errors due to hospital naming conventions, extended inpatient stays, individual dose calculations, preparation and administration of small medication doses, lack of appropriate commercially available dosage forms, drug exposure in utero or during lactation, immature organ systems, and limited quality evidence examining medication use in this population (National Association of Neonatal Nurses [NANN] Board of Directors, 2021). Unfortunately, several classic ADEs have occurred in neonates due to these challenges, including chloramphenicol-associated gray baby syndrome and benzyl alcohol–associated gasping syndrome. Knowledge of developmental differences in neonates and strategies to mitigate medication errors is essential to promote medication safety in the NICU.

Medication safety and error prevention strategies include collaborative efforts within a multidisciplinary healthcare team (providers, nurses, pharmacists, dietitians, respiratory therapists, and others), the use of computerized physician order entry systems, and barcode medication administration. The Institute for Safe Medication Practices (ISMP) publishes best practices for hospitals annually; several best practices are pertinent to the neonatal population (ISMP, 2024) (Box 21.1).

Use of standardized medication concentrations is recommended by both the ISMP and the Vermont Oxford Network (VON) for neonatal patients (VON, 2022). The American Society of Health-System Pharmacists (ASHP) began the Standardize 4 Safety initiative in 2008 to reduce medication errors, especially at transitions of care (ASHP, 2024b). This established national standards for both compounded oral medications and intravenous (IV) medications, including for pediatric patients. Standard medication concentrations should be implemented whenever possible.

The Pediatric Pharmacy Association published *Key Potentially Inappropriate Drugs in Pediatrics: The KIDS List* in 2020 (Meyers et al., 2020). A review of available literature

**BOX 21.1**

**2024 TO 2025 TARGETED MEDICATION SAFETY BEST PRACTICES FOR HOSPITALS**

Best Practice 3: Weigh each patient as soon as possible on admission and measure and document patient weights in metric units (kg) only.

Best Practice 5 (moved to Archived Status in 2022): Purchase oral liquid devices (oral syringes) that display only the metric scale (ml).

Best Practice 7: Segregate and differentiate neuromuscular blocking agents from other medications.

Best Practice 8: Administer all medication and hydration infusions via programmable infusion pump utilizing dose error-reduction systems.

Best Practice 11: When compounding sterile preparations, utilize workflow management systems.

Best Practice 16: Limit the variety of medications that can be removed from an ADC using the override function.

Best Practice 19: Layer numerous strategies throughout the medication-use process to improve safety with high-alert medications.

Best Practice 21: Implement strategies to prevent medication errors at transitions in the continuum of care.

Best Practice 22: Safeguard against errors with vaccines.

ADC, automated dispensing cabinet.

*Note:* Focus on those recommendations pertinent to the neonatal patient population.

*Source:* From Institute for Safe Medication Practices. (2024). Targeted medication safety best practices for hospitals. https://www.ismp.org/guidelines/best-practices-hospitals.

and expert recommendations was used to identify 67 medications or drug classes and 10 excipients (inactive ingredients in medication preparation) that may be inappropriate or harmful to pediatric patients. Many should be avoided or used cautiously, specifically in neonates and infants. Familiarity with this list and the known or potential harms associated with medications and excipients may help prevent future errors and ADEs (Table 21.2).

**TABLE 21.2**

**SELECT MEDICATIONS TO AVOID OR USE WITH CAUTION IN NEONATES OR INFANTS**

| Medication | Risk/Rationale |
|---|---|
| Benzocaine | Methemoglobinemia |
| Camphor | Seizures |
| Ceftriaxone, sulfonamides | Kernicterus |
| Chloramphenicol | Gray baby syndrome |
| Chlorhexidine | Chemical burn |
| Codeine | Respiratory depression, death |
| Daptomycin | Neuromuscular and skeletal adverse events |
| Dopamine antagonists (e.g., haloperidol, metoclopramide) | Acute dystonia; risk of respiratory depression, extravasation, and death with IV use |
| Loperamide | Ileus, lethargy |
| Macrolides (e.g., azithromycin, erythromycin) | Hypertrophic pyloric stenosis |
| Midazolam | Severe intraventricular hemorrhage, periventricular leukomalacia, death |
| Naloxone | Seizures |
| Nitrofurantoin | Hemolytic anemia |
| Paregoric | Gasping syndrome, seizures, CNS depression, hypoglycemia |
| Propofol | Propofol-related infusion syndrome |
| Salicylates | Reye syndrome |
| Tetracyclines (e.g., doxycycline) | Tooth discoloration, enamel hypoplasia, retardation of skeletal development and bone growth |
| Tramadol | Respiratory depression |
| Valproic acid | Pancreatitis, fatal hepatotoxicity |
| Verapamil | Asystole |

(*continued*)

**TABLE 21.2**

**SELECT MEDICATIONS TO AVOID OR USE WITH CAUTION IN NEONATES OR INFANTS (*continued*)**

CNS, central nervous system; IV, intravenous.

*Source:* Adapted from Meyers, R. S., Thackray, J., Matson, K. L., McPherson, C., Lubsch, L., Hellinga, R. C., & Hoff, D. S. (2020). Key potentially inappropriate drugs in pediatrics: The KIDs list. *Journal of Pediatric Pharmacology and Therapeutics, 25*(3), 175–191. https://doi.org/10.5863/1551-6776-25.3.175.

## DEVELOPMENTAL PHARMACOKINETICS

One reason the study and utilization of medications are challenging in neonates is that neonates respond to medications differently due to immature organ function. This can vary significantly between patients and based on GA. Terms used to describe these changes are *pharmacokinetics* and *pharmacodynamics*, which influence how medications are used in neonatal and pediatric patients. Pharmacokinetics is the study of the body's effects on a drug, while pharmacodynamics is the study of a drug's effect on the body. The four main processes included in the field of pharmacokinetics are absorption, distribution, metabolism, and elimination (ADME). There are notable changes in the ADME of drugs in different age groups, a phenomenon known as *developmental pharmacokinetics*. The following sections will discuss specific examples and challenges related to neonatal developmental pharmacokinetics. Standard pharmacokinetic terminology used to describe the ADME of medications is found in Table 21.3.

**TABLE 21.3**

**PHARMACOKINETIC TERMINOLOGY**

| Pharmacokinetic Term | Abbreviation | Definition |
|---|---|---|
| Bioavailability | F | The extent to which a drug enters the systemic circulation |
| Volume of distribution | Vd | The relation between the distribution amount of drug in the body and the measured plasma concentration |
| Clearance | Cl | The ability of eliminating organs to remove a drug from the blood or plasma |
| Elimination half-life | $t_{1/2s}$ | The time required for half the amount of drug present in the blood to disappear |
| Steady-state concentration | Cpss | A concentration at which the rate of drug administration is equal to the rate of drug elimination |

*Source:* Data from Soldin, O. P., & Soldin, S. J. (2002). Review: Therapeutic drug monitoring in pediatrics. *Therapeutic Drug Monitoring, 24*(1), 1–8. https://doi.org/10.1097/00007691-200202000-00001.

## Absorption

Medications must be absorbed from the site of administration into the systemic circulation. The extent to which a drug enters systemic circulation, or bioavailability, depends on the route of administration. IV administration results in 100% bioavailability, delivering the drug directly into the bloodstream. Medications administered via other routes have variable bioavailability depending on drug-specific properties and patient-dependent factors. Properties, including molecular weight, degree of ionization, and lipid solubility, affect a drug's ability to cross membranes and enter the systemic circulation. Age is a patient-dependent factor that affects medication absorption for many routes of administration, particularly for premature neonates.

### Enteral Routes

Enteral routes of administration include medications given by mouth and via feeding tubes that must be absorbed from the gastrointestinal (GI) tract. There are many differences in the GI tracts of neonates compared to older patients that affect the degree of medication absorption, including gastric acidity, gastric emptying time, bacterial colonization of the GI tract, intestinal transit time, biliary and pancreatic function, site of administration, and enteral feeding regimens. Neonates, regardless of birth GA, have an elevated gastric pH of approximately 7.0 at birth due to ingestion of amniotic fluid. The pH decreases steadily in the hours after birth to 1 to 3, then rises to reach neutral within the first 1 to 2 weeks of life before slowly decreasing to adult gastric pH values by 2 years of age (Lu & Rosenbaum, 2014; Neal-Kluever et al., 2019). The more basic environment of the neonatal GI tract can affect the bioavailability of acid-labile medications. Weak acids, such as phenytoin and phenobarbital, have decreased bioavailability, while weak bases, such as penicillin and ampicillin, have increased bioavailability. Gastric emptying time is prolonged, and intestinal motility is decreased in the neonatal period, which can result in delayed absorption of enterally administered medications (Lu & Rosenbaum, 2014). The enteral feeding regimen can also affect GI transit and medication absorption. For example, phenytoin absorption is significantly reduced when administered with enteral feedings (Phelps, 2012). Neonates receiving phenytoin and enteral feedings may require higher mg/kg phenytoin doses, more frequent therapeutic drug monitoring (TDM), or alterations in their feeding regimen to account for changes in medication absorption.

### Percutaneous Routes

Compared to older patients, newborn infants have a thinner and underdeveloped epidermal layer (stratum corneum), increased skin hydration, and a higher body surface area ratio to their body weight. These changes are particularly pronounced in premature infants and can increase the relative systemic absorption of medications administered topically. Systemic toxicity with the use of topical disinfectants, including iodine and isopropyl alcohol, has been reported in newborns; chlorhexidine gluconate may be a safer alternative for preterm infants, though this agent should still be used with care (Harris et al., 2024; Oranges et al., 2015). Topical nitroglycerin may be used in infants with ischemic injury but has been associated with adverse systemic effects such as hypotension and methemoglobinemia (Mosalli et al., 2021). Premature infants with poor skin should be monitored more closely if given topical medications that have potentially adverse systemic effects, including steroids, antimicrobials, and anesthetics/analgesics.

### Intramuscular Route

Neonates have decreased skeletal muscle mass, erratic muscle contractions, and blood flow (Kearns et al., 2003). This can result in delayed time to peak concentrations after intramuscular (IM) administration due to poor or unpredictable absorption. Some medications—such as phytonadione (vitamin K), given at birth and certain immunizations—must be given intramuscularly. Still, administration of other medicines via IM injection is often avoided unless the preferred IV or enteral routes are unavailable.

### Other Routes

Medications may be administered to neonates by several other routes, including rectal, intranasal, intratracheal, inhalation, and intraosseous (IO). Rectal absorption depends on regional blood flow and retention of the drug in the rectum; absorption may be less efficient than enteral routes, requiring higher mg/kg doses when administered rectally (Kearns et al., 2003). Intranasal administration results in bioavailability approaching that of IV administration and may be used for procedural sedation and seizures, particularly if it is difficult to establish IV access. Medications given IO are also well absorbed, but this route is reserved for emergencies without adequate IV access.

## Distribution

After a medication is absorbed into the systemic circulation, it will be distributed into organs, fluids, and tissues. Hydrophilic drugs mainly distribute into body water, while lipophilic drugs preferentially distribute into fat. The pharmacokinetic term used to describe the relation between the amount of drug in the body and the measured plasma concentration is the *apparent volume of distribution* (Vd) (Johnson, 2011). The volume of distribution is important to determine the need for loading doses. It is one of the parameters that determine a drug's half-life, or how long it takes for the drug to be eliminated from the body (Lu & Rosenbaum, 2014).

Total body water can be divided into intracellular and extracellular spaces. A full-term neonate is approximately 80% water at birth, with 45% as extracellular and 35% as intracellular fluid. Preterm neonates may have an even higher proportion of total body water. By 1 year of age, a child is approximately 60% water, with 20% extracellular and 40% intracellular fluid (Kearns et al., 2003). The high proportion of total body water means that water-soluble medications have a much higher volume of distribution in neonates than in adults. Aminoglycosides (such as gentamicin, tobramycin, and amikacin) and vancomycin are examples of highly water-soluble antibiotics that have a large Vd and, therefore, require higher mg/kg doses to achieve desired therapeutic effects in neonates. In comparison, body fat is approximately 1% of the total body composition of a premature infant at 29 weeks' GA, increases to approximately 15% at term, and is 25% of the total body composition between 1 and 2 years of age. Fat-soluble medications, such as fentanyl, have a much smaller Vd and require lower mg/kg doses in neonates than in adults (Kearns et al., 2003).

In addition to increased total body water, neonates have alterations in plasma proteins that affect drug distribution. Neonates have reduced formation of plasma proteins, including albumin, due to immature liver function, and there is decreased binding affinity and high concentrations of competing substances that can displace a drug from its binding site (Kearns et al., 2003; Lu & Rosenbaum, 2014). For highly protein-bound drugs such as phenytoin, this may result in high concentrations of unbound or free drugs. The unbound or free drug is the pharmacologically active component, so increased concentrations can lead to enhanced therapeutic and potential toxic effects. Phenytoin is a medication with a narrow therapeutic index requiring TDM, and phenytoin serum concentrations can be measured as either the free concentration or the total (free and protein-bound) concentration. Appropriate phenytoin monitoring in neonates should use the free concentration, or if only the total concentration is available, the level should be corrected based on the patient's albumin level (Bohannon et al., 2020). Finally, certain highly protein-bound drugs, such as sulfonamides and ceftriaxone, can compete for bilirubin-binding sites on albumin (Lu & Rosenbaum, 2014). When albumin levels are low, which often occurs in the neonatal period, this competition can increase unconjugated bilirubin levels and kernicterus risk, so most neonatal use of these medications is contraindicated.

## Metabolism

After distributing into tissues, drugs are metabolized into pharmacologically active or inactive compounds that will be eliminated from the body. Metabolism primarily occurs in the liver, and reactions occur in two phases. Phase I metabolism reactions are small structural alterations such as oxidation, reduction, methylation, hydrolysis, and hydroxylation. The cytochrome P450 (CYP) enzyme system is responsible for most phase I reactions. Phase II metabolism involves changes such as glucuronidation, sulfation, and acetylation. Enzymes and metabolic pathways for phase I and II reactions are immature in neonates and reach adult activity levels at varying times. Phase I reactions mature more rapidly, while some phase II reactions may not reach adult levels until 3 to 4 years of age (Cuzzolin, 2013). As a result, drug dosing, therapeutic or toxic effects, and drug metabolism pathways used in neonates may be different compared to adults, as described in the following examples.

Caffeine is a medication frequently used in the NICU for apnea of prematurity. It is metabolized by CYP1A2 in the liver, a phase I reaction that does not develop until 1 to 3 months of life (Aranda & Beharry, 2020). This results in more caffeine being excreted unchanged in the urine and prolonged pharmacologic activity, meaning has a much longer half-life in neonates (72–96 hours) than in adults (5 hours).

Many medications are substrates for the uridine 5-diphosphoglucuronic acid glucuronyl transferase (UGT) system as part of phase II metabolism. Uridine 5-diphosphoglucuronic acid glucuronyl transferase activity is low in neonates. Morphine is a substrate for UGT2B7, which forms the morphine 6-glucoronide metabolite that potentiates analgesic activity and is cleared renally. Chloramphenicol is also a UGT2B7 substrate; immature UGT activity can decrease glucuronidation and chloramphenicol clearance in neonates, causing "gray baby syndrome" (Craft et al., 1974). Acetaminophen is metabolized primarily via glucuronidation in older patients. In neonates, however, it is mainly converted into sulfate conjugates because this phase II reaction is better developed than glucuronidation at birth (Lu & Rosenbaum, 2014).

## Elimination

The final pharmacokinetic step is elimination, as the drug is removed from the body, primarily via the kidneys. Renal function changes with age. Nephrogenesis continues until 34 to 36 weeks GA, so the kidneys of premature neonates have decreased function and are at high risk of injury. Kidney function improves over time, with the function of young children surpassing that of adults. Elimination half-life, or the time it takes for half of the drug to be eliminated, is dependent on the volume of distribution and clearance of the drug. This helps determine the appropriate dosing frequency of medications. Poor renal function lengthens the half-life of drugs that are renally eliminated, meaning that they will need to be dosed less frequently. Aminoglycosides (such as gentamicin, tobramycin, and amikacin), vancomycin, and ampicillin are antibiotics commonly used in neonates that are renally eliminated. These medications are dosed less frequently in premature neonates compared to term infants and older children (Kearns et al., 2003).

Elimination half-life also helps determine the time to reach steady state concentration or the point at which drug administration and elimination rates are the same. Steady state is reached after approximately four to five half-lives of the drug. For medications with long half-lives, larger single doses known as *loading doses* are administered to help achieve steady-state and desired therapeutic effects faster. Neonates often receive loading doses of medications, including caffeine (as described previously), phenobarbital, levetiracetam, and fluconazole.

# THERAPEUTIC DRUG MONITORING

TDM uses serum drug concentrations and principles of pharmacokinetics and pharmacodynamics to determine dosing in individual patients. TDM is used for medications with a narrow therapeutic index and established concentrations correlating to efficacy or toxicity. This can be especially important in the neonatal population given the pharmacokinetic changes discussed previously, challenges with medication delivery due to small doses and volumes to be administered, blood volume available for measurement of serum drug concentrations, interference of endogenous substances with drug assays, extrapolation of therapeutic concentrations from adult data to the neonatal population, and rapid changes that can occur in neonatal pharmacokinetics as patients grow and mature (De Rose et al., 2020).

Medications used in the neonatal population that require TDM include aminoglycosides (gentamicin, tobramycin, and amikacin), vancomycin, unfractionated heparin, and low molecular weight heparin (enoxaparin), phenobarbital, and phenytoin. TDM may be used for other medications in certain institutions or situations, including caffeine and levetiracetam. TDM for most medications includes a measurement of the concentration of the drug or its metabolites in the blood, or it may include a measurement of the drug's physiologic activity.

Unless administered as a continuous infusion, medication concentration and activity are not static in the body and will vary based on the drug's ADME. Serum drug concentrations should generally be obtained when the medication reaches a steady state (after four to five half-lives when the rate of administration is approximately equal to the rate of elimination). The time at which serum drug concentrations are obtained is critical. Most serum drug concentrations are either peak levels (obtained after distribution has occurred when the serum concentration is highest) or trough levels (obtained shortly before another dose is administered when the serum concentration is lowest). Aminoglycosides are typically monitored using both peak and trough levels. Phenytoin and phenobarbital are monitored using trough levels. Enoxaparin is most often monitored using peak levels.

When serum drug concentrations are higher than the therapeutic target, medication doses are reduced by decreasing the mg/kg dose or giving the medication less frequently. When serum drug concentrations are lower than the therapeutic target, the opposite is done: Additional doses may be given to achieve therapeutic levels faster. After therapeutic drug levels are obtained, levels may be repeated if patients continue therapy for a prolonged period. Patients with rapidly changing clinical status, including their volume status and organ function, may require more frequent monitoring.

Finally, some medications, such as phenytoin, may be monitored as the total serum or free (unbound) concentration. For patients with hypoalbuminemia, as often occurs in the neonatal period, a therapeutic total concentration may be supratherapeutic if the free concentration is measured.

# MEDICATION ADMINISTRATION

Medications should be administered in ways that allow the drug to reach the site of absorption effectively while minimizing any potential harm from drug delivery. Many commercially available dosage forms must be manipulated for appropriate administration in the pediatric patient. Considerations regarding patient development and different routes of administration are discussed in the following section.

## Enteral Administration

Enteral medications given to neonatal and pediatric patients may be administered in several ways, including via a nipple, mixing into milk or formula feeds, directly into the mouth, or a feeding tube. Most enteral medications should be prepared as oral solutions or suspensions for appropriate dose measurements and ease of administration. However, many commonly used medications in the neonatal population are not commercially available as oral liquids, including hydrocortisone and ursodiol. Oral liquid medications are often compounded by pharmacies using tablet or capsule dosage forms mixed with other ingredients that may help dissolve, flavor, or preserve the drug. Compounding oral liquid medications can increase risk for medication errors due to manipulation of the drug, stability issues, and different concentrations that may be available (ASHP, 2024a, 2024b).

Both commercially available and compounded oral liquid medications can contain other ingredients that may be harmful to neonates. Highly concentrated oral liquids have a high osmolality, which may be associated with the development of necrotizing enterocolitis (Latheef et al., 2021). Other medications, such as phenobarbital and diphenhydramine elixirs, can contain alcohol content that may be harmless in older patients but can be a significant exposure for neonates. Most medications will be formulated with flavor or sweetening agents to improve palatability. These ingredients can be harmful for pediatric patients on the ketogenic diet, a specific type of diet used for patients with refractory epilepsy that requires minimal sugar and carbohydrates and can be disrupted by high carbohydrate content in some oral liquid medications.

Enteral medications given through feeding tubes must be compatible with the feeding system but should not be interchangeable with a nonenteral system such as an IV catheter. Serious medication errors have resulted from inadvertent administration of enteral medications connected to and administered via parenteral lines. Best practices published by ISMP include using oral or enteral syringes that comply with the International Organization for Standardization standard, such as ENFit, to reduce cross-connections risk (ISMP, 2024).

## Intravenous Administration

Administration of medications through the IV route is essential for many neonatal and pediatric patients, particularly in the NICU. Several of the same challenges and risks for medication errors with enteral medications exist with parenteral medicines, especially for extremely low birth weight neonates who often require very small medication doses and delivery volumes. Many commercially available IV medications must be diluted to draw up measurable doses for neonates. This can result in potential medication errors, increased infectious risk, or delayed care. Small medication volumes may also be lost in dead space in the syringe hub or IV tubing.

IV medications can be administered via IV push or an infusion device. The IV push method delivers medication rapidly but is inappropriate for many medications. Infusion devices with microbore tubing are used for medications that must be given over a longer duration or via continuous infusions. These devices allow precise control over the infusion rate, even with minimum infusion volumes, independent of the primary IV rate. Many infusion devices are considered "smart" pumps that incorporate technology to provide additional medication safety measures, including pump libraries that establish standard medication concentrations and soft and hard limits for infusion rates and durations (both minimum and maximum) (Lemoine & Hurst, 2012). Some smart pumps can also integrate with the electronic medical record. Syringe pumps have minimum infusion rates, such as 0.1 ml/hr, but vary based on the specific device and syringe size. Low infusion rates may limit the ability to administer certain medications for neonates, increase the time required to reach the patient through the drug delivery device and medication tubing, or necessitate the availability of multiple medication concentrations. This is often seen for medications used in critically ill neonates that are given as continuous infusions, such as sedatives, vasopressors, and inotropes.

IV medications are often formulated with preservatives or other ingredients to improve stability. However, these ingredients can harm neonates, and exposure should be limited (Meyers et al., 2020). Alternative, preservative-free formulations should be used when possible. Many medications must be diluted before administration, usually with either dextrose- or sodium-containing fluids. Diluents can contribute significantly to the total neonatal fluid, dextrose, or sodium provisions and must be considered.

Neonates may have limited IV access to administer medications. IV medications may be physically or chemically incompatible, meaning that they should be administered at different times through the same point of access. Compatibility is complex and dependent on many factors, including drug concentration, location and order of administration, pH, and temperature. Different drug information references may provide conflicting information about medication compatibility because of this. For example, calcium and phosphorus are two key components of parenteral nutrition for neonates but can precipitate when mixed in the same solution or coadministered (Anderson et al., 2022). The point at which they precipitate depends on the factors described above, including the amino acid formulation in the parenteral nutrition solution, which influences the pH. Limited compatibility information is available for many medications used in the NICU, making it challenging to determine the most appropriate way to administer complex IV medication regimens for some neonates.

Medication administration is also dependent on the type of IV access available. Neonates are at high risk for infiltration or extravasation of medications, that is, the leakage of IV fluids or medicines out of the vein and into the surrounding tissues. This can compromise circulation to the affected area, potentially resulting in functional or cosmetic defects. Medications including calcium, potassium, and vasopressors (such as dopamine) can cause tissue damage when extravasated or infiltrated. Certain medications with high osmolality, such as dextrose concentrations greater than 12.5% and many parenteral nutrition solutions, can also damage the injection site. Administration of these agents through superficial or tenuous venous access should be avoided. They should only be administer only through central lines unless alternative access is clinically necessary.

Treatment of injuries that result from medication extravasation or infiltration depends on the severity or degree of damage and the medication involved (Reynolds et al., 2014). Many medication extravasations (including calcium, potassium, parenteral nutrition, and other hyperosmolar fluids) can be treated with compresses and hyaluronidase, which helps distribute the infiltration into surrounding tissues to minimize injury. Vasoactive agents with extravasation properties can be treated with phentolamine, a vasodilatory medication. Topical nitroglycerin may be used to promote circulation to the affected limb.

## Medication Administration in Extracorporeal Membrane Oxygenation

Extracorporeal membrane oxygenation (ECMO) is a form of modified cardiopulmonary bypass that can be used to do the work of the heart, lungs, or both when conventional support methods are inadequate. Indications for ECMO in the neonatal population include persistent pulmonary hypertension of the newborn, meconium aspiration syndrome, congenital diaphragmatic hernia, and congenital heart disease. In general, ECMO is reserved for near full-term neonates with reversible or correctable causes of cardiac or respiratory failure; it is not feasible in most preterm neonates.

The ECMO circuit generally includes cannulas, tubing, a centrifugal pump, and an oxygenator. Patients on ECMO require many medications, including sedatives and analgesics, vasopressors and inotropes, antimicrobial agents, diuretics, and anticoagulants, all of which can be affected by substantial pharmacokinetic changes on ECMO. Notable changes include increased distribution volume, clearance alterations, and drug sequestration into the ECMO circuit. Neonates on ECMO require frequent administration of blood products, and significant volume is needed for priming the ECMO circuit, both of which lead to hemodilution and an increase in the volume of distribution. This is most observed with hydrophilic medications. Drug clearance is often reduced for patients on ECMO due to changes in renal and hepatic function during critical illness and the nonpulsatile flow of blood on the circuit associated with a decreased glomerular filtration rate (Raffaeli et al., 2019). Finally, medications can be sequestered in the tubing and other components of the ECMO circuit, particularly for lipophilic medications. Fentanyl, for example, has been shown to adsorb significantly to the tubing (Preston et al., 2007). Patients may require much higher doses of fentanyl, or many providers will change patients to an alternative agent such as morphine that is less affected by the ECMO circuit. Due to these pharmacokinetic changes, TDM can be of particular importance for neonates and infants on ECMO.

## FETAL AND INFANT EXPOSURE TO MATERNAL MEDICATIONS

Medication use during pregnancy is common, with approximately 90% of women reporting taking some type of medicine. About 70% take at least one prescription medication, and the use of prescription medications during the first trimester has increased over the past 20 years (Mitchell et al., 2011; Werler et al., 2023). Many medications will cross the placenta and expose the developing fetus to the medication, though the extent and therapeutic effects of this are often unknown (Hudson et al., 2023). Passage of drugs to the fetus depends on drug-specific properties and alterations to maternal pharmacokinetics during pregnancy. Maternal organ system changes include an increased volume of distribution and fat stores, lower protein binding, and increased renal function. Properties that make a drug more likely to cross the placenta and enter fetal circulation include a molecular weight of less than 500 Daltons, low protein binding, lipophilicity, and neutral pH. Other factors complicating fetal medication exposure include maternal serum drug concentrations, integrity of the placental barrier, and drug elimination from the fetus. Exposure to medications may result in little to no adverse effects for the developing fetus, or it may have deleterious effects.

Neonates and infants can also be exposed to medications while breastfeeding. The passage of medications into breastmilk depends on many of the same drug properties that affect placental crossing. Additional considerations that affect infant exposure to medications through breastmilk include the timing of medication administration in relation to breastfeeding or pumping and the volume of milk ingested. Few medicines are considered contraindicated during lactation, and strategies can be employed to minimize infant drug exposure to medications that could be harmful.

In 2014, the FDA amended regulatory requirements for prescription medication labeling regarding pregnancy and lactation risks, known as the Pregnancy and Lactation Labeling Rule or Final Rule (FDA, 2014). This removed the previous pregnancy categories A, B, C, D, and X from drug products. It established specific subsections required in drug labeling: "Pregnancy," "Lactation," and "Females and Males of Reproductive Potential". The "Pregnancy" subsection must include a statement about the existence of a pregnancy exposure registry for the drug, if applicable, as well as summarizing the available data for risks associated with using the drug during pregnancy from all relevant sources and clinical considerations for prescribers. The "Lactation" subsection similarly requires data for risks associated with using the drug during lactation and considerations to minimize drug exposure in the breastfed infant. The "Females and Males of Reproductive Potential" subsection requires relevant information for pregnancy testing or contraception recommendations surrounding drug therapy and data for drug-associated fertility effects. The final rule aimed to create consistent formatting to describe the risks of drug products during pregnancy or lactation and of reproductive potential and to assist prescribers in counseling patients regarding these risks.

## MEDICATION SHORTAGES

Medication shortages can contribute to disruptions in patient care for neonates and infants, especially because many shortages involve generic injectable products with limited suppliers (ASHP, 2017). Legislation enacted in 2012 aimed to curb drug shortages by requiring drug manufacturers to notify the FDA of changes in production expected to reduce the supply of medications. Despite this, medication shortages persist, with 156 new shortages in 2023 (ASHP, 2024a). Of the top 100 medications used in the NICU, 74 have been affected by 227 drug shortages from 2001 to 2016 (Ziesenitz et al., 2019). Most shortages are due to manufacturing problems. Natural disasters have also contributed, with hurricanes in 2017 and 2024 striking facilities responsible for supplying many parenteral products to hospitals in the United States. These shortages may affect the ability of institutions to provide IV fluids and parenteral nutrition to neonatal patients.

## SUMMARY

Neonates and infants are a unique population with specific challenges in pharmacotherapy. Medication use must be highly individualized. Drug dosing is most frequently calculated on a mg/kg basis, and appropriate dosing strategies depend on developmental pharmacokinetics—the changes in drug ADME related to patient age and organ development. There is a lack of quality literature and specific challenges with drug administration for this population. Strategies to improve medication safety, such as standardization of medication concentrations and using smart infusion pumps, are essential for optimal medication use in the NICU.

## ONLINE RESOURCES

CourseConnect

Resources for this chapter are online and available at www.springerpub.com/courseconnect.

## REFERENCES

References for this chapter are online and available at www.springerpub.com/courseconnect.

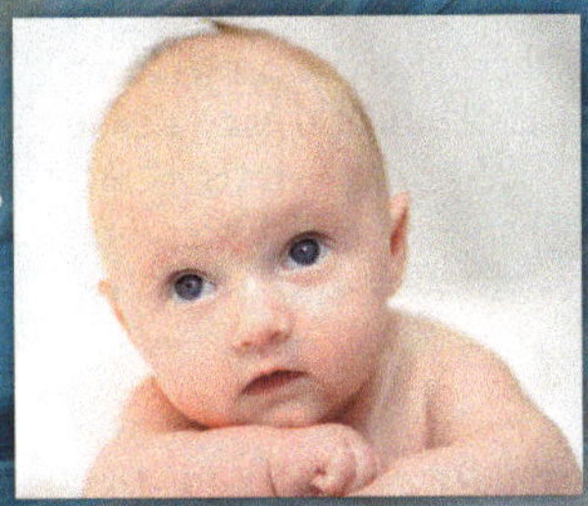

Source: Christian Jung/Adobe Stock

CHAPTER 22

# Pain in the Newborn and Infant

Marsha Campbell-Yeo and Mats Eriksson

## INTRODUCTION

All newborns and infants undergo pain related to health interventions, with those born preterm or sick often enduring significant repeated exposure. Despite known ways to assess and effectively manage newborn and infant pain, these interventions remain underutilized in clinical practice, leading to no or poorly managed pain in this population (Campbell-Yeo, Disher et al., 2024; Keels et al., 2016). Experiencing untreated pain in early life has been associated with immediate negative and long-term adverse outcomes affecting physiologic stability, pain perception, cognition, behavior, and neurodevelopment (Campbell-Yeo et al., 2022). In addition to adverse infant outcomes, parents report high levels of stress if effective pain management during medical procedures is not provided (Ullsten et al., 2024).

This chapter provides a definition and overview of the types of newborn and infant pain, a review of the developmental neurophysiology of pain, adverse effects associated with untreated pain in early life, factors that may influence the pain experience, valid pain assessment methods, and evidence-based interventions for managing infant pain and strategies for implementation. Evidence regarding the importance of parent engagement in newborn and infant pain care is also provided.

## DEFINING PAIN IN INFANTS

Through considerable work and collaboration across a diverse team in 2020, the International Association for the Study of Pain (IASP) released an updated definition for pain for neonates (younger than 1 month of age or 44 weeks post-conception) and infants (less than 1 year of age). Pain is defined as "an unpleasant sensory and emotional experience associated with, or resembling that associated with, actual or potential tissue damage" (Raja et al., 2020). This revision of the 1979 definition (IASP, 1979) addressed numerous concerns raised regarding the original definition. First, that the original definition did not fully consider that while pain is subjective and should be considered whatever the patient says it is, that nonverbal infants could not self-report pain. Another concern was that the assumption that pain was a learned experience was problematic for very young neonates who had not yet experienced pain. The original definition also lacked clarity regarding the possibility of pain or perceived pain due to allodynia, a condition common in newborns in which nonpainful touch can be perceived as painful due to alteration in immature pain processing following repeated untreated pain (Ilhan et al., 2022).

Despite the current definition's improvement, there remains a gap regarding the development and acceptance of consensus definitions of different types of pain in newborns and infants (Anand, 2017). Earlier work by van Ganzewinkel et al. (2014) attempted to categorize and define acute and chronic pain, yet some perceived gaps in the clarity and relevance remained. As such, a diverse international panel using a four-step process developed preliminary consensus definitions for acute episodic pain and chronic pain in neonates and infants (Ilhan et al., 2022). While continued work remains ongoing to achieve consensus regarding the definitions of different types of pain in newborns and infants, there does appear to be current agreement regarding the presumption and management of pain. Given the known short- and long-term risks associated with untreated pain, the primary principle of all providers should be that pain in the newborn or infant should be presumed in all situations usually considered to cause pain in adults and children, even in the absence of behavioral or physiologic signs (Altimier & Phillips, 2016).

## DEVELOPMENTAL NEUROPHYSIOLOGY OF PAIN

The fundamental mechanisms of pain perception in newborns and infants are like those of adults and include transduction and transmission and perception and modulation (Fitzgerald, 2015; Hatfield, 2014). While all basic anatomical components of the complex human pain processing system are present by approximately 20 weeks post-conception, because of neurophysiologic and cognitive immaturity, some differences exist (Goksan et al., 2015). Newborn pain pathways, especially those of infants born preterm, undergo significant changes postbirth, both developmentally and in response to environmental stimuli, highlighting the effect that untreated pain in early life can have on the normal development of pain processing in newborns and heightened risk for adverse long-lasting consequences (Gokulu et al., 2016; Tucker et al., 2023). A brief review is presented here and emphasizes the developmental and maturational changes that occur from birth and throughout infancy.

### Peripheral Transduction and Transmission

Nociception is perceived when noxious stimuli (mechanical, thermal, or chemical) excite primary afferent fibers, which leads to the transmission of information about the potentially damaging stimuli from the periphery to the dorsal horn of the spinal cord. Three primary afferent nerve fibers are involved with the transmission of pain stimuli. A-delta (large, myelinated, and fast-conducting) and C (small, unmyelinated, and slow-conducting) fibers are primarily responsible for pain impulse transmission (nociception). A-Beta (thickly myelinated) fibers, primarily responsible for transmitting pressure and touch in adults, have been reported to also transmit pain signals in newborns (Tucker et al., 2023).

These signals can be intensified or mitigated by the activation of adjacent neurons in the periphery and spinal cord. Tissue injury causes the release of inflammatory mediators (e.g., potassium, bradykinin, prostaglandins, cytokines, nerve growth factors, catecholamines, and substance P) that sensitize A-delta and C fibers and recruit other neurons (silent nociceptors) and result in hyperalgesia. Stimulation of A-beta fibers that signal nonpainful touch and pressure can compete with the transmission of nociception in the dorsal horn of the spinal cord, potentially leading to the modulation of the intensity of the perceived pain.

### Central Mechanisms and Modulation

Neurotransmitters in the spinal cord either amplify (e.g., substance P, calcitonin gene-related peptide, neurokinin A) or attenuate (e.g., endogenous opioids, norepinephrine, serotonin, gamma-aminobutyric acid [GABA], glycine) pain information from the periphery. Central sensitization occurs when excitatory amino acids act on *N*-methyl-D-aspartate (NMDA) receptors to induce prolonged depolarization and windup.

Nociceptive sensory input reaches the thalamus through second-order neurons in the spinothalamic, spinoreticular, and spinomesencephalic tracts and is then widely distributed throughout the brain. The perception, emotional interpretation, and cognitive meaning of nociceptive stimuli occur within a distributive neuromatrix; no one "pain center" exists. The sensory-discriminative, affective-motivational, and evaluative dimensions of pain perception are mediated by past experiences and the context of the painful event. For example, nociceptive stimuli activate areas of the limbic system to control emotion, particularly anxiety. Thus, differences in physiologic, biochemical, and psychologic factors influence the perception of pain, making it an individual phenomenon.

Descending modulation occurs when efferent projections from supraspinal areas such as the periaqueductal gray, raphe nucleus, and locus coeruleus release inhibitory neurotransmitters. The major neurotransmitters that mediate descending inhibition are norepinephrine, serotonin, endogenous opioids, GABA, and acetylcholine.

### Neurodevelopment of Pain Perception

Infants, even those born very preterm, have the neurologic capacity to perceive pain at birth (Walker, 2019). The peripheral and central structures necessary for nociception are present and functional early in gestation (between the first and second trimesters). Functional maturation of the cerebral cortex has been demonstrated by: (a) near-infrared spectroscopy and electroencephalogram (EEG) patterns that demonstrate alterations in cortical evoked potentials; (b) measurement of cerebral glucose use that shows maximal metabolic rates in sensory areas of the brain; and (c) well-defined periods of sleep and wakefulness that are regulated by cortical functioning from 28 weeks of gestation. The newborn infant possesses a well-developed hypothalamic–pituitary–adrenal (HPA) axis and can mount a fight-or-flight response with the release of catecholamines and cortisol.

Research suggests that some differences in nociceptive processes between infants and adults exist. For example, pain impulse transmission in neonates occurs primarily along nonmyelinated C fibers rather than myelinated A-delta fibers. The peripheral and central nervous systems in the preterm are also immature, leading to lower thresholds for activation, excitation, and transmission of nociceptive stimuli. Furthermore, the dorsal horn neurons in the spinal cord have large, overlapping cutaneous receptive fields that when stimulated amplify nociceptive signaling and can evoke long-term excitability within the spinal cord (Anand, 2017). Descending inhibitory neurotransmitters are also lacking, leading to decreased modulation of pain in the preterm neonate (Goksan et al., 2018). Thus, young infants may perceive pain more intensely than older children or adults because their descending control mechanisms are immature and thus limit their ability to modulate the experience (Hatfield, 2014).

Painful stimuli negatively influence the development of pain processing with direct tissue injury, leading to excessive nerve sprouting and hyperinnervation; hyperexcitation of the ascending pain fibers, leading to hypersensitivity to both painful and innocuous stimuli; maladaptive descending spinal tracts affecting endogenous analgesia; and reduced brain volume, leading to poor neurodevelopmental outcomes.

## CAUSES, PREVALENCE, AND CONSEQUENCES OF PAIN EXPOSURE

Given current prevention and screening of treatable medical conditions requiring needle-related interventions, ubiquitous exposure to pain in the first hours or days following birth is unavoidable for all newborns (World Health Organization [WHO], 2021). Moreover, recommended immunizations expose healthy infants to upwards of 20 intramuscular (IM) injections in the first 2 years of life. Infants born preterm or sick requiring neonatal care can undergo significantly higher repeated pain exposure. A synthesis of 18 global epidemiologic studies examining pain exposure and pain reducing practices demonstrated that infants undergo from 7 to 17 painful procedures in the neonatal intensive care unit (NICU) per day (Cruz et al., 2016).

While significant variability in pain exposure exists worldwide, there may be some reduction in exposure across some settings with Bueno et al. (2024) reporting that infants receiving care in four Canadian NICUs undergo an average of one to two procedures per day. Of note, this study reported on the entire hospital stay, whereas some of the included studies in the Cruz et al. (2016) review reported shorter durations following admission. Common painful NICU procedures can be found in Table 22.1.

Notwithstanding the substantial adverse effects related with untreated pain in early life, and evidence-based guidelines outlining effective interventions to prevent and manage pain, many infants continue to receive no or little treatment, and for those who do, most receive ineffective treatment (Cruz et al., 2016; Orovec et al., 2019).

In studies reporting predictors associated with effective pain care, infants who were less ill at birth and those receiving high-frequency ventilator support were the most likely to receive pharmacologic interventions (e.g., opiates) during tissue-breaking procedures. Parental presence significantly predicted the use of sweet taste or nonpharmacologic interventions (i.e., non-nutritive sucking [NNS], swaddling, rocking, positioning, skin-to-skin contact, breastfeeding) (Johnston et al., 2011). Although most of the previous work related to consequences of untreated pain has been done with preterm infants (i.e., < 37 weeks gestational age at birth) who experience greater exposure to pain, evidence suggests healthy newborns with less exposure still exhibit adverse effects, most notably related to neurologic processing of pain and altered perception of subsequent pain, as well as possible links with later needle phobia or aversion (Ozawa et al., 2011; Piira et al., 2007; Taddio et al., 1995, 1997, 2002, 2009).

**TABLE 22.1**

**COMMON PAINFUL PROCEDURES IN NEONATAL INTENSIVE CARE UNITS**

| | |
|---|---|
| Intramuscular (IM) and subcutaneous injections | Intubation |
| Heel lancing for blood collection | Lumbar puncture |
| Venipuncture and insertion of peripheral venous catheters | Insertion of arterial and venous umbilical catheters and peripheral arterial catheters |
| Naso- and endotracheal suctioning | Retinopathy of prematurity (ROP) eye examinations |
| Dressing changes or tape removal | Chest tube placement |

For infants born preterm, there is now convincing evidence that repeated exposure to untreated pain in early life has been linked with immediate and long-lasting adverse outcomes. Immediate effects have been associated with hemodynamic changes and increased intracranial pressure (ICP) (Craig et al., 1993; McGrath et al., 2009). Long-term negative effects include alteration in: later pain processing (Valeri et al., 2015), vision (Doesburg et al., 2013), HPA axis development (Brummelte et al., 2015; Grunau et al., 2004, 2010; McLean et al., 2023), mobility, and the ability to learn, control emotions, and behavior (Cook, 2023; McLean, 2022; Ranger, 2014; Vinall, 2013).

Repeated pain exposure in very preterm infants has also been linked to significant changes in overall brain growth and development (Vinall & Grunau, 2014), including reduced thalamic and cerebellar growth, frontal and partial brain width, and alteration in gray-to-white matter ratios and temporal lobe functional connectivity (Brummelte et al., 2015; Duerden 2018, 2022; Ranger 2013, 2015; Schneider, 2018). Lastly, there is some evidence that exposure to untreated pain can affect normal programming of epigenetic material and telomere length, also known to be affected in children exposed to childhood trauma (Chau et al., 2014; Provenzi et al., 2016).

## CLINICAL ASSESSMENT OF PAIN

### Factors That Influence Pain

While structural and functional maturity is reached at an early age, given the degree of plasticity in pain neurophysiology and anatomic and functional changes that occur throughout life, everyone's pain experience is unique. It is postulated that the experience of nociception and pain can be affected by multiple intrinsic and extrinsic factors. Newborns have complex neural networks (body-self neuromatrix) present at birth to perceive and respond to incoming painful stimuli and to be responsive to environmental conditions to modulate stressful experiences (Derbyshire, 2000; Melzack, 2001). This body-self neuromatrix, although genetically predisposed, is further shaped and developed by maturation, prior experiences, memory, and learning and sensory inputs. Specific factors include gestational age, postnatal age, gender, previous experiences of pain and inflammation, and environmental conditions such as noise and light. Most available methods to assess pain in infants do not adequately or quantitatively incorporate all aspects of the context of pain that influence the pain experience. As such, care providers should remain conscious of the ways in which perception of pain may be positively or negatively influenced by these factors. These factors do not influence pain in isolation but are listed separately for clarity.

**Behavioral State.** The behavioral state of the infant, ranging from deep sleep to awake and crying, acts as a moderator of behavioral pain responses. The behavioral state of the infant immediately before the painful stimulus affects the robustness of the response. Infants in awake states demonstrate more robust reactions to pain than infants in sleep states. Infants in a drowsy or deep sleep state will show less vigorous facial expression in response to a heel stick than infants who are alert or aroused before the heel stick (Grunau & Craig, 1987; Mathai et al., 2011; Stevens et al., 1994).

**Gestational Age and Gender.** Preterm neonates show lower tactile thresholds to painful stimuli (Fitzgerald & Beggs, 2001), increased sensitivity to non-noxious stimuli (Grunau et al., 2001; Johnston & Stevens, 1996), and higher baseline heart rate and lower heart rate variability (Sahni et al., 2000) when compared to more mature newborns. Gestational age affects infant pain responses, with younger infants displaying fewer and less vigorous behavioral responses to pain (Gibbins & Stevens, 2003; Johnston et al., 1995; Stevens et al., 1994, 1996). In addition, preterm neonates may demonstrate unique behaviors in response to noxious stimuli. Several researchers have used the Newborn Individualized Developmental Care and Assessment Program (NIDCAP®, Children's Hospital, Boston, MA) to examine responses of preterm neonates to a heel stick procedure and found that preterm neonates may uniquely respond to acute pain by increased flexion and extension of arms and legs, finger splay, fisting, frowning, and hand-on-face behaviors (Holsti et al., 2004). Gender influences are less well understood and only one study has demonstrated that postnatal female infants, regardless of gestational age, appear to show higher facial response to pain stimuli than male infants (Guinsburg et al., 2000).

The Premature Infant Pain Profile (Stevens et al., 1996) and the Premature Pain Profile–Revised (Stevens et al., 2014), a valid and reliable pain assessment tool for premature and full-term infants up to 1 month of age incorporates the contextual factors of behavioral state and gestational age when determining the infant pain score.

**Previous Experiences of Pain and Inflammation.** Early and repeated pain exposure especially in preterm infants can result in altered behavior and autonomic reactivity (Gibbins et al., 2008; Grunau et al., 2005) and structural and functional changes to pain pathways (Torsney & Fitzgerald, 2003). This potential influence on subsequent pain responses and regulation should be accounted for in any study examining these outcomes in this population.

**Caregiver Handling.** There is some evidence that preterm infants born between 30- and 32-weeks' gestational age show heightened states of arousal, greater behavioral responses to pain, and poor ability to modulate heart rate during recovery when a painful procedure was performed immediately following provision of routine clustered care (Holsti et al., 2006).

## Pain Assessment Tools

Pain assessment is a fundamental component of pain management. While self-report is considered the gold standard for non–cognitively impaired older children, youth, and adults, the use of valid, reliable, and age-appropriate observational pain assessment tools is essential for nonverbal populations (Eriksson & Campbell-Yeo, 2019). Infant pain assessment tools can be described as unidimensional, multidimensional, or composite, meaning that they include one or greater than one indicator of pain (e.g., behavioral and physiologic), or they can include multiple indicators as well as contextual indicators (e.g. behavioral state, gestational age). The latter, composite, tools are considered the most sensitive (Campbell-Yeo et al., 2022). Selection of an optimal tool should consider the validity and reliability of the tool related to the age of the newborn or infant, the type of pain being measured, the context in which it is being used, and the experience and educational preparation of the individual using the tool. The ideal pain assessment tool will be able to detect pain when pain is occurring (sensitivity) and differentiate true pain from nonpain conditions (specificity), distinguish the specific type of pain of pain being measured (validity), and provide the same results when being used by different providers (reliability) (Meesters et al., 2019). In a review of over 350 studies examining neonatal pain, the Premature Infant Pain Profile (PIPP) or Premature Infant Pain Profile—Revised (PIPP-R) were the most used ($n$ = 154 studies), followed by the Neonatal Infant Pain Scale (NIPS) ($n$ = 84 studies), the Neonatal Facial Coding System (NFCS) ($n$ = 33 studies) and the Douleur Aiguë Nouveau-Né (DAN; Carbajal, 1997) ($n$ = 20 studies) (Olsson et al., 2021).

Despite the robust body of evidence regarding the importance of biobehavioral pain assessment tools in newborns, there remain some challenges. As such, research is ongoing regarding the possible use of alternative ways to assess pain in newborns. Areas of research have focused on physiologic signs, and hormonal and neurophysiologic signs. Please see Table 22.2 regarding newborn and infant pain indicators and Table 22.3 for an overview of pain assessment tools with permission from Campbell-Yeo et al. (2022).

**TABLE 22.2**

**INDICATORS OF NEONATAL PAIN**

| Category | Description |
|---|---|
| ***Behavioral Signs*** | |
| ***Alertness and sleep–wake state*** | • A hyper-alert state is often seen during ongoing or prolonged pain.<br>• Younger or sicker infants can need longer time to comfort themselves and return to rest after a painful event. |
| ***Body movements and muscle tension*** | • Full-term infants withdraw limbs from pain, but in preterm infants these responses are more diffuse and harder to control.<br>• Strong infants can react with increased muscle tension in arms and legs.<br>• Younger or sicker infants can turn flaccid. |

(*continued*)

**TABLE 22.2**

## INDICATORS OF NEONATAL PAIN (*continued*)

| Category | Description |
|---|---|
| ***Crying*** | • Healthy, awake, and full-term newborn infants react with moaning or crying that gets more intense and with longer duration with increasing discomfort.<br>• Infants of lower gestational age, sick, in a sleeping state, or sedated will have difficulties showing a vocal reaction, so the absence of crying must not be taken for absence of pain; crying can often be noted as a weaker moaning sound. |
| ***Facial activity, grimacing*** | • The most used facial expressions that are indicators of pain:<br>o brow bulge<br>o squeezed eyes<br>o distinct furrows from the nose to the ends of the mouth<br>o tense and stretched mouth and tongue<br>o raised cheeks |
| ***Physiologic Signs*** | |
| ***Heart rate and heart rate variability (HRV)*** | • In healthy full-term infants, pain triggers an increased heart rate, which leads to increased blood pressure and a red skin color.<br>• Younger and sicker infants may react with an increase or decrease in heart rate, and possibly bradycardia.<br>• Pain reduces HRV.<br>• HRV is best suited for assessing prolonged pain. |
| ***Respiration rate*** | • In robust infants, the respiration rate will increase as a result of acute pain, whereas the opposite, and even apneas, can be seen in infants who do not have energy to trigger the fight-or-flight system.<br>• Pain in the thorax region can lead to impaired breathing. |
| ***Oxygen saturation*** | • Changes in oxygen saturation follows pain-associated changes in respiration and heart rate.<br>• Both an increase and decrease of oxygen saturation can be seen, depending on the context. |
| ***Cortisol*** | • Increased levels can be seen after surgery (Franck et al., 2011) and painful procedures (Mörelius et al., 2009).<br>• It is measured in plasma, saliva, or urine.<br>• There is high variability. It is more useful in research than clinically. |
| ***Neurophysiologic Signs*** | |
| ***Cerebral oxygenation*** | • Pain measured with NIRS is associated with cerebral activation and changes in oxygenated and deoxygenated hemoglobin concentration in the brain.<br>• An increase in oxygenated hemoglobin is assumed to reflect neuronal activation caused by pain.<br>• NIRS is sensitive to movement artifacts (Bembich et al., 2013; Pettersson et al., 2019). |
| ***EEG, evoked potentials*** | • Multi-channel EEG is used as a proxy for neuronal activity, with the majority of studies reporting on pain-related event-related potentials during acute painful procedures (Fabrizi et al., 2011; Jones et al., 2021),<br>• Primarily used in research, there is no standard clinical pain assessment method/tool. |
| ***fMRI*** | • It has shown which areas in the infant brain are activated by pain (Goksan et al., 2015; Hartley et al., 2017).<br>• It is not relevant as a bedside pain assessment tool.<br>• It can help in developing and validating other measures. |

fMRI, functional magnetic resonance; HRV, heart rate variability; NIRS, near-infrared spectroscopy.

*Source:* Adapted from Campbell-Yeo, M., Eriksson, M., & Benoit, B. (2022, February 11). Assessment and management of pain in preterm infants: A practice update. *Children (Basel). 9*(2), 244. https:doi.org/10.3390/children9020244.

**TABLE 22.3**

**PAIN ASSESSMENT TOOLS FOR TERM AND PRETERM INFANTS**

| Acronym/Name | Items |
|---|---|
| ***Acute Procedural Pain*** | |
| **ABC** (Bellieni, Bagnoli et al., 2007) | Acuteness, rhythmicity, and continuity of crying |
| **BIIP** (Holsti & Grunau, 2007)<br>Behavioral Indicators of Infant Pain | Behavioral state, brow bulge, eye squeeze, nasolabial furrow, horizontal mouth stretch, taut tongue, finger splay, fisting |
| **BPSN** (Schenk et al., 2019, 2020)<br>Bernese Pain Scale for Neonates | Alertness, duration of crying, time to calm, skin color, eyebrow bulge with eye squeeze, posture, breathing pattern |
| DAN (Carbajal et al., 1997) | Facial expressions, limb movements, vocal expressions |
| **FANS** (Milesi et al., 2010)<br>Faceless Acute Neonatal Pain Scale | HRV, acute discomfort, limb movements, vocal expressions |
| **FLACC** (Merkel et al., 1997)<br>Face, Legs, Activity, Cry, Consolability Scale<br>(validated birth to adolescence) | Face, legs, activity, cry, consolability |
| **NFCS** (& Craig, 1987)<br>Neonatal Facial Coding System<br>(some validation for postoperative pain) | Brow bulge, eye squeeze, nasolabial furrow, open lips, horizontal mouth stretch, vertical mouth stretch, lip purse, taut tongue, chin quiver |
| **NIPS** (Lawrence et al., 1993)<br>Neonatal Infant Pain Scale | Facial expression, cry, breathing patterns, arms, legs, state of arousal |
| **NIAPAS** (Pölkki et al., 2014)<br>Neonatal Infant Acute Pain Assessment Scale | GA, alertness, facial expressions, crying, muscle tension, breathing, respirator/CPAP, reaction to handling, heart rate, oxygen saturation |
| **PIPP, PIPP-R** (Gibbins et al., 2014; Stevens et al., 1996)<br>Premature Infant Pain Profile—Revised | GA, behavioral state, heart rate, oxygen saturation, brow bulge, eye squeeze, naso-labial furrow |
| ***Postoperative Pain*** | |
| **N-PASS** (Hummel et al., 2008)<br>Neonatal Pain, Agitation and Sedation Scale (some validation for acute procedural pain) | Crying/irritability, behavior state, facial expression, extremities tone, vital signs |
| **PAT** (Hodgkinson et al., 1994)<br>Pain Assessment Tool | Posture/tone, sleep pattern, expression, color, cry, respirations, heart rate, oxygen saturation, blood pressure, nurse's perception |
| ***Prolonged Pain*** | |
| **ALPS-Neo** (Lundqvist et al., 2014)<br>Astrid Lindgren and Lund Children's Hospital's Pain and Stress Assessment Scale for Preterm and Sick Newborn Infants | Facial expression, breathing pattern, tone of extremities, hand/foot activity, level of activity |

(*continued*)

**TABLE 22.3**

**PAIN ASSESSMENT TOOLS FOR TERM AND PRETERM INFANTS (*continued*)**

| Acronym/Name | Items |
|---|---|
| **COMFORT neo** (van Dijk et al., 2009)<br>(also validated for sedated infants) | Alertness, calmness/agitation, respiratory response, crying, body movement, facial tension, body muscle tone |
| **EDIN** (Debillon et al., 2001)<br>Échelle Douleur Inconfort Nouveau-né | Facial activity, body movements, quality of sleep, quality of contact with nurses, consolability |
| **MAPS** (Ramelet et al., 2007)<br>Multidimensional Assessment of Pain Scale<br>(validated birth to 31 months) | Vital signs, breathing pattern, facial expressions, body movement, state of arousal |

GA, gestational age; HRV, heart rate variability.

*Source:* Adapted from Campbell-Yeo, M., Eriksson, M., & Benoit, B. (2022, February 11). Assessment and management of pain in preterm infants: A practice update. *Children (Basel)*. *9*(2), 244. https:doi.org/10.3390/children9020244.

## MANAGEMENT OF NEONATAL PAIN

Leaving pain untreated or undertreated is considered unethical due to the availability of validated assessment tools, multimodal treatment options, and abundance of research on neonatal pain (Carter & Brunkhorst, 2017). Effective pain management is a modifiable factor that can improve newborn and infant outcomes. It should be considered standard of care and should be consistently provided (Campbell-Yeo et al., 2022). Pain management goals are to: (a) actively seek ways to prevent pain when possible; (b) assess pain regularly and routinely to help titrate up or reduce treatment to ensure infants receive effective treatment but are not overmedicated; (c) minimize the intensity and duration of the pain experience; and (d) maximize the infant's ability to cope with and recover from the painful experience.

Interventions to reduce newborn and infant pain can be grouped as nonpharmacologic, sweet-tasting solutions, and pharmacologic.

### Pain Prevention

Preventing pain exposure where possible is the optimal way to reduce the risk for long-term neurodevelopmentally adverse effects. Care providers should make conscious choices regarding the decision to conduct painful procedures, weighing the risk and benefits of each procedure. Emphasis should be placed on the incorporation of infant care practices to minimize the number of painful procedures in care as much as possible (e.g., by eliminating routine blood collections, clustering required bloodwork, and using noninvasive monitoring,). Of note, evidence supports that infants who undergo a painful procedure at night, or when their parent is not present, are significantly less likely to receive effective pain management (Johnston et al., 2011; Orovec et al., 2019). NICU policies should recommend that all nonemergent procedures should be conducted during the day and, where possible, when a parent can be present.

### Nonpharmacologic Interventions

Nonpharmacologic interventions are first-line therapies, and some can be used in isolation to reduce short-term mild-to-moderate pain and minimize stress during less invasive needle-related procedures such as a heel lance or venipuncture. Nonpharmacologic interventions can be combined to provide greater relief. They can also be combined with other pain-relieving modalities such as sweet-tasting solutions or pharmacologic agents for moderate or more severe pain (Campbell-Yeo et al., 2024). Most nonpharmacologic interventions are parent or nurse led, are easy to implement, and have not been demonstrated to have no or minimal risk.

#### Breastfeeding and Expressed Breast Milk

Direct breastfeeding, defined as when the infant latches onto the breast and actively sucks and swallows, before and during the painful procedure has been demonstrated to be as one of the most effective interventions to reduce needle-related pain in newborns and infants. In infants mature enough to achieve and sustain an effective latch, it has been shown to be more effective in reducing pain-related behavioral and physiologic responses when compared to no treatment, NNS, swaddling or containment, maternal holding, skin-to-skin contact, topical anesthetics, cooling spray, heel warming, and music therapy (Benoit et al., 2017; Shah et al., 2023). It is believed that the mechanisms contributing to its efficacy are multisensorial, including inputs associated with tactile touch, familiar smell, and gustatory (suckling and ingestion of breast milk) (Campbell-Yeo, MacNeil et al., 2024). There is some evidence that direct breastfeeding is likely superior to or at least equal to the provision of sweet-tasting solutions to newborns undergoing needle-related procedures (Shah et al., 2023; Yamada et al., 2023).

It appears that the mother (or birthing parent) is the most salient factor related to the pain-reducing effect of breastfeeding. This is demonstrated by the fact that while providing expressed breast in isolation of maternal contact provides a small amount of pain relief when compared to no treatment or placebo, it is significantly less effective than direct breastfeeding. It has been shown that while expressed breast milk alone without maternal contact provides some pain relief when compared to no treatment, it remains less effective than direct breastfeeding or sucrose administration (Shah et al., 2023). Despite the numerous benefits associated with breastfeeding, it is not a viable option for all infants cared for in the NICU, such as very preterm infants or those who are intubated and ventilated (Campbell-Yeo, MacNeil et al., 2024).

### Skin-to-Skin Contact

Skin-to-skin contact (SSC) is the upright holding of a diaper-clad infant on a mother or parent or family member's bare chest. Evidence from a Cochrane Database Review that included 25 clinical trials examining the effectiveness of SSC to reduce procedural pain in newborns demonstrates that SSC was highly effective in reducing biobehavioral signs of pain response in both full-term and very preterm infants undergoing a needle-related procedure such as heel lance or venipuncture (Johnston et al., 2017). In two other studies, SSC was shown to provide the same pain-reducing efficacy as sucrose and sustain its efficacy over repeated procedures (Campbell-Yeo et al., 2019; Gao et al., 2015).

While most studies examining the effects of SSC focus only on mothers, there is some evidence that fathers or other family members can provide similar pain reduction and are likely equally as effective as mothers (Johnston et al., 2017; Shukla et al., 2021). Nurses play a vital role in facilitating SSC for routinely performed procedures and should actively engage families in optimizing pain care. Given the high degree of effectiveness to reduce infant pain and the additional benefits to parents, healthcare providers should aim to promote parent-led pain reducing interventions to optimize parental involvement in their infants' care (Ferreira et al., 2021; Ullsten et al., 2024).

### Non-Nutritive Sucking

Non-nutritive sucking is the provision of a pacifier, gloved finger, or infant's digit in the mouth to promote sucking in the absence of a nutritional feeding with breast milk or formula. Results from a Cochrane systematic review of studies examining the effectiveness of nonpharmacologic interventions to reduce pain in newborns and infants demonstrated that NNS has some effect on reducing pain responses and improved regulation after painful procedures in both preterm and full-term neonates in undergoing immunization and heel stick procedures (Pillai Riddell et al., 2023). While NNS in isolation does not appear to provide sufficient effect, offering NNS as an effective paining adjuvant strategy in infants undergoing acute procedural pain is recommended (Campbell-Yeo, Disher et al., 2024). The combining of NNS with oral sucrose (Yamada et al., 2023) or "containment" (Peng et al., 2018) may result in greater effectiveness.

NNS is thought to produce analgesia through stimulation of orotactile and mechanoreceptors when a pacifier is introduced into the infant's mouth. NNS is hypothesized to modulate transmission or processing of nociception through mediation by the endogenous nonopioid system (Blass et al., 1987; Foster et al., 2016).

Breastfeeding or oral sucrose combined with NNS remain the preferred methods for pain from minor painful procedures in *full-term healthy* neonates or infants mature enough to achieve a latch (Campbell-Yeo, Disher et al., 2024).

### Facilitated Tucking or Swaddling or Containment

Facilitated tucking is a hand-swaddling technique that is defined as the placement of the hands of a parent or care provider to hold the infant's extremities flexed and contained close to the trunk or placed over the head, bottom, or feet of an infant to provide comfort, enhance regulation, and maintain the infant in a side-lying, flexed position (Axelin et al., 2006). In a review of 15 studies, facilitated tucking has been shown to attenuate pain responses in preterm neonates by decreasing heart rates, increasing oxygen saturation, decreasing crying time and sleep disruption times, and reducing pain scores during heel lance and endotracheal suctioning (Gomes Neto et al., 2020). Combining facilitated tucking with other interventions, such as sucrose, NNS, or both, appears to provide added relief (Bellieni, Cordelli et al., 2007; Cignacco et al., 2012; Liaw et al., 2012, 2013; Perroteau et al., 2018). There is some low-certainty evidence that there is little difference in pain response during a heel lance when facilitated tucking was compared with oral glucose or an oral opioid (Gomes Neto et al., 2020).

Swaddling is another simple and safe containment technique that can also be used as an adjuvant strategy in combination with other pain-reducing interventions by nurses and families to help regulate physiologic and pain-related responses in infants (Erkut & Yildiz, 2017). Swaddling, the gentle wrapping of an infant in a blanket while keeping the infant's limbs flexed, is believed to support infant self-soothing behaviors. Both swaddling and facilitated tucking are easy to do, cost effective, and developmentally supportive. Swaddling and facilitated tucking are more effective than no intervention in reducing pain in minor painful procedures in term and preterm infants; however, they are most effective when used in combination with other interventions such as sucrose (Gomes Neto et al., 2020; Ho et al., 2016; Perroteau et al., 2018; Pillai Riddell et al., 2023).

Other integrative therapies such as infant massage prior to the procedure may provide some added effect, though the certainty of this evidence is very low (Liu et al., 2022).

### Environmental Modifications

While the evidence is limited regarding environmental contextual factors such as light and noise, there is some evidence that infants who are sick or in pain will need changes in the environment to decrease stress and provide a healing atmosphere. These modifications generally include dim lighting, decreased noise, and activity around the bedside (Carter & Brunkhorst, 2017).

### Sweet-Tasting Solutions

Sweet-tasting solutions such as oral sucrose (a disaccharide comprised of fructose and glucose) or glucose provided with and without NNS are the most widely studied nonpharmacologic interventions for infant pain management.

Both oral sucrose and glucose have been reported to reduce needle-related procedural pain in preterm and term infants (Harrison et al., 2017; Yamada et al., 2023). A systematic review of 74 randomized control trials of full-term and preterm infants ($N = 7{,}049$) found that sucrose is safe and effective for reducing procedural pain in term and preterm neonates, particularly heel lance and venipuncture procedures and IM injections (Stevens et al., 2016). When only studies examining the effectiveness of sucrose in reducing pain associated with heel lance were included ($n = 55$), results supported that there was moderate certainty that oral sucrose reduced pain scores when compared to no treatment and some evidence that sucrose may be more effective compared to NNS, breastfeeding, laser acupuncture, facilitated tucking, and the effect of sucrose + NNS compared to NNS in reducing pain. There does not appear to be significant differences in efficacy when compared to breastfeeding, skin-to-skin contact, or expressed breast milk (Yamada et al., 2023). Although sucrose used alone is effective, there is evidence to support that sucrose used in combination with NNS may add additional benefit (Bellieni, Cordelli et al., 2007; Yamada et al., 2023).

Very few studies have examined the long-term effects of repeated sucrose administration. A systematic review of eight studies examining the efficacy and safety of repeated oral sucrose for procedural pain suggests that evidence is supportive of the safety and efficacy of repeated sucrose administration; however, results were mixed (Gao et al., 2015).

Although relatively few contraindications to the provision of swaddling and NNS for management of pain in neonates exist, the absolute safety of sucrose has not been determined. Rare instances of choking and decreased oxygen saturation, all resolving spontaneously, have been reported (Yamada et al., 2023). Although a study by Willis and colleagues (1977) reported a possible association between sucrose and necrotizing enterocolitis (NEC), subsequent research findings did not find any significant differences in incidence rates for NEC between infants who received repeated doses of sucrose over 28 days of life compared to control groups (Stevens et al., 2005). Furthermore, sufficient evidence of the safety of repeated doses of sucrose in neonates to recommend its widespread use for repeated painful procedures is lacking (Stevens et al., 2016). Johnston and colleagues reported that preterm infants less than 31 weeks postmenstrual age who received repeated doses of sucrose for painful procedures showed poorer neurodevelopmental scores at 36 and 40 weeks (Johnston et al., 2002). However, a later study failed to demonstrate significant differences on neurobiologic risk status outcomes between preterm infants who received sucrose plus pacifier, water plus pacifier, or the standard care group (Stevens et al., 2005).

Additional research is required to confirm the efficacy of sucrose used in extremely preterm infants, as well as the effect of sucrose on neurodevelopmental outcomes. Cumulative sucrose exposure for repeated procedural pain in preterm neonates was neither associated with a delay in neurodevelopment nor neuroprotective effects at 18 months of corrected gestational age (CGA) (Bueno et al., 2024).

While the exact mechanism of action of sucrose in unknown, it is believed to be mediated by the degree of sweet taste. The level of effectiveness of sucrose does appear to be associated with the concentration of sucrose. Concentrations less than 18% are not as effective as higher doses and doses greater than 50% do not appear to have added benefit. It is important to note that sucrose should be administered to the tip of the tongue 2 minutes prior to the procedure, may be repeated throughout the procedure, and should not be given via an oral or nasogastric (NG) tube. There is also some evidence that the pain-reducing effects are highest when provided 2 minutes before the painful stimulus and appear to coincide with endogenous opioid release triggered by the sweet taste of sucrose (Blass & Shah 1995). The effect of sucrose appears to last approximately 2 to 4 minutes; therefore, repeated doses may be necessary if procedures are prolonged (Stevens et al., 2016).

Dosing volumes for sucrose range from 0.05 to 2 ml of a 24% solution; however, the results of a large, randomized trial including four NICUs in Canada indicate that a dose of 0.1 ml provided 2 minutes prior to the procedure and repeated as needed throughout the procedure is effective (Stevens et al., 2018).

## Pharmacologic Management

Given the known detrimental effects of untreated pain exposure in early life including higher mortality and long-term alteration in normal development, consensus guidelines for the management of newborn pain recommend the use of pharmacologic agents to treat moderate or severe pain associated with invasive procedures, and surgical, chronic, or palliative conditions (Campbell-Yeo, Disher et al., 2024; Keels et al., 2016; Lago et al., 2009). However, the over-treatment of pain and unnecessary exposure to both opioid and non-opioid medications on the development of the brain is also a concern to clinicians. There remain ongoing questions related to the best choice of agents and the optimal balance between provision of effective pain management and excessive exposure to pharmacologic analgesic and sedation agents, most notably due to the off-label nature of most of these agents and a lack of clinical trial data examining their effectiveness and safety, and the uncertainty of possible long-lasting effects in both preterm and full-term populations (Campbell-Yeo et al., 2022; Squillaro et al., 2019).

### Analgesic Pain Reliever/Antipyretic

Acetaminophen (or paracetamol) is one of the most-used medications for newborns and infants. It can be provided via numerous routes—oral, rectal, or intravenously. Currently, there is a lack of evidence to support its use for infants less than a month of age for commonly performed needle-related procedures such as heel lance or for its use for procedures requiring a rapid onset of action (Ohlsson & Shah, 2016). There is evidence to support it as a potential opioid-sparing adjuvant treatment postoperatively and its use is recommended in the Enhanced Recovery After Surgery Society's guidelines (Brindle et al., 2020).

### Topical Anesthetics

While there is strong evidence regarding the use of topical anesthetics to reduce needle-related pain in young children and youth, a Cochrane review demonstrated that quality evidence is lacking to support its use in newborns during needle-related pain, most notably heel lance, during their first month after birth (Foster et al., 2017). Topical anesthetic was not associated with reduced pain scores associated with frenotomy (Shavit et al., 2017). Similarly, when used alone, topical anesthetic is insufficient in providing effective pain relief during circumcision (Labban et al., 2021).

In contrast, when compared to placebo, topical anesthetics (lidocaine or EMLA) may reduce neonatal pain scores during lumbar puncture (Pessano et al., 2023). Moreover, the use of topical anesthetic eye drops during routine eye examinations for retinopathy of prematurity (ROP) screening is recommended (Dempsey & McCreery, 2011). Current evidence demonstrates that the use of topical anesthetic eye drops combined with a multisensory intervention approach that includes 24% sucrose (or equivalent glucose solution) NNS, swaddling/containment, and parent voice when possible to achieve optimal pain management (Campbell-Yeo et al., 2022; Disher et al., 2018).

Caution is warranted when using topical anesthetics in extremely preterm infants, because there is a dearth of evidence to support their efficacy and safety. Further research is warranted.

### Opioids

Opioids, known to provide analgesia across the lifespan, are the first choice for the management of surgical or major painful procedures or conditions in the NICU, with morphine and fentanyl being the most widely used (Kinoshita, Olsson et al., 2023).

Due to the possible risk of adverse effects (e.g., respiratory depression, hypotension, urinary retention), close attention to safe and effective dosing is essential to achieve the optimal balance between effective pain management and opioid overuse, especially in infants born extremely preterm and infants requiring prolonged ventilation (Bellù et al., 2021) (Campbell-Yeo et al., 2022). A Cochrane review assessing the benefits and harms of opioids in preterm and term infants undergoing a painful procedure found that when compared to placebo, there is moderate evidence that opioids reduce pain scores during the procedure (Kinoshita, Olsson et al., 2023). The evidence was deemed uncertain about the effect of opioids when compared to nonpharmacologic measures or other analgesics for some procedures (Kinoshita, Olsson et al., 2023). Results from a 2023 Cochrane review regarding the association between intraventricular hemorrhage (IVH) and opioid exposure demonstrates that opioids have no or little effect on any degree of germinal matrix hemorrhage IVH, severe IVH, mortality, or major neurodevelopmental disability (Stróżyk et al., 2023).

While evidence exists to support that continuous IV infusions provide more effective pain management with fewer adverse effects than intermittent bolus, more research is warranted to inform a consensus recommendation on the optimal method of administration (Barrington et al., 2006; Roué, 2023).

Methadone, primarily classified as an opioid, also has weak activity as a noncompetitive NMDA receptor antagonist. Its use, as well as that of buprenorphine, a synthetic opioid, are emerging as potential agents to treat infants with in-utero opioid exposure. Their use as management for acute procedural pain remains rare and is understudied (Taleghani et al., 2019).

#### Iatrogenic Opioid Withdrawal

Newborns or infants who require opioid therapy for an extended period may develop physical dependence and withdrawal (Disher et al., 2019). Rapid weaning of opioids may lead to withdrawal symptoms such as irritability, crying, increased respiratory rate, jitteriness, hypertonicity, vomiting, diarrhea, sweating, skin abrasions, seizures, yawning, stuffy nose, sneezing, and hiccups. The goals of clinical management of opioid withdrawal are (a) to reduce withdrawal symptoms to promote regular sleep cycles and (b) to reduce agitation caused by care interventions (Anand et al., 2010).

There remains a lack of consensus regarding the optimal weaning rate of opioids to prevent withdrawal symptoms in neonates. There is some evidence that adhering to weaning guidelines that reduce the daily wean of rate of the opioid infusion based on duration of exposure is the optimal way to reduce reported adverse withdrawal symptoms (Muirhead & Kynoch, 2019). In one study authors reported that reduced rates of withdrawal were associated with daily rate reductions not exceeding 20% for infants who received opioids/benzodiazepines for 1 to 3 days; 13% to 20% for 4 to 7 days; 8% to 13% for 8 to 14 days; 8% for 15 to 21 days; and 2% to 4% for more than 21 days, respectively (Ducharme et al., 2005).

#### Prevention of Opioid Withdrawal Symptoms

Neonatal abstinence syndrome (NAS) is an overarching term used to describe any infant born to a mother/pregnant person with a substance use disorder who is experiencing signs of withdrawal (Jansson & Patrick, 2019). There has been a recent change to the common use of the term neonatal opioid withdrawal syndrome (NOWS) to incorporate a more specific term for infants experiencing signs of withdrawal primarily from exposure to opioids in utero (Jansson & Patrick, 2019). The diagnosis of both syndromes is made through careful assessment by healthcare providers of the infant following birth. Signs of withdrawal often present across multiple body systems, including the nervous and gastrointestinal systems (Grisham et al., 2019). Signs of withdrawal, such as irritability, increased tone, and poor feeding, are highly dependent on many interconnected factors: mono or polydrug use, duration of exposure in utero, use near the time of birth, and the gestational age of the infant at birth (Anbalagan et al., 2025; Dodds et al., 2019; Lacaze-Masmonteil & O'Flaherty, 2018).

Standardized scoring methods to evaluate the trend and severity of withdrawal symptoms are essential to guide the care of the infant with prenatal substance exposure. In most healthcare facilities, the modified Finnigan Scoring System continues to be used to assess infants diagnosed with NAS/NOWS, despite emerging evidence of challenges present in the use of this tool (Curran et al., 2020; Grossman et al., 2018; Schiff & Grossman, 2019; Singh & Davis, 2021). The Finnegan Neonatal Abstinence Scoring Tool (FNAST) has been used in clinical practice since 1974 and was the first objective measurement tool to assess the signs experienced by infants diagnosed with NAS/NOWS (Finnegan et al., 1975; Wachman et al., 2018). Although transformative for care at the time of its inception, the FNAST has been more recently criticized in the literature for its subjectivity, invasive and lengthy assessment, and lack of collaboration with the family (Anbalagan et al., 2025; Chin Foo et al., 2021; Cleveland & Bonugli, 2014). To address these concerns, a novel approach—the Eat, Sleep, Console (ESC) model of care—was developed (Grossman et al., 2018). The components of the tool are very simple and easy to use clinically and include the following:

- E = Eat: able to eat one or more ounces each feeding
- S = Sleeping: able to sleep for 1 hour or longer when uninterrupted
- C = Console: can be consoled within 10 minutes or less when upset

The implementation of the ESC model corresponds to another significant change in managing these infant(s) with the aim to reduce separation of mothers and their infants and provide as much care as possible on postpartum units rather than in the NICU setting. This change in care provision and use of the ESC scoring system has demonstrated promising improvements in the health of infants with NAS/NOWS, along with positive health system effects, including a significant decrease in the number of infants separated from their mothers, NICU admissions, length of hospital stays, and pharmacologic interventions (Grossman & Berkwitt, 2019; Grossman et al., 2017; Holmes et al., 2016). Moreover, the ESC model is fully aligned with family-centered care principles. The model emphasizes the parental role in care and provides mothers the opportunity to be the center of care for their infants who are withdrawing, improving communication and collaboration with the family, and ultimately decreasing stigma and discrimination experienced by this population (Grisham et al., 2019; National Institute for Children's Health Quality [NICHQ], 2019).

Although the ECS is a multidisciplinary healthcare innovation, this model is heavily dependent upon and driven by the nursing profession and specialized nursing care (Haaland et al., 2023). Registered nurses are responsible for assessment, education, and parent engagement in nonpharmacologic and pharmacologic interventions (Halloum et al., 2024; Phyu et al., 2024). As such, successful integration of the ESC model into clinical practice requires both healthcare provider and parent education to ensure competency and confidence in assessments and interventions (Haaland et al., 2023).

### Nonsteroidal Anti-Inflammatory Drugs

The use of nonsteroidal antiinflammatory drugs (NSAIDs) (e.g., ibuprofen, ketorolac, ketoprofen, indomethacin) is common among older children. However, its use in the neonatal population is less given the increased risk for kidney injury and possible gastrointestinal hemorrhage (Aldrink et al., 2011). Most NSAIDs are not approved, and many are contraindicated in infants less than 6 months of age (Ziesenitz et al., 2022). The populations at highest risk for potentially associated adverse outcomes are infants less than 3 weeks of postnatal age and those born preterm (Aldrink et al., 2011). Due to the considerable risks, no consensus recommendations can be made regarding the routine use of NSAIDs for procedural pain relief in newborns (Ziesenitz et al., 2022). There is some interest in the use of ketorolac in neonates and infants following cardiac surgery with some promise, although there are no large-scale studies to determine its safety and efficacy (Kiskaddon et al., 2024). Due to the substantial risks, no recommendations can be made regarding the use of NSAIDs for procedural pain relief (Campbell-Yeo et al., 2022).

### Sedatives

Sedatives are used to alter the level of consciousness in a patient and are commonly used as adjuncts to analgesics (Kinoshita, Stempel et al., 2023). Due to the lack of evidence to support the efficacy and safety associated with the use of sedatives in preterm and term populations, many are not used routinely in the NICU setting (Roué, 2023). Of major concern is the fact that sedatives do not provide significant analgesia while altering the infant's level of consciousness, and therefore may hide the clinical signs of pain (Donato et al., 2019; Roué, 2023). Midazolam is contraindicated for infants less than 34 weeks, due to the elevated risk associated for hypotension and neurologic injury (Ng et al., 2017). Therefore, sedatives should be used with caution, and never alone as a sole agent for neonatal pain (Kinoshita, Stempel et al., 2023).

### *N*-Methyl-D-Aspartate Receptor Antagonists

*N*-methyl-D-aspartate (NMDA) antagonists are a class of drug that inhibit the action of NMDA receptors. NMDA agents include medications such as ketamine, commonly used in older children, to provide sedative, analgesic, and amnesic effects (Carter & Brunkhorst, 2017). The literature is scarce related to the use of NMDA agents in newborns and infants, primarily due to concerns regarding potential side effects. A Cochrane review concluded that the trial evidence was of very low certainty about the effect of ketamine on pain scores and that no recommendations could be made about the use of ketamine for the treatment of procedural pain (Persad et al., 2023). To date, only two randomized controlled clinical trials have been conducted ($n$ = 269 infants). One study regarding pain management for circumcision compared oral ketamine (10 mg/kg body weight) versus sugar syrup (66.7% w/w at 1 ml/kg body weight). The other study compared IV ketamine versus fentanyl during laser photocoagulation for ROP. No other studies comparing NSAIDs with no treatment, placebo, sweet-tasting solutions, nonpharmacologic interventions, or different routes of administration for the same analgesics have been reported (Persad et al., 2023).

### Alpha-2 Adrenergic Receptor Agonists

#### Dexmedetomidine

IV dexmedetomidine has been shown that it may be an effective agent for pain treatment and sedation in neonates (Mantecón-Fernández et al., 2023). Dexmedetomidine is an alpha-2 adrenergic receptor agonist that produces sedation and analgesia and may be associated with fewer serious side effects such as respiratory depression (Ojha et al., 2022). A small animal study demonstrated showed that dexmedetomidine may also play a neuroprotective role but this has not been replicated in human studies (Maciel et al., 2019). To date, no large-scale randomized trials adequately powered to determine efficacy or safety have been done, nor have any studies have been conducted to determine the long-term neurologic outcomes of the use of dexmedetomidine in the neonatal period, which remains a considerable concern for healthcare providers (Mantecón-Fernández et al., 2023). Currently, there is insufficient evidence to determine the efficacy and safety of clonidine, also an alpha-2 agonist ($\alpha$2-agonist), for sedation and analgesia in term and preterm newborn infants receiving mechanical ventilation, postoperatively, or undergoing procedural pain (Kinoshita, Olsson et al., 2023; Kinoshita, Stempel et al., 2023; Romantsik et al., 2017). As such, no recommendations can be made for its use. A further review of commonly used agents for analgesia and sedation in newborns and infants can be found in Table 22.4.

**TABLE 22.4**

**COMMONLY USED AGENTS FOR ANALGESIA AND SEDATION IN NEWBORNS AND INFANTS**

| Agent | Onset of Action | Duration | Route | Comments |
|---|---|---|---|---|
| ***Sweet-Tasting Solutions*** | | | | |
| 24% Sucrose | 2 minutes | 2–5 minutes | PO (tip of the tongue) | Should be provided on tip of the tongue, may be repeated throughout the procedure to effect |
| 25%–30% Glucose | 2 minutes | 2–5 minutes | PO (tip of the tongue) | Should be provided on tip of the tongue, may be repeated throughout the procedure to effect |
| ***Analgesic/Antipyretic*** | | | | |
| Acetaminophen/ paracetamol | 30 minutes | 4 hours | PO, rectal, IV | Recommended postoperatively as an adjunct treatment |
| ***Topical or Local Anesthetic/Analgesic*** | | | | |
| Lidocaine/ prilocaineEMLA | 60 minutes | 1–2 hours | Topical | Apply and wrap with occlusive dressing; allow to remain intact for 60–90 minutes; remove and clean prior to procedure to avoid systemic absorption |
| Amethocaine gel | 30 minutes | 3 hours | Topical | Cover with occlusive dressing; do not spread or rub in; remove gel and dressing after 30 to 45 minutes; do not leave on for longer than 60 minutes; should not be used in premature infants or those younger than 1 month of age |
| Anesthetic eye drops | 30 seconds | 10–20 minutes | Topical | Drops applied to each eye prior to ROP screening |
| Lidocaine 1% | 1–5 minutes | 1–1.5 hours | Subcutaneous | Epinephrine should never be added to the lidocaine because of its vasoconstrictive properties and the risk of ischemia and necrosis; Infiltrate area using 25-G needle approximately 3–8 minutes prior to procedure |

*(continued)*

## TABLE 22.4

### COMMONLY USED AGENTS FOR ANALGESIA AND SEDATION IN NEWBORNS AND INFANTS (*continued*)

| Agent | Onset of Action | Duration | Route | Comments |
|---|---|---|---|---|
| ***NSAIDs*** | | | | |
| Ibuprofen, ketorolac, ketoprofen, indomethacin | | | | Due to the considerable risks, no consensus recommendations can be made for routine use |
| ***Opioid Analgesics*** | | | | |
| Morphine | IV—5–15 min<br>IM- 15–30 min<br>Oral—30 min | Half-life 10 hours<br>3–4 hours<br>3–6 hours | Intermittent IV<br>Continuous infusion<br>IM, subcutaneous<br>Oral/parenteral ratio | |
| Fentanyl | 1 minutes<br>5–7 minutes | Half-life 9.5 hours<br>1 hour | Intermittent IV<br>Continuous infusion<br>Intranasal | Bolus infections should be provided |
| Methadone | 5 minutes<br>30–45 minutes | 24–36 hours | IV<br>PO | Emerging use in infants with NOWS; little use for procedural pain |
| ***Sedatives*** | | | | |
| **Midazolam** | 30 minutes | 6 hours | PO | Contraindicated for infants < 34 weeks, due to the elevated rlsk associated wlth hypotension and neurologic injury |
| ***NMDA Antagonists*** | | | | |
| Ketamine | | | | Very low certainty about the effect of ketamine on pain scores and that no recommendations could be made about the use of ketamine for the treatment of procedural pain |
| ***Alpha-2 Adrenergic Receptor Agonists*** | | | | |
| Dexmedetomidine | 5–10 minutes<br>25–30 minutes | 60–120 minutes<br>55–100 minutes | IV<br>Intranasal | No large-scale randomized trials adequately powered to determine efficacy or safety |
| Clonidine | 5 minutes<br>30–60 minutes | 3–7 hours<br>6–8 hours | IV<br>PO | No large-scale randomized trials adequately powered to determine efficacy or safety |

IM, intramuscular; NOWS, neonatal opioid withdrawal syndrome; NSAIDs, nonsteroidal anti-inflammatory drugs; PO, by mouth.

## Pain Management at the End of Life

Compassionate care and relief of pain and suffering at the end of life (EOL) is a fundamental right of all individuals. According to the Institute of Medicine, "a decent or good death is one that is: free from avoidable distress and suffering for patients, families, and caregivers; in general accord with patients' and families' wishes; and reasonably consistent with clinical, cultural, and ethical standards" (Institute of Medicine et al., 2003, p. 40). The quality of the dying process in the NICU is affected by a complex interaction of infant, parent, caregiver, and contextual factors (Fortney & Steward, 2014). In 2013, the American Academy of Pediatrics published a policy statement on pediatric palliative care and hospice care, yet significant variation remains in protocols addressing comfort care in pediatrics at EOL (American Academy of Pediatrics Section on Hospice and Palliative Medicine and Committee on Hospital Care, 2013). Haug and colleagues (2018) reported that 45% of reporting institutions did not have neonatal comfort care guidelines and of those reporting, 19% did not address pain symptom management (Haug et al., 2018).

Pain assessment is extremely challenging in neonates at EOL. While the most-used neonatal pain assessment tools measure acute or postoperative pain, infants at the EOL predominately experience prolonged/chronic pain. Many neonatal care providers have limited experience measuring prolonged/chronic pain and this can create an additional frequent and challenging condition in the context of palliative care (Garten & Bührer, 2019). For prolonged/chronic pain, only three pain scores are currently validated for neonates: the Echelle Douleur Inconfort Nouveau-Né scale (EDIN scale) (Debillon et al., 2001); the Neonatal Pain, Agitation and Sedation Scale (N-PAS scale) (Hummel et al., 2008, 2010); and the COMFORTneo scale (van Dijk et al., 2009).

Pain management at EOL primarily centers on the provision of nonpharmacologic therapies to enhance the infant's comfort level, the use of opioids to minimize pain, and often the addition of sedatives or other agents to provide anxiolytic effects (Haug et al., 2020). Continuous infusions of opioid therapy such as morphine and fentanyl are often required to manage pain at EOL and should be titrated to desired clinical response (analgesia). Opioid doses well beyond those described for standard analgesia are often required for infants who are in severe pain or who have developed tolerance (decreasing pain relief with the same dosage over time) after the prolonged use of opioids (Carter & Brunkhorst, 2017). Physiologic comfort measures may modulate pain and distressing symptoms in infants at EOL and include reduction of noxious stimuli, organization of caregiving, and positioning and containment strategies (Garten & Bührer, 2019).

Institutions should implement a consistent guideline for neonatal EOL care to decrease variability of interventions and increase the use of appropriate symptom management. Pediatric palliative and advanced care teams can be an excellent support for both families and the healthcare team caring for an infant at EOL (Haug et al., 2020).

## PARENT ENGAGEMENT IN PAIN CARE

To protect the newborn brain from overwhelming sensory input, including stress and pain, eight principles of family- and patient-centered care for newborns have been formulated (Roué et al., 2017). They include psychological support for parents, a supportive environment, and—most importantly—free, 24-hour-a-day parental access with no limitations due to staff shift or medical rounds. This round-the-clock access that is the case in many European countries, while still not achieved in other regions, is a prerequisite for parents to be actively involved in their newborn's pain care in an optimal way (Greisen et al., 2009). Noteworthy though, also in neonatal units with a more limited parental access, parents can provide pain relief when they are at the unit, and they should be offered this opportunity.

Research has shown that parents are concerned by the pain their newborns are exposed to, and that they want to be involved in the pain care (McNair et al., 2024). There are many evidence-based pain-reliving methods that can be used by parents, alone but preferably in combination (Hasanul Huda et al., 2025). Most effective are breastfeeding and holding skin to skin, while facilitated tucking, massage, swaddling, or singing can be seen as adjuvant measures. If sweet solutions (sucrose or glucose) are given, parents can administer the dose and help their infant with NNS for an enhanced effect.

Breastfeeding is one of the most studied pain-relieving methods provided by mothers (Shah et al., 2023). It should be performed in a calm environment and the space should allow an ergonomic working position for the person performing the painful procedure. Breastfeeding protects against pain during venipuncture, heel stick, tape removal, or other moderate procedural pain. Skin-to-skin contact is also an effective way to reduce procedural pain and could, if provided by the mother, be combined with breastfeeding (Johnston et al., 2017).

Parents who can be present with their infant at the hospital can identify signs of pain and discomfort and communicate this to the hospital staff (Palomaa et al., 2023). By doing this and asking for adequate actions, the parents will serve as advocates for their infants in pain.

## THE NEONATAL NURSE'S ROLE AND RESPONSIBILITIES

All nurses have an ethical responsibility to prevent and relieve pain in the patients they are caring for (American Nurses Association [ANA], 2018). In a broader perspective, they should also strive to follow the latest evidence on pain management and advocate for evidence-based routines and guidelines on their workplace. In neonatal care this means that all nurses must do the following:

- Understand basic pain physiology.
- Know potential sources of pain for newborn infants.
- Recognize signs of pain and discomfort in newborns and be able to use an age-appropriate and validated pain assessment tool.
- Be able to use nonpharmacologic interventions to prevent and relieve pain.
- Work together with parents and with other professions at the unit to achieve good pain management.

Neonatal nurses are the healthcare professionals that are closest to the newborns and their families and therefore best suited to coordinate the multimodal interprofessional pain care at the unit. There are several resources nurses can use to keep a good pain management standard: textbooks (such as this one), online or in-person professional courses, and peer support from experienced colleagues. The IASP has a Special Interest Group for Pain in Childhood that promotes education about pain in children, organizes meetings, and publishes a pediatric pain letter. Many clinical and scientific organizations have Internet resources where nurses and other professionals can watch educational videos and download material.

Remember that it is not a once-achieved, forever-existing skill to be good at neonatal pain management. It is a constant, ongoing work to maintain the ability to manage neonatal pain and all neonatal nurses should have this as one of their main areas of focus at work.

## SUMMARY

Newborns and infants have high exposure to pain and most experience significant undertreatment. Ineffective treatment of pain in early life is linked with significant adverse short- and long-term health outcomes affecting later pain processing, cognition, and neurodevelopment. Preventing, assessing, and managing pain effectively is an essential part of optimal newborn and infant care. To ensure best outcomes, healthcare organizations should implement facility-wide pain management programs, with dedicated resources encompassing: comprehensive education for healthcare providers, practice uptake of pain prevention and control strategies, and quality improvement initiatives to reduce the amount of painful procedures; assess and reassess pain appropriately; lessen procedural, postoperative, and ongoing/chronic pain; and actively engage parents in pain care and shared decision making.

## CASE STUDY

**Identification of the Problem.** Female infant born very preterm with pain related to her condition and to care-related procedures.

**Assessment: History and Physical Examination.** Marie is a preterm girl, born at 30 weeks and 3 days gestational age, via elective cesarean section due to intrauterine growth retardation and signs of preeclampsia in the mother. Marie's birth weight was 1,150 g. Her mother is a 23-year-old woman with a 3-year-old boy, Glenn, at home. The father of both children lives with the family and is presently unemployed.

When Marie was born, she showed signs of respiratory distress with shallow breathing and low oxygen saturation (89%). Her upper airways were suctioned, and free-flow oxygen was provided over her mouth and nose. Her 5-minute Apgar score was 7, with a deduction for color, muscle tone, and respiration but after 10 minutes her color and saturation were better, and it was decided that she could be transferred to the NICU for neonatal care. She was placed skin to skin to her father, who was sitting in a wheelchair, and rolled to the NICU by two nurses. The father was provided a reclining chair where he could lie, with Marie on his bare chest.

**Development of Management Plan/Implementation.** After some hours at the NICU, Marie's breathing work became more labored with some audible grunting and visible chest retractions. She was first placed on continuous positive airway pressure (CPAP) with increasing oxygen needs up to 50% over the next few hours. Umbilical vessel catheters were inserted for blood sampling, medications, and nutrition. Given the worsening respiratory distress, high oxygen demand and chest x-ray findings, Marie was intubated, and surfactant was given in the trachea by the neonatal nurse practitioner.

Because the intubation was semi-elective, it was decided that there was time to give premedication. This was done with atropine, fentanyl, and succinylcholine (suxamethonium), in that order. Fentanyl was preferred over morphine due to a much shorter onset of action. When Marie was stable on the ventilator, her mother came to the NICU after her postoperative care, and the nurses helped to carefully place Marie skin to skin with her mother, ensuring that the endotracheal tube (ETT) tube and the umbilical catheters were secure.

Pain care for Marie at the NICU during this period included the following:

- Vital signs monitoring including heart rate, respiration rate, and blood pressure. Variations in all these can be signs of pain and distress.
- Observation of body tension and movements. Both vigorous movements and flaccid limps can be signs of pain. In a preterm and sick infant, flaccidness is more likely to occur than averting movements when the infant is in pain.
- Observation of skin color. A preterm infant who is in pain could show paleness.
- Observation and auscultation of the abdomen to detect early warnings of NEC, which is very painful.
- Most importantly, regular pain assessment with a valid pain assessment tool that is reliable for the gestational age and condition. Any signs of pain in this assessment should lead to interventions to alleviate the pain.

The ventilator was set to follow Marie's own spontaneous respiration attempts, and she tolerated the treatment well. Marie received nonpharmacologic support (e.g. skin-to-skin contact, reduced light and noise). She did not require any additional analgesia agents during the ventilation period. If she had needed opioids for more than 3 to 5 days, it would have been important to wean the opioids according to weaning guidelines to prevent and handle any signs of abstinence.

After 2 days, Marie's lungs were better and she could be extubated, going back to first CPAP for 3 days and then oxygen on a high-flow nasal cannula. Both her parents remained with her, both providing her skin-to-skin contact as much as possible. The grandparents helped to take care of Glenn at home, and sometimes he could visit his sister at the NICU. After 2 weeks, Marie can come off the oxygen cannula.

After 4 weeks at the unit, when everything was fine, Marie's condition worsened, with paleness, bradycardias, and increased oxygen demand. An infection was suspected, and she needed to undergo repeated blood samples and a lumbar puncture for diagnosis and required insertion of an IV cannula for antibiotics treatment. The cannula stopped functioning after 2 days and needed to be replaced.

Plan for Pain Management During the NICU Period

- Use a pain assessment tool designed for procedural pain during potentially painful procedures.

- Perform regular pain assessment with a tool designed for prolonged or ongoing pain. Any signs of pain in this assessment should lead to interventions to alleviate the pain.
- Use nonpharmacologic interventions to prevent and alleviate pain during procedures. Skin-to-skin contact and breastfeeding, best in combination, are effective methods that engage the parents in pain care. NNS, facilitated tucking, and a parent's voice are adjuvant strategies to help with pain management.
- Educate and encourage parents to be present and involved in providing pain care.
- Consider parent-led strategies as first-line treatments.
- If parents or a designated support person cannot be present, sweet-tasting solutions should be considered. Sweet-tasting solutions should be administered orally on the tip of the tongue with a pacifier being offered following.
- Avoid unnecessary tests and use noninvasive techniques when possible.
- Remove any adhesives carefully, using gentle technique, to avoid causing skin damage and pain.

**Outcome.** At a gestational age of 37+2 weeks, Marie can have full nutrition without gavage feeding and her vital signs were stable. She could go home to her family, who now have experience and were prepared to support her in future painful situations, such as vaccinations.

## EVIDENCE-BASED PRACTICE

### Reducing Pain Associated With Screening for Retinopathy of Prematurity

Infants born less than 1,500 g or less than 32 weeks' gestation are routinely subjected as part of standard neonatal care for necessary ophthalmologic screening for ROP, which is an eye disease that occurs in some premature infants and affects the retina. Unwanted blood vessels grow on the infant's retina and can cause serious eye and vision problems and even lead to blindness. Most infants born preterm undergo on average 6 to 10 ROP screening eye examinations, while the youngest and sickest can require many more. Screening examinations are a significant source of pain and discomfort and are associated with physiologic instability in preterm neonates. Documented pain scores demonstrate infants experience moderate-to-severe pain during these examinations (Laudiano-Dray et al., 2020). Despite concentrated efforts to find optimal ways to reduce the pain associated with eye examinations, none have been shown to consistently lower pain scores to low or no pain levels, with even those found to be effective only lowering pain scores to moderate levels (Disher et al., 2018). There remains a vital need to identify effective interventions for standard pain relief measures undertaken during ROP eye screening. In a Cochrane systematic review ($n$ = 2 studies) to determine the effect of instillation of topical anesthetic eye drops on pain responses of preterm neonates undergoing ROP screening, the authors concluded that the administration of topical anesthetic eye drops (proparacaine) at least 30 seconds prior to the examination was associated with a significant reduction in pain scores, but was not effective in eliminating or reducing pain to low pain scores (Dempsey & McCreery, 2011).

In a later systematic review and meta-analyses including 29 studies, Disher and colleagues (2018) reported that multisensory interventions including topical anesthetic drops, sweet-tasting solutions, swaddling, NNS sucking, and parent voice is currently the best treatment for reducing pain resulting from eye examinations in preterm infants. No known interventions were currently effective in eliminating or reducing pain to low levels. Findings from more recent studies demonstrate similar findings. In a study examining the effect of music combined with topical anesthetic drops compared to topical anesthetic drops alone, while infants receiving music had a slightly shorter crying time and lower pain scores, pain scores measured using the PIPP-R in both groups remained in a high-moderate pain range (11.2 ± 2.6, and 13.4 ± 2.1, respectively), indicating that neither treatment was effective (Çuhacı et al., 2024; Madvar et al., 2023). In another clinical trial including 105 preterm infants randomized to receive either acetaminophen drops, dextrose drops, or placebo, during a screening eye examination for ROP, no significant difference was found across groups and all infants demonstrated high-moderate pain scores (PIPP-R scores 11.39, dextrose 12.17, and placebo 11.54). None of the groups reported infants experiencing scores of 0 to 6, which would indicate low or no pain (Madvar et al., 2023). Similarly, in two studies examining the effectiveness of providing an intranasal opioid, either fentanyl or dexmedetomidine, in addition to recommended nonpharmacologic interventions and sweet taste, while some improvements in pain scores were reported, overall pain scores remained in the moderate range in both groups (Kara et al., 2023; Ozkan Zarif et al., 2024). Further research to investigate optimal pain reducing strategies during ROP eye screening in preterm infants is vital.

## ONLINE RESOURCES

CourseConnect

Resources for this chapter are online and available at www.springerpub.com/courseconnect.

## REFERENCES

References for this chapter are online and available at www.springerpub.com/courseconnect.

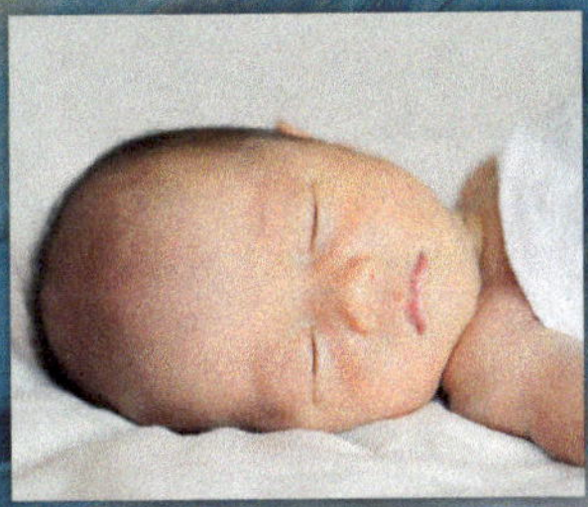

Source: Wong Sze Fei/Adobe Stock.

CHAPTER 23

# Identifying, Managing, and Caring for the Neonatal Organ and Tissue Donor

Justine Parsons

## INTRODUCTION

Internationally, the number of patients on waitlists for organ donation continues to grow. According to the Health Resources and Services Administration (HRSA), the United States has over 100,000 people listed, and over 700 of these are infants or children under 5 years. The Organ Procurement and Transplantation Network (OPTN) indicates that as of 2024, over 100 infants $<$ 12 months of age are waitlisted. These infants are primarily waiting for either a heart or a liver.

The situation is similar in many parts of the world. In Australia, the number of people waiting for organs exceeds supply significantly. Infants and children on waiting lists for solid organs are at substantially higher risk of dying while waiting, primarily due to the lack of available size-matched organs. Despite significant advances in the clinical management of infants and children on waitlists, an infant waiting for a donation of a heart has a mortality risk of between 8% and 17% (Klein et al., 2023).

In the United Kingdom (UK), in 2023, there were 39 children $<$ 18 years on the waitlist for solid organs. In the same year, there were only three donors in the same age bracket (National Health Service, Blood and Transplant).

Despite being recognized as a world leader in organ donation rates, Spain continues to experience challenges when considering organ donation for infants and children. At both the donor and transplantation levels, multiple barriers and considerations often result in poorer rates for pediatric donors and recipients (Núñez et al., 2020).

## ORGAN AND TISSUE DONATION POTENTIAL IN THE NEONATAL INTENSIVE CARE UNIT

Research has demonstrated that many infants who die in the neonatal intensive care unit (NICU) meet criteria that render them potential candidates for organ and tissue donation. Current evidence indicates that while there may be a large pool of potential neonatal donors, studies discussing neonatal organ utilization are relatively few (Bluhme et al., 2023). However, multiple case studies have presented successful kidney, heart, liver, and hepatocyte transplants.

Criteria for determining suitability for donation depend on each country's legislation, state laws and policies, and even health organization guidelines (Table 23.1). For example, in the UK, infants from 32 weeks corrected gestational age and $>$ 2.5 kg can be considered for tissue donation, and those from 37 weeks corrected gestational age for solid organ donation. The National Health Service Blood and Transplant division sets these criteria. In the United States, organ and tissue donation is governed by the OPTN, and in Australia, the Organ and Tissue Authority (OTA) is regulated by the Human Tissue Act. Specific gestational age, weight, and medical suitability are determined and overseen by these types of agencies.

Internationally, identifying and considering strategies that improve the pool of donors is critical. Multiple studies demonstrate that there are not insignificant numbers of infants dying in the NICUs who meet eligibility criteria (Trottier et al., 2021), and that infant families desire the opportunity to have all options offered to them, including the possibility of organ donation (Crouch et al., 2023).

Neonatal organs for infant recipients take advantage of the immaturity of each patient's immune system, often allowing for ABO-incompatible organs to be transplanted. Infants do not typically develop antibodies until approximately 6 months of age, and even then, only in low levels that permit ABO-incompatible transplants until approximately 12 months of age (Shaz et al., 2024).

### Clinical Exclusion Criteria

There are very few criteria that actually preclude organ and tissue donation. Generally, medical suitability screening weighs up risks and benefits to the recipient; therefore, infants should be consistently referred to donation specialist teams to make clinical suitability decisions (ANZICS, 2013). Table 23.2 lists a range of conditions that are commonly thought to exclude a patient from donation but may, in fact, be acceptable.

**TABLE 23.1**

**BROAD ELIGIBILITY CRITERIA INTERNATIONALLY—EXAMPLES**

| | United States | United Kingdom | Australia | Spain | Canada | Netherlands |
|---|---|---|---|---|---|---|
| Tissue donation | ≥ 36 weeks' gestation | ≥ 32 weeks' gestation and > 2.5 kg | ≥ 34 weeks' gestation | ≥ 34 weeks' gestation | ≥ 36 weeks' gestation | ≥ 37 weeks' gestation |
| Solid organ donation | ≥ 36 weeks' gestation and > 2 kg | ≥ 37 weeks' gestation | ≥ 34 weeks' gestation and > 3 kg (some flexibility on this) | ≥ 34 weeks' gestation and > 2 kg | ≥ 36 weeks' gestation and > 2.2 kg | ≥ 37 weeks' gestation and > 3 kg |

**TABLE 23.2**

**COMMON CONDITIONS AND DONATION ACCEPTABILITY**

| Common Conditions | Accepted or Excluded? |
|---|---|
| Infection (including CMV, or infants born to HIV +, mothers who are hepatitis B or C+) | Infants with treated infection, bacterial or viral, are accepted. |
| Organ dysfunction | Infants with acute organ dysfunction are accepted, particularly with previously normal organ function. Organs that have endured dysfunction in one infant, may not have dysfunction in a different patient. |
| History of hypoxia | Infants with hypoxic episodes at birth, but now resolved, are accepted. Neonatal organs and tissues demonstrate resilience in recovery. |
| Hematologic malignancy (such as leukemia) | Infants with an acute hematologic malignancy are excluded. |

CMV, cytomegalovirus.

## GOVERNING PRINCIPLES OF ORGAN DONATION IN THE NICU

- While the opportunity for neonatal organ donation is rare mainly due to improvements in infant/child mortality as well as advances in medical management, those infants who do meet eligibility criteria must be cared for by staff trained and confident in the process of identification, clinical management, and family support.
- Organ and tissue donation is an altruistic act that benefits patients in need and society. The process must always ensure patient rights, dignity, and the wishes of the family.
- Research demonstrates that families of infants who die in the NICU wish to be offered the opportunity to donate their infant's organs/tissues. Parents of infants who die have few opportunities to parent their children or make loving decisions for them, and they report that the donation conversation is a meaningful parenting experience for them (Crouch et al., 2023).
- Organ and tissue donation and transplantation processes must:
  - Demonstrate respect for all aspects of human dignity, including all involved individuals' worth, welfare, rights, beliefs, perceptions, customs, and cultural heritage.
  - Respect the dignity, rights, beliefs, and cultural heritage of all individuals.
  - Give priority to the potential donor and their family's needs over organ procurement.
  - Protect transplant recipients from harm.
  - Recognize the needs of the health professionals involved.
  - Ensure that just and transparent processes govern the organ and tissue allocation.
  - Ensure that those families who choose not to donate are treated with equal respect and understanding.

## GOALS OF CARE DURING NEONATAL ORGAN/TISSUE DONATION

- Infants deemed eligible to donate organs/tissues are identified promptly near the time that the infant is determined to be at the end of life.
- Dignified care is provided to the infant and their family at the end of life.
- Any decision to donate organs or tissue, or not, will be made without undue stress or influence.
- Any decision by the family to donate the infant's organs or tissue or not will not affect the care provided by staff to the infant or family.
- Staff involved in the care of the infant donating organs or tissue will provide support to the infant's family.
- Staff involved in providing care for the infant donating organs or tissue will receive appropriate support and opportunities to debrief, as well as further counseling if requested.
- If organ or tissue donation is pursued, an established clinical process that enables the retrieval of viable organs or tissues is followed.

## PATHWAYS TO ORGAN DONATION

Organ and tissue donation is a complex process involving multidisciplinary teams of health professionals. The most critical component in the organ donation process in the NICU is identifying eligible infants. Studies indicate that referral patterns for organ donation in the NICU may not be optimum. Timely referral to the organ and tissue donation service is rare (Aghion et al., 2020).

Generally, there are two pathways to organ and tissue donation: after neurologic death (or brain death) and after circulatory death, both rely on the patient being managed and supported in an intensive care or critical care area of the health facility.

### Donation After Neurologic Death

Donation after neurologic death (DND) refers to the donation of organs or tissues following the irreversible cessation of brain function. In adults or older children, this may be following a traumatic brain injury such as a hemorrhage or asphyxial event. The universally accepted determination of neurologic death relies on two separate medical assessments of the absence of brainstem reflexes, motor responses, and respiratory drive (without the presence of hypothermia, sedation, or metabolic derangement) from a known cause. The minimum age to confidently determine neurologic death varies by country but is somewhere in the vicinity of 36 to 37 weeks' gestation. Regardless of age, there are very few infants determined to be neurologically deceased, with adults outnumbering pediatric patients 100:1 (Spears et al., 2022).

Neurologic death is extremely rare in neonatal patients, even those with severe hypoxic encephalopathy, and subsequently, DND for NICU infants is also extremely rare. This is, in part, due to physiologic differences inherent in infants that complicate the required testing to determine brain death. Infants have open sutures and fontanelles that allow some brain parenchyma displacement, altered flow of cerebrospinal fluid, and tolerance to raised intracranial pressure from injury. Infants born before term may also have immature brainstem reflexes. This makes the interpretation of brain death test results challenging, creating a lack of confidence for the clinician.

It is also worth noting that one of the standard treatments for infants with encephalopathy is targeted hypothermia, often to temperatures considered moderately hypothermic for adults. Therapeutic cooling can dampen the neurologic response to some aspects of the required testing and delay sedatives' physiologic clearance. Due to the rarity of neurologic death in infants and a distinct paucity of research in this area, a conservative approach to testing is recommended, with a 24-hour waiting period between two neurologic death testing processes.

Infants determined to be neurologically deceased and consented to organ donation remain ventilated and supported throughout the process up until organ retrieval. Figure 23.1

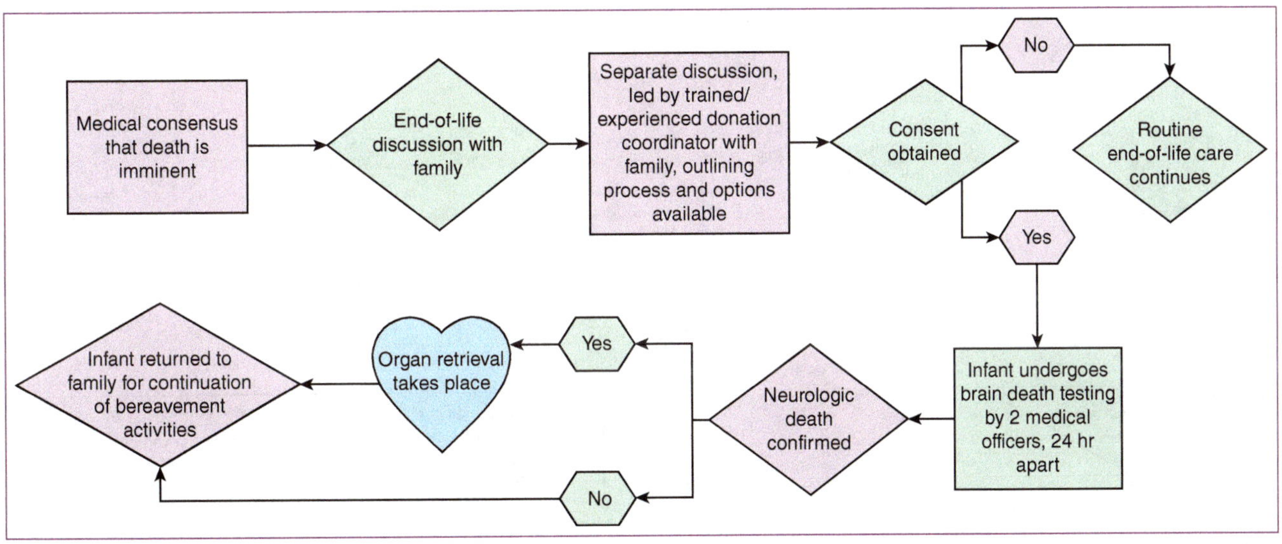


FIGURE 23.1 DND pathway for NICU infants.

outlines the process from the determination of end of life until organ retrieval.

### Donation After Circulatory Death

Donation after circulatory death (DCD) refers to the donation of organs or tissues following cessation of circulation, followed by a waiting period whereby circulation does not spontaneously restart. Patients are eligible for DCD where treatment is considered futile, are medically determined to be at the end of life, and withdrawal of life-sustaining measures has been discussed and agreed to with the next of kin. Research indicates that this is the most common pathway for infant patients in the NICU to meet the criteria for organ donation. Figure 23.2 outlines the process from end-of-life determination to organ donation retrieval.

## FAMILY CONVERSATION ON ORGAN AND TISSUE DONATION

Conversation on organ/tissue donation should not occur until the family and medical team have reached a consensus on the end-of-life status of the infant (da Silva Knihs et al., 2022). Raising the potential for organ or tissue donation should only proceed once the family has had an opportunity to discuss all end-of-life options available to them and consideration of all possible outcomes has taken place. This 'decoupling' of the end-of-life conversation from the potential for organ donation conversation is important in ensuring that no conflict of interest is perceived where families might question whether end-of-life care is proposed to obtain organ donation (AAP, 2023).

Research demonstrates that initial discussions with family on organ and tissue donation are ideally managed by an experienced donation specialist, separate from the treating team. This may be a donor-specialist medical practitioner or donor-specialist nurse with extensive training and knowledge in the nuances of raising the prospect of donation, answering questions regarding processes and pathways, and, critically, supporting family members throughout.

Research indicates that families, regardless of the decision made, welcome being approached about the possibility of organ and tissue donation (Darlington et al., 2019). The conversation validates their infant/child's existence. Where families are not approached, negative assumptions about the quality of their infant/child's organs might be made.

### Donation Specialist Teams

Doctors and nurses working exclusively in the field of organ and tissue donation have extensive training and experience in managing the donation process, from referral to organ retrieval and beyond. As a result, they offer unique skills and knowledge in supporting donor families throughout a traumatic time in their lives. Families during this time are vulnerable, and donation specialist staff navigate the family's needs while coordinating the practical aspects of the donation process with great skill and exquisite sensitivity (Aviles et al., 2022). By engaging the organ donation specialist team early, families are provided with the space, time, and information they require to make decisions that are right for them regarding the donation of their infant/child's organs or tissues.

### Family Decision Making About Organ and Tissue Donation

Studies demonstrate that complex factors can influence a family's view of organ or tissue donation for their infant/child and subsequent decision-making. Reported reasons for consenting or refusing organ donation are varied (Table 23.3).

Where a family indicates they wish to proceed with the organ/tissue donation process, the donation specialist will outline the following points during the conversation:

- organs/tissue that may be suitable for donation
- potential reasons donation might not proceed

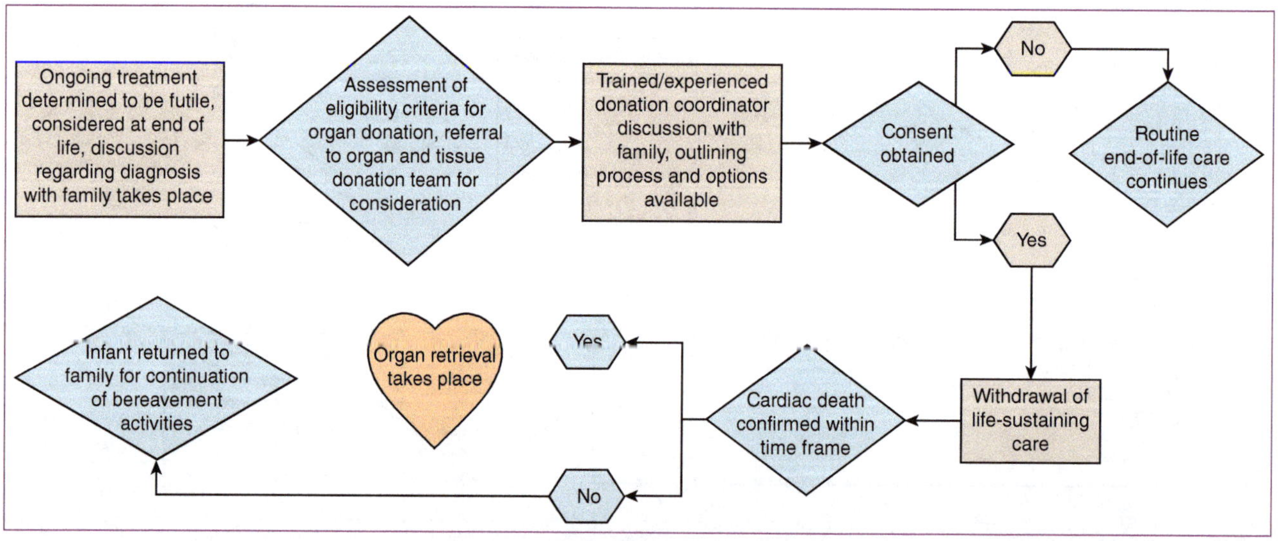


**FIGURE 23.2** DCD pathway for NICU infants.

**TABLE 23.3**

**FAMILY REASONS FOR CONSENT/REFUSAL FOR ORGAN DONATION**

| Reasons for Consenting | Reasons for Refusing |
|---|---|
| • Feelings of altruism, helping others<br>• Belief that their infant lives on in another<br>• Feelings of reciprocity<br>• Belief that donation is "the right thing to do"<br>• Validates the value and existence of their infant's life, provides meaning<br>• Pride in infant's ability to save the life of another | • Process interfering with end-of-life care<br>• Fear of infant's body being disfigured<br>• Belief that infant has "suffered enough"<br>• Overwhelming grief<br>• Timeframes too long<br>• Significant amounts of paperwork |

- timelines and expectations for the family during the process; typically, the end-of-life care processes can add 8 to 10 hours
- legal requirements for donation to proceed: written consent, completion of medical questionnaires, and so on
- comprehensive medical history of the infant and family to assess suitability
- discussion with other health providers regarding history (as applicable)
- consent for blood testing for screening, cross-matching, and tissue typing, which often includes maternal blood sampling
- plan for and location of removal of cardiorespiratory support (operating theaters, NICU)
- support for the family in the NICU environment throughout the process
- planning to update and advise the family of any changes affecting the donation process

## Family Refusal of Organ and Tissue Donation

In the event a family declines to donate organs or tissues, every effort should be made to explore the reasons behind the refusal. Then, offering condolences to the family and expressing gratitude for their consideration of donation, all care should continue as per routine end-of-life local practices. Families must be supported regardless of their decision regarding organ/tissue donation.

## PREDONATION NURSING CARE

The neonatal donor should be managed according to standard hemodynamic and respiratory strategies for neonates in the NICU.

- All vital observations should be within normal target ranges.
- Temperature to be maintained above 98.6°F (36°C). Therapeutic cooling is ceased after the end-of-life discussion, and rewarming commenced.
- The heart rate should be stable and appropriate for gestation. An arterial line should be in situ, where possible, for blood sampling and arterial blood pressure monitoring.
- Blood and mean arterial pressure are to be maintained as appropriate for gestation. Inotropes can be used to maintain blood pressure as per local policy.
- IV access for medications and hydration.
- Blood gas: aim for pH 7.35 to 7.45; $PCO_2$ 35 to 55; $PO_2$: 50 to 70 (term), 45 to 65 (preterm); $HCO_3$ 22 to 26 mEq/L; BE –2 to +2 mEd/L. Variations should be discussed with the donation specialist team.
- Maintain urine output > 1 ml/kg/hr.
- Blood collection as follows:
  - blood cross-match
  - full blood count
  - electrolytes
  - serology, with the donation specialist team advising on the minimum volume of blood required for testing after collaboration with hospital pathology services
- Ongoing care and assessment:
  - Continue antibiotics and all other medications.
  - Obtain chest x-ray, cardiac echocardiogram, and 3-lead electrocardiogram (ECG) if they are not complete.
  - Maintain hemodynamic stability.
  - Maintain normal electrolytes/blood gases.
  - Contact the donation specialist team when questions arise about donor management or changes in condition.

## PREDONATION FAMILY CARE

Parents who have consented to organ donation require intensive support throughout the entire process, but research indicates that some particularly critical moments benefit from extra care (Sarti et al., 2022). These include the immediate period following the decision to consent, during predonation clinical testing, and when the retrieval surgery time/plan is arranged.

Families who have provided feedback on the process and their experience of organ donation for their infant/child identify key factors that negatively or positively affect their perception of it (Table 23.4).

## INTRAOPERATIVE ORGAN DONATION NURSING CARE

Nursing care throughout the organ donation procedure is per local routine intraoperative care for other procedures. In conjunction with the operating team, scrub and scout nurses, and the donation specialist team, the team is usually in attendance and can provide regular updates to family members on the procedure's progress.

**TABLE 23.4**

**POSITIVE AND NEGATIVE FACTORS RELATED TO ORGAN DONATION**

| Positive Factors | Negative Factors |
|---|---|
| • Previous knowledge of organ donation concepts and programs<br>• Donor specialist team availability and communication<br>• Good rapport and open, trusting communication with bedside healthcare team<br>• Topic raised with sensitivity and care<br>• Availability of support person with shared experience (via donation networks) or specialist knowledge of donation<br>• Clear and simple information on how procedure is conducted, including what to expect when their infant is returned to them (suture lines, etc.)<br>• Advanced notification of clinical testing and required timeframes<br>• Provision of time to ask questions, identify fears<br>• Advanced notice of operating theater time for retrieval surgery where possible<br>• Ability to remain with infant/child until retrieval surgery, and accompany them to operating theaters<br>• Provision of support person while infant/child undergoing retrieval surgery<br>• Provision of updates throughout retrieval surgery, including organs successfully retrieved<br>• Ability for parents to spend time with their infant/child following retrieval surgery in a dedicated bereavement space | • No previous knowledge of organ donation concepts or programs<br>• Untrained/inexperienced staff member raising possibility of organ donation<br>• Topic raised without sensitivity<br>• Feeling pressured to make decisions<br>• Poor communication with bedside healthcare team<br>• Lack of information regarding process<br>• Lack of information regarding timeframes<br>• Organizational guidelines that do not encourage family involvement in processes<br>• Being left alone with no identified waiting space during retrieval surgery<br>• Lack of updates regarding retrieval surgery<br>• Inability to provide, or limiting time in, bereavement space for families following organ donation process |

Some families have found it comforting to send a special toy or memento to theaters with the infant to remain with them during the procedure. The donor specialist team can arrange this if required.

Donor infants are treated with utmost dignity and respect throughout the surgical procedure and its aftermath. At the completion of the procedure, the infant's surgical wound is neatly sutured and dressings applied. The donor specialist nurse will sponge the infant to remove disinfectants, etc., and dress/wrap the infant for return to their family.

## POSTOPERATIVE ORGAN DONATION NURSING CARE

The family should always be offered the opportunity to spend time with their infant following the organ donation operation. This can occur in the NICU, in a space dedicated to bereavement, or elsewhere in the hospital per local policy.

Then, usual bereavement care, such as bathing, hand/footprint collection, or other memory-making activities, can continue. It is important that the family continues to be supported throughout this time.

## DONATION SUPPORT FOLLOW-UP

Generally, organ and tissue donation programs offer specific follow-up services to support families both immediately after the donation and in the months and years to come. These may include phone contact, letters, or visits from the donor specialist nurse. Many programs also offer ongoing supportive counseling or remembrance ceremonies; however, this depends on the country.

Research demonstrates that many donor families are interested in contacting recipient families (Cignarella, et al., 2023). However, in most countries, anonymity and privacy are legal requirements of the organ donation process; therefore, deidentified written contact is generally the only method of contact using the organ donation specialist team as the intermediary. Internationally, many donor and recipient families have advocated for law reform to facilitate identifiable written contact or face-to-face contact between donor families and recipients where mutually requested (Cignarella et al., 2023). Studies indicate that there can be both benefits and burdens to this approach, although research is limited.

## HEALTHCARE STAFF AND ORGAN/TISSUE DONATION IN THE NICU

NICU staff are in pivotal positions of influence when considering organ and tissue donation for infants. The professional relationships and rapport built with families throughout the NICU admission can result in mutual feelings of trust and respect, which in turn can positively affect the family's experience of the organ donation process.

Given that the end-of-life care and the organ donation process overlap, healthcare staff can feel uncomfortable in this space. Staff often report that challenges in providing care for the dying infant, supporting family members, and managing tasks related to organ preservation require a delicate balance (Le Dorze et al., 2022).

### Education and Training

It is critical that healthcare staff are educated on the organ donation process and professionally and emotionally supported throughout to enable them to support a family throughout end-of-life care and potential organ donation.

Research indicates that staff finds raising the topic of organ donation extremely difficult (Darlington et al., 2019). While many healthcare professionals acknowledge that organ and tissue donation is vital, a lack of training and education can mean that staff avoids raising the prospect, creating delays in referral to specialist organ donation teams (Aghion et al., 2020). Another aspect for consideration is the relative rarity of organ donation in the NICU, creating staff who are not practiced in the skills required for family donation conversation. This results in health professionals with misinformation regarding donation practices and missing potential candidates who could be approached (Bursac et al., 2021).

Multiple studies outline the gap in donation education for health professionals, even those currently practicing in NICUs. A survey of intensive care physicians and nursing staff undertaken in Canada demonstrated that less than two-thirds of physicians reported a high level of comfort with the donation process, primarily attributed to a lack of education and training gaps (Bursac et al., 2021). A comprehensive training program should be provided to minimize doubts and fears for neonatal healthcare professionals (Caserio et al., 2022).

Easily accessible information and hospital guidelines need to be available to assist staff in confidently caring for an infant or child involved in the organ and tissue donation process (Simonsson et al., 2020). Education programs designed around a "high-stakes, low-frequency" philosophy that delivers training in multimodality are critical in eliminating the organ donation knowledge deficit barrier as it exists.

### Emotional and Psychological Support

Neonatal intensive care nurses are familiar with high-stress and complicated situations as part of their work; however, incorporating organ donation into their practice can add new layers of emotional and psychological complexity.

Studies have described nurses' experiences of caring for a patient and family throughout the process as emotionally demanding, multifaceted, and requiring a high level of responsibility (Simonsson et al., 2020). Nurses report needing intensive support from their managers and time to recover from the emotional strain experienced. Opportunities to reflect and debrief as a team after the donation experience were also seen as positive and supportive. Staff involved in the donation process should have a chance to receive information about the donation outcome and be provided with an opportunity to attend feedback sessions.

Any staff member who does not wish to participate in the donation process for religious or ethical reasons should be given the right to withdraw from caring for patients who may become organ donors. However, they must ensure that others are free to proceed with care.

## FUTURE DIRECTIONS FOR NEONATAL ORGAN DONATION

One of the main differences between DND and DCD relates to the warm ischemic time of the organ, between the time life support is withdrawn and the time circulatory death is confirmed. With DCD rates increasing internationally and within neonatal populations, researchers are monitoring patient and graft survival closely. So far, studies indicate that outcomes for DCD grafts are comparable to those of DND grafts, providing reassurance for clinicians (Kleinmahon et al., 2017).

Organ donation processes, optimization methods, and transplantation techniques continue to develop and improve globally. This includes organ selection, preserving organ tissues, managing organ transportation to the recipient site, and surgical methods.

At present, there are three standard methods of organ retrieval: direct procurement using machine perfusion (DP-MP), procurement after thoracic-abdominal-normothermic regional perfusion (TA-NRP) using either MP (NRP-MP) or traditional cold static storage (NRP-CS) (Fedson, 2024). Research into patient outcomes using these techniques continues, especially concerning minimizing warm ischemic time and further fine-tuning methods for surgical donation teams.

Another promising development is neonatal hepatocyte retrieval after DCD. Studies indicate that this is feasible and results in good graft maturation (Bluhme et al., 2023). Neonatal liver hepatocytes offer a greater viability and function compared to adult hepatocytes. Hepatocyte transplantation may prove to be a practical method for treating liver failure.

## ONLINE RESOURCES

**CourseConnect**

Resources for this chapter are online and available at www.springerpub.com/courseconnect.

## REFERENCES

References for this chapter are online and available at www.springerpub.com/courseconnect.

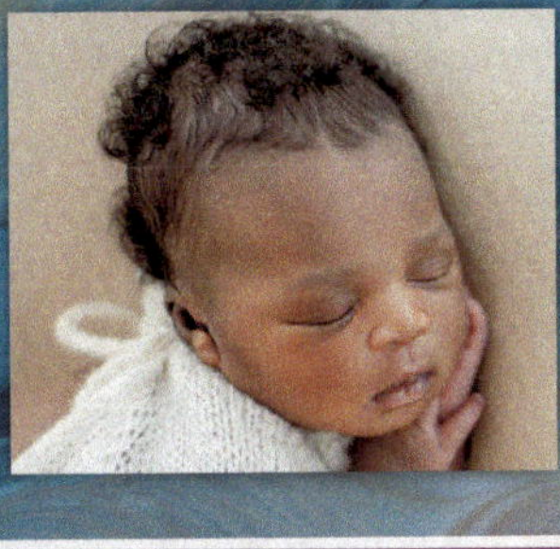
Source: tan4ikk/Adobe Stock.

CHAPTER 24

# Neonatal Abstinence Syndrome/Neonatal Withdrawal Syndrome

Gail A. Bagwell

## INTRODUCTION

Opiate/substance use disorder and neonatal abstinence syndrome (NAS)/neonatal opioid withdrawal syndrome (NOWS) are major health problems for pregnant persons and neonates in the United States. Neonatal intensive care units (NICUs) and special care units (SCNs) have been inundated with babies over the past 20 years who are withdrawing not only from opiates but from other licit and illicit substances that they were exposed to in utero. This chapter discusses the history, incidence, and diagnosis of NAS/NOWS, the screening tools and nonpharmacologic and pharmacologic management involved, the importance of nonjudgmental care of the parent–infant dyad, and the long-term outcomes of the NAS/NOWS neonate.

## HISTORY OF OPIATE/SUBSTANCE USE DISORDER

Opioid use during pregnancy is not a new phenomenon in the United States. Opioid use disorder in the United States is as old as our country: It dates back to the American Revolution, when both American and British soldiers were given opium for illness and injuries (Courtwright, 2001). With the discovery of morphine in 1803 and then the invention of the hypodermic syringe and needle in 1856, many feel that the first actual opiate use disorder (OUD) occurred with the Civil War in the United States. Morphine was used like opium in the American Revolution for the sick and injured soldiers but was also used to treat diseases of the uterus, ovaries, and nervous conditions of women. During this time, morphine did not require a prescription, so it was readily used. By 1895, one in 200 Americans had an OUD, with 60% of them being upper-class or middle-class White women (Courtwright, 2001). The use of morphine for women was largely due to a lack of understanding and training by physicians at the time; as medical education became more rigorous and knowledge of problems increased, and with the release of a new analgesic called aspirin in 1897, the use of morphine decreased. While the OUD problem did not go away, the OUD patient profile changed from war veterans and upper-class or middle-class White women to lower-class males and new immigrants with the opening of opium dens in America in the early 1900s. With the changing profile of the OUD, legal ramifications began to take hold in the United States, making possession of opium and heroin illegal, but these ramifications did not deter use.

In the 20th century, the heroin epidemic in the 1950s and 1960s brought attention to drug use by pregnant persons and concern about the effects of drugs on the developing fetus. In the late 1970s and the 1980s, heroin fell out of favor, and cocaine became an issue, but by the 2000s, heroin started to gain popularity again.

The resurgence of heroin is attributed in large part to the prescription drug abuse that began in the 1990s. Simultaneously, several events occurred that led to prescription drug abuse: The Joint Commission instituted the mandatory assessment of pain as the fifth vital sign; a new opiate medication, oxycodone, was promoted to practitioners as a nonaddictive opiate analgesic; insurance companies tightened their belts on what nonpharmacologic treatments that they would pay for, limiting what a practitioner could do for patients in acute pain; and healthcare practitioners and healthcare facilities began patient satisfaction surveys. These events resulted in practitioners overprescribing oxycodone and other narcotics to patients, which led many to a new generation of patients with OUD because we now know that oxycodone is as powerful as or more powerful than heroin (Quinones, 2015).

The Substance Abuse and Mental Health Services Administration (SAMHSA) estimated that in 2023, 47.7 million people were abusing illicit or prescription drugs. As in previous opiate epidemics, women were not immune to the problem. For women (ages 12 and older), SAMHSA (Center for Behavioral Health Statistics and Quality (CBHSQ), 2024) reported that in 2022, illicit substance use was admitted by 20.5 million females. Of the illicit substance use, 4.3 million females admitted to opioid misuse, both illicit and licit drugs. The largest category of misuse was prescription pain reliever misuse, being reported by 92.2% of female misusers. The most common misused prescription pain reliever was hydrocodone at 41.9%, followed by oxycodone at 28.6%. A 2021 study by Hirai et al. reported that from 2010 to 2017, maternal opioid-related diagnoses increased from 3.5/1,000 delivery hospitalizations to 8.2. This represented a 4.6/1,000 delivery hospitalizations increase.

## HISTORY AND EPIDEMIOLOGY OF NEONATAL ABSTINENCE SYNDROME

A consequence of the opiate epidemic is the exposure of the fetus in utero to opiates, which results in neonates withdrawing from the substance after birth. This is referred to as NAS or NOWS, which is not a new phenomenon. The term NAS was first coined by Dr. Loretta Finnegan and her colleagues in the early 1970s to describe neonates for whom they were caring who were withdrawing from heroin and other opiates, but the term now includes neonates withdrawing from other substances as well. More recently, the term NOWS was coined to describe the current group of neonates experiencing withdrawal in our current epidemic (Patrick et al., 2020). However, Finnegan was not the first description in the medical literature of neonates withdrawing from substances.

The first descriptions of this phenomenon appeared in medical publications as early as 1875 under the term *congenital morphinism* (Perlstein, 1947). With the morphine epidemic described earlier, there were documented cases of neonates dying several days after birth, even though they appeared normal at birth. The case reports described neonates displaying the signs of what we today call NAS/NOWS.

As the opioid epidemic increased in the early 2000s, NICUs and SCNs began to see an explosion of neonates being admitted for NAS/NOWS. In a first-of-its-kind article on the epidemic of NAS, Patrick et al. (2012) did a retrospective, cross-sectional analysis of data from the Centers for Medicare and Medicaid (CMS) of neonates diagnosed with NAS from 2000 to 2009 in the United States to determine the prevalence of NAS. The investigators found that the number of neonates experiencing NAS increased from approximately 1.3 per 1,000 births in 2000 to approximately 3.4 per 1,000 births in 2009. The number of neonates tripled in 9 years from approximately 4,000 to approximately 13,539 neonates, or approximately one neonate being born every hour with NAS (Patrick et al., 2012).

A follow-up study by Patrick et al. (2015) revealed that the numbers of infants being diagnosed with NAS continued to increase from 2009 to 2012. In the 2015 study, the investigators also looked at the regional prevalence of NAS and found that it varied from 2.6 per 1,000 births to 16.2 per 1,000 births based on geographic location. The overall incidence of NAS in 2012 was 5.8 per 1,000 births, equivalent to 21,732 births or one infant born every 25 minutes. In 2018, Winkelman et al. reported that in 2014, the overall incidence of NAS in the United States was 14.4 per 1,000 births, or one infant being born every 15 minutes. The most recent data demonstrated that from 2010 to 2017, NAS/NOWS increased significantly from 4.0/1,000 birth hospitalizations to 7.3/1,000 birth hospitalizations. This represented a 3.3/1,000 birth hospitalizations increase, but as in the 2015 study, the rate varied based on geographic location (Hirai et al., 2021).

As the number of babies being diagnosed with NAS/NOWS increased, mother/infant units were not equipped to care for the withdrawing infant, so the majority of the neonates affected were transferred to NICUs and SCNs to be observed and treated. Tolia et al. (2015) reported that the number of NICU admissions increased from seven per 1,000 admissions in 2004 to 27 per 1,000 admissions in 2013, putting a strain on NICUs and SCNs around the country by taking up valuable bed space and utilizing resources designed for ill neonates, neonates with congenital defects, and premature infants.

The increasing number of neonates with NAS that are being born in the United States has put a strain not only on hospitals but also on the healthcare system. In 2014, approximately 82% of all neonates with NAS were covered by Medicaid, up from 73.7% a decade earlier in 2004. Neonates with a NAS diagnosis who were Medicaid recipients had longer hospital stays than neonates with NAS who were covered by private insurance and neonates covered by Medicaid who did not have NAS. As a result of the increasing number of Medicaid-covered neonates, hospital costs increased from $65.4 million to $462 million during the 10 years from 2004 to 2014, putting a strain on many systems (Winkelman et al., 2018). The most recent data from 2017 demonstrated that the majority of infants with NAS, 84%, continue to be covered by Medicaid (Hirai et al., 2021).

## DIAGNOSIS

Diagnosis of NAS/NOWS begins with a thorough checking of the pregnant person's history of any substance usage during the pregnancy. A policy of universal screening for all pregnant persons should be in place in physician offices, hospitals, and birthing centers, because substance abuse occurs across all socioeconomic classes. Many confuse screening with testing pregnant people for a substance abuse problem and believe the terms are interchangeable, which they are not. Screening is different from testing, because it consists of interviewing the pregnant person for use of both licit and illicit substances, while testing involves checking for presence or absence of substances in biologic fluids.

### Pregnant Person Screening

When screening the pregnant person, the interview should be done in a nonjudgmental manner and in a private setting, away from family members and friends. This is done because many family members and friends may be unaware of the person's substance usage or may not want the person to divulge this information for fear of consequences. The interview questions should include the use of five types of substances: (a) prescription drugs; (b) over-the-counter drugs; (c) nutritional supplements, including herbal medications; (d) legal substances, such as alcohol, nicotine, and caffeine; and (e) illicit/illegal drugs. In addition to the type of substance/drug used, the length of use, the amount used, the method of use, the context of use, and any history of drug treatment are essential. For pregnant persons who do not admit to drug use, a history of drug habits of family members and friends should be obtained because often the person may admit to a family member's use/abuse but not to their own use/abuse.

There are many tools available to assist with screening patients with substance use disorders (SUDs), such as the Tolerance, Annoyed, Cutdown, Exacerbated (T-ACE); Substance Use Risk Profile—Pregnancy Scale (SURP-P); Pregnancy, Past, Partner, Parental Use (4Ps); Alcohol Use Disorders Intervention Test-C (AUDIT-C); National Institute on Drug Abuse (NIDA) Drug Use Screening Tool and Quick Screen; Opioid Risk Tool; Screening to Brief Intervention (S2BI); Brief Screener for Alcohol, Tobacco, and other Drugs (BSTAD); Cut down, Annoed, Guilty, Eye-opene (CAGE); and the Car, Relax, Forget, Friends, Trouble (CRAFFT). The BSTAD, CRAFFT, and S2BI are designed specifically for adolescents, and the remaining tools are designed for adults, though the NIDA test does have an adaptation for adolescents (NIDA, 2018). The choice of the correct tool is based on the age of the clientele and what the clinician needs to assess. Regardless of the tool chosen, it is important to use an evidence-based and validated tool and to ask questions nonjudgmentally.

One method to assist with obtaining information from a client is motivational interviewing (MI). MI was developed in the 1980s by Miller and Rollnick based on the work by Carl Rogers as a way to elicit information from a client and to begin the change process (Substance Abuse and Mental Health Services Administration-Health Resources and Services Administration [SAMHSA], 2021). MI utilizes the four principles of expressing empathy, avoiding arguing, developing discrepancy, rolling with resistance, and supporting self-efficacy. For the interviewer to be successful in using the MI technique, he or she must listen more than talk, be sensitive and open to the person's issue, invite the person to be open and to discuss and explore ideas of change, encourage the person to discuss reasons not to change, ask for permission to give them feedback, reassure the pregnant person/parent that ambivalence to change is normal, help them identify successes and challenges, seek to understand the person, summarize what they are hearing, value the person's opinion, and remind oneself that the person is capable of making their own choices (SAMHSA, 2021).

## Pregnant Person Biologic Testing

Urine drug testing can be ordered to help with the detection of a substance abuse disorder. Pregnant person urine toxicology is easy to obtain but is not always accurate. Persons with SUD have a fear of losing their babies and will go to great lengths to hide their substance use. The half-life of substances of abuse varies, so depending on the timing of the urine drug test, the urine may or may not be positive. Persons with SUD also know methods to ensure that the urine drug test has a false negative. A quick search online will show novel ways to pass a urine drug test, ranging from devices that could be used, information on how long substances are detectable, and how to clear the urine of substances. For these reasons, the pregnant person's urine drug test could be negative, even though there is a SUD. In addition, it is important to remember that pregnant person drug testing has legal implications if not all pregnant persons admitted to a hospital or a medical practice are tested because it could be considered profiling. Because of the legal issues of testing only certain individuals, many medical practices and hospitals are adopting universal drug testing protocols for all pregnant persons.

## Neonatal Testing

When an infant is symptomatic of NAS/NOWS, or there are indicators that the pregnant parent was abusing substances, laboratory tests can be ordered to help with the diagnosis of NAS/NOWS. Toxicology tests can be performed on neonatal urine, hair, meconium, or the umbilical cord. Each of these tests has its pros and cons related to their use and legal implications. Neonatal urine toxicology is the easiest to obtain but is not always accurate. Neonatal urine has several limitations, some of which are: (a) only recent drug use can be detected, so if the first urine is missed, the test may be negative; (b) if the pregnant parent was an infrequent user, the drug test may be negative; or (c) if the pregnant person has not used in the week before delivery of the infant, the test may be negative depending on the drug abused and its half-life (Hudak & Tan, 2012; Kocherlakota, 2014; Kwong & Ryan, 1997; Langman et al., 2023; Ostrea et al., 1976; Patrick et al., 2020; Sutter et al., 2014). If the urine drug test is positive, it is important to review the pregnant parent's medication record during delivery because narcotics given to the pregnant person during labor will show up in the neonate's urine.

Hair testing for drug use is more accurate than urine drug testing because it can detect in-utero drug usage for the last 3 to 4 months of pregnancy (Kwong & Ryan, 1997; Ostrea et al., 1976; Vinner et al., 2003). Hair testing is rarely used in the neonatal population because most newborns do not have the quantity of hair needed to perform the test, and for those who do, the mothers object to their newborns' hair being shaved (Kwong & Ryan, 1997).

Meconium analysis is the most common form of drug testing in the neonate and is considered the gold standard. Meconium analysis detects in-utero drug usage for the last two trimesters of pregnancy (Kocherlakota, 2014; Langman et al., 2023; Ostrea et al., 1976). Unfortunately, meconium is not always properly collected and stored in many units, leading to false-negative results. For meconium to be accurate, the entire column of meconium must be collected and stored in a specimen cup. Substance metabolites in meconium are stable for 2 weeks at room temperature but storing it in a refrigerator is preferable. When adding meconium to the specimen cup, the new meconium sample must be mixed with the existing sample to ensure that the metabolites are well distributed when the lab takes only one small sample for testing. **Quality and Safety:** **When the entire column of meconium has been passed and collected, the specimen is sent to the lab to be tested. The lab will only take a small sample (2–5 g) to be tested, so mixing all the meconium as it is added to the specimen cup is important.** While meconium is more accurate, it has its limitations. As stated before, false negatives will occur if it is not collected correctly. Second, if the infant is not suspected of being exposed in utero, not all of the meconium will be able to be collected. Thirdly, a specimen can be negative even if the mother abused drugs during pregnancy, depending on when and how often the mother abused drugs (Kocherlakota, 2014). Finally, meconium samples can be missed for infants who room-in with their mothers because the parents will throw the diapers away.

Umbilical cord testing for drug exposure in utero is a newer method of testing for pregnant parent drug usage. Like hair and meconium, the umbilical cord test is highly reliable and can detect the last 4 to 5 months of maternal drug usage (United States Drug Testing Laboratories [USDTL], 2024). The advantage of using the umbilical cord is the initial availability and ease of collection. A 6-inch segment of the umbilical cord is obtained at birth, drained of blood, cleansed per company protocol, labeled, sealed, and stored. The cord can be stored for a week at room temperature, refrigerated for up to 3 months, or frozen for up to 1 year (USDTL, 2024), so if an infant starts to show signs of withdrawal, the cord can be sent at that time. The disadvantage is that if the cord is not obtained at the time of birth, then it cannot be used.

**Quality and Safety: It is important to remember that no matter what type of specimen testing is done on a neonate, the appropriate chain of custody is maintained during the collection, labeling, and transport of the specimen from the unit to the laboratory. This is important for legal purposes.**

## Signs of NAS/NOWS

Of neonates exposed to substances in utero, approximately 55% to 96% will display signs of withdrawal (Hudak & Tan, 2012). For the majority of neonates, the onset of the acute signs of NAS can range from 12 to 96 hours after birth, though there are some cases reported of neonates beginning withdrawal only 7 days after birth. The wide range of time for withdrawal is related to the substance used, the timing of the last dose, the pregnant person's metabolism, the placental transport of the medication, as well as the neonatal gestation, metabolism, and excretion. The central and autonomic nervous system, the gastrointestinal system, and/or the respiratory system can be involved in the withdrawal process (Finnegan & MacNew, 1974; Hudak & Tan, 2012; Patrick et al., 2020). Table 24.1 outlines the most commonly seen signs of withdrawal in the neonate.

**TABLE 24.1**

**WITHDRAWAL SIGNS OF NAS/NOWS**

| Body System | Signs |
|---|---|
| Central nervous system | High-pitched continuous crying, irritability, tremors, hyperactive Moro reflex, sleep disturbances, increased muscle tone, skin excoriation, myoclonic jerking, and seizures |
| Autonomic nervous system | Fever, diaphoresis, mottling, sweating, and frequent yawning |
| Gastrointestinal system | Excessive sucking, poor feeding, regurgitation, vomiting, and loose or watery stools |
| Respiratory system | Tachypnea with or without retractions, frequent sneezing, nasal flaring, nasal stuffiness |

Not every neonate exposed to substances in utero will show signs of withdrawal. It has been well established that term neonates experience more significant withdrawal than preterm neonates, likely due to less exposure and a more mature nervous system (Hudak & Tan, 2012; Liu et al., 2010). However, other differences in withdrawal have been noted between males and females, between the type of substance exposure in utero, and, more recently, the finding of genetic polymorphisms. Studies are just beginning to be published on these differences. In a retrospective cohort study published in 2017, Charles et al. demonstrated that male neonates were more likely than female neonates to be diagnosed with NAS and require treatment; however, the severity of NAS was not affected by gender. Huybrechts et al. (2017) found in an observational cohort study that neonates exposed to antidepressants, benzodiazepines, and gabapentin had a 30% to 60% increase in NAS when compared to those infants not exposed.

In the past decade, there has been an increase in the number of studies in both addiction medicine and the study of NAS/NOWS, looking at the role of genetics and epigenetics. In adults, single nucleotide polymorphism (SNP) in the mu-opioid receptor (*OPRM1*), catechol-*o*-methyltransferase (*COMT*), and multidrug resistance (*ABCB1*) genes are associated with the risk of SUD (Vernovsky et al., 2024; Wachman et al., 2013; Wachman & Farrer, 2019). Wachman et al. (2013) did a multicenter prospective cohort study looking at DNA samples for variants in the SNPs of the *OPRM1*, *COMT*, and *ABCB1* genes of infants diagnosed with NAS. The results were that neonates with variants in the SNP of the *OPRM1* and *COMT* genes had significantly shorter lengths of hospital stay and a decreased need for medication therapy than those infants without. The *ABCB1* SNP did not make a difference in the length of stay or medication therapy. In another study, Mactier et al. (2017) looked for variations in neonate genotype of the *OPRM1*, *ABCB1*, *COMT*, *CYP2B6*, and *CYP2D6* genes as an explanation for the variation in the presentation of neonates whose mothers were maintained on methadone during pregnancy. The authors demonstrated that neonates treated for NAS were more likely to carry the homozygous allele of the *CYP2B6* gene. More recently, Vernovsky et al. (2024) looked at human studies on SNP, DNA methylation differences, and gene expression modifications seen in the placenta and body fluids of neonates with prenatal exposure versus those with non-prenatal exposure. The authors also reviewed animal studies that have identified the gene pathway that most likely contributes to the NAS/NOWS phenotype. As new information continues to emerge on how genes, epigenetics, and gene expression can influence how a neonate with NAS/NOWS will demonstrate signs of withdrawal and respond to therapy after in-utero exposure, it may lead to more tailored approaches in caring for the NAS/NOWS neonate soon.

With the increasing incidences of NAS/NOWS, it is easy to forget that the signs of NAS/NOWS are somewhat generalized and that other disease processes have similar signs. **Emergency Alert: Sepsis, hypoglycemia, and hypocalcemia have similar signs in newborns, so it is of utmost importance to rule these out before assuming that a neonate has NAS.**

## Tools for Assessing Signs of NAS

Several tools have been designed over the years to help quantify the onset and progression of signs of NAS/NOWS and judge the effectiveness of both nonpharmacologic and pharmacologic treatment. In the past, the most commonly used tool was the Finnegan Neonatal Abstinence Scoring System (FNASS), more commonly referred to as the Finnegan (Bagley et al., 2014; Gomez-Pomar & Finnegan, 2018), but the newer method for assessing is the Eat, Sleep, Console tool and has gained popularity because it is simpler to use and keeps the birthing parent–infant dyad together and out of the neonatal intensive care unit. The development of multiple tools over the years demonstrates the lack of agreement on how to best assess NAS/NOWS. The majority of tools have been validated for interrater reliability and sensitivity to diagnosing NAS/NOWS. Due to the subjective nature of the tools, especially the FNASS, it is essential for nurses to be trained on how to properly use a tool. One method for maintaining reliability in a nurse's assessment is to have nurses do dual scoring of an infant at least two times per day, which helps to maintain interrater reliability.

The tools range from the FNASS, which assesses for 21 different neurologic, autonomic, gastrointestinal, respiratory, and other signs to determine if a neonate is withdrawing, to a relatively simple newer tool called eat-sleep-console (ESC) that looks at three items to determine treatment for withdrawal, which includes whether the infant is eating at least 1 oz or breastfeeding well; whether the infant is sleeping greater than or equal to 1 hour; and whether the infant can be consoled within 10 minutes (Finnegan et al., 1975; Grossman et al., 2018). Table 24.2 compares the published tools for assessing NAS/NOWS. Studies looking at novel ways such as maternal vagal tone, fetal heart rate, skin conductance of the neonate, and brain-derived neurotropic factor levels within 48 hours of NICU admission have been done to assess and diagnose NAS/NOWS, but at this point these are not widely used (Wachman et al., 2018).

**TABLE 24.2**

**COMPARISON OF NEONATAL ABSTINENCE SCORING TOOLS**

| Name of Tool | Author | Year Published | Items Scored | Range of Scores | Treatment Score |
|---|---|---|---|---|---|
| FNASS | Finnegan et al. | 1975 | 21 | Severity ranges from 0 to 5 | Three continuous scores ≥8 or two continuous scores ≥12 |
| Narcotic Withdrawal Score | Lipsitz | 1975 | 11 | 0–3 | ≥4 |
| Neonatal Narcotic Withdrawal Index | Green & Suffett | 1981 | 7, with the seventh item being "other," which consists of 12 items | 0–2 | 5 or greater |
| Ostrea | Ostrea | 1976 | 6 | Ranking of symptoms | |
| Neonatal Withdraw Inventory | Zahorodny et al. | 1998 | 8 | 0–4 | Three continuous scores ≥8 or two continuous scores ≥12 |
| MOTHER NAS Scale | Jones et al. | 2010 | 19 | 0–8 | Two continuous scores ≥9 or one score ≥13 |
| FNASS—Short Form | Maguire, Cline, Parnell, & Tai | 2013 | 7 | 0–5 | Three continuous scores ≥8 or two continuous scores ≥12 |
| sFNASS | Gomez-Pomar et al. | 2017 | 10 | 0–5 | Three continuous scores ≥6 or two continuous scores ≥10 |
| ESC | Grossman et al. | 2018 | 3 | Yes or no to questions | Algorithm to determine treatment based on answers |

## MANAGEMENT

Once the infant is diagnosed with NAS/NOWS, management focuses on the prevention or worsening of withdrawal signs and the provision of comfort for the neonate. Both nonpharmacologic and pharmacologic treatment options are available to manage the neonate with NAS/NOWS. As more research becomes available on the detrimental effects of opioids and other medications on the developing newborn brain, the trend for treatment of babies with NAS/NOWS is to utilize nonpharmacologic treatment first, and only if that fails, then pharmacologic treatment would be utilized.

### Nonpharmacologic Treatment

Initially, nonpharmacologic interventions such as low lighting and noise levels, skin-to-skin contact by the birthing parent, as well as swaddling and holding the infant are utilized to help control the signs and provide comfort to the infant experiencing NAS/NOWS. Studies on nonpharmacologic interventions have been done, and many of the interventions, such as breastfeeding and rooming-in, demonstrate a decreased length of hospital stay and symptoms of NAS/NOWS. Still, it is important to remember that studies are usually small with low-quality evidence (Wachman et al., 2018). More recently, research has been done on baby-wearing by parents, healthcare providers, or volunteers for neonates with NAS/NOWS. The research demonstrates that baby-wearing decreases neonatal distress, promotes secure attachment, and decreases the infant's heart rate, especially when stroking of the head occurred (Rankin et al., 2024; Williams et al., 2020). Box 24.1 has a list of published nonpharmacologic interventions that are currently being used to help the NAS/NOWS neonate.

The method of feeding and type of feeding that the neonate receives has been shown to help alleviate the symptoms of NAS/NOWS and is considered a nonpharmacologic intervention. Research has demonstrated that breastfeeding can decrease the severity of signs of NAS and shorten the length of pharmacologic treatment and hospital stay. Breastfeeding, which is the optimal source of nutrition for all newborns, is recommended by the American Academy of Pediatrics (AAP) for newborns of mothers in methadone or buprenorphine treatment programs (Hudak & Tan, 2012; Patrick et al., 2020). Studies have shown that breastfeeding increases maternal attachment and compliance in drug treatment programs while it decreases the symptoms of NAS and the length of hospital stay for infants with NAS (Favara et al., 2019; McQueen et al., 2011; Pritham et al., 2012; Short et al., 2016). However, breastfeeding rates among this group of women are low. Wachman et al. (2010) found that of the 68% of women in a methadone treatment program who qualified for breastfeeding, only 24% breastfed their infants to some extent during hospitalization, and 60% discontinued in an average of 5.88 days. Reasons given for less breastfeeding among women in methadone treatment programs include (a) the lack of clear, consistent guidelines for breastfeeding mothers; (b) inconsistent advice from healthcare providers; (c) infant feeding problems due to drug withdrawal; (d) separation of the birthing parent–infant dyad because of hospitalization; (e) birthing parent's low self-esteem, lack of knowledge, and feelings of guilt; and (f) inadequate support from healthcare providers (Hicks et al., 2018; Jansson et al., 2008; McQueen et al., 2011;Yonke et al., 2019). Another factor that can affect a woman with a substance abuse disorder and her ability to breastfeed is her history of sexual abuse.

**BOX 24.1**

**NONPHARMACOLOGIC INTERVENTIONS FOR NAS**

- Swaddling—in a flexed position with hands midline against chest and legs loosely swaddled in lumbar flexion to decrease sensory stimulation
- Minimizing environmental and physical stimulation—low lighting and noise levels—do not use TV or mobile or personal electronic devices such as phones and tablets when attending to the neonate
- Avoidance of abrupt changes in infant's environment—handling neonate gently and keeping neonate close to the body to increase sense of security
- Skin-to-skin contact with the birthing parent or other family members
- Baby-wearing by parents, family members, nurses, or volunteers
- Gentle rocking—vertical rocking preferred over horizontal rocking
- Slow approach with a soft voice and gentle touching to awaken the infant and prepare for care
- Limiting all stimulation at first signs of distress
- Pacifiers for nonnutritive sucking
- Hand containment during care—involve the mother with this when present
- Use of soft shushing, singing, or humming
- Offering firm input to feet for bracing during feedings, your hand on the infant's chest to offer firm support and maintain flexion, which will increase organization for sucking, and applying firm pressure to palate to increase and improve quality of sucking
- Frequent, small feedings for infants with feeding difficulties or gavage feedings may be needed
- Avoid talking to the infant while feeding or rocking
- Clustering care with extended rest periods
- Encouraging mother to room-in with neonate
- Prone sleeping until stable, then transition to back sleeping for safe sleep at home
- Relaxation baths
- Acupuncture
- Massage therapy
- Aromatherapy using birthing parent's scent on a scent cloth

While breastfeeding is often perceived as a pleasurable experience for women, for those with a history of sexual abuse as a child, an adult, or during pregnancy, negative feelings and reflections of the past abuse can arise and deter breastfeeding (Jansson et al., 2017).

The advantages of breastfeeding (i.e., better birthing parent–infant bonding, fewer withdrawal symptoms, and a shorter length of hospital stay) fuel the recommendation of the AAP, the Academy of Breastfeeding Medicine (ABM), and the American College of Obstetricians and Gynecologists (ACOG) to encourage breastfeeding among mothers who are free of other drugs in methadone and buprenorphine treatment programs and are HIV negative or on HIV antiretroviral treatment (ACOG, 2017; Abuogi et al., 2024; Harris et al., 2023; Hudak & Tan, 2012; Patrick et al., 2020).

For those who are unable to breastfeed or choose not to breastfeed their infants, the choice of the formula that is offered to the infant, in terms of its calorie and lactose content, has generated some discussion among those treating such infants. While no randomized controlled trial studies have been done on this topic, observational studies, expert opinion, and quality improvement projects have been published. The Ohio Children's Hospital Consortium noted through observation that infants who were fed 22-calorie, low-lactose formula did better than those infants who were fed regular-lactose, 19-calorie formula (Hall et al., 2014, 2015).

In an orchestrated testing quality improvement project done by the Ohio Perinatal Quality Collaborative (OPQC), a 22 calorie/oz formula has been found to help with the alleviation of NAS symptoms, regardless of lactose content. The orchestrated testing comprised of putting the 54 hospitals participating in the quality improvement project into four types of feeding groups. The groups were low lactose 19 calorie, regular lactose 19 calorie, low lactose 22 calorie, and regular lactose 22 calorie. The neonates that had the 22-calorie formula, regardless of lactose concentration, had a decreased length of hospital stay and shorter medication treatment when compared to neonates in the 19-calorie groups (Kaplan et al., 2017). The higher concentration formula is needed to meet the higher metabolic demands of an infant going through active withdrawal. It also helps to decrease the weight loss seen in infants diagnosed with NAS. The higher calorie formula is only needed for the first week of life during the initial withdrawal period (Walsh et al., 2018).

## Pharmacologic

When nonpharmacologic treatments do not work, medication-assisted treatment will be needed to help alleviate the signs of withdrawal in the neonate. The recommendation of the AAP is to use the same medication class of the drug the neonate was exposed to in utero (Kocherlakota, 2014; Osborne et al., 2010). For narcotics and heroin, oral morphine, methadone, and buprenorphine are the most commonly used medications to help alleviate the withdrawal symptoms. Studies have been done comparing morphine to methadone for treatment in the neonate withdrawing from opiates, but to date, there is no consensus on which one is better. One of the issues when looking at the studies is that there is no national standard on how to prescribe or when to start the medication therapy (Sanlorenzo et al., 2018). Buprenorphine, which is a mainstay in treating pregnant persons with OUD, has been recently studied in neonates as an alternative to morphine and methadone. Studies showed that buprenorphine-treated neonates had a significantly decreased length of hospital stay and a decreased length of treatment than neonates treated with morphine (Anbalagan et al., 2024; Kraft et al., 2017).

For infants born to pregnant persons who are polysubstance abusers with drugs such as barbiturates, benzodiazepines, antidepressants, and/or antipsychotics and sedatives or hypnotics, phenobarbital and clonidine can be used in conjunction with the narcotic replacement medications (Kocherlakota, 2014). Table 24.3 lists the most commonly used medications in NAS treatment, including the route of administration and dosage.

No matter what pharmacologic agent is used, the standardization of a medication protocol has been shown to be beneficial in decreasing the length of treatment and hospital stay. The Ohio Children's Hospital Consortium, from 2012 to 2014, did a multicenter retrospective cohort study with 981 neonates on the implementation of a standardized NAS weaning protocol. Prior to forming the consortium, each of

**TABLE 24.3**

**COMMONLY USED MEDICATIONS TO CONTROL NEONATAL ABSTINENCE SYNDROME SYMPTOMS**

| Medication | Route | Dose Range |
|---|---|---|
| Morphine | PO | 0.03–0.05 mg/kg/dose q3–4h; increase by 0.03–0.05 mg/kg<br>Maximum dose: 0.2 mg/kg/d |
| Methadone | PO | 0.05–0.1 mg/kg/dose q6h, or 0.05–0.1 mg/kg/dose q4h.<br>Increase by 0.05 mg/kg q48h<br>Maximum dose: 1 mg/kg/d |
| Buprenorphine | Sublingual | 4.4–5.3 mcg/kg/dose q8h<br>Maximum dose: 60 mcg/kg/d |
| Phenobarbital | PO | Loading dose: 16 mg/kg<br>Maintenance dose:<br>5 mg/kg/dose q12h; usual required dose—2–8 mg/kg/d |
| Clonidine | PO | Initial dose: 0.5–1 mcg/kg, followed by 0.5–1.25 mcg/kg/dose q4–6h |

PO, by mouth.

*Source:* Data from LexiDrug. (2024). *UpToDate LexiDrug*. UpToDate Corp. Retrieved November 29. 2024. https://online.lexi.com.

the six children's hospitals treated NAS neonates in a different manner. Approximately halfway through the study, all the hospitals adopted a strict weaning protocol for either morphine or methadone. The adoption of the weaning protocol resulted in a shorter hospital stay, shorter duration of opioid treatment, and less need for adjunct therapy in the three centers that did not previously have a protocol (Hall et al., 2015).

## DEVELOPMENTAL OUTCOMES

While the acute signs of withdrawal can be ameliorated in days to weeks, subacute signs may last as long as 6 months, which can affect the neonate's development (Hudak & Tan, 2012). Studies have been published and are currently being done on the long-term outcomes of neonates diagnosed with NAS/NOWS. Still, the true effects are not totally known because it is difficult to determine the actual cause of developmental delays. Neonates diagnosed with NAS/NOWS usually have had exposure to more than one substance in utero, and many are raised in unstable home environments, shifting from one caretaker to another. Confounding factors such as low socioeconomic class, poor nutrition, lack of parenting skills due to the use of multiple drugs and/or psychiatric issues, and poor prenatal care, to name a few, are known to affect the development of a neonate. Furthermore, apart from NAS, most neonates are healthy, so long-term follow-up is often difficult because the parents do not see the need for developmental follow-up of their child if the child appears to be hitting their developmental milestones (Oei, 2018).

Outcomes explored in studies are the effects of chronic drug exposure in utero on vision and motor function; cognitive function and neurodevelopment; risk of OUD/SUD; emotional, behavioral, and social adjustment; resilience; physical health; academic outcomes; and potential criminal activity in adulthood, but all of them are contaminated by multiple drug exposures and adverse lifestyles, all of which cannot be discussed in this chapter.

Recent studies have been published on visual disturbances being observed in neonates exposed to opiates. Visual disturbances range from strabismus, nystagmus, reduced visual acuity, refractive errors, and cerebral visual impairment (Hamilton et al., 2010; Spiteri-Cornish et al., 2013). These disturbances are being noticed in the preschool-to-kindergarten age group and at this point it is undetermined if this will continue as the child grows and develops.

For cognitive function and neurobehavioral function, a study on opioid exposure demonstrated that those exposed had decreased cognitive and fine motor function when compared to nonexposed adults in both the early childhood period and adulthood. Again, confounding factors such as being in an adverse home situation with parents who lack parenting skills, poverty, and chaos at home affect developmental outcomes, which many of these subjects had been exposed to (Lisonkova et al., 2024; Nygaard et al., 2017; Oei, 2019; Ornoy, 2003; Ornoy et al., 2001).

With cannabis use becoming legal and more acceptable, it is important to look at the effects of cannabis exposure in utero on the long-term outcomes of the fetus. A study on the effects of prenatal cannabis exposure (PCE) on adults was done in Canada, which followed children until they were 22 years of age. Early concerns regarding behavioral issues had resolved by adulthood and the adults performed similarly to non–cannabis-exposed adults on cognitive testing. But a functional magnetic resonance imaging (MRI) demonstrated significantly different blood flow response to the posterior left brain, a side effect of the prenatal exposure (Smith et al., 2016).

A more recent study published in 2022 demonstrated that fetuses with PCE were more likely to be growth restricted at birth, and the exposure had subtle but long-term effects on memory and achievement in children and adolescents, as well as being more likely to have delinquency and substance use problems (De Genna et al., 2022). These authors also reported that in animal studies, PCE resulted in the endocannabinoid system being altered, causing alteration in neurotransmitters and modulators on brain plasticity, which can affect cognition, motivation, and behavior regulation (De Genna et al., 2022).

The risk of future addiction problems is of concern for neonates exposed in utero to any substance. It is now well known that there is a genetic component to addiction as well as environmental factors. **Quality and Safety:** **When comparing children of parents without SUD to children of parents who have SUD, the latter is two times more likely to develop a SUD to substances such as alcohol and/or drugs (Chasin et al. 1999).** A study on PCE demonstrated that the endocannabinoid system that modulates and influences neurodevelopment into adulthood is affected. This leads to an increased risk of poor social outcomes, criminal activity, higher failure rates in school, having children out of wedlock, unemployment, and psychiatric issues (Goldschmidt et al., 2004; Leech et al., 2006; Sonon et al., 2016).

## NONJUDGMENTAL NURSING CARE OF THE BIRTHING PARENT–INFANT DYAD

When caring for the infant diagnosed with NAS/NOWS, it is important to remember that you are not only caring for the neonate, but also for the birthing parent. Unfortunately, many healthcare providers view the birthing parent with SUD through a judgmental lens. Frequent comments from healthcare providers are: "The birthing parent shouldn't have gotten pregnant," "What a horrible thing they did to their baby!", "If they loved their baby, they would have just quit," or "They should be put in jail for what they did to their baby." The birthing parent often hears these statements or thoughts, or they will feel the judgment of the provider by their actions and attitude. When caring for the birthing parent–infant dyad, it is important to remember that up to 40% or more of persons with SUD/OUD have experienced child abuse, sexual abuse, or both (Konkolÿ-Thege et al., 2017). So, it is important when caring for the birthing parent–infant dyad that you confront your feelings about the fact that the infants were exposed to substances in utero. Remind yourself that addiction is a chronic disease of the brain and is similar to other chronic diseases such as diabetes and hypertension and that the birthing parent did not decide to have a SUD/OUD after becoming pregnant. The birthing parent of the NAS/NOWS neonate deserves to be treated with the same respect as any patient's birthing parent. To deal with birthing parents with

SUD/OUD, seeking education on trauma-informed care will help to care for them and their infants without judgment.

**Quality and Safety:** **Nursing care of the neonate requires careful ongoing physical assessments and always being mindful of potential seizure activity.** Documentation of the infant's tolerance to stimuli is important, as is monitoring the infant's fluid and electrolyte balance and daily weights. When caring for an infant requiring medication-assisted treatment, it is important to give the medication as ordered and on time.

When caring for the infant, you will also interact with the birthing parent, so you must develop a therapeutic relationship with the birthing parent and show them respect. This will encourage the birthing parent to be more open to teaching and interventions. The birthing parent is part of the caregiving team and needs to be taught how to provide supportive care to their infant. You can help the birthing parent bond with their infant by providing skin-to-skin contact opportunities, encouraging them to room-in with their infant, and providing positive feedback for all attempts to comfort them. Explaining to the birthing parent that the infant's behavior is not a reflection of them but a result of the drugs the infant was exposed to in utero and intervening early when the infant is fussy will also help them bond with their infant.

When providing information to the birthing parent, always provide clear, concise, and specific guidelines for expected behaviors. The education should be goal directed, and the educational materials must be presented nonjudgmentally and at an appropriate reading level.

Caring for infants diagnosed with NAS/NOWS and their birthing parent can be a difficult and tiring assignment. Acknowledging that the birthing parents and infants require flexibility in schedules, energy, patience, and a nonjudgmental attitude is vital. While it is good to provide consistent caregivers for these birthing parent–infant dyads, it is also important to take breaks to prevent burnout.

When the infant is ready for discharge, it is important to make the appropriate referrals if not done prior to discharge. A home health referral should be made, as well as a referral to an early intervention or Help Me Grow program. If the birthing parent is not already in a drug rehabilitation program, then a referral to a program should be done because this is a period where treatment can be most successful.

## SUMMARY

SUD/OUD in the United States has become a national epidemic. NAS/NOWS is a result of this epidemic and has increased in prevalence. Birthing parent SUD/OUD and NAS/NOWS is costing hospitals and the government millions of dollars each year in treatment costs. Improving the care of infants with NAS/NOWS and decreasing the length of stay in the hospital are two of the main issues facing hospitals and healthcare providers today. This chapter has attempted to discuss the many issues related to NAS/NOWS as we currently understand them. There are still many unanswered questions related to the care of the infant with NAS/NOWS regarding the best treatment strategy, the long-term outcomes, as well as why some infants do not show signs of withdrawal, even though there is known exposure in utero.

## CASE STUDY

**Identification of the Problem.** Baby girl Jones, a 1-day-old, is admitted to the NICU from an outside referring hospital for high-pitched crying, increasing irritability, tremors/jitteriness, increased muscle tone, poor feeding, emesis, and tachypnea requiring $O_2$ per nasal cannula.

**Assessment: History and Physical Examination.** The infant was born at 39 1/7 weeks' gestation at 3.2 kg to a 28-year-old gravida 4 para 4 AB 0, hepatitis B and C and HIV negative White birthing parent. The pregnancy was complicated by no prenatal care and a history of Graves' disease, with the birthing parent not adherent with medication therapy, unknown Group B bacterial streptococcal status, and opiate use. The infant was born by spontaneous vaginal delivery with clear amniotic fluid. The infant was vigorous at birth with Apgar scores of 8 and 8 and no resuscitation required. The mother's blood type was unknown and the infant's blood type was A positive. The infant was taken to the newborn nursery for tachypnea and $O_2$ administration and to be observed for signs of withdrawal. The infant was bottle-fed but had emesis with each feed. The course at the referring hospital was unremarkable except for increasing tachypnea with retractions, increasing irritability, poor feeding with emesis, tremors/jitteriness, and the requirement for continued $O_2$.

On admission to the NICU, the infant was noted to be alert and well hydrated. The infant was on a nasal cannula at 0.1 L/min for tachypnea with $O_2$ saturation at 99%. The infant's vital signs were within normal limits with an axillary temperature of 98.5°F (36.9°C), a heart rate of 150 beats/min, a respiratory rate of 55 breaths/min, and blood pressure of 60/36 mm Hg with a mean of 48 mm Hg. The infant's weight on admission was noted to be 2.88 kg, a 10% loss in 1 day. The infant's examination was nonremarkable, except for increased muscle tone. Finnegan scoring on the infant revealed a score of 8.

**Differential Diagnosis.** Several conditions in the neonate can cause the symptoms described in this infant. The most common are hypoglycemia, hypocalcemia, hypomagnesemia, neurologic insult, sepsis, and NAS/NOWS. With the mother's history of being nonadherent with medication for Graves' disease, neonatal Graves' disease must also be considered.

**Diagnostic Tests.** To determine the exact cause of the signs, a glucose, calcium, and a complete blood count (CBC) differential should be ordered as well as a $T_4$ and thyroid-stimulating hormone (TSH). The collection of meconium could be obtained from any remaining meconium that the infant passes and sent for toxicology. A call to the referring hospital to inquire if they collect umbilical cords at birth can also be made. If the cord was saved, then sending the cord for toxicology should be ordered.

**Working Diagnosis.** The infant's CBC and differential were normal, the glucose was 60, and the calcium normal at 9.0. The $T_4$/TSH was normal at 2.3 and 3.14. The infant continued to be irritable and a poor feeder, with jitteriness and increased muscle tone, as well as tachypnea. The infant started to develop excoriation on the cheeks from frequent rubbing on the mattress. Urine toxicology returned from the referral hospital was positive for opiates. The working diagnosis for the infant is NAS/NOWS secondary to in-utero exposure to opiates.

**Development of Management Plan.** The goal for the neonate with NAS/NOWS is to alleviate signs of withdrawal through nonpharmacologic and pharmacologic management. Wean the infant to room air (RA) from nasal cannula oxygen. Maintain $O_2$ saturation at 95% to 96%. Continue scoring the infant every 3 hours with the Finnegan Scoring Tool. Ensure that the neonate is swaddled with hands midline and legs flexed and placed in a dark, quiet environment to decrease stimulation. Encourage the mother to do skin-to-skin contact, baby-wear, or to hold the infant as much as possible. Feed the infant 22-calorie formula q3h, PO ad lib, because the mother is not yet in a treatment program. When the infant has three scores greater than 8 or two scores greater than 12, begin pharmacologic therapy of morphine at 0.05 mg/kg q3h and increase as needed based on scores.

**Implementation and Evaluation of Effectiveness.** The infant was weaned to RA over the next 2 hours, maintaining $O_2$ saturation between 95% and 96%. The infant's Finnegan scores began to escalate over the next 12 hours to three consecutive scores of 10, 12, and 14, respectively, despite maximizing nonpharmacologic interventions. The infant was started on morphine at 0.05 mg/kg/dose PO at 36 hours of age. Symptoms continued to escalate and the dose was increased to 0.07 mg/kg/dose PO by 48 hours of age. On day of life (DOL) 4, the infant had been stable on the morphine dose for 48 hours with Finnegan scores less than 8 and weaning of the morphine began. By DOL 10, the infant had been weaned off the morphine but Finnegan scoring continued for an additional 48 hours to ensure that the infant did not start to display signs of withdrawal after the discontinuation of the morphine. The infant did not display any signs of withdrawal, so this was discontinued on DOL 12.

**Outcome.** The infant was discharged home on DOL 13 on full PO feedings of 19 calorie formula with a weight of 3.2 kg. The infant was discharged to the care of a foster family and, after completing all discharge, newborn testing and education was completed with the foster family. A referral was made to Help Me Grow and the NAS/NOWS clinic at the regional referral center.

## ONLINE RESOURCES

CourseConnect

Resources for this chapter are online and available at www.springerpub.com/courseconnect.

## REFERENCES

References for this chapter are online and available at www.springerpub.com/courseconnect.

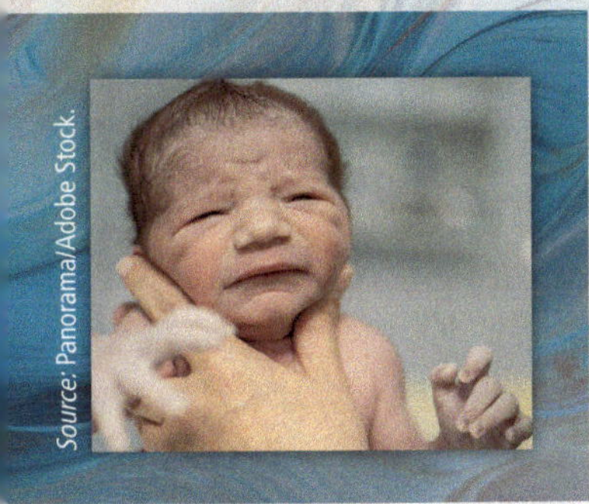

Source: Panorama/Adobe Stock.

# Unit V: Environmental Health and Family-Centered Care in the Neonatal Intensive Care Unit and Beyond

CHAPTER 25

# The Neonatal Intensive Care Unit Environment

**Leslie B. Altimier and Robert D. White**

## INTRAUTERINE VERSUS EXTRAUTERINE ENVIRONMENTS

Preterm infants have long been recognized as a population at high risk for mortality and adverse functional outcomes. Advances in neonatal intensive care practices have led to dramatic increases in the survival of preterm infants (Helenius et al., 2017; Younge et al., 2017). Over the last decades, the increasing survival rates of preterm infants admitted to the neonatal intensive care unit [NICU] have emphasized the importance of considering their neurodevelopmental outcomes (Aylward, 2014). Prematurity is associated with an increased risk of long-term health and neurodevelopmental problems. Preterm infants are more likely to have significant short- and long-term neurodevelopmental impairments because their brains go through a critical period of development and maturation between 24 and 40 weeks of gestation, occurring mainly during their NICU hospitalization (Pickler et al., 2010; Volpe et al., 2018). Preterm birth interrupts a critical period of intrauterine brain growth and increases the risk of brain injuries (Inder et al., 2023; Schneider & Miller, 2019). Significant neurodevelopmental disabilities associated with neurosensory, motor, behavioral, and cognitive outcomes may arise shortly after preterm infants' birth and beyond school age and adolescence (Rogers & Hintz, 2016), given that neurocognitive impairments in infants born preterm are still reported in adulthood (Eryigit Madzwamuse et al., 2015).

More attention is focused on environmental factors that can affect the long-term outcomes of preterm infants, particularly in light of the rapid maturation of the brain during these infants' early days of life (Cheong et al., 2020). The fact that the body systems of premature infants are not fully developed and that they are moving into an external environment that is not suitable for their development causes the infants to experience intense stress. In addition to biologic vulnerabilities conferred by preterm birth, the risk for neurodevelopmental delays may be compounded by environmental exposures in the NICU that are not conducive to infant development, including noise and a lack of exposure to language (Caskey et al., 2014; Santos et al., 2015; Stroustrup et al., 2019). To better understand the correlation of early environmental factors to the developmental problems associated with prematurity, examining (and frequently modifying) the environment in which these infants spend a critical period of their development is essential. Because NICU-related factors shape preterm infants' neurodevelopment during their hospitalization, evaluating which interventions are more beneficial for their neurodevelopment at this specific time is necessary. This chapter highlights differences in the intrauterine environment (maternal womb) compared with the extrauterine environment (NICU), the effects these differences have on fetal/infant neurosensory and neurobehavioral development, and what can be done to optimize the NICU environment to provide a healing, nurturing place for premature infants to grow, mature, and form secure bonds of attachments with their families.

From the first moments of life, the premature infant is abruptly separated from the dimly lit, temperature-controlled, fluid-filled womb of the mother in which it has been growing and is suddenly exposed to a significantly colder environment that often contains noxious smells and tastes, loud sounds, bright lights, and a multitude of painful and stressful procedures along with repetitive, non-nurturing handling. The mismatch between the NICU environment and the preterm infant's developing brain and neurologic system increases the risk for poor developmental outcomes, including emotional, cognitive, motor, and sensory abnormalities (Séassau et al., 2023).

More often than not, a full-term healthy infant has a consistent nurturing caregiver and an appropriate variety of stimulations. The full-term infant with 40 weeks of intrauterine development is ready for various sensory experiences, including tactile, gustatory, olfactory, auditory, and visual experiences. Appropriate patterns of adaptation, cognitive learning, and motor control are formed when sensory information interacts in developmentally appropriate ways with experience (Karlsson et al., 2022). Premature infants are typically exposed to numerous caregivers and high levels of inappropriate sensory input can alter adaptation patterns.

The neurologic and sensory systems do not exist as separate entities but are interdependent and comprise the neurobehavioral and neurosensory development of the infant. Every sensory experience is recorded in the brain, leading to a behavioral response and yet another sensory experience. The brain organization is incredibly complex: It is estimated that the human brain contains more than 200 billion neurons and non-neuron cells, 1 quadrillion connections, 100 km of nerve fibers, and 600 km of blood vessels (Silbereis et al., 2016). After birth, the "fetal" brain continues making synaptic connections at a rate of 40,000 per minute and must continue critical neurologic growth and maturation in the often-harsh extrauterine NICU environment (Keunen et al., 2017). While axons grow, facilitating significant connections in the white matter to find their cortical targets, the overlying cortex transforms its relatively smooth surface into a highly convoluted mantle with secondary and tertiary sulci that resembles the adult human brain (Chavoshnejad et al., 2021). Magnetic resonance imaging (MRI) studies in preterm infants have reported a fivefold increase in cortical surface area and a doubling of cortical curvature measures in the timeframe that coincides with the third trimester of pregnancy (Dimitrova et al., 2021) The ability of humans to perform complex mental activities, including thinking, reasoning, remembering, problem solving, decision making, and learning new information, depends on the ability of the brain to adapt to its environment and alter its functional and structural organization (Goyal et al., 2018). This is often referred to as brain, neuron, or synapse *plasticity* (Cirelli & Tononi, 2017; Lowe et al., 2017).

Brain development in the fetus, neonate, and infant includes sensory systems, motor systems, social/emotional systems, and the cognitive system, which are connected and integrated during development. The maternal womb, or intrauterine environment, is conducive to positive sensory input, which is crucial for normal brain development in a developing fetus. The intrauterine environment protects the developing fetus against harsh outside stimulation while providing a variety of tactile, vestibular, chemical, visual, and auditory sensory stimuli in an integrated, multimodal fashion (Lickliter, 2011). The intrauterine environment of a developing fetus is characterized by generalized extremity flexion and containment, limited light and noise exposure, sleep cycle preservation, and unrestricted access to the mother via somatosensory, auditory, and chemosensory pathways. The uterine wall provides secure boundaries for the developing fetus. Vestibular and tactile stimuli come from maternal and fetal movements, contact with warm amniotic fluid, and contact with body parts and the uterus wall. The hormonal cycles of the mother provide rhythmic and cyclical stimulation. Auditory input includes maternal voice, bowel sounds, blood flow through the placenta and umbilical cord, and filtered sounds from the extrauterine environment, transmitted through liquid and solid media.

Prematurely born neonates in the NICU are exposed to fluctuations in temperature, touch, light, sound, olfaction, oxygen, and nutrients that are very different from those they have experienced in utero. These negative sensory inputs replace the positive sensory inputs in the developing brain, which can permanently alter normal brain development. The architecture of connections in the brain is made with dendritic growth, synaptic networks, apoptosis, myelination, and pruning. Research shows that outside stimulation from the environment can induce changes in the pattern of brain development designed to occur in the last trimester of pregnancy and early life, altering the development and affecting the quality of these connections (Keunen et al., 2017).

MRI performed on the brains of infants born 10 weeks prematurely showed 30% less gray matter (the brain's thinking cells) and 40% less white matter (Inder et al., 2021; Keunen et al., 2017). Associative learning was derived by Donald Hebb in 1949 and includes what is now known as Hebb's law. While Hebb's law states that "neurons that fire together, wire together," it implies that "neurons that don't, won't," or that "neurons that fire apart, wire apart." This means that repeated experiences (positive or negative) reinforce particular patterns of synaptic connections (wiring), and a lack of appropriate experiences diminishes the firing of neurons, affecting the ability to "hardwire" synapses, thus altering the developing brain (Hebb, 1949).

When an infant is born prematurely, the still-developing brain and sensory systems are affected by the continuous interplay of stimuli in the NICU. Events, stimuli, and environmental factors can support the processes of sensory development or create significant interference. Sensory interference may occur when immature sensory systems are stimulated out of turn or with inappropriate stimuli. Background neurosensory stimulation must be kept at a level so sensory systems can discriminate and accommodate meaningful signals or stimulation. This observation is accurate for sound, touch, smell, position, and comfort, part of early neurosensory development and in-utero learning or NICU learning (Graven, 2006).

Prematurity deprives infants of the prenatal sensory stimulation essential to their correct development; in addition, the stressful environment of the NICU negatively affects their growth. Because the developing brain is extremely sensitive to the appropriate levels of sensory stimuli, alterations can result in abnormal structural and functional development of the brain. They could account for many premature infants' behavioral, cognitive, and functional deficits (Keunen et al., 2017; Ottolini et al., 2020; Vitale et al., 2021). Infants of low birth weight or very low birth weight (VLBW), many of whom are also small for gestational age, are at increased risk for auditory and visual impairment, including sensorineural hearing loss and deficits in visual acuity, color vision, and contrast sensitivity. Long-term alterations in retinal function and subtle deficits in neural conduction in auditory pathways have all been demonstrated (Bouyssi-Kobar et al., 2018; Di Fiore et al., 2024).

It is well documented that prematurely born infants have a high risk of developmental and behavioral disorders compared with those born at term (McGowan et al., 2024). Because sensory experience is the basis for much of learning in infancy, sensory problems that affect preterm infants may contribute to their high incidence of later developmental disorders (Beltrán et al., 2022; El-Metwally & Medina, 2020). Hearing and visual impairment, language delays, and sensory processing issues may also occur because fetal sensory development has been interrupted by preterm birth and exposed to the unpredictable sensory input of the NICU (Belanger et al., 2019; Papageorgiou & Pelausa, 2014). Although hearing and vision impairments are well-known sensory outcomes of prematurity, abnormalities in sensory processing, the organization of sensation for use, and sensory reactivity, an observable and immediate modulation of behavior in response to a sensory stimulus, are more challenging to identify and characterize (Papageorgiou & Pelausa, 2014).

Even the full-term neonate's neurologic system is in a highly active stage of development at birth. With volumes of research demonstrating long-term disabilities in preterm-born children, understanding how we can better support the infant's fragile neurologic system to minimize these impairments can guide us in helping the infant grow and thrive within the artificial extrauterine environment of the NICU. Part of this support is adopting the conceptual framework and philosophy of developmental care and neuroprotection. Neuroprotection has been defined as strategies to prevent cell death (McGrath et al., 2011). Advances in neuroimaging and research have provided broader insight into third-trimester brain development, and what traditionally has been viewed as simply developmentally supportive care is now recognized as neuroprotective care (Altimier & Phillips, 2016, 2018; McGrath et al., 2011; Soni et al., 2022). Validating the benefits of developmental care has been difficult because it is practiced in so many variations in different settings (Montirosso et al., 2016).

Pioneering work by Brazelton and Als found that assessing the individual infant's ability to cope with excessive stimulation provides the caregiver with information to modify each infant's environment and treatment strategies (Als, 1986; Brazelton, 1974; Brazelton et al., 1976). Infants born prematurely have demonstrated markedly improved outcomes when the stress of environmental overstimulation is reduced, and family bonds are supported. This can be accomplished by creating a supportive NICU environment utilizing innovative NICU design and by incorporating neuroprotective care into the care of high-risk neonates and their families. Neuroprotective interventions (NPIs) in the NICU are strategies used to support the developing brain or to facilitate the brain after a neuron injury in a way that allows it to heal through developing new connections and pathways for functionality and by decreasing neuronal death (Altimier & Phillips, 2013, 2016, 2020; Soni et al., 2022). NPIs that promote normal development and prevent disabilities include organizational, therapeutic, and environment-modifying measures, such as family-centered developmental care (Altimier & Phillips, 2013, 2016, 2018).

Along with the caregiving environment, the physical environment, including space, activity, temperature, humidity, smell, noise, and light, affects infant development (Altimier, 2015). The central circadian pacemaker is located in the brain and is entrained by environmental signals called *zeitgebers*. Zeitgebers, timekeeping cues given by the environment, such as a change in light or temperature, function to regulate the internal body clock (Van Gilst et al., 2023; White, 2017).

The Neonatal Integrative Developmental Care Model describes seven core measures of neuroprotective family-centered developmental care to support preterm infant development: (a) healing environment (physical, sensory, and emotional), (b) positioning and handling, (c) partnering with families, (d) minimizing stress and pain, (e) safeguarding sleep, (f) protecting skin, and (g) optimizing nutrition outline neuroprotective care related to each core measure (Altimier & Phillips, 2013, 2016). Each core measure has a related standard with defined infant characteristics, measurable goals, and corresponding NPIs. Although there are multiple models of developmental care, a common feature of each is the recognition that fragile preterm and sick infants and their families benefit from a specialized environment and care practices adapted to their specific developmental needs (Altimier & Phillips, 2020).

## PROVIDING A HEALING ENVIRONMENT

The concept of a "healing environment" dates back to the Crimean War and the work of Florence Nightingale, who needed little convincing as to the benefits of light, fresh air, and access to nature on recovery from illness and trauma (Nightingale, 1860). To make the NICU a place where premature and sick full-term infants can heal, it is important to pay close attention to temperature, touch, postural control, smell, taste, sound, and light, as well as the space, privacy, and safety (Altimier & Phillips, 2013, 2016; Green et al., 2019; White, 2018). The optimal healing environment for any infant is physical contact with his/her mother. Every effort should be made to keep mothers and newborns together in skin-to-skin contact (SSC) whenever possible. This is the developmentally expected habitat for all newly born infants where they can be coregulated by their mothers to achieve ongoing physiologic stability. Unless the infant or mother is medically unstable, this environment provides the highest level of support for optimal growth and development of preterm infants. In addition to the presence of an infant's mother (or other primary caregiver), a healing environment encompasses the physical environment (space, privacy, and safety), the sensory environment (touch, temperature, tastes, smells, noise, and light), and the social environment (families and staff). When the mother (or primary caregiver) cannot be present, or SSC is not an option (for maternal or infant reasons), more attention must be given to designing and maintaining the physical, sensory, and social environments.

The physical environment involves not only space but also characteristics of space that affect position, movement, and motor development. Privacy and safety are separate but equally important factors in the physical environment. The sensory environment includes the exposure and experience of touch/movement, temperature/thermoregulation, taste/gustation, smell/olfaction, noise/vocalization, light/vision, and nutritional and chemical exposure. All sensory stimuli carry social and emotional connections and characteristics and, in addition to creating cortical changes, directly affect social and emotional learning and memory, especially in the limbic system, where stress regulation, memory processing, and emotional development occur. The social environment includes family and staff and involves their availability for touch and emotional connections. Positive attitudes of compassion, caring, and love or negative attitudes of fear, anxiety, or anger are perceived by staff, family, and even the infants and affect the quality of interactions in the NICU environment.

There is considerable interaction between and within the physical, sensory, and social environments, and they are differentiated only to discuss opportunities for improvement in creating a holistic healing NICU environment for preterm and sick neonates and their families. Adverse physical, sensory, or social environmental factors can significantly interfere with growth, health, and appropriate neurodevelopment and neuroprocessing. They can lead to lifelong alterations in function and well-being (Graven & Browne, 2008), while a carefully designed, healing environment can provide the support needed for optimal physical, mental, and emotional development (Hendy et al., 2022; White, 2011; White, 2020a).

## The Physical Environment—Space, Privacy, and Safety

In 1976, the March of Dimes published *Toward Improving the Outcome of Pregnancy*, a landmark publication written by a multidisciplinary committee to provide a rationale, plan, and policy for regionalized perinatal care and details of facility design and staff roles. In 1992, a multidisciplinary NICU Committee, under the auspices of the Physical and Developmental Environment of the High-Risk Infant Project, reached a consensus on the first edition of recommended standards for NICU design. The purpose of this committee was to provide healthcare professionals, architects, interior designers, state healthcare facility regulators, and others involved in the planning of NICUs with a comprehensive set of minimum standards based on clinical experience and an evolving scientific database. The intent was to optimize design within the constraints of available resources and to facilitate excellent healthcare for the infant in a setting that supports the family's central role and the staff's needs. This group recognized that one way to promote the ideals of neurodevelopmental care and family-centered care (FCC) is through appropriate environmental modifications or the construction of new NICU facilities. NICU design should meet the neurodevelopmental needs of the infants, provide adequate space and facilities for FCC, and meet the needs of the NICU staff. This committee has continued updating the NICU design standards with the latest recommendations published in 2023, available at https://doi.org/10.1038/s41372-023-01784-4 (Altimier et al., 2023).

When designing a NICU's physical environment, attention should be given to the NICU configuration, the location within the hospital, minimum space, clearance, and privacy requirements for the infant space. Family, staff, administrative, and general support space must also be delineated. Attention should focus on illumination guidelines (ambient, daylighting, and procedural) and acoustic guidelines (floor, wall, and ceiling surfaces). Electrical, gas, mechanical, isolation, ambient temperature, humidity, and ventilation recommendations likewise are outlined in the recommended standards. While the Facility Guideline Institute (FGI) provides guidelines for hospitals that serve as building requirements for NICU design, the guidelines lack sufficient detail to aid in many design decisions, such as why a recommendation is included. The Recommended Standards for Newborn ICU Design aim to address the gaps in guidance by providing interpretations of the standards, which include contextual information for why the design features are essential (Altimier et al., 2023; FGI, 2018).

Research supports the concept that NICU design affects outcomes. One systematic review collectively linked a range of aspects of the physical environment of the NICU to the well-being of patients, family comfort, and the caregiving process. Single-family rooms (SFRs) were deemed superior to open-bay units for patient care and parent satisfaction (Fay et al., 2024; Franck et al., 2023). Others have demonstrated improved outcomes, including increased privacy, increased parental involvement in patient care, improved noise control, improved sleep, decreased length of hospital stay, decreased rehospitalizations, reductions in costly hospital-acquired infections, and lower direct costs of care (Feeley et al., 2019; Sadatsafavi et al., 2019; White, 2011, 2016; White, 2020a). A recent Lehtonen et al. (2020) study reported that single-family room care lowered the risk for bronchopulmonary dysplasia (BPD) (adjusted odds ratio 0.72, 95% confidence interval 0.61–0.86) (Lehtonen et al., 2020). A study by Silva et al., 2024) revealed that preterm neonates who were hospitalized in a NICU with an SFR design exhibited fewer stress behaviors and more self-regulation responses as compared to preterm neonates who were hospitalized in a NICU with an open-bay design (Feeley et al., 2019, 2020; Liu et al., 2019; Silva et al., 2024).

When considering NICU design and unit configuration, it is essential to remember that families and staff have different needs (Dunn et al., 2016). The primary function of early caregiver recognition and attachment is ensuring newborn infant closeness and survival (Sullivan et al., 2011). Families emphasize privacy and individualized care, whereas staff often emphasize efficiency and visibility. Parents prefer the intimacy of an SFR and the quieter atmosphere with decreased noise levels. Research shows that parental presence and holding in the NICU may promote healthy attachment and improve early neurobehavior in preterm infants, and the SFR provides an environment that supports longer parental stays (Barton & White, 2016; Browne, 2023; Reynolds et al., 2013). High maternal involvement is associated with improved 18-month neurodevelopmental outcomes, especially in infants cared for in an SFR NICU (Lester et al., 2016).

Newly born infants experience a burst of norepinephrine during birth, which facilitates learning their mother's odor and approach behaviors toward their mothers (Debiec & Sullivan, 2017). Many hormonal and neurotransmitter mechanisms have been developed to draw parents and their infants into close proximity and emotional closeness with each other (Debiec & Sullivan, 2017; Provenzi et al., 2021). Therefore, disturbances in these regulations may affect the infant's cognitive and emotional development. Nurtured attachment from parents plays an important role in the infant's stress regulation (Laurent et al., 2017). In a study by Vohr et al. (2017), infants cared for in SFR NICUs had higher Bayley III cognitive and language scores.

On the other hand, staff working in SFRs expressed concerns about higher workloads due to decreased visibility of infants and diminished opportunities for staff interaction and communication (Doede et al., 2018). NICU nurses are at high risk of developing compassion fatigue, secondary traumatic stress, and burnout (Kuper-Sassé et al., 2024). Grunberg et al. (2022) reported that 40% to 50% of parents in the NICU report elevated emotional distress, and 30% to 50% of staff report burnout (Grunberg et al., 2022).

The NICU at Beacon Children's Hospital in South Bend, Indiana, consists of beautiful, spacious, functional SFR NICU rooms. The SFRs have many elements that promote improved sensory development for the infant and family participation in care, which is the primary purpose of the SFR (White, 2011).

- Every patient room has a window. This important feature helps the infant, parents, and staff maintain circadian rhythms. Research shows that views of nature reduce stress and provide positive distraction for parents who may be distraught or depressed.
- Every SFR includes a family area with a toilet and shower that supports longer stays for families, encouraging their involvement in the care of their child.
- An interior garden courtyard is available that provides daylight and views of nature into the center of the unit.

Beacon Children's Hospital took the SFR concept a step further by introducing a new multipurpose patient care room called the NIC2 room. The innovative NIC2 room allows couplet care (care for the postpartum mother and the NICU infant) to occur in the same room, eliminating separation. This facilitates early mother–infant bonding, which historically has been limited during the first few days of the infant's life. At the center of every room, at the infant's bedside, is a kangaroo chair—a specialized recliner that allows the mother to lean back and hold her infant(s) safely, skin to skin. The NIC2 rooms have multiple purposes and functions beyond couplet care, such as accommodating multiples or group care, allowing for increased flexibility.

Like the SFR, the NIC2 room has a toilet room with a shower and sleeping space for two on a pull-out sofa bed. The toilet room has a sliding door, making it easy to access and reducing the inconvenience of the door swinging into the room. A breast pump is provided in every room, contained within the wardrobe on a dedicated shelf with a power outlet. Lockable drawers within the wardrobe are provided to secure personal valuables for the family. Also in the wardrobe is a refrigerator for the family to use. A separate refrigerator for breastmilk is located on the counter at the footwall of the room in every SFR. The NIC2 room has two breastmilk refrigerators if two unrelated infants are in the same room.

All lighting in the room is dimmable to control light levels at all times. No lights are located directly over the infant's bed, so there is no chance of direct light shining into the infant's eyes. The procedure light is mounted to the headwall on an adjustable arm. Colored light-emitting diode (LED) lights at the footwall of the room, in a hue chosen by the family, will wash the wall with color to personalize the room. The color can be easily changed to vary the room experience and suit daily mood. Wall sconces in the family area of the room provide a soft level of light for reading or conversation. Two solid-surface shelves on the wall provide space for families to personalize the room for the infant.

Specific guidelines around SFRs are outlined in Standard 6 (Altimier et al., 2023). The single-room NICU is a strategy that could address environmental concerns and minimize iatrogenic effects by reducing the risk of infection and stress on preterm infants while increasing opportunities for private parental interaction with their hospitalized infants. A mother's arms should be the preferred locus of neonatal care whenever possible (White, 2004). This concept has been enthusiastically endorsed by many and effectively applied in several healthcare settings. The NICU must be designed so families feel comfortable spending prolonged periods with their infants and are encouraged to engage in intimate, nurturing encounters (Dunn et al., 2016; Jaeger & Altimier, 2023).

The FGI: 2018 Guidelines for Design and Construction of Hospitals and Outpatient Facilities states that all patient rooms in the hospital setting must be single private rooms; yet why does the decision to build SFRs or bay/pod-type rooms in the NICU remain controversial? Cost savings associated with SFR units should be justified in terms of clinical outcomes, construction, and operation costs (Lester et al., 2014; Lester et al., 2016). Two types of expenses must be considered when analyzing the implications for SFRs compared to open-bay/pod NICUs: one-time construction and ongoing operating expenses. SFRs, compared to multiple-bed room designs, require additional square footage per bed (minimum 180 square feet in the clear versus 150 square feet [14 square meters] in the clear in the multiple-bed room) based on the Recommended Standards for Newborn ICU Design. The amount of space allocated beyond the minimum should be equivalent for both designs based on a NICU's functional needs.

Direct costs of NICU care in SFRs are no more significant than in traditional open-bay/POD NICUs (Stevens et al., 2014). In a theoretical business plan for an SFR NICU, using data from two independent studies, Shepley et al. (2014) demonstrated that the cost of constructing an SFR NICU may be recuperated within the first 12 months of operation (Shepley et al., 2014). NICU hospitalization is costly, and every day of maternal involvement has been associated with a 4.3-day decrease in the length of infants' hospitalization (Lester et al., 2016).

Specifications of materials used in the NICU also affect psychological, behavioral, physiologic, and environmental outcomes. Selected finishes should focus on safety and the ambient environment to provide psychological and physiologic outcomes for neonates, families, and caregivers. Mitigating hospital-acquired infections (HAIs) is crucial to improving neonatal outcomes. Other outcomes, such as social support and reducing stress, anxiety, and fatigue, become attainable through conscientious, evidence-based design in the NICU (Harris, 2016).

The number of NICUs designed to meet basic "green" design criteria is increasing (Shepley et al., 2016). LEED (Leadership in Energy and Environmental Design), a system authored by the U.S. Green Building Council, and the recommended standards for newborn ICU design provide information on building a NICU with an environmentally sustainable design (U.S. Green Building Council, 2009). Several actions are essential to accomplishing sustainable objectives (Gottlieb & Dickeman, 2007):

- evaluating medical devices, building materials, and electronics
- recycling and waste reduction
- conserving energy
- emphasizing sustainable foods
- specifying green cleaning products
- exploring the potential use of organic linens
- addressing staff transportation and climate change
- regulating pharmaceutical waste

Visual and physical access to nature and daylight are critical components of sustainability.

The U.S. Green Building Council also acknowledges the role of these environmental features and designates access to the natural environment as a source of points toward LEED certification.

While diurnal variation is important to infants, staff and families are the primary beneficiaries of the relationship with nature and daylight in the NICU. For example, studies have revealed that family satisfaction is associated with gardens, and nurses prefer access to natural conditions in lounge areas (Altimier, 2015).

## The Sensory Environment

Defining the optimal sensory environment in the NICU is an elusive task. There is conflicting data on the dangers of both overstimulation and sensory deprivation in premature infants. Replicating the in-utero environment is impossible in the NICU and is not the most appropriate. Continuation of the sensory environment found in utero can disadvantage the neurodevelopment of the preterm infant ex utero. For example, circadian rhythms are driven by endogenous processes and rely upon circadian time cues (zeitgebers) to remain appropriately oriented to the individual's environment and desired routine. The circadian rhythm of a fetus is guided by multiple maternal zeitgebers, none of which is readily available to the newborn infant. Instead, new zeitgebers must be established, most notably lighting cycles and breastmilk (White, 2018). Accomplishing this is not as easy as turning a light on and off at the appropriate time of day, nor is the solution to continuously leave the infant in a low-light environment. Sensory deprivation of any sense (touch, movement, taste, smell, sound, or light) is undesirable, as is overstimulation. It is also not as simple as getting the quantity of a particular stimulus right and giving it at the exact right time. Quality matters, and the target continually moves as the infant's medical condition, peripheral sensory apparatus, and brain maturity change almost daily (White, 2018).

**Tactile/Touch and Temperature/Thermoregulation.** One of the first principles of neonatal care is thermoregulation. At birth, the newborn moves from a warm, fluid-filled intrauterine environment to a cooler, dry environment. A significant goal of neonatal care is to provide a thermoneutral climate in which an infant's basal metabolic requirements are minimized.

The physical environment (macroenvironment) should incorporate the following factors:

- Temperature: 72°F to 78°F (22°C–26°C)
- Relative humidity: 30% to 60%
- Six air changes per hour (with two from outside air)
- All air filtered with at least the efficiency specified in the FGI Guidelines (FGI, 2018)

To enhance the development of the preterm infant, frequent attention is often paid to the thermoregulation (microenvironment) of the infant. The optimal environment for the infant is SSC with the mother, also known as kangaroo care (KC). SSC increases oxytocin levels in both mothers and fathers, a hormone that induces relaxation, facial recognition, and bonding. SSC also increases prolactin levels in the mother, which is linked to increased breastmilk production. Due to the proximity to the mother's breasts, SSC is associated with higher rates of breastfeeding. Thermal synchrony is observed when mothers or fathers hold their infants in SSC, making it possible to warm a cold infant or cool an overly warm infant. Free unrestricted parental access facilitates early and prolonged SSC and has been associated with higher KC and breastmilk feeding rates (Conde-Agudelo & Diaz-Rossello, 2016). SFR care is related to more frequent and longer SSC (Raiskila et al., 2017).

When parents are unavailable for SSC or SSC is not possible, thermoregulatory efforts should focus on the infant's individual bed space (microenvironment), whether it is a radiant warmer, incubator, or open crib. To maintain a constant central temperature within narrow limits of 97.7°F to 99.5°F (36.5°C–37.5°C), VLBW infants or premature infants need to be preferably cared for in a dual-function incubator or incubator (Altimier, 2012). The dual-function incubators include the incubator mode (closed-type incubator) and the radiant warmer mode (open-type incubator). This technology allows for caring for a critically ill premature infant in a highly humid environment (incubator mode), which can then be switched to the radiant warmer mode during a treatment or procedure.

Attention should be given to decibel (dB) levels inside and outside incubators. Much of the noise inside the incubator comes from sources outside the incubator. So, although the average noise level in most modern NICUs is around 62 decibels (A-weighted dBA), tests performed in NICUs show that the outside noise to the incubator reaches levels of 80.4 versus 79.1 dBA inside, despite educational programs carried out for noise reduction (Pinheiro et al., 2011; Shoemark et al., 2016; Tsunemi et al., 2012). Sound-absorbing incubator covers are available to minimize noise levels and prevent the light from reaching the infant's eyes. Positioning an infant in a midline, flexed, and contained position with the assistance of therapeutic positioning aids and swaddling decreases the surface area of the infant exposed to environmental air, thus reducing radiant and convective heat losses. A flexed and contained position offers additional temperature stability for the infant by minimizing extraneous movement and energy expenditure (Altimier, 2012).

**Chemosensory: Taste/Gustatory and Smell/Olfactory.** Among all senses from birth onward, olfaction plays a critical role in sensory communication. The gustatory and olfactory receptors of the infant begin to develop at 8 weeks into the pregnancy and finish maturing at 17 weeks and 24 weeks, respectively (Beker et al., 2017). Preferences for specific tastes or smells appear to begin from the stage of conception and continue right up until old age. The olfactory system is unique as a sensory system in its developmental neuroanatomy and function. Olfaction was reported to begin approximately the 24th week of gestation, and premature neonates show responses to olfactory stimulation after 28 weeks of gestation (Beker et al., 2019). At term, only 25% of neurons in the olfactory bulb are mature, and less than 10% of the olfactory tract is myelinated (Sarnat & Yu, 2015). Fetuses can process olfactory stimuli present in the womb and continue to prefer these odors for months after birth (Tristão et al., 2021).

Olfaction allows the newborn to adapt its suckling and feeding behaviors, to be attracted to maternal odors, and to improve mother–infant interactions.

Support for mothers and infants to be together early in the NICU supports olfactory and gustatory sensory development. Providing odors and the taste of the mother's milk facilitates infants' mouthing, sucking, arousal, and calming from irritability, especially in preparation for oral feeding (Yücel et al., 2024). Providing a pacifier with mother's milk increases non-nutritive sucking, intake, and growth and shortens the length of hospitalization (Orovou et al., 2022). Providing multisensory experiences (when developmentally appropriate), such as combining odor and taste with proprioceptive and kinesthetic visual and auditory input, can potentiate sensory organization during feeding. Holding the infant close to the caregiver's body provides this organized multisensory environment (Browne, 2008).

Olfaction (smell) is initiated by neural excitation in response to specific molecules in the immediate surroundings. Olfactory information (in the uterus for the fetus and at the breast for the neonate) is transmitted directly from the nose to the cerebral cortex. A mother's scent has been found to facilitate state regulation and optimal feeding experiences for both term and preterm infants. Because olfaction is functional in the second trimester, sensory stimuli from the NICU environment, rather than the mother, may interfere with the infant's development and other sensory development and attachment (Klaey-Tassone et al., 2021).

Unpleasant odors can negatively stimulate neonates' sense of smell. Various odorous products, such as cleaners, skin preparations, antibiotics, and alcohol (wipes and hand gels), are often present in the typical NICU environment. The neonate can also be exposed to fragrances, cologne, or aftershave worn by various staff members. Infants may respond to noxious olfactory stimuli with altered respirations, transient apnea, an increased heart rate (HR), and decreased cerebral blood flow (Gellrich et al., 2024).

Enhancing the olfactory environment can be achieved through the utilization of olfactory NPIs. These positive NPIs may include maternal breast scent via a breast pad or a soft scent cloth. SSC helps support the discrimination of maternal breast scent. Mouth care provided with the mother's milk helps the infant recognize the mother's smell and associates that smell with food and feeding when the infant can nipple feed. Staff should not wear perfume, cologne, or aftershave in the NICU. Available unscented procedure preparation products should be used. Alcohol wipes should not be opened near an infant's head, and preferably outside of the incubator environment. Cleaning products utilized in the NICU should be unscented. Laundry services should also use unscented products. The odor of tobacco on caregiver bodies and clothing and the odors of dry-cleaning chemicals should be avoided. NICU staff and parents should be educated on this topic to prevent olfactory overstimulation (Altimier & Phillips, 2016).

Tastebuds are observed by 8 weeks, and by 13 to 15 weeks, the tastebuds are similar to that of adults, and the fetus is sensitive to various tastes, including salty, bitter, sour, and sweet. Presenting the fetus with sour tastes results in them withdrawing and pulling faces, fussing, and changes in heart and respiratory rates. On the contrary, sweet tastes promote calming and prepare the fetus for feeding after birth. The fetus tastes what the mother tastes. For example, if a mother loves coffee during pregnancy, the coffee molecules are absorbed through the mucous membranes and move into the bloodstream. Then, it crosses the placenta, and the infant drinks up to 760 ml of amniotic fluid per day, getting to know the various tastes of the mother's diet. The intense sensory inputs of smell and taste are crucial for starting the metabolic pathways that help with digestion and metabolic control (Bloomfield et al., 2017).

**Noise/Auditory.** The hearing system is fully intact by 20 weeks, and a reaction to sound is observed at 24 weeks of gestation (6 months). At birth, ears are capable of discerning more than 300,000 sounds. The brain processes sounds a thousand times faster than images and registers sounds even during sleep. The constant bath of noise affects everything from concentration to health. The word *noise* comes from nausea, the Latin word for sickness. Arousal is important with premature infants who are unable to inhibit responses. Premature and sick neonates may require weeks of hospitalization in a noisy NICU environment with sound levels that may reach 120 dB. The American Academy of Pediatrics recommends a maximum sound level of 45 dB. Mean sound levels for day, evening, and night shifts were 83.5, 83, and 80.9 dB, respectively (Mayhew et al., 2022). Each time period exceeded the recommended guidelines 90% of the time and was almost double the American Academy of Pediatrics recommendation. A sound level of 45 dB is approximately equivalent to the sound level of rainfall, whereas a sound level of 120 dB is roughly equivalent to a thunderclap or an ambulance siren (Mayhew et al., 2022) Noise in hospitals has been a topic of concern for more than 160 years, dating back to the time of Florence Nightingale, who admonished, "Noise is the absence of care" (Nightingale, 1859).

Calikusu Incekar and Balci (2017) reported that the most prevalent noise sources in the NICU are monitor alarms and human voices. High noise levels in NICUs affect infants as well as staff and families. Stress reactions from loud noises in the NICU cause newborns to have bradycardia, tachycardia, increased systolic and diastolic blood pressure, apnea, hypoxemia, alterations in oxygen saturation, increased oxygen consumption, and elevated intracranial pressure, can increase the risk of problems such as growth delay, irregular sleep patterns, hearing loss, BPD, retinopathy of prematurity, intraventricular hemorrhage, periventricular leukomalacia, and developmental delay (Almadhoob & Ohlsson, 2020). Noise also contributes to sleep disturbance, hearing impairment, and decreased oxygen saturation, which can harm nervous system development (Reinke et al., 2020). It has been proven that moderate acoustic changes between 5 and 10 dBA can disrupt the sleep of very early preterm infants (Kuhn et al., 2011). Between 2% and 10% of infants born before their due date are diagnosed as hard of hearing, compared to only 0.1% of the general child population (Sibrecht et al., 2024).

The facility and operations in the NICU affect the acoustic environment. This noise comes from various structural and operational sources. Structural sources include heating, ventilation, and air conditioning (HVAC) systems, door openings and closings, and the hum generated by electrical equipment, such as computers and incubators. Operational sources encompass staff and visitor conversations, chair movement, the opening of disposable containers, medical equipment alarms, phones, and infant crying (Casey et al., 2020; Hernandez-Molina et al., 2020; Rodríguez-Montaño et al., 2024).

Much of the therapy provided in the NICU is noisy, making it challenging to facilitate developmentally beneficial auditory stimuli. These high noise levels are often a result of equipment, alarms, nonacoustic finishes, communication devices, and talking, as well as the underlying HVAC system. NICU sound levels vary based on the hour of day and are often related to shift changes and medical rounds (Hutchinson et al., 2020). SFRs and larger clinical patient areas help reduce environmental noise because sound transmission declines geometrically as distances are increased (Altimier et al., 2023).

Understanding baseline sound levels and contributing environmental factors is the first step in developing strategies to mitigate excessive noise in the NICU (Mayhew et al., 2022). Recommended guidelines for the acoustic environment state that infant rooms, staff work areas, and family areas shall be designed to produce minimal background noise and contain and absorb as much transient noise as possible.

The combination of continuous background sound and operational sound in the infant area/room shall not exceed an hourly local environmental quality (Leq) of 45 dBA, an hourly L10 (noise level exceeded for 10% of the time of the duration of the measurement) of 50 dBA, and transient sounds or Lmax (the RMS [root mean squared] maximum level of a noise source or environment) should not exceed A-weighted dBA of 65, slow response. In staff work areas, family areas, and staff lounge areas, the combination of continuous background sound and operational sound shall not exceed an hourly Leq of 50 dB and an hourly L10 of 55 dB levels, both A-weighted, slow response. Transient sounds or Lmax shall not exceed 70 dB, A-weighted, slow response in these areas (Altimier et al., 2023).

**Language Development.** One major morbidity associated with preterm birth is recessive and expressive language delay. Language outcomes are correlated with gestational age and birth weight and inversely correlated with the level of brain injury (Cristobal & Oghalai, 2008).

Extended hospitalization in the NICU causes missed opportunities for language exposure at critical developmental periods of neural pathways for language processing (Newnam & Muñoz, 2021). Achieving the desired sound levels can help promote infant sleep and allow the infant to hear human voices during normal conversations (Philben, 2004, 2017). Although it is known that alarms and high-decibel sounds are not good, soothing sounds and talking to the preterm infant are critical to auditory processing and language development. The acoustic environment in the NICU is particularly deleterious. This loud, highly pitched, unorganized, and unpredictable noise can contribute to the neurocognitive burden of preterm birth, leading to attention deficit disorders and potential alterations in early communicative skills (El-Metwally & Medina, 2020). Speech and language impairments of simple and complex language functions are shared among former preterm infants. Although incubator walls may protect against noxious noise levels, these findings reveal a potentially detrimental effect on language exposure for infants inside a NICU incubator (Monson et al., 2020). Risk factors include lower gestational age and increasing severity of illness, including severe brain injury. Even in the absence of brain injury, however, altered brain maturation and vulnerability imposed by premature entrance to the extrauterine environment are associated with structural and microstructural brain changes. These alterations are associated with language impairments, lasting effects in childhood and adolescence, and increased needs for speech therapy and education support (Vohr, 2014). Because nurses tend to be task oriented, this may need to be practiced to become "routine" during caregiving tasks.

One study by Pineda et al. (2012) showed that infants in SFRs with no parent present for significant periods had decreased verbal scores after NICU discharge (Pineda et al., 2012). Caskey and colleagues showed that infants whose parents talked to them had increased vocalizations in the NICU (Caskey et al., 2014; Filippa & Kuhn, 2024; Filippa et al., 2019; Filippa et al., 2020; Vohr et al., 2017). Healthcare providers (HCPs), particularly nurses, can be instrumental in providing infant-directed speech to improve neurodevelopmental outcomes. As frontline neonatal providers, nurses can be role models of infant-directed speech for parents, helping them gain comfort and understand the importance of speaking to their preterm infants. Nurses can also provide much-needed language nutrition to preterm infants when parents are absent (Newnam & Muñoz, 2021).

The noise in NICUs is louder than in our homes or most work environments. Reducing noise in the NICU to below 45 dB is recommended but very difficult to achieve (Sibrecht et al., 2024). Crowded rooms full of equipment can influence healthcare personnel's ability to provide environmentally appropriate care to premature infants. Noise equipment levels have been a challenge to minimize due to industrial design standards and alarm management parameters; however, more companies are focusing more attention on the noise levels generated by such equipment. Noise criterion ratings should be considered when selecting new equipment. Including this parameter in purchasing decisions is worthwhile.

Infant bed areas should be situated to produce minimal background noise and to contain and absorb as much transient noise as possible. Many sound control features should be considered when designing a NICU. Evidence-based sound-reducing strategies have decreased decibel levels by 4 to 6 dB when planning environmental management as part of a developmental, family-centered NICU (Rodríguez-Montaño et al., 2024). The current air duct and ventilation systems should be evaluated for noise and dust. Acoustic ceiling tiles in direct patient care areas should have a noise reduction coefficient (NRC) rating of at least 0.90 for 80% of the entire surface area or an average NRC of 0.85 for the whole ceiling, including solid and acoustically absorptive surfaces (Altimier et al., 2023). Porcelain sinks rather than stainless steel sinks can also minimize noise. Carpet decreases the noise level and promotes a homelike environment, yet rubber or vinyl flooring material directly at the bedside can ease routine cleaning. Carpeting should be avoided in direct patient care areas, around sinks, and in clean and soiled utility rooms. Other surfaces, such as sound-absorbing wall surfaces and acoustic partitions, may minimize noise (Altimier et al., 2023).

The thoughtful design of traffic patterns and workspaces can help remove unwanted noise. Beds built in a pod design rather than down a long hall can reduce staff travel time and decrease noise levels for the beds near the hallway's end (White, 2018). Additionally, strategically placing patient care supplies, linen, and trash on walls that access the hallway through sliding cupboards/doors is an innovative way to help reduce traffic into the patient room/care area.

Background sound levels in the NICU may interfere with an infant's ability to discriminate speech of parents and other caregivers. Neonates are also exposed to vibration and noise when transported and on high-frequency ventilation. Noise and vibration combined may have a synergistic effect. Telephones audible from the infant area should have adjustable announcing signals. Noise can be limited through communication devices such as wireless phones that are set to vibrate. This technology minimizes the need for hardwired phones placed close to the infant and can reduce the need for beepers, overhead paging systems, and intercoms.

Dampening sounds from equipment, such as waste receptacles, sinks, paper towel dispensers, and movable equipment, is suggested for sound containment. Eliminating radios and all other unnecessary sounds, transferring infants from warmers to incubators with quiet motors as soon after admission as possible, and covering incubators with thick quilts/blankets with sound-absorbent material will also assist with sound abatement. Fire alarms in the infant area should be restricted to flashing lights without an audible signal. The loud alarm level in other occupied areas must be adjustable.

Recently, Filippa et al. (2019) have provided an important and thorough review of the evidence supporting the behavioral orientation of the newborn to early vocal contact and music, assessed by functional neuroimaging techniques (Filippa, 2019; Filippa, et al., 2019). New evidence shows that music therapy has beneficial effects on vital signs when delivered to sleeping preterm infants (Kobus et al., 2021). Music therapy has been used in some NICUs to calm and soothe staff in the overall unit.

Sound exposure intensity and duration should be considered when evaluating the noise levels in a NICU. Some units place microphones in the ceiling above or on walls adjacent to infant care areas to determine the sound levels transmitted to the infant (decibel monitoring system). These microphones are wired to a monitoring device that feeds a signal to a visual alarm if the sound level exceeds a predetermined level. This visual system helps alert staff and parents to sounds that exceed a reasonable level. It provides a gentle reminder to lower the sound level to provide a quiet, healing environment for NICU infants, staff, and families (Altimier, 2015).

In addition to the effect on patient care, constant noise in the NICU also affects the health and well-being of nursing staff. Studies have shown that prolonged noise exposure can cause hearing fatigue, increase blood pressure, and contribute to the development of cardiovascular diseases and psychological disorders, such as anxiety and depression, difficulty communicating, work stress, decreased concentration, and increased risk of making mistakes, which in turn, can lead to decreased performance and negatively affect the quality of care they provide (Almadhoob & Ohlsson, 2020).

**Light/Vision.** Protecting the visual system's development is essential because visual problems continue to be common among NICU graduates who were born prematurely. Visual stimulation is not required at any point before term gestation because the visual system is the last sensory system to develop functionally at term. The eyelids and iris control the amount of light entering the eye. Infants at or before 32 weeks' gestation have thin eyelids and little or no pupillary constriction, thus allowing light to reach the retina much easier than more mature infants, children, and adults (Graven, 2011; LeVay et al., 1980). At 29 to 30 weeks' gestation, sleep partitions into rapid eye movement (REM) and non-REM (NREM; slow-wave) sleep. Transition to regular sleep occurs around 30 to 34 weeks' gestation. Protecting sleep cycles, especially REM sleep periods, is critical for healthy visual development because any event or drug that disrupts REM sleep can affect visual development (Graven, 2011).

Endogenous brain activity stimulation (activity independent) is created by spontaneous firing of neural cells in the retina, lateral geniculate nucleus (LGN), spinal cord, hippo campus, pons, cerebellum, cerebral cortex, and auditory systems, which occurs at a particular time in their development. The endogenous stimulation of the visual system prepares the retina, LGN, and visual cortex for exogenous or outside stimulation (Graven, 2006). At 40 weeks' gestation, the human visual system has intact retinal development and pathways to the visual cortex. At this time, the visual system must have regular visual stimulation. Visual experiences for healthy visual development require ambient light (not direct light), focus, attention, novelty, movement, and color after 2 to 3 months. The visual system develops in utero in almost a total absence of light, and therefore, the visual system is not developmentally ready for external visual stimuli until birth at term. Three main areas of care in the NICU that can adversely affect visual development are interference with endogenous brain cell activity, sleep deprivation, and intense light exposure (Graven, 2006).

Lighting in the NICU should be adjusted to support each infant's best sleep and awake organization and to deliver care without impinging on other infants' development, comfort, and care. Additionally, light needs adjusted to the infant's developmental stage with a balance between dimmed ambient lighting, natural lighting, and brighter task lighting (Lawhon & Als, 2010). A preterm infant should never be positioned facing directly into a light source. Only indirect ambient lighting should be utilized for preterm infants who cannot block light through their thin eyelids, turn away from light, and communicate their needs (Rodríguez & Pattini, 2016; White, 2018). The focus of care for preterm infants of 22 to 28 weeks' gestation and VLBW infants should be on protecting the eyes from direct light and keeping ambient light exposure to low levels. Care of preterm infants at 28 to 36 weeks' gestation should focus on safeguarding sleep cycles, especially REM sleep. During this time, intense stimulation from NICU noises, vibrations, and other disturbing stimuli of different sensory systems can significantly interfere with the processes of visual system development (Lickliter, 2011).

Ambient lighting levels in the infant care spaces shall be adjustable through a range of at least 10 to no more than 600 Lux (the international symbol unit of illuminance), with a color rendering index (CRI) greater than 80 and a gamut area index (GAI) greater than 80 and less than 100. Both natural and electric light sources need to have controls that allow immediate, sufficient darkening of any bed space for transillumination when necessary. No direct view of the electric light source or sun shall be permitted in the infant space. Using multiple switches with individual dimmers to allow different illumination levels is helpful. Procedural lighting should be available at each bedside to enable caregivers to evaluate an infant or to perform a procedure. This increased illumination should not increase the light levels of adjacent infants. Illumination of support areas such as charting, medication preparation, and reception areas should be adequate to allow essential or critical tasks. This light level should conform to Illuminating Engineering Society specifications (www.iesna.org). Independent controls should be used to accommodate sleeping infants and working staff (Altimier et al., 2023; Rea & Figueiro, 2016).

Each infant room, care area, or adjacent staff work area should have at least one daylight source visible. Windows provides a psychological benefit to NICU staff as well as families. Daylighting is desirable for charting and the evaluation of infant skin tone. Exterior windows provide the recommended natural light and assist with diurnal cycling. However, serious problems with radiant heat loss or gain and glare can occur if infants are placed too close to external windows. External windows should be at least 2 feet from the infant's bed and may be placed away from direct patient areas—for example, high up on the walls, as skylights, or in other locations that provide indirect light to the patient area. The latter might be a window in a hallway that secondarily allows light to pass into the NICU. All windows, including skylights, should have retractable covers for times when light is not desired. These windows should be insulated and have shading devices in a neutral color to minimize color distortion from transmitted light. Significant flexibility in lighting levels is required to accommodate the disparate needs of infants at various stages of development and at different times of the day, as well as the needs of caregivers (Altimier et al., 2023).

## Safeguarding Sleep

Sleep is essential for life. Sleep is not simply a period of physical and mental rest; like wakefulness, it is an active physiologic process during which complex changes occur in the brain. Sleep in early life is essential for proper functional brain development, which is necessary for the brain to integrate and process information. Sleep is one of the primary activities of the brain during early development and plays an essential role in healthy cognitive and psychosocial development in early life (Chaput et al., 2017). Sleep serves multiple purposes for ensuring brain health, including maturation of the central nervous system, learning and memory consolidation, emotional processing, secretion of growth hormones, energy storage, illness recovery, and, most importantly, maintaining neural networks and synaptic plasticity (Als et al., 1994; Cirelli & Tononi, 2017; Graven & Browne, 2008). Sleep plays a critical role in regulating emotional brain function, which is the ability of the human brain to generate, regulate, and be guided by emotions in daily life (Kurth et al., 2015).

Sleep organization begins during fetal life when it is influenced by multiple maternal zeitgebers (White, 2018). Preterm infants are deprived of these maternal factors, so they develop a sleep structure based on the environment of the NICU. Preterm infants typically sleep less and have seriously disrupted and fragmented patterns of sleep (Levy et al., 2017).

The chaotic environment of the NICU can interfere with infants' ability to modulate their sleep–wake states. Preterm infants need caregivers' assistance regulating their sleep–wake states by reducing environmental stress and adjusting nursing care activities (Als, 1986). Therefore, it is important to develop supportive interventions to facilitate infants' sleep and mitigate the negative influences of sleep disruption in the NICU.

As the primary behavioral state of the newborn infant, sleep (REM and NREM sleep cycling) is a prerequisite for normal neural network development, synaptogenesis, and synaptic plasticity, particularly during the accelerated period of brain development that occurs in the last trimester (Cirelli & Tononi, 2017; Graven, 2006; Lowe et al., 2017). In neonates, the sleep cycle is frequently categorized into three stages: active, quiet, and indeterminate. Quiet sleep plays a role in energy restoration and cerebral maturation, particularly in developing thalamocortical and cortical pathways and synaptogenesis. It stabilizes neuronal connections, increases protein synthesis, and releases growth hormones. A high level of endogenous neuronal activity characterizes active sleep. It contributes to the central nervous system's maturation, memory consolidation, and axonal connections, especially between the retina and the brain, and is accompanied by REM (Graven, 2006; Tarullo et al., 2011).

Zores et al. (2018) found that small light-level increases led to sleep disruption in very preterm infants. Combined with their previous results, which documented the physiologic responses of very preterm infants to changes in light levels, their current findings demonstrate that very preterm infants are visually sensitive to small changes in light levels. Notably, these behavioral and physiologic responses occurred when small light-level changes were within the range recommended by the American Academy of Pediatrics. The primary determinant of awakening was the initial light level. The physiologic and behavioral responses were more remarkable, and awakening events were more common under medium light protection than high light protection conditions. Thus, very preterm infants reacted more strongly to a slight change in light level when the baseline light level was greater (White, 2020b; Zores-Koenig et al., 2020). The Cochrane review on cycled lighting also included randomized controlled trials demonstrating improved outcomes for infants in a cycled lighting environment (Morag & Ohlsson, 2016).

Sleep states in the human fetus are expressed as different behavioral states during the earliest weeks of development, driven by activity from deeper brain structures (Uchitel et al., 2022); at approximately 28 weeks' gestation, individual sleep patterns emerge characterized by REM and NREM sleep periods. These periods become constant by 36 to 38 weeks gestational age. REM sleep dominates in the initial sleep cycles; REM and NREM are nearly equal as the infant approaches term, and by 8 months of age, NREM sleep occupies almost 80% of sleep time (Hobson, 1995). REM and NREM sleep cycling are essential for early neurosensory development, learning and memory, and preservation of brain plasticity for the individual's life. For the visual system, the need for visual experiences only occurs near term or 40 weeks gestational age. The environment of the fetus in utero and the preterm infant in the NICU require appropriate levels of specific neurosensory stimuli for healthy early brain development (Graven, 2006; Graven & Browne, 2008).

The preservation of "brain plasticity," the ability of the brain to change its structure and function constantly in response to environmental changes, is an essential process throughout childhood and adult life. Alterations in sleep architecture correlate with measurable structural changes in the brain (Benders et al., 2015). Sleep deprivation (REM and NREM) results in a loss of brain plasticity, manifested by smaller brains, altered subsequent learning, and long-term effects on behavior and brain function. Facilitation and protection of sleep and sleep cycles are essential to long-term learning and continuing brain development by preserving brain plasticity (Graven & Browne, 2008).

Because REM sleep is essential for neurosensory as well as visual development, neuroprotective strategies for the NICU infant include the following:

- Protect the eyes from direct light exposure and maintain low levels of ambient light when not needed for care and procedures.
- Provide some daily exposure to light, preferably including shorter wavelengths, for entrainment of the circadian rhythm.
- Protect sleep cycles, and especially REM sleep; avoid sleep interruptions, bright lights, loud noises, and unnecessary physical disturbing activities.
- Avoid high doses of sedative and depressing drugs, which can depress the endogenous firing of cells, thus interfering with visual development, REM, and NREM sleep cycles.
- Provide developmental care appropriate for the age and maturation of the infant (Graven, 2011).

Continuous bright lights in the NICU can disrupt sleep–wake states. Patients of any age who are trying to sleep find direct light unpleasant. Premature infants are photophobic; however, they will open their eyes with dim lights. Infants never experience the diurnal rhythm necessary for development if the light levels never change. Reducing light levels may facilitate rest and subsequent energy conservation and promote organization and growth.

Particular attention should be given to lighting for caregivers who work night shifts. Staff's visual and circadian needs are quite different from those of patients. Five characteristics of light essential for both human visual and circadian systems are quantity, spectrum, timing, duration, and distribution. The visual system responds well to a light stimulus at any time of the day or night and does not depend on light timing. Timing of the light exposure, however, is critical for circadian development. The visual system responds to a light stimulus in milliseconds, yet the duration of light exposure necessary to stimulate the circadian system can take minutes (Figueiro, 2020; White, 2017).

Most infants should remain in a dimly lit environment at night, yet some staff may have difficulty staying alert, which could cause safety concerns. Shift work disorder (SWD) is a circadian rhythm sleep–wake disorder characterized by insomnia and excessive sleepiness with a shortened total sleep time that occurs due to a recurring work schedule that overlaps with one's habitual sleep period. SWD is associated with decreased productivity, impaired safety, diminished quality of life, and adverse effects on health, such as increased risk for metabolic syndrome, diabetes, cardiovascular disease, ischemic stroke, depression, obesity, gastrointestinal dysfunction, and ulcers, reproductive problems, and cancer (Sachdeva & Goldstein, 2020). Both caregivers' health and infants' safety need to be considered in all unit designs.

Light levels should be regularly monitored and reported to staff for self-assessment and to provide interventions and opportunities for improvement. Both intensity and duration of light exposure should be considered when evaluating the light levels in a NICU. Some units place visual sensors in the ceiling above or on walls adjacent to infant care areas to determine the light levels transmitted to the infant. This can help alert staff and parents to light levels that exceed a reasonable level and provide a gentle reminder to lower the light level to provide a dimmed healing environment for NICU infants, staff, and families.

## Positioning, Handling, and Clustering Care

Even as we focus on the macroenvironment in most of this chapter, we must remember the microenvironment. Positioning (or nesting) the neonate in midline, flexion, and containment is an important NPI that minimizes the effect of environmental stimuli from the NICU, promoting comfort and sleep. Nesting facilitates the transformation of the sleep pattern from erratic disturbed spells to deep, peaceful periods of sleep, which has been shown to conserve energy and minimize weight loss. A study by Mony et al. (2018) observed the effect of nesting on sleep patterns among preterm infants admitted to NICUs. Results demonstrated a significantly higher (113 minutes) total duration of sleep time among infants with nesting as compared to routine care (86 minutes), which was highly significant ($t = 4.930$, $p < .001$) (Mony et al., 2018).

Newborn infants admitted to the NICU are constantly handled, which disturbs their sleep patterns. Therefore, to ensure that infants get enough undisturbed sleep, daily routines such as cleaning, changing diapers, oil massage, weighing, putting caps, gloves, and socks, giving antibiotics, and feeding can be easily done by the nurse together in a cluster when the infant is awake instead of disturbing the infant's sleep by doing these activities at different times (Greenspan et al., 2021). Clustered care represents clustering nursing care procedures and several routine practices performed together instead of spacing them out over time. The main goal of clustering care is to allow premature infants to rest longer by improvements in state/sleep organization (Hendy et al., 2024; Mizan, 2021).

## Minimizing Stress and Pain

Prolonged exposure to high levels of noise can increase the risk of sleep disorders and stress. Additionally, preterm infants typically cared for in NICUs undergo repeated invasive procedures, which can result in pain and stress and, in turn, disturb infants' sleep cycles and sleep quality, all of which influence their growth and overall health (Lan et al., 2018; Lan et al., 2019; Valeri et al., 2015).

Large numbers of painful procedures in preterm infants (gestational age ≤ 29 weeks) are associated with delayed postnatal growth, poor early neurodevelopment, high cortical activation, long-term abnormalities in white matter microstructure, brain development, and lower IQ in toddlers born very preterm (gestational age ≤ 32 weeks). Furthermore, more significant numbers of painful neonatal experiences cumulatively have been associated with a poor quality of cognitive and motor development at 1 year of age and changes in cortical rhythmicity and cortical thickness in children at 7 years of age (Valeri et al., 2015).

The procedures involved in neonatal intensive care are considered stressful to varying degrees, regardless of the postconceptional age of preterm neonates. Such exposure can trigger toxic stress responses in the body, leading to irritability, increased blood pressure, and HR, increasing the risk of physiologic instability and bleeding in cranial and intravascular regions (McPherson et al., 2020; van Dokkum et al., 2021). The utilization of supportive care bundles (modulation of the infants' states, nonnutritive sucking, facilitated tucking, and oral sucrose) during intrusive procedures not only significantly increases sleep efficiency and total sleep time but also significantly decreases the duration of sleep latency and frequency of wake bouts ((Lan et al., 2018). Bundled developmental care lowers newborns' pain, stress, and recovery time (Chuang et al., 2019).

### The Social Environment—Staff and Family Partnerships

The admission of an infant to the NICU is frequently a crisis for the family. The delivery is usually unexpected, and the family unit is often separated. Their infant is attached to wires, cables, and equipment in a harsh NICU environment that is far different from the newly decorated home nursery they had planned. The environment can become comforting and inviting, with attentive and compassionate caregivers who provide a welcoming environment to initiate effective partnerships with parents.

Partnering with families in the NICU offers a philosophy of care acknowledging that, over time, the family has the most significant influence over an infant's health and well-being. Creating an effective partnership between professionals and families has shown benefits such as decreased length of stay (LOS), increased satisfaction for both staff and parents, and enhanced neurodevelopmental outcomes for infants (Segers et al., 2018). A recent study by Welch et al. (2017) strengthened the conclusion that family-nurturing interventions (FNI) promote cerebral cortical development in preterm infants (Welch et al., 2017).

Establishing family–professional partnerships in the NICU environment can be challenging; yet, because families are the constant in the infant's life, helping families achieve a positive outcome from their NICU experience should be a priority while providing care. The family is integral to developmental care, and NICU design should include accommodations and considerations for the comfort and support of families. Parents must be viewed as partners in the care of their infant rather than visitors to the NICU, and spaces should be created in the NICU environment that are welcoming and encourages their presence in the NICU and participation in their infant's care. Consideration should be given to attractive and clear signage in the primary languages spoken by the populations served by the hospital. Adequate and convenient storage of personal belongings should be made available to parents who will spend considerable time in the NICU. Comfortable chairs should be present at every bedside to facilitate prolonged SSC between parents and infants because early SSC is associated with a reduced risk of BPD development, cholestasis, and nosocomial infections (Casper et al., 2018). Providing parents with computer and Internet access, educational materials, and space for parents to socialize supports the emotional and psychosocial needs of NICU parents. It is ideal to have spaces with equipment for parents to make meals, wash clothes, shower, and sleep near their infant. Private spaces for therapeutic interactions with NICU mental health providers will facilitate psychosocial support for NICU parents who are at significantly increased risk for postpartum depression, anxiety disorders, and posttraumatic stress disorder.

The well-being of NICU staff is equally important. NICU staff often suffer from caregiving fatigue and secondary posttraumatic stress. Prioritizing equipment and workspace in the NICU design that optimizes staff workflows will support NICU staff in providing the best care efficiently. NICU design that includes spaces for rest in a pleasant environment during work breaks will give NICU staff tangible evidence of the value placed on their well-being.

Promoting a healing social environment requires a NICU design that prioritizes the need to support all members of the multidisciplinary team involved in caring for preterm and sick infants in the NICU, including medical, nursing, therapy staff, and parents. Equilateral respect and support among all members involved in this partnership will promote optimal patient care, enhance family satisfaction, and engage the healthcare team.

## THE FUTURISTIC NICU

Premature and ill full-term infants require complex, real-time clinical decision support correlating medical data from multiple sources because there are many potential complications of prematurity.

Neonatal intensive care is a complex environment that must support collaborative decision making among various care providers. Clinical decision support utilizing "Big Data" in the NICU can benefit from online health analytics platforms that leverage high-speed physiologic data and other electronic health record data (Cole, 2021; Zimmet et al., 2021).

Infants in the NICU are frequently attached to many different medical devices, such as cardiorespiratory monitors, mechanical ventilators, temperature probes via incubators, smart infusion pumps, and neurologic monitors, all of which display constantly changing sensed data, usually at second-by-second intervals, generating over a billion data points per patient per day. Caregivers, typically NICU nurses, must translate this data into actionable information.

Recent and upcoming technologies are changing how we deliver neonatal intensive care and support infants and their parents through their NICU journey. Technology has long been the backbone of modern neonatal intensive care, yet with the overwhelming amounts of data generated by technology and electronic medical records, there is a need to view the infant and infant parameters holistically to support clinical decision making. Clinical rule-based engines and deep learning combined with comprehensive, integrated platforms can address current issues of NICUs, such as tedious workflows and the integration of big data generated by multiple devices at once.

## SUMMARY

The NICU is where an extraordinary period of growth and development will take place for premature infants. Because preterm infants are no longer protected in the uterus, their physiologic and neuroprotective needs have dramatically changed. To meet the unique developmental needs of preterm and sick neonates, efforts must be made to modify the usual hospital environment to create a specialized healing environment that supports their ongoing neurosensory and neurobehavioral development. Whenever possible, the optimal healing environment for infants in the NICU is in SSC with their mothers (or other primary caregivers). It also encompasses the physical environment (space, privacy, and safety), the sensory environment (touch, temperature, tastes, smells, noise, and light), and the social environment (families and staff). While aiming for a gentler approach, continually assess and reevaluate the treatments and routines because sometimes "less" is best, while at other times, "less" might not be enough.

## CASE STUDY

**Identification of the Problem.** A 24-week gestational age newly born premature infant girl weighing 650 g

**Assessment: History and Physical Examination.** Upon delivery, the infant was limp, cyanotic/pale, and apneic. The infant was successfully resuscitated following Neonatal Resuscitation Program© (NRP) guidelines; required 2 minutes of positive pressure ventilation by T-piece resuscitator to initiate effective ventilation when spontaneous respirations were noted; the infant received 10 minutes of continuous positive airway pressure (CPAP) via the T-piece resuscitator, prior to being transferred to the NICU.

### Physical Examination on Admission to the NICU

- TEMPERATURE: 96.26°F (35.7°C), axillary HR 180 beats/min; respiratory rate (RR): 56, shallow; saturations 88% to 92% in room air
- HEAD, EARS, EYES, NOSE, AND MOUTH (HEENT): Within normal limits (WNL)
- RESPIRATORY: lung fields bilaterally clear and equal to bases; grunting
- CARDIOVASCULAR: rate regular with no murmur noted; good peripheral perfusion, capillary blood refill less than 3 seconds, and strong peripheral pulses noted
- ABDOMEN: abdomen soft, flat, and nontender with no masses palpable; three-vessel cord; the anus appeared patent
- GENITOURINARY: normal female infant genitalia
- NEUROLOGIC: appropriate responses, eyes open, and infant blinks; extremities well formed; decreased muscle tone
- SKIN: pale pink, thin, transparent, yet intact skin
- EXTREMITIES: well-formed; 10 digits per extremity; low tone
- Umbilical arterial and venous catheters were placed for fluid management and laboratory specimen draws

**Differential Diagnosis.** The differential diagnosis includes the following:

1. Prematurity
2. Perinatal hypoxic-ischemic injury
3. Shock
4. Congestive heart failure
5. Sepsis screen

**Diagnostic Tests.** Head ultrasound at 24 hours of age

**Working Diagnosis.** Extreme prematurity

### Development of a Management Plan

- Place the infant in 80% humidified incubator.
- Position the infant in the midline, flexed, and contained position utilizing positioning aids.
- Continuously monitor vital signs (VS) every 2 to 4 hours.
- Maintain fluid support; total parenteral nutrition (TPN) within 24 hours of life.
- Provide respiratory support with CPAP as needed.
- Administer antibiotics until cultures are negative for 72 hours.

**Implementation.** Implementation of Management Plan (Immediately After Initial Assessment in the NICU)

- Mother was transferred with infant to a Couplet Care Room for her care as well as the care of her infant with father assisting.
- Infant was placed on a CPAP setting of five within the first half hour of life.

### Evaluation of Effectiveness

- Temperature was 98.06°F (36.7°C) at 1 hour of life.
- Respiratory status was stable by 2 hours of life.
- Blood pressure was normal within 2 hours of life.

**Outcome.** Extremely premature white female infant with stable VS. Anticipate lengthy NICU stay. Neuroprotective family-centered developmental care will be individualized to meet the infant's and family's needs at each developmental stage. Exogenous stimuli will be limited, with positive neuroprotective strategies introduced as tolerated and warranted.

## EVIDENCE-BASED PRACTICE

The design and operation of NICUs have evolved from the 1960s to the 2020s to support and accommodate the changes in technology involved in meeting the physical and caregiving needs of preterm infants and their families. The equipment has changed, the space has enlarged, and caregiving practices have changed. Units historically were designed as large, open areas with visibility for the caregivers. Infants were in rows, close to each other, with open space between bays. Technology has advanced with the ability to keep smaller and smaller infants alive. Small infants—those who are less than 1,500 g—occupy most patient days, with many stays being 3 months and longer. Although the survival rate has improved, the number of infants with evidence of neurologic and learning problems continues to increase.

The focus on the environment of preterm infants and young neonates began in the 1970s but made little progress in changing the environment of the fetus or infant until the 1990s. Even in 2025, it is estimated that less than half of the more than 1,500 NICUs in the United States, and even fewer in Europe and Asia, are able to maintain an environment and care practices that are supportive of early neurosensory and neuromotor brain development. These units support the physiology of care, but many fail to support the needs for healthy brain development.

Although preterm birth accelerates the maturation of the lungs, kidneys, and gastrointestinal tract, it does not accelerate neuroprocesses, and under most conditions of care, it can seriously alter these processes. Processes under genetic control are thought to be important but not altered by the environment. With the studies of epigenetics, it is now clear that environmental factors can alter the expression of genes related to brain development without altering the DNA structure or code for the gene.

Alterations in the sensory environment including excess noise, bright lights, sleep deprivation, and poorly timed caregiving all affect neurosensory development in the preterm infant. The physical environment, the nutritional environment, and the social/emotional environment also influence the processes involved in the early development of the neurosensory systems. Neuroprotective family-centered developmental care provided in an environment that supports early brain development is essential for optimal outcomes and the best possible long-term development. It is essential that NICUs make changes necessary to have a healing environment along with care practices that support and protect the processes of early brain development (Altimier & White, 2020; Altimier et al., 2023).

### References

Altimier, L., & White, R. (2020). The neonatal intensive care unit (NICU) environment. In C. Kenner Boykova & J. Altimier (Eds.), *Comprehensive neonatal nursing care* (6th ed., pp. 2–6). Springer Publishing.

Altimier, L., Barton, S. A., Bender, J., Browne, J., Harris, D., Jaeger, C. B., Johnson, B. H., Kenner, C., Kolberg, K. J. S., Loder, A., Martin, G. L., Mohammed, S., Oelrich, T., Wilson Orr, L., Philbin, M. K., McCuskey Shepley, M., Shultz, J., Smith, J. A. ... White, R. D. (2023). Recommended standards for newborn ICU design. *Journal of Perinatology*, *43*(Suppl. 1), 2–16. https://doi.org/10.1038/s41372-023-01784-4

## ONLINE RESOURCES

**CourseConnect**

Resources for this chapter are online and available at www.springerpub.com/courseconnect.

## REFERENCES

References for this chapter are online and available at www.springerpub.com/courseconnect.

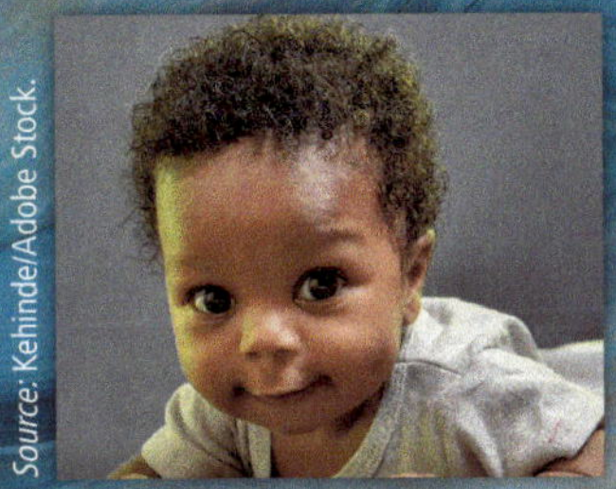


CHAPTER 26

# Touching Lives, Impacting Lifetimes: Trauma-Informed Developmental Care in the Neonatal Intensive Care Unit

Mary Coughlin, MS, NNP-NCC-E

## INTRODUCTION

In the neonatal intensive care unit (NICU), life begins in an environment where the first experiences of infants, families, and even clinicians are shaped by high stakes, stress, and hope. These early experiences leave profound imprints, influencing not only short-term outcomes but also the lifelong trajectory of every infant and family member. For clinicians, the cumulative exposure to trauma within the NICU can be equally impactful, underscoring the need for sustainable, compassionate care.

The Adverse Childhood Experiences (ACE) framework provides critical insights into how early adversity disrupts development and creates lasting physiologic, emotional, and relational consequences (Holuka et al., 2024; Swedo et al., 2023; Zhou & Ryan, 2023). The experience of early life adversity is not restricted to "other" people but to all people. In the NICU, early life adversity affects not only the infants and their families but also the clinicians, administrators, environmental service staff, cafeteria workers, security team, greeters, volunteers—everyone. While the ripple effects of adversity touch everyone in the NICU and beyond, the experiences of infants, families, and clinicians are uniquely intertwined, forming the core of trauma-informed developmental care efforts.

NICU infants face stressors such as separation from caregivers, painful procedures, and sensory overload—experiences that parallel those highlighted in the ACE research (Felitti et al., 1998). In a ground-breaking paper, Montirosso and Provenzi (2015) indicate that preterm birth is indeed "an early adverse experience characterized by exposure to high levels of stress and altered buffering effects of maternal care." These stressors disrupt neurodevelopment and can leave biologic imprints, predisposing infants to long-term challenges in cognitive, emotional, and physical health (Chung et al., 2020; Malin et al., 2024; Ramos et al., 2024). Families, too, are profoundly affected by the NICU experience. The uncertainty and trauma of having a critically ill infant can compound preexisting adversities, creating ripple effects that affect mental health, parental confidence, and attachment (Ciciolla et al., 2021; Mackle et al., 2023; Williams et al., 2023). Parents with higher ACE scores may be particularly vulnerable as unresolved trauma can influence their ability to navigate the NICU environment and bond with their child. Clinicians, while offering critical care, are not immune to the effects of trauma. The repeated exposure to suffering and high-pressure decision-making inherent in the NICU places them at risk for secondary trauma, empathic distress, and burnout (Beck, 2020; Beck et al., 2017; Benz et al., 2023; Dowling, 2018; Gannot et al., 2022). These outcomes mirror those seen in ACE populations, emphasizing the need for strategies that foster resilience and mitigate the emotional toll of care.

Trauma-Informed Developmental Care (TIDC) emerges as a compassionate and evidence-based response to these interconnected challenges. By integrating the ACE framework with advances in neuroscience and the principles of Dr. Jean Watson's Caring Science, TIDC offers a holistic approach to mitigating trauma and promoting healing. This model aligns the art and science of neonatal nursing, creating a framework where infants, families, and clinicians can thrive.

## MATERNAL CHILDHOOD ADVERSITY: RISK FOR PERINATAL COMPLICATIONS

Mothers' health profoundly shapes their children's outcomes, particularly during the perinatal period (Nolvi et al., 2023; Ramiro-Cortijo et al., 2021). Research on ACEs has highlighted how maternal early-life adversity contributes to a cascade of biologic, psychological, and social challenges that increase the risk of perinatal complications, including preterm birth, low birth weight, and NICU hospitalization (Barclay et al., 2023; Souch et al., 2022).

### Maternal Adverse Childhood Experiences and Perinatal Risk

Women with high adverse childhood experience (ACE) scores are at greater risk for complications during pregnancy, labor, and delivery. Studies indicate that maternal ACEs are associated with increased rates of hypertension, gestational diabetes, and preterm labor (Hardcastle et al., 2022; Mamun et al., 2023; Swedo et al., 2023). These complications are linked to the physiologic wear and tear of chronic stress, often referred to as *allostatic load*, which disrupts hormonal, immune, and vascular systems crucial for healthy pregnancy outcomes. The dysregulation of the hypothalamic–pituitary–adrenal (HPA) axis—a hallmark of ACE-related stress—can also influence placental function and fetal development, increasing the likelihood of preterm delivery and neonatal complications (Duffy et al., 2023; George et al., 2024).

Beyond physical health, maternal ACEs affect mental health during the perinatal period. Mothers with higher ACE scores are more likely to experience prenatal and postpartum depression, anxiety, and posttraumatic stress disorder (PTSD), which can hinder attachment and caregiving behaviors (Ciciolla et al., 2021; Williams et al., 2023). These challenges not only affect maternal well-being but also create an environment of heightened stress for the developing infant, compounding risks for adverse outcomes.

### Transgenerational Effects of Early Life Adversity

Early life adversity does not end with the individual; it ripples across generations. Epigenetic studies have shown that maternal stress and trauma can alter gene expression in offspring, influencing their vulnerability to chronic disease and developmental challenges (Hari et al., 2024; Hodge et al., 2024; Malin et al., 2023; Mascheroni et al., 2022; Provenzi et al., 2018). For instance, heightened maternal cortisol levels during pregnancy—linked to ACE-related stress—have been associated with changes in fetal brain development, including altered connectivity in regions responsible for emotion regulation and attachment (Nolvi et al., 2023; Stoye et al., 2020; Wu et al., 2020).

The transgenerational transmission of adversity is not limited to biologic mechanisms. Behavioral and relational pathways also play a critical role. Mothers with unresolved trauma may struggle to provide the consistent, nurturing care needed for secure attachment, unintentionally perpetuating cycles of dysregulation and adversity (Ishikawa et al., 2022; Kostova & Matanova, 2024; Sakti et al., 2023). This phenomenon, often referred to as "intergenerational trauma," underscores the importance of addressing maternal ACEs as part of neonatal care.

### Implications for Neonatal Intensive Care Unit Care

The NICU provides a unique opportunity to disrupt the transgenerational cycle of adversity. TIDC integrates an understanding of maternal ACEs into practices that support both the infant and the family. Strategies such as empowering parents to participate in caregiving, fostering skin-to-skin contact (SSC), and offering mental health resources for mothers can help mitigate the effects of trauma. These practices support maternal mental health and promote the parent–infant bond, laying a foundation for resilience.

Clinicians in the NICU must also be aware of the hidden vulnerabilities associated with maternal ACEs. Providing compassionate, nonjudgmental care creates a healing environment where mothers feel safe sharing their experiences and seeking support. This relational approach aligns with Watson's Caring Science—emphasizing the interconnectedness of the caregiver and the cared-for in the healing process.

### The Path Forward: Healing Across Generations

Addressing maternal childhood adversity is not just about improving individual outcomes—it is about breaking cycles of trauma and fostering resilience across generations. By recognizing the transgenerational effect of ACEs, NICU clinicians can advocate for care models that prioritize the holistic well-being of both the infant and the family. Trauma-informed practices, enriched by Caring Science principles, offer a pathway to healing that acknowledges the profound interplay between past experiences and future possibilities.

## THE CLINICIAN'S EARLY LIFE EXPERIENCES: SHAPING PROFESSIONAL PRESENCES

Just as early life adversity (ELA) shapes the trajectories of infants and families, it also influences the clinicians who care for them (Bryce et al., 2023; Icekson et al., 2024a, 2024b). A clinician's personal history—whether marked by security and resilience or adversity and trauma—affects their emotional responses, interpersonal dynamics, and overall approach to care. Understanding this interplay is critical for fostering self-awareness and cultivating trauma-informed professional practice.

### The Effect of Clinicians' Adverse Childhood Experiences on Care Delivery

Clinicians with higher ACE scores may find their own experiences of childhood adversity resurfacing in the emotionally charged NICU environment (Bouchard & Rainbow, 2021; Clark & Aboueissa, 2021). For some, witnessing the distress of families or the fragility of preterm infants may trigger unresolved trauma or feelings of helplessness. Others may unconsciously adopt hypervigilant or emotionally detached coping mechanisms, which can affect their ability to build authentic, empathetic connections with families and colleagues.

For example, a clinician with a history of unmet childhood needs may overidentify with a struggling parent, potentially leading to emotional overinvestment or burnout (Icekson et al., 2024b). Conversely, clinicians who experienced neglect or rejection in their own lives may unintentionally avoid deep emotional engagement with families to protect themselves from feelings of vulnerability (Coughlin McNeil, 2018). Though rooted in self-preservation, these reactions can create barriers to relational care and compromise the clinician's well-being.

### Building Resilience: Clinicians as Trauma-Informed Professionals

Acknowledging and addressing the potential influence of a clinician's ACEs is a key component of trauma-informed professional development (Graham, 2021; Mercer et al., 2023; Wolotira, 2022). Self-reflection and awareness are foundational for recognizing how past experiences shape present behaviors and reactions. Training programs that include modules on ACEs and self-care equip clinicians to identify triggers and adopt healthy coping strategies that enhance their professional presence.

Supportive NICU cultures also play a vital role in mitigating the effect of clinicians' ACEs (Fink-Samnick, 2022; Greer, 2023; Lauridsen & Munkejord, 2022). Structured opportunities for peer support, reflective practice, and mentorship allow clinicians to process challenging experiences and foster a sense of shared humanity. For instance, a clinician who feels emotionally overwhelmed by a parent's distress can benefit from debriefing with colleagues, where shared perspectives and support help reframe the experience as part of the collective caregiving journey.

### Trauma-Informed Self-Care as Professional Practice

Trauma-informed self-care is not a luxury but a necessity for clinicians in high-stress environments such as the NICU. Mindfulness practices, such as grounding exercises and meditation, can help clinicians regulate their stress responses and reconnect with their sense of purpose (Crego et al., 2021; Green & Kinchen, 2022 Riedl et al., 2024). Watson's Caring Science principles emphasize the importance of cultivating personal wholeness, encouraging clinicians to nurture their well-being as a prerequisite for compassionate care (Delgado-Galeano et al., 2023; Perkins, 2021; Watson, 2020).

Furthermore, understanding one's ACEs can deepen a clinician's empathy and resilience. When clinicians bring self-awareness to their practice, they can engage more authentically with families, fostering relationships built on mutual respect and understanding. This relational approach benefits families and reinforces the clinician's sense of meaning and fulfillment in their work.

### Transforming Adversity Into Strength

Clinicians' early life experiences, including adversity, can become a source of strength when integrated with intention and reflection. By acknowledging and addressing the influence of their past, clinicians can develop a deeper connection to their work and the families they serve. Trauma-informed care becomes a framework for healing others and a pathway for clinicians to heal themselves and grow as professionals.

In this way, clinicians embody the duality of resilience and vulnerability, modeling the courage and authenticity that lie at the heart of TIDC. Their ability to recognize and transform their own adversity becomes a powerful tool for breaking cycles of trauma and fostering a culture of healing in the NICU.

## THE INFANT IN THE NEONATAL INTENSIVE CARE UNIT AND ADVERSE CHILDHOOD EXPERIENCES

The earliest days of life for infants in the NICU are marked by stressors that parallel those identified in the ACE framework. While these infants are born into an environment designed to save lives, the unavoidable interventions and separations inherent in NICU care can introduce developmental adversity (Forkey et al., 2021; Montirosso & Provenzi, 2015; Sanders & Hall, 2018). Applying the lens of ACEs to the NICU experience highlights the importance of TIDC in mitigating stress and fostering resilience.

### Neonatal Intensive Care Unit Experiences as Early Adversity

The NICU experience for infants often involves invasive procedures, separation from caregivers, disrupted sleep patterns, and sensory overload. These stressors, though necessary for survival, activate a chronic toxic stress response that derails a healthy developmental trajectory and contributes to long-term physiologic and psychological consequences (Duffee et al., 2021; Forkey et al., 2021).
For example:

- Painful procedures: Frequent medical interventions activate the infant's stress response, increasing cortisol levels and altering stress regulation pathways (Melchior et al., 2022; Zhao et al., 2022, 2024).
- Caregiver separation: Prolonged physical separation from parents disrupts bonding and can impair the infant's emotional security (Bergman, 2019; Bergman et al., 2019).
- Sensory overload or deprivation: The high-tech NICU environment, with its constant alarms, bright lights, and limited opportunities for natural stimulation, can overwhelm or understimulate an infant's developing sensory systems (Beltran et al., 2022; Pavlyshyn et al., 2024; Pineda et al., 2021, 2023).

These early disruptions compound the infant's primary traumatic experience of maternal separation, which forms the backdrop for all subsequent traumatic experiences. Without intentional interventions aimed at buffering and/or ameliorating the infant's lived experience of the NICU, the accumulation of these stressors leaves biologic imprints that increase their risk for developmental delays, learning challenges, and emotional dysregulation later in life (Cong et al., 2017; Montirosso et al., 2017; van Dokkum et al., 2021; Zhang et al., 2022).

## THE BIOLOGIC IMPRINT OF STRESS

Advances in neurodevelopmental science and epigenetics have illuminated how early stress influences the developing brain. Toxic stress—the prolonged activation of stress response systems without adequate buffering—has been shown to disrupt the HPA axis, impairing the development of brain regions responsible for regulation, memory, and attachment, such as the prefrontal cortex, hippocampus, and amygdala (Malin et al., 2023; van Dokkum et al., 2021; Weber & Harrison, 2019).

Repeated stress exposure alters epigenetic markers influencing gene expression and predisposing vulnerable infants to chronic illness, anxiety, and behavioral challenges across the lifespan. These findings align with ACE research linking early adversity to long-term health outcomes such as cardiovascular disease, depression, chronic pulmonary disease, obesity as well as psychopathology that may lead to suicide (Crump, 2020; Risnes et al., 2021; Robinson et al., 2020; Wolke et al., 2019).

## The Effect of Adverse Childhood Experiences on the Infant: A Polyvagal Perspective

The Polyvagal Theory offers a profound lens for understanding how ACEs shape infant physiologic and behavioral responses in the NICU (Sanders & Hall, 2018). By examining the autonomic nervous system (ANS) and its role in trauma and regulation, the theory illuminates how ELA influences an infant's capacity for safety, connection, and resilience (De Bellis & Zisk, 2014). ACE and trauma leave a lasting imprint on the neurodevelopmental trajectory of individuals whose ANS is still maturing (Lammertink et al., 2021; Mulkey et al., 2018; Schlatterer et al., 2021).

Polyvagal Theory describes three primary states of autonomic functioning: the ventral vagal state, associated with feelings of safety and social connection; the sympathetic state, activating the fight-or-flight response; and the dorsal vagal state, corresponding to immobilization and shutdown behaviors (Table 26.1) (Porges, 2021, 2022). In a healthy environment, the autonomic system dynamically shifts between these states based on external cues, enabling the infant to navigate stress and safety adaptively. However, in infants exposed to ACEs or ELA, the ANS becomes dysregulated, defaulting to survival-oriented states such as fight or flight or shut down due to the absence of consistent safety signals.

This dysregulation is exacerbated by the stressors inherent in the NICU environment. Painful medical procedures, separation from caregivers, and sensory overstimulation can overwhelm the infant's immature autonomic system, pushing them into prolonged states of sympathetic hyperarousal or dorsal vagal withdrawal. This disruption can manifest as excessive crying, irritability, gastrointestinal disturbances, lethargy, and withdrawal, reflecting the infant's struggle to achieve physiologic stability and regulation (Als, 1982, 1986). Over time, these patterns may interfere with the development of the ventral vagal state, which supports social engagement, attachment, and emotional regulation.

**TABLE 26.1**

**POLYVAGAL STATES AND TIDC IN THE NICU**

| Polyvagal State | Description | Signs in Infants | TIDC Strategies |
|---|---|---|---|
| Ventral vagal | The state of safety, connection, and social engagement. Supports growth, healing, and bonding. | • Calm and alert demeanor<br>• Regular heart rate<br>• Engaged in social interactions (e.g., eye contact, sucking) | • Encourage SSC (kangaroo care) to promote bonding and regulate autonomic function.<br>• Maintain a predictable, soothing environment with dim lighting and soft voices.<br>• Use a gentle, responsive touch during caregiving activities. |
| Sympathetic | The fight-or-flight state activated by perceived threats. Prioritizes survival responses over growth and connection. | • Excessive crying or irritability<br>• Rapid breathing or increased heart rate<br>• Difficulty feeding or calming | • Minimize sensory stressors, such as loud noises and sudden disruptions.<br>• Use parent-mediated nonpharmacologic pain/stress management strategies such as SSC, swaddling and nonnutritive sucking.<br>• Adopt a responsive caregiving strategy to meet the moment-to-moment needs of the infant. |
| Dorsal vagal | The freeze or shutdown state triggered by overwhelming stress. Associated with withdrawal and energy conservation. | • Lethargy or reduced responsiveness<br>• Irregular breathing<br>• Decreased muscle tone | • Engage parents in comforting activities, such as SSC, singing, or gentle rocking.<br>• Create a quiet, low-stimulation environment to support recovery.<br>• Foster coregulation by ensuring consistent, predictable caregiving routines. |

NICU, neonatal intensive care unit; TIDC, trauma-informed developmental care. SSC, skin-to-skin contact.

The inability to access the ventral vagal state can have profound implications for an infant's social engagement system (Kolacz & Porges, 2024). In the NICU, a infant experiencing sympathetic hyperarousal may exhibit heightened sensitivity to stress, responding to caregiver cues with hypervigilance rather than comfort. Conversely, a infant in a dorsal vagal state may withdraw, showing minimal responses to caregiving efforts. Both patterns disrupt the coregulation process, where caregivers help the infant achieve emotional and physiologic balance. These disruptions not only affect immediate bonding and attachment but also carry long-term neurodevelopmental consequences, increasing the risk for anxiety, emotional dysregulation, and cognitive challenges later in life.

From a polyvagal perspective, addressing ACEs in the NICU requires creating an environment that supports autonomic regulation and fosters a sense of safety for the infant (Porges, 2022; Yoshida & Funato, 2021) (Figure 26.1). Minimizing stressors such as noise and bright lights helps reduce sensory overload, allowing the infant to transition more easily into the ventral vagal state. Pain management is critical because both pharmacologic and nonpharmacologic

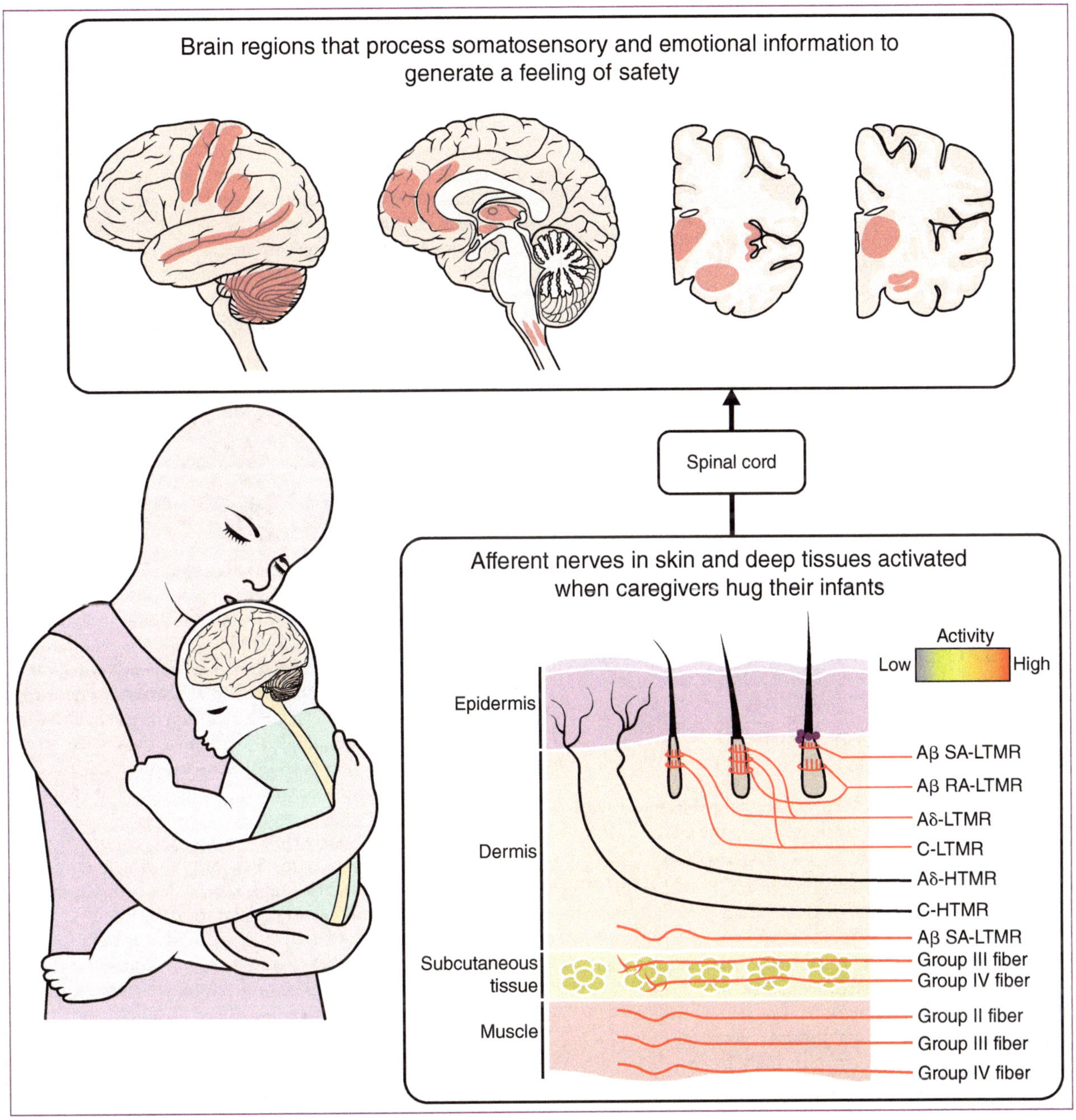


**FIGURE 26.1 Somatosensory perceptions and feelings of safety.**

*Source:* From Yoshida, S., & Funato, H. (2021). Physical contact in parent–infant relationship and its effect on fostering a feeling of safety. *iScience, 24*(7), 102721. https://doi.org/10.1016/j.isci.2021.102721. Licensed under CC BY 4.0 (https://creativecommons.org/licenses/by/4.0/deed.en).

interventions buffer the physiologic stress response and mitigate the cumulative effect of trauma.

Coregulation with caregivers is the gold standard in buffering infant and parental trauma (Buhler-Wassmann & Hibel, 2021; Graf et al., 2022; Naeem et al., 2022;). Practices such as SSC provide critical cues of warmth, rhythm, and touch, activating the ventral vagal system and reinforcing the infant's sense of safety (Feldman & Eidelman, 2003; Sanders & Hall, 2018). Empowering consistent caregiving interactions, where parents participate in activities such as mealtimes or diaper changes, further supports a neuroception of safety—the nervous system's unconscious detection of safety or threat—and helps the infant develop trust in their environment (Porges, 2004).

Protected sleep is another cornerstone of autonomic regulation. Sleep allows the ANS to recover and recalibrate, promoting neurodevelopment and emotional stability (Bennet et al., 2018; Petty & van den Hoogen, 2022). Structuring care schedules to prioritize uninterrupted sleep cycles protects the infant's physiologic development and contributes to their capacity for self-regulation.

Promoting the development of the social engagement system is equally essential. Gentle eye contact, soothing vocal tones, and nurturing touch during caregiving moments help the infant transition from survival-oriented states into a place of connection and calm. Recognizing and responding to the infant's cues of engagement and disengagement reinforces their autonomy and fosters their ability to interact with caregivers safely and meaningfully (Beebe et al., 2018; Feldman, 2007; Tronick, 1989).

By integrating the principles of Polyvagal Theory into TIDC, NICU teams can buffer the effect of ACEs, supporting the infant's ability to achieve autonomic balance and develop a robust social engagement system. This mitigates the immediate effects of adversity and establishes a foundation for lifelong emotional, social, and physiologic resilience. When care is informed by the understanding of safety, regulation, and connection, infants and their families are given the best chance to survive and thrive (Coughlin, 2016; Porges et al., 2019; Sanders & Hall, 2018).

### The Role of Trauma-Informed Developmental Care

TIDC provides a framework for addressing the unique vulnerabilities of NICU infants while reducing the adverse effects of early stress. By incorporating practices that buffer against trauma and promote coregulation, TIDC seeks to transform the NICU from a space of survival to one of healing and resilience. Key components of TIDC include:

- **Protecting sleep:** Uninterrupted sleep cycles are critical for brain development and stress recovery.
- **Pain and stress management:** Minimize the effect of painful procedures through pharmacologic and nonpharmacologic strategies that include sucrose, facilitated tucking, and SSC.
- **Parental engagement:** Encourage parental involvement in caregiving activities to reinforce bonding and support neurodevelopment, including feeding, diapering, and kangaroo care.
- **Creating a healing environment:** Reduce sensory overload by dimming lights, minimizing noise, and fostering a calm atmosphere that supports regulation.

These interventions align with the principles of TIDC, prioritizing safety, trust and transparency, healthy relationships and interactions, empowerment, voice and choice, equity, antibias efforts, and cultural/gender affirmation (Massachusetts Childhood Trauma Task Force, 2020) as foundational elements of care. By addressing the stressors inherent in the NICU experience, clinicians can mitigate the biologic imprint of adversity and promote healthy developmental trajectories for infants.

The NICU experience represents a pivotal period of neuroplasticity, where both risk and opportunity are heightened. Without trauma-informed care, the stressors of the NICU may contribute to developmental vulnerabilities that echo throughout a child's life. However, when intentional buffering strategies are employed, the NICU can be a launching pad for resilience, equipping infants and families with a stronger foundation for future health and well-being.

This recognition reinforces the critical role of NICU teams as buffers against trauma and advocates for the lifelong success of their patients. TIDC, grounded by the ACE framework, not only addresses the present challenges but also lays the groundwork for healthier, more connected futures for the most vulnerable among us.

## THE SOUL OF TRAUMA-INFORMED DEVELOPMENTAL CARE

### The Foundation of Caring Science: Jean Watson's Vision

Caring Science, developed by Dr. Jean Watson, offers a transformative approach to healthcare that emphasizes the integration of humanistic values, relational presence, and transpersonal care (Watson, 2021, 2018). Grounded in the belief that caring is central to healing, Watson's work extends beyond traditional biomedical frameworks, encouraging clinicians to view their practice as a sacred science that honors the interconnectedness of all human beings. At its core, Caring Science challenges clinicians to embrace love, compassion, and authentic presence as foundational elements of their care.

Watson's work is structured around the Theory of Human Caring and the Ten Caritas Processes®, which guide holistic, patient-centered care (Table 26.2) (Watson Caring Institute, 2025). These processes promote practices that balance the technical aspects of healthcare with the relational and spiritual needs of patients and families. Watson posits that caring is not just an emotional response but a deliberate, evidence-informed practice that fosters healing environments for care recipients and caregivers (Watson, 2018, 2021).

The concept of transpersonal care is central to Caring Science (Delgado-Galeano et al., 2023: Clark, 2016; Watson, 2002). Transpersonal care emphasizes connections that transcend healthcare's physical and technical dimensions, focusing instead on the deeper, spiritual dimensions of human experience. In this model, the clinician–patient relationship

**TABLE 26.2**

**WATSON'S 10 CARITAS PROCESSES**

| Caritas Process | Description |
|---|---|
| 1. Embrace (*Loving-Kindness*) | Sustaining humanistic-altruistic values by the practice of loving-kindness, compassion and equanimity with self/others |
| 2. Inspire (*Faith-Hope*) | Being authentically present, enabling faith/hope/belief system; honoring subjective inner, life-world of self/others |
| 3. Trust (*Transpersonal*) | Being sensitive to self and others by cultivating own spiritual practices; beyond ego-self to transpersonal presence |
| 4. Nurture (*Relationship*) | Building strong, mutual trust with patients and colleagues to enhance care and connection |
| 5. Forgive (*Holding Space*) | Allowing for expression of positive and negative feelings—authentically listening to another person's story |
| 6. Deepen (*Creative Self*) | Creatively problem solving/"solution seeking" through the caring process; full use of self and artistry of caring and healing practices via the use of all ways of knowing/being/doing/becoming |
| 7. Balance (*Learning*) | Engaging in transpersonal teaching and learning within the context of caring relationship; staying within other's frame of reference; shifting toward coaching model for expanded health/wellness |
| 8. Co-create (*Caritas Field*) | Creating a healing environment at all levels; subtle environment for energetic authentic caring presence |
| 9. Minister (*Humanity*) | Reverentially assisting with basic needs as sacred acts, touching mind–body–spirit of spirit of other; sustaining human dignity |
| 10. Open (*Infinity*) | Opening to spiritual, mystery, unknowns—allowing for miracles |

*Source:* Data from Watson, J. (n.d.). 10 Caritas Processes®. Watson Caring Science Institute. https://www.watsoncaringscience.org/about-wcsi/jean-bio/caring-science-theory/10-caritas-processes/.

becomes a mutual exchange of energy, where the clinician's presence and intention create a space for healing that encompasses body, mind, and spirit.

## Caring Science and Its Relevance to Trauma-Informed Developmental Care

TIDC shares profound synergies with Caring Science because both frameworks recognize the importance of relational, holistic, and compassionate approaches to care. TIDC focuses on mitigating the effects of trauma while promoting resilience and healing for NICU infants, families, and clinicians. When integrated with Caring Science, TIDC extends beyond the physical needs of patients to address the emotional, psychological, and spiritual dimensions of healing.

Both frameworks underscore the sacredness of caregiving, emphasizing that every interaction is an opportunity to promote healing and connection. The alignment between Caring Science and TIDC is particularly evident in their shared principles of safety, trust, empowerment, and collaboration. For example, TIDC's commitment to creating healing environments resonates with Watson's emphasis on cultivating environments that honor the dignity and humanity of every individual (Table 26.3).

Integrating Caring Science into TIDC enhances the trauma-informed approach by embedding practices prioritizing relational care, authentic presence, and acknowledging each family's unique journey. This holistic perspective supports the well-being of NICU families and infants and nurtures clinicians, ensuring that they can sustain their practice with purpose and resilience.

**TABLE 26.3**

**KEY PARALLELS BETWEEN CARING SCIENCE AND TIDC**

| Caring Science Principle/Caritas Process (CP) | TIDC Principle/Core Measure | Connection |
|---|---|---|
| Cultivating Authentic Presence (CP #2) | Trust & Transparency (Principle) | Both frameworks emphasize the importance of relational care, where trust is built through genuine, open communication and mutual respect. |
| Creating Healing Environments (CP #8) | The Healing Environment (Core Measure) | Caring Science and TIDC both prioritize environments that support emotional and physical safety, reducing stress for infants, families, and clinicians. |
| Promoting and Accepting Emotions (CP #5) | Empowerment, Voice, & Choice (Principle) | Caring Science encourages caregivers to hold space for emotional expression, aligning with TIDC's focus on empowering families to advocate for their needs and choices. |
| Developing Helping-Trusting Relationships (CP #4) | Compassionate Collaborative Relationships (Core Measure) | Watson's emphasis on authentic connections complements TIDC's goal of fostering collaborative partnerships between clinicians and families. |
| Ministering to Humanity (CP #9) | Activities of Daily Living (e.g., posture and play, mealtimes, bathing) (Core Measure) | Both frameworks integrate technical expertise with relational care, ensuring that even routine tasks honor the individuality and dignity of the patient. |
| Caring for the Caregiver (CP #1 & #3) | Addressing Clinician Well-Being (Core Measure) | Both Caring Science and TIDC recognize the importance of supporting clinicians through reflective practice, mindfulness, and organizational cultures that value emotional safety and well-being. |

TIDC, trauma-informed developmental care.

## Operationalizing Caring Science in Trauma-Informed Developmental Care Practices

**Relational Care and Authentic Presence.** A cornerstone of Caring Science and TIDC is recognizing that authentic presence creates the foundation for healing relationships. In the NICU, this can take the form of clinicians actively engaging with families, listening to their fears and hopes, and providing reassurance through words and actions. By intentionally fostering these connections, clinicians create a safe and trusting family environment.

**Creating Healing Environments.** Caring Science views the environment as a crucial component of healing. In the NICU, this principle aligns with TIDC measures such as reducing sensory stress, protecting sleep, and ensuring a calm, supportive atmosphere. For instance, dimmed lighting, soft sounds, and SSC support neurodevelopment and reflect the sacredness of the caregiving space.

**Emphasizing Holistic Healing.** Caring Science encourages clinicians to see beyond the immediate medical needs of patients, addressing their emotional, relational, and spiritual well-being. In the context of TIDC, this translates to practices such as partnering and empowering parents in caregiving routines, offering mental health resources, and holding space for rituals or moments of reflection. These practices honor the individuality of each family's journey, fostering resilience and hope.

**Nurturing the Caregiver.** Just as Caring Science emphasizes the importance of self-care for clinicians, TIDC recognizes that the caregiver's well-being directly affects the quality of care. Reflective practices, peer support, and mindfulness interventions help clinicians navigate the emotional demands of the NICU, ensuring that they can sustain their work with compassion and purpose.

## Caring Science as a Transformative Lens for Trauma-Informed Developmental Care

Integrating Caring Science into TIDC enriches the trauma-informed framework, providing a philosophical and practical foundation for addressing the holistic needs of infants, families, and clinicians. By emphasizing love, compassion, and authentic presence, Caring Science transforms the NICU into a space where healing transcends physical outcomes, fostering resilience and connection for all who enter.

Caring Science and TIDC together remind us that the art of caregiving is as vital as its science. By aligning these frameworks, NICU clinicians mitigate trauma and create a legacy of care that honors the sacredness of life and the profound effect of every caring moment.

## ELEMENTS OF TRAUMA-INFORMED DEVELOPMENTAL CARE

### Core Measures of Trauma-Informed Developmental Care

The Core Measures of TIDC serve as actionable frameworks that prioritize infants' physiologic, developmental, and emotional needs while supporting families and clinicians (Coughlin, 2021, 2024; Coughlin et al., 2022, 2023). Each measure provides specific guidance for creating an environment that buffers trauma and promotes healing.

**Healing Environment.** The healing environment core measure includes the environment's physical, human, and organizational elements. Creating a healing environment mitigates the sensory overload typical of the NICU, offering a sense of calm, safety, and consistency. This could include minimizing noise and light exposure, maximizing parental presence, and fostering predictability for infants. Families benefit from private spaces for bonding, emotional processing, and role validation. At the same time, clinicians thrive in a supportive atmosphere that reduces stress and burnout and ensures that the highest quality of care is consistently maintained (Coughlin, 2021, 2024; Coughlin et al., 2022, 2023) (Table 26.4).

**Protected Sleep.** Sleep is critical for infants' brain development, immune function, and growth. The protected sleep core measure includes assessment of sleep–wake cycles, supporting uninterrupted sleep, and promoting sleep safety. Aligning caregiving schedules with natural sleep–wake cycles ensures uninterrupted sleep for infants. Educating families on the importance of sleep empowers them to advocate for restful environments. In contrast, clinicians who respect sleep schedules enjoy significant compassion satisfaction (Coughlin, 2021, 2024; Coughlin et al., 2022, 2023) (Table 26.5).

**Pain and Stress Prevention and Management.** Unmanaged pain and stress disrupt neurodevelopment and emotional regulation. Core criteria for this core measure include preventing pain and stress, assessing and managing pain and stress, and using parent-mediated nonpharmacologic strategies and routines. Clinicians employ pharmacologic and nonpharmacologic strategies in partnership with parents to reduce pain and promote a sense of safety and comfort. A proactive approach to pain management supports a culture of compassionate care (Coughlin, 2021, 2024; Coughlin et al., 2022, 2023) (Table 26.6).

**Activities of Daily Living.** Activities of daily living (ADLs) such as posture and play, mealtimes and nourishment, bathing, and skin care activities are opportunities to support development, cultivate safe, stable, and nurturing relationships, and foster family empowerment. Ensuring that ADLs are developmentally appropriate for infants reinforces parents' confidence and competence as caregivers (Coughlin, 2021, 2024; Coughlin et al., 2022, 2023) (Table 26.7).

**Compassionate Collaborative Relationships.** Strong relationships among caregivers, families, and clinical teams are essential for trauma-informed care. The key components for this core measure include emotional well-being, self-efficacy, and compassionate communication. Compassionate, collaborative relationships are built on trust, mutual respect, and a shared commitment to the infant's well-being, fostering an environment where families feel valued as integral members of

**TABLE 26.4**

**ASPECTS AND APPLICATIONS FOR THE HEALING ENVIRONMENT CORE MEASURE**

| Aspect | Application in Practice |
|---|---|
| Infants | Dim lighting, noise control, gentle touch, and SSC |
| Families | Private bonding spaces and welcoming, family-centered design |
| Clinicians | Structured quiet times, mindfulness spaces, and team support to reduce caregiver stress |

SSC, skin-to-skin contact.

**TABLE 26.5**

**ASPECTS AND APPLICATIONS FOR PROTECTED SLEEP CORE MEASURE**

| Aspect | Application in Practice |
|---|---|
| Infants | Nonemergent care is guided by the infant's sleep–wake cycle. |
| Families | Education on the value of sleep and encouragement to participate in soothing routines validates role identity. |
| Clinicians | Care plans built around sleep cycles to foster teamwork and reduce unnecessary sleep fragmentation and disruptions. |

**TABLE 26.6**

**ASPECTS AND APPLICATIONS FOR THE PAIN AND STRESS PREVENTION AND MANAGEMENT CORE MEASURE**

| Aspect | Application in Practice |
|---|---|
| Infants | Consistent use of appropriate pain scales and nonpharmacologic interventions such as SSC, breastfeeding and/or oral administration of a sweet solution during painful and distressing events/ procedures. |
| Families | Empowering parental comforting activities, such as SSC or singing to infant during procedures. |
| Clinicians | Proactive pain assessments and individualized pain management and comfort plans for each infant. |

SSC, skin-to-skin contact.

**TABLE 26.7**

**ASPECTS AND APPLICATIONS FOR THE ADLS CORE MEASURE**

| Aspect | Application in Practice |
|---|---|
| Infants | Developmentally appropriate and enjoyable mealtime interactions; playful encounters with family, and soothing bathing and hygiene rituals and routines |
| Families | Facilitating and empowering parents in role validating ADLs, such as diaper changes, mealtimes, play and postural support to strengthen bonding |
| Clinicians | Collaborative planning of ADLs to respect both infant needs and family preferences |

ADLs, activities of daily living.

the care team and clinicians experience a sense of connection and purpose (Coughlin, 2021, 2024; Coughlin et al., 2022, 2023) (Table 26.8).

**TABLE 26.8**

**ASPECTS AND APPLICATIONS FOR THE COMPASSIONATE COLLABORATIVE RELATIONSHIPS CORE MEASURE**

| Aspect | Application in Practice |
|---|---|
| Infants | Consistent caregivers provide stability and foster safe, stable and nurturing relationships. |
| Families | Parents are essentials personnel and integral to the multidisciplinary team |
| Clinicians | Regular team debriefings and open communication foster a culture of trust and emotional support among colleagues. |

## Principles of Trauma-Informed Developmental Care

The principles of TIDC provide a philosophical foundation toward a culture of safety, respect, and empowerment in the NICU (Massachusetts Childhood Trauma Task Force, 2020). Principles guide implementation of the Core Measures by addressing relational and systemic aspects of care (Table 26.9).

**Safety.** Safety forms the cornerstone of TIDC, ensuring that physical and emotional well-being are prioritized for all who inhabit the NICU space. For infants, this involves creating an environment free from excessive sensory stimuli, such as bright lights and loud noises, while ensuring gentle touch and parental presence. Parents are empowered primary caregivers and receive education and support to foster confidence and competence. For clinicians, a culture of safety includes predictable protocols, structured workflows, and emotional safety through supportive teamwork—reducing stress and enhancing the quality of care.

**Trust and Transparency.** Building trust and maintaining transparency is essential for fostering authentic relationships. Infants benefit from having consistent caregivers—helping them feel secure and promoting stable neurodevelopment. Families experience trust through regular, honest updates about their infant's condition and care plan and by having opportunities to actively participate in decision making. For clinicians, fostering trust requires clear communication and collaborative practices among team members, ensuring reliability and mutual respect across all levels of care.

**Healthy Relationships and Interactions.** The NICU is a relational environment and nurturing healthy interactions is critical for trauma-informed care. Infants thrive through practices such as SSC, which promotes bonding, emotional regulation, and neurodevelopment. Families build confidence and

**TABLE 26.9**

**PRINCIPLES OF TIDC IN ACTION**

| Principle | Infant | Family | Clinician |
|---|---|---|---|
| Safety | Parental presence, gentle touch, consistent routines and minimizing sensory stressors (e.g., light, noise) | Parents are empowered primary caregivers and receive education and support to foster confidence and competence. | Commitment to evidence-based practice standards in trauma-informed developmental care ensures consistent, high-quality care delivery. |
| Trust and transparency | Consistent caregivers provide stability and support for the infant's sense of security. | Parents experience regular, clear updates about their infant's condition and participate in care planning and decision-making. | Open communication within the care team fosters trust and reliability among colleagues. |
| Healthy relationships and interactions | Maximize SSC and parent caregiving to ensure optimal outcomes. | Recognize parents as the primary caregiver through empowerment and education. | Interdisciplinary collaboration fosters mutual respect and enhances team dynamics. |
| Empowerment, voice, and choice | Cue-based care ensures the infant's natural rhythms and preferences are respected. | Parents are encouraged to incorporate family and/or cultural rituals and routines into their caregiving repertoire, reinforcing their role identity. | Clinicians are encouraged to share insights and advocate for trauma-sensitive practices. |
| Equity, antibias efforts, and cultural/ gender affirmation | Care is individualized to align with the infant's unique needs and developmental stage. | Families have unrestricted access to culturally congruent resources and interpreter services throughout their hospital stay. | Training on cultural humility equips clinicians to provide inclusive, equitable, and respectful care. |

NICU, neonatal Intensive care unit; TIDC, trauma-informed developmental care.

strengthen relationships with their infants through hands-on caregiving activities such as mealtimes, bathing, and soothing. Clinicians, in turn, benefit from fostering collegial relationships built on mutual respect, empathy, and shared goals, creating a cohesive and supportive care team.

**Empowerment, Voice, and Choice.** Empowerment in the NICU means respecting the individuality and preferences of infants, families, and clinicians alike. For infants, this involves recognizing and responding to their cues, ensuring care aligns with their natural rhythms and needs. Families are recognized as the primary caregivers of their infants and empowered to incorporate family rituals and routines into their caregiving repertoire, reinforcing their role identity. For clinicians, empowerment includes advocating for trauma-sensitive practices and contributing their professional insights to enhance care delivery and team collaboration.

**Equity, Antibias Efforts, and Cultural/Gender Affirmation.** Equity ensures that every infant and family receives care that is individualized, respectful, and inclusive of their unique backgrounds and identities. For infants, this means tailoring care to align with their developmental stage and specific needs. Families benefit from culturally congruent resources, access to interpreter services, and respect for their traditions and values, ensuring that they feel understood and included. For clinicians, training in cultural humility and implicit bias awareness fosters the ability to provide equitable and unbiased care, ensuring a truly inclusive environment in the NICU.

**The B.U.F.F.E.R. Framework: A Soulful Approach to Care.** The B.U.F.F.E.R. Framework (Caring Essentials Collaborative, 2023) integrates the soul of caregiving into TIDC practices, addressing the relational and emotional dimensions that mitigate the effect of ACEs in the NICU and beyond (Table 26.10). Each value within the framework emphasizes the importance of connection, compassion, and holistic healing. By centering on the human spirit and authentic relationships, the B.U.F.F.E.R. Framework serves as a guide for fostering an environment where trauma is buffered, and resilience is nurtured.

**TABLE 26.10**

**THE B.U.F.F.E.R. FRAMEWORK IN PRACTICE**

| Value | Description | Application in the NICU |
|---|---|---|
| Belonging | Fostering inclusion and unity within the care team and with families | Involving families in decision making and caregiving and cultivating a supportive workplace culture for clinicians |
| Understanding | Recognizing and honoring each individual's unique narrative and perspective | Tailoring care to reflect families' cultural, emotional, and relational contexts; fostering empathy within the team |
| Forgiveness | Encouraging self-compassion and grace, reducing guilt and interpersonal tension | Supporting clinicians in processing secondary trauma and encouraging forgiveness to resolve conflicts within teams or families |
| Frameworks | Grounding care in structured, evidence-based practices while maintaining relational focus | Applying TIDC principles and Watson's Caritas Processes to create consistent, compassionate care plans |
| Equanimity | Cultivating balance and fairness, approaching challenges with calm and compassion | Training clinicians in mindfulness and emotional regulation to navigate stressful NICU situations |
| Respect | Treating every person with inherent dignity, recognizing their unique contributions to the NICU ecosystem | Listening to families' voices, respecting cultural differences, and ensuring interdisciplinary collaboration among clinicians |

NICU, neonatal intensive care unit.

- **Belonging** emphasizes inclusion and unity—creating spaces where infants, families, and clinicians feel connected and valued: zero separation for infants and continuous parental presence, recognizing families as essential members of the care team, and having clinicians foster a supportive workplace culture that prioritizes connection over isolation.
- **Understanding** encourages caregivers to honor each individual's unique narrative and experiences—acknowledging the infant's personhood while recognizing the diverse perspectives of families and colleagues. This value promotes empathy and tailored care.
- **Forgiveness** supports self-compassion and interpersonal grace—reducing internalized stressors such as guilt or resentment. It reminds clinicians to extend kindness to themselves and others, acknowledging the shared humanity of all involved in the NICU journey.
- **Frameworks** ensure caregiving practices are grounded in structured, evidence-based models—providing reliable care delivery while allowing space for relational and spiritual connection.
- **Equanimity** cultivates balance and fairness by encouraging caregivers to approach challenges calmly and compassionately—reinforcing resilience amidst the high-stakes NICU environment.
- **Respect** honors the inherent dignity of each individual, from the tiniest patient and their family to the most seasoned clinician. It calls for recognition of the unique roles everyone plays within the NICU ecosystem.

By embodying the principles of the B.U.F.F.E.R. Framework, clinicians weave the soul of caregiving into every interaction, creating a space where trauma is mitigated and transformed into opportunities for connection and growth. This approach aligns seamlessly with Watson's Caring Science, emphasizing the centrality of the human spirit in healing and the profound effect of authentic connection. Through the B.U.F.F.E.R. Framework, clinicians foster environments rich in inclusion, empathy, and respect, ensuring that infants, families, and clinicians alike are supported and empowered in their healing journeys.

## THE CONNECTION BETWEEN TRAUMA-INFORMED DEVELOPMENTAL CARE AND DIVERSITY, EQUITY, AND INCLUSION EFFORTS IN THE NEONATAL INTENSIVE CARE UNIT

In the NICU, where vulnerability and resilience intersect, the integration of TIDC with diversity, equity, and inclusion (DEI) efforts is essential for addressing the multifaceted challenges faced by infants, families, and clinicians. Both frameworks aim to create an environment fostering safety, trust, and healing while actively addressing the systemic inequities and cultural barriers disproportionately affecting marginalized communities.

Families from diverse backgrounds navigate complex medical, emotional, and logistic challenges in a high-stakes, technologically oriented environment. Infants in the NICU are uniquely vulnerable to trauma, and families often face compounding stressors such as racial bias, language barriers, and financial hardship. TIDC provides a relational, healing-centered approach to mitigate trauma and promote resilience. However, without a DEI lens, implementing TIDC risks perpetuating inequities by failing to account for the structural barriers and implicit biases that shape families' experiences.

For example, the Principle of Safety in TIDC emphasizes the creation of a predictable and nurturing environment for infants and families. DEI efforts enrich this principle by addressing how safety is perceived differently across cultural contexts, ensuring that families feel both physically and emotionally secure. Similarly, the Core Measure of Compassionate Collaborative Relationships highlights the importance of family engagement, which is only achievable when communication is equitable, inclusive, and culturally affirming. DEI initiatives support this measure by advocating for interpreter services, culturally congruent resources, and staff training on implicit bias.

From a clinician perspective, integrating TIDC and DEI helps create a workplace culture where diversity is valued and team members feel empowered to address systemic inequities. This alignment supports reflective practices that reduce bias, enhance cultural humility, and improve relational care for families. For example, clinicians who understand the intersection of trauma and systemic racism are better equipped to recognize how historical and structural inequities may amplify a family's distress in the NICU.

By aligning TIDC with DEI efforts, the NICU becomes more than a space of medical intervention—it transforms into a relationally centered, inclusive environment where the needs of infants, families, and clinicians are met with compassion, cultural humility, and justice. This connection ensures that trauma-informed practices are effective and equitable, addressing the root causes of disparities while promoting healing for all.

## Disparities in the Neonatal Intensive Care Unit: Challenges and Opportunities for Equity

The NICU is a critical environment where lifesaving interventions meet complex social and systemic challenges. Despite advancements in neonatal care, significant disparities persist, disproportionately affecting marginalized communities. These inequities stem from socioeconomic barriers, systemic bias, and cultural misunderstandings, affecting not only medical outcomes but also the emotional and psychological experiences of families. Addressing these disparities is a core tenet of TIDC, which emphasizes equity, antibias efforts, and cultural humility.

## Challenges Surrounding Disparities in the Neonatal Intensive Care Unit

Families navigating economic challenges often encounter barriers to accessing NICU care, such as limited transportation, financial strain, and workplace inflexibility (Lechner et al., 2024; McCarty et al., 2024; Pang et al., 2021) (Table 26.11). These obstacles reduce parental involvement, which is critical for bonding and promoting infant development. Similarly, racial and ethnic disparities in neonatal outcomes are well documented, with Black, Hispanic, and Indigenous infants

**TABLE 26.11**

**CHALLENGES OF NICU DISPARITIES AND THEIR EFFECTS**

| Challenge | Impact on Families | Effect on Infants |
|---|---|---|
| Socioeconomic inequities | Reduced parental presence due to logistical barriers | Delayed bonding and developmental milestones |
| Racial and ethnic disparities | Feelings of exclusion, mistrust in care systems | Higher rates of preterm birth, mortality, and inequities in care |
| Communication barriers | Misunderstandings in care planning; feelings of alienation | Inconsistent or suboptimal care |
| Cultural and gender bias | Withdrawal from caregiving roles due to lack of cultural alignment | Less individualized and developmentally appropriate care |
| Limited access to follow-up | Missed therapy sessions and interventions postdischarge | Increased risk of developmental delays and health complications |

NICU, neonatal intensive care unit.

experiencing higher rates of preterm birth, low birth weight, and mortality compared to White infants (Edwards et al., 2021; Johnson et al., 2023; Sigurdson et al., 2019; Witt et al., 2022). Implicit bias within healthcare systems can exacerbate these disparities, leaving families feeling excluded or misunderstood (McCarty, 2023; Shaikh et al., 2023; Vela et al., 2022). Communication barriers also play a significant role, particularly for families whose primary language is not English (Fisher et al., 2024; Kynoe et al., 2020; Kyno & Hanssen, 2022; Palau et al., 2019; Patriksson et al., 2019; Reddy et al., 2024). Without access to interpreters or culturally appropriate resources, families may struggle to engage with care teams, leading to suboptimal care plans for their infants. Additionally, cultural and gender biases can result in the dismissal of diverse parenting styles or emotional expressions, further alienating families (Nyaloko et al., 2023; Sigurdson et al., 2018; Yinger et al., 2024). Postdischarge disparities compound the problem, as families from underserved communities face challenges in accessing follow-up care and early intervention services.

## Opportunities to Address Disparities Through Trauma-Informed Developmental Care

A trauma-informed approach provides a framework for addressing these inequities through intentional practices that prioritize trust, respect, and collaboration (Berring et al., 2024; Duffee et al., 2021; Huo et al., 2023; Kimberg & Wheeler, 2019) (Table 26.12). By building partnerships with families, fostering cultural humility, and advocating for systemic change, NICU teams can help mitigate disparities and improve outcomes for all. To build trust and inclusion, healthcare teams must actively recognize and address systemic inequities. Equity efforts in the NICU begin with acknowledging implicit bias and training staff in cultural humility and antiracist practices (Brown-Madan et al., 2023). For instance, offering culturally relevant resources and interpreter services ensures families can engage fully in their infant's care. Policies that support continuous family presence and family-centered care planning empower parents to participate meaningfully, even amidst logistic challenges (Franck et al., 2023; Urbina et al., 2024). Collaboration with community organizations is also essential for addressing social determinants of health. Providing resources such as housing support, financial assistance, and transportation options reduces barriers families face during their NICU journey (Cordova-Ramos et al., 2022). Postdischarge, these efforts can extend to ensuring equitable access to early intervention programs, therapy services, and developmental follow-up care (Harris et al., 2024; Hebballi et al., 2021).

## Moving Toward Equity in the Neonatal Intensive Care Unit

Addressing disparities in the NICU requires a holistic approach that integrates trauma-informed practices, systemic advocacy, and cultural humility. By prioritizing equity through the principles of TIDC, NICU teams can create a more inclusive and supportive environment where every infant and family has the opportunity to thrive. While the challenges are significant, the opportunities to transform care are equally profound. Through sustained commitment to compassionate, equitable care, we can mitigate the effect of disparities and foster resilience in even the most vulnerable populations.

**TABLE 26.12**

**OPPORTUNITIES FOR EQUITY IN THE NICU**

| Opportunity | Action Step | Expected Outcome |
|---|---|---|
| Build trust through equity and inclusion | Provide staff training on implicit bias and cultural humility; use interpreters and culturally appropriate materials. | Families feel respected, valued, and engaged in care processes. |
| Strengthen family-centered partnerships | Include families in decision making; establish flexible visitation policies. | Increased parental involvement and advocacy |
| Address social determinants of health | Collaborate with social workers and community organizations to provide logistical and financial support. | Reduced barriers to accessing care, both during and after NICU hospitalization |
| Advocate for systemic change | Participate in institutional and policy-level advocacy efforts. | Broader healthcare reforms that reduce disparities and improve neonatal outcomes |

TIDC, trauma-informed developmental care; NICU, neonatal intensive care unit.

# THE SKILLS OF TRAUMA-INFORMED DEVELOPMENTAL CARE

## Buffering Trauma Through Caring Science and Trauma-Informed Developmental Care

In the NICU, TIDC intersects with the relational and spiritual framework of Caring Science to buffer trauma for infants, families, and clinicians. Caring Science emphasizes the sacredness of caregiving and the healing potential of love, connection, and intentional presence. Through her 10 Caritas Processes®, Watson provides a structured approach to fostering resilience, trust, and holistic healing.

At its core, Caring Science aligns with TIDC's Principles and Core Measures by viewing care as a relational act that honors the interconnectedness of all beings. It extends beyond tasks and protocols, asking clinicians to cultivate an authentic presence that nurtures the soul of every interaction. Together, Caring Science and TIDC offer a framework that mitigates trauma and transforms the NICU into a sanctuary of healing.

## Integrating Caring Science Into Trauma Buffering

**For Infants: A Sacred Start.** For infants whose neurodevelopment is profoundly shaped by early experiences, buffering trauma begins with intentional practices that promote safety, regulation, and connection. Caring Science enriches TIDC's Core Measures by framing caregiving activities as sacred acts of healing.

- **Healing environment:** A quiet, dimly lit NICU reduces overstimulation and fosters a sense of safety. Watson's 8th Caritas Process, "Creating a Healing Environment," reminds us that these adjustments are practical and profoundly relational, honoring the infant's need for safety, stability, and nurturance.
- **Protected sleep:** Uninterrupted sleep is critical for brain maturation. Guided by the 9th Caritas Process, "Reverently Assisting with Basic Needs," clinicians can approach sleep as a sacred time for restoration, ensuring that caregiving schedules respect the infant's sleep–wake cycles and circadian rhythms.
- **Pain/stress assessment and management:** Pain relief is both a medical necessity and a moral imperative. The 1st Caritas Process, "Practicing Loving-Kindness and Equanimity," invites clinicians to assess and manage pain and stress consistently and compassionately, treating even the smallest interventions as opportunities to alleviate suffering.

**For Families: Relational Healing.** Families in the NICU often face emotional and psychological trauma compounded by feelings of helplessness and guilt. Caring Science emphasizes the relational nature of healing—aligning with TIDC's focus on empowerment and trust building.

- **Compassionate collaborative relationships:** Building strong relationships with families fosters a sense of belonging. The 4th Caritas Process, "Developing a Helping-Trusting Relationship," underscores the importance of mutual respect and authenticity in these interactions.
- **Empowerment, voice, and choice:** Facilitating parental partnerships in caregiving helps them reclaim their role as primary caregivers. This aligns with the 6th Caritas Process, "Creative Use of Self," which honors the strengths and contributions of every individual.
- **Healthy relationships and interactions:** SSC and other bonding activities support attachment and reflect the 5th Caritas Process, "Promoting Expression of Positive and Negative Feelings." These moments help parents navigate their emotional journey with greater confidence and connection.

**For Clinicians: Sustaining Compassionate Practice.** Caring Science speaks directly to the needs of clinicians who often experience secondary trauma, empathic distress, and burnout in the NICU. Watson's work provides a pathway for self-care and resilience, recognizing that healing begins with the caregiver.

- **Reflective practice:** Regular mindfulness and team debriefing opportunities allow clinicians to process emotions and reconnect with their purpose. The 3rd Caritas Process, "Cultivating One's Own Spiritual Practices," encourages clinicians to integrate practices that sustain their emotional and spiritual well-being.
- **Team collaboration:** A culture of mutual respect and collaboration enhances the team's ability to navigate the challenges of NICU care. The 7th Caritas Process, "Engaging in Genuine Teaching-Learning Experiences," fosters shared growth and learning among colleagues.
- **Self-compassion:** Clinicians who treat themselves with kindness and patience embody the 1st Caritas Process, "Practicing Loving-Kindness and Equanimity," extending the principles of care inward and outward.

# THE ATTRIBUTES OF A TRAUMA-INFORMED PROFESSIONAL: A FOUNDATION FOR COMPASSIONATE CARE

Becoming a Trauma-Informed Professional (TIP) is not just about mastering skills—it is a profound commitment to self-awareness, intentional presence, and fostering compassionate connections. In the NICU, where vulnerability and resilience intersect, clinicians who embody trauma-informed attributes create an environment that buffers trauma and promotes healing for infants, families, and themselves. The eight attributes of a trauma-informed professional—knowledge, healing intention, personal wholeness, courage, advocacy, role modeling, scholarship, and leadership for change—serve as a guide for professionals to align their practice with the principles of Caring Science and TIDC (Table 26.13) These attributes represent a dynamic blend of science, soul, and skills, empowering clinicians to provide care that is both effective and compassionate (NANN, 2022).

## TABLE 26.13

### TIDC, TIP ATTRIBUTES, AND WATSON'S CARITAS PROCESSES—PARALLELS AND SYNERGY

| TIDC Element | Watson's Caring Science Caritas Processes | Parallels and Synergy |
|---|---|---|
| ***Principle:*** Safety | 1. Cultivating the Practice of Loving-Kindness and Equanimity | Both prioritize creating an environment where the patient feels emotionally and physically safe. In TIDC, safety is crucial for the infant's healing, while Watson emphasizes the caregiver's responsibility to provide a nurturing, safe, and loving space. |
| ***Principle:*** Trust and Transparency | 4. Developing and Sustaining a Helping-Trusting, Authentic Caring Relationship | TIDC focuses on clear communication and building trust with the family and infant. Similarly, Watson's Caring Science highlights the creation of trusting, genuine relationships between the caregiver and patient. |
| ***Principle:*** Healthy Relationships and Interactions | 2. Being Authentically Present | TIDC advocates for responsive, nurturing relationships that support infant development. Watson emphasizes being fully present with the patient, fostering authentic and caring connections. |
| ***Principle:*** Empowerment, Voice, and Choice | 6. Creative Use of Self and All Ways of Knowing | TIDC empowers families by respecting their voice and choices. Watson supports this by encouraging nurses to use creativity and intuition, as well as honoring patients' choices and individuality in their care. |
| ***Principle:*** Equity, Antibias Efforts and Cultural/Gender Affirmation | 8. Creating Healing Environments at All Levels | TIDC promotes equity and cultural/gender affirmation, creating environments that honor and respect diversity. Watson's process of creating healing environments also reflects this, ensuring that the care space is emotionally, culturally, and spiritually supportive. |
| ***Core Measure:*** Healing Environment | 7. Engaging in Genuine Teaching-Learning Experiences | Both frameworks emphasize the creation of environments that support not only physical healing but also emotional and psychological well-being. TIDC's focus on healing environments parallels Watson's teaching-learning approach, where mutual respect and shared knowledge foster deeper healing. |
| ***Core Measure:*** Protected Sleep | 5. Promoting and Accepting Expression of Positive and Negative Feelings | TIDC emphasizes the importance of protecting infants' sleep as a foundational aspect of healing. In Watson's framework, allowing emotional expression and rest contributes to an overall healing process, including the restful states necessary for recovery. |
| ***Core Measure:*** Pain and Stress Prevention and Management | 9. Administering Sacred Acts of Caring with Presence | Both frameworks focus on relieving distress and preventing harm. TIDC includes managing pain and stress for infants, while Watson highlights the sacredness of caring, which includes attentively alleviating suffering. |
| ***Core Measure:*** Activities of Daily Living | 3. Cultivating One's Own Spiritual Practices and Transpersonal Self, Going Beyond Ego-Self | In TIDC, ADLs for infants—such as posture, play, feeding, bathing, and skin care—are essential for supporting physical growth and development. Watson's Caritas Process encourages caregivers to connect with their transpersonal self, aligning with the nurturing and attentive care required for ADLs. This focus on compassionate, mindful actions in daily routines supports the infant's holistic development. |

(*continued*)

**TABLE 26.13**

**TIDC, TIP ATTRIBUTES, AND WATSON'S CARITAS PROCESSES—PARALLELS AND SYNERGY (*continued*)**

| TIDC Element | Watson's Caring Science Caritas Processes | Parallels and Synergy |
|---|---|---|
| ***Core Measure:*** Compassionate Collaborative Relationships | 10. Opening to Spiritual-Mysterious and Existential Unknowns | Both TIDC and Watson's Caring Science emphasize the power of relationships in healing. TIDC includes compassionate collaboration between care providers and families, while Watson opens to the spiritual dimension, where deep human connections foster profound healing experiences. |
| ***Attribute:*** Knowledgeable | 7. Engaging in Genuine Teaching-Learning Experiences | TIDC's Knowledgeable attribute, which emphasizes using all ways of knowing, aligns with Watson's Balance (Learning) by valuing shared knowledge, continuous learning, and mutual respect, ultimately fostering holistic understanding in care. |
| ***Attribute:*** Healing Intention | 1. Cultivating the Practice of Loving-Kindness and Equanimity/Embrace (Loving-Kindness) | Healing Intention in TIDC emphasizes compassionate, intentional care, resonating with Watson's Embrace (Loving-Kindness) process, which sustains humanistic, altruistic values and centers the patient in a space of loving presence. |
| ***Attribute:*** Personal Wholeness | 2. Being Authentically Present—Inspire (Faith-Hope) | TIDC's Personal Wholeness encourages caregivers to foster well-being within themselves, aligning with Watson's Inspire (Faith-Hope), which stresses the caregiver's inner peace and faith, allowing them to connect authentically with patients. |
| ***Attribute:*** Courage | 5. Promoting and Accepting Expression of Positive and Negative Feelings—Forgive (Holding Space) | TIDC's Courage attribute involves advocating for vulnerable patients despite challenges. Watson's Forgive (Holding Space) supports this by allowing space for resilience, self-compassion, and strength when providing trauma-informed care. |
| ***Attribute:*** Advocacy | 6. Creative Use of Self and All Ways of Knowing—Deepen (Creative Self) | Advocacy in TIDC is about empowering families and supporting patient autonomy, much like Watson's Deepen (Creative Self), which encourages the caregiver to respect patients' voices, choices, and individuality in the caregiving process. |
| ***Attribute:*** Role Model and Mentor | 4. Developing and Sustaining a Helping-Trusting, Authentic Caring Relationship—Nurture (Relationship) | Role Model and Mentor in TIDC aligns with Watson's Nurture (Relationship), emphasizing modeling supportive, compassionate behavior for both patients and colleagues, creating a relational environment that inspires trust and authenticity. |
| ***Attribute:*** Scholarly | 9. Administering Sacred Acts of Caring with Presence—Minister (Humanity) | TIDC's Scholarly attribute emphasizes using research and evidence to inform care, which aligns with Watson's Minister (Humanity) as caregiving is treated as a sacred act, highlighting the importance of evidence-informed, compassionate care. |
| ***Attribute:*** Leader for Change | 10. Opening to Spiritual-Mysterious and Existential Unknowns/Open (Infinity) | Leader for Change in TIDC reflects a commitment to collaborative, innovative care, paralleling Watson's Open (Infinity) process, which embraces mystery, spirituality, and openness to new possibilities in healing and care transformation. |

ADLs, activities of daily living; TIDC, trauma-informed developmental care; TIP, trauma-informed professional.

## Foundational Attributes

- **Knowledgeable:** Staying informed about the effects of trauma on neurodevelopment, family dynamics, and clinician well-being equips professionals with tools to respond empathetically and effectively and ensures that relationally focused care is grounded in the latest evidence.
- **Healing intention:** Bringing a mindful, purposeful presence to each interaction transforms routine care into moments of connection and trust. Healing intention aligns with Watson's 1st Caritas Process, "Practicing Loving-Kindness and Equanimity," inviting clinicians to approach their work with a sense of sacred responsibility.
- **Personal wholeness:** Clinicians must care for themselves to bring their best selves to care for others. Personal wholeness emphasizes the importance of self-reflection, resilience, and self-compassion, allowing professionals to sustain their ability to provide trauma-informed care.

## Empowering Attributes

- **Courage:** Advocating for vulnerable patients, challenging systemic inequities, and pushing for cultural shifts within healthcare systems require boldness and perseverance. Courage enables clinicians to confront difficult truths and foster environments that prioritize safety and equity.
- **Advocacy:** Beyond individual courage, advocacy involves empowering families to participate in their infant's care, ensuring their voices are heard and respected. Advocacy mirrors the Principle of Empowerment, Voice, and Choice in TIDC, building a foundation for collaboration and trust.
- **Role modeling and mentorship:** TIPs serve as exemplars of compassionate care, inspiring colleagues to integrate these principles into their own practice. This attribute reflects the 7th Caritas Process, "Engaging in Genuine Teaching-Learning Experiences," which values mutual growth and shared learning.

## Visionary Attributes

- **Scholarly:** A commitment to continuous learning and evidence-based practice ensures that care evolves alongside advancements in the field. Scholarship bridges the art and science of caregiving, emphasizing the importance of integrating research with relational care.
- **Leadership for change:** TIPs are agents of transformation, advocating for systemic improvements that enhance outcomes for infants, families, and clinicians. This attribute aligns with Watson's 10th Caritas Process, "Opening to Spiritual Unknowns," embracing innovation and possibility in the pursuit of healing.

When clinicians cultivate these attributes, they elevate their capacity to deliver compassionate, relational care while addressing the complex needs of the NICU environment. These qualities empower professionals to create healing connections with families, buffer the effects of secondary trauma in themselves, and foster resilience across the NICU community. By embracing these attributes, TIPs honor their role as caregivers and advocates. They transform the challenges of NICU work into opportunities for growth and healing, touching lives in ways that resonate far beyond the bedside.

# TOOLKIT FOR TRAUMA-INFORMED DEVELOPMENTAL CARE AND DIVERSITY, EQUITY, AND INCLUSION ACTIVISM

Integrating TIDC with DEI activism in the NICU requires practical tools and templates that guide clinicians and teams in operationalizing these principles. Here are several suggestions for tools, templates, and strategies that can support this integration (Table 26.14).

**TABLE 26.14**

**OVERVIEW OF TIDC–DEI TOOLS AND TEMPLATES**

| Tool/Template Name | Purpose | Key Feature |
|---|---|---|
| DEI-TIDC Integration Checklist | Evaluate alignment with TIDC and DEI principles. | Sensory regulation, equitable policies, staff training |
| Cultural Humility Reflection Guide | Encourage clinicians to reflect on biases and assumptions. | Prompts for self-awareness, curiosity, collaborative care |
| Family Engagement Toolkit | Empower families and foster collaboration in caregiving. | Welcome packet, care participation plan, postdischarge resources |
| Equity and Bias Audit Tool | Identify disparities in outcomes, policies, and resources. | Clinical outcome analysis, family feedback, resource allocation |

(continued)

TABLE 26.14

OVERVIEW OF TIDC–DEI TOOLS AND TEMPLATES (*continued*)

| Tool/Template Name | Purpose | Key Feature |
|---|---|---|
| Reflective Practice Template | Support clinician growth and promote accountability in practice. | Case reflection, team feedback, actionable steps |
| TIDC-DEI Training Modules | Educate staff on trauma-informed and equitable care principles. | Implicit bias, cultural humility, trauma-informed communication |
| TIDC-DEI Alignment Tracker | Track progress in integrating TIDC and DEI principles into the NICU. | Metrics for training, family satisfaction, and disparity reduction |
| NICU Vision Statement Template | Co-create a shared vision reflecting TIDC and DEI values. | Core values, commitments, community goals |

DEI, diversity, equity, and inclusion; NICU, neonatal intensive care unit; TIDC, trauma-informed developmental care.

## Diversity, Equity, and Inclusion: Trauma-Informed Developmental Care Integration Checklist

Following is a comprehensive checklist to evaluate how well NICU practices align with TIDC and DEI principles.

*Sections:*

- **Environment:** Is the NICU designed to support diverse cultural practices (e.g., private spaces for religious or cultural rituals)? Are sensory stressors minimized to create a healing environment?
- **Policies:** Are visitation policies equitable, accommodating work schedules, transportation challenges, and nontraditional family structures?
- **Communication:** Are interpreters readily available? Are care plans and updates provided in a language and format accessible to all families?
- **Staff training:** Have clinicians received training on implicit bias, cultural humility, and trauma-informed care?
- **Follow-up:** Are there plans to connect families to culturally appropriate community resources after discharge?

*Purpose:* This tool provides a starting point for NICU teams to identify strengths and gaps in TIDC-DEI integration.

*Example in practice:* A NICU team uses the checklist to identify a gap in culturally appropriate family resources. As a result, they develop multilingual educational materials and hire an interpreter dedicated to family consultations.

## Cultural Humility Reflection Guide

Following is a reflective practice template for clinicians to examine their biases, assumptions, and interactions with families.

*Prompts:*

- **Self-Awareness:** Reflect on a recent interaction with a family. Based on my background, did I assume anything about their values, preferences, or needs?
- **Curiosity:** Did I invite the family to share their cultural or personal preferences regarding their infant's care?
- **Communication:** Did I provide information that respected their language and literacy level? How did I make space for their voice and choice?
- **Collaboration:** How did I ensure that the family was an equal partner in the care plan?

*Purpose:* Encourage clinicians to approach care with openness and humility, fostering stronger connections with diverse families.

*Example in practice:* A nurse reflects on a missed opportunity to involve a father in caregiving. In future interactions, the ensures that the father is included, actively building his confidence and trust.

## Family Engagement Toolkit

Following is a set of tools designed to empower families and build trust, incorporating both TIDC and DEI principles.

*Components:*

- **Welcome packet:** This includes NICU practices, family rights, and culturally appropriate care resources.
- **Care participation plan:** This is a template where families outline their caregiving preferences, such as feeding methods, involvement in procedures, and cultural or spiritual needs.
- **Daily communication log:** This is a simple form for clinicians to provide updates and invite questions from families, ensuring transparent and collaborative communication.

- **Postdischarge resource map:** This is a list of local organizations, early intervention services, and support groups tailored to diverse cultural and socioeconomic needs.

*Purpose:* Create a partnership model where families feel informed, respected, and actively involved in their infant's care.

*Example in practice:* A parent, initially hesitant to perform SSC, gains confidence after reviewing the toolkit. They report feeling more connected to their infant and better supported by the care team.

## Equity and Bias Audit Tool

Following is a framework for evaluating NICU policies, practices, and outcomes to identify and address disparities.

*Sections:*

- **Clinical outcomes:** Analyze disparities in preterm survival rates, pain management, breastfeeding support, and follow-up care across demographic groups.
- **Resource allocation:** Assess whether all families have equal access to resources, such as lactation support, interpreters, or financial aid.
- **Workforce diversity:** Evaluate staff demographics and efforts to recruit and retain a culturally representative workforce.
- **Family feedback:** Collect and analyze family feedback about their experience in the NICU, with specific questions about equity and inclusion.

*Purpose:* Provide actionable insights into systemic disparities and guide improvements.

*Example in practice:* An audit reveals lower breastfeeding rates among Hispanic families. The NICU has introduced Spanish-speaking lactation consultants and is seeing significant improvement.

## Reflective Practice and Peer Debriefing Template

Following is a structured template for reflective practice sessions focused on TIDC and DEI principles, supporting clinicians' emotional and professional growth.

*Sections:*

- **Case reflection:** Share a case where DEI or trauma-informed care felt particularly challenging or successful.
- **Lessons learned:** What biases, barriers, or strengths emerged? How can they inform future care?
- **Team feedback:** Invite input from peers on strategies to improve equitable and trauma-informed care delivery.
- **Action steps:** Outline specific, measurable actions to integrate lessons into practice.

*Purpose:* Build a culture of accountability, learning, and mutual support within the NICU team.

*Example in practice:* A team reflects on a case involving miscommunication with a non–English-speaking family. They commit to prioritizing interpreter services for all care discussions.

## Trauma-Informed Developmental Care: Diversity, Equity, and Inclusion Training Modules

Following are interactive training templates for ongoing education on trauma-informed care and DEI principles.

*Modules:*

- **Implicit bias in the NICU:** Role-play scenarios to explore how bias influences care and decision-making.
- **Cultural competence versus cultural humility:** Perform activities that highlight the difference and importance of relational, adaptive care.
- **Trauma-informed communication:** Perform techniques for building trust and collaboration with families from diverse backgrounds.
- **Advocacy for equity:** These are strategies for clinicians to address systemic barriers and promote inclusive policies within their organization.

*Purpose:* Equip clinicians with practical skills and knowledge to enhance their practice.

*Example in practice:* After completing a training session, clinicians implement new communication strategies, such as asking open-ended questions to better understand family needs.

## Trauma-Informed Developmental Care: Diversity, Equity, and Inclusion Alignment Tracker

Following is a dynamic template to track progress on integrating TIDC and DEI principles into the NICU.

*Metrics:*

- **Training completion:** Percentage of staff who have completed TIDC and DEI training
- **Family satisfaction:** Results from surveys that assess family experiences of respect, inclusion, and empowerment
- **Disparity reduction:** Changes in clinical outcomes or access to care across demographic groups
- **Workplace culture:** Feedback from staff on their sense of belonging and alignment with trauma-informed principles

*Purpose:* Provide a measurable framework for accountability and continuous improvement.

*Example in practice:* A NICU uses the tracker to identify and address a gap in staff training, leading to improved family feedback scores.

## Neonatal Intensive Care Unit Vision Statement Template

Following is a template to help NICU teams co-create a shared vision statement that integrates TIDC and DEI values.

*Sections:*

- **Core values:** What principles guide our care (e.g., safety, equity, compassion)?
- **Commitments:** What specific actions will we take to uphold these values?

- **Community goals:** How will we ensure that infants, families, and staff thrive in our care ecosystem?

*Purpose:* Anchor the team's work in a unifying vision that reflects their commitment to trauma-informed and equitable care.

*Example in practice:* The NICU team collaboratively develops a vision statement that prioritizes equitable care and trauma-informed principles, reinforcing their shared mission.

### Integrating Lessons: Building a Culture of Buffering

These tools and templates provide practical pathways for integrating TIDC with DEI efforts in the NICU. By fostering reflection, collaboration, and accountability, they empower NICU teams to create environments where every infant, family, and clinician feels valued and supported.

By embedding these practices into the NICU culture, clinicians can buffer trauma effectively while fostering resilience for infants, families, and themselves. Reflective practice, grounded in the Caritas Processes®, encourages continual growth and adaptation in the face of complex challenges.

## CONCLUSION: TRANSFORMING CARE, TOUCHING LIVES, AFFECTING LIFETIMES

The NICU is a unique space where the fragility of life and boundless healing potential coexist. Infants, families, and clinicians navigate profound challenges here, shaped by ELA, emotional vulnerability, and the demands of critical care. However, within this complexity lies an extraordinary opportunity: the chance to buffer trauma and foster resilience through intentional, compassionate, and trauma-informed care.

Integrating Caring Science, Principles and Core Measures of TIDC, Attributes of a TIP, and the B.U.F.F.E.R. approach provides a holistic framework for meeting these challenges. Together, these models elevate NICU care beyond technical expertise, grounding it in relational, humanistic, and healing-centered practices. This means creating environments that support neurodevelopment and emotional regulation for infants, laying a foundation for lifelong health. For families, it means fostering empowerment, trust, and connection, breaking cycles of adversity, and nurturing hope. For clinicians, it means cultivating self-awareness, resilience, and authenticity, sustaining the ability to care with integrity and compassion.

The work of buffering trauma is not merely a task—it is a sacred responsibility and a profound privilege. Every interaction in the NICU has the potential to leave an indelible mark, not only on the individuals involved but on the interconnected web of relationships that extend beyond the hospital walls. By embodying trauma-informed care, NICU teams create ripples of healing that touch generations.

Reflecting on the interplay between science, soul, and skills, this chapter invites us to reimagine the NICU as a healing sanctuary. Here, the art and science of caregiving converge, honoring the humanity of every infant, every family, and every clinician. Through practices grounded in love, authenticity, and intentional presence, trauma is buffered, resilience is cultivated, and lives are transformed.

In this work, we are reminded of the profound truth: care is not only about what we do but who we are. By embracing the transformative power of TIDC, we fulfill a shared mission—to touch lives, affect lifetimes, and create a legacy of healing that echoes far beyond the NICU.

## ONLINE RESOURCES

**CourseConnect**

Resources for this chapter are online and available at www.springerpub.com/courseconnect

## REFERENCES

References for this chapter are online and available at www.springerpub.com/courseconnect.

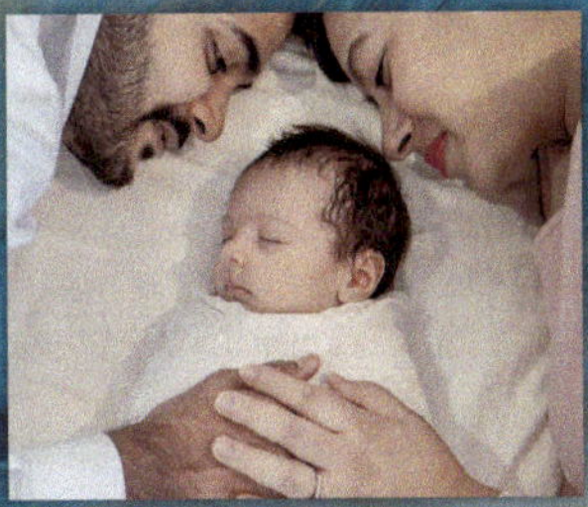

*Source:* paulaphoto/Adobe Stock.

**CHAPTER 27**

# Family: Essential Partner in Care

**Dorothy Vittner and Jacqueline M. McGrath**

## INTRODUCTION

Parents are essential to the growth and development of their infant. Parents are a child's avenue for interfacing with society and the conduit for the child over time to take on their own role in the community and within the larger society. Parents need to be more than just present; they must actively participate and engage in all aspects of the care of their infant, even in hospital settings. While extraordinary advances have been made in the medical care of critically ill newborns, facilitating the family's role in the care of their infant has been much slower and inconsistent (White et al., 2023). Evidence is increasingly providing direction for how best to fully engage parents in the neonatal intensive care unit (NICU). To continue to advance this work, NICU health professionals need to find and create opportunities for reducing separation of parents and infants during hospitalizations (McGlothen-Bell & McGrath, 2024). These opportunities must include increasing both physical and emotional closeness within parent–infant interactions and caregiving activities as well as within caregiving, decision making, and management (Vittner et al., 2025; White et al., 2023). *Parent engagement* is defined as a dynamic process focused on enhancing and supporting the parent–infant experience, specifically enhancing the acquisition of skills for problem solving and the provision of appropriate infant care based on the infant's unique needs at a particular point in time (Makris et al., 2019; Vittner et al., 2019).

The premise of parent engagement in the care of their infant develops through a parent's self-motivation to set goals and to utilize informational resources about the unique care necessary for their child; parents can increase their engagement while simultaneously improving the progression of their infant's health (Makris et al., 2019). Defining parent engagement facilitates the identification of factors related to parent risks and needs for intervention to optimize outcomes for premature infants (Vittner et al., 2019). A paradigm shift in caregiving practices is essential to ensure infant–family nonseparation and acknowledge the critical importance of nurturing human interaction for optimal infant health and well-being. Supporting and facilitating parent engagement is one means of decreasing what has been recently documented as posttraumatic stress disorder (PTSD) experienced by parents who must traverse the unfamiliar and chaotic NICU environment in partnership with their high-risk infant (Garfield et al., 2018; Malin et al., 2023a). The NICU environment has been repeatedly documented as traumatic to parents, which creates toxic stress, and parents need increasing support depending on their reactions to the environment (Malin et al., 2023a). Increasing parent engagement has the potential to enhance parent confidence, competence, and self-efficacy, which ultimately has the potential to improve their ability to self-manage their child's care after discharge to optimize the health and developmental outcomes for the child (Amin et al., 2018; Malin et al., 2023b; Vance & Brandon, 2017). Even more importantly, the unique needs of the infant's developing brain demand that caregiving delivered by both parents and health providers be neuroprotective, matching the "expectations" for experiences that "nurture" their short- and long-term neurocognitive development (McGrath & Vance, 2022; Vittner et al., 2025; White et al., 2023). Trauma-informed care has been increasingly implicated in caregiving in the NICU, and we as caregivers need to continue to acknowledge that care is traumatic to all involved (D'Agata et al., 2018; Malin et al., 2023b).

Mothers who give birth prematurely sometimes feel disconnected from their infant because the birth is so unexpected and can often be traumatic. These ambivalent feelings decrease the mother's ability to be appropriately responsive and sensitive to her infant's needs, potentially leading to dyssynchrony within mother–infant interactions and poorer attachment (Flacking et al., 2016; Franck et al., 2023). Sometimes, prenatal diagnosis provides the opportunity to enter and learn about the environment of the NICU prior to the birth of a high-risk infant. Although providing this information to families is helpful, if the birth is traumatic, the context for what information the parents were offered prior to the birth may have less of an effect than the traumatic experiences (Beck, 2020).

Regardless of how a family enters the NICU, it is important to remember that immediately on admission, a partnership must be formed between the family and professionals providing care for the infant (Vittner et al., 2025). Parent-driven organizations, such as the NICU Parent Network, advocate for all NICUs to consider parents as their infant's primary caregivers and essential, equal, and integral healthcare team members. Hospital policies and bedside care must encourage and support continuous and uninterrupted family presence, participation, and engagement from admission through discharge. The relationship between parents and health professionals must continue as a true collaborative partnership for as long as it is in the best interest of the child (Lechner et al., 2024; Urbina et al., 2024). Even though the integration of family-centered care (FCC) has become increasingly prioritized and is prevalent in most NICUs today, families continue to report being extremely distressed by the environment and their inability to parent their child in the way they had planned or the way they would at home (Lechner et al., 2024; Stremler et al., 2017; Urbina et al., 2024). These reports by families must be heard and continue to drive the delivery of infant care practices in the NICU.

Partnerships exist when there is a relationship between two or more parties with a shared goal. Effective partnerships between NICU health professionals and families are based on mutual respect, valuing of family expertise, fully shared information, and collaborative decision making (Urbina et al., 2024). When parents are considered partners who are consistently well-informed and involved within the NICU team, ethical dilemmas can be potentially lessened, and care decisions can be optimized in the best interest of the infant and the family (Lechner et al., 2024). Partnership and collaboration between families and health professionals are essential and are the crux of caregiving interventions.

Change is the most certain event throughout a person's life. A family experiencing the birth of an infant faces many changes. Some variations in lifestyle occur in the areas of employment, financial security, daily activities, relationships with others, and roles within the family. These changes have a major effect on each parent, family member, and on the family as a whole. When medical needs require admission of the infant to an intensive care nursery, the changes experienced by families become even more significant because, for the most part, the complex needs of this unique infant or complicated birth have not been planned for or expected. For the family, these changes can be devastating and challenging. The more fully integrated the family is within the NICU caregiving team, the more unlikely these events will be considered insurmountable or as challenging. During this difficult time, parents need more than support; they need to be true partners and an integral part of the process of caring for and parenting their child (McGlothen-Bell & McGrath, 2024). The environment of the NICU needs to be considered as more than the physical context but the social and emotional context. Thus, it is wholly impossible to provide excellent care to the infant without partnering with the family in every aspect of care (Vittner et al., 2025; White et al., 2023).

Families provide the foundation for health and are the child's entrance to the healthcare system. Family beliefs and individual health values are highly correlated. Families are the constant for the child. The provision of individualized developmental care (IDC), of which FCC is a core principle, is pivotal to optimizing long-term medical and developmental outcomes for the child (O'Reilly et al., 2020; Vittner et al., 2025). IDC effects are documented into school age, adolescence, and young adulthood (McAnulty et al., 2013; Sullivan et al., 2022). Understanding the many influences of the context of the family on the mental health status of each of its members is essential for those caring for infants and children (Box 27.1) (Beck, 2020; D'Agata et al., 2017; Garfield et al., 2018). Most professionals collaborating with children and families believe that a family-centered approach is essential and the best option because this type of care supports optimal outcomes for the child in concert with those derived from high-quality professional and technical care (Bansal et al., 2024;). Fundamental to the infant's developmental trajectory

**BOX 27.1**

### FUNDAMENTAL CHARACTERISTICS OF FAMILY-CENTERED CARE

The practice of FCC involves the following:

1. recognizing the family as the constant in a child's life, whereas the service systems and those who work within each are always changing
2. facilitating family–professional partnerships and collaborations at all levels of healthcare provision
3. providing care for the individual child and his or her unique characteristics
4. families partnering and participating in program development, implementation, and evaluation
5. collaborating with families to contribute to policy formation
6. honoring the racial, ethnic, cultural, religious, and socioeconomic diversity of families
7. recognizing family strengths and individuality and celebrating those differences as valuable
8. respecting and supporting different methods of family coping with difficult situations and information
9. partnering with families, on a continuing basis and in a supportive manner, complete and unbiased information with full transparency
10. encouraging and facilitating family-to-family supports and networking opportunities
11. incorporating the unique developmental needs of infants, children, and their families into healthcare systems
12. implementing comprehensive policies and programs that provide emotional and financial support to meet the unique needs of families
13. designing accessible healthcare systems that are flexible, culturally competent, and responsive to family-identified needs

*Sources: Adapted from:* Institute for Family-Centered Care and Institute for Healthcare Improvement; Institute for Patient- and Family-Centered Care. (2017). *Advancing the practice of patient- and family-centered care in hospitals: How to get started*. Author. http://www.ipfcc.org/resources/getting_started.pdf.

is early parent–infant contact. Parent–infant contact through nurturing touch, especially during skin-to-skin contact (SSC), has the potential to reduce the adverse consequences of critically ill infants (Kamphorst et al., 2018; Olsson et al., 2017). These benefits occur through physiologic changes in the infant and parents, which facilitate increased feelings of comfort, attachment, and physiologic stability (Campbell-Yeo et al., 2017; Casio et al., 2018; Vittner et al., 2018). SSC is an evidence-based holding strategy that increases the opportunity for parental proximity and provides a continuous interactive environment known to enhance infant physiologic stability and affective closeness within the parent–infant dyad (Kuo et al., 2022; Linnér et al., 2020; Vittner et al., 2018, 2019).

Clear definitions of family and the philosophy of FCC are critical to the foundation of the concepts presented in this chapter. Role theory is used to explain the issues families face during this challenging time. Factors that influence parenting behaviors include personal experiences, medical and nursing professional expectations, environmental influences, and peer relationships. These factors can either promote or interfere with the development of a robust family unit (Vittner et al., 2025). The birth of a critically ill newborn complicates the attachment process (Browne, 2023), and the learning of parenting skills, and thus, an evidence-based framework is provided for understanding what families need in terms of appropriate support and facilitation in the neonatal setting. Several different models of FCC are presented. The chapter concludes with evidence-based FCC strategies that support optimal family functioning during the hospital experience and promote the discharge of intact families as the crisis of newborn intensive care begins to resolve. These strategies also include issues related to sibling adaptation and the involvement of extended family members in the care and decision making related to the infant.

## FAMILY-CENTERED CARE

FCC is a philosophy of care in which the family's pivotal role in children's lives is recognized and respected (IPFCC, 2017). According to this philosophy, families are supported in their natural caregiving and decision-making roles by building on their unique strengths as people and then extending this same examination of strengths to the family unit. FCC recognizes and promotes the normal patterns of a family's life at home and in the community (Franck & O'Brien, 2019). Rather than expecting the family to take on the medical culture of the institution, healthcare professionals recognize and reinforce the family's culture through a partnership formed in the child's best interests. Parents and professionals are equals in a partnership committed to the child and to the development of optimum quality in the delivery of all levels of healthcare (IPFCC, 2017). FCC strengthens the family unit through empowerment and advocacy by enabling the family to nurture and support their child's development (Box 27.2) (IPFCC, 2017; White et al., 2023).

From the child's perspective, FCC is safe and familiar; the infant/child is first and foremost a member of a family, and care that is individualized to the family is also individualized to the infant (Hill et al., 2018). When the framework of FCC is the foundation for caregiving, the family is visible, available, and supportive of their infant's needs. They are an integral part of every decision that affects their child, even if they are not present at the bedside 24 hours a day like any other member of the health professional team (Browne, 2023; Miyagishima et al., 2017). Thus, their presence is noted in all aspects of care. The family members are empowered partners in the caregiving practices of their child within the healthcare setting (Vittner et al., 2025). FCC begins wherever and whenever a family enters the healthcare system and continues throughout the hospitalization to discharge. Families should encounter this philosophy of care before birth in antenatal care and continue it into the delivery room and beyond into the postpartum period (Franck, & O'Brien, 2019). It is important to remember that families are not replaceable at any level in the child's overall development. Within the implementation of the philosophy of FCC, their effect always supersedes that of the healthcare system (Foster et al., 2018, White et al., 2023).

IDC organizes infant care to minimize separation of parents and infants, which provides infant care practices that integrate a foundation in bonding and attachment theory that supports parents and infants directly or indirectly. Nonseparation of infants and parents also has ethical and legal support (McGlothen & McGrath, 2024). The United Nations Convention on the Rights of the Child from 1989 states in Article 7: "The child ... shall have the right from birth to ... be cared for by his or her parents" and in Article 9: "Parties shall ensure that a child shall not be separated from his or her parents against their will...." Couplet care is an emerging concept within neonatal care that provides facilities for

**BOX 27.2**

### FOUNDATIONAL PRINCIPLES OF FAMILY-CENTERED CARE

- **Enabling:** Building on family strengths to create opportunities and ways for families to use the abilities and competencies they already have to learn new ones to meet the infant's unique needs
- **Empowering:** Acknowledging and respecting families have existing strengths and capabilities and building on those strengths by supporting the family in meaningful decision making about issues that affect their well-being. Professionals who empower families interact collaboratively and form partnerships with families in ways such that the family develops and maintains a sense of control over their own lives and are able to make positive changes to reinforce their own strengths, abilities, and actions.

*Sources:* Adapted from Institute for Family-Centered Care and Institute for Healthcare Improvement; Institute for Patient- and Family-Centered Care. (2017). *Advancing the practice of patient- and family-centered care in hospitals: How to get started*. Author. http://www.ipfcc.org/resources/getting_started.pdf.

parents to live in the neonatal intensive care nursery along with their infants throughout the hospitalization by coupling the care of the infant with the care of the newly delivered mother. This model has been practiced in Sweden for over 10 years. It includes postpartum care after a normal delivery and care of mothers with more advanced needs. After the immediate postpartum period, approximately half of all mothers with infants born prematurely have a prolonged need for medical care and would otherwise be separated from their infants during the very important first days of bonding and attachment (Westrup, 2015). When introducing couplet care, it is important to adjust the design and structure of the nursery appropriately. It is essential to build structures for a close collaboration with obstetrics because they must still have the medical responsibility for the mothers; for example, do rounds, prescribe medications, and decide if the mother is receiving adequate care. FCC cannot happen in a vacuum; it must be supported by organizational policies and procedures that optimize the strengths of the family (Milette et al., 2017a, 2017b). Delivery requires a whole team approach where everyone has the same beliefs and attitudes toward the importance of families to ensure that all families receive this type of care.

## DEFINITION OF FAMILY

The concept of who and what comprises a family in North America is defined best by each specific family unit. Families expand, contract, and realign rapidly to keep up with the rapidly changing demands of our world. Today, dual-career families; single-parent households; unmarried couples; lesbian, gay, bisexual, queer, and transgender (LGBQT) couples; remarried couples; and sole-parent adoptions are all accepted models of family, in addition to the "traditional" family units common a century ago.

The term *family* is a broad term that is best defined by the individual; however, in general, a family is made up of those people, both related and unrelated, who provide support, structure beliefs, and define values. Family has also been defined as a social system composed of two or more people who coexist in the context of expectations of reciprocal affection, mutual responsibility, and temporal duration (Lechner et al., 2024). Families provide the framework through which individuals enter and interact with society at large. For infants and children, families are the means to resources, education, and society. Again, it is important to remember that families bring their children to the healthcare system for care. No matter how an infant comes to us, it comes with a family.

A family is defined by its members; the concept of family is an internal concept of how that unique group defines itself. It may be composed of blood relations or friends; it may not depend on a blood bond but on the emotional tie of closeness felt among its members. It also may be an extended family that includes parents, grandparents, other relatives, and friends. Families today are not necessarily defined as they have been in the past and not according to gender-specific roles. Families can also be defined by considering the degree to which the following five attributes are present (these attributes also depend on the family's societal and cultural orientation).

1. A family is a social system or unit.
2. Family members may or may not be related by birth, adoption, or marriage.
3. A family may or may not include dependent children.
4. Families involve commitment and attachment.
5. Family members usually have roles and caregiving functions (e.g., protection, nourishment, and socialization).

## ROLE THEORY

In the context of better understanding family dynamics, reviewing and examining role theory is important. Role theory, which first appeared in the literature in the 1930s, offers a framework for understanding families and identifying individuals' roles within the family. As a broad term, role theory represents a collection of concepts, subtheories, and research addressing aspects of social behavior that are relevant to families. Roles are social contexts with patterned behaviors that develop over time and are predetermined by social forces. Roles are dynamic, interactional, and reciprocal relationships among individuals; therefore, values, attitudes, and behaviors influence these relationships. Each role has specific behaviors and expectations placed on it by society. These expectations guide individuals as to when, where, and how to perform within the role.

Each role within a family has specific demands. An individual learns these demands by maturing and advancing through the middle to later stages of the life cycle: (a) adolescence, (b) adulthood, (c) marriage and parenthood, and (d) middle and old age. Individuals respond to the demands of a role differently based on their maturity and current developmental stage in the life cycle. For example, a single adolescent girl would be expected to perform the maternal role differently from a married adult woman.

Within role theory, seven areas of distress have been identified: (a) role ambiguity, (b) role conflict, (c) role incongruity, (d) role overload, (e) role underload, (f) role overqualification, and (g) role underqualification. These terms are defined in Table 27.1. Distress is often responsible for producing role stress and strain. Role stress is defined as either internal or external pressure that generates role strain. Consequently, feelings of frustration, tension, or anxiety are produced in the individual or the reciprocal partners. When problems occur within a role or a person, the group members may need to modify or completely change roles. Changing roles can be stressful for the individual and the group. However, not changing roles can result in intrapersonal and interpersonal role conflict, which can lead to further stress and anxiety. Parenting in the NICU can lead to role conflict because parents may feel they are not the ones parenting their child (Makris et al., 2019).

The working mother is an example of role conflict and role overload; she may struggle with her dual professional and maternal roles. Deciding to quit work and devote all her time to mothering may contribute to a lack of self-worth or identity. A decision to continue both roles may generate feelings of guilt because the new mother feels that she is neglecting her family's needs. Reducing her work hours is a behavioral change she may make to allow more time for her family.

**TABLE 27.1**

**POTENTIAL ROLE CHALLENGES EXPERIENCED BY PARENTS**

| Role | Potential Challenges |
|---|---|
| Ambiguity | Role expectations are vague or lack clarity. |
| Conflict | Role expectations are incompatible (conflicts exist between reality and expectations). |
| Incongruity | Self-identity and subjective values are grossly incompatible with role expectations. |
| Overload | Too much is expected in the time available. |
| Underload | Role expectations are minimal and underuse the role occupant's abilities. |
| Overqualification | Occupant's motivation, skills, and knowledge far exceed those required. |
| Underqualification | Incompetence: The role occupant lacks one or more of the necessary resources (commitment, skill, knowledge). |

*Source:* Data from Dibble, S. L., Hayre-Kwan, S., & Lipson, J. G. (Eds). (2019). *Culture and clinical care* (3rd ed.). Independently published.

She thus receives the positive reinforcement of employment yet has more time for family and her maternal role. If she does not modify her roles, she may experience further stress and anxiety. To be effective, role change requires several steps. Such change develops through gradual, continuous, and dynamic processes based on the individual's needs and those of relevant others. The steps to successful role change include identifying the role of the relevant other (or others), identifying the expectations of the new role, developing the abilities for it, taking on the new role, and modifying it.

## PARENTAL ROLE

Certain behaviors define the role of the parent. It is also important to remember that not all families today are composed of mothers and fathers, so identifying who is taking on the parenting role is important to understand how to best support families. Several factors influence these behaviors: cultural background, personality, previous parenting and life experiences, degree of attachment to the infant, and expectations that parents have of themselves and the infant. Parents must take on a new role; they are not just partners sharing a relationship; they are now mothers and/or fathers as well. Feelings of inadequacy, conflict, and fatigue are often apparent during the transition and may adversely affect existing relationships and those developing between parent and child (Treyvaud et al., 2019). Parenting remains the only major role for which our society has little systematic preparation. Difficulties encountered in the early stages of parenting may adversely affect all relationships, especially the relationships between partners (Jackson et al., 2016). These difficulties can arise even if the new child is not the first child in the family unit; each additional member of the family brings unique joys and challenges.

The situation in which a person must parent also influences behaviors. Parents faced with a crisis must modify their roles and adapt to the necessary changes encountered with the crisis. Role and behavior changes can cause considerable stress, mainly if these changes occur abruptly (Browne, 2023). Maternal depression is a well-known phenomenon encountered by many mothers both during pregnancy and in the postpartum period. Mothers who must experience the NICU are at exceptionally high risk for developing depression (Lechner et al., 2024). Parents experiencing mental or physical illness or those who are chemically dependent can have limited coping abilities and social support (McGlothen-Bell et al., 2024). Screening at admission and throughout the infant's stay in the NICU is essential to provide support and treatment for at-risk mothers (McGlothen-Bell et al., 2024). Other interventions might include enhancing the mother's ability to become more engaged in her infant's care, helping her connect with other mothers in similar situations, and finding resources for them in the community (Makris et al., 2019; Vittner et al., 2019).

Single, adolescent, or first-time parents are also at a disadvantage. They may lack maturity and coping skills because of limited life experiences and unavailable or inappropriate social support systems. These disadvantaged situations may inhibit the development of the parent–infant relationship and thus impair parenting behaviors regardless of whether the infants are high-risk, preterm, or full-term (Malin et al., 2022). In addition, people parent differently and take on roles differently (Malin, 2024). These differences are not wrong or right; they are just differences that must be acknowledged and accepted. Parents who have experienced a previous loss or utilizing infertility may also have more difficulties parenting their infant in the NICU because their investment in having a child may be causing role strain accompanied by increased stress and anxiety (Bellizzi et al., 2024; Treyvaud et al., 2019). Sensitivity to these experiences and previous losses is vital in understanding how best to support these parents in the NICU. Lastly, in the NICU, it is important to focus on supporting fathers and non–birth parents, which can easily be overlooked and not well understood or supported (Treyvaud et al., 2019). The care of men in this high-risk situation is changing, but it is still an area where we need to improve and provide optimal care and support (Kim, 2018).

Infant-related factors can also interfere with parental attachment and subsequent parenting behaviors. An example is an infant born with a congenital anomaly (Neel et al., 2018). Many of these infants may be mentally or physically disabled for a lifetime, which interferes with the parent's expectations of their infant (Bansal et al., 2024; Flacking et al., 2016). A visible anomaly is particularly difficult for parents because society emphasizes appearance. An infant with an easily correctable anomaly is tentatively unacceptable to society until the anomaly has been corrected. A visible, noncorrectable anomaly has a more significant effect on the parents and other family members. This stigma may include preterm infants who have deficits related to their untimely birth, such as blindness, deafness, or severe respiratory compromise. Parents may struggle with prognostic uncertainty, the need to make complex medical decisions, and navigating new hopes and fears (Bansal et al., 2024; Coughlin & Sethares, 2017). It may be helpful to connect these families with support groups or other families with children with similar disabilities or diagnoses (Al Maghaireh et al., 2016; Bansal et al., 2024; Stefana & Lavelli, 2017).

A life-threatening or terminal illness in a child is another situation that may interfere with parenting attachment and behaviors (Pelentsov et al., 2016). Parents may hold back their feelings for the child to try to protect themselves from loss and pain if the child dies (Currie et al., 2016; Rodrigues et al., 2024). This inability to attach to their infant interferes with the parenting experience and may affect the child's development if the child lives past the previously expected lifespan.

At any birth or other interaction between a parent and his or her child, the nurse must identify adaptive and maladaptive parenting behaviors. Adaptive behaviors indicate that both the infant's and parent's needs are met and the parent–child relationship can be established. Parents may express their parental roles differently based on gender differences (Rodrigues et al., 2024). Table 27.2 identifies parenting behaviors the nurse can use as a foundation for assessing adaptive or maladaptive behaviors. It is important to remember that these guidelines must be adapted individually to each parent based on his or her personality and the specific situation.

**TABLE 27.2**

**GUIDELINES FOR ASSESSING PARENTING BEHAVIORS**

| Attachment and Bonding Behaviors | Detachment and Challenging Infant Behaviors |
|---|---|
| ***Delivery*** | |
| Attempts to turn head to see infant as soon as delivered and while infant is on warming table | Approaches infant from behind, does not look toward or change head position to see infant |
| When shown infant:<br>• Smiles<br>• Keeps eyes on infant, looking at all parts exposed<br>• Attempts a face-to-face position<br>• Uses fingertip touch on face and extremities<br>• Asks to hold infant<br>• Partly opens blanket to see more of infant<br>• Talks to infant<br>• Asks questions about infant | When shown infant:<br>• Frowns or appears distressed<br>• Stares at ceiling or focuses on technology/phone<br>• May not look at infant<br>• Stares at infant without expression<br>• Does not assume *en face* position<br>• Does not touch infant<br>• Does not ask to hold infant<br>• Declines offer to hold infant<br>• If infant is placed in her arms, lies still, and does not touch or stroke infant's face or extremities<br>• Does not talk to infant<br>• Asks few or no questions |
| Makes positive statements about infant: "She's so cute!" "He's so soft!" | Makes no comments or makes only negative statements: "She looks awful." "He looks funny." |
| May cry out of joy or relief that infant is normal or of desired sex | May cry, appearing unhappy or depressed |
| May smile and cry at the same time (to differentiate from crying out of disappointment, note facial expressions and verbal statements) | When asked why she is crying, states she is disappointed in infant |

(*continued*)

**TABLE 27.2**

**GUIDELINES FOR ASSESSING PARENTING BEHAVIORS (*continued*)**

| Attachment and Bonding Behaviors | Detachment and Challenging Infant Behaviors |
|---|---|
| Expresses satisfaction with or acceptance of infant's gender: "We really wanted a girl, but it's more important that he's healthy." "I can't believe it's a boy, at last!" | Expresses dissatisfaction with infant's gender: "Not another girl. I should have known better than to try again for a boy." "I don't even want to see him." May use profanity when told gender |
| Predominant affect: appears pleased and happy | Predominant affect: appears sad, angry, or expressionless |
| Suddenly decides she wants to breastfeed | Suddenly decides against breastfeeding |
| ***First Week*** | |
| Initially uses fingertips on head and extremities; progresses to using fingers and palm on infant's trunk; eventually draws infant toward her, holding infant against her body | Uses fingertip touch without progressing to palm on trunk or drawing infant toward her body |
| Snuggles infant to neck and face | Does not hold infant to neck or face |
| Makes spontaneous movements, kissing, stroking, and rocking | Makes few or no spontaneous movements with infant |
| Talks to infant with positive manner and tone, uses appropriate language, speech, and content | Uses curt language or content |
| Attempts to establish eye contact by moving infant, assuming *en face* position, or shielding infant's eyes from light | Does not use *en face* position or attempt to establish eye-to-eye contact |
| Handles and holds infant at times other than when giving direct care | Handles infant only as necessary to feed or change diapers |
| Relaxed with child; relaxed posture, muscle tone | Rigid posture, tension, fidgeting, seems somewhat agitated |
| Smiles at infant frequently; changes affect appropriately, such as when infant cries | Rarely smiles at infant or smiles all the time without change in affect |
| Makes many specific observations of infant: "Her eyes look like they might turn brown." "One foot turns in just a bit." | Makes no observations or makes few observations that are either general or negative |
| Discusses infant's characteristics, attempting to relate them to others in the family: "He has my ears but his daddy's chin." "She really doesn't look like either of us, she just looks like herself." | Does not discuss infant's characteristics in relation to characteristics of family members |
| With a positive manner, uses animal characteristics to describe infant: "She's just like a cuddly little kitten." "His hair feels like down." | In a negative or hostile manner, uses animal characteristics to describe: "She looks awful, just like a drowned rat." "He looks like an ape to me." |
| Asks questions about caring for infant discharge | Asks no questions about care |

(*continued*)

**TABLE 27.2**

**GUIDELINES FOR ASSESSING PARENTING BEHAVIORS (*continued*)**

| Attachment and Bonding Behaviors | Detachment and Challenging Infant Behaviors |
|---|---|
| Seeks information about the child; asks appropriate questions | Does not ask questions or questions are not appropriate |
| ***First Few Weeks (if infant remains hospitalized after mother has been discharged)*** | |
| Calls every day or every other day | Calls less frequently than every other day or not at all |
| Is present at bedside a minimum of twice a week | Is unable to be present at least twice a week, or is not present at all |
| Stays at bedside for a minimum of 30 minutes | Stays at bedside for < 30 minutes |
| Asks specific questions about infant's condition | Asks no specific questions |
| Asks appropriate questions frequently | Asks inappropriate questions |
| Spends most of the time at bedside participation in care while looking at and handling infant | Spends most of the time at bedside observing unit activities and other infants (this may be normal behavior for the first few times the parent is in the NICU); has little or no interaction with infant even though she/he does participate in caregiving with encouragement |
| Becomes involved with care when encouraged and supported by staff | When encouraged by staff to participate in care, refuses, or decides to leave the NICU, or performs only minimal care |
| Although the parent is not able to be at the bedside often, when is able to be present, the time at the bedside lasts longer than 30 minutes; makes statements about missing infant (e.g., says that she misses infant at home or that she/he wishes she/he could be present more often and stay longer) | Makes no statements about missing infant, or states that she/he misses infant at home and wishes she could be present more often, but comments are not validated by frequent or lengthy time spent at bedside with infant |
| Expresses reluctance to terminate time at the bedside; is reluctant to leave | Leaves nursery with little hesitation |
| Waits until infant is asleep before leaving; touches or talks to infant just before leaving; may stand outside window and look at infant before leaving unit | Frequently asks nurse to complete feeding or to change and settle infant |
| Expresses a desire to participate in holding the infant | Seems afraid to hold infant or participate in care |
| Expresses a desire to participate in SSC | Finds it difficult or refuses to participate in SSC |
| Expresses desire to protect the child, aware of environmental hazards, actively protects | Protective behaviors not exhibited |
| Is available and willing to learn new things to better care for the child | Is unwilling to learn caregiving skills |

(*continued*)

**TABLE 27.2**

**GUIDELINES FOR ASSESSING PARENTING BEHAVIORS (*continued*)**

| Attachment and Bonding Behaviors | Detachment and Challenging Infant Behaviors |
|---|---|
| Supportive of partner in caring for the child and participating in caregiving, holding, and so on | Communication between partners is distant or nonexistent |
| ***First Months*** | |
| Holds infant close to her/his body | Does not hold infant securely against body |
| Supports infant's trunk and head in position of comfort | Head and body of infant are not well supported |
| Muscles in her/his arms and hands are relaxed and conform to curvature of infant's body | Shoulder, arm, and hand muscles appear tense; hands and fingers do not conform to infant's body |
| During feedings, holds infant in well-supported position against her body | Holds infant away from her body during feedings or props infant or bottle |
| Positions during feeding so eye-to-eye contact can occur | Position during feeding prevents eye-to-eye contact |
| Minimizes talking to infant while infant is sucking | Continues talking to infant during feeding even though infant is distracted and stops sucking |
| Refers to infant using given or affectionate name | Refers to infant in impersonal way (e.g., "the baby," "she," or "it") |
| Plays with infant at times unrelated to direct care | Handles infant mainly during caretaking activities |
| When infant is in infant seat, playpen, or crib, frequently interacts with infant | Leaves infant for long periods in infant seat or crib, interacting only after infant becomes fussy |
| Places infant, when awake, in an area where infant can observe and interact with others | Leaves infant, when awake, alone for long periods in bedroom or isolated area |
| Occasionally leaves infant with someone else | Frequently leaves infant with someone else or refuses to leave infant with someone else |
| Uses discretion in selecting babysitter and provides instructions on infant's routines, likes, and dislikes | Does not use good judgment in selecting babysitter; provides inadequate or no instructions for care |
| Provides infant with routine well-baby care; carries out medical plan for management of specific problems or conditions (e.g., thrush, anemia, or ear infection); makes additional phone calls or additional visits to physician | Fails to provide infant with well-baby care, seeking medical assistance only after problems, or keeps all appointments and makes emergency room visits for imagined or insignificant problems |
| Remains close to infant during physical examinations and attempts to soothe infant if infant becomes distressed | Remains seated at a distance from the examination table; does not soothe infant during examination; frequently arranges for someone else to take infant for medical appointments |
| Makes positive statements about parenting role | Makes negative statements about parenting role |

*Source:* Data from Hall-Johnson, S. (1986). *Nursing assessment and strategies for the family at risk* (2nd ed.). Lippincott William & Wilkins.

## PARENTING DURING CRISIS

Taking on the parenting role is a significant life task for a couple. The crisis of having a critically ill newborn in the NICU compounds the stress of that task. Whether the family unit attains growth from a positive resolution of this crisis or splinters because of a maladaptive adjustment largely depends on the partnership formed with caregiving and the quality of support provided (Bansal et al., 2024; Treyvaud et al., 2019). The memory of what happens in the first days after a traumatic birth often stays with a family forever. Consider inquiring with a mother to describe her birth experience, and she will talk for hours, explaining every detail (Rodrigues et al., 2024; Treyvaud et al., 2019). Consequently, the relationships formed and interventions provided during the initial trauma can be critical to the adjustment and continued growth of the family unit (Bansal et al., 2024; Rodrigues et al., 2024).

### Parent Responses

A *crisis* can be defined as an upset of a steady state, a period of disequilibrium precipitated by an inescapable demand to which the person is temporarily unable to respond adequately. The birth of a critically ill infant represents two types of crises for parents. The birth of any infant is a developmental crisis, a natural transitional phase in parents' lives. When the infant is premature or ill, parents also experience an accidental and unexpected crisis. The meaning of the event for the family and the resources available to deal with the event are variables that determine the scope of the crisis. With the technological advances in medicine, some families can better prepare for and make decisions about their child's prognosis and medical needs before birth. For example, many infants with gastroschisis or other anomalies are diagnosed during a prenatal ultrasound examination. In such cases, families can better plan for the birth and make decisions with the healthcare team in a more conducive and supportive environment. The ability to anticipate the needs of the child reduces the sense of crisis for these families with the birth of the child.

Families of premature or sick newborns react in different and individual ways. Some common responses are anxiety, guilt, fear, resentment, and anger. During the illness of a newborn, the parents must face many issues; two important ones are the loss of the perfect child they have anticipated and the fear that their infant may die (Bansal et al., 2024; Rodriguez et al., 2024). In general, excitement and a flurry of preparation surround the birth of a child. Family celebrations help parents share the anticipation of a new infant with friends and extended family members. Parents spend much time imagining what this child will look like and dreaming about the joys of parenting. The parents experience disappointment when the infant or pregnancy is not as anticipated. They may feel a sense of isolation from other parents who have a normal pregnancy or infant. They may even feel isolated from each other or close family members. The inability to produce a healthy infant or to protect the infant from the invasive and painful environment necessary to sustain the child's life may cause feelings of inadequacy. For some parents, the role they believed they would assume seems impossible to attain in the environment of the NICU, where often it seems that everyone else is making decisions about the fate of their infant (Bansal et al., 2024; Treyvaud et al., 2019). Parents seldom have had experience with the NICU before, and the intensity of the situation is heightened even more by the fact that they and their infant are center stage.

To move forward with the attachment process, parents must reconcile their idealized image of the child with the actual infant. They mourn the loss of the perfect child that was expected and encounter anticipatory grief for the infant whose life may now be in jeopardy (Bansal et al., 2024; Treyvaud et al., 2019). The birth of an ill or premature infant often places parents in a state of disequilibrium; nothing is as it was before. Hope is an important emotional concept for many parents during this crisis (Ingram et al., 2017). Hope provides some equilibrium that will improve things for their infant and themselves. However, hope can also lead parents to develop high expectations for their child that may conflict with the healthcare team's expectations (Nordheim, Rustøen et al., 2018). These different expectations can lead to more conflict and role strain as families are trying to maneuver the difficult situation of the NICU and understand how to assume their parenting role and best support their child (Rodrigues et al., 2024).

Mothers of premature infants have had the emotional work of pregnancy cut short and thus are often psychologically unprepared for the birth (Rodrigues et al., 2024). If the mother had felt ambivalent about the pregnancy, she may believe that the infant's illness is somehow punishment for those emotions. A mother may also feel guilty that she could not carry the infant to term, even if no reason can be found for the infant's premature birth.

Many parents of sick newborns go through identifiable stages of grief and loss with very emotional reactions (Currie et al., 2016). The initial response is usually one of overwhelming shock, characterized by irrational behavior, crying, and feelings of helplessness and despair. Families at this stage have difficulty with organization because the unexpected birth has disrupted their lives. They may feel that everything is in chaos and the situation is out of their control. Substance abuse, adolescent pregnancy, clinical depression, and domestic violence can increase the chaos and vulnerability of these families (Malin et al., 2024). Parents also may feel guilt over the premature delivery or the infant's illness. Self-blame often characterizes these feelings (e.g., "If only I had stayed home the day I noticed the spotting"). Parents may try to escape the situation through denial (e.g., "Everything will be fine in just a few days"). At the bedside in these initial days, parents may focus on facts they can understand and avoid issues they do not. To healthcare professionals, this may seem as if the parents are not listening or are unwilling to hear the information provided. Yet, the parents are trying to cope with what to them is an overwhelming situation (Malin et al., 2024).

Intense feelings of resentment and anger follow denial. Parents may direct these feelings at themselves, the infant, healthcare team members, God, or even each other as parents. They may also experience feelings of ambiguity and may fear the infant's physical and mental outcome. For these reasons, they may avoid emotional involvement with the infant to protect themselves from the pain of possible loss. A lessening of the intense emotional reactions and an increased ability to begin caring for their infant's emotional and physical needs are characteristics of adaptation and taking on the parenting role. Reorganization is the final stage; at this point, parents come to terms with their infant's problems. This can take from a few days to several months. Sometimes, these feelings of loss and grief may never be resolved (Currie et al., 2016). Throughout these stages, hope often helps parents move forward and believe that a new day will bring better outcomes for their child (Nordheim, Rustøen et al., 2018).

## Factors That Affect Parenting Skills

Certain factors affect a person's ability to acquire parenting skills during the NICU experience (Box 27.3). Parental presence and active participation in infant care are essential (Bansal et al., 2024; Vittner et al., 2025). Parents are unable to attach and detach at the same time; these two tasks are incongruent. Parents need time to detach or grieve for the lost perfect child before they can begin to attach to the ill infant. This adjustment may take days or even weeks, and for some parents, attachment may never occur (Rodrigues et al., 2024; Treyvaud et al., 2019).

Parents in the NICU environment face physical, mechanical, psychological, and emotional obstacles during this difficult time. In this chapter, we refer primarily to the psychosocial behaviors of parenting and becoming a family. Still, it is important to note that these behaviors also have implications for the parent's health and personal well-being (Treyvaud et al., 2019). These physiologic issues cannot be ignored because parents who do not attend to their personal and physical needs are not as able to attend to the needs of their child (Bansal et al., 2024). Evidence supports that an infant's appearance and experience of painful procedures, as well as the perceived severity of the child's illness, all contribute to the degree of stress experienced by parents (Bansal et al., 2024). A nurse who can properly identify the specific stressors with each parent or family has the opportunity to assist them in reducing those stressors and promoting adaptation for the family unit (Bansal et al., 2024; Treyvaud et al., 2019).

The nurse is potentially the principal barrier to parenting in the NICU because the nurse can be seen as the gatekeeper of the infant (Treyvaud et al., 2019). In reality, the infant belongs to the family, not the healthcare team. For parents to attach to their infant, a welcoming, calming environment in which they feel comfortable is essential in the NICU (Box 27.4) (Venkataraman et al., 2018). This kind of environment encourages parents to grow in their primary caregiver role to develop the skills needed to advocate for their child. This advocacy is essential for the infant's continuing development, especially if the child has special needs (Rodrigues et al., 2024). Meiers et al. (2007) developed the Family Nurse Caring Belief Scale to examine nurses' beliefs about FCC activities. This instrument can be used to understand how nursing staff perceive their own delivery of FCC and as a means to examine changes in FCC in a particular NICU environment over time.

Parents react to stress and grief differently (Rodrigues et al., 2024). A man may isolate himself, become engrossed in his work, and not share his feelings with a woman. A man often tries to be strong for the woman and may become protective, sometimes shielding her from painful information (Treyvaud et al., 2019). A wife may view her husband's stoic behavior as cold and unfeeling. Both may have difficulty discussing the child because of their grief or guilt feelings.

### BOX 27.3

**FACTORS THAT INFLUENCE FAMILY REACTIONS TO A CHILD'S HOSPITALIZATION OR ILLNESS**

- severity of the illness and the threat to the child
- previous experience with illness or hospitalization (or both)
- familiarity with the medical procedures involved in diagnosis and treatment
- available support systems
- available coping strategies of family members
- number and degree of other family stresses
- cultural or religious beliefs
- communication patterns of family members

### BOX 27.4

**CREATING A WELCOMING ENVIRONMENT IN THE HOSPITAL FOR FAMILIES**

1. When the opportunity presents before the birth, prepare the family for the infant's admission to the NICU and hospital course. This may include a tour of the NICU and the opportunity to meet with staff and discuss some of the potential procedures the infant may encounter.
2. Provide a special orientation for families who have undergone an emergency admission.
3. Provide for the needs of families who have traveled long distances.
4. Make sure fathers are as welcome as mothers. Strategies include communicating with both parents and making sure the father's voice is heard.
5. Meet the needs of siblings and other family members.
6. Enable families to be together as much as possible; have open visiting hours 24 hours a day.
7. Encourage families to bring items from home to create a personalized environment that makes their child feel more at home.
8. Provide privacy for the family when present at the bedside.
9. Encourage family participation in the child's care.
10. Help the family stay in touch with extended family members and support-givers in the community.

*Source:* Adapted from Institute for Patient- and Family-Centered Care. (2017). *Advancing the practice of patient- and family-centered care in hospitals: How to get started.* Author. http://www.ipfcc.org/resources/getting_started.pdf.

Normal postpartum blues can increase the mother's sensitivity to this situation and lead to further depression (Malin et al., 2024). She may cry for no real reason and feel embarrassed about irrational behavior. Existing weaknesses in their relationship are often magnified. Parents are frequently separated in their feelings at this time, and fears may arise that their relationship is falling apart at a time when they each need the other. Lack of communication can lead to isolation and feelings of resentment in each of the partners. Each may make assumptions about the other's feelings, resulting in misconceptions. The need to communicate and share in each other's experiences is especially true if the child has special needs or a developmental disability. These misconceptions, along with gender differences in coping, may continue for a lifetime if they are not recognized and addressed during the neonatal period (Bansal et al., 2024). Helping parents understand that their feelings are not unusual is essential to facilitate sharing these feelings with their partner. Some people may require counseling during this time.

Other stressors in the family, such as the needs of other children, financial concerns, illness of family members, or marital stress, can complicate the situation (Curtis et al., 2016). For example, factors that can influence the degree of stress perceived by the family include the availability of appropriate emotional and psychological support among family members and from friends and the availability and use of community resources (Curtis et al., 2016; Wang et al., 2016). Maintaining a support system and using community resources and professional assistance are excellent coping strategies for dealing with the crisis. Coping abilities demonstrated during previous crises often can predict how parents will cope with the current situation. In an acute crisis, the family may be unable to use the resources available adequately because of lowered self-esteem, reduced family cohesiveness, and impaired family communication. Interventions during this time should focus on helping parents recognize and use available coping strategies. Communication patterns could be impaired because of anger or emotion derived from the crisis situation (Curtis et al., 2016). Therefore, at times, the family may require outside assistance; they may be unable to use or maintain the community resources required without this support (IPFCC, 2017).

A stressful situation has a specific meaning for each family and each member of the family because of previous experiences and the family's perceptions of these demands and their personal capabilities. For example, a sepsis workup may not seem particularly stressful to the healthcare team but may be very stressful to parents and families (Rodrigues et al., 2024). For some families, the least hint that their infant is sicker or more unstable can be devastating. Certain personality types thrive on stress and deal effectively with any crisis. Others are unable to deal with even the smallest crisis. For example, if a family acknowledges a stressor as a challenge or can bestow meaning on the situation, such as believing that "it is the Lord's will," adaptation will likely be more successful. Maladaptation results if the family interprets the stressor as threatening or undesirable. The family's expectations for themselves and this new child affect parenting skills (Giambra et al., 2017). Each partner draws on his or her own childhood experience for parenting role models. The stressor's meaning to the family also depends on the family's identity, cultural beliefs, and worldview. The family's identity comprises the values of the family, which are seen in the routines and rituals that develop in individual families. Stressors may disrupt these routines and rituals, threatening the family system's development, maturation, and stability (IPFCC, 2017). The family's worldview is based on how they interpret reality, its core belief system (religious and cultural beliefs), and its purpose in life. How a family handles its problems or changes is often based on the family identity and worldview. The family worldview is the most stable of the three levels of meaning, but even this can be shattered by a severe crisis (Treyvaud, et al., 2019).

The coping strategies are cognitive and behavioral components of the effort to handle the stressful event, that is, what the family "does" to handle the stress. These strategies can be emotion focused (i.e., strategies for controlling the emotions the crisis has engendered, such as denial or anger) or problem focused (i.e., action-oriented strategies to manage the crisis). Coping behaviors are learned, and families can use any or all major coping functions in a crisis. Emotion-focused strategies are used most often in the adjustment phase of a crisis, and problem-focused strategies are used more in the adaptation phase (Foster et al., 2018).

## CULTURAL PERSPECTIVES

### Definitions

Some key definitions are important to an understanding of cultural perspectives, as follows.

- Ethnicity: a common ancestry through which individuals have evolved shared values and customs
- Culture: socially inherited characteristics, such as rituals, thoughts, beliefs, behavior patterns, and traits inherent within a particular racial, religious, or social group
- Acculturation: changing one's cultural patterns and assimilating behaviors consistent with those of the society in which one lives; this task can be done by learning the language, intermingling socially, developing friendships, or through marriage or relationships formed in school or workplaces
- Religion: a belief in divine powers; a system of beliefs, practices, and rituals

The family has always been the critical social unit for passing on beliefs and values in our society. Healthcare professionals must recognize and be sensitive to the influence of culture and ethnicity on a child's development and the family's response to illness or a chronic condition (Lipson & Dibble, 2005). The family's cultural ties provide support and stability during upheaval and stress.

The meaning of family varies with the ethnic or cultural background of the family (Bansal et al., 2024). Differences exist across cultures; although there are similarities, it is important not to generalize them across social groups. Examples provided here are just that: examples. Nurses should work with each family as individuals who may or may not exhibit these characteristics. The concept of immediate family among Anglo-Americans often means the nuclear family of mother, father, and children. However, this is changing as other definitions of family are becoming increasingly acceptable in our society. Lesbian, gay, and same-sex partners are now more common, and they may be raising children who may need care in the NICU. Parents who are unmarried but living together are becoming increasingly commonplace. Families should not be stereotyped, and all must embrace their unique characteristics. Families must be recognized as essential members of the healthcare team.

Examples of how family ethnicity and composition vary are provided to consider these differences fully. For Black families, the definition of family often includes extended family members within the community. For Italians, family can often include a very strongly knit group of family and friends extending over three or four generations. The Chinese family can often be defined as all their ancestors and descendants. Mexican-American families often include close-knit members and multigenerational supportive communities. Family hierarchy differences can positively and negatively influence young parents (Al Maghaireh et al., 2016). Understanding and appreciating the uniqueness and differences in the meaning of family across cultures and ethnic groups can assist the healthcare professional in promoting the family's health and supporting the family in times of illness or debilitating conditions (Treyvaud et al., 2019). No judgments should be made, and the child's parents should be able to choose who they believe is their family and support system, particularly in this time of stress.

Ethnic or cultural groups also differ in the meaning they give to illness and disability and when seeking healthcare (Condon et al., 2022; Treyvaud et al., 2019). Although the nurse must recognize that each family and situation must be assessed individually, some general characteristics may help understand differences among ethnicities. For example, generally, members of an Italian family rely on the family for help when they are ill and seek medical help only as a last resort. They use words and emotions to convey the meaning of an experience to others. The close-knit family is vital; the nurse must respect the family as a cohesive unit. In general, Blacks often have an underlying distrust of the healthcare system. To effectively work with Black families, the nurse must support or empower the family to solve their own problems, providing as much information as possible. Racism and oppression have left their marks on these families, and healthcare providers must facilitate the family to be advocates for the ill child, to cope constructively with problems, and to deal with an unknown future if disabilities persist (Al Maghaireh et al., 2016). The process of delivering FCC is influenced by factors across six domains: equitable relationships, building trust, knowledge sharing, family empowerment, environment and culture, and regulations (Kutahyalioglu et al., 2023). The illness is part of the whole person. Native American Hawaiians may view illness as an imbalance in the energy or harmony within the family. The illness is part of wellness, and this disharmony is a normal part of life. Anglo-Americans may view illness as stemming from a scientific cause outside the family. The illness is foreign and intrusive to the individual and the family. Considering these traditional characteristics may help understand the context of culture.

When a child is hospitalized, several important issues must be discussed with the family:

- what support does the family want to be provided by the caregiving team
- what their unique degree of participation in decision making will be
- preferences regarding language, holding, food, holidays, religion, and kinship
- beliefs about health, illness, and technological advances
- health practices (e.g., immunizations, annual physical examinations)
- habits, customs, and rituals that could affect health

Understanding cultural differences can help the nurse provide care, determine the meaning of the illness or disability to the family, and assist the family in interventions appropriate to their culture (Treyvaud et al., 2019). This understanding also shapes parent and staff expectations of each other and how care is provided. Taking the time to ask questions and understand the cultural influences on families cared for in the NICU can facilitate communication between families and healthcare professionals (Bansal et al., 2024). Language can often be a barrier to providing care and understanding the needs of families. It is important to provide appropriately supportive interpreters to facilitate families to understand the needs of their infant, yet this is not an individual initiative; rather, it involves a complex set of interrelationships between care teams to enhance communication (Condon et al., 2022; Kutahyalioglu et al., 2023).

## PROMOTING PARENTING IN THE NEONATAL INTENSIVE CARE UNIT

A major nursing goal in the NICU for the care of the family is to optimize parent engagement and active participation in the infant to increase the parent's confidence and competence (Makris et al., 2019; Novak & Vittner, 2021). There are different ways to ease parental anxiety during the NICU experience. Open visiting policies encourage unrestricted parent presence throughout the 24 hours and provide parents more opportunities to be with their infant while allowing them to manage other responsibilities outside the NICU (Raiskila et al., 2017). Parental presence with their infant facilitates developing relationships and the parenting processes (Vittner et al., 2025).

### Facilitating the Attachment Process

The attachment process for most parents begins at birth, or perhaps before birth, during the pregnancy process. With a sick or premature infant, this process can be delayed until the parents can establish eye contact with and begin touching and caring for their infant. Bonding and attachment are enhanced by supporting parents to touch and hold their infant as soon as the child's condition allows, especially SSC (Casio et al., 2018; D'Agata et al., 2016; Kutahyalioglu et al., 2023). The preterm neonate's physical appearance, disorganized behavioral responses, and variable physiologic responses to touch can cause much anxiety in the parents as they attempt to interact with their infant. However, it is important that the bedside nurse, well versed in what the sick or premature infant will tolerate, explains those maturational limitations to the parents. Parents must understand an infant's immaturity and inability to navigate often overwhelming sensory experiences; otherwise, parents may misinterpret the infant's behavioral cues or detach from their infant in an effort to not bother or overstimulate the infant. Interventions that focus on helping parents to understand and respond sensitively to infant cues have been found to facilitate both the infant and the family (Moradi et al., 2018; Treyvaud et al., 2019). It is also important for the nurse to work with the parents to help them recognize an infant's distress behaviors (e.g., hiccups, unsteady breathing, twitching, or tremors) so that parents can gauge their caregiving interactions by their infant's unique cues and behavior (Vittner et al., 2025).

Parent participation in caregiving must begin at admission (Vittner et al., 2019). Soothing touch, providing containment, gentle infant massage, holding the infant, bathing, and SSC or kangaroo care are just a few opportunities to promote parent engagement with their infant (Butler et al., 2024; Casio et al., 2018;). These supportive strategies should be provided to all infants in the NICU and reserved for families to implement with their infants. When parents are providing these interventions, there are physiologic and behavioral benefits for the infant as well as benefits to parents, including early bonding, increased confidence in parenting skills, and a sense of control (Nordheim, Anderzen-Carlsson, et al., 2018; Vance & Brandon, 2017). Parents who have the opportunity to participate in caregiving and get to know their infant begin to have a sense of confidence that their infant is well cared for and may survive (Amin et al., 2018; Condon et al., 2022). Nurses can use several key techniques to prepare parents for working with their infant and the technology in the NICU:

- Build all communication and education on parents' strengths.
- Ask parents what they want to be able to do with their infant and how they would like to be supported.
- Ask parents how they learn best so all education can be tailored to their needs.
- Encourage and avoid constructive criticism.
- Encourage parents to observe infant cues and behaviors to guide care interactions.
- Encourage parents to discuss their concerns and emotions.
- Provide parents with information specific to their infant's care or condition.
- Clarify information that parents have received through other channels.
- Draw the parents' attention to positive points about their infant, including how the child responds to the parents.
- Use transparent communication strategies.
- Embody motivational interviewing strategies by remaining open and nonjudgmental.

Interventions with families must acknowledge each member's individuality and the family as a unit. Understanding that the needs of the whole are not equal to, greater than, or less than those of the parts is often a difficult concept for the neonatal nurse, who sometimes sees his or her role as involved more specifically with the care of the high-risk infant. Researchers repeatedly have found that hospital-based neonatal nurses view caring for families as not within their realm of practice (and certainly not a priority in their practice), but as something extra they do "when there is time" (Vittner, DeMeo, et al., 2022). These views are not congruent with developmentally supportive FCC practices. Optimal care requires that healthcare providers adopt a family-centered philosophy (Bansal et al., 2024). Full implementation of a family-centered approach depends upon the support of the unit leadership and the institution (Milette et al., 2017a, 2017b). One way to facilitate greater involvement of families is to form parent advisory boards that guide implementation of practices in the NICU (IPFCC, 2018). Staffing plans that allow healthcare providers, especially nurses, time in their schedules to work collaboratively with families must be a priority if developmentally supportive family-centered practices are truly fundamental to the philosophy of care in the NICU (IPFCC, 2017).

Parents have repeatedly reported that they felt that healthcare professionals did not recognize them as the expert caregivers of their child and the constant in their child's life (Bansal et al. 2024; Kutahyalioglu et al., 2023). This perception may lead to mistrust in the developing partnership between the caregivers and the professionals and may intensify the stress for the parent and, ultimately, the child during the hospitalization (Aagaard et al., 2018). Acknowledging that parents are the experts and nurses are the consultants to whom parents come to for information or support is a shift that remains difficult for some professionals (IPFCC, 2017). Parents are empowered by nurses when they are respected; involved in the plan of care; provided with complete, unbiased information; and given a sense of control in the healthcare setting (IPFCC, 2017; Kutahyalioglu et al., 2023). To support full integration and implementation, see Table 27.3 for evidence-based strategies and interventions that empower and support families during newborn intensive care.

Caretaking is a normal part of parenting. However, parents of sick or premature infants are often deprived of the time to prepare psychologically for caring for a high-risk infant and to develop the caretaking skills to feel confident (Amin et al., 2018; Novak & Vittner, 2021). Parents may feel inadequate or resent the nurses if nurses do not allow the family to become regularly involved in caretaking tasks. Positive reinforcement builds self-confidence in parenting abilities. Family empowerment interventions are important to infant and family short- and long-term outcomes (Bansal et al., 2024).

## Providing Information

Throughout the infant's illness, parents need accurate, timely information about their child's condition (Box 27.5). If the information provided is not timely and does not anticipate the parents' needs related to their relationship with their infant, it may not be helpful and may hamper the care (Vittner, DeMeo, et al., 2022). Information should be direct and honest and not contradictory, so limiting the number of professionals

## TABLE 27.3

### EVIDENCE-BASED FAMILY-CENTERED CARE STRATEGIES TO SUPPORT INFANTS AND FAMILIES IN THE NICU

| Intervention | Level of Evidence | References |
|---|---|---|
| Encourage the family to spend as much time with their infant as possible; support nonseparation | III | Condon et al. (2022) |
| | I | Browne et al. (2023) |
| | V | D'Agata et al. (2017) |
| | III | Feeley et al. (2016) |
| | V | McGlothen-Bell and McGrath (2024) |
| Facilitate and maintain a true collaborative partnership with families | I | Adama et al. (2022) |
| | V | Craig et al. (2015) |
| | I | Browne (2023) |
| | IV | Butler et al. (2024) |
| | V | McGlothen-Bell and McGrath (2024) |
| Assist the family in resolving feelings of guilt | V | McGlothen-Bell and McGrath (2024) |
| | I | Adama et al. (2022) |
| | IV | Coughlin and Sethares (2017) |
| Facilitate and provide opportunities for families to develop and sustain hope | V | Bally et al. (2018) |
| | IV | Nordheim et al. (2018) |
| | I | Adama et al. (2022) |
| | I | Bally et al. (2018) |
| | IV | Ingram et al. (2017) |
| Provide the family with opportunities to learn about infant cues and behaviors to facilitate attachment and decrease a sense of vulnerability | V | McGlothen-Bell and McGrath (2024) |
| | IV | Makris et al. (2019) |
| | IV | Moradi et al. (2018) |

*(continued)*

## TABLE 27.3

### EVIDENCE-BASED FAMILY-CENTERED CARE STRATEGIES TO SUPPORT INFANTS AND FAMILIES IN THE NICU (*continued*)

| Intervention | Level of Evidence | References |
|---|---|---|
| | I | Vittner et al. (2025) |
| | IV | Aita et al. (2021) |
| | II | Peyrovi et al. (2015) |
| Provide the family with opportunities to hold and touch their child early in the NICU stay | IV | Casio et al. (2018) |
| | III | Campbell-Yeo et al. (2017) |
| | I | Bansal et al. (2024) |
| Provide parents the choice to be present during procedures to support their child | V | McGlothen-Bell and McGrath (2024) |
| | V | Garfield et al. (2018) |
| | I | Treyvaud et al. (2019) |
| | IV | Kamphorst et al. (2018) |
| Facilitate parent presence and infant care through communication that is welcoming and supportive | I | Adama et al. (2022) |
| | I | Bansal et al (2024) |
| | III | Flacking et al. (2016) |
| | III | Provenzi et al. (2015) |
| | IV | Raiskila et al. (2017) |
| | IV | Vittner et al. (2018) |
| Provide parents opportunities to participate in care through scheduling of caregiving to increase their presence | V | McGlothen-Bell and McGrath (2024) |
| | I | Amin et al. (2018) |
| | VI | Gasparini et al. (2015) |
| | III | Kjellsdotter et al. (2018) |
| Provide support to fathers and encourage them to participate in care | IV | Kim (2018) |
| | VI | Merritt (2021) |

(*continued*)

**TABLE 27.3**

**EVIDENCE-BASED FAMILY-CENTERED CARE STRATEGIES TO SUPPORT INFANTS AND FAMILIES IN THE NICU (*continued*)**

| Intervention | Level of Evidence | References |
|---|---|---|
| Screen often and regularly for maternal depression and provide resources to support women (men) as needed | I | Bellizzi et al. (2024) |
| | VI | Beck (2020) |
| Provide care that is culturally sensitive | V | Al Maghaireh et al. (2016) |
| | II | Condon et al. (2022) |
| Introduce the family to support systems in the form of families with children who are undergoing or have undergone similar experiences | V | McGlothem-Bell and McGrath (2024) |
| | I | Al Maghaireh et al. (2016) |
| | II | Stefana and Lavelli (2017) |
| Provide the family with resources from the community (e.g., spiritual, economic, and social help, as well as information) | V | Al Maghaireh et al. (2016) |
| | V | Bos et al. (2018) |
| | IV | Hägi-Pedersen et al. (2017) |
| Assist the family in recognizing and using their strengths and coping skills or facilitating development of new coping strategies to decrease stress in the NICU; encourage the family to explore positive ways of coping with the situation | IV | Aagaard et al. (2018) |
| | IV | Amin et al. (2018) |
| | IV | Garfield et al. (2018) |
| | VI | Nordheim et al. (2018) |
| Facilitate positive perceptions of staff by families through staff communication styles | III | Feeley et al. (2016) |
| | III | Franck et al. (2020) |
| | VI | Dykes et al. (2016) |
| | IV | Foster et al. (2018) |
| | V | Giambra et al. (2017) |
| | IV | Miyagishima et al. (2017) |
| Provide education for families that meets their needs and is provided in a supportive style | IV | Bracht et al. (2013) |
| | IV | Aagaard et al. (2018) |

(*continued*)

## TABLE 27.3

### EVIDENCE-BASED FAMILY-CENTERED CARE STRATEGIES TO SUPPORT INFANTS AND FAMILIES IN THE NICU (*continued*)

| Intervention | Level of Evidence | References |
|---|---|---|
| | I | Altimier et al. (2023) |
| | V | Hill et al. (2018) |
| | IV | Neel et al. (2018) |

Rating System for the Hierarchy of Evidence

| | |
|---|---|
| Level I: | Evidence from a systematic review or meta-analysis of all relevant RCTs, or evidence-based clinical practice guidelines based on systematic reviews of RCTs |
| Level II: | Evidence obtained from at least one well-designed RCT |
| Level III: | Evidence obtained from well-designed controlled trials without randomization |
| Level IV: | Evidence from well-designed case-control and cohort studies |
| Level V: | Evidence from systematic reviews of descriptive and qualitative studies |
| Level VI: | Evidence from a single descriptive or qualitative study |
| Level VII: | Evidence from the opinion of authorities and/or reports of expert committees |

RCT, randomized controlled trial.

*Source:* Data from Melnyk, B., & Fineout-Overholt, E. (2023). *Evidence-based practice in nursing and healthcare* (5th ed.). Wolters-Kluwer.

## BOX 27.5

### GUIDELINES FOR PROVIDING INFORMATION TO FAMILIES OF ILL INFANTS

Focus the information session so as to build confidence and foster independence in the family. Build from strengths of the parents; do not focus on weaknesses.

1. Begin by assessing what the family members already know.
2. Establish a working rapport with the family; work to ease their anxiety and fear and to convey confidence and assurance to family members. Direct communication is essential.
3. Ask family members what they expect to learn from the session and provide information directed toward their concerns. Also ask about what strategies work best for their learning.
4. Initially, focus information on the diagnosis or current crisis.
5. Use language the family understands; avoid medical jargon.
6. Include the key characteristics of the plan of care and treatment.
7. Explain the ways in which the illness or medication regimen will affect daily life.
8. Use a variety of information strategies, materials, and styles. All information should first be provided orally and reinforced with handouts to be taken home.
9. Keep the information simple and concrete; reinforce oral communication with handouts. Expect to repeat the information and do so readily.
10. Avoid fear tactics while providing information on both benefits and detrimental effects.
11. Use praise to instill confidence.
12. Include anticipatory guidance.

*Sources:* Data from Baker, B. J., & McGrath, J. M. (2011). Maternal infant synchrony: An integrated review of the literature. *Neonatal, Paediatric, and Child Health Nursing, 14*(3), 2–13.

providing information can be helpful. Parents also appreciate the use of drawings and diagrams when their infant's condition is explained to them, and they appreciate being encouraged by healthcare team members to ask questions. Consider asking parents how best they learn and what questions they may have at the end of every session. Presenting this information with some optimism allows the family some hope, and, as discussed earlier, hope is an essential concept for coping with the NICU (Ingram et al., 2017; Nordheim, Rustøen et al., 2018). Ideally, the information should be presented to both parents simultaneously. It should be expressed in simple terms with short explanations. The parents are stressed, and this information may be unfamiliar (Bansal et al., 2024; Treyvaud et al., 2019). Facts may need to be repeated several times before they are absorbed. Parents need a clear understanding of the information provided to make informed decisions about their infant's care. Family-friendly language in understandable terms in common English should be used when delivering care and information (Kutahyalioglu et al., 2023). Medical information from a primary caregiver, such as a neonatal nurse practitioner or primary physician, provides consistency, especially when the news is difficult or may be considered bad (Box 27.6). Consistency in caregiving and information sharing is vital so that families are not confused by the different information they receive, adding to their distress and sense of distrust of healthcare providers (Carroll et al., 2018; Kutahyalioglu et al., 2023). Families also need information about unit policies, equipment, procedures, and treatments their infant receives. Direct telephone access allows an update from their nurse or physician at all times. In support of oral communication, written information helps parents remember essential facts. In addition, written communication also provides a place to refer to later when the information is more relevant to the care of the infant or when there are more questions (Bansal et al., 2024; Kutahyalioglu et al., 2023). Information can also be reinforced with digital, online materials or apps as appropriate. Providing multiple avenues for information sharing provides better support to families who may not always be ready to take in information when shared but have other ways to obtain the information later.

## Family Presence During Rounds

In many NICUs, inviting family members to participate in medical rounds is becoming common (Butler et al., 2024). Families are part of the decision-making process and, as such, are provided information so that they can, in collaboration with the medical/nursing team, decide when they would like to be present and make decisions for their child and when they feel they would rather not be involved (Bansal et al., 2024; Treyvaud et al., 2019). Through their presence in rounds, families are involved in assessing and planning for their child (Butler et al., 2024). Caregiving issues related to the scheduling of rounds, the teaching of medical staff, and confidentiality for families during rounds can be a concern for healthcare professionals, yet many hospitals have embodied family participation in medical rounds (Butler et al., 2024). These family-centered practices are now common and have found that the collaboration and partnership between the family and the healthcare team is worth the effort required to implement such decision-making relationships (Butler et al., 2024; Vittner et al., 2022). Providing for and facilitating the family's role as the constant in the infant's life is the best approach for the infant's long-term development. Critical pathways (see Supporting Families With Caregiving Protocols later in this chapter) can also be used as an excellent means of providing education and anticipatory guidance to parents and families, especially when the provision of information with skill building must be completed over an extended hospitalization or by several healthcare team members (Butler et al., 2024).

**BOX 27.6**

### PROVIDING DIFFICULT INFORMATION

Although difficult information is most often provided by physicians, nurses often are part of the team, especially if the information will be painful to the family. Nurses must know how to support families in these difficult situations. Unexpected news is sometimes considered bad news, yet healthcare professionals' approaches can change the perspective for the family receiving the news.

1. Whenever possible, difficult information should be delivered with both parents present and/or supportive family members as deemed by the family. Crafting the conversation as sharing unexpected news, rather than bad news, can shape what families hear and understand.
2. Remember that the language you use will be how the family shares the news with others, so choose your words carefully. Provide unbiased information that is clear, direct, detailed, and understandable; get to the focus of the discussion quickly.
3. Provide the information with compassion and care in a gentle but confident style; a private, quiet place free of distractions should be used for the discussion.
4. Personalize the information to this infant or child and this family. Use the child's name whenever possible. Begin the conversation by sharing with the family what is going well and congratulating them on their child's successes or strengths.
5. Allow the family time to express feelings and ask questions. Provide support for those feelings and questions. Offer hope about the next phase of the child's journey. Do not personalize families' responses.
6. Provide information about resources and anticipatory guidance. Speak with the family about what you expect will happen next.
7. Arrange an opportunity for the family to meet another family who has experienced a similar situation or crisis.
8. Follow up with the family after an appropriate time to answer any latent questions or provide further support.

*Source:* Adapted from Carroll, C., Carroll, C., Goloff, N., & Pitt, M. B. (2018). When bad news isn't necessarily bad: Recognizing provider bias when sharing unexpected news. *Pediatrics, 142*(1), e201–e204. https://doi.org/10.1542/peds.2018-0503

## Family Presence and Participation in Procedures

One of the fundamentals of FCC is the belief that from birth, the family is an active member of the caregiving team. Members of the caregiving team are not visitors. Parents should be integrated into medical rounds or procedures to be essential healthcare team members. Parents can be as involved during procedures as they feel comfortable; the degree of involvement will vary from parent to parent and family to family (Bansal et al., 2024). Parents need to have enough information to feel welcome and supportive of their infant during procedures to be present (Palomaa et al., 2016). Presence during resuscitation is another area where organizations support families in being present and supportive of their infant. However, this means that someone from the healthcare team needs to support the parents during the event (Treyvaud et al., 2019). Healthcare professionals may resist including families in these interventions because of the degree of risk to the infant (Vittner et al., 2022). Nurses must also consider that even though parent participation may be challenging with competing demands, active partnerships with families are in the best interest of the infant and family. Established protocols and education of both staff members and parents help with the transition to increase parental participation in the NICU (Vittner et al., 2022).

## Supporting Families With Caregiving Protocols

Critical pathways and caregiving protocols have been developed to aid in organizing and evaluating nursing assessments and interventions with infants and families. These pathways help promote continuity of care and assist the nurse in prioritizing the infant's and family's needs. They are outcome oriented and provide an excellent means of documenting nurses' actions. They can enhance interaction between parents and their critically ill infants. The pathway serves as a means to support parents with the changing needs of their developing infant. Implementing the pathway increases parents' knowledge and responsiveness to their infant's behavior and helps parents develop independent, cue-based care interactions (Vittner et al., 2025). Other pathways have been created with five areas of emphasis: (a) environmental organization; (b) infant care practices; (c) feeding (all of which relate more to the infant); (d) family involvement; and promotion of FCC (Vittner et al., 2025). Involving families in developing and testing these protocols is important (Celenza et al., 2017). Outcomes for infants include physiologic stability, behavioral organization, and establishing predictable behavioral patterns; outcomes for the family include enhancing social support, increasing knowledge, and increasing engagement of parents in the infant's care while preparing for discharge (McGlothen-Bell & McGrath, 2024). Critical pathways are also an excellent means of providing education and anticipatory guidance to parents and families, especially when teaching must be done over an extended hospitalization or by several staff members.

## Family Integrated Care

Recently, the concept of delivering supportive care to the infant and family in the NICU has been reconceptualized as the Family Integrated Care (FICare$^{TM}$) model in which parents provide all care for their infant, except the most advanced medical care, with support from the healthcare team (Franck et al., 2020). First introduced in Canada, the premise of this model is based on the fact that parents must be an integral part of the healthcare team. Parents participating in this program must be in the NICU at least 6 hours a day, 5 days each week, to care for their infant. Parent participation is facilitated by parent education programs that provide the content and facilitation for parents to provide complete care to their infants successfully. Educational tools and self-directed learning approaches increase parental confidence and decrease parental stress (Franck et al., 2020). The educational programs encompass materials that empower parents to recognize infant cues and behaviors through engagement in their unique role in their infant's life. Ongoing dialogues among the team are encouraged to accommodate a variety of learning styles and remain flexible to adapt materials to meet the diverse needs of families (Franck et al., 2020). A recent scoping review concluded that family-integrated care shows a positive effect on increasing breastfeeding rates at discharge (Ding et al., 2023). The outcomes of this research have been very positive, with more studies now in progress in Canada and the United States. One research limitation to date is the high refusal rate (> 50%) related to the degree of parent presence required if parents choose to participate. In addition, there are no true measures of the degree of parent engagement in the studies, and there is yet little support for whether this dose (6 hours a day for 5 days each week) is the correct dose to achieve the desired outcomes. While more research is needed to better understand how to implement FICare best, this model of care is propelling caregiving that increases the family's true partnership in caring for their infant in the NICU.

## Family Conferences

Family conferences can be used to evaluate the intervention strategies and how well they met the family's goals. Collaboration during conferences allows all present the opportunity to examine individual perspectives and goals while negotiating and reevaluating strategies to increase satisfaction with the treatment plan (Mooney et al., 2024; Urbina et al., 2024). The type of information communicated is also an important consideration. Healthcare professionals have often provided families with a lot of information about their infant in the here and now; what is sometimes missing is the "so what?" of that information (Mooney et al., 2024; Urbina et al., 2024). The result is that parents are not always provided with all the information they need to understand the whole situation for their child now and in the future so that appropriate participation in decision making can occur (McGlothen-Bell & McGrath, 2024).

## Facilitating Transfer to Another Facility

If the infant is transported from another facility or transferred to another hospital, parents need time to be with their infant before the move and should go on the transport whenever possible (Bansal et al., 2024). These brief interactions before

**BOX 27.7**

**PRINCIPLES OF FAMILY–PROFESSIONAL COLLABORATION**

Family–professional collaboration accomplishes the following:

- promotes a relationship in which family members and professionals work together to ensure the best services for the infant and family
- recognizes and respects the knowledge, skills, and experience that families and professionals bring to the relationship
- acknowledges that the development of trust is an integral part of a collaborative relationship
- facilitates open communication so that families and professionals feel free to express themselves
- creates an atmosphere in which the cultural traditions, values, and diversity of families are acknowledged and honored
- recognizes that negotiation is essential in a collaborative relationship
- brings to the relationship the mutual commitment of families, professionals, and communities to meet the requirements of children with special health needs and their families

*Source:* Adapted from Institute for Patient- and Family-Centered Care. (2017). *Advancing the practice of patient- and family-centered care in hospitals: How to get started*. Author. http://www.ipfcc.org/resources/getting_started.pdf.

**BOX 27.8**

**LANGUAGE THAT FACILITATES COLLABORATION**

"What would you prefer us to call you?"

"Here's what I'm thinking, but I'm wondering how this will work for you."

"Tell me how I can help you."

"Our institution usually does it this way. Would that work for you?"

"These are the things I plan to provide for your child today. Would you like to provide some of these activities?"

"What goals do you have for your child's care?"

"How does your child look to you today?"

"Do you have any questions or suggestions about your child's care?"

"This sounds important; help me to understand your concern."

"Who would you like to have included in discussions about your child's care?"

"Let's talk about how much you want to be consulted."

*Source:* Adapted Fox, S., Platt, F. W., White, M. K., & Hulac, P. (2005). Talking about the unthinkable: perinatal/neonatal communication issues and procedures. *Clinics in Perinatology, 32*(1), 157–viii. https://doi.org/10.1016/j.clp.2004.11.011.

transport reduce anxieties about the status of the neonate and promote bonding and attachment behaviors (Aagaard et al., 2018). Occasionally, the mother's condition is unstable, and she or a family member cannot be present in the NICU. Instant pictures can be taken and given to the mother as soon as possible or digitally through apps. Some NICUs also use video monitoring to connect families to their infant better.

The number of nursing or medical professionals who interact with the parents in nondescript surgical scrub outfits can be overwhelming. Therefore, introductions by name and position are essential to families, and personnel should wear name tags to help further identify each staff member. Many institutions have adopted a primary nursing style of care where the number of caregivers is limited to a small group of professionals to increase consistency of caregiving and information sharing. Families often feel more secure knowing that one nurse or team of nurses direct their infant's nursing care throughout the hospitalization, which establishes a trusting, collaborative relationship (Box 27.7). A friendly approach facilitates open communication and demonstrates openness and approachability.

Using language that invites participation is also important (Box 27.8). The primary nurse can act as liaison between the family and the healthcare team. The liaison ensures that information about the infant's current condition, any changes in condition, and long-term outcomes for the infant are communicated to the family. The liaison role becomes essential if the infant is transported back to a community hospital or to another unit in the same facility (Aagaard et al., 2018). Parents need to know what to expect in the new unit and understand how this new environment is now better suited to meet the changing needs of their infant. Otherwise, undue parental stress and perhaps mistrust may develop (Aagaard et al., 2018).

**Preparing for Discharge.** As nurses prepare the infant for discharge from the NICU, it is vital that the parents feel prepared to care for their infant (Bos et al., 2018; Smith et al., 2022). For lesbian, gay, bisexual, transgender, queer, or other sexual and gender minority identity (LGBTQ+) parents, this stress may be compounded by health disparities and fear of stigma and discrimination (Yinger et al., 2024). Sources of strength and resilience, and the provision of FCC can help diffuse these disparities and discrimination (Yinger et al., 2024). Building on the already established relationship, parents can be provided one last boost in confidence by allowing them to room-in with high-risk newborns before discharge (Toral-López et al., 2016). Structured education has also been found to increase parent confidence and caring knowledge prior to discharge, which could make the transition from hospital to home more manageable for families (Smith et al., 2022; Yinger et al., 2024). Parents feel secure knowing that nurses are close by if they are needed. This process also assures parents that they can care for their infants adequately.

Many times, neonatal intensive care hospitalization is the beginning of chronicity for the infant and the family (Bally et al., 2018). Parenting a chronically ill child is qualitatively different from parenting a normal child. Nurses must promote the parent's and family's role as caregivers for the child by determining the family's mode of coping and supporting those strategies while promoting family adaptation to the chronic illness and parent learning of self-management skills (Hägi-Pedersen et al., 2022). A major goal of care for these families is to integrate the child back into the family unit rather than to make the child with a chronic illness a "special nucleus" that becomes the only priority or focus of family needs (Nightingale et al., 2017).

FCC of an infant or child with any chronic illness is based on the premise that the family is the primary source of support and caregiving for the child. Thus, FCC can be achieved through specific nursing strategies to create opportunities for families to use their strengths and abilities to meet the infant's and family's needs (Adama et al., 2022; Bally et al., 2018). Ultimately, family-centered interventions empower families to develop and maintain healthy lifestyles, improving the family's quality of life.

### Providing Support for Parents and Families

Parent networking can be a vital tool for promoting parenting. Knowing that other families have survived this crisis can be reassuring. Support groups are generally helpful but only appropriate for some situations (Griffith et al., 2022). Some couples need counseling to feel more comfortable with decision making and participation in care. The primary nurse plays a key role in assessing signs that the family is not coping and needs therapeutic counseling. Support groups or counseling help families examine problems objectively and learn alternative behaviors for adaptive coping (Ardal et al., 2011; Hall et al., 2015). The nurse also can assist parents in identifying additional means of support. Ideally, parents should be permitted to define their "family" as needed to provide support during this crisis, allowing family members to be present as unit policy dictates. Grandparents, extended family, neighbors, and friends may constitute this group (Stefana & Lavelli, 2017).

Grandparents are a source of support for many parents. However, grandparents may be forced into an uncomfortable role by seeing their child in pain without a way to relieve that pain. Understanding intergenerational dynamics is important in providing the best support to families. Grandparents are also trying to cope with this new crisis. They may relive their own birthing experiences, which could result in associated anxieties and prevent them from being available to support the parents (Frisman et al., 2012). Extended family members may be more helpful if discord exists between grandparents and the nuclear family (Greisen et al., 2009). Friends of the family can be an asset if they are effective listeners. They can offer to provide transportation for the mother and child care for siblings, or they can take over housekeeping chores to help alleviate family responsibilities. Just having someone to make telephone calls to other friends and family to update them on the infant's condition can be a great relief for the family.

Social workers involved early in the hospital stay provide parents with an objective person to discuss caregiving options and provide contact with community resources. Families are often reluctant to express dissatisfaction with their child's care to nurses. Social workers can help parents express concerns without fear of retaliation against their child. Clergy provide spiritual support for a family. Families often turn to religion for comfort and support in times of crisis. It is important to offer these resources to parents and to provide the appropriate privacy to exercise their religious freedom. Recently, it has been recommended that we reconceptualize the neonatal intensive care environment to be the neonatal intensive parenting unit (NIPU) (Hall et al., 2017; Hynan et al., 2015). This reconceptualization places the parent with the infant at the center of caregiving. The evolution of caregiving, such that care providers are for the support of parents and infants, is one that needs increasing support because the family is the constant and the long-term care provider for the infant.

## PARENT AND STAFF EXPECTATIONS

When parents have a sick infant in the NICU, they have expectations. They expect excellent medical and nursing care for their child (Latour et al., 2010). They expect accurate and timely information throughout their child's illness and to be involved in decision making about the infant's care (McGlothen-Bell & McGrath, 2024). They expect that this developing relationship with the healthcare team will be a partnership and that the partnership will be honored in every interaction. The medical and nursing healthcare team members, who support each other and the family, can instill confidence in parents through this partnership (Vittner, Young, et al., 2022). Parents develop advocacy skills through collaborative communications with the nursing and medical team (McGlothen-Bell & McGrath, 2024). Conversely, members of the medical and nursing staff have expectations of the infants and families within this partnership related to the care of the infant. Expectations for the family may include regular presence and participation in caregiving, respecting the routines of the NICU setting, and sharing information that may be helpful in the care of the infant (McGlothen-Bell & McGrath, 2024). Sometimes, these expectations are unrealistic. The staff may expect parents to be present and more active in caregiving more often, even though the parents live far from the hospital, have other children, must return to work, and have other responsibilities that may prevent more frequent presence and participation in caregiving (Craig et al., 2015). Parents may also feel their role is diminished or not as important in the NICU if a collaborative partnership has not been established and the environment is not welcoming (Treyvaud et al., 2019). Healthcare professionals' expectations for the infant may include wanting the infant to nipple-feed more often or be weaned from oxygen faster. It can be distressing to parents to think that the medical staff is not pleased with their infant's progress, even though this attitude may not be verbalized. For this reason, incongruities should be avoided in actions and communications (McGlothen-Bell & McGrath, 2024). It seems reasonable to assume that parents who are partners, well informed, and participating in the care are less likely to experience these concerns (Hopwood et al., 2017).

Healthcare team members' attitudes are an essential part of the development of positive parenting (Box 27.9). Staff behaviors and attitudes can inhibit or encourage parenting skills. Conflict about parenting roles can exist between parents and healthcare team members, which may escalate into a struggle for control. Parents may view healthcare team members as acting as the infant's parents or the infant as belonging to the nurses because nurses provide most of the infant care (Vittner, Young, et al., 2022). The staff members' pet names for the infant further reinforce parents' apprehensions. Nursing staff can help the family by encouraging them to personalize the infant's care and following their lead with naming and dressing. Parents contribute to caretaking by bringing in clothes, toys, and pictures of other family members and making recordings of family voices.

Nurses who care for families need to provide support and promote the family as a unit; however, the overinvolvement of nurses can be detrimental to the family unit. Establishing appropriate relationships with families in our care can sometimes be challenging. It is necessary to identify inappropriate nursing behaviors and correct them. Educating nursing professionals about the parenting process facilitates the identification of inappropriate nursing behaviors (Box 27.10). The education can be initiated during the orientation of new healthcare team members and reinforced at intervals with continuing education workshops on the subject. Nurses must provide support while always acknowledging the boundaries of the family. Some families build walls and are so private about family matters that it is difficult to obtain enough information to meet family needs. In contrast, other families become overly dependent on the nursing staff, needing their support at every moment. Interventions that promote independent family decision making include the following (IPFCC, 2017):

- respecting the family as a unique unit
- providing unbiased care to all families
- providing as much continuity in the care provider as possible to promote family strengths
- allowing the family to determine the implementation of the plan of care

With adequate staffing, nurses can better promote parenting in the NICU. Overworked nurses can become frustrated and stressed, overwhelmed by competing demands that inhibit FCC implementation (Vittner, DeMeo, et al., 2022, Vittner, Young, et al., 2022). These feelings may impede their ability to interact calmly and therapeutically with a fragile family unit. Nursing management considerations should include the

**BOX 27.9**

### KEY CONTENT OF FAMILY-CENTERED TRAINING PROGRAMS FOR HEALTH PROFESSIONALS

- principles of family-centered care
- cultural competence
- child development
- family systems
- fostering communication with children and families
- building collaborative relationships with families
- support for and strengthening of families in their caregiving roles
- effect of hospitalization, illness, and injury on children and families, including the effect of healthcare costs on family resources
- support for the developmental and psychosocial needs of children and families through hospital policies and programs
- function and expertise of each discipline in the medical setting
- multidisciplinary collaboration and team building
- ethical issues and decision making
- community resources for children and families

*Source:* Adapted from Institute for Patient- and Family-Centered Care. (2017). *Advancing the practice of patient- and family-centered care in hospitals: How to get started.* Author. http://www.ipfcc.org/resources/getting_started.pdf.

**BOX 27.10**

### BEDSIDE CAREGIVER BEHAVIORS THAT MAY BECOME BARRIERS TO POSITIVE PARENTING

- Using language that states the infant "belongs" to the nurse and the NICU rather than to the family; for example, the nurse refers to her assignments or primaries as "my babies."
- Family is not considered a member of the caregiving team; for example, they are asked to leave for rounds and shift reports.
- Family is not asked about the characteristics of their infant or included in discussions related to the infant. Families are not seen as the experts on their infant. They are talked *about* rather than talked *with*. Families are either not actively included in medical rounds or their voice is considered secondary to those of health professionals.
- Care is task oriented and staffing is acuity based rather than based on meeting the needs of families. Families are not included as active participants in the child's care.
- Infant's schedule belongs to the nurse and the NICU rather than to the family, so that feeding and caregiving might occur when the family is unavailable to participate. Scheduling is inflexible and fixated on the clock rather than the infant's behavior (sleep and wakefulness).
- Family is seen as an adjunct to infant care. They are not the client or patient. Spending time with families is not considered a priority but rather a luxury. Spending time with families is not seen as essential to providing care for the infant.

*Source:* Data from Institute for Patient- and Family-Centered Care. (2017). *Advancing the practice of patient- and family-centered care in hospitals: How to get started.* Bethesda, MD

provision of adequate staffing to allow nurses the time and emotional energy to meet the needs of parents in crisis. Patient assignments should be evaluated not only for the technical care an infant requires but also for the psychosocial demands of the family. Institutional policies should be carefully assessed to determine how they meet the needs of families. Rationing or missed care must be regularly evaluated and considered to deliver optimal care to all infants and families (Tubbs-Cooley et al., 2017). FCC activities are the ones most likely to be listed as missed caregiving tasks. These could include family teaching, breastfeeding education, discharge planning, holding, and SSC.

## SIBLINGS

Siblings have needs because they are vital to the new infant's life. Sibling visits may help relieve anxieties and make the birth a reality. Siblings have a variety of responses to a newborn's arrival in the home, especially after a lengthy hospitalization. A typical birth disrupts family routines, which are further disturbed by admission to the NICU and then again at the time of discharge (Aita et al., 2021). Siblings may feel displaced while parents are at the NICU participating in the caregiving of the ill infant. Siblings are often left with babysitters when they rarely have experience with caretakers outside the immediate family. Fathers who may be uncertain about their family role may embrace their familiar work role and spend more time on the job. In these ways, routines are disrupted, and parents are less available for their other children (Merritt, 2021). There are comprehensive and clinical tools for nurses to use to enhance family participation in infant care. Parents may benefit from website resources, and storybooks for siblings may promote a family's adaptation to help parents support their older children during a NICU hospitalization (Aita et al., 2022).

The birth of a new infant precipitates a family upheaval and the need for a realignment of relationships and positions within the family constellation. Becoming a sibling is a stressful or "crisis" experience for young children and can affect their mental, emotional, and social development. The birth of a preterm or critically ill neonate who requires intensive care constitutes a further crisis for parents and consequently disrupts the equilibrium of the family system (Morrison & Gullon-Rivera, 2017; Stefana & Lavelli, 2017). Parents are reported to experience feelings of anxiety, grief, fear, anger, and guilt in response to the unanticipated events. Siblings are also affected and may experience helplessness, powerlessness, guilt, and anger in addition to the disruption of their daily routines and separation from their parents. The siblings may feel very alone because their worried parents are preoccupied with the newborn. Siblings feel like forgotten family members when they need attention most (Morrison & Gullon-Rivera, 2017).

Addressing the needs of the families of hospitalized infants has gained acceptance and support among nurses since the advent of the concept of FCC (IPFCC, 2017; Vittner, DeMeo, et al., 2022). All family members, parents, and siblings may exhaust their coping strategies and feel unsupported by those usually available emotionally and physically. The philosophy of FCC in the NICU is reported to encourage parent participation and the involvement of the well sibling or siblings in the family process. This involvement allows children to see their new sibling and feel like they are a part of the family process. Feelings of isolation may engender fantasies about what is taking place in the NICU. At any age, it is easier to cope with reality than with what can be imagined. Increasing numbers of hospitals encourage children's participation at a sibling's birth, in the postpartum unit, and in intensive care nurseries (Aita et al., 2021).

For nurses facing these challenges, the philosophy of FCC can provide a firm foundation in striving toward excellence in caring for children and families (IPFCC, 2018; Stefana & Lavelli, 2017). Developing a sibling–infant bond is vital to establishing and enhancing the relationship within the family unit. Holistic care surrounding childbirth may set up patterns or pathways that dramatically affect subsequent family interactions.

Some families feel that they cannot be part of the care team. They either do not desire to provide care or cannot do so. Sometimes, there is a tendency to label them as noncompliant with what the healthcare professional believes the family should do or how they should act. Before a label is used, it is important to learn from the parents because they may want to refrain from participating. Is it because they fear they will hurt the infant? Is it because they want to be parents and not be responsible for the care? Is it a lack of understanding of what is being asked of them? Based on their response, an individualized plan of care can be developed. For example, for parents fearful about providing care, the healthcare team can provide education and psychological support and be present to support caregiving activities. The key to success is to talk to the family, listen to their concerns/perspectives, and then tailor a plan to increase their participation as a care team member.

### Sibling Participation in the Neonatal Intensive Care Unit

Sibling participation in the hospital after delivering a newborn has become common. However, limited recent research examines the consequences of permitting and prohibiting sibling visits in the NICU despite the argument that sibling involvement is consistent with the concept of family-centered perinatal care. Early studies of NICU sibling visitation programs provided valuable descriptive data on siblings' responses to the sick neonate (Aita et al., 2021). Sibling participation allows the older brother or sister to see, touch, and talk to the newborn. This exposure was reported to help the children integrate the reality of the experience, to prepare for the possible loss of the newborn, and, in some cases, to reverse regressive behavior that had begun during the newborn's hospitalization. However, the findings of these studies reflected the perceptions of professionals and not necessarily those of the parents or siblings (Vittner, DeMeo, et al., 2022). More research is needed in this area. Some NICUs restrict sibling participation during respiratory syncytial virus (RSV) season. In contrast, some do not have a strict policy for how visiting might still occur during this time of the year. The same is true for varicella exposures and how to safeguard infants. The COVID-19 pandemic provides many opportunities for improvement because FCC practices were halted (Litmanovitz et al., 2021). Although restrictions on family presence go against psychological and neuroscientific evidence in support of unrestricted parental presence for hospitalized infants, many families were prohibited from being with their hospitalized infants during the pandemic (Litmanovitz et al., 2021). Family presence and active participation in infant care throughout the hospitalization are associated with better medical and developmental outcomes (Lv et al., 2019).

## Implications for Practice

Nurses have a unique opportunity to support the development of positive sibling relationships in the NICU environment. Evolving models of comprehensive care no longer overlook or delegate the care and needs of the whole family. Research on the families of NICU neonates has demonstrated parents' desire for a family-centered approach to care (Miyagishima et al., 2017). Siblings are an integral part of any family; their adjustment or lack of adjustment to the birth of a newborn greatly affects the whole family's well-being. Siblings' adjustment to the once-sick infant needs further exploration.

When the birth of a sibling is further complicated by the infant's being ill or at risk, professionals caring for the infant are in a position to reassure parents that siblings will respond in various ways based on each child's personality, age, and interests. The parent's ability to accept their older children's competitive feelings and continue to love them helps them integrate ambivalence. Support through this ambivalence facilitates acceptance of the infant and the infant's incorporation into the family. Increasing parents' knowledge about promoting positive sibling relationships through parent education programs may influence parental attitudes, enhancing future sibling relationships. Many hospitals have implemented sibling visitation and educational programs in response to consumer demand. This preparation can help siblings deal with the realities of the experience. Special attention from the NICU staff can also help siblings feel recognized, supported, and appreciated during this time of stress. Encouraging the sibling to gently touch and talk to the infant and allowing gifts of toys or even a drawing of themselves to be kept with the infant may foster attachment and a growing connection with the newborn.

The death of a sibling usually has profound and lasting effects on surviving children. Surviving siblings, however young, may need some evidence that the infant existed—a visit to see the ill newborn in the incubator, a photograph, or a chance to participate in the funeral. Regardless of the child's age, it seems that the level of care offered to these siblings is crucial to determining the psychological and life adjustment of the bereaved child. Nurses need to be alert to the range and depth of childhood reactions. Many research findings discussed here can serve as invaluable guides to help NICU nurses promote and facilitate effective sibling interactions and positive involvement between the sick neonate and the siblings. An appropriate environment in which nurses can assist children in coping with the profound changes that affect the sibling bond should also be provided. Such efforts help siblings fully integrate this significant event into their young lives.

## Environmental Effects

A calm, welcoming atmosphere with low lighting helps calm both infants and their families. External stimuli in the NICU must be controlled; unnecessary stimuli aggravate these infants' already overwhelmed immature nervous systems, and loud monitor alarms and excessive staff noise can be upsetting and unnerving to parents (D'Agata & McGrath, 2016; Vittner et al., 2025). Sometimes, the equipment and technology overwhelm families and can be challenging to navigate. A family's discomfort inhibits interactions with the infant and delays their participation in infant care practices. Researchers suggest changes in the NICU's technology, such as using different kinds of alarm signals with diminished volume, wireless, handheld information terminals, and remote monitoring. Some of this technology is already appearing in the NICU. The technology used in the NICU must be continually reevaluated and designed with a parent- and consumer-based perspective (D'Agata & McGrath, 2016). Achieving a balance between the high-technology environment and the need for parents to touch their infant frequently helps foster parental self-confidence. This balance must be a priority for the neonatal nurse.

Recommendations for single rooms in the NICU and other acute care areas throughout the hospital setting are now included in the Guidelines for the Design and Construction of Hospital and Healthcare Facilities (Altimier et al., 2023). These guidelines are based on several significant research studies where single rooms throughout the healthcare setting were found to offer higher occupancy rates, reduced transfer costs, and lower labor costs, even when the cost of new construction was calculated into the equation (Altimier et al., 2023; Browne 2023).

In addition, hospital-acquired infection and medication errors were reduced in these settings. Most patients and families also report better communication with healthcare professionals in single rooms because the provider often spends more time, answers questions more thoroughly, and is more compassionate and caring. Patient length of stay has been documented as shorter in private single rooms, which also adds to the decrease in costs (Brown, 2023).

So, how do these guidelines affect the NICU? Most units across the United States have always been equipped with a few isolation rooms that have been used for infants with highly infectious diseases and, more recently, to isolate extremely low birth weight preterm infants who appear to be most overstimulated by the big open room environment of the NICU. With new construction and a greater emphasis on individualized family-centered developmentally supportive care, more units have added these single rooms, and some units have chosen to move to an entirely single-room design (Altimier et al., 2023; Brown et al., 2020).

Research to support a less stressful NICU environment with lower lights and less noise and activity has demonstrated shorter lengths of stay, decreased iatrogenic effects, and increased deep sleep and alerting behaviors in the infant, which may provide greater opportunities for more normal cognitive development. Moreover, in changing the environment to meet the needs of infants and families, the less stressful environment is oftentimes more positive for healthcare professionals and families and should have a positive effect on patient outcomes and a decrease in medication errors (Browne, 2023). The challenge in providing care in these designs is finding a balance between the needs of infants, families, and healthcare professionals in the NICU. Couplet care of the mother and NICU infant in the same room is a new, rapidly evolving option for caring for NICU infants (White, 2024). Evidence-based design standards for the NICU do exist and should be considered with any remodeling or new construction project (Altimier et al., 2023; Browne, 2023; White, 2024). These guidelines should be used as a standard, especially when data are needed to support the need to invest upfront in more space, better traffic patterns, multiple kinds of lighting, and noise reduction materials. Paying attention to design is especially important for vulnerable infants who are at risk of developing disabilities. Research data also exist and should be used to support the need to choose colors and textures that increase health and well-being for all who interface in healthcare settings. For staff to transition to and work with ease in single-room designs, they must have access to and become comfortable with central monitoring and communication systems that provide them with knowledge about patient status even from remote locations. Work areas for nurses must also be near the private rooms and allow for interaction and teamwork among staff. More research is needed in this area and should be a focus for the future.

## SUMMARY

The birth of any infant produces tremendous change in the lives of each member of the family. Normal adaptation can be complicated by the birth of a premature, critically ill infant, or one with congenital anomalies requiring admission to the NICU. If the family does not have adequate coping strategies or resources, this crisis has the potential to produce much role stress and strain that ultimately can weaken or destroy the family unit. The nurse plays an integral role in supporting and guiding the family to appropriate resources and services. By promoting adaptive roles, the nurse can ensure an intact family unit after the crisis of intensive care.

### EVIDENCE-BASED PRACTICE

John Jones was born at 33 weeks' gestation. The nurses described him as a typical preemie with respiratory distress syndrome and intermittent apnea and bradycardia. He required continuous positive airway pressure (CPAP) for several days and then hood oxygen for a week. After being weaned to room air, he was moved to the transitional nursery, where he stayed for another week until he matured to suck, swallow, and breathe safely. John's mother was present often and actively participated in his daily care. Mrs. Jones kept John supplied with breastmilk and the latest drawings from his two sisters, Suzie, age 6, and Becky, age 4. John's father was present in the NICU irregularly. He tried to make the time to be present on his way home from work but did not take an active role in John's daily care practices. He said that he was afraid to hold John but that he would as soon as John got bigger and stronger. John was a cuddly little guy who had an uneventful recovery and was discharged after 3 weeks in the NICU.

Several days before discharge, John's mother confided in his primary nurse that she was at the end of her rope because her husband was working longer hours and her daughters were acting up in ways they never had before. Becky had demonstrated regression behaviors of bed-wetting and thumb-sucking. She had also started carrying around her blanket again, something she had stopped doing long ago. Becky was particularly close to her mother, and after her mother's daily trips to the NICU, Becky would hit her mother, crying, "I hate you! I wish the baby would go away!" Mrs. Jones said that when she tried to console Becky, the child ran and hid under her bed, crying, "Leave me alone! You only love that baby!" If that were not bad enough, Suzie had begun waking up with stomachaches and refusing to go to school. Suzie had always loved her teacher and classmates and now was frequently in trouble for misbehaving in class. When Mrs. Jones would make Suzie go to school, the little girl would cry and say, "I hate that baby! I'd like to run over him with Daddy's car!" Mr. Jones had withdrawn from family life and was spending long hours at work. Mrs. Jones was beside herself.

The nurse reassured Mrs. Jones that the behaviors of her husband and daughters were typical. Although this reassurance did not immediately alter the situation, at least Mrs. Jones knew that many families respond to NICU hospitalization in this way and that, given time, the family would reestablish equilibrium. She spent a couple of special days with her daughters and engaged her husband in life outside the worries of the NICU.

However, this did not provide Mrs. Jones with emotional support or help with her feelings of being overwhelmed and depressed. The nurse listened to her concerns and then put her in touch with a parent organization that had been formed to help support families through the transition home. The parent organization offered peer support from parents who had been through the experience.

The girls had enjoyed their weekend with their mother and were in a better frame of mind for the homecoming. Peer support helped Mrs. Jones so that she could in turn be available to her family. John was about ready for discharge and had progressed well. Once John was home, Mrs. Jones included the girls in the infant's routine as much as possible by asking them to get his diapers and having them feed their dollies while she fed John. Suzie brought pictures of John to school for show and tell, and after Mrs. Jones called to speak to the teacher to explain the disruptions at home, Suzie gradually quit misbehaving. Becky continued with thumb-sucking and bed-wetting for several months while incorporating John into the family and establishing a new family routine.

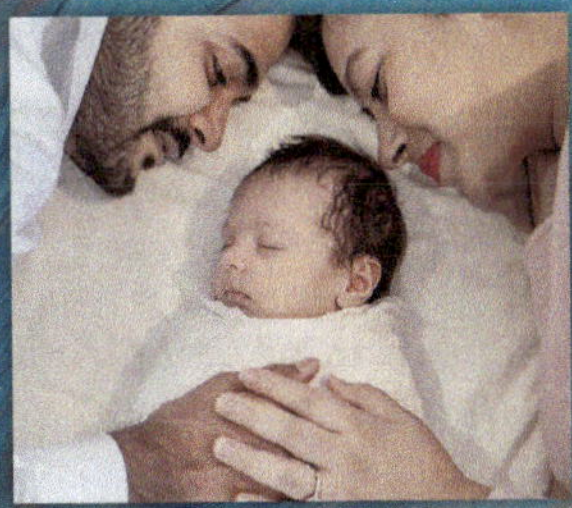
*Source:* paulaphoto/Adobe Stock.

## PARENT VOICES

### Ali Dunn

Allowing someone you have just met to care for your tiny, sick baby is one of the hardest things a parent can do. Having to rely on the nurses to tell me how my babies were doing, to show me how to care for them, and to give me permission to hold them was heartbreaking, as I had waited so long to be a mother. But over the days and months that my babies stayed in the NICU, the good nurses helped me realize that the nights spent apart or the feeds you missed did not diminish your mothering heart. The good nurses empowered me to change tiny diapers without assistance, so for brief moments I could feel like a normal parent. The good nurses waited for me to do the next feed, even if it meant putting themselves behind schedule, so I could momentarily forget about the wires and tubes, the monitors and machines, and just enjoy a nurturing moment with my child. The good nurses know that even though parents do not always say it, we are forever grateful to them for loving our children when we were not there, and for caring for our babies when we could not.

### Jennifer M. Driscoll

Both of my children were both prematurely, Lilian Hope in 2007 and Aidan Patrick in 2013. Lily spent just under a month in the NICU, and Aidan only a few days. Being discharged from the hospital with Lily was probably one of the most nerve-racking days of my life. Fortunately, when Aidan came home, I had that "mom" confidence, and having been in the NICU before, I knew what to expect.

I personally need a lot of information and dialog when it comes to caring for my children. I learned that I need to visualize what this new "normal" would look like and have a clear understanding before taking on this big change. I remember asking tons of questions, taking advantage of infant CPR classes, apnea monitor classes, reading all the literature from the hospital, and even staying over in the hospital NICU with Lily the night before she was discharged for practice. I'm a rule-follower by nature, so when coming home with Lily, I tried to instill the rules and guidelines that the NICU staff suggested. These were things like limiting the number of visitors, having hand sanitizer at every sink, no touching the baby until they washed their hands and used hand sanitizer, not taking the baby out in public if you can avoid it, and more. And I listened, which was great and tough. I felt lonely and nervous because I was a new mom caring for this 3-lb, 11-oz baby that had just entered our lives so abruptly.

Home became a learning experience. Where do I buy preemie clothing, diapers, and this special formula? I don't think I was ever even in a Babies R Us but to register for my shower, Amazon Prime wasn't even a thing in 2007. We went day by day, spending time doting on her, learning about her, and trying to comfort and nurture her as best we could. Home brought new challenges like severe reflux, visiting nurses waking her up from nap times, severe lack of sleep, a husband that worked a swing shift and caring for this little infant alone, a dog that barked every time she cried, and much more. We learned to roll with the punches, stay flexible, but yet always be in tune with what the baby was "telling" us.

### Katie Reginato Cascamo, MA

Neonatal staff who truly transform families begin with their own wellness first. The metaphor of putting on one's own breathing mask before caring for others is more critical than ever before in healthcare. As healthcare providers become more whole and fill their own emotional bucket, they effortlessly pour that out to families in crisis. As clinicians grow as healthcare leaders, they build the container skills for families who will need to take a leadership role in their family. Even the most difficult families respond well to healthcare providers who have invested in their wellness and leadership development. As you engage in your work holistically, you are equipping parents to take the initiative to transform their lives. So, take that hike. Do yoga. Develop a spiritual practice. Participate in wellness programs. Create meaningful connections with your coworkers. Care first for yourself so we can depend on you to care for us.

Our NICU was organizationally healthy and committed to transforming our lives. Our NICU served a large geographic area of nine counties and we lived 100 miles away over a snowy pass in the middle of winter. We did not trust our local, rural hospital primarily due to the lack of interpersonal development of the staff. The day after our NICU discharge and our return home, our son desaturated to 82% $O_2$ that I believed had to do with a 3,000-foot elevation change. I took him to our local dysfunctional emergency room simply because

(*continued*)

## PARENT VOICES (*continued*)

I had no other choice and we spent three more days in the hospital that redefined my mission to transform dysfunctional healthcare. The local healthcare staff refused to believe that the elevation change played any role in his desaturation and drastically changed how we perceived the community we called home. One year later we moved to a healthy, thriving community with world-class healthcare solely based on our experience in a healthy, engaged healthcare system and its counterpart, a toxic, dysfunctional healthcare system. Through our relocation to a community with high-quality healthcare came a world-class education system, commitment to the integration of children with special needs into society, and my ability to retrain for a job in healthcare practice administration.

All parents that come into the NICU have a story. Be willing to listen to our story and discover our strengths. Most of us have professional experience and are equipped to care for our babies. We are often fearful of touching our babies and experiencing trauma and it is the very act of learning how to care for our babies that heals us. The best amenities for families are parent-led resources. The world's best, most empathetic resources are those resources written for parents and by parents who have experienced a NICU stay. Our resources are very high quality, have the oversight of neonatal professionals, and are trusted by healthcare systems.

Integrating families into the care processes of the NICU is a win-win for everyone involved. For nursing staff, investing in our skill development is one more item to check off the healthcare checklist. As we learn to do nonessential tasks such as diapering, feeding, and dressing, we help you manage your workload better. We want to care for our baby and need guided instruction so we can take over nonessential tasks. Most importantly, when we leave the NICU, the skills you are teaching us are skills we will need when we return home. As we learn these skills, we become leaders in our families and we make sure that we engage in ongoing developmental therapies for our children through early intervention. As we broadly became the primary caretakers from birth throughout childhood, we are ensuring successful developmental outcomes of our preemies.

## ONLINE RESOURCES

**CourseConnect**

Resources for this chapter are online and available at www.springerpub.com/courseconnect.

## REFERENCES

References for this chapter are online and available at www.springerpub.com/courseconnect.

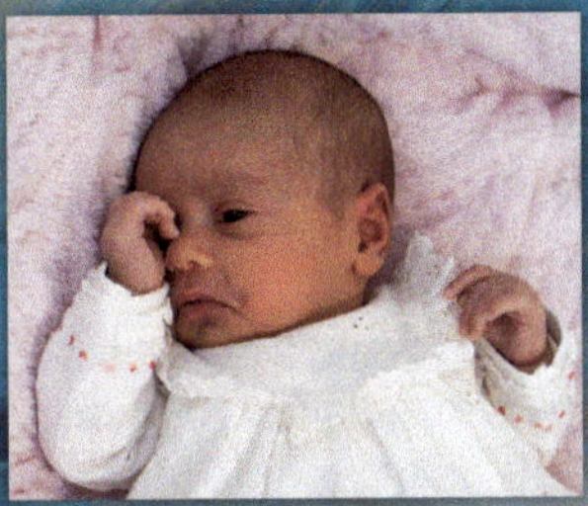


CHAPTER 28

# Postdischarge Care of the Newborn, Infant, and Families

Marina V. Boykova, Carole A. Kenner, and Deborah A. Discenza

## INTRODUCTION

The multiple problems that bring an infant to a neonatal intensive care unit (NICU) have been described, in depth, throughout the preceding chapters. Upon hospital discharge, high-risk infants require no less care than in the hospital because the healthcare needs of the initially sick infant often remain numerous and complex. Postdischarge and follow-up care focuses on the convalescing infant's growth, development, health promotion, disease prevention, chronic disease management, and care coordination. Importantly, parents also need care after their infant's hospital discharge. The transition from hospital to home for infants and their families is a very important and crucial period. This transition starts when the family begins to accept the role of the full-time caregiver outside the safety net of the hospital. The focus of this chapter is on the infant and parental care after hospital discharge.

## POSTDISCHARGE CARE FOR HIGH-RISK INFANTS

The American Academy of Pediatrics (AAP) and the American College of Obstetricians and Gynecologists (ACOG) recommend that healthcare professionals give special considerations to the following four groups of high-risk newborn infants before discharge: (a) preterm infant, (b) infant with special healthcare needs or dependence on technology, (c) infant at risk because of family issues, and (d) infant with anticipated early death (AAP & ACOG, 2017). Discharge criteria as well as the postdischarge care both depend on the different needs of these patient categories. For high-risk infants to be discharged, they must be physiologically stable; the decision to discharge is based on the clinical judgment of health professionals and determination of the infant's medical status.

The first category, preterm infants, can be discharged when oral feedings are sufficient to support appropriate and stable growth. Also, they must maintain normal body temperature in a homelike environment without supplemental heat and their respiratory control is mature and sufficient (e.g., no apnea) (AAP Committee on Fetus and Newborn, 2008). Most preterm infants achieve major physiologic milestones by 36 to 37 weeks' postmenstrual age (AAP & ACOG, 2017); however, feeding and adequate respiratory control are often achieved last and small for gestational age (SGA) infants also achieve the milestones later than term infants (Bakewell-Sachs et al., 2009; Hoffman et al., 2024). Apneic episodes are common in preterm infants before discharge; feedings and weight gain are also challenging issues (Cardin et al., 2023; Walton et al., 2022). Up to 7 days without apnea and with a stable pattern in feeding/gaining weight before discharge from a NICU is recommended; the readiness in these physiologic functions will depend on the gestational age.

For NICU infants before discharge, weight gain of 15 to 40 g/d must continue over a reasonable time (several days to 1 week); milk fortification, iron, vitamins, foliate, and vitamin D supplementation are often necessary after discharge to monitor the infants' growth by measuring weight, length, and head circumference (Bala et al., 2024; De Rose et al., 2024; Talebiyan & Belfort, 2023). Weight gain should occur in an open environment (dressed, in a crib, no supplemental heat) and should continue during the first 3 to 4 months of life and then decline to 5 to 15 g/d by the age of 12 to 18 months. For larger and healthier infants, 108 kcal/kg/d can be sufficient for adequate growth. For preterm infants, 110 to 130 kcal/kg/d can be required with increased protein and fat intake—approximately 4 g/kg of protein and 3.5 g/kg of fat daily (Kumar et al., 2017). In the postdischarge period, there is also a need to avoid excessive weight gain, which may result in health problems such as obesity, hypertension, and cardiovascular disease later in life (Gnawali, 2021). Nutritional requirements will vary depending on the infant's past medical problems, status, and tolerance of feedings; thus, individualized postdischarge feeding instructions are necessary. Available and widely used growth charts are not always valid for preterm infants or infants with continuing health problems, but some recent research-based information is available for infants of different gestational ages (Fenton et al., 2024; Viswanathan et al., 2022).

Length, head circumference, and weight should always be considered together, and nutritional assessment of the infant is more than just body measurements and may even require indirect calorimetry. The increase in the frontal-to-occipital head circumference in preterm infants should be 0.7 to 1 cm/wk (in term infants 0.5 cm/wk) in the immediate postnatal period; by 12 to 18 months of age, it should decline to 0.1 to 0.4 cm/mo. Increase in crown-to-heel length should be approximately 0.8 to 1.1 cm/wk in preterm infants (0.7–0.75 in term infants) in the immediate postnatal period; by 12 to 18 months of age, it should decline to 0.75 to 1.5 cm/mo. Consultation with a pediatric dietitian or an infant nutrition specialist should be obtained if there are concerns about growth failure and catch-up because the adherence to the nutrition guidelines can be low and feeding problems in the preterm infants can persist over a long period of time (Kamity et al., 2021). Additional information on specific formulas, nutrition aspects, and standardized growth charts are presented in Chapter 20, "Nutrition Management of Premature Infants".

In the second category, the infant with special healthcare needs or dependence on technology will have differing needs than the average NICU graduate. Depending on the exact health condition (e.g., chronic lung disease [CLD], genetic condition, congenital heart disease [CHD], and postsurgical and late preterm infants), the infant may require more calories due to the "work of breathing" such as in a case with CLD or CHD. With CLD (e.g., bronchopulmonary dysplasia [BPD]), the infant may require 120 to 150 kcal/kg/d plus increased protein intake (4.0–4.5 g/kg/d in infants having a birth weight of < 1,000 g and at 3.5 to 4.0 g/kg/d in neonates with a birth weight of 1,000–1,800 g), fluid restriction (no more than 150 ml/kg/d), electrolyte management, and control of vital functions (Karatza et al., 2022). While solid research evidence regarding nutrition in the CLD patients is still lacking (Bauer et al., 2022), it is recommended that the total lipid intake should be 4.8 to 6.6 g/kg/d with 12 to 30 mg/kg/d of arachidonic acid and 18 to 42 mg/kg/d of docosahexaenoic acid in these patients (Karatza et al., 2022). An infant with CLD will often require home oxygen therapy, so the appropriate parental teaching on the use of oxygen and monitoring health of the infant should be done before discharge. A pediatric pulmonologist should also be involved in postdischarge management of CLD/BPD patients; periodic evaluation of electrolyte status should be performed due to the use of diuretics in such infants. An infant with cardiac health issues will also often require fluid restriction and may need increased caloric intake as well. A pediatric cardiologist should be involved in postdischarge management of such infants; periodic evaluation of electrolyte status also should be performed due to the use of diuretics in these patients as well.

The third category of infants who should receive special attention after discharge are infants who are at health risk because of family issues. The infant may or may not be premature, or having specific health needs, and the family may have problems in adjusting to having a once-sick infant at home who now is ready for discharge (discussed later in this chapter). For infants in the fourth category—infants with anticipated early death—the aspects of the care are described in Chapter 29, "Palliative and End-of-Life Care."

## Follow-Up of High-Risk Infants

Adequate and effective postdischarge care should be provided to any NICU graduate. The attention to taking a preterm infant home was set forth almost 100 years ago (Lundeen, 1937). The follow-up appointments with primary care providers for high-risk infants should occur in accordance with the needs of the patient (AAP & ACOG, 2017). For preterm infants (including late preterm) and healthy term infants with early discharge from the maternity unit (< 48 hours after delivery), AAP and ACOG (2017) recommend that the first appointment with the primary healthcare provider should occur in the first 24 to 48 hours after discharge. In the immediate period after discharge, some of the high-risk infants should be examined by the primary healthcare provider weekly or semimonthly (AAP & ACOG, 2017). In NICU graduates, the neurodevelopmental, behavioral, and sensory status should be assessed more than once during the first year "to ensure early identification of problems and referral for the appropriate interventions" (AAP & ACOG, 2017, p. 471). Infants born with birth weight < 1,500 g, as well as infants with hypoxic–ischemic encephalopathy (HIE), seizures, hypoxic cardiorespiratory failure, and multiple congenital anomalies should have standard neurodevelopmental tests at 1 and 2 years of corrected age (CA) (AAP & ACOG, 2017). It has been shown that infants who underwent major and minor surgeries (e.g., repairs for diaphragmatic hernia, major heart defects, pyloric stenosis, inguinal hernia) may have some degree of developmental delays (Berken et al., 2024; Culbreath et al., 2024; Kikuchi et al., 2024; Serrano et al., 2024). Purdy and Melwak (2012) have also suggested the following "red flags" when a very thorough high-risk infant follow-up care is required:

- low Apgar score at 5 minutes (< 4)
- intraventricular hemorrhage more than Grade II, hydrocephalus
- HIE, abnormal neurologic examination (tremors, hypotonia/hypertonia), seizures
- hyperbilirubinemia close to exchange transfusion levels
- severe infections (sepsis, meningitis)
- hypoglycemia requiring treatment
- persistent pulmonary hypertension, extracorporeal membrane oxygenation, and use of inhaled nitric oxide
- discharge on apnea monitor and caffeine
- infant of substance-abusing mother
- congenital birth defects (such as trisomy 21 or Down syndrome) (Purdy & Melwak, 2012)

Frequency of follow-up visits for the *well infant* varies with the state, local and community practices; however, it should be consistent with AAP's guidelines (AAP & ACOG, 2017) on preventive pediatric healthcare (Figure 28.1). *The Bright Futures* online resource provides guidance, tools, and schedules for promoting health in the neonatal and pediatric populations (see https://brightfutures.aap.org/Pages/default.aspx). The follow-up visit can take place at home or clinic;

American Academy of Pediatrics
DEDICATED TO THE HEALTH OF ALL CHILDREN®

## Recommendations for Preventive Pediatric Health Care

Bright Futures/American Academy of Pediatrics

Bright Futures. prevention and health promotion for infants, children, adolescents, and their families™

Each child and family is unique; therefore, these Recommendations for Preventive Pediatric Health Care are designed for the care of children who are receiving nurturing parenting, have no manifestations of any important health problems, and are growing and developing in a satisfactory fashion. Developmental, psychosocial, and chronic disease issues for children and adolescents may require more frequent counseling and treatment visits separate from preventive care visits. Additional visits also may become necessary if circumstances suggest concerns.

These recommendations represent a consensus by the American Academy of Pediatrics (AAP) and Bright Futures. The AAP continues to emphasize the great importance of continuity of care in comprehensive health supervision and the need to avoid fragmentation of care.

Refer to the specific guidance by age as listed in the *Bright Futures Guidelines* (Hagan JF, Shaw JS, Duncan PM, eds. *Bright Futures: Guidelines for Health Supervision of Infants, Children, and Adolescents.* 4th ed. American Academy of Pediatrics; 2017).

The recommendations in this statement do not indicate an exclusive course of treatment or serve as a standard of medical care. Variations, taking into account individual circumstances, may be appropriate.

The Bright Futures/American Academy of Pediatrics Recommendations for Preventive Pediatric Health Care are updated annually.



| | INFANCY | | | | | | | | EARLY CHILDHOOD | | | | | | |
|---|---|---|---|---|---|---|---|---|---|---|---|---|---|---|---|
| **AGE[1]** | **Prenatal[2]** | **Newborn[3]** | **3-5 d[4]** | **By 1 mo** | **2 mo** | **4 mo** | **6 mo** | **9 mo** | **12 mo** | **15 mo** | **18 mo** | **24 mo** | **30 mo** | **3 y** | **4 y** |
| **HISTORY** Initial/Interval | ● | ● | ● | ● | ● | ● | ● | ● | ● | ● | ● | ● | ● | ● | ● |
| **MEASUREMENTS** | | | | | | | | | | | | | | | |
| Length/Height and Weight | | ● | ● | ● | ● | ● | ● | ● | ● | ● | ● | ● | ● | ● | ● |
| Head Circumference | | ● | ● | ● | ● | ● | ● | ● | ● | ● | ● | ● | | | |
| Weight for Length | | ● | ● | ● | ● | ● | ● | ● | ● | ● | ● | | | | |
| Body Mass Index[5] | | | | | | | | | | | | ● | ● | ● | ● |
| Blood Pressure[6] | | ★ | ★ | ★ | ★ | ★ | ★ | ★ | ★ | ★ | ★ | ★ | ★ | ● | ● |
| **SENSORY SCREENING** | | | | | | | | | | | | | | | |
| Vision[7] | | ★ | ★ | ★ | ★ | ★ | ★ | ★ | ★ | ★ | ★ | ★ | ★ | ● | ● |
| Hearing | | ●[8] | ●[9] ⟶ | ⟶ | ⟶ | ★ | ★ | ★ | ★ | ★ | ★ | ★ | ★ | ★ | ● |
| **DEVELOPMENTAL/SOCIAL/BEHAVIORAL/MENTAL HEALTH** | | | | | | | | | | | | | | | |
| Maternal Depression Screening[11] | | | | ● | ● | ● | ● | | | | | | | | |
| Developmental Screening[12] | | | | | | | | ● | | | ● | | ● | | |
| Autism Spectrum Disorder Screening[13] | | | | | | | | | | | ● | ● | | | |
| Developmental Surveillance | | ● | ● | ● | ● | ● | ● | | ● | ● | | ● | | ● | ● |
| Behavioral/Social/Emotional Screening[14] | | ● | ● | ● | ● | ● | ● | ● | ● | ● | ● | ● | ● | ● | ● |
| Tobacco, Alcohol, or Drug Use Assessment[15] | | | | | | | | | | | | | | | |
| Depression and Suicide Risk Screening[16] | | | | | | | | | | | | | | | |
| **PHYSICAL EXAMINATION[17]** | | ● | ● | ● | ● | ● | ● | ● | ● | ● | ● | ● | ● | ● | ● |
| **PROCEDURES[18]** | | | | | | | | | | | | | | | |
| Newborn Blood | | ●[19] | ●[20] ⟶ | ⟶ | ⟶ | | | | | | | | | | |
| Newborn Bilirubin[21] | | ● | | | | | | | | | | | | | |
| Critical Congenital Heart Defect[22] | | ● | | | | | | | | | | | | | |
| Immunization[23] | | ● | ● | ● | ● | ● | ● | ● | ● | ● | ● | ● | ● | ● | ● |
| Anemia[24] | | | | | | ★ | | | ● | ★ | ★ | ★ | ★ | ★ | ★ |
| Lead[25] | | | | | | | ★ | ★ | ● or ★[26] | | ★ | ● or ★[26] | | ★ | ★ |
| Tuberculosis[27] | | | | ★ | | | ★ | | ★ | | | ★ | | ★ | ★ |
| Dyslipidemia[28] | | | | | | | | | | | | ★ | | | ★ |
| Sexually Transmitted Infections[29] | | | | | | | | | | | | | | | |
| HIV[30] | | | | | | | | | | | | | | | |
| Hepatitis B Virus Infection[31] | | ★ ⟶ | ⟶ | ⟶ | ⟶ | ⟶ | ⟶ | ⟶ | ⟶ | ⟶ | ⟶ | ⟶ | ⟶ | ⟶ | ⟶ |
| Hepatitis C Virus Infection[32] | | | | | | | | | | | | | | | |
| Sudden Cardiac Arrest/Death[33] | | | | | | | | | | | | | | | |
| Cervical Dysplasia[34] | | | | | | | | | | | | | | | |
| **ORAL HEALTH[35]** | | | | | | | ●[36] | ●[36] | ★ | | ★ | ★ | ★ | ★ | ★ |
| Fluoride Varnish[37] | | | | | | | ⟵ | ⟵ | ⟵ | ⟵ | ● | ⟶ | ⟶ | ⟶ | ⟶ |
| Fluoride Supplementation[38] | | | | | | | ★ | ★ | ★ | | ★ | ★ | ★ | ★ | ★ |
| **ANTICIPATORY GUIDANCE** | ● | ● | ● | ● | ● | ● | ● | ● | ● | ● | ● | ● | ● | ● | ● |

| | MIDDLE CHILDHOOD | | | | | | ADOLESCENCE | | | | | | | | | | |
|---|---|---|---|---|---|---|---|---|---|---|---|---|---|---|---|---|---|
| **AGE[1]** | **5 y** | **6 y** | **7 y** | **8 y** | **9 y** | **10 y** | **11 y** | **12 y** | **13 y** | **14 y** | **15 y** | **16 y** | **17 y** | **18 y** | **19 y** | **20 y** | **21 y** |
| **HISTORY** Initial/Interval | ● | ● | ● | ● | ● | ● | ● | ● | ● | ● | ● | ● | ● | ● | ● | ● | ● |
| **MEASUREMENTS** | | | | | | | | | | | | | | | | | |
| Length/Height and Weight | ● | ● | ● | ● | ● | ● | ● | ● | ● | ● | ● | ● | ● | ● | ● | ● | ● |
| Head Circumference | | | | | | | | | | | | | | | | | |
| Weight for Length | | | | | | | | | | | | | | | | | |
| Body Mass Index[5] | ● | ● | ● | ● | ● | ● | ● | ● | ● | ● | ● | ● | ● | ● | ● | ● | ● |
| Blood Pressure[6] | ● | ● | ● | ● | ● | ● | ● | ● | ● | ● | ● | ● | ● | ● | ● | ● | ● |
| **SENSORY SCREENING** | | | | | | | | | | | | | | | | | |
| Vision[7] | ● | ● | ★ | ● | ★ | ● | ★ | ● | ★ | ★ | ● | ★ | ★ | ★ | ★ | ★ | ★ |
| Hearing | ● | ● | ★ | ● | ★ | ● | ⟵ | ⟵ | ●[10] | ⟶ | ⟵ | ● | ⟶ | ⟵ | ⟵ | ● | ⟶ |
| **DEVELOPMENTAL/SOCIAL/BEHAVIORAL/MENTAL HEALTH** | | | | | | | | | | | | | | | | | |
| Maternal Depression Screening[11] | | | | | | | | | | | | | | | | | |
| Developmental Screening[12] | | | | | | | | | | | | | | | | | |
| Autism Spectrum Disorder Screening[13] | | | | | | | | | | | | | | | | | |
| Developmental Surveillance | ● | ● | ● | ● | ● | ● | ● | ● | ● | ● | ● | ● | ● | ● | ● | ● | ● |
| Behavioral/Social/Emotional Screening[14] | ● | ● | ● | ● | ● | ● | ● | ● | ● | ● | ● | ● | ● | ● | ● | ● | ● |
| Tobacco, Alcohol, or Drug Use Assessment[15] | | | | | | | ★ | ★ | ★ | ★ | ★ | ★ | ★ | ★ | ★ | ★ | ★ |
| Depression and Suicide Risk Screening[16] | | | | | | | | ● | ● | ● | ● | ● | ● | ● | ● | ● | ● |
| **PHYSICAL EXAMINATION[17]** | ● | ● | ● | ● | ● | ● | ● | ● | ● | ● | ● | ● | ● | ● | ● | ● | ● |
| **PROCEDURES[18]** | | | | | | | | | | | | | | | | | |
| Newborn Blood | | | | | | | | | | | | | | | | | |
| Newborn Bilirubin[21] | | | | | | | | | | | | | | | | | |
| Critical Congenital Heart Defect[22] | | | | | | | | | | | | | | | | | |
| Immunization[23] | ● | ● | ● | ● | ● | ● | ● | ● | ● | ● | ● | ● | ● | ● | ● | ● | ● |
| Anemia[24] | ★ | ★ | ★ | ★ | ★ | ★ | ★ | ★ | ★ | ★ | ★ | ★ | ★ | ★ | ★ | ★ | ★ |
| Lead[25] | ★ | ★ | | | | | | | | | | | | | | | |
| Tuberculosis[27] | ★ | ★ | ★ | ★ | ★ | ★ | ★ | ★ | ★ | ★ | ★ | ★ | ★ | ★ | ★ | ★ | ★ |
| Dyslipidemia[28] | | ★ | | ★ | ⟵ | ● | ⟶ | ★ | ★ | ★ | ★ | ★ | ⟵ | ⟵ | ⟵ | ● | ⟶ |
| Sexually Transmitted Infections[29] | | | | | | | ★ | ★ | ★ | ★ | ★ | ★ | ★ | ★ | ★ | ★ | ★ |
| HIV[30] | | | | | | | ★ | ★ | ★ | ★ | ● ⟶ | ⟶ | ⟶ | ⟶ | ⟶ | ⟶ | ⟶ |
| Hepatitis B Virus Infection[31] | ⟶ | ⟶ | ⟶ | ⟶ | ⟶ | ⟶ | ⟶ | ⟶ | ⟶ | ⟶ | ⟶ | ⟶ | ⟶ | ⟶ | ⟶ | ⟶ | ⟶ |
| Hepatitis C Virus Infection[32] | | | | | | | | | | | | | | ● ⟶ | ⟶ | ⟶ | ⟶ |
| Sudden Cardiac Arrest/Death[33] | | | | | | | ★ ⟶ | ⟶ | ⟶ | ⟶ | ⟶ | ⟶ | ⟶ | ⟶ | ⟶ | ⟶ | ⟶ |
| Cervical Dysplasia[34] | | | | | | | | | | | | | | | | | ● |
| **ORAL HEALTH[35]** | ★ | ★ | | | | | | | | | | | | | | | |
| Fluoride Varnish[37] | ⟶ | | | | | | | | | | | | | | | | |
| Fluoride Supplementation[38] | ★ | ★ | ★ | ★ | ★ | ★ | ★ | ★ | ★ | ★ | ★ | ★ | | | | | |
| **ANTICIPATORY GUIDANCE** | ● | ● | ● | ● | ● | ● | ● | ● | ● | ● | ● | ● | ● | ● | ● | ● | ● |

1. If a child comes under care for the first time at any point on the schedule, or if any items are not accomplished at the suggested age, the schedule should be brought up to date at the earliest possible time.
2. A prenatal visit is recommended for parents who are at high risk, for first-time parents, and for those who request a conference. The prenatal visit should include anticipatory guidance, pertinent medical history, and a discussion of benefits of breastfeeding and planned method of feeding, per "The Prenatal Visit" ( https://doi.org/10.1542/peds.2018-1218).
3. Newborns should have an evaluation after birth, and breastfeeding should be encouraged (and instruction and support should be offered).
4. Newborns should have an evaluation within 3 to 5 days of birth and within 48 to 72 hours after discharge from the hospital to include evaluation for feeding and jaundice. Breastfeeding newborns should receive formal breastfeeding evaluation, and their mothers should receive encouragement and instruction, as recommended in "Policy Statement: Breastfeeding and the Use of Human Milk" (https://doi.org/10.1542/peds.2022-057988). Newborns discharged less than 48 hours after delivery must be examined within 48 hours of discharge, per "Hospital Stay for Healthy Term Newborn Infants" (https://doi.org/10.1542/peds.2015-0699).
5. Screen, per "Clinical Practice Guideline for the Evaluation and Treatment of Children and Adolescents with Obesity" (https://doi.org/10.1542/peds.2022-060640).
6. Screening should occur per "Clinical Practice Guideline for Screening and Management of High Blood Pressure in Children and Adolescents" (https://doi.org/10.1542/peds.2017-1904). Blood pressure measurement in infants and children with specific risk conditions should be performed at visits before age 3 years.
7. A visual acuity screen is recommended at ages 4 and 5 years, as well as in cooperative 3-year-olds. Instrument-based screening may be used to assess risk at ages 12 and 24 months, in addition to the well visits at 3 through 5 years of age. See "Visual System Assessment in Infants, Children, and Young Adults by Pediatricians" (https://doi.org/10.1542/peds.2015-3596) and "Procedures for the Evaluation of the Visual System by Pediatricians" (https://doi.org/10.1542/peds.2015-3597).
8. Confirm initial screen was completed, verify results, and follow up, as appropriate. Newborns should be screened, per "Year 2007 Position Statement: Principles and Guidelines for Early Hearing Detection and Intervention Programs" (https://doi.org/10.1542/peds.2007-2333).
9. Verify results as soon as possible, and follow up, as appropriate.
10. Screen with audiometry including 6,000 and 8,000 Hz high frequencies once between 11 and 14 years, once between 15 and 17 years, and once between 18 and 21 years. See "The Sensitivity of Adolescent Hearing Screens Significantly Improves by Adding High Frequencies" (https://www.sciencedirect.com/science/article/abs/pii/S1054139X16000483).
11. Screening should occur per "Incorporating Recognition and Management of Perinatal Depression Into Pediatric Practice" (https://doi.org/10.1542/peds.2018-3259).
12. Screening should occur per "Promoting Optimal Development: Identifying Infants and Young Children With Developmental Disorders Through Developmental Surveillance and Screening" ( https://doi.org/10.1542/peds.2019-3449).
13. Screening should occur per "Identification, Evaluation, and Management of Children With Autism Spectrum Disorder" (https://doi.org/10.1542/peds.2019-3447).

*(continued)*

KEY: ● = to be performed ★ = risk assessment to be performed with appropriate action to follow, if positive ⟵ ★ or ● ⟶ = range during which a service may be provided

BFNC.2025.PSMAR
3-372/0325

**FIGURE 28.1** American Academy of Pediatrics (2024) recommendations for well-child follow-up care appointments.

*Source:* With permission from the American Academy of Pediatrics. (2024). *Recommendations for preventive pediatric health care.* https://www.aap.org/en/practice-management/care-delivery-approaches/periodicity-schedule/.

physical examination and measurements, developmental surveillance, psychosocial, and behavioral assessments are recommended at the infancy period at 1, 2, 4, 6, and 9 months of age. In early childhood, developmental surveillance should take place at 12, 15, and 24 months of age and then at 3 and 4 years of age. Developmental screening (tests) is recommended at 9, 18, and 30 months of age (AAP, 2024a). NICU graduates and high-risk infants might require additional health checkups; thus, every infant should be managed on the individual basis.

Due to risks of visual impairments in NICU patients (i.e., retinopathy of prematurity [ROP]), ophthalmic examinations should be performed. Recent studies show that the incidence of ROP increased in the last decades (especially in Black and Hispanic infants) and while ROP screening has improved through the years, approximately 10% of infants have not receive recommended screening (Bhatnagar et al., 2023; Prakalapakorn et al., 2021). All infants weighing less than or equal to 1,500 g or less than or equal to 32 weeks of gestation, infants with unstable clinical course, should have retinal screening at the hospital. The first fundal examination in infants above 22 weeks of gestation should occur at 31 weeks' postmenstrual age or between 4 and 9 weeks of chronological age, depending on the gestational age at birth; follow-up appointments should occur in 1- to 3-week intervals depending on the initial fundal examination (Fierson et al., 2018). It had also been recommended that preterm infants with or without ROP should be evaluated at 4 to 6 months of age and then yearly (Fierson et al., 2018). Special attention should be given to parents of preterm infants with low health literacy and limited English language proficiency because these parents often lack knowledge about ROP (Eneriz-Wiemer et al., 2018). Providing educational materials that adhere to the health literacy guidelines to parents had been shown to be an effective measure to improve follow-up compliance (McCahon et al., 2023; Mullane & Gaffar, 2023; Ndukwe et al., 2022).

Hearing screening is vitally important because hearing-impaired children experience irreversible delays in speech and language development; not only NICU graduates but all infants should be screened for hearing impairment regardless of the risk (Shah & Lotke, 2023). Permanent hearing loss remains a serious complication of prematurity, certain neonatal diseases such as hyperbilirubinemia, congenital cytomegalovirus or Zika infections, meningitis, or prolonged oxygen and antibiotic use (Shah & Lotke, 2023). Hearing screening should be performed before discharge in any infant who was hospitalized for more than 5 days; auditory brainstem response (ABR), automated ABR (AABR), and otoacoustic emissions (OAEs) are the widely used methods for newborn hearing screening (NHS) (Shah & Lotke, 2023). After discharge, an infant should be evaluated at 1, 2, 4, 6, and 9 months of age (AAP Early Hearing Detection and Intervention, 2020) and enrolled in early intervention (EI) programs by 6 months of age (AAP Early Hearing Detection and Intervention, 2020). The AAP periodicity schedule for the current hearing screening schedule as well as other health evaluations can be found at https://downloads.aap.org/AAP/PDF/periodicity_schedule.pdf. Early hearing screening (by 1 month of age), diagnosis in the first 3 months, and enrollment into EI programs before 6 months of age are beneficial for infants with hearing loss in terms of language and cognition development as well as socioemotional outcomes (Bower et al., 2023; AAP Early Hearing Detection and Intervention, 2020). In 2022, 86.8% of infants diagnosed with hearing problems were referred to EI (60.3% enrolled); only 40.9% of infants were enrolled in EI before 6 months of age (Centers for Disease Control and Prevention [CDC], 2024a). Special attention should be given to the family caregivers with low educational levels, underserved families, families geographically distanced/residing in rural areas, and families with inadequate insurance because such factors are associated with missed follow-up and readmissions (Atherton et al., 2023; Feister et al., 2024; Nicholson et al., 2022; Warner-Czyz et al., 2024). It was found that during the COVID-19 pandemic, some patients were lost for follow-up (Rockwell et al., 2023). The systematic review by Mackey et al. (2022) identified key protocol and program factors influencing referral and loss to follow-up (LTFU) rates in NHS. The review included 101 studies, with 58 reporting on referral rates, 8 on LTFU rates, and 35 on both. Key findings include (Mackey et al., 2022) the following:

1. Screening method: Automated auditory brainstem response (aABR) generally resulted in lower referral rates compared to transient-evoked otoacoustic emissions (TEOAE) for well babies (WB). Combining both methods (two-technology screening) also reduced referral rates compared to using TEOAE alone.
2. Rescreening: Rescreening before hospital discharge and screening after 3 days of age reduced referral rates.
3. Infant age: Screening performed at 3 days of age or later had lower referral rates compared to earlier screenings.
4. Screener experience: More experienced screeners had lower referral rates, particularly with OAE.
5. Program organization: Programs with audiologist involvement, no fees for follow-up steps, integration into larger regional or national programs, and accessible follow-up locations had lower LTFU rates.
6. Infant group: Higher LTFU rates were observed for infants from the NICU compared to WB, especially in programs with low overall LTFU.

The review highlights the importance of considering multiple factors and local contexts to improve NHS outcomes effectively. Early hearing detection and intervention (EHDI) guidelines for pediatric medical home providers can be located at https://www.aap.org/en/patient-care/early-hearing-detection-and-intervention/early-hearing-and-detection-resources/.

## Immunizations

Appropriate immunizations should be given at discharge from a hospital (AAP, 2024b). The full schedule can be found at https://publications.aap.org/redbook/resources/15585. Vaccinations for preterm infants should be given according to the chronological age; routine immunization schedules are not changed, but some catch-up schedules should be acknowledged (please see AAP resource mentioned earlier). Some specifics related to the hepatitis B (HepB) immunizations in infants weighing less than 2,000 g are as follows: The first HepB vaccine is given at 1 month of age or at discharge and then three vaccines are given at 1, 2, and 6 (up to 18) months of age (AAP, 2025a, 2025b). AAP (2024b) recommends adding HepB immunoglobulin to HepB vaccine in infants of mothers with unknown or positive HBsAg status. In infants who are heavier than 2,000 g and those mothers who are HBsAg positive, immunoglobulin should be added to HepB vaccine within 12 hours after birth.

Vaccinations can be delayed if needed (e.g., due to the present medical conditions, transient illnesses, and rehospitalizations). Careful attention should be given to the immunization schedule of NICU graduates: Some studies highlight that while some NICUs achieve high immunization rates at discharge, others face challenges, with a significant proportion of infants being underimmunized. Factors influencing these rates include the infant's age at discharge, medical conditions, and the implementation of quality improvement measures within the NICU (Bryan et al., 2022; Flannery & Wade, 2021; Macintosh et al., 2017; Sadeck & Kfouri, 2023). The schedule for the recommended vaccinations and catch-up schedule for patients who start late, or more than 1 month behind, can be found at the Red Book online resource mentioned previously (AAP, 2024b). Please see some recommended schedules for immunizations in Figure 28.2.

To prevent respiratory syncytial virus (RSV) infection, a leading cause of hospitalization among U.S. infants (Jones et al., 2023), an RSV vaccine (a recombinant human IgG1κ monoclonal antibody such as nirsevimab-alip [brand name Beyfortus], a cost-saving and long-lasting replacement vaccine for palivizumab [brand name Synagis], both made by Astrazeneca AB) can be administered to neonates and infants born during or entering their first RSV season at the time of birth [AAP, 2025]). For infants born outside the RSV season, the vaccine can be administered once prior to the start of the RSV season—the duration of protection provided by single dose of nirsevimab-alip is 5 months. A single dose of 50 or 100 mg intramuscularly is recommended for those infants who weigh < 5 kg and ≥ 5 kg, respectively (https://www.fda.gov/drugsatfda), in most of the continental United States from October through the end of March (Jones et al., 2023). Infants and children aged 8 to 19 months who are at the increased risk for RSV infection (infants with CLD, children with severe immunocompromise, children with cystic fibrosis who have manifestations of severe lung disease, and American Indian or Alaska Native) should receive 1 dose of nirsevimab-alip 200 mg, administered as two 100-mg injections given at the same time at different injection sites (Jones et al., 2023). There is no need for nirsevimab for most infants aged < 8 months whose pregnant parent received RSV vaccine ≥ 14 days before giving birth; however, administering this vaccine may be considered in certain cases (based on the clinical judgment of the healthcare provider): When an infant born to a pregnant parent who might not have developed a proper adequate immune response due to HIV or other immunosuppression, when an infant was on cardiopulmonary bypass or extracorporeal membrane oxygenation (ECMO), or when an infant has hemodynamically significant CHD or requires oxygen at hospital discharge (AAP, 2024b).There is a visual guide for administration of the RSV vaccine (see Figure 28.3 below [AAP, 2024b]).

If both nirsevimab and palivizumab are available for eligible high-risk patients, they should receive nirsevimab (O'Leary et al., 2025). If palivizumab is administered, a proper use and adequate number of doses are of vital importance. Palivizumab is given monthly during RSV season; typically, 5 doses are given, spaced about 28 to 30 days apart (intramuscularly, 15 mg/kg/dose). Palivizumab can be given at 48 to 72 hours before discharge or as soon as possible after discharge, preferably 1 month before RSV season. Infants with CLD or CHD who are younger than 12 months of age and on medical therapy, as well as preterm infants born before 29 completed weeks of gestation, are eligible for maximum 5 monthly doses. For preterm infants with CLD or CHD, immunizations usually start on November 1st for most geographic locations of the United States. For Florida and Alaska, timing for vaccination may vary due to differences in the length of RSV season. The detailed dosage and timing can be found at the Red Book online resource (AAP, 2024b). Importantly, RSV seasons may vary from country to country and region to region; the reference to appropriate professional guidelines should be made.

The timing of COVID-19 vaccination for an infant who was in the NICU depends on multiple factors, including their age, medical condition, and vaccine eligibility guidelines at the time. Here are general considerations based on current recommendations:

- COVID-19 vaccines are typically recommended for children starting at 6 months of age in many regions, including the United States (CDC, 2023). At least one dose of updated 2024 to 2025 vaccine should be given, with additional doses of Moderna vaccine or Pfizer-BioNTech vaccine (AAP, 2025).
- All vaccine doses should be from the same manufacturer (AAP, 2025).
- Infants younger than 6 months are not eligible for COVID-19 vaccination.
- Premature infants and those with underlying medical conditions, such as CLD or congenital heart defects, may be more vulnerable to severe COVID-19. These infants should receive the vaccine as soon as they meet the age requirement and are medically stable.
- NICU graduates who meet age and eligibility criteria can safely receive COVID-19 vaccines once they are discharged or as advised by their pediatrician.
- The COVID-19 vaccines authorized for young children, such as those by Pfizer-BioNTech and Moderna, are given in *age-appropriate* doses. The dosing schedule is available at https://publications.aap.org/redbook/resources/15585 (AAP, 2025; CDC, 2023, 2024b).
- COVID-19 vaccines can generally be administered alongside other routine childhood vaccines, though healthcare providers may space them out in some cases for prematurely born infants or those with complex health needs.

Consultation with the infant's pediatrician or a pediatric infectious disease specialist for personalized guidance is recommended to evaluate the infant's health, vaccination schedule, and local guidelines to determine the best timing. Helpful family-friendly information and infographics can be found at https://www.aap.org/en/patient-care/immunizations/maternal-and-infant-immunization-discussion-guides/. There are still high

# Table 1 Recommended Child and Adolescent Immunization Schedule for Ages 18 Years or Younger, United States, 2025

**These recommendations must be read with the notes that follow.** For those who fall behind or start late, provide catch-up vaccination at the earliest opportunity as indicated by the green bars. To determine minimum intervals between doses, see the catch-up schedule (Table 2).

| Vaccine and other immunizing agents | Birth | 1 mo | 2 mos | 4 mos | 6 mos | 9 mos | 12 mos | 15 mos | 18 mos | 19–23 mos | 2–3 yrs | 4–6 yrs | 7–10 yrs | 11–12 yrs | 13–15 yrs | 16 yrs | 17–18 yrs |
|---|---|---|---|---|---|---|---|---|---|---|---|---|---|---|---|---|---|
| Respiratory syncytial virus (RSV-mAb [Nirsevimab]) | 1 dose depending on maternal RSV vaccination status (See Notes) | | | | | 1 dose (8 through 19 months), See Notes | | | | | | | | | | | |
| Hepatitis B (HepB) | 1st dose | ←— 2nd dose —→ | | | ←— 3rd dose —→ | | | | | | | | | | | | |
| Rotavirus (RV): RV1 (2-dose series), RV5 (3-dose series) | | | 1st dose | 2nd dose | See Notes | | | | | | | | | | | | |
| Diphtheria, tetanus, acellular pertussis (DTaP <7 yrs) | | | 1st dose | 2nd dose | 3rd dose | | | ←— 4th dose —→ | | | | 5th dose | | | | | |
| *Haemophilus influenzae* type b (Hib) | | | 1st dose | 2nd dose | See Notes | | ← 3rd or 4th dose (See Notes) → | | | | | | | | | | |
| Pneumococcal conjugate (PCV15, PCV20) | | | 1st dose | 2nd dose | 3rd dose | | ←— 4th dose —→ | | | | | | | | | | |
| Inactivated poliovirus (IPV) | | | 1st dose | 2nd dose | ←— 3rd dose —→ | | | | | | | 4th dose | | | | | See Notes |
| COVID-19 (1vCOV-mRNA, 1vCOV-aPS) | | | | | 1 or more doses of 2024–2025 vaccine (See Notes) | | | | | | | | | | | | |
| Influenza (IIV3, ccIIV3) | | | | | 1 or 2 doses annually | | | | | | | | 1 dose annually | | | | |
| or | | | | | | | | | | | | | or | | | | |
| Influenza (LAIV3) | | | | | | | | | | | 1 or 2 doses annually | | 1 dose annually | | | | |
| Measles, mumps, rubella (MMR) | | | | | See Notes | | ←— 1st dose —→ | | | | | 2nd dose | | | | | |
| Varicella (VAR) | | | | | | | ←— 1st dose —→ | | | | | 2nd dose | | | | | |
| Hepatitis A (HepA) | | | | | See Notes | | 2-dose series (See Notes) | | | | | | | | | | |
| Tetanus, diphtheria, acellular pertussis (Tdap ≥7 yrs) | | | | | | | | | | | | | | 1 dose | | | |
| Human papillomavirus (HPV) | | | | | | | | | | | | | | See Notes | | | |
| Meningococcal (MenACWY-CRM ≥2 mos, MenACWY-TT ≥2years) | | | See Notes | | | | | | | | | | | 1st dose | | 2nd dose | |
| Meningococcal B (MenB-4C, MenB-FHbp) | | | | | | | | | | | | | See Notes | | | | |
| Respiratory syncytial virus vaccine (RSV [Abrysvo]) | | | | | | | | | | | | | | Seasonal administration during pregnancy (See Notes) | | | |
| Dengue (DEN4CYD: 9–16 yrs) | | | | | | | | | | | | | Seropositive in endemic dengue areas (See Notes) | | | | |
| Mpox | | | | | | | | | | | | | | | | | |

Range of recommended ages for all children | Range of recommended ages for catch-up vaccination | Range of recommended ages for certain high-risk groups or populations | Recommended vaccination can begin in this age group | Recommended vaccination based on shared clinical decision-making | No Guidance/ Not Applicable

Page 2

**FIGURE 28.2** American Academy of Pediatrics immunization schedule, 2025.

*Source:* With permission from the American Academy of Pediatrics. (2025). *Recommended child and adolescent immunization schedule for ages 18 years or younger, United States, 2025.* https://publications.aap.org/redbook/resources/15585

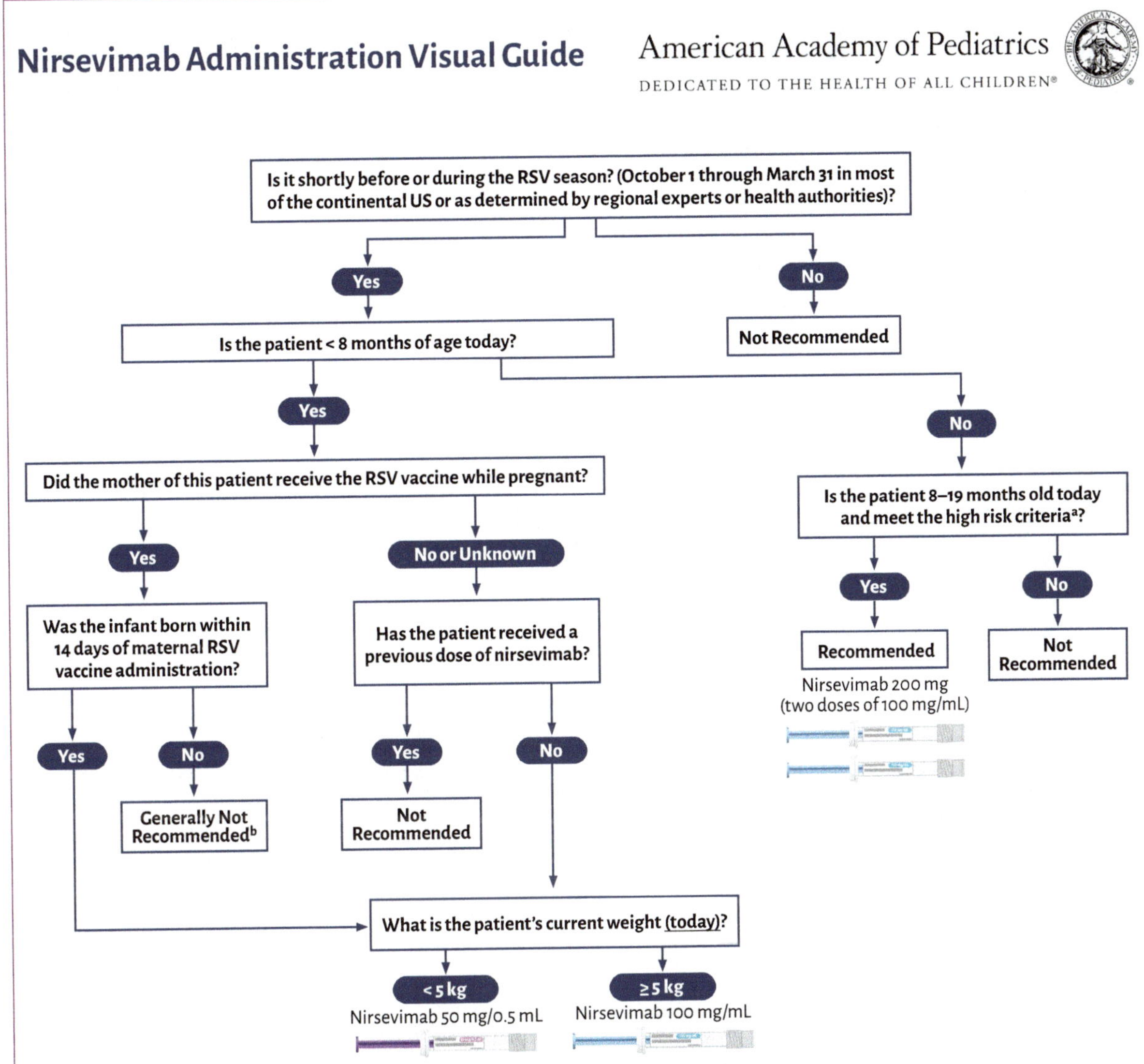


a. Children 8 through 19 months of age who are recommended to receive nirsevimab when entering their second RSV season because of increased risk of severe disease.

- Children with chronic lung disease of prematurity who required medical support (chronic corticosteroid therapy, diuretic therapy, or supplemental oxygen) any time during the 6-month period before the start of the second RSV season.
- Children who are severely immunocompromised.
- Children with cystic fibrosis who have manifestations of severe lung disease (previous hospitalization for pulmonary exacerbation in the first year of life or abnormalities on chest imaging that persist when stable) or have weight-for-length that is <$10^{th}$ percentile.
- American Indian and Alaska Native children (note that this is a new group for whom second-season prophylaxis is recommended in contrast to the current palivizumab recommendations).

b. Nirsevimab can be considered when, per the clinical judgement of the healthcare provider, the potential incremental benefit of administration is warranted, including but not limited to the following rare circumstances:

- Infants born to pregnant people who may not mount an adequate immune response to vaccination or have conditions associated with reduced transplacental antibody transfer.
- Infants who have undergone cardiopulmonary bypass or extracorporeal membrane oxygenation leading to loss of maternal antibodies.
- Infant with substantial increased risk for severe RSV disease (eg, hemodynamically significant congenital heart disease, requiring oxygen at discharge following an intensive care admission).

Last updated Sept. 10, 2024

**FIGURE 28.3 Nirsevimab administration.**

*Source:* American Academy of Pediatrics. (2024). *AAP recommendations for the prevention of RSV disease in infants and children.* https://publications.aap.org/redbook/resources/25379?autologincheck=redirected.

# Nirsevimab Administration Visual Guide

American Academy of Pediatrics
DEDICATED TO THE HEALTH OF ALL CHILDREN®

## Immunization Administration Tips

At the time of administration, affirm the 7 rights to reduce errors:

1. Right patient
2. Right time (age, in RSV season)
3. Right immunization (correct medication)
4. The right dosage (based on weight)
5. The right route, needle length, and technique

**Intramuscular (IM) injection**
Use a 22–25 gauge needle. Choose the injection site and needle length that is appropriate to the person's age and body mass.

| Age | Needle length | Injection site |
|---|---|---|
| Newborns (1st 28 days) | ⅝"[a] | Anterolateral thigh muscle |
| Infants (1–12 months) | 1" | Anterolateral thigh muscle |
| Toddlers (1–2 years) | 1–1¼" | Anterolateral thigh muscle[c] |
| | ⅝[b]–1" | Deltoid muscle of arm |

6. Right site
7. The right documentation

## Co-administration and Suggested Injection Volumes

In accordance with the CDC's General Best Practice Guidelines for Immunization, simultaneous administration of nirsevimab with age-appropriate vaccines is recommended. CDC does not address the issue of maximum volumes that can be injected into each muscle group in different age groups. CDC is in the process of creating a job aid for healthcare providers to help address the issue and offers the suggested volumes as follows:

- **Deltoid muscle of arm:** Average 0.5 mL (range 0.5–2 mL)
- **Anterolateral thigh muscle (Vastus Lateralis):** Average 1–4 mL (range 1–5 mL)

Infants and toddlers would fall at the lower end of the range, whereas adolescents and adults would generally fall on the higher end of the range. Strategies healthcare providers can use to decrease the number/injection volume include:

- Healthcare providers should always use professional judgement when administering injections. Muscle size can vary greatly from one patient to another.
- Include an age-appropriate combination vaccine in the facility's inventory (Pentacel, Pediarix, Vaxelis).
- Use an alternate route (other than IM) if possible. IPV (single component, NOT a combination vaccine), MMR (toddlers and infant travelers only), Varicella-containing vaccines (toddlers only), and PPSV23 (high-risk toddlers only) can be administered subcutaneously.
- Take advantage of recommended age ranges some of the routinely recommended vaccines have. For example, the 3rd dose of HepB can be given as late as 18 months of age.

a. If skin is stretched tightly and subcutaneous tissues are not bunched.

b. Alternate needle lengths may be used if the skin isstretched tightly and subcutaneous tissues are not bunched, as follows: a) a 5/8" needle in toddlers, children, and patients weighing less than 130 lbs (less than 60 kg) for IM injection in the deltoid muscle only, or b) a 1" needle for administration in the thigh muscle for adults of any weight

c. Preferred site

NOTE: Always refer to the package insert included with each biologic for complete vaccine administration information. CDC's Advisory Committee on Immunization Practices (ACIP) recommendations for the particular vaccine should be reviewed as well. Access the ACIP recommendations at www.immunize.org/acip.

Last updated Sept. 10, 2024

**FIGURE 28.3** (*continued*)

levels of vaccination errors present (Institute for Safe Medication Practices, 2023); thus, an adequate attention should be given to the vaccinations of any infant, and especially a NICU graduate.

## Early Intervention Services

Early intervention services and programs aim to prevent or improve cognitive, behavioral, developmental, and physical outcomes in infants and preschoolers; these services also provide family support and decrease parental stress, improving mother–infant interactions and feeding practices, and having positive effects on both maternal and infant outcomes (Bernabe-Zuñiga et al., 2024; Elvrum et al., 2024; Fan et al., 2021; Fontana et al., 2020; Øberg et al., 2023; Orton et al., 2024a; Silveira et al., 2024). Globally, there are 53 million children under the age of 5 with developmental disabilities (Olusanya et al., 2018). Early intervention services are provided to children from birth to 5 years of age to foster child health, development, adapting parenting and family functions and, in general, include physical, occupational, and speech therapies and developmental interventions (McManus et al., 2020; Øberg et al., 2023). In the United States, EI service is covered under the Individuals with Disabilities Education Act (IDEA), Part C, and infants are eligible to participate (U.S. Department of Education, 2011). However, these programs are expensive (Hunter et al., 2023), and referral to them can be problematic, especially during and after the COVID-19 pandemic (Atkins et al., 2020; David et al., 2024; Ortinau et al., 2022; Ponnapakkam et al., 2021). Nationally, for the U.S. 2016 cohort, costs of the EI services and special education was estimated at $1.3 billion only for prematurely born infants (Waitzman et al., 2021). Additionally, criteria for these programs vary by state, and not all high-risk infants and their families are referred to EI services (Dempsey et al., 2020; Gallegos et al., 2021; McManus et al., 2020; Peacock-Chambers et al., 2019; Reynolds et al., 2023; Seppänen et al., 2024). A recent retrospective cohort study ($N = 14,710$) found that only 18.7% of EI-eligible children were referred for services, with just 26% of those receiving them, while referral likelihood was higher for children with severe developmental conditions and lower for Black, non-Hispanic children and those with a diagnosed condition (McManus et al., 2020). Regional variation in EI participation/utilization has been also shown to be significant (Mussatto et al., 2018).

Another important issue is that some health professionals do not feel prepared to assess the high-risk infant and their families; thus, referral may be inadequate because of insufficient knowledge and training of health professionals (Altman et al., 2018; Petty et al., 2022; Williams et al., 2024). While the reported use of standardized developmental screening tools among pediatricians tripled in recent decades and referrals to EI programs increased, further efforts are needed to strengthen referral systems, improve EI programs, and track child outcomes (Lipkin et al., 2020; Meurer et al., 2022). Research focusing on caregiver perspectives highlighted challenges in accessing EI services postdischarge, gaps in communication and support from healthcare providers, suggesting a need for better provider knowledge and resources to facilitate timely EI referrals and services (Lakshmanan et al., 2022). The Zero to Three National Center for Infants, Toddlers, and Families is a nonprofit organization that provides training and education to professionals and families (www.zerotothree.org).

Long-term measurable outcomes of EI programs are sometimes not precisely detectable through the months after NICU discharge, yet beneficial effects have been found in the most vulnerable children with complications (Orton et al., 2024a). Many high-risk infants are discharged with home oxygen, specific medications and feeding tubes and may experience long-term consequences of initial disease. Thus, health professionals should carefully consider all the problems with provision of adequate postdischarge care and undertake appropriate actions to help NICU graduates, such as appropriate referral to specific treatments or EI services. Additional resources for information on EI services can be found at the national Early Childhood Technical Assistance Center (ECTA; http://ectacenter.org/Default.asp).

Parents often encounter stressful challenges with EI services trying to access services and make numerous appointments; connecting and scheduling an EI visit should start before discharge (Lakshmanan et al., 2022). Recent studies showed that having a family/care navigator helped parents from marginalized communities overcome systemic and structural barriers and increased participation in EI (Feinberg et al., 2023; Mirzaian et al., 2024; Thevathasan et al., 2022). Healthcare professionals should also consider family factors when referring to EI, especially in high-risk categories: One study found that less than half of infants with neonatal abstinence syndrome (NAS) were enrolled in EI services, with referral more likely among those discharged to biologic parents and enrollment more strongly associated with longer hospital stays (Peacock-Chambers et al., 2019). Also, Black, Asian, Latino, and Hispanic infants are less likely to receive EI services; rural families often experience delayed responses from healthcare providers, leading to an average diagnosis delay of 5 months (Barnard-Brak et al., 2021; Gallegos et al., 2021). Another study connected higher parental socioeconomic status with the EI receipt while limited parental awareness of EI services, language barriers, and in some cases religious and cultural values, were found to be barriers to EI participation (Sapiets et al., 2021). In summary, EI programs play a crucial role in supporting the developmental trajectory of infants post-NICU discharge, leading to improved cognitive, motor, and overall health outcomes.

## Cerebral Palsy

One of the complications of newborn health issues is cerebral palsy (CP). Globally, there are approximately 8 million children under 5 years of age are estimated to have CP and 16.1 million having intellectual disability, mostly in low-income and middle-income countries (Olusanya et al., 2022). The prevalence of CP at present is decreasing (McIntyre et al., 2022); even extremely low birth weight (ELBW) infants have only minor functional impairments. However, this is an important topic in postdischarge care that deserves attention from healthcare professionals.

Cerebral palsy is defined as a group of neurologic disorders of movement, muscle coordination, and posture that cause activity limitations (National Institute of Neurological

Disorders and Stroke, 2024). Brain damage contributing to CP can result from white matter injury (periventricular leukomalacia [PVL]), abnormal brain development (cerebral dysgenesis), brain bleeding (intracranial hemorrhage), or oxygen deprivation (asphyxia). Risk factors during pregnancy include low birth weight, premature birth, multiple births, maternal infections (e.g., rubella, Zika), toxic exposures, and maternal conditions such as thyroid disorders or seizures. Labor and delivery risks include breech presentation, complicated labor, small size for gestational age, jaundice, and neonatal seizures. While these factors increase CP risk, not all affected infants develop the condition (National Institute of Neurological Disorders and Stroke, 2024).

The four main types of CP are spastic, dyskinetic, ataxic, and mixed. Spastic CP is the most common, causing stiff muscles and awkward movements. It includes hemiplegia (affecting one side), diplegia (mainly affecting the legs), and quadriplegia (severe stiffness in all limbs, often with intellectual disability and seizures). Dyskinetic CP leads to involuntary, jerky, or writhing movements, often affecting speech and coordination but not intelligence. Ataxic CP affects balance and depth perception, causing unsteady walking and difficulty with fine motor skills. Mixed CP combines symptoms of different types, leading to varied muscle stiffness and control issues (National Institute of Neurological Disorders and Stroke, 2024).

The motor disorders of CP are often accompanied by associated impairments such as epilepsy, speech, vision and hearing impairments, and some form of intellectual impairment. Most injury occurs in the perinatal period; however, CP does occur in early childhood and for many infants, the complete causal pathway remains unclear.

In 2017, the landmark international guidelines provided contemporary evidence-based data on optimal early diagnosis and intervention for children with CP. These guidelines state that CP can be predicted with a high degree of accuracy in infants < 5 months of age using the General Movements Assessment, the Hammersmith Infant Neurological Assessment (HINE), and neuroimaging with magnetic resonance imaging (MRI) (Novak et al., 2017). They also provide data to guide early detection of infants in low- and middle-income countries where imaging may not be available. Neonatal nurses should be aware of these guidelines because increasing evidence supports the value of EI in improving outcomes: The earlier the CP is identified, the more optimal are the outcomes (Morgan et al., 2021).

The average age at which a child receives a diagnosis of CP is approximately 15 to 18 months; however, it can be diagnosed by 12 months of age (Hornby et al., 2024) and evidence-based assessments (MRI, General Movements Assessment [GMA], HINE) are helpful for earlier diagnosis (Sutter et al., 2024). Earlier identification is important as the optimal time for neuroplasticity, and therefore, the opportunity for targeted EI. One diagnostic study of high-risk infants found that early neurodevelopmental assessments at 3 to 4 months' CA reliably predicted CP and its severity by 24 to 36 months' CA, highlighting their importance in enabling EI (Razak et al., 2024). Referral of infants deemed to be "at risk" of CP is preferable. It is important, therefore, that neonatal nurses should have knowledge of the risk factors and tools available for early identification of infants with CP or those in the neonatal units deemed to be "at high risk" of CP. Neonatal nurses have an integral role, not only in saving the lives of small and sick neonates but also in preventing disability and in the early identification of these "at-risk" infants.

The implementation of GMA in neonatal units has highly predictive accuracy for CP (Hadders-Algra et al., 2024). The GMA is a noninvasive, video-based tool used to evaluate spontaneous movements in infants, helping to predict CP and other neurodevelopmental disorders. Conducted in two phases—Writhing Movements (preterm to 6–9 weeks postterm) and Fidgety Movements (9–20 weeks postterm)—GMA assesses movement quality rather than strength or reflexes. Normal, varied movements suggest typical development, while poor repertoire, cramped-synchronized, or absent fidgety movements indicate a higher risk of CP. With 90% to 98% predictive accuracy, GMA is a crucial early screening tool that facilitates timely intervention and improves long-term motor outcomes (Hadders-Algra et al., 2024). Another reliable tool (with three subscales: a neurologic, developmental and socio-emotional) that can be used for infants from 6 weeks to 12 months CA to predict CP and intellectual disability is the Standardized Infant NeuroDevelopmental Assessment (SINDA) (Hadders-Algra et al., 2020). One study showed that atypical scores on the neurologic scale predicted atypical outcomes with a sensitivity of 83% and specificity of 96%, while atypical developmental scores predicted intellectual disability with a sensitivity of 77% and specificity of 92% (Hadders-Algra et al., 2020). SINDA serves as a comprehensive screening instrument, enabling early detection of infants at risk for neurodevelopmental disorders, thereby facilitating timely interventions.

The HINE is a standardized tool designed to assess neurologic function in infants aged 2 to 24 months (Haataja et al., 1999; Romeo et al., 2022) that was built upon the foundational work of Dr. Lilly Dubowitz and Dr. Victor Dubowitz in the 1980s to 1990s (Dubowitz et al., 1980, 1999). It evaluates cranial nerve function, posture, movements, tone, and reflexes through 26 items, each scored from 0 to 3, culminating in a maximum score of 78. A score below 57 at 6 months indicates a high risk of CP, while scores above 73 suggest typical neurodevelopment. The HINE is particularly valued for its simplicity, quick administration (approximately 5–10 minutes), and high interrater reliability, making it a practical choice in various clinical settings. Additionally, an asymmetry score (a subcomponent used to assess differences between the left and right sides of the infant's body) exceeding 5 is effective in identifying infants with hemiplegic CP, facilitating EI (Romeo et al., 2022).

Cerebral palsy has no cure, but early and individualized treatment improves a child's abilities and quality of life. A team of specialists, including neurologists, therapists, and orthopedic surgeons, should develop a tailored plan addressing motor, communication, and daily function challenges. Therapies such as physical, occupational, and speech therapy help improve mobility, posture, and communication, while recreation therapy (participation in art and cultural programs, sports) enhances social and cognitive skills. Drug treatments include muscle relaxants such as baclofen and botulinum toxin (BT-A) injections to manage spasticity. Surgical options such as orthopedic surgery for mobility (lengthening muscles and tendons) or selective dorsal rhizotomy (SDR, cutting selected overactivated nerves at the at the base of the spinal column) for severe spasticity are considered when other treatments are ineffective (National Institute of Neurological Disorders and Stroke, 2024).

CP is a lifelong condition, so parents require accurate information regarding the outcomes, interventions, and supports available (Harniess et al., 2022, 2024). Neonatal nurses must consider that the priority is not only saving lives but consistently implementing neuroprotective strategies to prevent or minimize disability in the early days and months of an infant life. These include, but are not limited to, adequate skills and knowledge, gentle handling and positioning, minimizing stressors and reducing pain, optimizing nutrition and growth, and supporting families in the care of their infant. Infants identified as "at risk" for CP should be referred to EI services while in the NICU, and families should be referred/scheduled to CP-specific services when they leave the neonatal unit; parents' active and direct involvement in EIs is associated with improved parent–infant relationships, bonding, increased parental confidence and empowerment, and improved understanding processes (Øberg et al., 2023). Quality neonatal intensive care transcends from the immediate focus on survival to the long-term well-being and nurturing of an infant.

## Rehospitalizations and Readmissions

The postdischarge health issues of NICU graduates can be complex and numerous, especially in prematurely born infants. The associated costs of the hospital and posthospital care, readmissions, and rehospitalizations are substantial as well (Hua et al., 2023; Mowitz et al., 2021; Pai et al., 2024; Rolnitsky et al., 2023; Siffel et al., 2022a, 2022b; van Hasselt et al., 2024; Welke et al., 2024; Yang et al., 2023a, 2023b). In one recent study that investigated the healthcare utilization in NICU graduates, 16% of NICU graduates had an unplanned hospital visit within 90 days of discharge and 7% had required readmission; the mean cost per readmission and standalone emergency department (ED) visit were $25,624 and $475, respectively, while unplanned hospital visits of recent NICU graduates in a single hospital system cost the healthcare system nearly $1 million (Hebballi et al., 2023). It was also estimated that the total costs for these infants with unplanned hospital visits were estimated to be $785,804 with a mean of $1,898 per patient; hospital readmissions accounted for 98% ($768,718) of the total costs and ED visits for 2% ($17,086) (Hebballi et al., 2023). Previously, it had been estimated that 37% of the NICU graduates ($N$ = 4973) readmit during the first year after discharge and 64% had been admitted to emergency departments (Kuo et al., 2018). Readmissions in the NICU graduates, especially in extremely preterm infants, can be twice as high as those in the term group, even when there is good follow-up care (Siffel et al., 2022). However, being a term infant can also be a risk factor for readmission, in the case of earlier discharge (Bernardo et al., 2023). The rates of readmission in preterm infants can be much higher (up to 40%) depending on the initial neonatal health problems, gestational age, comorbidities (such as BPD, presence of ventriculoperitoneal shunt), and adequacy of postdischarge and follow-up care, especially in the first 3 months after discharge (Amsalu et al., 2022; Bernardo et al., 2023; Hannan et al., 2020; Kuo et al., 2018; Mowitz et al., 2021). Readmission rates (as well as the types of mothers' insurance) are also related to postdischarge mortality rates (Feister et al., 2024; Johnson et al., 2023; Rubinos et al., 2022; Siffel et al., 2022). Preterm infants (including late preterm) are likely to require readmission more often than their term counterparts (Alsaif et al., 2023; Amsalu et al., 2023; van Hasselt et al., 2024). In this group, respiratory infections (such as RSV, bronchiolitis), feeding problems and jaundice are the prevalent reasons for readmission (Amsalu et al., 2022; Siffel et al., 2022; Stevenson et al., 2023). Surgical patients also have a high incidence of readmissions (Marquart et al., 2023; Rubinos et al., 2022; Welke et al., 2024). One recent study showed that 40% of infants with gastroschisis readmitted at least one time during the first year after initial discharge, with multiple operations and the presence of a feeding tube or central line at discharge being associated with readmission (Marquart et al., 2023). Another study showed that 12% of infants with CHD readmitted within 1 month after discharge (Berry et al., 2021), confirming that the first few months after discharge is a high-risk period for unplanned hospital readmissions after CHD surgery.

The majority of NICU graduates readmit to pediatric intensive care units (PICUs), where they usually stay for longer periods of stay and consume a large amount of PICU resources (Boerman et al., 2023; Seaton et al., 2024; Sharp et al., 2023; van de Riet et al., 2022). ED visits are much more costly than primary care visits, yet families often feel they need the expertise of an acute care facility. The use of the hospital versus primary care services needs further research, as does the effect of parents' readiness for the transition to home on readmissions. Providing care for parents after discharge is just as important as providing family-centered care in the NICU.

# THE NICU EXPERIENCE

The NICU experience is stressful and traumatic to parents (van Wyk et al., 2024). Parents often fear of death of a new family member, a vulnerable infant whose birth should be celebrated and yet a sense of doom clouds the birth experience. For the most part, parents lack knowledge about the medical diagnosis, equipment, treatments, and routines necessary to support sick or small newborn infants. In the past few decades, research has repeatedly shown that the NICU environment is extremely stressful for parents and can lead to depression, distress, and anxiety, both inside and outside the hospital, that can last a lifetime if there is no attention/intervention (Bozzette & Holditch-Davis, 2015; Klein & McDonald, 2024; Raines, 2013; Rodrigues et al., 2024; Schuetz Haemmerli et al., 2020; Shetty et al., 2024; van Wyk et al., 2024).

Giving birth to a sick or small infant often interferes with the parental role development (Caporali et al., 2020). Guiding parents to take care of their child, proper and timely communication helps parents of NICU infants process their experiences, feel validated, and strengthen their well-being, emphasizing the need for early family support in the NICU (Åberg Petersson et al., 2021; Petersson et al., 2023). The support needs of parents are numerous: There are informational, emotional, and practical care needs; needs for hands-on support; as well as the need for the emotionally intelligent healthcare providers. All of these needs emphasize the importance of staff communication, empathy, and tailored interventions to improve parental well-being and outcomes (Adama et al., 2022). While psychotherapeutic support interventions to support NICU parents are not well researched nor used (Jane et al., 2024), some interventions such as physical contact with the infant during the live music therapy or implementing "listening visits" (empathic listening and problem-solving sessions provided by a psychologist or a nurse, face-to-face or online) were shown to reduce the stress of the NICU environment and distress symptoms in NICU parents (Dewan et al., 2024; Scabia et al., 2024; Segre et al., 2024).

With the infant in the NICU, the mothers must also make a physiologic and psychological postpartum adjustment (Schobinger et al., 2022). They are also in need of care, yet most mothers when asked to express their own needs, they put aside their own time for healing to focus on their infants. Often, mothers of NICU infants experience significantly higher stress, anxiety, and depression than fathers; they usually participate more in caregiving. For the fathers who are often the first parent to visit their infant in the NICU (Saxton et al., 2021), the NICU experience is also stressful (Merritt, 2021; Webber et al., 2025) and their depressive symptoms might have a different trajectory in the NICU and after discharge (Garfield et al., 2021). While paternal anxiety does not interfere with mother–infant bonding, maternal depression increases paternal anxiety (Ettenberger et al., 2024). The need to run between two units (the postpartum and the NICU) is an added stress even if these units are in the same institution (Beck & Vo, 2020). Constraints of work are also impressive—being a breadwinner, a husband, and a father at the same can put a lot of pressure on a NICU father (Lian et al., 2020; Noergaard et al., 2017, 2018; Schmid et al., 2024). The parents' concern for their partners and their children often forces them between the two. For the family with other children at home, the stress becomes even greater. Who can take charge of the children? How long will it be necessary for another person to help with family responsibilities? Is someone who can or will step in to help even be available? These are very real family concerns to exist during the NICU hospitalization of an infant, and gender-sensitive support and staff training are essential for improving parental well-being and family-centered care (Bua et al., 2024). Research suggests that, for fathers, skin-to-skin contact (SSC) and eye contact play a crucial role in bonding; fathers feel more engaged in caregiving when physically present, but their infant's fragile appearance can heighten stress levels (Holm et al., 2022; Koliouli et al., 2022). The fathers express the need to be assured and informed about their infant health (Govindaswamy et al., 2020).

## POSTDISCHARGE FAMILY CARE

Parenting and caring of the vulnerable infant upon coming home can be very challenging for parents. The concept of the family as a unit is another important issue for providing adequate care for infants after discharge. New challenges occur for parents after discharge—questions about care to give to the infant, infant development, and the future. Along with these concerns comes the assumption of the new parental role and a change in family functioning. The parental role adjustment occurs for both first-time and experienced parents. It requires a change from a previous functional pattern to a new one. This change marks a developmental passage or transition.

Postdischarge care should focus not only on the mother but other family members as well. The father and siblings are often forgotten during discharge preparation and afterward despite the stress they experience (Baldoni et al., 2021; Cyr-Alves et al., 2018). Most fathers want to participate in the care and decision making for a healthy or sick/premature newborn, which improves their mental health (Filippa et al., 2021); however, they require the same support (e.g., social) as mothers. The responses of fathers are sometimes different from those of mothers, but fathers also get stressed to a large extent while the infant is in the NICU and afterward; they also may have decreased levels of parental self-efficacy (Vance et al., 2021; Webber et al., 2025). Siblings must also adjust to the infant, who may not seem real to them, until they are able to visit the infant in the NICU (Mooney-Doyle et al., 2022; Silva et al., 2022; Trajkovski & Tehrani, 2025). Many units now encourage sibling visits to help ease the infant into the family well before the actual discharge. The change in NICU design to more single-family rooms and the inclusion of family areas or transition areas afford the family more opportunities to stay together as a family unit. This design provides the family with more of a homelike atmosphere while offering more privacy to them and increasing their confidence in parenting and satisfaction with care (Crump et al., 2023; Fay et al., 2024; Machry et al., 2023; Mann & Stansfield, 2024). This concept of care needs to continue following the discharge.

The AAP Committee on the Fetus and Newborn (2008) guidelines for discharge of the high-risk infant's state that the "infant may be discharged before one of the infant's physiologic competencies has been met, provided the healthcare team and the parents agree that it is appropriate, and suitable plans have been made to provide the additional support needed to ensure safe care at home" (p. 1121). These guidelines also state that parents should be actively involved and prepared for caring for an infant at home. Preparedness of parents for discharge and postdischarge infant care as well as professional support are vital to ensure a successful transition home (AAP & ACOG, 2017). The most commonly prioritized and implemented practices include providing standardized comprehensive handoffs to primary care practitioners (PCPs) at least 1 day before discharge, using a single source for discharge checklists and sharing it with the parents/healthcare team, and early discharge planning meetings with the parents at least 1 week before discharge for infants with complex needs (Bourque et al., 2023). Other practices, such as assessing families' social determinants of health and screening parental mental health, are recognized as priorities but, unfortunately, less frequently integrated into routine practice (Bourque et al., 2023).

While many parents are ready for their infant's discharge and may have reported high self-efficacy at discharge (Franck et al., 2023), stress related to their infant's hospitalization and discharge can make advice and teaching overwhelming and some parents may not recall all the information given to them by health professionals within the hospital or at discharge (Weiss et al., 2017). Smith and colleagues found that 7% of families felt unprepared for discharge; those families were more likely to have sicker infants, to be raising the infant alone, or of Black race (Smith et al., 2021). Another study found that even when parents felt prepared for the discharge, almost one-half of them still had unplanned use of health services during the first month after discharge (Rio et al., 2021). Parental levels of health literacy and discharge plan complexity may affect adherence to discharge instructions (Glick et al., 2019). The hospitalization and discharge of high-risk and preterm newborn infants always hold certain risks for the health of the infant. These times should be considered as serious challenges for parents.

## Transition

Throughout life, events necessitate change. These life changes are often viewed as turning points. In the case of a NICU family, these turning points are the birth of a sick or preterm infant, hospitalization, discharge from the hospital, and the transition to home. All these events require a new role acceptance (to accept the reality, facts about their infant's health), an adjustment or change in a role, a setting of new priorities, and an examination of expectations. Taking on a new role requires energy, commitment, and, most of all, a change in the pattern of functioning—thus, a transition. Transition involves change—leaving behind the familiar and trying something new. There are at least three transition processes for parents of NICU infants: transition to parenthood, transition to home, and transition to primary healthcare settings.

### Transition to Parenthood

The parental role development is a good example of the transition process. For parents of a NICU infant, the transition to parenthood may have two time points—one associated with becoming parents at the time of birth and the other occurring at the time of discharge. Three important processes can be impeded in NICU parents, specifically mothers, while in the hospital: maternal role attainment (MRA), attachment, and bonding. These disturbances have consequences that may extend beyond the immediate posthospital discharge period, and both mothers and fathers can be struggling with certain problems, such as psychological distress, and lower parenting self-efficacy and confidence in parenting (Fernández Medina et al., 2018; Frese & Nguyen, 2022; Pisoni et al., 2024; Rodrigues et al., 2025).

Once a pregnancy is confirmed, both mother and father begin the task of examining their individual roles. For first-time parents, this means considering what it will be like to be a mother or father to a dependent infant. For parents with other children, the new infant will bring a unique personality and another dimension to the already formed family unit. This infant, too, will require role adjustment on the part of the parents. Acquisition of the maternal role and maternal identity, as described by Rubin (1984) and Mercer (1995), focused on mothers of healthy, term infants (Mercer, 1995; Rubin, 1984). When the infant is premature or sick and does not fit the image of the desired child, women lose their normal frame of reference for the development of their own role expectations and the expectations of their infants as well. Later, MRA had been replaced with the new term, "Becoming a Mother" (BAM), as a more inclusive and comprehensive concept where maternal confidence and identity continue to grow or can be disrupted with a child's developmental challenges and life's realities (Mercer, 2004). Decreased MRA was observed with medically fragile infants due to high levels of worry in mothers and less responsiveness of infants (Miles et al., 2011); parenting quality has been shown to be influenced more by MRA than by child illness severity (Holditch-Davis et al., 2011).

The immediate process of attachment, a formation of a relationship between a parent and her or his newborn infant, occurs with wanting the pregnancy, positive maternal feelings, seeing the infant soon after birth, and immediate contact with the infant after birth (Bialoskurski et al., 1999). Delayed and problematic attachment may occur with a premature infant; uncertain outcomes; a handicapped child; poor maternal health; prolonged care that limits the family's ability to touch, hold, and protect their infant; a poor attitude in the partner; a lack of social support; drug dependency; and a taking-1-day-at-a-time attitude (Givrad et al., 2021; Ionio et al., 2024). Attachment, which is considered a dyadic process, becomes a triadic relationship in the NICU, in which NICU personnel—especially nurses—can alter the process. The mother of a premature infant is also a premature mother. Not only are the binding-in and claiming processes affected, but the mother herself is a "preemie" as well. Her pregnancy has ended before her own expectations were met and needs were fulfilled. The interactive and therapeutic relationships between a nurse and a mother foster the process of BAM. Nurses can hinder or facilitate a mother's attachment to her infant and facilitate bonding by encouraging mother–infant touch or by forbidding it. Attachment- and relationship-based interventions in the NICU (parent education and involvement in care, provision of accurate information about the infant's care and health status, early psychological parent–infant interventions and ongoing communication that can facilitate the formation of attachment and bonding) proved effective in reducing maternal traumatic stress and depression, while also promoting infant weight gain and development (Kim & Kim, 2022; Leppänen et al., 2024). While nurses at the NICU were named as the best source of information that helped parents to understand infants' medical conditions (Kowalski et al., 2006) and, from parent's perspectives, the value of nurse–parent relationships is of vital importance for parental well-being (DiGregorio, 2024), there is still a need for nurses training in communication with families (Bry et al., 2023). Numerous research in recent decades has also shown that a decrease in maternal stress as well as a decrease in early separation during hospitalization can prevent the development of distorted attachments in mothers of sick or preterm infants. Also, those mothers can form balanced attachments with their infants, and maternal–infant interaction may be more positive and of higher quality than in mothers of full-term infants if maternal stress is managed and their interaction is fostered prior to and following discharge (Bieleninik et al., 2021; Leppänen et al., 2024).

In addition to possible affected attachment and development of parental role, the actual assumption of the new parental role can be quite overwhelming. Even when a healthy newborn is brought into a family, stress and even crisis can occur (Miller & Sollie, 1980). Some researchers and clinicians viewed transition to parenthood as a *crisis* rather than just a developmental passage to a new functional level. Since the 1960s, research has shown that families see birth hospitalization and bringing home a premature or ill infant who has been in the NICU as a crisis (Affleck & Tennen, 1991; Affleck et al., 1986; Caplan et al., 1965). Even parents of low-risk premature infants experience distress. During hospitalization, parents and siblings often experience psychological distress (van Wyk et al., 2024; Worrall et al., 2024) that may exist for a longer time after discharge as posttraumatic stress disorder (PTSD) (Laccetta et al., 2023; Malouf et al., 2022; McKeown et al., 2023; Sandnes et al., 2024). PTSD is characterized by intrusive memories, avoidance of trauma-related stimuli, negative alterations in cognition and mood, and heightened arousal (such as irritability, startling easily, anger, and difficulties with sleeping), persisting for more than 1 month after exposure to a traumatic event (Bryant, 2019). One recent review found that up to one-third of NICU parents experience PTSD (McKeown et al., 2023). Even if the infant requires no special equipment postdischarge or does not experience the initial neonatal disorder, the family may still experience PTSD related to the initial hospitalization and long-term consequences of initial psychological trauma for the family. Parenting of high-risk neonates may also lead to fewer years of education of family members, higher unemployment, lower incomes, distortion of marital relationships, and family strain. Fortunately, the negative effects of neonatal hospitalization on family functioning, quality of life, and child behavior have been shown to decrease with time, and the family may adjust well and have a posttraumatic positive growth (a positive response to the trauma) (Koivula et al., 2022; Wang et al., 2023; Xingyanan et al., 2025). In Saigal et al.'s (2010) study that examined the effect of illness in young adults born with extremely low birth weight at age 20, mothers reported that caring for their child with neurosensory impairment had even brought their family closer together (Saigal et al., 2010). What is important is helping families to cope with initial transitions after hospital discharge—and many young adults who were born preterm are contributing members to society despite initial problems at birth (Saigal et al., 2020).

Two other major problems can occur when parenting high-risk and preterm infants after discharge. These are vulnerable child syndrome (VCS) and compensatory parenting. Parental responses to their infant are mediated by the infant's illness, the hospitalization, and "near-miss" events. The VCS is one such response that has an effect on both the infant and parents. Green and Solnit (1964) hypothesized that, when children are expected to die prematurely or were seriously injured, the result is a disturbed psychosocial development of the family, based on the parent–child relationship (Green & Solnit, 1964). Because the child is seen as "vulnerable" parents overprotect the child, make more visits to healthcare providers for relatively minor illnesses, and may discipline the child in a gentler manner, which may result in behavior problems (Adama et al., 2016; Hoge et al., 2021; Shaw et al., 2023). What is important is the fact that VCS is a family disorder cyclically affecting both parents and children. Maternal adaptation during the neonatal period and maternal self-inefficacy beliefs about caring and feeding the infant can affect the mother's later perceptions of the infant's vulnerability. Thus, maternal attachment, development of the parental role, and perception of the infant health influence the entire post-discharge well-being of the family and infant.

Compensatory parenting is another disturbance when parenting an initially hospitalized child. This parenting style is compensation for feeling sorry for or guilty about having an infant in the NICU (Miles & Holditch-Davis, 1995). Parents try to provide special experiences for their infants born preterm and avoid other experiences; sometimes more stimulation to foster development with these children is provided. At the same time, they have shielded their children from other life situations to protect them from further hurt, viewing them as "special" and "normal" at the same time (Miles & Holditch-Davis, 1997).

Disturbances in parenting are tightly related to parental psychological well-being. Anxiety and depression have been documented in parents of high-risk and preterm infants, both in the hospital and postdischarge, and especially in low-income families (Enlow et al., 2017; Malouf et al., 2022; Shaw et al., 2023). One recent review revealed that in the first 2 years, depression, anxiety, posttraumatic stress symptoms, and parenting stress were present in ~20% of mothers of extreme and very low birth weight infants (Sandnes et al., 2024). Fortunately, it has also been reported that parental distress, depression, and anxiety decrease over time while parenting self-efficacy increases (Klein & McDonald, 2024; Vance et al., 2020) and sometimes have no negative effect in terms of parenting. However, often parents are still in need of supports (social, professional, peer) after a hospital discharge.

"Searching for normalcy" and grief are other aspects of parental challenges after hospital discharge (Bright et al., 2020; Golish & Powell, 2003; Laverty et al., 2024; May, 1997). Mothers are searching for normalcy in their lives through caring of their infants when they are at home; learning caregiving, maintaining vigilance for their infant's progress, normalizing with caregiver burden, and help seeking are the main themes (May, 1997). Contradictory feelings of joy and grief are also present in parents of preterm infants who lost the "ideal child" and are often unable to communicate that feeling of loss (Golish & Powell, 2003; Shaw et al., 2023). Unresolved grief may lead to insecure attachment and inadequate interactions between mother and infant. What is important here is that the normal grief response can become a chronic sorrow in parents who have a child with permanent, progressive, or cyclic health problems; this chronic sorrow can even become a pathologic grief (Gordon, 2009).

## Transition to Home

Although the NICU discharge is the overriding goal for the healthcare professional and the family, the actual transition to home can be a time of crisis for the family. Transition to home can be even more difficult for parents than the period of the infant's hospitalization because parents are moving from a safe hospital environment to home and taking all the responsibilities for the care of their vulnerable infant while losing the support for the NICU staff (Klein & McDonald, 2024; Spence et al., 2023). For many parents, the NICU reinforces learned helplessness. Parents express the need to understand their role and what is expected of them in relationship to their infants' care needs; yet they feel "in the way" and unable or incapable of caring for their infants. Thus, they learn to be helpless. The picture changes, however, at the time of discharge when parents move from the safety net of the hospital to independent caregiving at home and accepting total responsibility for their infants. The parents are told, "Now it is your turn." It is no wonder that this discharge can be cognitively appraised as being a stressor and that early parenting problems, possible risks in relationship development, can affect both the family and the infant (Sandnes et al., 2024). Parents should be a part of the NICU healthcare team to fully understand what is wrong with their infant and to feel able to make decisions. When given the opportunity to discuss their concerns, parents are vocal about their feelings regarding their NICU care and preparation for discharge—and their voices should be considered by the health professionals seriously.

Preparedness for discharge is vital. Information is critical to the successful transition home. Recent studies show that families are not always well prepared for discharge, and especially those with limited English proficiency (Franck et al., 2023; Smith et al., 2022; Taylor & Hambridge, 2025). Even when parents report that they are prepared at discharge (Franck et al., 2023), parents can be naively confident in caregiving and, in fact, be unable to provide proper care at home. It can be assumed that inadequacy of caregiving and skills when caring for vulnerable infants may affect the health status of an infant and lead to readmissions or overuse of healthcare services postdischarge. This assumption needs further research.

Transition to home can be especially challenging for parents if the infant requires technology at home or has specific healthcare needs. All the healthcare needs of the infant often require advanced knowledge and skills from parents and primary healthcare providers. Infants with special needs tend to use the ED and were hospitalized more often (Lasby et al., 2023). All the ongoing healthcare needs require additional support and education of parents postdischarge. Feeding issues (such as tube feedings, food intolerance, breastfeeding problems, and formula selection) as well as developmental concerns bring enormous stress on parents (Bater et al., 2022; Spence et al., 2023). More than three decades of research showed that the needs for informational support in parents of infants is very high, both when healthy and sick, both in the hospital and afterward (Boykova, 2016b; Boykova & Kenner, 2012; Kenner & Lott, 1990; McKim et al., 1995; Spence et al., 2023; Tajalli et al., 2025). Parents often feel unprepared for this specific transition (Taylor & Hambridge, 2025), and especially adolescent mothers (Orr et al., 2020). Importantly, knowledge and skills needed by parents sometimes differ from those provided by health professionals (Flierman et al., 2024; Lebel et al., 2024), and fulfilling individual information needs of parents is vital. Even if some infants must be rehospitalized due to medical conditions and parent education might have little effect in such cases, transition from hospital to home remains to be dependent on the levels of parental knowledge and skills, competency and confidence in caring for an infant, and the availability of professional and social supports. Often, parents do not trust the available Internet knowledge/mobile applications (while it has been found useful [Kermani et al., 2023; Suir et al., 2022]) or peer support (Fratantoni et al., 2022; Sunshine et al., 2023)—instead, they prefer professional advice from healthcare providers (face-to-face or online) as well as home visits that help with transitional challenges and promote infant health (Edwards et al., 2024; McKelvey et al., 2021; Quinn et al., 2025). Yet there is limited research on transitional problems in parents of NICU patients, as well as solid theoretical frameworks and validated measurement tools. Some concepts of transition for parents of NICU infants are presented in Figure 28.4. One of the available models and instruments is described as follows.

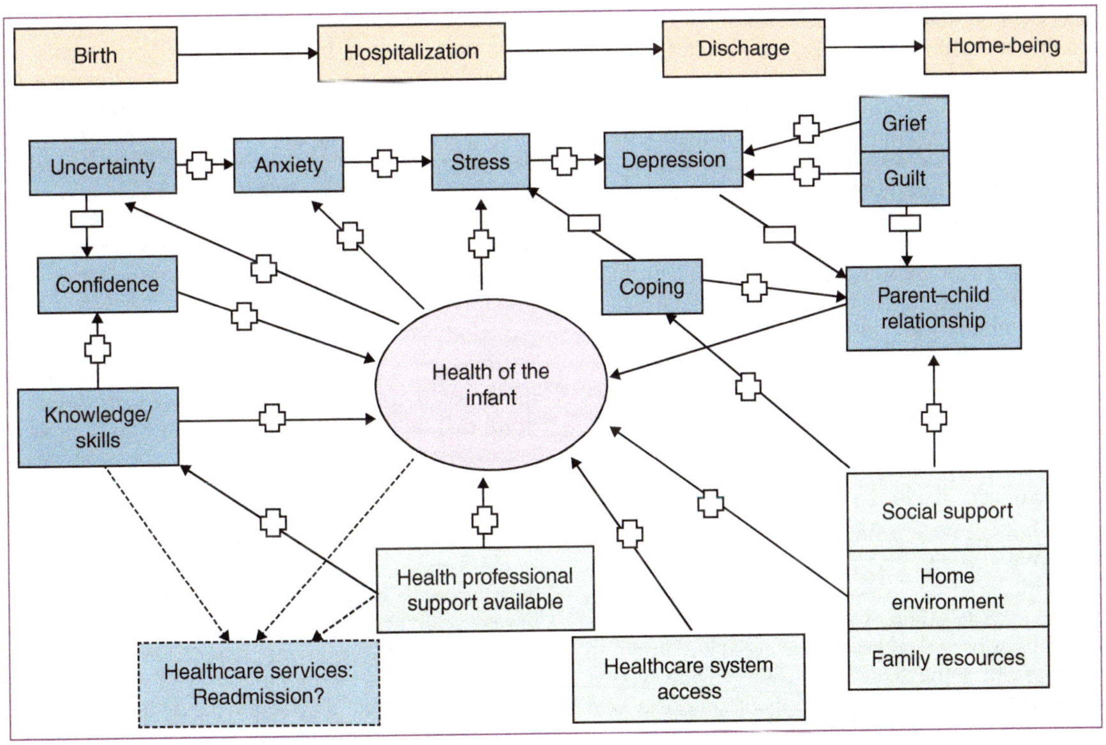


**FIGURE 28.4** **Concepts involved in transition derived from the literature and possible relationships among parental challenges, knowledge, infant health, professional support, and readmissions.**

### Example of Theoretical Framework on Parental Transition From NICU to Home

One theoretical model has been developed in the 1990s for parents of NICU patients who transitioned from hospital to home—the Transition Model developed by Kenner and colleagues (Flandermeyer et al., 1992a, 1992b; Kenner, 1988, 1990; Kenner & Lott, 1990). A series of studies were conducted on parents of both term and preterm infants after hospital discharge. Five main parental transitional challenges were identified in the immediate postdischarge period: Informational Needs, Parent–Child Role Development, Stress and Coping, Social Interaction, and Grief. Despite the changes in neonatal intensive care and health provision, these concepts are still standing for transitional concerns of parents of high-risk infants who were hospitalized after birth.

### Informational Needs

The informational needs of parents include the following:

1. how to provide routine newborn care (e.g., feeding, bathing)
2. how to recognize normal newborn characteristics, both physical and behavioral (amount of "normal" crying) as well as any warning signs
3. how to keep the infant healthy after discharge (i.e., immunizations)
4. how to recognize sleeping and awake periods, and if their infant is not well
5. infant development and prognosis for future
6. equipment used on their infant at home if any; during home follow-up, parents, particularly mothers, want more information about feeding, formula, breastfeeding, elimination patterns, weight gain, and the infant's breathing pattern

Parents seek online sources for information on infant development and play, with a preference for websites, though those with at-risk infants. favor home visits or classes (Cohen et al., 2024; Lopez et al., 2012; Orlando et al., 2023). While EI providers rarely inquire about parents' information sources and perceive existing developmental resources as higher quality than those on play, healthcare professionals should engage parents in discussions about their preferred information sources to ensure access to high-quality educational resources (Orlando et al., 2023). One study assessed the health literacy of EI providers and found that they struggled most with appraising health information and navigating the healthcare system (Leslie et al., 2022). Higher health literacy was associated with older age, higher education, licensure, and more EI experience. Findings of this study highlight the need for targeted professional development to enhance EI providers' health literacy skills, improving their ability to support families effectively (Leslie et al., 2022).

### Parent–Child Role Development

This category refers to parents and children's role expectations that are influenced by the development of relationships and interactions with an infant, which can be impaired by the infant's initial illness or special healthcare needs and interfere with the development of the parental role. For anyone making a transition or entering a new level of functioning or a new stage of life, certain expectations about what is to come exist. New parents of healthy infants adjust in how they carry out the tasks of daily living once their newborn is at home. When a problem with the infant who requires more attention or special care arises, parents may have to set aside their expectations of their roles and feel inadequate in parenting and making healthcare decisions for the infant. The parents may feel that they are not "real" parents and not capable of parenting and caring for their infant and that the physician's permission is necessary to make even the smallest change in the infants' routines that had been established in the hospital.

### Stress and Coping

Stress and coping are related to alterations in parental role, uncertainty and anxiety caused by health problems of the infant, and parental perceptions of their abilities to care for and cope with challenges at home. The expected feelings of joy and the months of anticipation of discharge to home are replaced by sharply contrasting feelings of fear, anxiety, caregiver's tiredness, and overwhelming stress. Coping abilities that must be present to overcome the stress of discharge depend on resources available (informational, material, and social).

### Social Support and Interaction

The Social Interaction category includes parents' ability to socialize after their infant is born sick or preterm. Often, parents isolate themselves due to healthcare risks for their infant (such as RSV infection) or limit their social activities because of misunderstanding about their infant's health issues or if their infant is technology dependent; the feeling of isolation related to protection of a infant is prominent in contemporary research as well (Barthel et al., 2020; Berlin et al., 2024; Lakshmanan et al., 2017; Spence et al., 2023). On the other hand, family and friends may be frightened to approach the parents for fear of doing or saying the wrong thing, thus isolating parents of a vulnerable infant. Social interaction depends on social support from the parental informal network, and the recipient determines support from healthcare professionals, which can be viewed positively or negatively. Support from healthcare professionals improves competency and confidence in care because parenting a high-risk or preterm infant can be socially disruptive, increases parent–infant relationship, promotes emotional and social support, and reduces unplanned hospital visits and parental stress (Boykova, 2016b; Griffith et al., 2022). Such interventions include in-person home visits, phone/video calls, text messages, periodic email questionnaires, and mobile/website applications ("apps") (Griffith et al., 2022).

### Grief

Grief found in parents of NICU infants is related to loss of the image of an "ideal" infant and fear of the infant's ultimate death that influences relationships between the parent and infant within the family as a whole and social interaction (Shaw et al., 2023). Parents express the loss of their expected child once the reality of the neonatal problem shatters their hopes and fantasies. As time goes on, parents continue to grieve but in the form of anticipating that the infant would eventually die if he or she would be sick enough to require special care or have developmental problems. The process of grief and the period of mourning begin once the infant does not meet the parents' expectations of the fantasy or ideal child. If the parents have other children, they may speak of how different this child is from their other children or how different the infant is from their expectations. Another component of grief is the loss of the expected parenting role—that is, their normal role. Some or all of the social rituals that socialize mothers into their impending role and prepare them for their new responsibilities—such as baby showers, parenting classes, and birth announcements—may often have been absent with the birth of a premature or ill infant. Friends and family who would normally be happy to help celebrate the joyous occasion of birth with the exuberant parents may feel uncomfortable and helpless around them, thus withdrawing needed psychological support.

These categories form the basis for transition to home and have not changed in almost four decades (Affleck et al., 1986; Boykova, 2016a, 2016b, 2018; Boykova & Kenner, 2012; Bruder & Walker, 1990; DiBari & Rouse, 2023; Eriksson et al., 2024; Flandermeyer et al., 1992a, 1992b; Garfield et al., 2021; Hutchinson et al., 2012; Kenner, 1988, 1990; Kenner et al., 1992; Kenner & Lott, 1990; Klein & McDonald, 2024; Lebel et al., 2024; McKim et al., 1995; Namnabati et al., 2017; Phillips-Pula et al., 2013; Salomè et al., 2022; Spence et al., 2023; White et al., 2017; Williams & Williams, 1997). These five categories of parental concerns represent the taxonomy for transitional care follow-up. All concepts are interrelated, and relationships between them are reciprocal, with Informational Needs being the core category. The main feature of the model is that transition is viewed as a process, not the product or outcome of changes that were brought to parents with the birth of a vulnerable child. Hospitalization of an infant is the key factor that might influence the postdischarge transition to home. This assumption was confirmed in other studies through the years: Kenner (1988) and Bagwell (1990) found that parents from Level II and III units had similar concerns after hospital discharge. Boykova (2008) did not find any correlation between parental transitional concerns and birth weight or gestational age of former NICU infants (see the depiction of the model in Figure 28.5) (Bagwell, 1990; Boykova, 2008; Kenner, 1988). Research studies continue to confirm the presence and importance of the information needs in parents of high-risk infants (Davis-Strauss et al., 2021; Flierman et al., 2024; Gaskin et al., 2024; Lebel et al., 2024).

The Transition Model has a specific multidimensional tool for the measurement of transition challenges in parents of NICU infants—the Transition Questionnaire.

## Transition Questionnaire

The original Kenner Transition Questionnaire (Boykova & Kenner, 2012) consisted of four parts:

1. thirty-seven statements in Likert-scale format that measure parental concerns and perceptions postdischarge
2. three multiple-choice–format items considering certain informational needs in parents
3. three open-ended questions related to parental concerns after discharge that they might have had
4. demographic information part of the tool, consisting of 21 items about the parent and infant

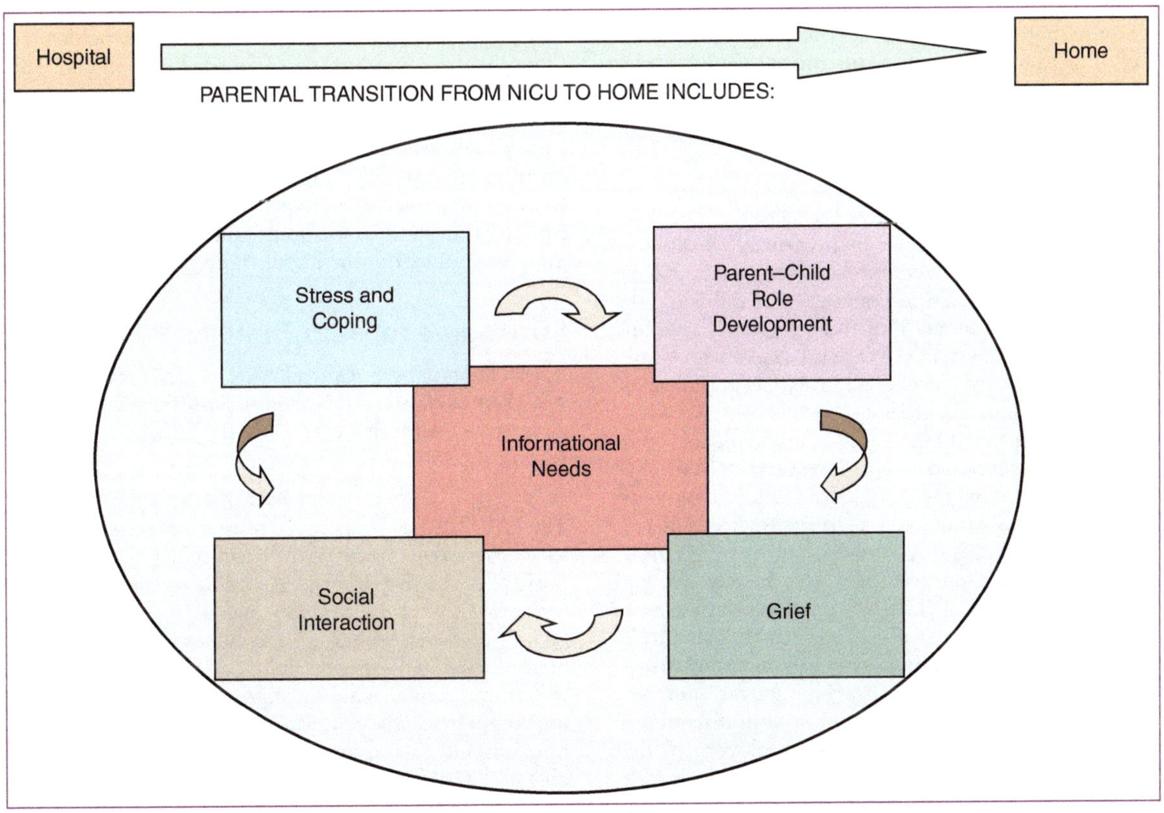


**FIGURE 28.5 Hypothesized depiction of the concepts in the Kenner Transition Model.**

*Sources:* From Kenner, C. (1988). *Parent transition from newborn intensive care unit to home* [Doctoral dissertation, Indiana University, Indianapolis, IN, USA]. http://openlibrary.org/works/OL2733775W/PARENT_TRANSITION_FROM_THE_NEWBORN_INTENSIVE_CARE_UNIT_(NICU)_TO_HOME; Kenner, C. (1990). Caring for the NICU parent. *Journal of Perinatal and Neonatal Nursing, 4*(3), 78–87. https://doi.org/10.1097/00005237-199012000-00010.

Several items are negatively worded to decrease response bias; 17 items must be reversed when scoring. Scores on each item of the Likert-scale format are summed for the total score, as well as for subscales. The possible range of scores is 37 to 185, with the larger score reflecting fewer problems after discharge. The dimensions of the instrument are Informational Needs (6 items), (Boykova, 2016a) (15 items), Parent–Child Role Development (9 items), Grief (4 items), and Social Interaction (3 items). The item readability level is the fifth grade; time to complete the tool is approximately 15 to 25 minutes. Examples of the items are (a) "I feel competent in caring for my child," (b) "I have trouble sleeping at night because I worry about my child," (c) "I believe no one really understands how I feel," (d) "The people I live with have been supportive of me," (e) "I cannot control my child's health." The development of the instrument has been described elsewhere; both the Transition Model and instrument warrant further development and validation (Boykova & Kenner, 2012).

This questionnaire was revised, updated, and tested (Boykova, 2018). Based on three studies conducted from 2012 to 2015, the items were revised, and exploratory factor analysis (principal axis factoring with oblimin rotation) on the construct of transition in parents was performed. The original version of the questionnaire was reduced to 17 items in four major dimensions, as reported by parents ($N$ = 704): *Isolation*, *Worry*, *Confidence*, and *Professional Support*. It seems that in the era of a vast amount of online resources, parental informational needs to be transformed into a more prominent (and more important for parents) need for professional support after discharge. The revised instrument demonstrated adequate psychometric characteristics (Boykova, 2018); however, the tool requires further testing and validation as well as five major factors revealed in the study.

### Transition to Primary Healthcare

The third type of transition in parents and infants in the postdischarge period is the transition to the primary healthcare settings. Continuity of care, comprehensiveness, timeliness, and appropriateness of posthospital care can influence the health of an infant and family tremendously. Often, parents have difficulties in finding primary care providers who would be experienced and knowledgeable about NICU populations' needs and risks (Toole et al., 2024).

The linkage between patient readmissions, avoidable complications, and appropriateness of postdischarge care has been well documented in the population of adult patients. The Transitional Care Model of Dr. Mary Naylor and colleagues from the University of Pennsylvania is an example of a practice model that has been proven to be effective and efficient in the population of elder/older patients with various medical conditions (Naylor et al., 2004, 2011). This model provides in-hospital planning and home follow-up for chronically ill high-risk patients, with a transitional care nurse as an assigned leader and coordinator for a multidisciplinary transitional care team of medical doctors, social workers, discharge planners, pharmacists, and other members of healthcare teams (Naylor et al., 2009). A more recent study on the transition to home in high-risk NICU infants also showed that home visits by social workers and registered nurses may reduce readmissions and thus healthcare use and medical spending (Lewis et al., 2023).

Less is known about parents of NICU infants after discharge, but evidence is growing. An online survey on parents of preterm infants ($N$ = 52; 99.9 were mothers) conducted with the help of the moderator of the blog from PreemieWorld, Deb Discenza, revealed that only 44.2% of parents participated in transitional care/follow-up programs (Boykova, 2016b). Parents often had difficulties with navigating the healthcare system, getting appointments, and finding specialists who would manage their infant's medical problems after discharge (such as pulmonologists, pediatricians, dietitians, developmental specialists, and lactation specialists). Despite the expansion of developmental and family care principles all over the world during recent decades, in this pilot study, 77.1% of parents had been separated from their infants during the hospital stay, and 41.7% could do only a small amount of caregiving while in the hospital. At least one rehospitalization after discharge occurred in 52.4% of cases. However, parents who were participating in transitional care programs were very satisfied with the provided care. And yet, attendance in follow-up programs can be a problem due to various reasons—perceived necessity to maintain participation from the parents' side, logistics, residing in rural and distant areas, financial burden, health literacy, and so forth (McCahon et al., 2023; Nantsi et al., 2024; Rosenfeld et al., 2023). One recent study showed that only 29% of eligible toddlers with complex CHD attended neurodevelopmental evaluations, with hospital-initiated scheduling being the strongest predictor of attendance (Ortinau et al., 2023). Unpreparedness for discharge, in addition to inadequate continuity of care and limited knowledge of primary healthcare providers, can be related to the overuse of services or avoidable readmissions. These findings dictate better continuity of care in the postdischarge period. Better care coordination of postdischarge services and multidisciplinary approach to the follow-up care is needed to provide support to the family unit, ease the transition to the home, and promote positive growth and development of the infant (Bouwmeester et al., 2024).

## Strategies to Help Families Postdischarge

Many interventions can alleviate a crisis for a family of a NICU or premature infant in a postdischarge period. Some approaches and strategies are described in the following section.

### Discharge Teaching and Information Giving

The NICU nurse—in the role of primary nurse, clinical nurse specialist, or neonatal nurse practitioner—can advocate for positive parental discharge. Recognizing parents' need for information about their infants and the required at-home care facilitates development of a collaborative, interdisciplinary plan of care, including discharge and follow-up. This type of collaborative plan should include the parents' demonstrating competence and comfort with routine newborn care. The nurse should ensure that the parents are completely comfortable with bathing, feeding, and diapering their infant and with administering any special care procedures, such as medication or oxygen therapy. Information given to parents about feeding patterns of preterm infants should include differences and similarities between term and preterm infants. Preterm infants often have shorter periods of sustained sucking, whether receiving feedings from the breast or bottle. Signs of adequate intake are similar for both groups: exhibiting feeding cues on a regular basis, seven to 10 feeds per 24 hours, and five to six wet diapers and two to three stools per 24 hours. If available, a board-certified lactation consultant (BCLC) should assist the mother because continued support of the breastfeeding mother is essential to decreasing the risk of early weaning. The parents also need to be taught how the NICU infant's temperament may differ from that of a healthy newborn. Parents need to be informed and reminded that even though their infant is 6 months old by chronological age, she or he may be only 3 months old by conceptional age. Thus, the infant may act more like a 3-month-old infant than like a 6-month-old infant.

Comprehensive discharge teaching has also been advocated in NICUs for a long time. Quality of discharge teaching provided by nurses is vital. Good discharge teaching includes all things mentioned earlier as well as information on infant development. Decades ago, Melnyk and coworkers have developed a specific educational-behavioral program for parents of NICU infants, the Creating Opportunities for Parent Empowerment (COPE) for the use in the hospital and postdischarge. The program consisted of audiotaped information and workbooks for parents; parents were taught about behavior and development and caring for their infant. Teaching parents occurred in four phases, the first of which started at a NICU. This program has been proven to be effective and efficient; the cost savings for healthcare systems are estimated at more than $2 billion per year if the program were routinely implemented in NICUs across the country (Melnyk et al., 2004, 2008; Melnyk & Feinstein, 2009). More recently, the COPE program was shown to produce better learning and coping in parents and improve parental self-efficacy (Hirter et al., 2024). Parenting Preemies was another program that helped parents to ease the transition to home, with educational materials, follow-up telephone calls, and home visits lasting 10 weeks (Willis, 2008). Such programs bring needed support and reassurance to parents, as well as contributing to continuity of care. Importantly, advice on financial issues, insurance coverage, and available programs is often needed, too (Discenza, 2009). Use of technology, for example, a smartphone application, may also provide support to parents of vulnerable infants, in the NICU and beyond (Chua & Shorey, 2022; Garfield et al., 2022; Phillips et al., 2024; Wagenaar et al., 2024; Yang et al., 2023).

### Communication and Continuity of Care

Parents often report that they feel supported and reassured if a professional healthcare provider, in addition to family or friends, advises them. However, many parents also express the frustration of trying to build rapport with medical and nursing staff in primary healthcare settings. Follow-up care nurses and nurse practitioners should recognize that it could be difficult to build trust and rapport with parents who have suffered and been traumatized by their infant's hospitalization and health problems. Communication is the key element to successful relationships. Nurses are expert communicators because the art of nursing has revolved around the ability to convey care and personal attention to the patient. Unfortunately, because of today's healthcare crisis, nursing shortages have resulted in staff mixes and use of unskilled personnel, coupled with economic constraints resulting in shortened hospital stays; nurses are also falling into the trap of assembly-line healthcare delivery. However, nurses have the advantage of being able to identify and assess a family's needs and to convey these needs to other healthcare team members. Being an advocate for the family is an essential part of preparing a family for discharge. Follow-up, in essence, is allowing an open line of communication among healthcare professionals, the healthcare delivery system, and the family. It allows a partnership to develop between the healthcare team and the family. It gives the family back some control. Follow-up moves the family away from the learned helplessness acquired in the hospital to a more participative role. Families who want to vent feelings and concerns often seek out nurses—as long as the family feels that the nurses care enough to be concerned. Parents need to be able to openly express their concerns without fear of being judged as "bad" parents. Nonverbal cues can get in the way of communication. The nurse's expertise, knowledge, and use of medical terminology without explanations all convey the nurse's need to be in control. Someone must be in control, but relinquishing some control to the family does not lessen one's credibility as a professional. It conveys to the family that they have a role in their infant's care and that they are important, too. Importantly, nurses also need to convey information and coordinate the data between physicians, social workers, counselors, and other members of the healthcare team who work with the family. Application of the nursing process may sound trite, but it is important in terms of not only collecting data but also using the data to identify problems, make nursing diagnoses, and develop a plan of care before and after discharge. Communication among the healthcare team members, including the parents, has a positive effect on the parents before and after discharge. Collaboration among pediatric medical follow-up, parent support or psychosocial assessments at home, and obstetrical follow-up for the mother is essential. Each healthcare professional has something to contribute to the family's overall well-being. It is essential not to compete but to work with other professionals for the good of the family. It also means that each profession must share information that it receives from the family.

### Social and Material Support

After discharge, social support from family members, relatives, and friends (informal social networks) is vital. Social support is an important aspect of coping and managing stress; if support is not provided, family functioning and health may suffer. Once the social support needs of the NICU family have been identified, a plan of action must be implemented. Helpful resources might be parent support groups, parent hotlines, referral to financial resources, or home care agencies. Balancing infant care with other demands is difficult, at best, and maternal fatigue is often a major issue that is associated with depression when the infant comes home. Acknowledgments of the mother's own physical discomfort convey a caring and supportive attitude. The caring attitude by healthcare professionals, the friendly hug, and the taking time to talk with the parents, even if it was about something other than their infant's problems, can have positive effects on parental well-being and ease their stress. The availability of a phone number and the potential for a home visit serve as additional sources of support for parents. For many parents, the home visit provides a way to vent feelings that otherwise might be suppressed around family and friends; home visits also provide needed reassurance for parents in caring. Unfortunately, with the current healthcare insurance coverage in the United States, few home visits are made, but are still available in some places and countries. In many cases, parents appreciate even a telephone call from NICU personnel.

## Screening

Another important aspect of postdischarge care could be screening for depression, PTSD, and parenting disturbances. Screening for depression, PTSD, anxiety, and stress in NICU parents has been long recommended because depression is a known risk following a high-risk birth. As described in this chapter, continued stress, feelings of failure, and grieving for the loss of the fantasy child all have the potential to lead to maternal and paternal depression. Parental anxiety and the depressive symptoms should be assessed in the postdischarge period and be part of routine follow-up care. Psychological counseling and other needed treatments should be available for parents.

## Home Care

With the shift from acute care hospitals to providing home care for infants, even technology-dependent infants, the postdischarge transitions can be even more challenging for parents than before. Some families are expected to set up a "mini" intensive care unit in the home, even providing lung ventilation or intravenous medications. There are several types of home care.

### Types of Home Care

Home care, for most practical purposes, is classified as short-term, long-term, or hospice care. Other programs involve respite care, which is relief care for parents; day care, which is at a specialized place that provides care for high-risk infants during daylight hours; and foster care, which refers to a family or individual who takes in a child to live in their house that is not their own when the birth family cannot provide care.

#### *Short-Term Care*

Short-term care is considered by many healthcare services to be < 6 months in duration. Short-term care of an infant at home may include phototherapy for hyperbilirubinemia, administration of supplemental oxygen to treat respiratory distress, home monitoring for apnea of the premature infant, medication administration for various neonatal conditions, and alternative feeding methods such as gavage for nutritional support. The primary caregivers in the home usually attend to these treatment modalities. Parents and families are carefully instructed about the use of any equipment placed in the home to administer healthcare. Extensive teaching before hospital discharge must convey the precise reasons for the therapy, the necessity for close observation of the infant by the caregivers, and the importance of communication and supervision by the primary care physician. In situations of short-term home care, the condition is usually self-limiting, and the home therapy can be discontinued at a predetermined endpoint.

#### *Long-Term Care*

The point at which care becomes long term is determined by the nature of the healthcare needs of the individual. The providers of extended care and the insurers paying for the care also arbitrarily set the period for long-term care. In general, long-term care indicates that the duration of the condition and the need for care will exceed 6 months. Long-term home care addresses situations for children with disease processes such as BPD, short bowel or short gut syndrome, CHD, physical and cosmetic defects, neurologic and metabolic disorders, and numerous other prolonged pathologic conditions. On discharge, these children may require home care services performed by professional home care agencies or programs. Families gradually become integrated into the healthcare routine. The family's responsibility changes as the infant's condition changes. The primary care physician must be closely involved and should be able to rely comfortably on the caregiver's judgment for making assessments and alterations in the home care plan. Long-term home care requires open communication among the family, community physicians, tertiary resources, community healthcare providers, home medical equipment providers, and financial providers. Many hospital records are now incorporating discharge notes, especially nursing case management notes or orders for the actual discharge and home care follow-up plan. These notes are a good vehicle for communication among the community healthcare providers and the discharging hospital.

#### *Hospice Care*

Congenital anomalies are the leading cause of infant mortality in the United States and are also a major contributor to childhood morbidity, long-term disability, and loss of years of potential life. The proportion of infant deaths attributed to birth defects has remained significantly high. The HIV epidemic is improving, but it still takes its toll on the neonatal population. Those infants require specialized home care and, in some instances, palliative care. In addition, with technological advances, the ability to prolong lives has increased. Infants who are born dying do go home, where they need end-of-life (EOL) or palliative care, the care concepts that still require improvement in the neonatal field. When it becomes clear that an infant will no longer benefit from acute intervention, plans for healthcare should focus on physical and emotional comfort. The transition from acute care to palliative care involves the concept of hospice. Hospice care is a philosophy of caring when cure is no longer a reasonable expectation. This care is not strictly a kind of terminal care, but rather an effort to maximize current quality of life without giving up all interest in a cure. Hospice provides comfort measures and emphasizes alleviation of symptoms. Whether the infant is terminally or chronically ill, the goal is to provide an environment that comforts the child and supports the family.

## Criteria for Home Care

Some hospitals throughout the country are developing specialized outreach and home care services as an extension of their inpatient services. Regardless of how services are to be provided, the decision to facilitate early discharge from hospital care to home care must be based on standards that are safe and that provide effective ongoing therapy. The infant, the family, the home equipment must meet criteria for discharge to home care.

### Infant Criteria

The infant's home healthcare needs must be assessed as to technical feasibility and medical requirements. Nutritional support must be evaluated. How does the infant feed and how frequently? How often does the infant require gavage feedings and which feeding techniques are required? Pharmacologic support assessment must be evaluated. What medication does the infant need and how often? What are the desired and adverse effects of these drugs? Does the infant require supplemental oxygen, respiratory therapy treatments, or chest physical therapy? The assessment of the level of care required must be matched to the ability and skills of the home care providers. It must be determined before discharge so that care in the home will be safe and meet the needs of the infant and family.

The specific criteria for discharge of special groups of children—such as those with BPD,short bowel or short gut syndrome, neurologic disease, cardiac disease, and other pathologic conditions—are addressed in the preceding chapters.

### Family Criteria

The assessment of the family's commitment to home care is perhaps the most critical factor determining the success or failure of home healthcare. After extensive discharge teaching, skills development, and repeated occasions of caregiving, the family must want the child at home and under their care. They must be willing and able to devote the time and energy required to meet the physical and emotional needs of the child. These factors are essential for the well-being of the family unit. To prepare families for the discharge of their sick or high-risk infant, NICU personnel must begin teaching them as soon as the neonate is admitted to the unit. Once the family is confident and capable of meeting the needs of the infant, a home assessment should be completed. Basic facilities such as heat, water, telephone, electricity, and transportation must be available. Appropriate support systems must be set up in the home, including the technology necessary for the delivery of care. The operation of phototherapy lights or blankets, oxygen delivery systems, portable suction equipment, respiratory and cardiac monitoring systems, ventilators, and numerous other devices must be thoroughly understood by the caregivers. Clear instructions need to be given to the family members by the providers of the home care technology. Ideally, the parents should bring the equipment to the hospital, or the equipment company can help transport it to the hospital before discharge. The rationale is that the parents can be taught on their own equipment. If a problem arises, it can usually be identified before the infant's discharge. The parents should spend at least 24 hours providing total care before discharge. This time under a health professional's supervision helps the family gain confidence in their caregiving abilities. They can also be reassured that they have the proper equipment.

### Home Equipment Criteria

The most common equipment needs for neonates are cardiopulmonary monitoring, oxygen, suction, and feeding implements. The family's first decision is how to select a home care equipment company. Hospital discharge planners or the nurse responsible for the discharge can make recommendations. Once the supplier has been selected and the necessary equipment identified, parent education can begin, including neonatal cardiopulmonary resuscitation (CPR). The parents should be given written instructions to take home and a checklist for the CPR procedure that can be clearly posted. If the parents cannot read, visual charts outlining the steps should be made available.

A cardiopulmonary monitor is the most common equipment needed in the home. Infants who should be placed on this type of monitoring are those whose sibling died of sudden infant death syndrome (SIDS) or who are at risk for SIDS, such as premature infants. These infants are usually monitored for several months. An infant on home oxygen or one who has neurologic impairment is at risk for apneic or bradycardic episodes or desaturation, thus requiring pulse oximetry. Most of the cardiopulmonary monitors have built-in memory or pneumographic capabilities that allow trends and strips to be viewed by home care nurses. Often, parents struggle with alarm limits and sounds, so appropriate teaching should be done before discharge. Online educational modules might be effective and improve parental knowledge on SIDS and promote change in parental behavior. Parents need to understand alarm delays or oversensitivity, when to change probes, and how to respond.

If parents have an infant who requires home respiratory support, the family will need a ventilator, with oxygen and air tanks. An air compressor and oxygen concentrator may also be needed. Portable or stationary oxygen devices vary in size and the amount of time that they will last. Humidification and suctioning equipment are needed for patients with ventilation support or tracheostomies. Parents should be taught how to perform suctioning, how often, and how to adjust suction when an illness occurs that may put the infant at risk for cross-contamination. Suctioning should be performed according to individual needs of a patient and to the physician or nurse practitioner's orders. Signs that indicate the need for suctioning are the same as those used by health professionals in the NICU: restlessness, decreased color, coughing, increased respiratory effort, or sounds of congestion. Humidification of the airway is necessary for infants with artificial airways, regardless of whether they are on oxygen. If the airway is not humidified, mucous membranes may dry and crack, creating areas that may become infected.

These examples of home care and monitoring are the most common. Specific instructions are needed regarding which equipment is necessary and how to use it in each situation; the equipment should be obtained from the home healthcare agency that is to provide care, the hospital equipment vendors, and the home healthcare equipment vendors. Information on home use of ventilators can be obtained from the Home Mechanical Ventilation Resource Center of the American College of Chest Physicians (www.chestnet.org). If parents are primary caregivers, they should keep a log of the timing of the suctioning and the type of secretions obtained. The time of medication administration and feedings also should be recorded. An emergency backup unit must be available—whether it is housed in the home or at immediate dispatch from the equipment company does not matter, as long as it is available for times when equipment failures occur with the portable device. Battery backup is also necessary. Ideally, the nurse should make a home visit before the discharge to assess the home environment for safety hazards. For example, is the house/apartment too hot or cold? Either condition can lead to apneic spells. Are there exposed wires in the house? Peeling paint? Open flames used for cooking when oxygen is going to be used in the house? Are there any strong or chemical odors that may be harmful to a child with respiratory compromise?

Is there an emergency phone? Have utility companies been notified? Is there a backup plan in case of a power outage? Is there a plan for continued health promotion, such as immunizations? All aspects of the home and the community setting should be considered when discharging the infant and family.

## SUMMARY

Postdischarge care is vital for an infant and family, and no less so than intensive care provided in the hospital. Former NICU infants may experience numerous health problems and may have numerous healthcare needs. Parents are in need as well. The crisis of hospitalization and discharge has no time limit because it is so individual. Three major transitions can be identified in parents of former NICU and preterm infants: transition to parenthood, transition to home, and transition to primary healthcare settings; all transitions can bring challenges to the infant and family. Parental role alteration, anxiety, depression, and an increased need for professional and social supports are tremendous. Medical follow-up of NICU infants as well as helping parents to deal with postdischarge challenges are vital to promote infant health, development, and family well-being. The outcome of transition (i.e., readmissions, health status of the infant, and parenting style disturbances) will depend on whether resources are available to support the individuals undergoing postdischarge challenges and may influence the whole lifespan of the infant and family. Application of the interventions as close to the time of the discharge as possible is vital. The crisis of neonatal hospitalization and difficulties in caregiving and parenting of an initially sick or small infant can be alleviated by appropriate interventions and strategies. These are appropriate discharge teaching, parental participation in transitional care programs, adequacy and timeliness of follow-up, access and attendance to transitional programs and follow-up, provision of timely and appropriate resources for family and infant, continuity and coordination of care, case management, and access to home care, to name a few. Close collaboration and open communication between healthcare providers and family is required, as well as informational and technical assistance. The absence of these can lead to a less than optimal environment for the infant and child to grow.

## KENNER TRANSITION MODEL AND THE TECHNOLOGY-DEPENDENT INFANT: A CASE STUDY

This case study applies the Kenner Transition Model to the care of a technology-dependent infant.

In recent years, the number of technology-dependent infants discharged home has increased, because of the many early discharge programs available and the survival of ELBW infants with chronic conditions. Although a fair amount has been written about setting up early discharge programs and the positive financial rewards associated with early discharge, little research is available to look at the effects of having a technology-dependent infant at home.

Spangler-Torok (2001) studied mothers receiving and caring for their technology-dependent infants in the home and applied the concepts of transition to this unique population. The experiential descriptions were from eight mothers, aged 17 to 42, who were the primary caretakers of their technology-dependent infants. All the mothers were interviewed within the first 4 weeks of receiving their infant into the home. Although this was a phenomenologic study, it provides support for the concepts of the Kenner Transition Model (Spangler-Torok, 2001).

**Information Needs.** Mothers in this study understood the need to learn about care and equipment so that the infant could be discharged. Mothers described moving from learning care to making judgments regarding the infant's health. Gathering information is a way of seeking control of the situation. The mothers in this study sought information to make an overwhelming experience more manageable. The mothers described their initial fear of caring for the infant at home and their ability to move beyond the fear and do what needed to be done. As more information was gathered, mothers described using their judgment in making infant health decisions. When receiving and caring for a technology-dependent infant in the home, more information seems to give mothers more control, confidence, and peace of mind.

**Grief.** The mothers in this study feared the infant becoming ill and requiring rehospitalization. Several of the mothers voiced concern that the infant might die. Mothers grieved over the loss of the "ideal" pregnancy and infant. Mothers would report that they were managing the home care experience, "but this is not what I planned for." Mothers grieved about the life their infants would have and vowed to give them "as normal a life as possible." Mothers worried about what others would think: "Will they think it was something I did while I was pregnant that caused this to happen to the infant?" Mothers felt the need to "warn" others that the infant was different before they approached the infant.

**Parent–Child Role Development.** Once they were at home, mothers in this study believed that they were getting to know their infants and that their infants were getting to know them as their mothers. Mothers reported learning things about their infants that they did not know until they were home, such as when their fussy times were. Mothers believed that as they learned more about infant preferences and health-related behaviors, they were able to make appropriate adjustments to infant care. Regardless of whether they had other children, the mothers saw a need to adjust the parenting role and expectation to accommodate the premature infant. They realized that this infant was different and required special care—in some instances, more vigilant care. They discussed how the increased needs of this infant took time away from other children and spouses, but acknowledged that being home was easier than extended hospital visits. Most of the mothers in this study quit their jobs or school to care for the infant, which they would not have planned to do if the infant had been healthy. The mothers discussed lifestyle changes since the infant came home from the hospital, such as decreased number of outings, staying indoors more, and limiting visitors to the home.

**Stress and Coping.** Mothers in this study acknowledged that receiving and caring for a technology-dependent infant in the home is a lot of work. One mother stated it is "a ton of work ... 10 times more work than a normal infant." Mothers report that more time is needed with infant care as well as with supplemental tasks, such as dealing with insurance companies, managing supplies, and checking equipment. A lot of time is required to prepare the infant for outings, and time is needed for the infant to readjust to home after outings. Mothers reported problems with infant digestion and temperament when away from home. "She may require 2 or 3 days to recover from an outing to the doctor's office." All of the mothers described the extra work and time the infant required, but most felt it was worth it to have the infant home with them. This initial anxiety decreases as the infant's respiratory status improves and the infant becomes less dependent on oxygen therapy.

Two mothers described being overwhelmed with infant care in the home and felt they faced too many demands. One mother felt torn between caring for the infant and spending time with her other children. She was "only one person" and could "only be in one place at a time." She appreciated the break the home nurses provided but felt guilty that her infant received care from others. Another mother described frustration in dealing with the equipment. She had a "hard time looking" at the feeding tube but was less bothered by the tracheotomy. She got angry when her husband gravitated toward Holly, the "normal" twin, and left all the work for Grace to her. This mother was afraid that her infant would pick up on her frustration with the equipment and feel that she did not love her.

**Social Interaction.** Several mothers in this study attributed their ability to care for this infant at home to the support of family and friends. Mothers stated they could focus on infant care because others were handling household chores and running errands for them. One mother described how strangers who heard of their situation were delivering food to them. The same mother felt that their experience was probably easier than others because "so many people have pitched in to do things." In describing her experience, one mother stated, "We just needed a lot of family." Having people come and help seemed to make the experience more manageable for some of the mothers. One mother described being supported by the home care nurses. "It's wonderful to have the nursing staff here, because when you want to break down and cry, they're there to tell you, rub your hand, or your shoulder and say, 'you're doing a good job, don't think that you're not; you are'." She was thankful for them and used the nurses for other things so that she could spend time with the infant.

Although some mothers spoke of the assistance they received, others described the lack of support from family and friends. A mother spoke of being "annoyed" with her husband. She discussed how supportive they were of each other during their infant's hospitalization and that she had assumed that would continue once they were home. She was disappointed by her husband's lack of support and assistance with infant care and home management. "Hey, we have special circumstances here, this isn't just your average baby, and you need to help me," she said. Another mother described a lack of support from her husband, children, and friends. She said her husband helped with the cooking, but it took her three times as long to clean up. Although her 12-year-old daughter was old enough to help, she did not. She also wondered why friends had not come to see her. She believed they were afraid to see the infant and, therefore, did not visit. She sometimes felt alone in her responsibility for the infant.

The experiences of the mothers caring for infants who require technology support lend credence to the Kenner Transition Model. The mothers reported a need for information, grieved for the loss of the healthy child, and found they needed to adjust their parenting roles. They felt stressed and overwhelmed. These are all concepts in the Kenner Model. Other studies report similar findings.

## EVIDENCE-BASED PRACTICE

For more than 30 years, issues around the transition home, discharge coordination, and follow-up care have been researched. The reality is that for parents of a premature or sick newborn, life changes with a NICU stay. The discharge, while anticipated, is not easy. The transition to home—even with follow-up appointments and programs in place and written discharge instructions given—is not easy for most families. There is fear that the infant will become sick again; fear that the infant might die; and fear that the health professionals in primary care or the community will not know what to do the way NICU professionals do. Social and professional support needs are high. Published research studies continue to support the need for more research in the area of transition from hospital to home and the need for a clearer understanding of the actual and needed follow-up approaches, including adherence to suggested follow-up visits and programs (Bouwmeester et al., 2024; Boykova, 2018; DiBari & Rouse, 2023; Klein & McDonald, 2024; Postier et al., 2024; Spence et al., 2023). One or more of these themes have been reported in transition research studies for more than three decades. In light of healthcare reform and the emphasis on health promotion, the time is right to use this evidence to create better follow-up programs and improve postdischarge care.

### References

Bouwmeester, D., Anolda Naber, F. B., Heyman, H., Hoffmann-Haringsma, A., Lens, A., & Brunt, T. M. (2024). Follow-up care and support to parents of premature children: Multidisciplinary versus regular follow-up care. *Child: Care, Health and Development*, *50*(1), e13185. https://doi.org/10.1111/cch.13185

(*continued*)

## EVIDENCE-BASED PRACTICE (*continued*)

Boykova, M. (2018). Transition from hospital to home in parents of preterm infants: Revision, modification, and psychometric testing of the questionnaire. *Journal of Nursing Measurement*, *26*(2), 296–310. https://doi.org/10.1891/1061-3749.26.2.296

DiBari, J. N., & Rouse, L. (2023). Parent perspectives: Part 2—Considerations for the transition home post-NICU discharge. *Children*, *10*(12), 1835. https://www.mdpi.com/2227-9067/10/12/1835

Klein, C. C., & McDonald, N. M. (2024). Parenting stress following a neonatal intensive care unit hospitalization: A longitudinal study of mothers and fathers. *International Journal of Environmental Research and Public Health*, *21*(8), 970. https://doi.org/10.3390/ijerph21080970

Postier, A. C., Foster, L. P., Remke, S., Simpson, J., Friedrichsdorf, S. J., & Brearley, S. G. (2024). Predictors of improvement in parental stress after the first three months at home with a medically fragile infant. *Maternal & Child Health Journal*, *28*(2), 303–314. https://doi.org/10.1007/s10995-023-03827-w

Spence, C. M., Stuyvenberg, C. L., Kane, A. E., Burnsed, J., & Dusing, S. C. (2023). Parent experiences in the NICU and transition to home. *International Journal of Environmental Research and Public Health*, *20*(11), 6050. https://doi.org/10.3390/ijerph20116050

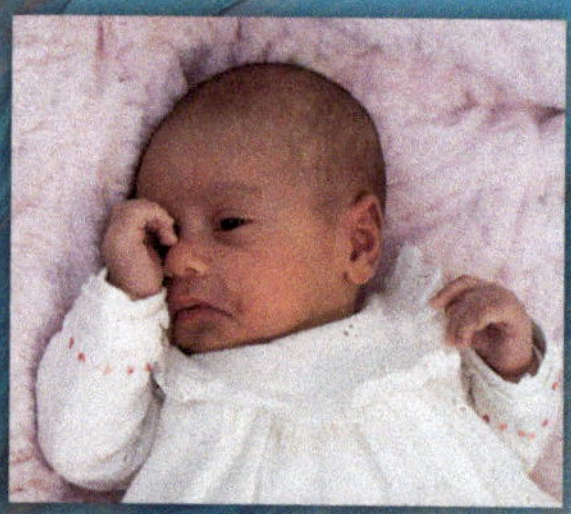

*Source:* lotharnahler/Adobe Stock.

## PARENT VOICES

### Deborah A. Discenza

**I always tell my families that they should rely on their parent instincts. If something does not seem right with their child, they should absolutely check out the problem with the pediatrician, or with a specialist. Early identification can mean a dramatic change in their child's outcomes and identifiable supports when it comes to developmental delays and diagnosed disabilities. Yet as a parent of a 30-week premature infant girl now 15 years old, I can honestly say that the parent instinct is truly the common denominator among all of the specialties outside the NICU. The parent is the expert of his or her child starting from conception. They notice tiny but crucial nuances where others would assume no general concern mainly because of their continued presence in that child's life throughout every day. And they carry the knowledge with them from doctor to doctor even when the communication between specialists is used.**

**I know this all too well having watched my own daughter's progression from NICU to home and into the school years being challenging at best. Even despite my best efforts to vocalize thoughts while partnering with the pediatrician and with the specialists at hand, no one saw what I saw very early on—concerns about CP. At various points throughout my daughter's childhood and early adolescence, I sought out help for her increasingly complicated walk, her difficulty with running. This is a child who went through EI, through therapies for other conditions along the way (autism, attention deficit-hyperactivity disorder [ADHD], motor coordination). It was the orthopedic surgeon who fitted my daughter for orthotics (for the "squishy ankles" I noticed as my daughter trained on an elliptical machine) that finally listened and contemplated my concerns. Two years later, at the same practice, despite my assuming that they weren't going to diagnose her, they did. My daughter was 13.5 years old and, while mild, had spasticity and was really struggling. I felt let down by the medical and therapeutic systems in place.**

**If I as a mother with strong advocacy skills could not get my daughter's diagnosis in place until 13.5 years old, imagine how many families are out there with less capability and no diagnosis. Outcomes data are dependent on many factors, and it should include parents' and, at one point, the patient's own reporting to help drive better information, better advocacy, and proper diagnoses.**

## ONLINE RESOURCES

CourseConnect

Resources for this chapter are online and available at www.springerpub.com/courseconnect.

## REFERENCES

References for this chapter are online and available at www.springerpub.com/courseconnect.

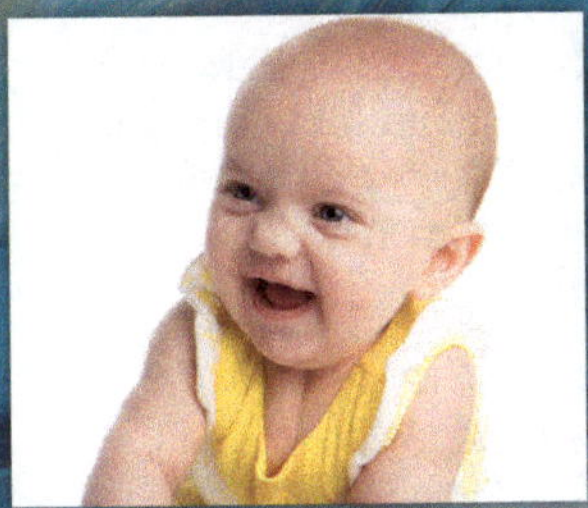

Source: Benjamin Simeneta/Adobe Stock.

CHAPTER 29

# Palliative and End-of-Life Care

Jennifer M. Burford and Monica Muir

## INTRODUCTION

While the neonatal intensive care unit (NICU) is often a place where the most advanced medical technologies are aggressively employed daily to ensure the survival of the most fragile infants, it is important to recognize the human beings that exist at the center of this advanced care and that not all outcomes are what is desired. Not every NICU journey is smooth or without grief, and deaths do occur in the NICU. All families facing the uncertainty of a prolonged NICU course deserve the opportunity to receive specialized care to help them navigate and process this often difficult journey. This specialized care frequently comes in the form of highly skilled palliative care. Palliative care specialists help families navigate difficult decisions and turning points in the NICU journey and assist with end-of-life (EOL) care planning and implementation if such services are required. This chapter will focus on specialized care for infants and their families in the NICU facing life-altering or life-limiting conditions that can ultimately lead to death during the perinatal period.

## DESCRIPTION OF PALLIATIVE CARE

Pediatric Palliative Care is a full spectrum of care designed to support patients and families with complex, life-altering, and life-limiting illnesses or diagnoses. The approach to implementing Pediatric Palliative Care includes comprehensive, holistic care to address patients' and their caregivers' physical, mental, emotional, spiritual, and psychosocial needs. While the primary tenant of palliative care supports a patient's needs as an individual, another primary facet includes pain and symptom management. Pediatric Palliative Care "is the art and science of patient and family-centered care, aimed at evaluating and minimizing suffering in all domains (physical, psychosocial, and spiritual), promoting shared decision-making, and coordinating the care of all children with life-threatening conditions as well as their families" (Verhagen, 2024, p. 119). Overall, palliative care focuses on ensuring patient comfort and providing psychosocial and spiritual support, all while supporting the family and honoring the individual values and needs of both the infant and the family (Sieg et al., 2018). The essential concepts for delivering quality palliative care include compassion, commitment to providing palliative care, dignity, integrity, respect, open communication, parental decision making, and teamwork (Sieg et al., 2018). "It is important for palliative care to be seen as a standard of care and not as an additional service that may or may not be offered when an infant is diagnosed with a life-altering or life-limiting condition" (Sieg et al., 2018, p. E10).

Palliative care is a benchmark for holistic, patient-centered care. This holistic approach led the American Academy of Pediatrics (AAP) to establish five principles of palliative care: (a) respect for the dignity of patients and families, (b) access to competent and compassionate palliative care, (c) support for the caregivers, (d) improved professional and social support for pediatric palliative care, and (e) continued improvement of pediatric palliative care through research and education. A section on Hospice and Palliative Medicine within the AAP is updated regularly. This section upholds the AAP (2000, 2025) guidelines and reinforces the need to enhance the child's and family's quality of life. It also stresses care coordination and a team approach while carrying out the five previously listed principles of care (Linebarger et al., 2022).

The Institute of Medicine also identified five core competencies that guide patient care. These are patient-centered care, interdisciplinary teams, evidence-based medicine, quality improvement, and information technology (Greiner & Knebel, 2003). All these competencies are relevant to palliative care because it is patient and family focused and requires an integrated interprofessional team approach to provide quality care.

### Access to Competent and Compassionate Palliative Care

Compassionate neonatal palliative care extends beyond the prescription or administration of medications to encompass holistic support for the infant, family, and healthcare team throughout the journey of life-limiting illness or end-of-life care (Sieg et al., 2018). While pain and symptom management includes alleviation of physical pain and other symptoms, it also includes alleviation of mental, emotional, and spiritual pain by providing families with access to supportive therapies, such as grief counseling and spiritual support. This principle can also include the provision of adequate respite care for parents when available (AAP, 2000; Goldman et al., 2012). This all translates to the idea that newborns should be respected as human beings and comfort ensured through family-centered care (Kim et al., 2024).

## EMPOWERING PARENTS AND GUARDIANS

It can be daunting for parents to know how to care for seriously ill children, especially in the NICU setting. Mullins et al. (2012) conducted a study funded by the National Institute for Nursing Research (NINR; 1 R21 NR010103-01A1) that examined the needs of parents of children newly diagnosed with cancer. Findings supported the parents' need for clear messages from the healthcare team and information to support positive coping and decrease stress (Mullins et al., 2012). The healthcare team's job is to empower parents to participate actively in their child's care. In the NICU, parents should be supported and encouraged to care for their infants. Before their direct involvement, they must be provided with sufficient information about the uncertainties ahead, what their role will involve, and how they can meaningfully participate in their infant's care. It is also essential to acknowledge and respect the social, cultural, religious, and personal diversity of each family (Kim et al., 2024)." Regular meetings between providers and parents must occur so that parental needs can be acutely identified, parents can be permitted to participate optimally, and cultural and religious beliefs can be followed and respected (Sieg et al., 2018). It is often emphasized that parents should have the opportunity to create meaningful memories throughout the NICU stay, especially when infant survival is uncertain or death is expected (Sieg et al., 2018). The desire for these opportunities should be explored on an ongoing basis. Furthermore, providing emotional support through a multidisciplinary approach is crucial. It is essential to consider the physical and emotional vulnerability of both the neonate and the parents during the postpartum period (Kim et al., 2024).

### Improved Professional Support for Pediatric Palliative Care

Many barriers can prevent families from obtaining pediatric palliative care, and healthcare professionals are burdened with helping families overcome these obstacles (AAP, 2000). This can lead to burnout, moral distress, compassion fatigue, and decreased job satisfaction. There is an ongoing need to provide adequate education and comprehensive physical and mental health support to medical staff, including nurses, to enable the delivery of high-quality palliative care (Kim et al., 2024). The AAP recognizes the importance of supporting healthcare professionals involved in the care of seriously ill children. This support may include paid funeral leave, peer counseling, or remembrance ceremonies (AAP, 2000). "Mindfulness training programs that strengthen nurses' resilience and self-compassion" can help minimize compassion fatigue (Gibson et al., 2018, p. 472). There is a need for the support of nurses when caring for these patients and an acknowledgment that it is difficult (Gibson et al., 2018).

## PALLIATIVE CARE NATIONALLY AND GLOBALLY

Palliative care is a global issue, especially in the pediatric population. In 2016, the National Institutes of Health (NIH) estimated that there were 21 million children annually in the world who require palliative care (Connor et al., 2016). These numbers will likely continue to expand as medical technologies allow infants and children with complex medical needs to survive much longer than historically predicted. These children and families would undoubtedly benefit from longitudinal care that is holistic, patient centered, and focused primarily on improving and sustaining quality of life (Lenington et al., 2024). Early palliative care involvement provides for the opportunity to support these families through the course of their child's illness or condition, and, ideally, that longitudinal care that helps their child live life to their fullest potential and has availability of a trusted care team if or when their child's condition progresses. They require complex medical decisions to be made or need EOL care. The key benefit of early palliative care involvement in these settings is that goals of care can be established, and discussions regarding limitations of care can take place prior to an urgent or emergent situation that requires decisions to be made under duress. Tan et al. (2012) found that "anticipatory support initiated prior to the death of an infant can help parents experience a smoother transition from caring for their ill infant to coping with the actual death and aftermath" (p. 579). The death of an infant "disrupts the natural order of events as most parents" do not expect to outlive their children, and pediatric palliative care can help parents find a balance between bonding with their infant and processing their anticipatory grief (Sieg et al., 2018, p. E11). A study of childhood deaths in Canadian hospitals found that the acuity of care was high before death and that most of the decisions about EOL issues were made very close to the actual time of death (McCallum et al., 2000). In that study, most of the children were intubated at death (73%), and most died in the intensive care unit (ICU; 83%); this is a trend that remains largely unchanged today. In the United States, most pediatric deaths also occur in hospital ICUs (Kerr, 2001), and there is evidence that children often suffer needlessly before death (Wolfe et al., 2000). According to the Centers for Disease Control and Prevention (CDC), the infant mortality rate in the United States in 2023 was 5.61 deaths per 1,000 births (CDC, 2024). These figures have implications for neonatal care because many infants in the NICU frequently die while still intubated and connected to various pieces of equipment.

Fortunately, some progress has been made in creating consensus recommendations, policies, and procedures (Carter et al., 2004) regarding pediatric palliative care. Books are available to guide the practitioner in working with children and their families with life-altering and life-limiting illnesses (Carter et al., 2011). Catlin and Carter (2002) developed a palliative care protocol that has assisted many perinatal and neonatal centers in developing policies to help with EOL and palliative care issues. Rogers et al. (2008) developed an education program to address the problems of moral distress in NICU nurses. In 2010, the National Association of Neonatal Nurses (NANN, 2016) published a position statement, "NICU Nurse Involvement in Ethical Decisions (Treatment of Critically Ill Newborns)."

Additionally, NANN (2015), in their 2015 position statement "Palliative and EOL Care for Newborns and Infants," Kenner et al. (2015) and the AAP (Linebarger et al., 2022) have recommended practices for neonatal palliative care. Despite all of these resources available to health professionals, many providers remain uncomfortable discussing palliative care with families because their focus has always been on saving lives (Kenner et al., 2015). Frequently, they worry that discussing adverse outcomes might destroy hope or diminish therapeutic relationships. As a result, "palliative care is still an option often offered too late and rarely delivered in an integrated approach" (Kenner et al., 2015, p. S10). Often, many disciplines offer advice, unaware of what has already been conveyed to parents (Kenner et al., 2015), proving that care for critically ill pediatric patients remains poorly coordinated, with a failure to approach the patient holistically and in a way that incorporates the big picture. Cortezzo et al. (2013) found that palliative care education was deemed essential and needed among healthcare providers and discovered that barriers included emotional difficulties, staff disagreements, and difficulty forming palliative care teams. Cortezzo et al. (2013) further reported that when palliative care teams or staff bereavement groups were willing and able to initiate palliative care or bereavement support, it led to more positive views or experiences among healthcare providers. They recommended that further exploration of differing views of palliative care among interdisciplinary teams is needed. A study that implemented a quality-of-life program to evaluate moral distress in healthcare providers found that after implementing the Pediatric Quality of Life Program, nurses and other providers encountered morally distressing situations less often (Brandon et al., 2014). The researchers further discovered that providers felt they had greater comfort with, and competence in, providing care focused on patients' quality of life after completing the program. Brandon et al. (2014) recommended that because most "palliative care programs include many activities that reduce moral distress, nurses should actively participate in debriefing sessions and staff education to maximize their work quality of life" (p. 189). Nurses who work in a NICU with a Neonatal Palliative Care policy and who have received palliative care education demonstrated more favorable attitudes toward neonatal palliative care. Policy and educational programs are essential strategies to promote high-quality care for high-risk infants and their families (Chin et al., 2021).

Regardless of the setting, the goal should be to provide family-centered perinatal and neonatal palliative care and support to families experiencing anticipated or unanticipated life-altering/life-limiting conditions or death of their infant (Kenner et al., 2015). Wolfe (2000) identified the "principle of family" in pediatric care: an obligation to treat the whole family. Wolfe (2000) emphasized that healthcare staff have an ethical obligation to pursue comfort aggressively and to fully involve parents in the decision-making process regarding their child's care.

Conversations regarding goals of care need to be had early and revisited often for families with critically ill infants in the NICU, and palliative care teams are uniquely poised to have these conversations effectively. The interprofessional teams can then be fully informed of the parents' choices so that care can be coordinated, and the family's wishes can be fulfilled (Kenner et al., 2015). Additionally, perinatal loss needs to be acknowledged as a unique type of grief that requires specialized bereavement care. "Advances in genetics and technology enable many families to know well in advance that their fetus has a potentially life-limiting condition" (Kenner et al., 2015, p. S20). In either anticipated or unanticipated diagnosis, efforts should be made to include families as part of the decision making.

## INCORPORATING PEDIATRIC PALLIATIVE CARE INTO THE NICU

It is important to note that palliative care is not synonymous with EOL care, and this is especially true in the NICU. Care for dying patients is often a very small part of the broad spectrum of support that palliative care provides to families. Key to this recognition is that the clinical course for critically ill infants in the NICU is often unpredictable, and there will likely be many junctures in an infant's hospitalization that call for complex decision making or increased support for families and caregivers. The establishment of a trusted provider–family relationship is vital to allowing palliative care teams to fully support families through these more difficult moments in their child's NICU journey. The AAP recommends that palliative care begins at the time of diagnosis or identification of a life-altering, life-threatening, or terminal condition (AAP, 2000). In the NICU, particularly for extremely premature neonates and for neonates with life-threatening anomalies, palliative care should begin at the time of admission. During the early diagnostic phase, palliative care can and should be provided along with advanced technologic care; this arrangement allows the staff to focus on symptom management and pain control while weighing the benefits and harm of aggressive treatments and interventions. It also provides a space for interdisciplinary team members to engage with the family and support their needs from a holistic standpoint. "Therefore, when choosing the appropriate medical intervention or planning care, it is necessary to consider not only the potential clinical outcomes but also the emotional and psychological consequences to the infant and family" (Sieg et al., 2018, p. E10).

## END-OF-LIFE CARE IN THE NICU

New approaches must be taken to establish compassionate EOL care for all infants in the NICU. This challenge is intensified in a system where healthcare professionals are oriented toward active intervention with technological devices rather than accepting death (Jecker & Pagon, 1995; Kenner & Boykova, 2010). Death should not necessarily be viewed as "failure" but rather a natural part of life, and even in the most distressing and heartbreaking of situations, such as the death of an infant in the NICU, comprehensive EOL care should not be delayed or avoided simply because the circumstances are particularly distressing or uncomfortable.

Often, when a neonate is born at the edge of viability, the clinical course rarely follows a purely optimistic path. The neonate's physiologic parameters can cause concern as evidence mounts that organ systems are failing. This scenario represents the inevitable point at which intensive efforts to prolong life merely serve to prolong the infant's death. In such cases, infants and their families would benefit from a smooth transition to an intensive comfort-focused rather than survival-focused approach. This requires a level of care that is not always present in the NICU. Care providers must quickly recognize the futility of sustained therapies and be experts at providing palliative care to infants and families (Gibson et al., 2018). Unfortunately, all too often, infants and children die while still intubated (McCallum et al., 2000), with pain inadequately controlled (Kenner & Boykova, 2010), and no palliative care support. NANN, the Association of Pediatric Oncology Nurses (APON), and the Society of Pediatric Nurses (SPN) have stated that this area of neonatal care is very important. National leaders in pediatric palliative care have developed guidelines for healthcare providers that incorporate recommendations for how pediatric EOL care is approached and delivered. They have also developed recommendations on appropriate language use for cases where an infant is "born dying" or is not expected to survive and ways to support the unique needs of families in such cases (https://caringcommunity.org/topics/resources/children-pediatrics/). The development of such guidelines stands as an important milestone in efforts to recognize that neonatal and pediatric patients and their families deserve the same level of care that adults receive.

Palliative care options for neonates are necessary because neonates have the highest death rate in the pediatric population (Kiman & Doumic, 2014). Palliative care can be delivered within the NICU or special care unit, an ambulatory care center in the community, or the home. Despite the reality that very few pediatric hospice groups exist and fewer for neonates and families, Catlin found that many infants stay 6 months or longer in the hospital, with 20% of the NICU infants transferred to the pediatric intensive care unit (PICU) to die, even when care is deemed futile (as cited in Thaxton et al., 2016).

## Ethical Obligation to Provide Optimum End-of-Life Care

It can be argued that all healthcare team members have an ethical obligation to plan and implement EOL care; to always provide highly skilled care, *except* at the EOL, is to ignore the essence of comprehensive healthcare. The ethical dimensions of neonatal EOL care include an obligation to provide compassionate care, autonomy, and beneficent and nonmaleficent care. This is especially true regarding infant pain, respecting family values in the provision of treatment options, justice in ensuring equitable access to care and resources, dignity in being treated with respect and honor, and truthfulness and honesty in providing information in a gentle, sensitive, and compassionate manner (Thaxton et al., 2016).

## Cultural Influences

Variations in how children with life-threatening illnesses are treated are sometimes linked to cultural values and beliefs around the concepts of disability and death. To provide culturally competent care, the nurse must be sensitive to cultural, ethnic, and religious values and must adapt and individualize care (Thaxton et al., 2016). Families should be provided with memory-making options and asked if a ritual is important to their cultural or belief system (Kenner et al., 2015). Footprints, handprints, a lock of hair, a receiving blanket, heartbeat recordings, and special keepsake boxes are examples of mementos related to the baby's hospital stay and provide parents with options for remembering their baby. However, some cultures may not accept these options (Kenner et al., 2015). Photographs provide visual proof of the reality of their baby's life and can be valuable in the mourning process (Kenner et al., 2015). "Dressing the baby is important, so the family has a photo or mental picture of their baby and not one that is naked connected to tubes and wires" (Kenner et al., 2015, p. S21). Clothing can include items of cultural or spiritual significance. Community spiritual and cultural leaders should be permitted to be present at the request of parents to support parents and perform specific cultural practices as appropriate. Parents should also be offered peer-to-peer support or referred to a regional or national parent support organization if there are no regional functioning peer support programs (Kenner et al., 2015).

## Obligation to Provide Beneficent Care

The widely accepted ethical principle of beneficence requires that healthcare professionals actively provide care that benefits their patients. As defined by Beauchamp and Childress (2001), the principle of beneficence encompasses both positive beneficence and actively providing benefit and utility, which requires balancing benefits and adverse effects. Professional codes of ethics require that nurses and physicians act to benefit those entrusted to their care. Healthcare professionals, therefore, are obligated to examine their actions regarding intended beneficial outcomes while simultaneously considering the drawbacks or adverse consequences of their actions.

## Obligation of Nonmaleficence

Healthcare professionals also have a legal and moral obligation to avoid causing harm to their patients (Beauchamp & Childress, 2001). Adherence to this ethical principle, nonmaleficence, may encompass the provision of life-sustaining treatments and the cessation of such treatments. For example, when a therapy ceases to provide the intended benefit for a patient, it may be considered futile or even harmful, and the healthcare professional should, therefore, no longer be obligated to continue that treatment (Beauchamp & Childress, 2001). It also refers to adequately managing pain and not inflicting undue harm from inadequate management.

Healthcare professionals who continue to provide futile and burdensome treatments may be viewed as doing more harm than good. The distinction is made by meticulously balancing the benefits and burdens to the patient. For critically ill infants in the NICU, procedures or treatments can be considered inhumane if they inflict pain or discomfort on the infant without actual or perceived benefits (Jecker & Pagon, 1995). Terminally ill or medically fragile infants discharged home using technology can sometimes cause more harm than good (Carnevale et al., 2006).

Despite these arguments for humane care, burdensome, futile treatments are sometimes still given in the NICU. Weir (1984, 1995) has argued that death should not be considered the worst outcome for some infants, mainly when the chances for survival are remote or when physiologic survival is accompanied by unrelieved pain and suffering. In such cases, healthcare providers may be merely prolonging dying. Healthcare providers are ethically obligated not to offer interventions that will provide no benefit or cause undue harm.

### Recognition of Parents' Moral Authority

Parents have both the legal and moral authority to serve as surrogate decision makers for their infants. As Catlin and Carter (2002) point out, the real need in these instances is clear communication with parents of risks, benefits, and possible outcomes and an understanding of how they wish to be involved in these decisions.

When all appropriate life-sustaining therapies have been exhausted, parents and professionals often are uncertain about how to provide EOL care. The following quote is from Robert Stinson, father of Andrew, who was born in 1976 at 24 weeks' gestation. Andrew's survival was unprecedented. He received ICU support for 6 months, was critically ill throughout this time, and was resuscitated numerous times before his death.

> *"What they never understood was that one can care deeply enough about a child like Andrew to want his misery ended. Allowing Andrew to die naturally was what we wanted for him, not just for him. I thought often, when I did go in to see him, about his massive pain. He was sometimes crying then; a nearly soundless, aimless cry of pain, undirected and unlistened to except, I sometimes thought, by me. As often as I wanted to gather him into my arms, I wanted him to be allowed to die. What is the name for that?" (Stinson & Stinson, 1979).*

Although the Stinsons' experience occurred many years ago, evidence suggests that similar scenarios continue today. Professionals do not always incorporate the parental perspective into care decisions, particularly regarding burdensome, futile treatments (Yellin et al., 1998).

### Burden of Treatment

The burden of treatment experienced by extremely premature infants in the NICU, especially those with minimal chance for survival, requires further ethical examination. In a national survey of physicians certified in neonatal–perinatal medicine, Yellin et al. (1998) found that many neonatologists believe that "there is an ethical or legal obligation to perform treatments that are not in the infant's best interests, regardless of parental preference." Yellin and coworkers concluded that because some neonatologists are unwilling to withdraw treatments, they may be overtreating some infants in the NICU. Unfortunately, this situation has not changed much today (Kenner & Boykova, 2010).

Penticuff (1998) identified harm that ensues for infants, families, the healthcare team, and society when there is no accepted definition of futility. Such harm may include needless infant suffering caused by the prolongation of the dying process, as well as the psychological entrapment of both the medical team and the family—where initial aggressive interventions escalate into increasingly intensive treatments, with death becoming the only eventual stopping point. An example is the controversy around treatment options for children with trisomy 13 and 18, where mixed opinions exist about how far treatment should go and how parents must be included in decision making, including decisions about palliative care (Carey, 2012). It is important to note that infants with previously termed lethal diagnoses (such as trisomy 13 and 18) are surviving far beyond what has historically been expected and that a diagnosis alone should not preclude the standard of care interventions being offered when otherwise deemed appropriate.

## COMFORT CARE AT THE EOL

Palliative care includes optimum symptom relief for the neonate, regardless of the length of life or where life is lived (Thaxton et al., 2016). Brody et al. (1997) call for compassionate clinical management during the withdrawal of intensive life-sustaining treatment for adult patients using a strategic approach with well-defined goals that dictate the plan of care. Once the goals have been identified, the team examines both the benefits and burdens of the proposed treatment plan with the family. With this approach, any treatment that is more burdensome than beneficial is limited or eliminated. Brody et al. (997) and coworkers identified pain and discomfort as components of treatment burden and said there is "no sound rationale for withholding adequate analgesia or sedation" during EOL care. This approach should serve as the standard of care in the NICU, just as it is when caring for adult patients.

Physicians and nurse practitioners should follow the guidelines outlined by the AAP when engaging in discussions with parents about whether to initiate or continue intensive care of an infant who may not survive (American Academy of Pediatrics Committee on Fetus and Newborn, 2007; Cummings & American Academy of Pediatrics, Committee on Fetus and Newborn, 2015).

Interventions can always be used to promote comfort during EOL for infants with complex chronic conditions (Thaxton et al., 2016). Unfortunately, there is limited research on the provision of analgesia and sedation for infants at the EOL. One study focused on medications administered during life-support (e.g., ventilator) withdrawal. Partridge and Wall (1997) conducted a retrospective chart review to examine the practice of opioid analgesia administration in one NICU at the time of life-support withdrawal. **Emergency Alert: Despite growing concern over opioid use, pain management, including opioids, is essential for infants who are potentially dying.** They found that of infants who had a known painful condition (e.g., acute abdominal or surgical pain) who were receiving analgesia before the decision was made to withhold further life-sustaining treatment, 84% received opioid analgesia during life-support withdrawal. An interesting finding of this study was that the infants who did not receive any analgesia at the time of life-support withdrawal had also not received any pain medication before the decision was made to discontinue life support. These findings suggest that analgesia is not being given to ease the possible suffering associated with withdrawal of life support but rather to manage specific disease processes or only to manage symptoms after they become overtly apparent rather than anticipating discomfort through such a process. (Additional aspects of neonatal pain management are discussed in Chapter 22.) Even the smallest of patients have rights, including compassionate EOL care and pain management.

## PEDIATRIC HOSPICE CARE

The use of hospice and palliative care has made a significant difference in EOL care for adults. Its primary focus while still supporting life is care, not cure (Friebert & Williams, 2015). According to the National Hospice and Palliative Care Organization (NHPCO, 2001, 2018a), hospice care can be provided in select hospitals, individual hospice facilities, or a person's home. In 2013, the AAP Section on Hospice and Palliative Medicine and Committee on Hospital Care published a paper outlining the care commitments and recommendations for pediatric palliative and hospice care programs. These recommendations included that interdisciplinary trained teams can provide this care if the child is in a large institution (AAP, 2013). These were updated in 2022 (Linebarger et al., 2022). This type of care is considered a critical component of quality care and facilitates safe care. **Quality and Safety:** **Family support and compassionate care with consideration of family wishes and cultural values are important.**

Reliable statistics for children who receive pediatric palliative care or hospice care services still need to be made easier to parse from existing sources. It is also challenging to characterize children who might be appropriate or eligible for services because this characterization is a moving target. Variations in chronological, definitional, and prognostic criteria, as well as accessibility to establish programs, hinder accurate descriptions of this population (Friebert & Williams, 2015, p. 4).

There is still a lot of headway to be made regarding pediatric EOL and hospice care nationally. A study conducted by Children's International Project on Palliative/Hospice Service (ChiPPS, now referred to as Children's Project on Palliative/Hospice Services) found that only a small percentage of children who could have benefited from palliative or hospice care were provided this care (5,000 out of 53,000) and most very late in their disease (NHCPO, 2001). Awareness of the need for hospice and palliative care in the neonatal/pediatric population is growing. Some settings are developing a connection with perinatal hospices when a problem is detected before delivery that may result in a stillborn or "born dying" infant. One example is Alexander's House in Kansas City, Missouri (Pearce, 2006). Children's Hospital Medical Center, Cincinnati, Ohio, developed a perinatal hospice program called "Star Shine Hospice," another example of a hospice specifically focused on children (for more information, see www.cincinnatichildrens.org/service/s/starshine/default). Many families can now decide to take their infant home to die. Assessment of the family's wishes, ability to cope, support systems in place, and whether palliative care or hospice care for families and neonates is available in their community is recommended before being discharged from the hospital (Kenner et al., 2015). About 80% of the U.S.-based children's hospitals have palliative care teams, and 31% offer home visits (NHPCO, 2023).

### Barriers to Pediatric Hospice Service

Unfortunately, there are many barriers to the availability and provision of hospice care to ill children and families who could benefit from it. The NHPCO (2000) described psychological, financial, educational, and regulatory barriers to pediatric palliative care. One of the psychological barriers is the association of palliative care with the concept of giving up or going against hope (Kenner & Boykova, 2010). Hope has long been considered essential to humans in several disciplines, including nursing. At the EOL, hope is a complex and dynamic emotion, and there have been different interpretations and conceptions of hope (Guedes et al., 2021). The concept's consequences were quality of life, survival, acceptance, and a peaceful death (Guedes et al., 2021). Hope in palliative care is a determinant of quality of life, survival, acceptance, and peaceful death (Silveira et al., 2023). Families often avoid palliative care rather than identifying with the life-enhancing benefits it offers. Financial barriers arise because home-based, multidisciplinary care is frequently not reimbursed. The educational barriers for care providers are evident in the lack of palliative care training for most physicians and the avoidance of discussing hospice care with parents (Moody et al., 2011). These training issues can be addressed through simulated difficult conversations (Brown et al., 2012).

Regulatory barriers also exist because the reimbursement system is based on the needs of adults. Ignoring the differences in care needs between children and adults creates barriers to hospice as an option for many families. With the enactment of the Affordable Care Act (ACA) in 2010, there is now a stipulation for what is known as Concurrent Care, which allows patients under the age of 21 to receive life-sustaining interventions and treatments, along with hospice support (Manchikanti et al., 2011). This has improved enrollment, but more education is needed on all fronts before the full benefits of the Concurrent Care provision can be realized (NHPCO, 2023).

## BEREAVEMENT

Grief is unique to everyone and varies in expression, duration, and meaning. Parents often move through the grief process differently. The infant's mother may express her grief by crying, whereas the father may express his grief by isolating himself. There can also be differences between mothers and fathers in their reaction to the loss of their infant. Mothers often feel like they failed as a woman to produce a healthy child, or they feel guilty because they blame themselves even if they did not do anything to cause the premature delivery or congenital anomaly. Fathers often feel they failed to protect their families (Kenner et al., 2015). Either mother or father may be reluctant to share their feelings, and mothers may be more accepting of support groups and counseling than fathers (Kenner et al., 2015). Healthcare providers should also take into consideration the bereaved families that may lack support during a sudden and unexpected perinatal loss (Gold et al., 2017), and any lack of agreement that might exist among health professionals and parents regarding palliative care.

For many parents, grief is a lifelong process. Significant life events can trigger grieving, as can such routine childhood milestones as seeing a neighbor's child get on the school bus for her first day of kindergarten or, many years later, receiving a high school graduation announcement for what would have been their child's class.

As parents progress through the first year after their loss, it is essential to prepare them for the grief they are likely to experience in the future and to help them develop a plan for themselves. Every family is unique and determines their milestone days, which bring special remembrance of their child. Milestone days may include the child's birthday, the anniversary of the child's death, or holidays. It is sometimes helpful for parents to schedule time off on these milestone days so that they can plan a unique activity. Some parents may want to be alone and take a quiet walk together. Others may prefer to be surrounded by relatives or a few close friends. Still, others may want to spend the day with another parent who has experienced similar grief.

Nurses should stress three essential points to bereaved families: (a) grief is individualized; (b) grief is a process; and (c) family members should not hesitate to seek assistance with their grief, even years after the child's death.

## CONTINUED IMPROVEMENT OF PEDIATRIC PALLIATIVE CARE THROUGH RESEARCH AND EDUCATION

Healthcare professionals need continuing education on ways to provide comprehensive palliative care. There is a need for research that specifically focuses on the effectiveness of palliative care interventions and models of pediatric palliative care delivery (AAP, 2000). The creation of the End-of-Life Nursing Education Consortium (ELNEC) training through the City of Hope and the American Association of Colleges of Nursing (AACN, 2018) has helped facilitate hospital-based nurses, nurse faculty, and, in turn, students to learn palliative care principles. The ELNEC modules can be used in undergraduate and graduate curricula as a part of any clinically based management course or in a standalone elective. The NHPCO (2018b) has a similar program called EPEC EOL care, focusing on interdisciplinary palliative care training. Both of these programs are train-the-trainer models.

Worldwide recognition of the need for neonatal and pediatric palliative care is growing, thanks to funding from the Soros Foundation, the Robert Wood Johnson Foundation, City of Hope, Johns Hopkins University, AACN, and other organizations that support educational efforts about EOL and palliative care. Nursing curricula are being revised to include content and competencies on EOL care. Training programs such as the ELNEC (www.aacn.nche.edu/elnec) broaden nurses' knowledge in this specialty. One ELNEC training focuses specifically on the neonatal/pediatric population (AACN, 2018). Modules that focus specifically on developmental issues regarding the concept of death and dying, as well as how to assess for pain in the neonatal population and nonverbal children, help health professionals adapt materials to their settings. Organizations such as the International Association of Hospice and Palliative Care, the NHPCO, and the Hospice and Palliative Care Nurses Association, which traditionally focused on adult issues, have begun incorporating pediatric palliative care concerns into their initiatives. Including a chapter (Kenner & Boykova, 2010) on palliative care in the NICU in Dr. Betty Ferrell's palliative care textbook—the gold standard in palliative care—will increase awareness of the need for EOL care in this population. All these actions bode well for integrating EOL care into customary pediatric and neonatal care as a standard that is expected and demanded.

In 2015, the National Perinatal Association, under the leadership of Drs. Sue Hall and Michael Hynan, invited neonatal/perinatal specialists and parents to develop program standards for psychosocial support of parents and infants admitted to a NICU (Hall et al., 2015). Part of these recommendations focused on palliative and bereavement care (Hall et al., 2015; Hynan & Hall, 2015; Kenner et al., 2015). Recommendations for NICU bereavement and palliative care (Kenner et al., 2015) can be found in Boxes 29.1 to 29.3.

**BOX 29.1**

### ANTENATAL RECOMMENDATIONS

Perinatal and neonatal Palliative Care is a coordinated care strategy that encompasses actions in obstetric and neonatal care, focusing on maximizing the quality of life and comfort for fetuses and newborns with conditions considered life limiting (Quinn et al., 2020). Parents anticipating a perinatal loss should be offered the following:

1. An antenatal interdisciplinary conference should be held to develop the following plans, which should be individualized according to parents' desires and cultural, spiritual, and religious beliefs:
   a. A birth plan should include parents' preferences regarding the conduct of labor, the circumstances surrounding delivery, and the care for the infant and parents after the infant's birth.
   b. The plan should include the extent of resuscitation to be performed and whether to allow a natural death.

*(continued)*

**BOX 29.1**

## ANTENATAL RECOMMENDATIONS (*continued*)

c. A palliative care plan should be developed as indicated and desired when infants are not expected to survive. This plan should include parents' preferences on where the infant's care will be delivered, how nutrition will be provided, and how the infant's pain and discomfort will be managed (Craig & Goldman, 2003; Craig & Mancini, 2013).

2. Parents should be encouraged to bond with their infant and to create memories throughout the pregnancy whenever feasible, recognizing the barriers parents may face in bonding.
3. Psychosocial support should be provided for all family members, including grandparents and the infant's siblings.
4. Both practical and psychosocial support should be provided to help parents cope with their infant at home when infants with life-limiting conditions survive hospital discharge (American Academy of Pediatrics Section on Hospice and Palliative Medicine and Committee on Hospital Care, 2013).

*Source:* From Wool, C., & Northam, S. (2011). The Perinatal Palliative Care Perceptions and Barriers Scale Instrument©: Development and validation. *Advances in Neonatal Care, 11*(6), 397–403. https//doi.org/10.1097/ANC.0b013e318233809a

**BOX 29.2**

## NICU RECOMMENDATIONS FOR BEREAVEMENT CARE

1. Parents who lose an infant before, during, or shortly after birth or later in the NICU should be offered the following:
   a. Anticipatory guidance should be offered regarding the grieving process, including how mothers, fathers, and other family members may grieve differently (Wallerstedt & Higgins, 1996). This anticipatory guidance should begin antenatally if a life-limiting diagnosis has been determined (Bennett et al., 2011; Calhoun et al., 2003).
   b. Participation in bereavement rituals, including those that meet their spiritual, religious, and cultural preferences, should also be offered. These rituals may include a variety of practices and items that will help them remember their infants, such as the provision of handprints, footprints, and photographs (Carter, 2004; De Lisle-Porter & Podruchny, 2009). Smooth communication should be facilitated between parents and the staff of the NICU and obstetric units throughout the dying process; a perinatal social worker or other designated person can assist with this (National Association of Perinatal Social Workers, 2007).
   c. Psychosocial support should be provided for all family members, including but not limited to grandparents and the infant's siblings (American Academy of Pediatrics Section on Hospice and Palliative Medicine and Committee on Hospital Care, 2013; Pearson, 1997).
   d. Peer-to-peer support and referral to community or Internet support organizations should be provided.
   e. Counseling should be provided regarding both the physical and psychological considerations of attempting another pregnancy (American Academy of Pediatrics Section on Hospice and Palliative Medicine and Committee on Hospital Care, 2013).
   f. Posthospital follow-up should be provided in a variety of forms, including individual contact by a staff member at various time periods as well as a conference 4 to 6 weeks after the infant's death to review the autopsy and other results that will help parents understand what happened to their infant (Levitown, 2008).
2. When intensive care is not provided, a collaborative, interdisciplinary approach should be used to provide palliative and EOL care, including bereavement care, to any family whose fetus or neonate is facing a life-limiting condition or imminent death (Aladangady & de Rooy, 2012).
3. Physicians and nurse practitioners should follow the guidelines outlined by the AAP when engaging in discussions with parents about whether to initiate or continue intensive care for a infant who may not survive (American Academy of Pediatrics Committee on Fetus and Newborn, 2007; Cummings & American Academy of Pediatrics, Committee on Fetus and Newborn, 2015); neonatal nurses and perinatal social workers should be included in the decision-making process as well (National Association of Neonatal Nurses, 2016; National Association of Perinatal Social Workers, 2007). Intensive care should be provided only if the infant is believed to benefit. The infant's best interests should be the guiding standard

(*continued*)

**BOX 29.2**

**NICU RECOMMENDATIONS FOR BEREAVEMENT CARE (*continued*)**

(American Academy of Pediatrics Committee on Fetus and Newborn, 2007; Cummings & American Academy of Pediatrics, Committee on Fetus and Newborn 2015).

4. In cases where there are disagreements between parents and the healthcare team when making EOL decisions, particularly around the futility of further care for an infant, a bioethics consult should be obtained, and the case should be presented to the hospital Bioethics Committee (American Academy of Pediatrics Committee on Fetus and Newborn, 2007).
5. Parents whose infants with life-limiting conditions survive and are discharged from the hospital should be offered both practical and psychosocial support to help them prepare for discharge and learn how to both care for and cope with their infant at home and/or they should be referred to a hospice with experience caring for infants. Their infant's primary care provider, neonatal specialist, medical home, or subspecialists should be fully involved in making and carrying out home care plans and providing follow-up support.

*Source:* From Kenner, C., Press, J., & Ryan, D. (2015). Recommendations for palliative and bereavement care in the NICU: A family-centered integrative approach. *Journal of Perinatology, 35*, S19–S23. https://doi.org/10.1038/jp.2015.145

**BOX 29.3**

**HEALTH SYSTEM RECOMMENDATIONS**

1. All health professionals who work with pregnant women, neonates, and their families should receive education and demonstrate competence in palliative and bereavement care that is appropriate within their scope of practice. This education should include training in how to communicate effectively and empathetically with families (American Academy of Pediatrics Section on Hospice and Palliative Medicine and Committee on Hospital Care, 2013; Boss et al., 2009; National Association of Neonatal Nurses, 2015).
2. Policies for palliative care and bereavement practices in any part of a healthcare system should be in place and easily accessible to all staff to ensure a standard of care for all families. Standardized guidelines should be implemented with the goal of achieving a state of comfort for newborns throughout the course of illness (Parravicini, 2017).
3. Palliative and bereavement care resources in the community should be available to anyone who is providing care to a neonate and family facing a life-threatening condition or imminent death or has experienced a loss, whether there is a palliative care team or program at a specific institution or not.
4. Hospitals should work in partnership with their local organ donation organizations to determine whether specific infants are eligible to become organ donors and assess, in collaboration with the family, whether organ donation is the right choice.
5. Healthcare staff who provide palliative and/or bereavement care should receive psychosocial support and engage in self-care (Sanchez-Reilly et al., 2013), to enable them to provide optimal care to the families they serve, as well as to prevent burnout, compassion fatigue, or secondary traumatic stress (American Academy of Pediatrics Section on Hospice and Palliative Medicine and Committee on Hospital Care, 2013). The perinatal social worker (De Lisle-Porter & Podruchny, 2009), NICU psychologist (Gold et al., 2007), or pastoral care staff (Sharp, 1991) can be instrumental in providing this support.

*Source:* From Kenner, C., Press, J., & Ryan, D. (2015). Recommendations for palliative and bereavement care in the NICU: A family-centered integrative approach. *Journal of Perinatology, 35*, S19–S23. https://doi.org/10.1038/jp.2015.145

## SUMMARY

An ever-growing, broad spectrum of patients could and should benefit from comprehensive pediatric palliative care, especially in the NICU. As technology advances, more infants will survive the immediate perinatal period and require ongoing, specialized care. For these infants and their loved ones, it is vital to establish trusted relationships with healthcare teams, receive coordinated care, discuss goals of care, discuss how specific interventions can and will affect the life of both the infant and family, and receive culturally competent care. And when death approaches in the NICU, measures can and should be taken to ease the infant's transition and adequately assist the family. It is no longer enough to provide either invasive, technology-burdened, aggressive support or bereavement and postmortem care to infants and their families; we must also provide holistic, patient-focused care that aligns with the overall goals and beliefs of families. Ongoing research and evaluation of care guidelines are needed so that infants can receive the same quality of holistic care throughout an illness course afforded to other members of society. Palliative care is the benchmark of this care. Neonatal nurses have been at the forefront of this movement and now can serve as leaders in designing and implementing exemplary neonatal palliative care programs.

## CASE STUDY

**Identification of the Problem.** An infant was born at 24 weeks' gestation to a family that had just moved to a new city and had no relatives in the area. This was the first baby in the family. Shortly after birth, it was recognized that the infant would probably not survive because, in addition to being premature, overwhelming sepsis was present. The care team (without the family) met. Some felt that the family needed to be given options immediately, such as calling the palliative care team for a discussion of treatment options.

**Assessment: History and Physical Examination.** In contrast, other team members believed that the infant should be given a few more days to see how the infant would respond to ventilation and antibiotic therapy.

**Development of Management Plan.** A consultation was done with the palliative care team that convinced the neonatal team to talk with the family, describe the infant's status, discuss the possible course, and ask them to be part of the team to make decisions about palliative care and in what form—in other words, how aggressive they wanted the treatment to be, how in either case palliative care would be provided, how care would be coordinated, and how they as a family would be supported regardless of the outcome. Over the next week, the infant continued to get progressively sicker. The palliative care team supported the family, and relatives were contacted via the Internet to ensure they could help the family and see the infant.

**Implementation.** The family planned the care and eventually decided to take the infant, whom they named Sarah Elizabeth, off the ventilator. They held and rocked the infant surrounded by staff they selected until the moment of death. The death was peaceful, and the palliative care team continued to follow up with the family over the next month. The team also debriefed the neonatal caregivers who worked closely with the family to ensure they were supported. The principles of dignity, respect, and need for caregiver support for both the family and professional staff were upheld.

## EVIDENCE-BASED PRACTICE

Much progress has been made since the early 2000s when protocols for perinatal and neonatal palliative care appeared. Drs. Charlotte Wool and Sally Northam developed the Perinatal Palliative Care Perceptions and Barriers Scale Instrument. This instrument was developed and validated for use with nurses and physicians over time. The focus is to determine the perceptions of health professionals to develop staff/faculty training programs to provide better support to patients and families. This instrument can be used in various ways and needs further testing to broaden its use.

*Source:* From Wool, C., & Northam, S. (2011). The perinatal palliative care perceptions and barriers scale instrument©: Development and validation. *Advances in Neonatal Care*, *11*(6), 397–403. https://doi.org/10.1097/ANC.0b013e318233809a

## PARENT VOICES

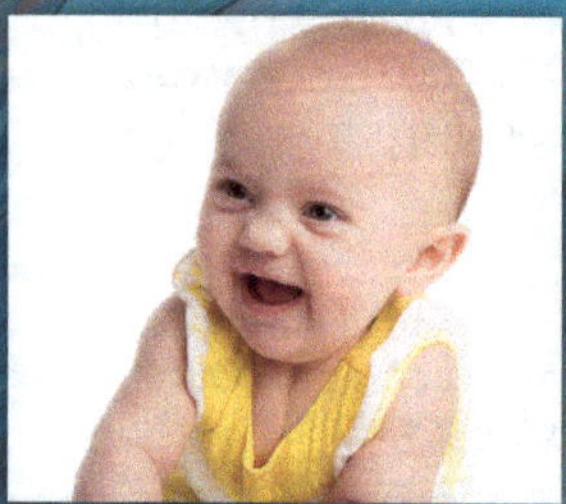

*Source:* Benjamin Simeneta/Adobe Stock.

### Amy Blanchard

**After we realized our daughter was not going to get better, my husband and I met with the palliative care team. This team included the chaplain, the pain management team, and the social worker. The most important thing for nurses to do is not to act like the baby has already passed away. Know that she is still alive and the parents are making life decisions for their child. We had some phenomenal nurses who treated our daughter like their own. That meant the world to us. We were comfortable leaving our daughter in their capable hands. Having a care team of nurses was one of the most important aspects of Molly's nursing care. These nurses cared for and loved our daughter and us (her parents).**

**During palliative care, we would ask for the nurses' opinions. They knew our daughter almost as well as we did. They knew how certain medications affected her and if she was in pain. We valued their opinion regarding some of the care that she received during the end. They wanted Molly to be pain free and as comfortable as we wanted her to be.**

*(continued)*

## PARENT VOICES (*continued*)

I will never forget the last day of my daughter Molly's life; it feels like it was yesterday. Discontinuing care was the hardest decision my husband and I have ever had to make. On that day, we were able to call two of our favorite nurses from Molly's care team. They were not scheduled to work but came to Molly's room to say their goodbyes. They sat with us and cried with us while we held our daughter for the last time. These two nurses gave my sweet baby girl her last bath when I could not. They were angels who flew in and took over when I was an emotional wreck. I'll be forever grateful for Molly's loving nurses.

To some families, like mine, NICU nurses should know that they are not just "a nurse." They are also caretakers to the baby's parents. They will cry along with mothers and fathers, and when a baby passes away, they are the first ones the parents may want to see. A strong bond forms when your baby spends 4 to 5 months with a nurse. I hope these nurses know that they will forever be a part of some family's lives, even if the baby passes away and the family no longer visits. These nurses will be remembered always.

## ONLINE RESOURCES

CourseConnect

Resources for this chapter are online and available at www.springerpub.com/courseconnect.

## REFERENCES

References for this chapter are online and available at www.springerpub.com/courseconnect.

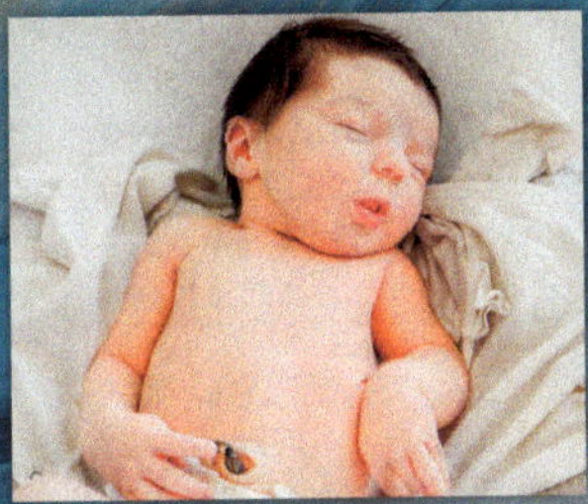

*Source:* Amelie/ Adobe Stock.

APPENDIX A

# Conversion Table to Standard International Units

| Component | Present Unit | × | Conversion Factor | = | SI Unit |
|---|---|---|---|---|---|
| *Clinical Hematology* | | | | | |
| Erythrocytes | per $mm^3$ | | 1 | | $10^6$/L |
| Hematocrit | % | | 0.01 | | (1)vol RBC/vol whole blood |
| Hemoglobin | g/dL | | 10 | | g/L |
| Leukocytes | per $mm^3$ | | 1 | | $10^6$/L |
| MCHC | g/dl | | 10 | | g/L |
| MCV | $\mu m^3$ | | 1 | | fL |
| Platelet count | $10^3/mm^3$ | | 1 | | $10^9$/L |
| Reticulocyte count | % | | 10 | | $10^{-3}$ |
| *Clinical Chemistry* | | | | | |
| Acetone | mg/dl | | 0.1722 | | mmol/L |
| Albumin | g/dl | | 10 | | g/L |
| Aldosterone | ng/dl | | 27.74 | | pmol/L |
| Ammonia (as nitrogen) | mcg/dl | | 0.7139 | | μmol/L |
| Bicarbonate | mEq/L | | 1 | | mmol/L |

(*continued*)

| Component | Present Unit | × | Conversion Factor | = | SI Unit |
|---|---|---|---|---|---|
| Bilirubin | mg/dl | | 17.1 | | μmol/L |
| Calcium | mg/dl | | 0.2495 | | mmol/L |
| Calcium ion | mEq/L | | 0.50 | | mmol/L |
| Carotenes | mcg/dl | | 0.01836 | | μmol/L |
| Ceruloplasmin | mg/dl | | 10.0 | | mg/L |
| Chloride | mEq/L | | 1 | | mmol/L |
| Cholesterol | mg/dl | | 0.02586 | | mmol/L |
| Complement, $C_3$ or $C_4$ | mg/dl | | 0.01 | | g/L |
| Copper | mcg/dl | | 0.1574 | | μmol/L |
| Cortisol | mcg/dl | | 27.59 | | nmol/L |
| Creatine | mg/dl | | 76.25 | | μmol/L |
| Creatinine | mg/dl | | 88.40 | | μmol/L |
| Digoxin | ng/ml | | 1.281 | | nmol/L |
| Epinephrine | pg/ml | | 5.458 | | pmol/L |
| Fatty acids | mg/dl | | 10.0 | | mg/L |
| Ferritin | ng/ml | | 1 | | mcg/L |
| α-Fetoprotein | ng/ml | | 1 | | mcg/L |
| Fibrinogen | mg/dl | | 0.01 | | g/L |
| Folate | ng/ml | | 2.266 | | nmol/L |
| Fructose | mg/dl | | 0.05551 | | mmol/L |
| Galactose | mg/dl | | 0.05551 | | mmol/L |
| *Gases* | | | | | |
| $PO_2$ | mm Hg (= torr) | | 0.1333 | | kPa |
| $PCO_2$ | mm Hg (= torr) | | 0.1333 | | kPa |
| Glucagon | pg/ml | | 1 | | ng/L |

*(continued)*

| Component | Present Unit | × | Conversion Factor | = | SI Unit |
|---|---|---|---|---|---|
| Glucose | mg/dl | | 0.05551 | | mmol/L |
| Glycerol | mg/dl | | 0.1086 | | mmol/L |
| Growth hormone | ng/ml | | 1 | | mcg/L |
| Haptoglobin | mg/dl | | 0.01 | | g/L |
| Hemoglobin | g/dl | | 10 | | g/L |
| Insulin | mcg/L | | 172.2 | | pmol/L |
| | mU/L | | 7.175 | | pmol/L |
| Iron | mcg/dl | | 0.1791 | | µmol/L |
| Iron-binding capacity | mcg/dl | | 0.1791 | | µmol/L |
| Lactate | mEq/L | | 1 | | mmol/L |
| Lead | mcg/dl | | 0.04826 | | µmol/L |
| Lipoproteins | mg/dl | | 0.02586 | | mmol/L |
| Magnesium | mg/dl | | 0.4114 | | mmol/L |
| | mEq/L | | 0.50 | | mmol/L |
| Osmolality | mOsm/kg $H_2O$ | | 1 | | mmol/kg $H_2O$ |
| Phenobarbital | mg/dl | | 43.06 | | µmol/L |
| Phenytoin | mg/L | | 3.964 | | µmol/L |
| Phosphate | mg/dl | | 0.3229 | | mmol/L |
| Potassium | mEq/L | | 1 | | mmol/L |
| | mg/dl | | 0.2558 | | mmol/L |
| Protein | g/dl | | 10.0 | | g/L |
| Pyruvate | mg/dl | | 113.6 | | µmol/L |
| Sodium ion | mEq/L | | 1 | | mmol/L |
| *Steroids* | | | | | |
| 17-hydroxycorticosteroids | mg/24 h | | 2.759 | | µmol/d |

(*continued*)

| Component | Present Unit | × | Conversion Factor | = | SI Unit |
|---|---|---|---|---|---|
| 17-ketosteroids | mg/24 h | | 3.467 | | μmol/d |
| Testosterone | ng/ml | | 3.467 | | nmol/L |
| Theophylline | mg/L | | 5.550 | | μmol/L |
| *Thyroid tests* | | | | | |
| Thyroid-stimulating hormone | μU/ml | | 1 | | mU/L |
| Thyroxine ($T_4$) | mcg/dl | | 12.87 | | nmol/L |
| Thyroxine free | ng/dl | | 12.87 | | pmol/L |
| Triiodothyronine ($T_3$) | ng/dl | | 0.01536 | | nmol/L |
| Transferrin | mg/dl | | 0.01 | | g/L |
| Triglycerides | mg/dl | | 0.01129 | | mmol/L |
| Urea nitrogen | mg/dl | | 0.3570 | | mmol/L |
| Uric acid (urate) | mg/dl | | 59.48 | | μmol/L |
| Vitamin A (retinol) | mcg/dl | | 0.03491 | | μmol/L |
| Vitamin $B_{12}$ | pg/ml | | 0.7378 | | pmol/L |
| Vitamin C (ascorbic acid) | mg/dl | | 56.78 | | μmol/L |
| *Vitamin D* | | | | | |
| Cholecalciferol | mcg/ml | | 2.599 | | nmol/L |
| 25 OH-cholecalciferol | ng/ml | | 2.496 | | nmol/L |
| Vitamin E (alpha-tocopherol) | mg/dl | | 23.22 | | μmol/L |
| D-xylose | mg/dl | | 0.06661 | | mmol/L |
| Zinc | mcg/dl | | 0.1530 | | μmol/L |
| Energy | kcal | | 4.1868 | | kJ (kilojoule) |
| Blood pressure | mm Hg (= torr) | | 1.333 | | mbar |

MCHC, mean corpuscular hemoglobin concentration; MCV, mean corpuscular volume.

*Source:* Modified from Young D. S. (1987). Implementation of SI units for clinical laboratory data. Style specifications and conversion tables. *Annals of Internal Medicine, 106, 114–129.* https://doi.org/10.7326/0003-4819-106-1-114.

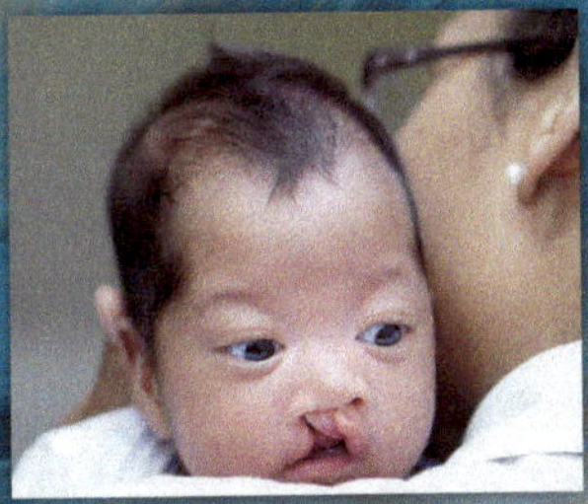

*Source:* Thomas Talkner/ peopleimages.com/Adobe Stock.

# APPENDIX B

# Frequently Used Reference Values and Conversions

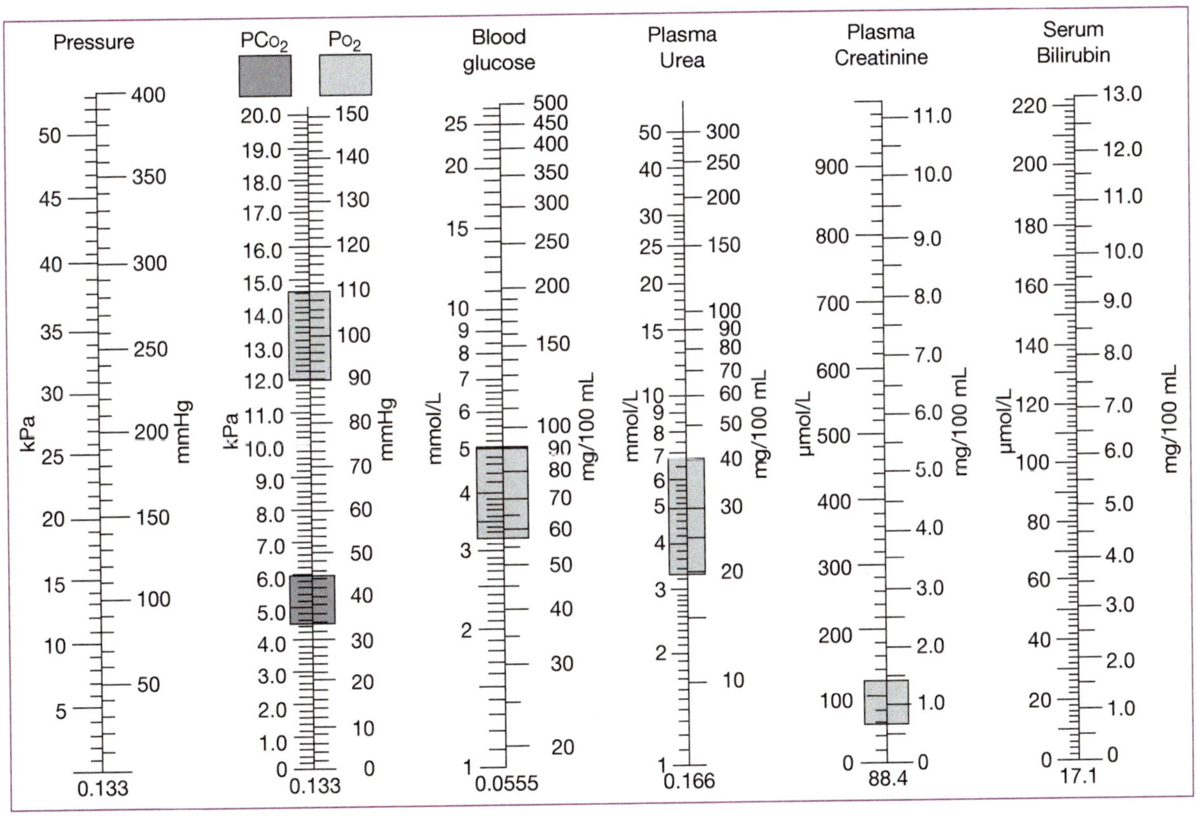


*Note:* Shading indicates the normal range where appropriate. To convert "old" to "new" units, multiply by the conversion factor at the foot of each column.

*Source:* Modified from Halliday, H. L., McClure, G., & Reid, M. (1985). *Handbook of neonatal intensive care* (2nd ed.). WB Saunders.

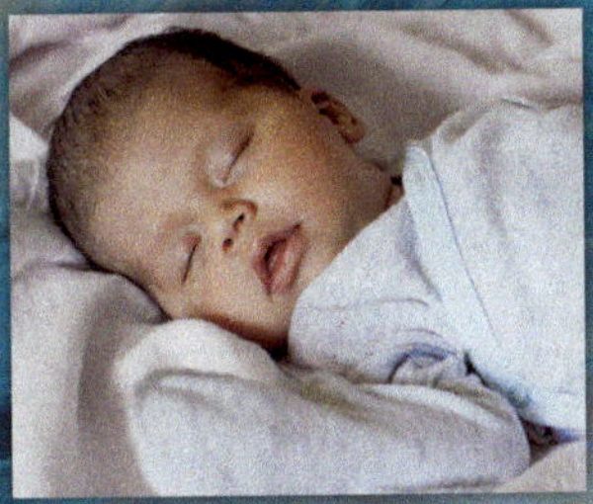


APPENDIX C

# International Standards for Newborn Weight, Length, and Head Circumference by Gestational Age and Sex

UNIVERSITY OF OXFORD

INTERGROWTH-21st

Boys

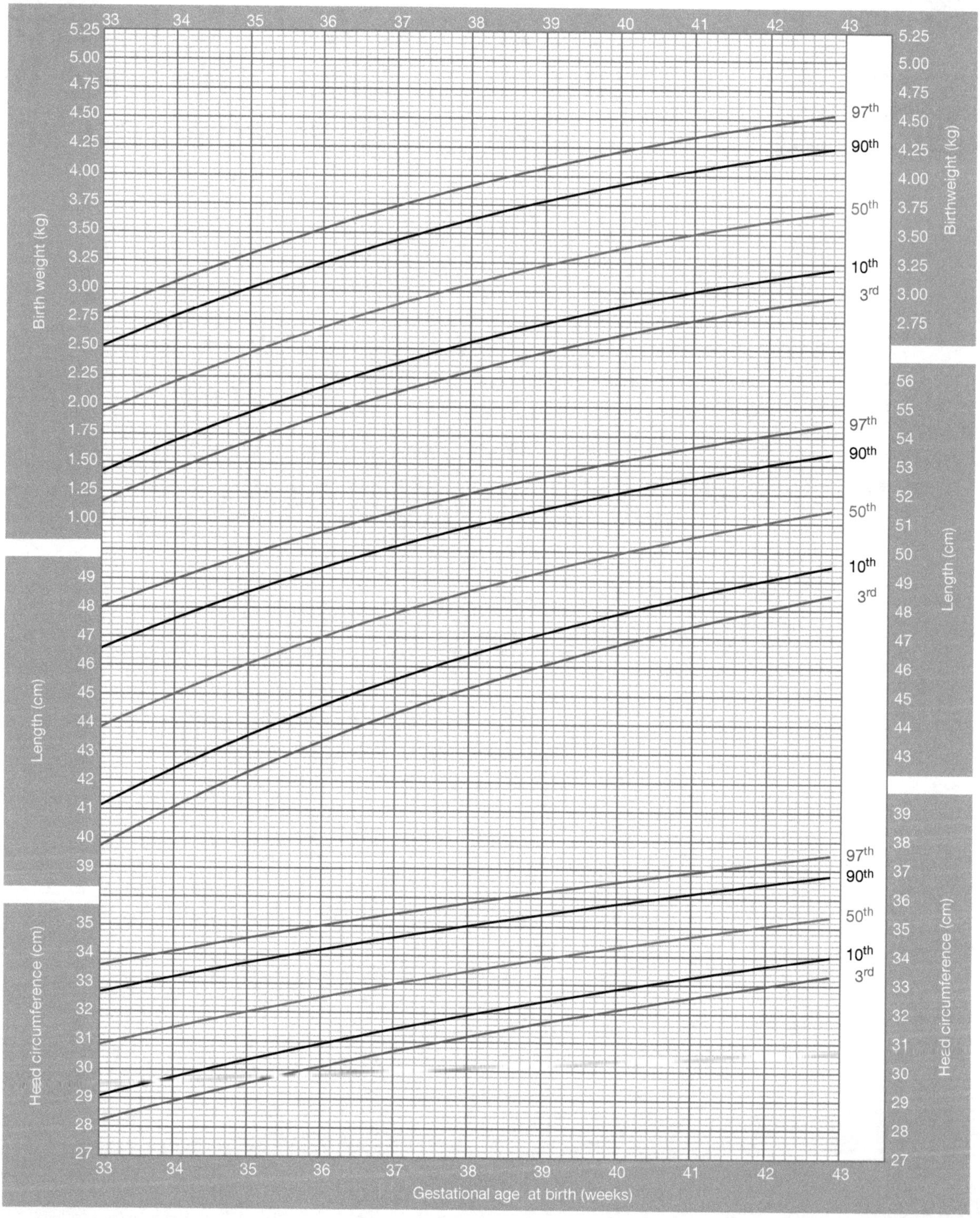


*Source:* INTERGROWTH-21st newborn size at birth standards. Reprinted by permission from Intergrowth-21st © 2009–2016. hhttps://intergrowth21.com/tools-resources/newborn-size.

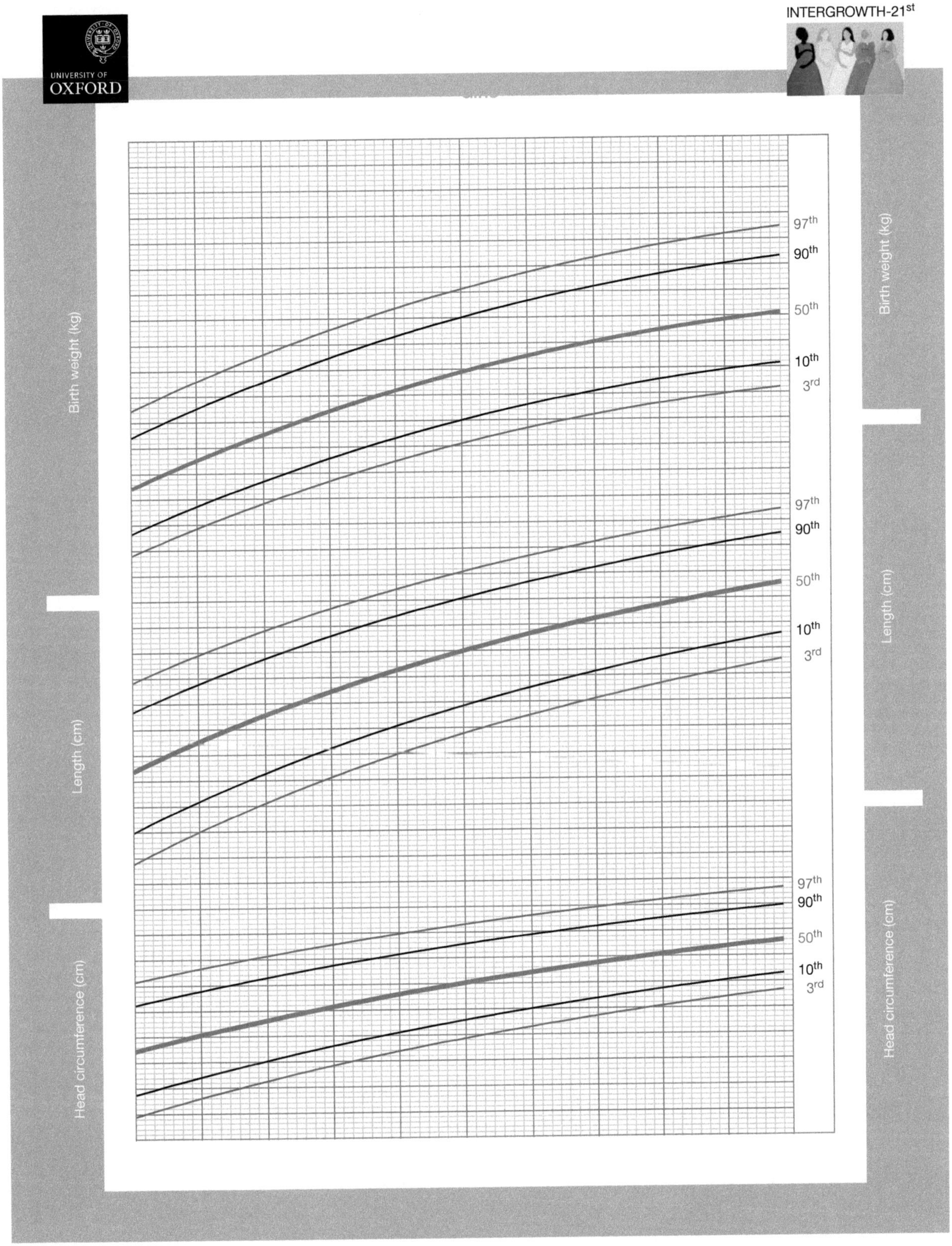


*Source:* INTERGROWTH-21st newborn size at birth standards. Reprinted by permission from Intergrowth-21st © 2009–2016. https://intergrowth21.com/tools-resources/newborn-size.

# Index